VARCAROLIS'
Foundations of Psychiatric-Mental Health Nursing
A Clinical Approach

ABOUT THE COVER ARTWORK

"Butterfly Abstract" is by Bradley D. Rankin of Cuyahoga Falls, Ohio. Bradley created this painting for the 2020 annual Art of Recovery event in Akron, Ohio. This event highlights artwork of clients from a local community mental health center. Bradley comments, "The abstract background with the more realistic butterflies depicts the confusion that sometimes overpowers our environment." Bradley's recovery from mental illness has led to a full-time job and the enjoyment of creating art.

In his own words: "Art has given me confidence and pride in my work and life. My grandmother is a retired professional artist and is my teacher. We enjoy working together even though sometimes we disagree on the subject I'm painting." The artist was given the opportunity to address the nursing students who will use this book. Bradley responded by saying, "Mental illness recovery is possible with help from family, friends, and professionals. Never give up on a patient."

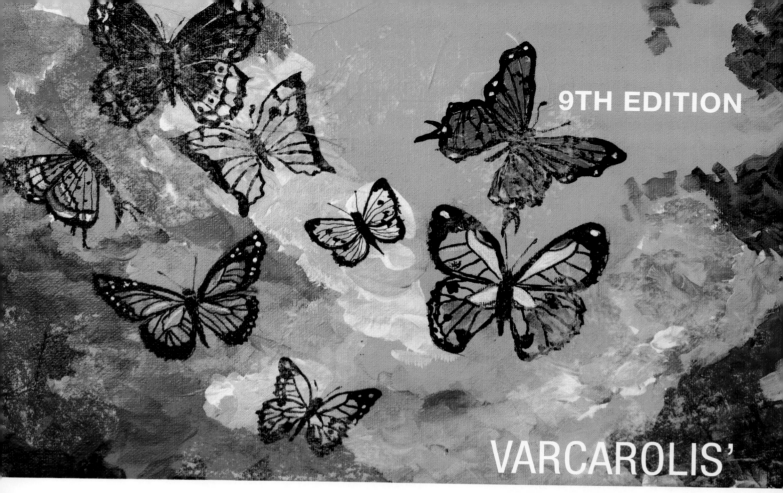

9TH EDITION

VARCAROLIS'
Foundations of Psychiatric-Mental Health Nursing
A Clinical Approach

Margaret (Peggy) Jordan Halter, PhD, APRN
Editor, *Manual of Psychiatric Nursing Care*
Former Clinical Nurse Specialist, Cleveland Clinic Akron General, Akron, Ohio
Former Faculty, Malone College, Canton, Ohio; University of Akron, Akron, Ohio;
    Ohio State University, Columbus, Ohio
Former Associate Dean, Ashland University, Mansfield, Ohio

ELSEVIER

Elsevier
3251 Riverport Lane
St. Louis, Missouri 63043

VARCAROLIS' FOUNDATIONS OF PSYCHIATRIC-MENTAL
HEALTH NURSING: A CLINICAL APPROACH, EDITION 9

ISBN: 978-0-323-69707-1

Notice

Practitioners and researchers must always rely on their own experience and knowledge in evaluating and using any information, methods, compounds or experiments described herein. Because of rapid advances in the medical sciences, in particular, independent verification of diagnoses and drug dosages should be made. To the fullest extent of the law, no responsibility is assumed by Elsevier, authors, editors or contributors for any injury and/or damage to persons or property as a matter of products liability, negligence or otherwise, or from any use or operation of any methods, products, instructions, or ideas contained in the material herein.

Previous editions copyrighted 2018, 2014, 2010, 2006, 2002, 1998, 1994, and 1990.

Library of Congress Control Number: 2021939107

Executive Content Strategist: Yvonne Alexopoulos
Senior Content Development Manager: Lisa P. Newton
Publishing Services Manager: Julie Eddy
Book Production Specialist: Clay Broeker
Design Direction: Brian Salisbury

Printed in the United States of America

Last digit is the print number: 9 8 7 6 5 4 3 2

Working together
to grow libraries in
developing countries

www.elsevier.com • www.bookaid.org

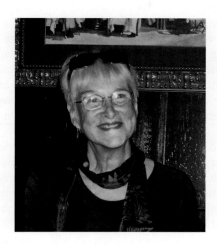

In memory of my friend and mentor, Betsy Varcarolis, who developed and edited five editions of this textbook. Her life's work in psychiatric nursing has influenced generations of future nurses, touched the lives of countless people, and profoundly changed my life.
December 8, 1940 - May 31, 2020

This book is also dedicated to people who are being treated for and recovering from mental illness and to the future nurses who will support their treatment and recovery.

ACKNOWLEDGMENTS

While revising the 9th edition of *Foundations of Psychiatric-Mental Health Nursing,* there were virtually none of the usual distractions for me. There was no "Let's meet for lunch," "It's time for the gym," or lure of retail therapy. The global coronavirus pandemic resulted in a muffled solitude that was conducive to researching, developing, and revising. Much of this edition was written during an Ohio shelter-in-place order.

The period of 2020–2021 was a time of an unprecedented change in life as usual, not to mention unprecedented suffering and loss of life. While many of us adapted to stay-at-home orders by working and being educated in our residences, countless essential workers faced the invisible danger of COVID-19. Healthcare providers, especially nurses (who are the largest group of direct 24/7 caregivers), risked their own well-being to deliver urgently needed care. There are no adequate words to express appreciation, but heartfelt thanks and tremendous admiration goes out to them.

The year 2020 also marked a milestone in the history of psychiatric nursing. After 80 years of a life well lived, Elizabeth (Betsy) Merrill Varcarolis, the creator of this and other leading psychiatric nursing textbooks, died. It has been 3 decades since Betsy achieved the publication of her first edition of this textbook. I believe that *Foundations* became popular mainly due to her communication style and commitment to effective communication. She had the unique ability to talk *with* nursing students as they read her words and not *at* them.

In this 9th edition of the book, Elizabeth Varcarolis will continue to be honored by the positioning of her last name at the beginning of the book's title. I am beyond grateful to Betsy for enriching my life through her mentoring and entrusting me with *Foundations.* The profession of psychiatric nursing and countless students and recipients of psychiatric-mental health care felt the influence that her words had on patient care. Countless people have benefited from her wisdom. Betsy leaves behind an inspiring legacy to a life well lived.

My heartfelt appreciation also goes out to the talented group of writers who contributed to the 9th edition. Some of these writers are veterans of earlier editions whose knowledge and passion continue to influence psychiatric nursing. New writers whose expertise was both recognized and sought out agreed to join us in this edition. It has been a joy working with each of you. Thanks for the countless hours you spent researching, writing, and rewriting!

A huge debt of gratitude goes to the many educators and clinicians who reviewed the manuscript and offered valuable suggestions, ideas, opinions, and even criticisms. All comments were appreciated and helped refine and strengthen the individual chapters and the textbook as a whole.

Throughout this project, an expert team at Elsevier has provided superb support. I am grateful for Clay Broeker, our Book Production Specialist, who nudged me to meet deadlines, and Brian Salisbury, a talented and creative designer. I have worked with Yvonne Alexopoulos, Senior Content Strategist, and Lisa Newton, Senior Content Development Manager, for over a decade. These women are cutting-edge experts in publishing whose planning, guidance, and support are essential. Their friendship during this revision and over the years has been an added bonus. My deep appreciation goes out to the whole Elsevier team!

Peggy

CONTRIBUTORS

Lois Angelo, MSN, APRN
Case Manager
Emergency Department
Newton-Wellesley Hospital
Newton, Massachusetts
Former Professor of Nursing
Berkshire Community College
Howard University
Washington, DC
Massachusetts College of Pharmacy and
    Health Sciences
Boston, Massachusetts

**Audrey M. Beauvais, DNP, MSN, MBA,
RN**
Associate Dean and Associate Professor
Egan School
Fairfield University
Fairfield, Connecticut

**Rachel Childs, MS, MA, MSSA,
PMHNP**
Psychiatric Nurse Practitioner
Pediatric Psychiatry
Mary Bridge Children's Hospital
MultiCare Health System
Tacoma, Washington

**Alison M. Colbert, PhD, PHCNS-BC,
FAAN**
Associate Professor
School of Nursing
Duquesne University
Pittsburgh, Pennsylvania

**Jessica B. Emshoff, BS, PharmD, BCPS,
BCGP**
Associate Professor, Pharmacy Practice
Northeast Ohio Medical University
Rootstown, Ohio
Clinical Pharmacy Specialist, Palliative
University Hospitals Portage Medical Center
Ravenna, Ohio

Chyllia D. Fosbre, MSN, PMHNP-BC
Psychiatric Nurse Practitioner
District Medical Group
Children's Rehabilitative Service
Phoenix, Arizona

**Emily Fowler, MSN, APRN,
PMHNP-BC**
Psychiatric Nurse Practitioner
Native American Community Clinic
Lyn-Lake Psychotherapy and Wellness
Minneapolis, Minnesota

Christina Fratena, MSN, APRN-CNS, BC
Instructor of Nursing
Malone University
Canton, Ohio
Clinical Nurse Specialist
SpringHaven Counseling Center
Dundee, Ohio

Faye J. Grund, PhD, APRN
Psychiatric Nurse Practitioner
Ohio Health Mansfield
Mansfield, Ohio
Adjunct Professor
Dwight Schar College of Nursing and Health
    Sciences
Ashland University
Mansfield, Ohio

**Margaret (Peggy) Jordan Halter, PhD,
APRN**
Editor
*Foundations of Psychiatric-Mental Health
    Nursing*
Elsevier
St. Louis, Missouri

**Monica J. Halter, MSN, APRN,
PMHNP-BC**
Nurse Practitioner
Psychiatry
PsychBC
Beachwood, Ohio

**Edward A. Herzog, MSN, PMH, APRN-
CNS**
Faculty Emeritus
College of Nursing
Kent State University
Kent, Ohio

Lorann Murphy, MSN, PMHCNS, BC
Clinical Nurse Specialist
Behavioral Health
Advanced Recovery Concepts
Beachwood, Ohio
Adjunct Professor
Nursing
Baldwin Wallace University
Berea, Ohio

Chris Paxos, PharmD, BCPP, BCPS, BCGP
Director, Pharmacotherapy
Associate Professor, Pharmacy Practice
Associate Professor, Psychiatry
Northeast Ohio Medical University
Rootstown, Ohio

**Donna Rolin, PhD, APRN, PMHCNS-
BC, PMHNP-BC**
Clinical Associate Professor
School of Nursing
University of Texas at Austin
Austin, Texas

**L. Kathleen Sekula, PhD, PMHCNS-BC,
FAAN**
Professor
School of Nursing
Duquesne University
Pittsburgh, Pennsylvania

**Jane Stein-Parbury, BSN, MEd, PhD,
FRCNA**
Emeritus Professor
Faculty of Health
University of Technology, Sydney
Sydney, Australia

**Kathleen Wheeler, PhD, PMHNP-BC,
APRN, FAAN**
Professor
Egan School of Nursing and Health Studies
Fairfield University
Fairfield, Connecticut

Kathryn Witner, MSN, RN, PCCN
Registered Nurse
Progressive Care
University of Colorado Hospital
Clinical Faculty
Denver College of Nursing
Aurora, Colorado

Kimberly M. Wolf, PhD, PMHCNS-BC
Lead Psychiatric Advanced Practice
    Provider
Psychiatry
Hennepin County Medical Center
Minneapolis, Minnesota
Psychiatric Provider
Outpatient Psychology Clinic
Associated Clinic of Psychology
Minneapolis, Minnesota
Adjunct Faculty
School of Nursing
Duquesne University
Pittsburgh, Pennsylvania

Sandra S. Yaklin, APRN, PMHNP-BC
PhD Student
School of Nursing
University of Texas at Austin
Austin, Texas

Rick Zoucha, PhD, PMHCNS-BC, CTN-A, FAAN
Professor and Joseph A. Lauritis, C.S.Sp.
    Endowed Chair for Teaching
    and Technology and Chair of Advanced
    Role and PhD Programs
School of Nursing
Duquesne University
Pittsburgh, Pennsylvania

ANCILLARY WRITERS

Linda Turchin, RN, MSN, CNE
Professor Emeritus of Nursing
Fairmont State University
Fairmont, West Virginia
Test Bank
Pretests/Posttests
Student Review Questions

Linda Wendling, MA, MFA
Learning Theory Consultant
University of Missouri—St. Louis
St. Louis, Missouri
*TEACH for Nurses and PowerPoints Case
Studies and Nursing Care Plans*

Rachel M. Childs, MS, MA, MSSA, PMHNP
Psychiatric Nurse Practitioner
Pediatric Psychiatry
Mary Bridge Children's Hospital
MultiCare Health System
Tacoma, Washington

Melinda Cuthbert, RN, BScN, MSc, MSN, PhD
Assistant Professor, School of Nursing
University of California at San Francisco
San Francisco, California

Andrea Kwasky, DNP, PMHNP-BC, PMHCNS-BC
Clinical Professor
McAuley School of Nursing
University of Detroit Mercy
Detroit, Michigan

Suzanne Lugger, DNP, RN, FNP-BC
Assistant Professor
School of Nursing
University of Michigan at Flint
Flint, Michigan

Becky McDaniel, MSN, RN-BC
Assistant Professor of Nursing
North Dakota State University
Fargo, North Dakota

Christie Obritsch, MSN, RN
Assistant Professor of Practice
School of Nursing
North Dakota State University
Fargo, North Dakota

Chris Paxos, PharmD, BCPP, BCPS, BCGP
Director, Pharmacotherapy
Associate Professor, Pharmacy Practice
Associate Professor, Psychiatry
Northeast Ohio Medical University
Rootstown, Ohio

Kathryn Witner, MSN, RN, PCCN
Registered Nurse
Progressive Care
University of Colorado Hospital
Clinical Faculty
Denver College of Nursing
Aurora, Colorado

TO THE INSTRUCTOR

We are living in an age of fast-paced discoveries in neurobiology, genetics, and pharmacotherapy. Researchers continue to seek the most effective evidence-based approaches for patients and their families. Legal issues and ethical dilemmas faced by the healthcare system are magnified accordingly. Given these challenges, keeping up and knowing how best to teach our students and serve our patients can seem overwhelming. With contributions from many knowledgeable and experienced nurse educators, our goal is to bring to you the most current and comprehensive trends and evidence-based practices in psychiatric-mental health nursing.

NEW TO THIS EDITION

- One of the most important changes to this edition is the addition of specific types of case studies to the clinical chapters. This change stems from a 2013–2014 National Council of State Boards of Nursing (NCSBN) Strategic Practice Analysis that considered the complexity of decisions new nurses make while doing patient care. This analysis led to the question: Is the national licensure exam for registered nurses (RNs) (NCLEX®) measuring the right things? To answer this question, the NCSBN launched the Next Generation NCLEX® (NGN®), a research project to determine whether clinical judgment and decision making in nursing practice can reliably be assessed (https://www.ncsbn.org/next-generation-nclex.htm). The conclusion was a need for more research and the use of new item types on the NCLEX®.
- The NCSBN projects that a revised NCLEX® exam will be rolled out in 2023. It is important to prepare nursing students for the licensure examination and to support faculty who prepare them even as the new test is in the development phase. To this end, new item types are included at the end of patient and clinically oriented chapters. These item types may be single episode or unfolding case studies and include:
  - *Enhanced hot spot:* Data are highlighted that are relevant to answer the question.
  - *Cloze:* Two or more blanks are filled into complete statements or tables. Options that provide the missing information are listed for each blank.
  - *Extended multiple response or select all that apply:* Select all of the choices that answer the question. Up to 10 choices may be provided.
  - *Matrix:* Choose the status of multiple actions or assessments as part of a grid or table.
  - *Extended drag and drop:* Choose from a list of options to match them with selected complications, medications, or client or nurse responses.
- These item types are part of the NCSBN's Clinical Judgment Measurement Model and are focused on patient care. They

are designed to measure how the nurse recognizes cues, analyzes cues, prioritizes hypotheses, generates solutions, takes actions, and evaluates outcomes.

OTHER CHANGES TO THE 9TH EDITION

The following changes reflect contemporary nursing practice and psychiatric-mental healthcare and are considered in detail in this edition:
- A transition was made to nursing diagnoses based on the International Classification for Nursing Practice (ICNP) by the International Council of Nurses. This nomenclature promotes interprofessional collaboration through a familiar set of terms that are used by nurses and other healthcare professionals across the world.
- Full *Diagnostic and Statistical Manual of Mental Disorders, 5th edition (DSM-5)* diagnostic criteria are provided for major disorders within the clinical chapters.
- Genetic underpinnings of psychiatric disorders and genetic implications for testing and treatment choices are emphasized.
- Advanced practice treatment modalities are addressed separately from the nursing process in categories of biological treatments (e.g., pharmacotherapy, brain stimulation therapies) and psychological therapies (e.g., cognitive-behavioral therapy, interpersonal therapy).
- Thoroughly updated US Food and Drug Administration–approved medications and treatments are featured in all clinical chapters.
- Due to the near-universal experience of trauma in individuals with psychiatric disorders and conditions, an increased emphasis is given to adverse childhood experiences, trauma, and trauma-informed care.
- Screenings and severity rating scales, introduced in Chapter 1 and included throughout most clinical chapters, provide quantifiable data to supplement categorical criteria.
- Increased attention is given to opioid use disorder and associated disorders such as neonatal abstinence syndrome.
- Refer to the To the Student section of this front matter for examples of thoroughly updated familiar features with a fresh perspective, including Evidence-Based Practice boxes, Considering Culture boxes, Health Policy boxes, Key Points to Remember, Assessment Guidelines, Vignettes, and other features.

ORGANIZATION OF THE TEXT

Chapters are grouped in units to emphasize the clinical perspective and facilitate location of information. The order of the clinical chapters approximates those found in the *DSM-5*. All clinical chapters are organized in a clear, logical, and consistent format with the nursing process as the strong, visible framework. The basic outline for clinical chapters is:

- Introduction: Provides a brief overview of the disorder and identifies disorders that fall under the umbrella of the general chapter name.
- Clinical Picture: Presents an overview of the disorder(s), *DSM-5* criteria for many of the disorders, and strong source material.
- Epidemiology: Helps the student understand the extent of the problem and characteristics of those who may be more likely to be affected. This section includes information such as 12-month prevalence, lifetime prevalence, age of onset, and gender differences.
- Comorbidity: Describes the most common conditions that are associated with the psychiatric disorder. Knowing that comorbid disorders are often part of the clinical picture of specific disorders helps students as well as clinicians understand how to better assess and care for their patients.
- Risk Factors: Provides current views of causation. This section is being updated to increasingly focus on genetic and neurobiological factors in the etiology of psychiatric diagnoses.
- Application of the Nursing Process: Provides a summary of the steps used to provide care for patients with certain classifications of disorders or specific disorders.
  - Assessment:
    - General Assessment: Identifies assessment for specific disorders, including assessment tools and rating scales. The rating scales that are included help to highlight important areas in the assessment of a variety of behaviors and mental conditions.
    - Self-Assessment: Discusses the nurse's thoughts and feelings that should be addressed to enhance self-growth and provide the best possible and most appropriate care to the patient.
    - Assessment Guidelines: Provides a summary of specific areas to assess by disorder.
  - Nursing Diagnosis: The International Classification for Nursing Practice (ICNP) is published by the International Council of Nurses (ICN) as part of the World Health Organization (WHO) family of classifications. The ICNP diagnoses are both logical and intuitive and can be used to create multidisciplinary health vocabularies within information systems. This classification system is used to support the nursing process throughout the clinical chapters in this textbook.
  - Outcomes Identification: Overall desired outcomes are based on the nursing diagnosis and reflect the desired change. Shorter-term goals help to achieve the outcomes.
  - Planning: Encourages students to develop patient-centered priorities in conjunction with patients, families, and others.
  - Implementation: Interventions follow the standards set forth in the *Psychiatric-Mental Health Nursing: Scope and Standards of Practice* (2014). This publication was developed collaboratively by the American Nurses Association, the American Psychiatric Nurses Association, and

the International Society of Psychiatric-Mental Health Nurses. These standards are incorporated throughout the chapters.
  - Evaluation: Addresses evaluation of nursing care as essential to support current planning and intervention. Evaluation also provides direction in modifying the plan of care and updating priorities.
- Treatment Modalities: Addresses treatments that are ordered and/or practiced by advanced practice professionals such as nurse practitioners, psychiatrists, medical doctors, and physician assistants. Treatment modalities fall within two major categories: biological treatments that include pharmacotherapy, brain stimulation therapies, and exercise; and psychological therapies such as cognitive-behavioral therapy.

TEACHING AND LEARNING RESOURCES

For Instructors

Instructor Resources on Evolve, available at http://evolve.elsevier.com/Varcarolis, provide a wealth of material to help you make your psychiatric nursing instruction a success. In addition to all of the Student Resources, the following are provided for faculty:

- **TEACH for Nurses Lesson Plans**, based on the textbook chapter Learning Objectives, serve as ready-made, modifiable lesson plans and a complete roadmap to link all parts of the educational package. These concise and straightforward lesson plans can be modified or combined to meet your particular scheduling and teaching needs.
- **PowerPoint presentations** are organized by chapter, with approximately 750 slides for in-class lectures. The slides are detailed and include customizable text and images to enhance learning in the classroom or in web-based course modules. If you share them with students, they can use the note feature to help them with your lectures.
- **Audience Response Questions for iClicker and other systems** are provided with two to five multiple-answer questions per chapter to stimulate class discussion and assess student understanding of key concepts.
- **Next Generation NCLEX® (NGN)–Style Case Studies for *Varcarolis' Foundations of Psychiatric-Mental Health Nursing*** are available.
- The **Test Bank** has more than 1800 test items, complete with the correct answer, rationale, cognitive level of each question, corresponding step of the nursing process, appropriate NCLEX® Client Needs label, and text page reference(s).
- A *DSM-5* **Webinar** explains the changes in structure and changes to disorders from the *DSM-IV-TR*.

For Students

Student Resources on Evolve, available at http://evolve.elsevier.com/Varcarolis, provide a variety of valuable learning assets. The Evolve page inside the front cover lists log-in instructions.

- **Animations** of the neurobiology of select psychiatric disorders and medications make complex concepts come to life with multidimensional views. You can find these illustrations in the textbook with the icon ▶ next to them.

- **Answer Keys to Critical Thinking Guidelines** provide possible outcomes for the Critical Thinking questions at the end of each chapter.
- **Case Studies and Nursing Care Plans** provide detailed case studies and care plans for specific psychiatric disorders to supplement those found in the textbook.
- The **Glossary** provides an alphabetical list of nursing terms with accompanying definitions.
- **NCLEX® Review Questions,** provided for each chapter, will help students prepare for course examinations and for the RN licensure examination.

- **Pretests** and **Posttests** provide interactive self-assessments for each chapter of the textbook, including instant scoring and feedback at the click of a button.
- **Answers and Rationales for NGN Case Studies and Questions** provides answers for the NGN case studies in the textbook's clinical chapters.

We are grateful to educators who send suggestions and provide feedback and strive to incorporate these ideas from this huge pool of experts into reprints and revisions of *Foundations*. We hope this 9th edition continues to help students learn and appreciate the scope and practice of psychiatric-mental health nursing.

Peggy Halter

Psychiatric-mental health nursing challenges us to understand the complexities of the brain and human behavior. We focus on the origin of psychiatric disorders, including biological determinants and environmental factors. In the chapters that follow, you will learn about people who experience psychiatric disorders and how to provide them with quality nursing care in any setting. As you read, keep in mind these special features.

READING AND REVIEW TOOLS

Objectives and **Key Terms and Concepts** introduce the chapter topics and provide a concise overview of the material discussed.

Key Points to Remember at the end of each chapter reinforce essential information.

Critical Thinking activities at the end of each chapter are scenario-based critical thinking problems for practice in applying what you have learned. **Answer Guidelines** can be found on the Evolve website.

Ten multiple-choice **Chapter Review** questions at the end of each chapter help you review the chapter material and study for exams. **Answers** are conveniently provided following the questions. **Answers** along with **rationales** and textbook **page references** are located on the Evolve website.

ADDITIONAL LEARNING RESOURCES

Your **Evolve Resources** at *http://evolve.elsevier.com/Varcarolis* offer more helpful study aids, such as additional Case Studies and Nursing Care Plans.

CHAPTER FEATURES

Vignettes are short stories that describe the unique circumstances surrounding individual patients with psychiatric disorders.

Self-Assessment sections explore thoughts and feelings you may experience working with patients who have psychiatric disorders. These thoughts and feelings may need to be addressed to enhance self-growth and provide the best possible and most appropriate care to patients.

Assessment Guidelines in the clinical chapters provide summary points for patient assessment.

Evidence-Based Practice boxes demonstrate how current research findings affect psychiatric-mental health nursing practice and standards of care.

Considering Culture boxes reinforce the importance of incorporating culturally sensitive care as part of patient-centered care.

Health Policy boxes promote the vital topic of healthcare advocacy and the role of nurses in influencing and determining the political process.

FDA-Approved Drug tables present the latest information on medications used to treat psychiatric disorders.

Patient and Family Teaching boxes underscore the nurse's role in helping patients and families understand psychiatric disorders, treatments, complications, and medication side effects, among other important issues.

Case Studies and Nursing Care Plans present individualized histories of patients with specific psychiatric disorders following the steps of the nursing process. Interventions with rationales and evaluation statements are presented for each patient goal.

CONTENTS

Deinstitutionalization and Transinstitutionalization, 592
Inadequate Access to Care, 592
Key Points to Remember, 592
Critical Thinking, 593
Chapter Review, 593

33 Forensic Nursing, 596
L. Kathleen Sekula and Alison M. Colbert
Forensic Nursing, 596
Education, 597
Roles and Functions of Forensic Nurses, 598
Forensic Psychiatric Nursing, 599
Roles and Functions of Forensic Psychiatric Nurses, 599
Correctional Nursing, 602
Key Points to Remember, 604
Critical Thinking, 604
Chapter Review, 605

UNIT VII Other Intervention Modalities

34 Therapeutic Groups, 607
Donna Rolin and Emily Fowler
From Group to Therapeutic Group, 607
Concepts Common to All Groups, 608
Therapeutic Factors, 608
Group Content and Process, 609
Phases of Group Development, 609
Planning Phase, 609
Orientation Phase, 610
Working Phase, 610
Termination Phase, 610
Evaluation and Follow-up, 611
Roles of the Group Members, 611
Theoretical Frameworks for Groups, 611
Virtual Groups, 611
Nurses as Group Leaders, 612
Styles of Leadership, 613
Group Leader Supervision, 613
Ethical Issues in Group Therapy, 614
Dealing With Challenging Member Behaviors, 614
Monopolizing Group Member, 615
Disruptive Group Member, 615
Silent Group Member, 615
Expected Outcomes, 615
Key Points to Remember, 615

Critical Thinking, 616
Chapter Review, 616

35 Family Interventions, 619
Christina Fratena and Laura G. Leahy
Family Structure, 619
Family Functions, 620
Management, 620
Boundaries, 620
Communication, 621
Emotional Support, 621
Socialization, 621
Overview of Family Therapy, 622
Concepts Central to Family Therapy, 623
The Identified Patient, 623
Triangulation, 623
Application of the Nursing Process, 623
Assessment, 623
Genograms, 624
Self-Assessment, 624
Nursing Diagnosis, 624
Outcomes Identification, 625
Planning, 625
Intervention, 626
Family Psychoeducation, 626
Evaluation, 626
Treatment Modalities, 627
Psychological Therapies, 627
Key Points to Remember, 627
Critical Thinking, 628
Chapter Review, 628

36 Integrative Care, 630
Christina Fratena
Integrative Care in the United States, 630
Consumers and Integrative Care, 631
Integrative Nursing Care, 631
Integrative Care Education and Certification, 632
Classification of Integrative Care, 632
Natural Products, 632
Mind and Body Approaches, 633
Other Complementary Therapies, 636
Historical Notes Regarding CAM, 638
Key Points to Remember, 638
Critical Thinking, 639
Chapter Review, 639

Index, 642

Mental Health and Mental Illness

Margaret Jordan Halter

Visit the Evolve website for a pretest on the content in this chapter: http://evolve.elsevier.com/Varcarolis

OBJECTIVES

1. Define mental health and mental illness.
2. Describe the continuum of mental health and mental illness.
3. Discuss risk and protective factors for mental illness and mental health.
4. Explore the role of resilience in the prevention of and recovery from mental illness and consider resilience in response to stress.
5. Identify how culture influences the view of mental illnesses and behaviors associated with them.
6. Discuss the nature/nurture origins of psychiatric disorders.
7. Summarize the social influences of mental healthcare in the United States.
8. Discuss the role of public policy on mental health funding.
9. Explain how epidemiological knowledge supports mental healthcare.
10. Identify how the *Diagnostic and Statistical Manual, Fifth Edition (DSM-5)* is used for diagnosing psychiatric conditions.
11. Describe the specialty of psychiatric-mental health nursing.
12. Discuss future challenges and opportunities for mental healthcare in the United States.

KEY TERMS AND CONCEPTS

clinical epidemiology
comorbid condition
cultural competence
Diagnostic and Statistical Manual of Mental Disorders, Fifth Edition (DSM-5)
diathesis-stress model
electronic healthcare
epidemiology

incidence
mental health
mental health continuum
mental illness
phenomena of concern
prevalence
psychiatric-mental health advanced practice registered nurse (PMH-APRN)

psychiatric-mental health nursing
psychiatric-mental health registered nurse (PMH-RN)
recovery
resilience
stigma

If you are a fan of vintage films, you may have witnessed a scene similar to this: A doctor, wearing a lab coat, carrying a clipboard, and displaying an expression of deep concern, enters a hospital waiting room. He approaches an obviously distraught gentleman seated there. The doctor says, "I'm afraid your wife has suffered a nervous breakdown."

From that point on in the film, the woman's condition is only vaguely hinted at. The husband dutifully drives through the asylum gates and enters the stately building. Sounds of sobbing or shrieking patients are heard. Patients are rocking on the floor or shuffling down the hall.

As he nears his wife's room, the staff regard him with sad expressions and keep a polite distance. He may find his wife lying in her bed motionless, standing by the window and staring vacantly into the distance, or sitting with other patients in the hospital's garden. The viewer can only speculate about the actual nature of the woman's illness.

MENTAL HEALTH AND MENTAL ILLNESS

We have come a long way in acknowledging and addressing mental illness since the days of nervous breakdowns. In your

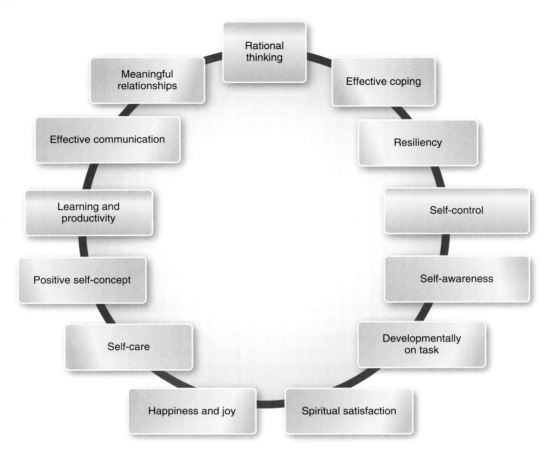

Fig. 1.1 Some attributes of mental health.

psychiatric-mental health nursing course, you will learn about psychiatric disorders, associated nursing care, and treatments. As a foundation for this learning, we will begin by exploring what it means to be mentally healthy.

First, overall health is not possible without good mental health. The World Health Organization (2019) describes health as "a state of complete physical, mental, and social well-being and not merely the absence of disease or infirmity." There is a strong relationship between physical health and mental health: Poor physical health can lead to mental distress and disorders, and poor mental health can lead to physical problems.

What does it mean to be mentally healthy? The World Health Organization (2018a) again provides us with a useful definition. **Mental health** is a state of well-being in which individuals reach their own potential, cope with the normal stresses of life, work productively, and contribute to the community. Mental health provides people with the capacity for rational thinking, communication skills, learning, emotional growth, resilience, and self-esteem. Some of the attributes of mentally healthy people are shown in Fig. 1.1.

Society's definition of mental illness evolves over time. It is a definition shaped by the prevailing culture and societal values, and it reflects changes in cultural norms, social expectations, political climates, and even reimbursement criteria by third-party payers.

In the past, the term *mental illness* was applied to behaviors considered "strange" and "different," behaviors that occurred infrequently and deviated from established norms. Such criteria are inadequate because they suggest that mental health is based on conformity. Applying that definition to nonconformists and independent thinkers such as Abraham Lincoln, Mahatma Gandhi, and Florence Nightingale might result in a judgment of mental illness. Although the sacrifices of a Mother Teresa or the dedication of Martin Luther King, Jr. are uncommon, virtually none of us would consider these much-admired behaviors to be signs of mental illness.

Mental illness refers to all psychiatric disorders that have definable diagnoses. These disorders are manifested in significant dysfunctions that may be related to developmental, biological, or psychological disturbances in mental functioning. The ability to think may be impaired—as in Alzheimer's disease. Emotions may be affected—as in major depressive disorders. Behavioral alterations may be apparent—as in schizophrenia. People may experience some combination of the three alterations.

Mental illness is such a common problem that most of us know someone with a disorder. You may even have one yourself. According to the Substance Abuse and Mental Health Services Administration (SAMHSA, 2020), in 2019:

- One in five, or nearly 21%, of American adults experienced a mental health illness.
- Young adults aged 18 to 25 had the highest level of mental illness, with a prevalence of about 24%.

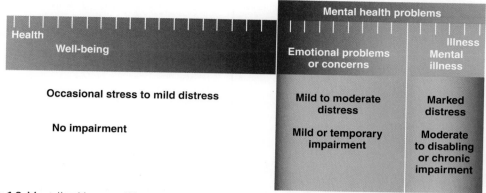

Fig. 1.2 Mental health–mental illness continuum. (From University of Michigan, "Understanding U." [2007]. *What is mental health?* Retrieved from https://hr.umich.edu/benefits-wellness/health/mhealthy/mental-emotional-well-being/understanding-mental-emotional-health/mental-emotional-health-classes-training-events/online-tutorial-supervisors/section-1-what-you-need-know-about-mental-health-problems-substance-misuse.)

- About 5.2% of Americans lived with a serious mental illness, such as schizophrenia, bipolar disorder, or major depressive disorder.
- Approximately 0.06% of adults attempted suicide, and 1.2% of young adults aged 18 to 25 attempted suicide.

MENTAL HEALTH CONTINUUM

You may wonder if there is some middle ground between mental health and mental illness. After all, it is a rare person who does not have concerns regarding mental functioning at one time or another. The answer is that there is definitely a middle ground. In fact, mental health and mental illness can be conceptualized as points along a mental health continuum (Fig. 1.2).

On one end of the continuum is mental health. A sense of well-being describes the general state of people in this category. Well-being is characterized by adequate to high-level functioning. Although individuals at this end of the continuum may experience stress and discomfort resulting from problems of everyday life, they experience no serious impairments in daily functioning.

For example, you may spend a day or two in a gray cloud of self-doubt and recrimination over a failed exam, a sleepless night filled with worry about trivial concerns, or months of genuine sadness and mourning after the death of a loved one. During those low times, you are fully or vaguely aware that you are not functioning well. However, time, exercise, a balanced diet, rest, interaction with others, and mental reframing may alleviate these problems or concerns.

At the opposite end of the continuum is mental illness. Individuals may have emotional problems or concerns and experience mild to moderate discomfort and distress. Mild impairment in functioning such as insomnia, lack of concentration, or loss of appetite may be felt. If the distress increases or persists, individuals might seek professional help. Problems in this category tend to be temporary, but individuals with mild depression, generalized anxiety disorder, and attention-deficit disorder may fit into this group.

The most severely affected individuals fall into the mental illness portion of the continuum. At this point, individuals experience altered thinking, mood, and behavior. It may include relatively common disorders such as depression and anxiety, as well as major disorders such as schizophrenia. The distinguishing factor in mental illness is typically chronic or long-term impairments that range from moderate to disabling.

All of us fall somewhere on the mental health–mental illness continuum and experience gradual or sudden shifts. Many people will never experience the mental illness stage. On the other hand, many people who do reach a more severe level of impairment can experience recovery that ranges from a glimmer of hope to leading a satisfying and fulfilling life.

People who have experienced mental illness can testify to the existence of changes in functioning. The following comments of a 40-year-old woman illustrate the continuum between illness and health as her condition ranged from deep depression to mania to well-being (recovery):

Depression	*It was horror and hell. I was at the bottom of the deepest and darkest pit there ever was. I was worthless and unforgivable. I was as good as—no, worse than—dead.*
Mania	*I was incredibly alive. I could sense and feel everything. I was sure I could do anything, accomplish any task, and create whatever I wanted if only other people wouldn't get in my way.*
Well-being (recovery)	*I am much calmer. I realize now that, when I was manic, it was a pressure-cooker feeling. When I am happy now, or loving, it is more peaceful and real. I have to admit that I sometimes miss the intensity—the sense of power and creativity—of those manic times. I never miss anything about the depressed times, but of course the power and the creativity never bore fruit. Now I do get things done, some of the time, like most people. And people treat me much better now. I guess I must seem more real to them. I certainly seem more real to me (Altrocchi, 1980).*

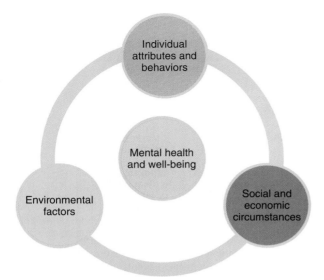

Fig. 1.3 Contributing factors to mental health and well-being. (From World Health Organization. (2013). Mental health: An action plan 2013-2020. Retrieved from https://apps.who.int/iris/rest/bitstreams/424776/retrieve.)

RISK AND PROTECTIVE FACTORS

Many factors can affect the severity and progression of a mental illness, as well as the mental health of a person who does not have a mental illness. Individual characteristics and attributes influence mental health and well-being (WHO, 2013). Socioeconomic circumstances and the environment also influence mental health (Fig. 1.3).

Individual Attributes and Behaviors

Individual attributes refer to characteristics that are both inborn and learned that make us who we are. We all have unique ways of managing thoughts and feelings and navigating the everyday pressures of life. The ability to respond to social cues and participate in social activities influences our view of ourselves and how others view us.

Biological and genetic factors can also influence mental health. Prenatal exposure to alcohol and oxygen deprivation at birth are two examples of biological factors. Genetic factors are huge predictors of mental health and are implicated in nearly every psychiatric disorder.

What makes some people adapt to tragedy, loss, trauma, and severe stress better than others? The answer may be the individual attribute of resilience. Resilience is the ability and capacity for people to secure the resources they need to support their well-being. It is a quality found in some children of poverty and abuse who seek out trusted adults. These adults provide them with the psychological and physical resources that allow them to excel.

Being resilient does not mean being unaffected by stressors. People who are resilient are effective at regulating their emotions and not focusing on negative, self-defeating thoughts. You can get an idea of how good you are at regulating your emotions

BOX 1.1   Brief Resilient Coping Scale

Consider how well the following statements describe your behavior and actions:

1. I look for creative ways to alter difficult situations.
   1 = Does not describe me at all
   2 = Does not describe me
   3 = Neutral
   4 = Describes me
   5 = Describes me very well
2. Regardless of what happens to me, I believe I can control my reaction to it.
   1 = Does not describe me at all
   2 = Does not describe me
   3 = Neutral
   4 = Describes me
   5 = Describes me very well
3. I believe that I can grow in positive ways by dealing with difficult situations.
   1 = Does not describe me at all
   2 = Does not describe me
   3 = Neutral
   4 = Describes me
   5 = Describes me very well
4. I actively look for ways to replace the losses I encounter in life.
   1 = Does not describe me at all
   2 = Does not describe me
   3 = Neutral
   4 = Describes me
   5 = Describes me very well

The possible score range on the Brief Resilient Coping Scale is from 4 (low resilience) to 20 (high resilience). According to the authors of the scale, scores can be interpreted as follows:

Score	Interpretation
4-13	Low resilient copers
14-16	Medium resilient copers
17-20	High resilient copers

From Sinclair, V. G., & Wallston, K.A. (2004). The development and psychometric evaluation of the Brief Resilient Coping Scale. *Assessment, 11*(1), 94-101.

and coping with difficult situations by using the Brief Resilient Coping Scale in Box 1.1.

Social and Economic Circumstances

Your immediate social surroundings impact personal attributes. The earliest social group, the family, has tremendous effects on developing and vulnerable humans. The family sets the stage in promoting confidence and coping skills or for instilling anxiety and feelings of inadequacy.

The social environment extends to schools and peer groups. Again, this environment has the ability to affect mental health positively and negatively. For example, socioeconomic status dictates the sort of resources available to support mental health and reduce concerns over basic needs such as food, clothing, and shelter. Educational advancement is a tremendous supporter of mental health by providing opportunities for a satisfying career, security, and economic benefits.

Environmental Factors

The overall environment that affects mental health relates to the political climate and cultural considerations. Access and lack of access to basic needs and commodities such as healthcare, water, safety services, and a strong highway system have a profound effect on community mental health. Social and economic policies, which are formed at the global, national, state, and local government levels, also impact mental health. For example, in the United States, laws have been gradually shifting toward better reimbursement for mental health services. This shift makes it easier to access and improve mental healthcare.

Predominant cultural beliefs, attitudes, and practices influence mental health. There is no standard measure for mental health, partly because it is culturally defined. One approach to differentiating mental health from mental illness is to consider what a particular culture regards as acceptable or unacceptable. In this view, those with mental illness are those who violate social norms and thus threaten (or make anxious) those observing them.

Throughout history, people have interpreted health or sickness according to their own current views. A striking example of how cultural change influences the interpretation of mental illness is an old definition of *hysteria*. According to *Webster's Dictionary* (Porter, 1913), hysteria was:

> A nervous affection…in women, in which the emotional and reflex excitability is exaggerated, and the will power correspondingly diminished, so that the patient loses control over the emotions, becomes the victim of imaginary sensations, and often falls into paroxysm or fits.

Treatment for this condition, thought to be the result of sexual deprivation, often involved sexual activity. Thankfully, this diagnosis fell into disuse as women's rights improved, the family atmosphere became less restrictive, and societal tolerance of sexual practices increased.

Cultures differ not only in their views regarding mental illness but also the types of behavior categorized as mental illness. Culture-bound syndromes seem to occur in specific sociocultural contexts, and people in those cultures easily recognized them. For example, one syndrome recognized in parts of Southeast Asia is running amok, in which a person (usually a male) runs around engaging in almost indiscriminate violent behavior. In the United States and other developed countries such as those in Europe and Australia, anorexia nervosa is recognized as a disorder characterized by voluntary starvation. Until recently, this disorder was unheard of in third-world countries. However, social media may be contributing to the proliferation of anorexia through increased awareness of its existence.

Perceptions of Mental Health and Mental Illness
Mental Illness Versus Physical Illness

People often make a distinction between mental illnesses and physical illnesses. This is a peculiar distinction. *Mental* refers to the brain, the most complex part of the body, responsible for the higher thought processes that set us apart from all other creatures. Surely the workings of the brain—the synaptic connections, the areas of functioning, the spinal innervations and connections—are *physical*.

One problem with this distinction is that it implies that psychiatric disorders are "all in the head." Most damaging is the belief that these disorders are under personal control and indistinguishable from a choice to engage in bad behavior. These beliefs support the stigma to which people with mental illness are often subjected. Stigma, the belief that the overall person is flawed, is characterized by social shunning, disgrace, and shame.

Perhaps the difference between mental and physical illness lies in the tradition of explaining the unexplainable through superstition. Consider that the frightening convulsions of epilepsy were once explained as demon possession or a curse. Unfortunate individuals with epilepsy were subjected to horrible treatment, including shunning, imprisonment, and exorcisms. We now recognize that seizures are the result of electrical disturbances in the brain and not under personal control. How do we know? Because we can *see* epilepsy on brain scans as areas of overactivity and excitability.

There are no specific biological tests to diagnose most psychiatric disorders—no cranium culture for major depressive disorder and no magnetic resonance imaging (MRI) for obsessive-compulsive disorder (OCD). However, researchers are convinced that the root of most mental disorders lies in intercellular abnormalities. We can now see clear signs of altered brain function and/or structure in several psychiatric disorders, including schizophrenia, OCD, anxiety, and depression.

Nature Versus Nurture

For centuries, people believed that extremely unusual behaviors resulted from supernatural (usually evil) forces. In the late 1800s, the mental health pendulum swung briefly to a biological focus with the "germ theory of diseases." Germ theory explained mental illness in the same way other illnesses were being described (i.e., a specific agent in the environment caused them). This theory was abandoned rather quickly because clinicians and researchers could not identify causative factors for mental illnesses. There was no "mania germ" that could be viewed under a microscope and subsequently treated.

Although biological treatments for mental illness continued to be explored, psychological theories dominated and focused on the science of the mind and behavior. These theories explained the origin of mental illness as faulty psychological processes that could be corrected by increasing personal insight and understanding. For example, a patient experiencing depression and apathy could be assisted to explore feelings from childhood when overly protective parents strictly discouraged attempts at independence.

This psychological focus was challenged in 1952 when chlorpromazine (Thorazine) was found to have a calming effect on patients experiencing agitation and feeling out of control. Imagine what this discovery must have been like for clinicians. Out of desperation they had resorted to every biological treatment imaginable, including wet wraps, insulin shock therapy, and psychosurgery (in which holes were drilled in the head of a patient and probes inserted into the brain) as attempts to change behavior. The scientific community began to believe that if psychiatric problems respond to medications that alter neurochemistry, then a disruption of intercellular components must already be present.

A **diathesis-stress model**—in which diathesis represents biological predisposition and stress represents environmental stress or trauma—is the most accepted explanation for mental illness. This nature-*plus*-nurture argument asserts that most psychiatric disorders result from a combination of genetic vulnerability and negative environmental stressors. One person may develop major depressive disorder largely as the result of an inherited and biological vulnerability that alters brain chemistry. Another person with little vulnerability may develop depression as a result of a stressful environment that causes changes in brain chemistry.

Social Influences on Mental Healthcare
Consumer Movement and Mental Health Recovery

More than 100 years ago, tremendous energy was directed toward improving equality in the United States. Black men were given the right to vote in 1870, as were women, finally, in 1920. Treating people fairly and challenging labels became a focus of the American culture.

With regard to treatment of people with mental illness, decades of institutionalization had created significant political and social concerns. Groups of people with mental illnesses—frequently called mental health consumers—began to advocate for their rights and fought against discrimination and forced treatment.

In 1979, people with mental illnesses and their families formed a nationwide advocacy group, the National Alliance on Mental Illness (NAMI). In the 1980s, individuals in the consumer movement organized by NAMI began to resist the traditional arrangement of mental healthcare providers dictating treatment without the input of the patient. This paternalistic relationship was demoralizing, and it also implied that patients were not competent to make their own decisions. Consumers demanded increased involvement in decisions concerning their treatment.

The consumer movement also promoted the concept of **recovery**, a new and an old idea. On one hand, it represents a concept that has been around a long time: that some people—even those with the most serious illnesses such as schizophrenia—recover. One recovery was depicted in the movie *A Beautiful Mind*. In this film, a brilliant mathematician, John Nash, seems to have emerged from a continuous cycle of devastating psychotic relapses to a state of stabilization and recovery (Howard, 2001).

A newer conceptualization of recovery evolved into a consumer-focused process. According to the SAMHSA (2012), recovery is "a process of change through which individuals improve their health and wellness, live a self-directed life, and strive to reach their full potential." The focus is on the consumer and the consumer's abilities. A real-life example of recovery follows in the vignette.

VIGNETTE: Jeff began hearing voices when he was 19 and was diagnosed with schizophrenia the same year. He dropped out of college, lost his part-time job at a factory, and began collecting Social Security Disability Income. For 20 years, Jeff was told what medication to take, where to live, and what to do.

At the community health center where he received services, he met a fellow patient, Linda, who was involved with a recovery support group. She gave him a pamphlet with a list of the 10 guiding principles of recovery:

1. **Recovery emerges from hope:** Recovery provides the essential motivating message of a better future: That people can and do overcome the barriers and obstacles that confront them. Hope is the catalyst of the recovery process.
2. **Recovery is person driven:** Self-determination and self-direction are the foundations for recovery. Consumers lead, control, exercise choice over, and determine their own path of recovery.
3. **Recovery occurs through many pathways:** Individuals are unique with distinct needs, strengths, preferences, goals, culture, and background (including past trauma) that affect their pathways to recovery. Recovery is nonlinear and may involve setbacks. Abstinence from the use of alcohol, nonprescribed medications, and tobacco is essential. A supportive environment is essential, especially for children.
4. **Recovery is holistic:** Recovery encompasses an individual's whole life, including mind, body, spirit, and community.
5. **Recovery is supported by peers and allies:** Mutual support and aid groups play an invaluable role in recovery. Peers improve social learning, provide experiential knowledge and skills, and a sense of belonging. Helping others helps one's self.
6. **Recovery is supported through relationships and social networks:** The presence and involvement of people who believe in the person's ability to recover; who offer hope, support, and encouragement; and who suggest strategies and resources for change are important.
7. **Recovery is culturally based and influenced:** Culture and cultural background are keys in determining a person's journey and unique pathway to recovery. Services should be culturally grounded, attuned, sensitive, congruent, and competent, as well as personalized to meet unique needs.
8. **Recovery is supported by addressing trauma:** Trauma (e.g., physical or sexual abuse, domestic violence, war, disaster) is associated with substance use and mental health problems. Services and supports should be trauma-informed to foster safety and trust, as well as promote choice, empowerment, and collaboration.
9. **Recovery involves individual, family, and community strengths and responsibility:** Individuals, families, and communities have strengths and resources that serve as a foundation for recovery.
10. **Recovery is based on respect:** Community, systems, and societal acceptance and appreciation of consumers—including protecting their rights and eliminating discrimination and stigma—are crucial in achieving recovery.

Jeff's involvement in the recovery support group changed his view of himself, and he began to take the lead role in his own care. According to Jeff, "Nobody knows your body better than you do, and some, maybe some mental health providers or doctors, think, 'Hey, I am the professional, and you're the person seeing me. I know what's best for you.' But technically, it isn't true. They only provide you with the tools to get better. They can't crawl inside you and see how you are."

Jeff asked for and received newer, more effective medications. He moved into his own apartment and returned to community college and focused on information technology. Jeff now attends recovery support groups regularly and has taken up bicycling. He has his high and low days but maintains goals, hope, and a purpose for his life.

Adapted from Substance Abuse and Mental Health Administration. (2012). *SAMHSA's working definition of recovery updated.* Retrieved from http://blog.samhsa.gov/2012/03/23/defintion-of-recovery-updated/#.VpQInpMrLBl.

Decade of the Brain

In 1990, President George H.W. Bush designated the last decade of the 1900s as the Decade of the Brain. The overriding goal of this designation was to make legislators and the public aware of the advances that had been made in neuroscience and brain research. This US initiative stimulated a worldwide growth of scientific research. Advances and progress made during the Decade of the Brain include:

- Understanding the genetic basis of embryonic and fetal neural development
- Mapping genes involved in neurological illnesses, including mutations associated with Parkinson's disease, Alzheimer's disease, and epilepsy
- Discovering that the brain uses a relatively small number of neurotransmitters but has a vast assortment of neurotransmitter receptors
- Uncovering the role of cytokines (proteins involved in the immune response) in such disorders as depression
- Refining neuroimaging techniques
- Bringing together computer modeling and laboratory research, which resulted in the new discipline of computational neuroscience.

Surgeon General's Report on Mental Health

The first Surgeon General's report on the topic of mental health was published in 1999 (US Department of Health and Human Services, 1999). This landmark document was based on an extensive review of the scientific literature in consultation with mental health providers and consumers. The two most important messages from this report were that (1) mental health is fundamental to overall health and (2) there are effective treatments. The report is reader-friendly and a good introduction to mental health and illness. You can review the report at http://www.surgeongeneral.gov/library/mentalhealth/home.html.

Human Genome Project

The Human Genome Project was a 13-year project that lasted from 1990 to 2003 and was completed on the 50th anniversary of the discovery of the DNA double helix. The project has strengthened biological and genetic explanations for psychiatric conditions. The goals of the project (US Department of Energy, 2008) were to do the following:

- **Identify** the approximately 20,000 to 25,000 genes in human DNA.
- **Determine** the sequences of the 3 billion chemical base pairs that make up human DNA.
- **Store** this information in databases.
- **Improve** tools for data analysis.
- **Address** the ethical, legal, and social issues that may arise from the project.

Researchers are continuing to make progress in understanding genetic underpinnings of diseases and disorders. You will be learning about these advances in the clinical chapters that follow.

President's New Freedom Commission on Mental Health

The President's New Freedom Commission on Mental Health chaired by Michael Hogan released its recommendations for

---

BOX 1.2   Goals for a Transformed Mental Health System in the United States

Goal 1
Americans understand that mental health is essential to overall health.
Goal 2
Mental healthcare is consumer and family driven.
Goal 3
Disparities in mental health services are eliminated.
Goal 4
Early mental health screening, assessment, and referral to services are common practice.
Goal 5
Excellent mental healthcare is delivered, and research is accelerated.
Goal 6
Technology is used to access mental healthcare and information.

Data from US Department of Health and Human Services, President's New Freedom Commission on Mental Health. (2003). *Achieving the promise: Transforming mental health care in America.* USDHHS Publication No. SMA-03–3832. Retrieved from http://www.mentalhealthcommission.gov/reports/finalreport/fullreport-02.htm.

---

mental healthcare in America in 2003. This was the first commission since First Lady Rosalyn Carter's (wife of President Jimmy Carter) in 1978. The report stated that the system of delivering mental healthcare in America was in shambles. It called for a streamlined system with less fragmentation in the delivery of care. The commission advocated for early diagnosis and treatment, adoption of principles of recovery, and increased assistance in helping people find housing and work. Box 1.2 describes the goals necessary for such a transformation of mental healthcare in the United States.

Institute of Medicine

The *Improving the Quality of Health Care for Mental and Substance-Use Conditions: Quality Chasm Series* was released in 2005 by the Health and Medicine Division (HMD) of the National Academies of Medicine, formerly the Institute of Medicine (IOM, 2005). It highlighted effective treatments for mental illness and addressed the huge gap between the best care and the worst. It focused on such issues as the problem of coerced (forced) treatment, a system that treats mental health issues separately from physical health problems, and lack of quality control. The report encouraged healthcare workers to focus on safe, effective, patient-centered, timely, efficient, and equitable care.

Another important and related publication issued by the IOM in 2011 is *The Future of Nursing: Focus on Education.* This report contends that the old way of training nurses is not adequate for the 21st century's complex requirements. It calls for highly educated nurses who are prepared to care for an aging and diverse population with an increasing incidence of chronic disease. They recommended that nurses be trained in leadership, health policy, system improvement, research, and teamwork.

Quality and Safety Education for Nurses. Recommendations from both documents were addressed by a group called Quality and Safety Education for Nurses (QSEN; pronounced *Q-sen*) and were funded by the Robert Wood

Johnson Foundation. They developed a structure to support the education of future nurses who possess the knowledge, skills, and attitudes to continuously improve the safety and quality of healthcare.

QSEN principles improve patient care and even save lives. The case of Betsy Lehman, a health reporter for the Boston Globe who was married to a cancer researcher, helps to illustrate the role of QSEN principles. When she herself was diagnosed with cancer, she was prescribed an incorrect, extremely high dose of an anticancer drug. Ms. Lehman sensed something was wrong and appealed to the healthcare providers, who did not respond to her concerns. The day before she died, she begged others to help because the professionals were not listening (Robert Wood Johnson Foundation, 2011).

How could her death have been prevented? Consider the key areas of care promoted by QSEN and how they could have prevented Ms. Lehman's death:

1. **Patient-centered care:** Care should be given in an atmosphere of respect and responsiveness, and the patient's values, preferences, and needs should guide care.
2. **Teamwork and collaboration:** Nurses and interprofessional teams need to maintain open communication, respect, and shared decision making.
3. **Evidence-based practice:** Optimal healthcare is the result of integrating the best current evidence while considering the patient/family values and preferences.
4. **Quality improvement:** Nurses should be involved in monitoring the outcomes of the care that they give. They should also be care designers and test changes that will result in quality improvement.
5. **Safety:** The care provided should not add further injury (e.g., nosocomial infections). Harm to patients and providers are minimized through both system effectiveness and individual performance.
6. **Informatics:** Information and technology are used to communicate, manage knowledge, mitigate error, and support decision making.

Brain Research Through Advancing Innovative Neurotechnologies Initiative

In 2013, President Barack Obama announced that $300 million in public and private funding would be devoted to the Brain Research through Advancing Innovative Neurotechnologies (BRAIN) Initiative. This money would be used to develop innovative techniques and technologies to unravel the mystery of how the brain functions. The goal is to uncover new ways to prevent, treat, and cure psychiatric disorders, epilepsy, and traumatic brain injury.

According to the National Institutes of Health (2016) more than $70 million is going to over 170 researchers working at 60 different institutions. These researchers are examining such topics as:

- Developing computer programs that may help researchers to detect and diagnose autism and Alzheimer's disease from brain scans
- Building a cap that uses ultrasound waves to precisely stimulate brain cells
- Creating a "neural dust" system made of tiny electric sensors for wirelessly recording brain activity

- Improving current rehabilitation technologies for helping the lives of stroke patients
- Studying how the brain reads and speaks

Research Domain Criteria Initiative

In other specialty areas, symptom-based classification has been replaced by more scientific understanding of the problem. For example, physicians do not make a cardiac diagnosis depending on the type of chest pain a person is having but rather on diagnosing the specific problem, such as myocarditis. Psychiatry continues to rely heavily on symptoms in the absence of objective and measurable data.

In 2013, the National Institute of Mental Health (NIMH) announced that it would no longer fund *Diagnostic and Statistical Manual (DSM)* diagnosis-based studies. Instead, it would put all of its time, effort, and money into something called the Research Domain Criteria (RDoC) Initiative. This initiative challenges researchers to seek causes for mental disorders at the molecular level. NIMH hopes to transform the current diagnostic procedure by using genetics, imaging, and fresh information to create a new classification system.

LEGISLATION AND MENTAL HEALTH FUNDING

Mental Health Parity

Imagine insurance companies singling out a group of disorders such as digestive diseases for reduced reimbursement. Imagine people with colon cancer being assigned higher copays than other cancers. Imagine limiting the number of treatments for which patients could be reimbursed for Crohn's disease over a lifetime. People would be outraged by such discrimination. Yet this is exactly what happened with psychiatric disorders. Too often, insurance companies:

- Did not cover mental healthcare at all
- Identified yearly or lifetime limits on mental health coverage
- Limited hospital days or outpatient treatment sessions
- Assigned higher copayments or deductibles

In response to this problem, advocates fought for parity, a term that refers to equivalence or equal treatment. The Mental Health Parity Act was passed in 1996. This legislation required insurers that provide mental health coverage to offer annual and lifetime benefits at the same level provided for medical/surgical coverage. Unfortunately, by the year 2000, the Government Accounting Office found that although 86% of health plans complied with the 1996 law, 87% of those plans actually imposed new limits on mental health coverage.

The Wellstone-Domenici Parity Act was enacted in 2008 for group health plans with more than 50 employees. The law required that any plan providing mental health coverage must do so in a manner that is functionally equivalent or on par with coverage of other health conditions. This parity pertains to deductibles, copayments, coinsurance, and out-of-pocket expenses, as well as treatment limitations (e.g., frequency of treatment and number/frequency of visits).

Patient Protection and Affordable Care Act of 2010

Parity laws were a good first step in providing more equitable coverage for mental healthcare. However, parity laws do not *require* health plans to cover psychiatric care. Furthermore, the parity laws only applied to large insurers. The Patient Protection and Affordable Care Act (ACA) of 2010 improved coverage for most Americans who are uninsured through a combination of expanded Medicaid eligibility (for the very poor) and the creation of Health Insurance Exchanges in the states to serve as a broker to help uninsured consumers choose among various plans. The so-called "insurance mandate" added a requirement that people without coverage obtain it. The ACA improved mental healthcare coverage in several ways:

- Eliminated medical underwriting in the individual and small group markets, so medical history no longer resulted in enrollment denials for preexisting conditions or higher premiums.
- Required all individual and small group health plans to cover 10 essential health benefits with no annual or lifetime dollar limits. Mental health and addiction treatment were among the essential benefits.
- Made health insurance with mental health benefits available for many individuals who previously had been uninsured. Significant numbers of these (mostly low-income) persons had untreated mental health problems.
- Allowed young adults to remain on their parents' health plans until age 26. This is important to mental health since most psychiatric disorders emerge in adolescence or early 20s.

Insurance regulation changes have occurred since the 2016 presidential election. One of the most significant changes has been expanded access to short-term health insurance plans. These plans are not subject to parity rules for mental health coverage. Individuals may not be aware of this until they are faced with treatment for psychiatric conditions or substance use.

EPIDEMIOLOGY OF MENTAL DISORDERS

Epidemiology, as it applies to psychiatric-mental health, is the quantitative study of the distribution of mental disorders in human populations. Understanding this distribution helps to identify high-risk groups and risk factors associated with illness onset, duration, and recurrence. In clinical chapters (i.e., Chapters 11 to 24) such as schizophrenia spectrum disorders and depressive disorders, epidemiology is consistently addressed. Understanding epidemiological terms will be helpful in interpreting those statistics.

According to SAMHSA (2020), nearly 52 million adults in the United States experienced a diagnosable mental illness in 2019. Major depressive disorder is the leading cause of disability worldwide, with more than 300 million people affected (World Health Organization, 2018b).

Individuals may have more than one mental disorder or another medical disorder. The presence of two or more disorders is known as comorbidity. They can occur at the same time or in sequence. For example, schizophrenia is frequently comorbid with diabetes due to side effects of antipsychotic medications. The interactions between the illnesses can worsen the course of both.

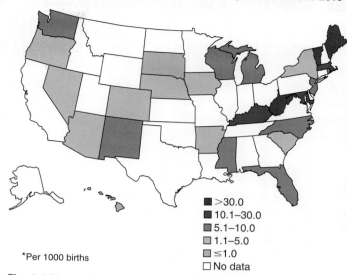

Neonatal Abstinence Syndrome Incidence, 25 States 2012-2013*

- ■ >30.0
- ■ 10.1–30.0
- ■ 5.1–10.0
- ■ 1.1–5.0
- ■ ≤1.0
- ☐ No data

*Per 1000 births

Fig. 1.4 Neonatal abstinence syndrome incidence. (Data from Ko, J. Y., Patrick, S. W., Tong, V. T., Patel, R., Lind, J. N., & Barfield, W. D. (2016). The incidence of neonatal abstinence syndrome—28 states, 1999–2013. *Morbidity and Mortality Weekly Report, 65,* 799–802.)

Two different but related words used in epidemiology are incidence and prevalence. *Incidence* conveys information about the risk of contracting a disease. It refers to the number of new cases of mental disorders in a healthy population within a given period of time, usually annually. An example of incidence pertains to the result of opioid use in pregnancy. The incidence of neonatal abstinence syndrome was 32,000 in 2014, a fivefold increase over the course of a decade (Winkelman et al., 2018). These numbers help to reveal a disturbing public health trend that should be addressed by healthcare providers and policy makers (Fig. 1.4).

Prevalence describes the total number of cases, new and existing, in a given population during a specific period of time, regardless of when they became ill. An example of prevalence is the number of 8-year-olds from 11 states with autism spectrum disorder. In 2014, 16.8 children out of 1000 (1 in 59) screened positively for these disorders at specific clinical sites (Baio et al., 2018). This prevalence rate of nearly 2% was higher than previously demonstrated at these clinical sites. Because these sites do not provide a representative sample of the entire United States, the results are not generalizable to all 8-year-olds.

A disease with a short duration such as the common cold tends to have a high incidence (many new cases in a given year) and a low prevalence (not many people suffering from a cold at any given time). Conversely, a chronic disease such as diabetes will have a low incidence because people will be dropped from the list of new cases after the first year (or whatever time increment is being used) and a high prevalence (given the long-term nature of the illness).

Lifetime risk data, or the risk that one will develop a disease in the course of a lifetime, will be higher than both incidence and prevalence. According to Kessler, Berglund, and colleagues (2005), 46.4% of all Americans will meet the criteria for a

TABLE 1.1 Twelve-Month Prevalence of Psychiatric Disorders in the United States

Disorder	Prevalence Over 12 Months (%)	12 Month % Receiving Treatment	Comments
Schizophrenia	1.1	45.8	Affects men and women equally
Major depressive disorder	6.7	51.7	Leading cause of disability in United States and established economies worldwide Nearly twice as many women (6.5%) as men (3.3%) suffer from major depressive disorder every year
Bipolar disorder	2.6	48.8	Affects men and women equally
Generalized anxiety disorder	3.1	43.2	Can begin across life cycle; risk is highest between childhood and middle age
Panic disorder	2.7	59.1	Typically develops in adolescence or early adulthood Approximately one in three people with panic disorder develop agoraphobia
Obsessive-compulsive disorder	1	No data	First symptoms begin in childhood or adolescence
Posttraumatic stress disorder (PTSD)	3.5	49.9	Can develop at any time Approximately 30% of Vietnam veterans experienced PTSD after the war; percentage high among first responders to September 11, 2001, US terrorist attacks
Social phobia	6.8	40.1	Typically begins in childhood or adolescence
Agoraphobia	0.08	45.8	Begins in young adulthood
Specific phobia	8.7	32.4	Begins in childhood
Any personality disorder	9.1	No data	Antisocial personality disorder more common in men
Alzheimer's disease	10 (65+) 50 (85 years+)		Rare, inherited forms can strike in the 30s–40s

Data from Kessler, R. C., Chiu, W. T., Demler, O., & Walters, E. E. (2005). Prevalence, severity, and comorbidity of twelve-month DSM-IV disorders in the National Comorbidity Survey Replication (NCS-R). *Archives of General Psychiatry, 62*(6), 617–627.

psychiatric disorder in their lifetimes. Table 1.1 shows the prevalence of some psychiatric disorders in the United States.

Originally, epidemiology meant the study of epidemics. Clinical epidemiology is a broad field that examines health and illness at the population level. Studies use traditional epidemiological methods and are conducted in groups usually defined by the illness or symptoms or by the diagnostic procedures or treatments given for the illness or symptoms. Clinical epidemiology includes the following:

- Studies of the natural history—what happens if there is no treatment and the problem is left to run its course—of an illness
- Studies of diagnostic screening tests
- Observational and experimental studies of interventions used to treat people with the illness or symptoms

Analysis of epidemiological studies can reveal the frequency with which psychological symptoms appear together with physical illness. For example, epidemiological studies demonstrate that depression is a significant risk factor for death in people with cardiovascular disease and premature death in people with breast cancer.

Classification of Mental Disorders

Nursing care, as opposed to medical care, is care based on responses to illness. Registered nurses do not diagnose, prescribe, and treat major depressive disorder. They treat the problems associated with depression, such as insomnia or hopelessness. Nurses provide effective care using the nursing process as a guide to holistic care. Nurses, physicians, and other healthcare

providers are part of an interprofessional team. When the team is well coordinated, it can provide optimal care for the biological, psychological, social, and spiritual needs of patients.

To carry out their diverse professional responsibilities, educators, clinicians, and researchers need clear and accurate guidelines for identifying and categorizing mental illness. For clinicians in particular, such guidelines help in planning and evaluating their patients' treatment.

Currently, there are two major classification systems used in the United States: the *Diagnostic and Statistical Manual, Fifth Edition (DSM-5)* and the *International Classification of Disease, Tenth Revision, Clinical Modification (ICD-10-CM)* (WHO, 2016). Both are important in terms of planning patient care and determining reimbursement for services. However, the *DSM-5* is the dominant method of categorizing and diagnosing mental illness in the United States and is the framework for clinical disorders in this textbook.

The *DSM-5*

The *Diagnostic and Statistical Manual (DSM)* is a publication of the American Psychiatric Association (APA). First published in 1952, the latest 2013 edition describes criteria for 157 disorders. The development of the *DSM-5* was influenced by clinical field trials conducted by psychiatrists, psychiatric-mental health advanced practice registered nurses, psychologists, licensed clinical social workers, licensed counselors, and licensed marriage and family therapists.

The *DSM* identifies disorders based on specific criteria. It is used in inpatient, outpatient, partial hospitalization, consultation-liaison, clinics, private practice, primary care, and community settings. The *DSM* also serves as a tool for collecting epidemiological statistics about the diagnosis of psychiatric disorders.

The following is a list of disorder categories in the *DSM-5*. You may notice that the order of the list is similar to the way the chapters are organized in this textbook.

1. Neurodevelopmental Disorders
2. Schizophrenia Spectrum Disorders
3. Bipolar and Related Disorders
4. Depressive Disorders
5. Anxiety Disorders
6. Obsessive-Compulsive Disorders
7. Trauma and Stressor-Related Disorders
8. Dissociative Disorders
9. Somatic Symptom Disorders
10. Feeding and Eating Disorders
11. Elimination Disorders
12. Sleep-Wake Disorders
13. Sexual Dysfunctions
14. Gender Dysphoria
15. Disruptive, Impulse Control, and Conduct Disorders
16. Substance-Related and Addictive Disorders
17. Neurocognitive Disorders
18. Personality Disorders
19. Paraphilic Disorders
20. Other Disorders

A common misconception is that a classification of mental disorders classifies *people*, when the *DSM* actually classifies *disorders*. For this reason, the *DSM* and this textbook avoid the use of stigmatizing labels such as he is "a schizophrenic" or "an alcoholic." Viewing the person as a person and not an illness requires more accurate terms such as "an individual with schizophrenia" or "my patient has major depressive disorder."

The *ICD-10-CM*

In an increasingly global society, it is important to view the United States' diagnosis and treatment of mental illness as part of a bigger picture. The international standard of disease classification is the *International Classification of Diseases, Tenth Revision (ICD-10)* (WHO, 2016). The United States has adapted this resource with a "clinical modification," hence its title of *ICD-10-CM*.

PSYCHIATRIC-MENTAL HEALTH NURSING

In most clinical settings, nurses work with people going through a variety of crises. These crises may be based on physical, psychological, mental, and spiritual distress. Most of you have already come across people going through difficult times in their lives. Although you may have handled these situations well, there may have been times when you wished you had additional skills and knowledge.

The psychiatric nursing rotation will greatly increase your insight into the experiences of others with mental health alterations. Exploring mental health and mental illness may even help you to increase insight into yourself. You will learn

essential information about psychiatric disorders and hopefully have the opportunity to develop new skills for dealing with a variety of behaviors associated with them. The rest of this chapter is devoted to psychiatric nursing—what psychiatric nurses do, their scope of practice, and the challenges and evolving roles for the future healthcare environment.

What Is Psychiatric-Mental Health Nursing?

Psychiatric-mental health nursing is the nursing specialty that is dedicated to promoting mental health through the assessment, diagnosis, and treatment of behavioral problems, mental disorders, and comorbid conditions across the life span (American Nurses Association [ANA] et al., 2014). Psychiatric-mental health nurses work with people throughout their life span: children, adolescents, adults, and older adults.

Psychiatric-mental health nurses assist people who are in crisis or who are experiencing life problems, as well as those with long-term mental illness. These nurses work with patients with dual diagnoses (e.g., a mental disorder and a comorbid substance disorder), homeless persons and families, forensic patients (i.e., people in jail), and individuals who have survived abusive situations. Psychiatric-mental health nurses work with individuals, couples, families, and groups in every nursing setting. They work with patients in hospitals, in their homes, in halfway houses, in shelters, in clinics, in storefronts, on the street—virtually everywhere.

The *Psychiatric-Mental Health Nursing: Scope and Standards of Practice* defines the specific activities of the psychiatric-mental health nurse. This publication—jointly written in 2014 by the American Nurses Association (ANA), the American Psychiatric Nurses Association (APNA), and the International Society of Psychiatric-Mental Health Nurses (ISPN)—defines the focus of psychiatric-mental health nursing as "promoting mental health through the assessment, diagnosis, and treatment of human responses to mental health problems and psychiatric disorders" (p. 14).

The psychiatric-mental health nurse uses the same nursing process you have already learned to assess and diagnose patients' illnesses, identify outcomes, and plan, implement, and evaluate nursing care. Box 1.3 describes phenomena of concern—human experiences and responses—for psychiatric-mental health nurses.

Classification of Nursing Diagnoses

While the *DSM-5* is used to diagnose a psychiatric disorder, a well-defined nursing diagnosis provides the framework for identifying appropriate nursing interventions for dealing with the patient's reaction to the disorder. To provide the most appropriate and scientifically sound care, the psychiatric-mental health nurse uses standardized classification systems developed by professional nursing groups. These systems provide standardized diagnoses, many of which are related to psychosocial/psychiatric nursing care. The diagnoses provide a common language to aid in the selection of nursing interventions and ultimately lead to outcome achievement. The *International Classification for Nursing Practice (ICNP)*, developed by the

International Council of Nurses (ICN, n.d.), provides standardized nursing diagnoses that are used to guide care in this textbook.

Psychiatric-Mental Health Nurse Education Levels

Psychiatric-mental health nurses are registered nurses educated in nursing and licensed to practice in their individual states. Psychiatric nurses are qualified to practice at two levels, basic and advanced, depending on educational preparation.

BOX 1.3 Phenomena of Concern for Psychiatric-Mental Health Nurses

Phenomena of concern for psychiatric-mental health nurses include:
- Promotion of optimal mental and physical health and well-being
- Prevention of mental and behavioral distress and illness
- Promotion of social inclusion of mentally and behaviorally fragile individuals
- Co-occurring mental health and substance use disorders
- Co-occurring mental health and physical disorders
- Alterations in thinking, perceiving, communicating, and functioning related to psychological and physiological distress
- Psychological and physiological distress resulting from physical, interpersonal, and/or environmental trauma or neglect
- Psychogenesis and individual vulnerability
- Complex clinical presentations confounded by poverty and poor, inconsistent, or toxic environmental factors
- Alterations in self-concept related to loss of physical organs and/or limbs, psychic trauma, developmental conflicts, or injury
- Individual, family, or group isolation and difficulty with interpersonal relations
- Self-harm and self-destructive behaviors, including mutilation and suicide
- Violent behavior, including physical abuse, sexual abuse, and bullying
- Low health literacy rates contributing to treatment nonadherence

From American Psychiatric Nurses Association, International Society of Psychiatric-Mental Health Nurses, & American Nurses Association. (2014). *Psychiatric-mental health nursing: Scope and standards of practice* (2nd ed.). Silver Spring, MD: NursesBooks.org.

Table 1.2 describes basic and advanced psychiatric nursing interventions.

Basic Level

Basic level registered nurses are professionals who have completed a nursing program, passed the state licensure examination, and are qualified to work in most any general or specialty area. The **psychiatric-mental health registered nurse (PMH-RN)** is a nursing graduate who possesses a diploma, an associate degree, or a baccalaureate degree and chooses to work in the specialty of psychiatric-mental health nursing. At the basic level, nurses work in various supervised settings and perform multiple roles, such as staff nurse, case manager, home care nurse, and so on.

After 2 years of full-time work as a registered nurse, 2000 clinical hours in a psychiatric setting, and 30 hours of continuing education in psychiatric nursing, a baccalaureate-prepared nurse may take a certification examination administered by the American Nurses Credentialing Center (the credentialing arm of the ANA) to demonstrate clinical competence in psychiatric-mental health nursing. After passing the examination, a board-certified credential is added to the RN title, resulting in RN-BC. Certification gives nurses a sense of mastery and accomplishment, identifies them as competent clinicians, and satisfies a requirement for reimbursement by employers in some states.

Advanced Practice

One of the first advanced practice nursing roles in the United States was the psychiatric clinical nurse specialist (CNS) in the 1950s. These expert nurses were originally trained to provide individual therapy and group therapy in state psychiatric hospitals and to provide training for other staff. Eventually they, along with psychiatric nurse practitioners (NPs) who were introduced in the mid-1960s, gained diagnostic privileges, prescriptive authority, and the ability to provide psychotherapy.

Currently, the **psychiatric-mental health advanced practice registered nurse (PMH-APRN)** is a licensed registered

---

TABLE 1.2 Basic Level and Advanced Practice Psychiatric-Mental Health Nursing Interventions

Basic Level Intervention	Description
Coordination of care	Coordinates implementation of the nursing care plan and documents coordination of care
Health teaching and health maintenance	Individualized anticipatory guidance to prevent or reduce mental illness or enhance mental health (e.g., community screenings, parenting classes, stress management)
Milieu therapy	Provides, structures, and maintains a safe and therapeutic environment in collaboration with patients, families, and other healthcare clinicians
Pharmacological, biological, and integrative therapies	Applies current knowledge to assessing patient's response to medication, provides medication teaching, and communicates observations to other members of the healthcare team
Advanced Practice Intervention	**Description**
All of the Above Plus:	
Medication prescription and treatment	Prescription of psychotropic medications with appropriate use of diagnostic tests; hospital admitting privileges
Psychotherapy	Individual, couple, group, or family therapy using evidence-based therapeutic frameworks and the nurse-patient relationship
Consultation	Sharing of clinical expertise with nurses or those in other disciplines to enhance their treatment of patients or address systems issues

Data from American Psychiatric Nurses Association, International Society of Psychiatric-Mental Health Nurses, & American Nurses Association. (2014). *Psychiatric-mental health nursing: Scope and standards of practice.* Silver Spring, MD: NurseBooks.org.

nurse with a Master of Science in Nursing (MSN) or Doctor of Nursing Practice (DNP) in psychiatric nursing. This DNP is not to be confused with a doctoral degree (PhD) in nursing, which is a research degree, whereas the DNP is a practice doctorate. The PMH-APRN functions with various levels of autonomy depending on the state and is eligible for specialty privileges. Some advanced practice nurses continue their education to the PhD level.

Unlike other specialty areas, there is no significant difference between a psychiatric NP and a CNS as long as the CNS has achieved prescriptive authority. Certification is required and is obtained through the American Nurses Credentialing Center. Only one examination—the Psychiatric-Mental Health Nurse Practitioner—Board Certified (PMHNP-BC)—is currently available. Three other examinations have been discontinued:

- Adult Psychiatric-Mental Health Nurse Practitioner—Board Certified (PMHNP-BC)
- Adult Psychiatric-Mental Health Clinical Nurse Specialist—Board Certified (PMHCNS-BC)
- Child/Adolescent Psychiatric-Mental Health Clinical Nurse Specialist—Board Certified (PMHCNS-BC)

Although these examinations are no longer given, you will still find many nurses who practice in these roles. Their credentials will continue to be renewed if professional development and practice hour requirements are met.

TRENDS AFFECTING THE FUTURE OF PSYCHIATRIC-MENTAL HEALTH NURSING

Significant trends will affect the future of psychiatric nursing in the United States. These trends include educational challenges, a shortage of mental health professionals, an aging population, increasing cultural diversity, and technological opportunities.

Educational Challenges

As with other specialty areas in a hospital setting, psychiatric nurses are caring for more acutely ill patients. In the 1980s, it was common for patients who were depressed and suicidal to have insurance coverage for approximately 2 weeks. Currently, patients are lucky to be covered for 3 days, if they are covered at all. This means that nurses need to be more skilled and be prepared to discharge patients for whom the benefit of their care will not always be evident.

Providing educational experiences for nursing students is challenging as a result of this level of acute care and also due to the declining inpatient populations. Clinical rotations in general medical centers are becoming more difficult to obtain. Faculty are fortunate to secure rotations in state psychiatric hospitals, veterans administration facilities, and community settings.

Community psychiatric settings also provide students with valuable experience, but the logistics of placing and supervising students in multiple sites has required creativity on the part of nursing educators. Some schools have established integrated rotations that theoretically allow students to work outside the psychiatric setting with patients who have psychiatric disorders. For example, a student may provide care for a person with major depressive disorder on an orthopedic floor. Some faculty are concerned that without serious commitment, this type of specialty integration may water down a previously rich clinical experience.

A Demand for Mental Health Professionals

The growth of the psychiatric workforce has not been keeping pace with demand. As previously stated, in 2019, nearly 52 million US adults older than the age of 18 had a mental illness. This number represents approximately 21% of all adults (SAMHSA, 2020). During the same year, about 16% of adults received treatment. Lack of treatment results in disability, impaired relationships, and, in the case of suicide, mortality.

Nurse-led medical/health homes and clinics are becoming increasingly common. Community nursing centers that can secure funding serve low-income and uninsured people. In this model, psychiatric-mental health nurses work with primary care nurses to provide comprehensive care, usually funded by scarce grants from academic centers. These centers use a nontraditional approach of combining primary care and health promotion interventions. Advanced practice psychiatric nurses have also been extremely successful in setting up private practices where they provide both psychotherapy and medication management.

An Aging Population

As the number of older adults grows, the prevalence of Alzheimer's disease and other neurocognitive disorders requiring skilled nursing care in inpatient settings is likely to increase. Healthier older adults will need more services at home, in retirement communities, or in assisted living facilities. Psychiatric-mental health nurses will be on the forefront in managing care for older adults. For more information on the needs of older adults, refer to Chapters 23, 28, and 31.

Cultural Diversity

Cultural diversity is steadily increasing in the United States. The US Census Bureau (2015) notes that the United States will have a majority minority population by 2044. Psychiatric-mental health nurses will need to increase and maintain their **cultural competence**. Simply put, cultural competence means that nurses adjust *their* practices to meet their patients' cultural beliefs, practices, needs, and preferences. Chapter 5 provides a more thorough discussion of the cultural implications for providing psychiatric nursing care.

Science, Technology, and Electronic Healthcare

Genetic mapping from the Human Genome Project has resulted in a steady stream of research discoveries concerning genetic markers implicated in a variety of psychiatric illnesses. This information could be helpful in identifying at-risk individuals and in targeting medications specific to certain genetic variants and profiles. However, the legal and ethical implications of responsibly using this technology are staggering. For example:

- Would you want to know you were at risk for a psychiatric illness such as bipolar disorder?
- Who should have access to this information—your primary care provider, insurer, future spouse, or a lawyer in a child-custody battle?
- Who will regulate genetic testing centers to protect privacy and prevent 21st-century problems such as identity theft and fraud?

Despite these concerns, the next decade holds great promise in the diagnosis and treatment of psychiatric disorders, and nurses will be central as educators and caregivers. Scientific advances through research and technology are certain to shape psychiatric-mental health nursing practice. MRI research, in addition to comparing healthy people to people diagnosed with mental illness, is now focusing on the development of preclinical profiles of children and adolescents. The hope of this type of research is to identify people at risk for developing mental illness, which allows earlier interventions to try to decrease impairment.

Electronic healthcare services provided from a distance are gaining wide acceptance. In the early days of the internet, consumers were cautioned against the questionable wisdom of seeking advice through an unregulated medium. However, the internet has transformed the way we approach healthcare needs and allows people to be their own advocates.

In 2020, the coronavirus pandemic resulted in fears of contagion from in-person meetings. As with other healthcare providers, many psychiatric professionals adopted telehealth in order to support their patients and also to continue working. The pandemic will likely alter the healthcare landscape for the foreseeable future because some providers have opted to continue telehealth in the future, even when the danger has passed.

Telepsychiatry through audio and visual media is an effective way to reach underserved populations and those who are homebound. Providing healthcare in this private setting also destigmatizes the experience by offering greater privacy. It allows for assessment and diagnosis, medication management, and even group therapy. Psychiatric nurses may become more active in developing websites for mental health education, screening, or support, especially to reach geographically isolated areas. Many health agencies hire nurses to staff help lines or hotlines, and as provision of these cost-effective services increases, so too will the need for bilingual resources.

ADVOCACY AND LEGISLATIVE INVOLVEMENT

Through direct care and indirect action, nurses advocate for the psychiatric patient. As a patient advocate, the nurse reports incidents of abuse or neglect to the appropriate authorities for immediate action. The nurse also upholds patient confidentiality, which has become more of a challenge with the use of electronic medical records. Another form of nursing advocacy is supporting the patient's right to make decisions regarding treatment.

On an indirect level, the nurse may choose to be active in consumer mental health groups (such as NAMI) and state and local mental health associations to support consumers of mental healthcare. The nurse can also be vigilant about reviewing local and national legislation affecting healthcare to identify potential detrimental effects on the mentally ill. Especially during times of fiscal crisis, lawmakers are inclined to decrease or eliminate funding for vulnerable populations who do not have a strong political voice.

The APNA devotes significant energy to monitoring legislative, regulatory, and policy matters affecting psychiatric nursing and mental health. As the 24-hours-a-day, 7-days-a-week caregivers and members of the largest group of healthcare professionals, nurses have the potential to exert tremendous influence on legislation.

However, when commissions and task forces are developed, nurses are not usually the first group to be considered to provide input and expertise for national, state, and local decision makers. In fact, nursing presence is often absent at the policymaking table. Consider the President's New Freedom Commission for Mental Health, which included psychiatrists (medical doctors), psychologists (PhDs), academics, and policymakers—but no nurses. It is difficult to understand how the largest contingent of mental healthcare providers in the United States could be excluded from a group that would determine the future of mental healthcare.

It is in the best interest of consumers of mental healthcare that all members of the collaborative healthcare team, including nurses, be involved in decisions and legislation that will affect their care. Current political issues that need monitoring and support include mental health parity, discriminatory media portrayal, standardized language and practices, and advanced practice issues, such as autonomous practice and government and insurance reimbursement for nursing care.

KEY POINTS TO REMEMBER

- Overall health is not possible without good mental health.
- Mental illness refers to all psychiatric disorders with definable diagnoses that cause significant dysfunction in developmental, biological, or psychological disturbances.
- A mental health and mental illness continuum is a useful representation for demonstrating how functioning may change over time. Mental health and illness are not either/or propositions but are instead endpoints on a continuum.
- Risk factors such as inborn vulnerability, a poor social environment, economic hardship, and poor health policy may increase the risk of adverse mental health outcomes.
- Protective factors such as resiliency improve a person's ability to respond to stress, trauma, and loss.
- The distinction between mental and physical illness is artificial. Mental illness is brain based and is therefore a physical illness.

- Psychiatric disorders are generally the result of nature and nurture. A diathesis-stress model—in which diathesis represents biological predisposition and stress represents environmental stress or trauma—is the most accepted explanation for mental illness.
- The recovery movement has shifted the focus of decision making from a paternalistic system, where compliance is emphasized, to a focus on self-determination and self-direction.
- Government programs and initiatives such as the Decade of the Brain, the Human Genome Project, Brain Research through Advancing Innovative Neurotechnology, and RDoC are expanding our knowledge of the brain and will provide the basis for future treatments.
- Until recently, funding for psychiatric care had not been equal to that of other medical care. Mental health parity refers to equality in funding.

- The study of epidemiology can help to identify high-risk groups and behaviors. In turn, this can lead to a better understanding of the causes of some disorders. Prevalence rates help us to identify the proportion of a population experiencing a specific mental disorder at a given time.
- The *DSM-5* provides criteria for psychiatric disorders and a basis for the development of comprehensive and appropriate interventions.
- A standardized nursing classification system, the *International Classification for Nursing Practice,* is used to form and communicate nursing diagnoses and patient problems.
- As a result of social, cultural, scientific, and political factors, the future holds many challenges and opportunities for psychiatric-mental health nurses.

CRITICAL THINKING

1. Brian, a college sophomore with a grade-point average of 3.4, is brought to the emergency department after a suicide attempt. He has been extremely despondent since the death of his girlfriend 5 months ago, when the car he was driving crashed. His parents are devastated, and they believe that taking one's own life prevents a person from going to heaven.

   Brian has epilepsy and has had more seizures since the auto accident. He says he should be punished for his carelessness and does not care what happens to him. He has stopped going to classes and no longer shows up for his part-time job tutoring young children in reading.
   a. What might be a possible *DSM-5* (medical) diagnosis?
   b. What are some factors that you should assess regarding aspects of Brian's overall health and other influences that can affect mental health?
   c. If an antidepressant medication could help Brian's depression, explain why this alone would not meet his multiple needs. What issues do you think have to be addressed if Brian is to receive a holistic approach to care?
   d. Formulate two potential nursing diagnoses for Brian.
   e. Would Brian's parents' religious beliefs factor into your plan of care? If so, how?

2. In a small group, share experiences you have had with others from unfamiliar cultural, ethnic, religious, or racial backgrounds, and identify two positive learning experiences from these encounters.

3. Would you feel comfortable referring a family member to a mental health clinician? What factors influence your feelings?

4. How could basic and advanced practice psychiatric-mental health nurses work together to provide the highest quality of care?

5. Would you consider joining a professional group or advocacy group that promotes mental health? Why or why not?

CHAPTER REVIEW

1. When providing respectful, appropriate nursing care, how should the nurse identify the patient and his or her observable characteristics?
   a. The manic patient in room 234
   b. The patient in room 234 is a manic
   c. The patient in room 234 is possibly a manic
   d. The patient in room 234 is displaying manic behavior

2. Recognizing the frequency of depression among the American population, the nurse should advocate for which mental health promotion intervention?
   a. Including discussions on depression as part of school health classes
   b. Providing regular depression screening for adolescent and teenage students
   c. Increasing the number of community-based depression hotlines available to the public
   d. Encouraging senior centers to provide information on accessing community depression resources

3. Which statement made by a patient demonstrates a healthy degree of resilience? *Select all that apply.*
   a. "I try to remember not to take other people's bad moods personally."
   b. "I know that if I get really mad, I'll end up being depressed."
   c. "I really feel that sometimes bad things are meant to happen."

   d. "I've learned to calm down before trying to defend my opinions."
   e. "I know that discussing issues with my boss would help me get my point across."

4. Which statement demonstrates the nurse's understanding of the effect of environmental factors on a patient's mental health?
   a. "I'll need to assess how the patient's family views mental illness."
   b. "There is a history of depression in the patient's extended family."
   c. "I'm not familiar with the patient's cultural view on suicide."
   d. "The patient's ability to pay for mental health services needs to be assessed."

5. When considering stigmatization, which statement made by the nurse demonstrates a need for immediate intervention by the nurse manager?
   a. "Depression seems to be a real problem among the teenage population."
   b. "My experience has been that the Irish have a problem with alcohol use."
   c. "Women are at greater risk for developing suicidal thoughts than acting on them."
   d. "We've admitted several military veterans with posttraumatic stress disorder this month."

6. A nursing student new to psychiatric-mental health nursing asks a peer what resources he can use to figure out which symptoms are present in a specific psychiatric disorder. The best answer would be:
   a. National Institute of Mental Illness
   b. National Alliance on Mental Illness
   c. International Classification for Nursing Practice
   d. DSM

7. Epidemiological studies contribute to improvements in care for individuals with mental disorders by:
   a. Providing information about effective nursing techniques.
   b. Identifying risk factors that contribute to the development of a disorder.
   c. Identifying individuals in the general population who will develop a specific disorder.
   d. Identifying which individuals will respond favorably to a specific treatment.

8. Which of the following activities would be considered nursing care and appropriate to be performed by a basic level nurse for a patient suffering from mental illness?
   a. Treating major depressive disorder
   b. Teaching coping skills for a specific family dynamic
   c. Conducting psychotherapy
   d. Prescribing antidepressant medication

9. Which statement about mental illness is true?

   a. Mental illness is a matter of individual nonconformity with societal norms.
   b. Mental illness is present when irrational and illogical behavior occurs.
   c. Mental illness changes with culture, time in history, political systems, and the groups defining it.
   d. Mental illness is evaluated solely by considering individual control over behavior and appraisal of reality.

10. The World Health Organization describes health as "a state of complete physical, mental, and social well-being and not merely the absence of disease or infirmity." Which statement is true in regard to overall health? *Select all that apply.*
    a. There is no relationship between physical and mental health.
    b. Poor physical health can lead to mental distress and disorders.
    c. Poor mental health does not lead to physical illness.
    d. There is a strong relationship between physical health and mental health.
    e. Mental health needs take precedence over physical health needs.

1. d; 2. b; 3. a, d, e; 4. c; 5. b; 6. d; 7. b, d; 8. b; 9. c; 10. b, d

Visit the Evolve website for a posttest on the content in this chapter: http://evolve.elsevier.com/Varcarolis

REFERENCES

Altrocchi, J. (1980). *Abnormal behavior.* New York, NY: Harcourt Brace Jovanovich.

American Nurses Association, American Psychiatric Nurses Association, & International Society of Psychiatric-Mental Health Nurses. (2014). *Psychiatric-mental health nursing: Scope and standards of practice.* Spring, MD: NursesBooks.org.

American Psychiatric Association. (2013). *Diagnostic and statistical manual of mental disorders* (5th ed.). Washington, DC: Author.

Baio, J., Wiggins, L., Christensen, D. L., Maenner, M. J., Daniels, J., Warren, Z., & Dowling, N. F. (2018). Prevalence of autism spectrum disorder among children age 8 years. *Surveillance Summaries, 67*(6), 1–23.

Department of Health and Human Services. (2003). *New Freedom Commission on Mental Health.* Publication number SMA-03-3831. Rockville, MD: Author.

Howard, R. (director) (2001). *A beautiful mind* [film]. Los Angeles: Universal Pictures.

Institute of Medicine (IOM). (2005). *Improving the quality of health care for mental and substance-use conditions: Quality chasm series.* Washington, DC: National Academies Press.

Institute of Medicine (IOM). (2011). *The future of nursing: Focus on education.* Retrieved from http://nationalacademies.org/hmd/reports/2010/the-future-of-nursing-leading-change-advancing-health/report-brief-education.aspx.

International Council of Nurses. (n.d.). About ICNP. Retrieved from. https://www.icn.ch/what-we-do/projects/ehealth-icnptm/about-icnp.

Johnson Foundation, Robert Wood (2011). *QSEN branches out.* Retrieved from http://www.rwjf.org/humancapital/product.jsp?id=72552.

Kessler, R. C., Berglund, P., Demler, O., Jin, R., & Walters, E. E. (2005). Lifetime prevalence and age-of-onset distributions of DSM-IV disorders in the national comorbidity survey replication. *Archives of General Psychiatry, 62*, 593–602.

National Institutes of Health. (2016). *NIH nearly doubles investment in BRAIN Initiative research.* Retrieved from https://www.nimh.nih.gov/news/science-news/2016/nih-nearly-doubles-investment-in-brain-initiative-research.shtml.

Porter, N. (Ed.). (1913). *Webster's revised unabridged dictionary.* Boston, MA: Merriam.

Substance Abuse and Mental Health Services Administration. (2012). *SAMHSA announces a working definition of "recovery" from mental disorders and substance use disorders.* Retrieved from http://www.samhsa.gov/newsroom/advisories/1112223420.aspx.

Substance Abuse and Mental Health Services Administration. (2020). *Key substance use and mental health indicators in the United States: Results from the 2019 National Survey on Drug Use and Health.* Retrieved from http://www.samhsa.gov/newsroom/press-announcements/201411200115.

United States Census Bureau. (2015). *Projections of the size and composition of the US population: 2014 to 2060.* Retrieved from http://www.census.gov/content/dam/Census/library/publications/2015/demo/p25-1143.pdf.

United States Department of Energy. (2008). *The Human Genome Project.* Retrieved from http://www.ornl.gov/sci/techresources/Human_Genome/home.shtml.

United States Department of Health and Human Services. (1999). *Mental health: A report of the Surgeon General.* Washington, DC: US Government Printing Office.

Winkelman, T. N. A., Villapiano, N., Kozhimannil, K. B., Davis, M. M., & Patrick, S. W. (2018). Incidence and costs of neonatal abstinence syndrome among infants with Medicaid: 2004-2014. *Pediatrics, 141*(4), e20173520.

World Health Organization. (2013). *Mental health: An action plan 2013-2020.* Retrieved from https://apps.who.int/iris/rest/bitstreams/424776/retrieve.

World Health Organization. (2016). *ICD-10: International Statistical Classification of Diseases, tenth revision, clinical modification.* New York, NY: Author.

World Health Organization. (2018a). *Mental health: A state of well-being.* Retrieved from https://www.who.int/news-room/fact-sheets/detail/mental-health-strengthening-our-response.

World Health Organization. (2018b). *Depression.* Retrieved from https://www.who.int/news-room/fact-sheets/detail/depression.

World Health Organization. (2019). *Constitution.* Retrieved from https://www.who.int/about/who-we-are/constitution.

Theories and Therapies

Margaret Jordan Halter

Visit the Evolve website for a posttest on the content in this chapter: http://evolve.elsevier.com/Varcarolis

OBJECTIVES

1. Describe the evolution of theories of psychiatric disorders and conditions.
2. Distinguish between dominant theories and associated therapies for psychiatric alterations.
3. Identify how psychiatric theories and therapies are applied in nursing care.
4. Discuss the major components of Peplau's Theory of Interpersonal Relationships.
5. Describe the biological model and its impact on the treatment of psychiatric disorders.
6. Explain the value of developmental theories to patients across the lifespan.

KEY TERMS AND CONCEPTS

automatic thoughts
behavioral therapy
biofeedback
classical conditioning
cognitive behavioral therapy (CBT)
cognitive distortions
conditioning
conscious

countertransference
defense mechanisms
ego
extinction
id
interpersonal therapy
negative reinforcement
operant conditioning

positive reinforcement
preconscious
psychodynamic therapy
punishment
reinforcement
superego
transference
unconscious

Every professional discipline, from math and science to philosophy and psychology, bases its work and beliefs on theories. Most of these theories can be best described as explanations, hypotheses, or hunches rather than testable facts.

The word *theory* may conjure up some dry, conceptual images. You may vaguely recall the physicists' theory of relativity or the geologists' plate tectonics. However, compared with most other theories, psychological theories are filled with familiar concepts and terms. Psychological theories have filtered their way into parts of mainstream thinking and speech. For example, advertisers use the behaviorist trick of linking a seductive woman to the utilitarian minivan. And who has not attributed language mistakes to subconscious motivation? As the fictional king greets his queen: "Good morning, my beheaded...I mean my beloved!" we comprehend the Freudian slip.

Dealing with other people is one of the most universally anxiety-provoking activities, and psychological theories provide plausible explanations for perplexing behavior. Maybe the guy at the front desk who never greets you in the morning does not really despise you. Maybe he has an inferiority complex because his mother was cold and his father was absent from the home.

This chapter will provide you with snapshots of some of the most influential psychological theories. It also gives you an overview of the treatments, or therapies, that the theories inspired. We will also address the contributions that the theories have made to the practice of psychiatric-mental health nursing.

PSYCHOANALYTIC THEORIES AND THERAPIES

Psychoanalytic Theory

Sigmund Freud (1856–1939), an Austrian neurologist, revolutionized thinking about mental health disorders. He introduced a groundbreaking theory of personality structure, levels of awareness, anxiety, the role of defense mechanisms, and the stages of psychosexual development.

Originally, he was searching for biological treatments for psychological disturbances and even experimented with using cocaine as medication. He soon abandoned this physiological approach and focused on psychological treatments. Freud came to believe that the vast majority of mental disorders resulted from unresolved issues that originated in childhood.

Levels of Awareness

Freud believed that there were three levels of psychological awareness in operation. He used the image of an iceberg to describe these levels of awareness (Fig. 2.1).

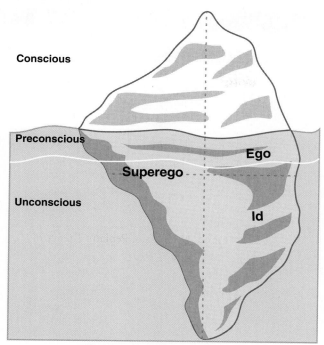

Fig. 2.1 The mind as an iceberg.

Conscious. The conscious part of the mind is the tip of the iceberg. It contains all the material a person is aware of at any one time, including perceptions, memories, thoughts, fantasies, and feelings.

Preconscious. Just below the surface of awareness is the preconscious, which contains material that can be retrieved rather easily through conscious effort.

Unconscious. The unconscious includes all repressed memories, passions, and unacceptable urges lying deep below the surface. Memories and emotions associated with trauma may be stored in the unconscious because the individual finds it too painful to deal with them. The unconscious exerts a powerful yet unseen effect on the conscious thoughts and feelings of the individual. The individual is usually unable to retrieve unconscious material without the assistance of a trained therapist.

Personality Structure

Freud (1960) delineated three major and distinct but interactive systems of the personality: the id, ego, and superego.

Id. At birth, we are all id. The id is totally unconscious and impulsive. It is the source of all drives, instincts, reflexes, and needs. The id cannot tolerate frustration and seeks to discharge tension and return to a more comfortable level of energy. The id lacks the ability to problem solve and is illogical. A hungry, screaming infant is the perfect example of id.

Ego. Within the first few years of life as the child begins to interact with others, the ego develops. The ego resides in the conscious, preconscious, and unconscious levels of awareness. The problem solver and reality tester, the ego attempts to navigate the outside world. It is able to differentiate subjective experiences, memory images, and objective reality.

The ego follows the reality principle, which says to the id, "You have to delay gratification for right now," then sets a course of action. For example, a hungry man feels tension arising from the id that wants to be fed. His ego allows him not only to think about his hunger but also to plan where he can eat and to seek that destination. This process is known as reality testing because the individual is factoring in reality to implement a plan to decrease tension.

Superego. The superego, which develops between the ages of 3 and 5, represents the moral component of personality. The superego resides in the conscious, preconscious, and unconscious levels of awareness. The superego consists of the conscience (all the "should nots" internalized from parents and society) and the ego ideal (all the "shoulds" internalized from parents and society). When behavior falls short of ideal, the superego may induce guilt. Likewise, when behavior is ideal, the superego may allow a sense of pride.

In a mature and well-adjusted individual, the three systems of the personality—the id, ego, and superego—work together as a team under the administrative leadership of the ego. If the id is too powerful, the person will lack control over impulses. If the superego is too powerful, the person may be self-critical and suffer from feelings of inferiority.

Defense Mechanisms and Anxiety

Freud (1969) believed that anxiety is an inevitable part of living. The environment in which we live presents dangers and insecurities, threats and satisfactions. It can produce pain and increase tension or produce pleasure and decrease tension. The ego develops defenses, or defense mechanisms, to ward off anxiety by preventing conscious awareness of threatening feelings.

Defense mechanisms share two common features: (1) they all (except suppression) operate on an unconscious level and (2) they deny, falsify, or distort reality to make it less threatening. Although we cannot survive without defense mechanisms, it is possible for our defense mechanisms to distort reality to such a degree that we experience difficulty with healthy adjustment and personal growth. Chapter 15 provides a full list and description of defense mechanisms.

Psychosexual Stages of Development

Freud believed that human development proceeds through five stages from infancy to adulthood. He believed that experiences during the first 5 years determined an individual's lifetime adjustment pattern and personality traits. By the time a child enters school, subsequent growth consists of elaborating on this basic structure. Freud's psychosexual stages of development are in Table 2.1.

Psychoanalytic Therapy

Classical psychoanalysis, as developed by Sigmund Freud, is seldom used nowadays. Freud's premise that early intrapsychic conflict is the cause for all mental illness is no longer widely thought to be valid. Such therapy requires an unrealistically lengthy period of treatment (i.e., three to five times a week for many years), making it prohibitively expensive and uncovered by insurance.

TABLE 2.1   Freud's Psychosexual Stages of Development

Stage (Age)	Source of Satisfaction	Primary Conflict	Tasks	Desired Outcomes	Other Possible Personality Traits
Oral (0–1 year)	Mouth (sucking, biting, chewing)	Weaning	Mastery of gratification of oral needs; beginning of ego development (4–5 months)	Development of trust in the environment, with the realization that needs can be met	Fixation at the oral stage is associated with passivity, gullibility, and dependence; the use of sarcasm; may develop orally focused habits (e.g., smoking, nail-biting).
Anal (1–3 years)	Anal region (expulsion and retention of feces)	Toilet training	Beginning of development of a sense of control over instinctual drives; ability to delay immediate gratification to gain a future goal	Control over impulses	Fixation at the anal stage is associated with anal retentiveness (stinginess, rigid thought patterns, obsessive-compulsive disorder) or anal-expulsive character (messiness, destructiveness, cruelty).
Phallic (oedipal; (3–6 years)	Genitals (masturbation)	Oedipus and Electra	Sexual identity with parent of same sex; beginning of superego development	Identification with parent of the same sex	Fixation may result in reckless, self-assured, and narcissistic person. Lack of resolution may result in inability to love and difficulties with sexual identity.
Latency (6–12 years)	—	—	Growth of ego functions (social, intellectual, mechanical) and the ability to care about and relate to others outside the home (peers of the same sex)	The development of skills needed to cope with the environment	Fixations can result in difficulty identifying with others and in developing social skills, leading to a sense of inadequacy and inferiority.
Genital (12 years and beyond)	Genitals (sexual intercourse)	—	Development of satisfying sexual and emotional relationship; emancipation from parents—planning of life goals and development of a sense of personal identity	The ability to be creative and find pleasure in love and work	Inability to negotiate this stage may derail emotional and financial independence, may impair personal identity and future goals, and disrupt ability to form satisfying intimate relationships.

Data from Gleitman, H. (1981). *Psychology.* New York, NY: W. W. Norton.

The purpose of classical psychoanalytic sessions is to uncover unconscious conflicts. Specific tools include:

- Free association—Analysts actively encourage patients to freely share whatever thoughts or words come to mind to access the unconscious.
- Dream analysis—Patients are encouraged to share the content of dreams, which the therapist analyzes for symbolic meanings (e.g., "I was falling" could be interpreted as the patient feels unable to control situations).
- Defense mechanism recognition—The analyst assists the patient in recognizing and subsequently changing the overuse of maladaptive defense mechanisms, such as denial, projection, and rationalization (see Chapter 15 for a discussion of defense mechanisms).

These tools support the analyst in providing an educated guess, or hypothesis, of the meaning of dominant unconscious conflict. These educated guesses are known as interpretation and are the basis of psychoanalysis.

Two important concepts from classic psychoanalysis are transference and countertransference (Freud, 1969). **Transference** refers to unconscious feelings that the patient has toward a healthcare worker that were originally felt in childhood for a significant other. The patient may say something like, "You remind me exactly of my sister." The transference may be positive (affectionate) or negative (hostile). Psychoanalysis actually encourages transference as a way to understand original relationships. Such exploration helps the patient to better understand certain feelings and behaviors.

Countertransference refers to unconscious feelings that the healthcare worker has toward the patient. For instance, if the patient reminds you of someone you do not like, you may unconsciously react as if the patient were that individual. Strong negative or positive feelings toward the patient could be a red flag for countertransference. Such responses underscore the importance of maintaining self-awareness and seeking supervisory guidance as therapeutic relationships progress. Chapter 8 talks more about countertransference and the nurse-patient relationship.

Psychodynamic Therapy

Psychodynamic therapy is rooted in traditional psychoanalysis and uses many of the same tools, such as free association and dream analysis, and concepts such as transference and countertransference. However, the therapist has increased involvement and interacts with the patient more freely than in traditional psychoanalysis. The therapy is oriented toward the here and now and makes less of an attempt to reconstruct the developmental origins of conflicts. Psychodynamic therapy tends to last longer than other common therapeutic modalities and may extend for more than 20 sessions, which insurance companies often reject.

The best candidates for psychodynamic therapy are relatively healthy and well-functioning individuals, sometimes referred to as the "worried well" who have a clear area of difficulty and are intelligent, psychologically minded, and well-motivated for change. Patients with psychosis, severe depression, borderline personality disorders, and severe personality disorders are not appropriate candidates for this type of treatment.

At the start of treatment, the patient and therapist agree on what the focus will be and concentrate their work on that focus. Sessions are held weekly, and the total number of sessions to be held is determined at the outset of therapy. There is a rapid, back-and-forth pattern between patient and therapist with both participating actively. The therapist intervenes constantly to keep the therapy on track, either by redirecting the patient's attention or by interpreting deviations from the focus to the patient.

Implications of Freudian Theory for Nursing Practice

Freud's theory offers a comprehensive explanation of complex human processes. It emphasizes the importance of childhood experiences on personality development. Nurses can be sources of support and education for both parents and children to promote a healthy emotional environment.

Freud's theory of the unconscious mind is particularly valuable as a baseline for considering the complexity of human behavior. By considering conscious and unconscious influences, a nurse can identify and begin to think about the root causes of patient suffering. Freud emphasized the importance of individual talk sessions characterized by attentive listening with a focus on underlying themes as an important tool of healing in psychiatric care.

INTERPERSONAL THEORIES AND THERAPIES

Interpersonal Theory

Harry Stack Sullivan (1892–1949), an American-born psychiatrist, developed a model for understanding psychiatric alterations that focused on interpersonal problems. Sullivan (1953) believed that human beings are driven by the need for interaction. Indeed, he viewed loneliness as the most painful human condition. He emphasized the early relationship with the primary parenting figure, or significant other (a term he coined), as crucial for personality development.

According to Sullivan, the purpose of all behavior is to get needs met through interpersonal interactions and to reduce or avoid anxiety. He defined anxiety as any painful feeling or emotion that arises from social insecurity or prevents biological needs from being satisfied. Sullivan coined the term security operations to describe measures the individual uses to reduce anxiety and enhance security. Collectively, all of the security operations an individual uses to defend against anxiety and ensure self-esteem make up the self-system.

Interpersonal Therapy

Interpersonal therapy is an effective short-term therapy. The assumption is that psychiatric disorders are influenced by interpersonal interactions and the social context. The goal of interpersonal therapy is to reduce or eliminate psychiatric symptoms (particularly depression) by improving interpersonal functioning and satisfaction with social relationships.

Interpersonal therapy has proven successful in the treatment of major depressive disorder. Treatment is based on the notion that disturbances in important interpersonal relationships (or a deficit in one's capacity to form those relationships) can play a role in initiating or maintaining clinical depression. In interpersonal therapy, the therapist identifies the nature of the problem to be resolved and then selects strategies consistent with that problem area. Three types of problems in particular respond well to interpersonal therapy (Weissman et al., 2007):

1. **Grief and loss:** Complicated bereavement after death, divorce, or other loss
2. **Interpersonal disputes:** Conflicts with a significant other
3. **Role transition:** Problematic change in life status or social or vocational role

Implications of Interpersonal Theory to Nursing

Hildegard Peplau (1909–1999) (Fig. 2.2), influenced by the work of Sullivan and learning theory, developed the first systematic theoretical framework for psychiatric nursing in her groundbreaking book *Interpersonal Relations in Nursing* (1952). Peplau not only established the foundation for the professional practice of psychiatric nursing but also continued to enrich psychiatric nursing theory and work for the advancement of nursing practice throughout her career.

Peplau was the first nurse to identify psychiatric-mental health nursing both as an essential element of general nursing and as a specialty area that embraces specific governing principles. She was also the first nurse theorist to describe the nurse-patient relationship as the foundation of nursing practice. She also shifted the focus from what nurses do *to* patients to what nurses do *with* patients.

Her theory is mainly concerned with the processes by which the nurse helps patients to make positive changes

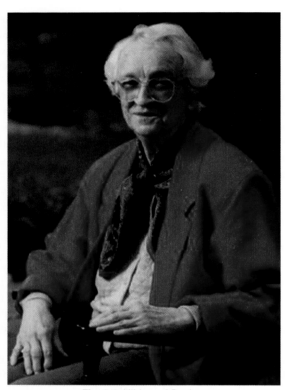

Fig. 2.2 Hildegard Peplau.

in their healthcare status and well-being. She believed that illness offered a unique opportunity for experiential learning, personal growth, and improved coping strategies. Psychiatric nurses play a central role in facilitating this growth.

Peplau proposed an approach in which nurses are both participants and observers in therapeutic conversations. She believed it was essential for nurses to observe the behavior not only of the patient but also of themselves. This self-awareness on the part of the nurse is essential in keeping the focus on the patient and in keeping the social and personal needs of the nurse out of the nurse-patient conversation.

Perhaps Peplau's most universal contribution to the everyday practice of psychiatric-mental health nursing is her application of Sullivan's theory of anxiety to nursing practice. She described the effects of different levels of anxiety (mild, moderate, severe, and panic) on perception and learning. She promoted interventions to lower anxiety with the aim of improving patients' abilities to think and function at more satisfactory levels. Chapter 15 presents more on the application of Peplau's theory of anxiety and interventions.

Table 2.2 lists selected nursing theorists and summarizes their major contributions and the impact of these contributions on psychiatric-mental health nursing.

TABLE 2.2   Selected Nursing Theorists, Their Major Contributions, and Their Impact on Psychiatric-Mental Health Nursing

Nursing Theorist	Focus of Theory	Contribution to Psychiatric-Mental Health Nursing
Patricia Benner	Caring as foundation for nursing	Benner encourages nurses to provide caring and comforting interventions. She emphasizes the importance of the nurse-patient relationship and the importance of teaching and coaching the patient and bearing witness to suffering as the patient deals with illness.
Dorothea Orem	Goal of self-care as integral to the practice of nursing	Orem emphasizes the role of the nurse in promoting self-care activities of the patient; this has relevance to the seriously and persistently mentally ill patient.
Sister Callista Roy	Continual need for people to adapt physically, psychologically, and socially	Roy emphasizes the role of nursing in assisting patients to adapt so that they can cope more effectively with changes.
Betty Neuman	Impact of internal and external stressors on the equilibrium of the system	Neuman emphasizes the role of nursing in assisting patients to discover and use stress-reducing strategies.
Joyce Travelbee	Meaning in the nurse-patient relationship and the importance of communication	Travelbee emphasizes the role of nursing in affirming the suffering of the patient and in being able to alleviate that suffering through communication skills used appropriately through the stages of the nurse-patient relationship.

Data from Benner, P., & Wrubel, J. (1989). *The primacy of caring: stress and coping in health and illness.* Menlo Park, CA: Addison-Wesley; Leddy, S., & Pepper, J. M. (1993). *Conceptual bases of professional nursing* (3rd ed., pp. 174–175). Philadelphia, PA: Lippincott; Neuman, B., & Young, R. (1972). A model for teaching total-person approach to patient problems. *Nursing Research, 21,* 264–269; Orem, D. E. (1995). *Nursing: Concepts of practice* (5th ed.). New York, NY: McGraw-Hill; Roy, C., & Andrews, H. A. (1991). *The Roy adaptation model: The definitive statement.* Norwalk, CT: Appleton & Lange; Travelbee, J. (1961). *Intervention in psychiatric nursing.* Philadelphia, PA: F. A. Davis.

BEHAVIORAL THEORIES AND THERAPIES

Behavioral theories developed as a protest to Freud's assumption that a person's destiny was carved in stone at a very early age. Behaviorists have no concern with inner conflicts but argue that personality simply consists of learned behaviors. Consequently, personality becomes synonymous with behavior—if behavior changes, so does the personality. Behaviorists believe that behavior can be influenced through a process referred to as conditioning. Conditioning involves pairing a behavior with a condition that reinforces or diminishes the behavior's occurrence.

Classical Conditioning Theory

Ivan Pavlov (1849–1936) was a Russian physiologist. He won a Nobel Prize for his outstanding contributions to the physiology of digestion, which he studied through his well-known experiments with dogs. In incidental observation of the dogs, Pavlov noticed that the dogs were able to anticipate when food would be forthcoming and would begin to salivate even before actually tasting the meat.

Pavlov formalized his observations of behaviors in dogs in a theory of classical conditioning. Pavlov (1928) found that when a neutral stimulus (a bell) was repeatedly paired with another stimulus (food that triggered salivation), eventually the sound of the bell alone could elicit salivation in the dogs. A human example of this response is a boy becoming ill after eating spoiled coleslaw at a picnic. Later in life, he feels nauseated whenever he smells coleslaw. It is important to recognize that classical conditioned responses are *involuntary*—not under conscious personal control—and are not spontaneous choices.

Behavioral Theory

John B. Watson (1878–1958) was an American psychologist who rejected the unconscious motivation of psychoanalysis for being too subjective. He developed the school of thought referred to as *behaviorism*, which he believed was more objective or measurable. Watson (1919) contended that personality traits and responses—adaptive and maladaptive—were socially learned through classical conditioning. In a famous (but terrible) experiment, Watson stood behind Little Albert, a 9-month-old who liked animals, and made a loud noise with a hammer every time the infant reached for a white rat. After this experiment, Little Albert became terrified at the sight of white fur or hair, even in the absence of a loud noise. Watson concluded that controlling the environment could mold behavior and that anyone could be trained to be anything, from a beggar man to a merchant.

Operant Conditioning Theory

B. F. Skinner (1904–1990) represented the second wave of behavioral theorists. Skinner (1987) researched operant conditioning, a method of learning that occurs through rewards and punishment for *voluntary* behavior. Behavioral responses are elicited through reinforcement, which causes a behavior to occur *more* frequently.

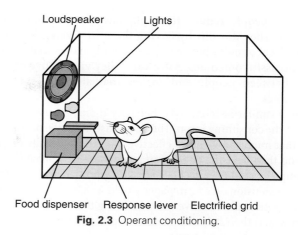

Fig. 2.3 Operant conditioning.

Skinner conducted experiments with laboratory animals in what is now referred to as a Skinner Box. The contents of this box included a lever and an electric grid (Fig. 2.3). To cause behavior *more* frequently, Skinner used two methods. When a hungry rat pressed the lever, it would receive a food pellet. He learned to go straight to the lever for food. This is positive reinforcement of the behavior. Another rat was placed in the cage with an electrical charge on the grid under his feet. If he accidentally pressed the lever, the charge would turn off. He learned to go straight to the lever to eliminate the shock. This removal of an objectionable or averse stimulus is negative reinforcement.

Other techniques can cause behaviors to occur *less* frequently. One technique is an unpleasant consequence, or punishment. Driving too fast may result in a speeding ticket, which—in mature and healthy individuals—decreases the chances that speeding will occur.

Absence of reinforcement, or extinction, also decreases behavior by withholding a reward that has become habitual. For example, if a person tells a joke and no one laughs, the person is less apt to tell jokes because his joke-telling behavior is not being reinforced. Teachers use this strategy in the classroom when they ignore acting-out behavior that had previously been rewarded by more attention.

Behavioral Therapy

Behavioral therapy assumes that changes in maladaptive behavior can occur without insight into the underlying cause. This approach works best when it is directed at specific problems and the goals are well defined. Behavioral therapy is effective in treating people with phobias, alcohol use disorder, schizophrenia, and many other conditions. Five types of behavioral therapy are discussed here: modeling, operant conditioning, exposure and response prevention, aversion therapy, and biofeedback.

Modeling

In modeling, the therapist provides a role model for specific identified behaviors, and the patient learns through imitation. The therapist may do the modeling, provide another person to model the behaviors, or present a video for the purpose. Bandura, Blanchard, and Ritter (1969) were able to help people reduce their phobias about nonpoisonous snakes. They did this by having them first view closeups of filmed encounters between people and snakes that resulted in successful outcomes. Afterward, they viewed live encounters between people and snakes that also had successful outcomes.

In a similar fashion, some behavior therapists use role playing in the consulting room. They demonstrate patterns of behavior that might prove more effective than those usually engaged in and then have the patients practice these new behaviors. For example, a student who does not know how to ask a professor for an extension on a term paper would watch the therapist portray a potentially effective way of making the request. The clinician would then help the student to practice the new skill in a similar role-playing situation.

Operant Conditioning

Operant conditioning is the basis for behavior modification and uses positive reinforcement to increase desired behaviors. For example, when desired goals are achieved or behaviors are performed, patients might be rewarded with tokens. These tokens can be exchanged for food, small luxuries, or privileges. This reward system is known as a *token economy*.

Operant conditioning has been useful in improving the verbal behaviors of children who are mute, autistic, and developmentally disabled. In patients with severe and persistent mental illness, behavior modification has helped to increase levels of self-care, social behavior, group participation, and more. You may find this a useful technique as you proceed through your clinical rotations.

A familiar case in point of positive reinforcement is the mother who takes her preschooler along to the grocery store, and the child starts acting out, demanding candy, nagging, crying, and yelling. Here are examples of three ways the child's behavior can be reinforced:

Action	Result
1. The mother gives the child the candy.	The child continues to use this behavior. This is positive reinforcement of negative behavior.
2. The mother scolds the child.	Acting out may continue, because the child gets what he really wants—attention. This positively rewards negative behavior.
3. The mother ignores the acting out but gives attention to the child when he is acting appropriately.	The child gets a positive reward for appropriate behavior.

Exposure Therapy

Exposure therapy is used for people who experience anxiety due to fears, phobias, or traumatic memories. To manage or eliminate this anxiety, they avoid anything that reminds them of the feared object, activities, or situation. This avoidance may help in

the short term, but in the long term, it can make the fear more powerful by leading to obsessive thinking.

In exposure therapy, patients are encouraged to face their fears and emotionally process them in a safe environment. The goal of this therapy is the elimination, or extinction, of these responses. Exposure therapy is used for phobias, panic disorder, social anxiety disorder, obsessive-compulsive disorder, posttraumatic stress disorder, and generalized anxiety disorder.

There are several variations of exposure therapy. They include:

- Imaginal exposure: In this type of therapy, patients are encouraged to imagine and confront the fear or situation. For example, a person with arachnophobia (fear of spiders) is asked to recall responses to spiders and describe associated thoughts and feelings.
- In vivo exposure: Patients actually confront their fears in a real-world setting. For example, a patient with fear of flying may go to an airport and begin by simply watching planes take off and then discuss his or her feeling.
- Virtual reality exposure: This therapy is a combination of imaginal and in vivo exposure. A patient with a fear of elevators may use virtual reality goggles and audio that provides the sights and sounds of elevators (Fig. 2.4). Gradually the patient can explore approaching and then entering the virtual elevator in safety.

Exposure can be paced in different ways depending upon the patient and the problem. Graded exposure moves in a hierarchy from least feared to most. Systematic desensitization is similar to exposure and response prevention, but incorporates

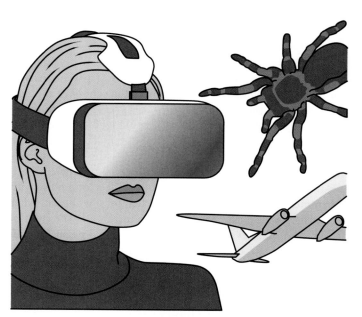

Virtual reality exposure: This therapy is a combination of imaginal and in vivo exposure. A patient with a fear of elevators may use virtual reality goggles and audio that provides the sights and sounds of elevators. Gradually the patient can explore approaching and then entering the virtual elevator in safety.

Fig. 2.4 Virtual reality exposure. (Courtesy of Fenichel, 2000.)

the incremental exposure of graded exposure along with relaxation techniques such as slow, deep breathing. Flooding, the most extreme method, relies upon confronting the most feared object, situation, or event and then managing and processing it.

Aversion Therapy

Aversion therapy is used to treat conditions and behaviors such as alcohol use disorder, paraphilic disorders, shoplifting, aggressive behavior, and self-mutilation. Aversion therapy is pairing a target behavior with a negative stimulus, to extinguish undesirable behavior. This treatment may be used when other less drastic measures have failed to produce the desired effects.

A simple example of aversion therapy is applying bitter substances on the fingernails of nail biters or the thumbs of thumb suckers. Other examples of aversive stimuli are chemicals that induce nausea and vomiting, unpleasant odors, unpleasant verbal stimuli (e.g., descriptions of disturbing scenes), costs or fines in a token economy, and denial of positive reinforcement (e.g., isolation).

Aversion therapy is somewhat controversial, partly due to a scarcity of research support. A dramatic use of aversive measures focused on sexual preferences. Before the American Psychiatric Association eliminated homosexuality as a disorder, gay individuals were subjected to forms of aversion therapy to alter their sexual preferences. One treatment consisted of a slide projector connected to a shock generator. When neutral slides were displayed, nothing happened. However, when a slide portrayed "deviant" sexual behavior, a shock was administered.

While initiating any aversive protocol, the therapist, treatment team, or society *must* answer the following questions:

- Is this therapy in the best interest of the patient?
- Does its use violate the patient's rights?
- Is it in the best interest of society?

If the therapist believes aversion therapy is the most appropriate treatment, ongoing supervision, support, and evaluation of those administering it must occur.

Biofeedback

Biofeedback is another form of behavioral therapy and is successfully used nowadays, especially for controlling the body's physiological response to stress and anxiety. This feedback helps people to make changes, such as relaxing certain muscles to reduce or eliminate pain. Clinicians have used technology to monitor brain waves, respirations, heart rate, muscle contraction, perspiration, and body temperature.

Technology has expanded and allowed individuals access to sophisticated wearables such as smart watches, bands, garments, and patches with embedded sensors. Small portable devices and mobile applications record and provide users with a variety of feedback on physical responses and performance. An example of a US Food and Drug Administration

(FDA)-approved biofeedback device is RESPeRATE, for lowering blood pressure by promoting slow, deep breathing. A computerized control unit, a breathing sensor, and a set of earbuds coach individuals to pace breathing and prolong exhalation.

Chapter 10 discusses biofeedback in further detail.

Implications of Behavioral Theory to Nursing

Behavior and health are inextricably linked. Consider the toll that such behaviors as smoking, overeating, alcohol and substance use problems, and inactivity take on the body and mind. A behavioral model provides a concrete method for modifying or replacing undesirable behaviors. An example of a nurse teaching a behavioral technique is smoking cessation by modifying routines to reduce smoking cues, such as avoiding bars.

Nurses may work in units based on behavioral principles, particularly with children and adolescents. *Token economies* represent extensions of Skinner's thoughts on learning. In a token economy, patients' positive behaviors are reinforced with tokens. These tokens may be small plastic disks, checkmarks, or coins with no real value that can be used in exchange for materials (e.g., candy, gum, books) or services (e.g., phone calls, time off the unit, recognition).

COGNITIVE THEORIES AND THERAPIES

While behaviorists focused on increasing, decreasing, or eliminating measurable behaviors, they did not focus on the thoughts, or cognitions, that were involved in these behaviors. Rather than thinking of people as passive recipients of environmental conditioning, cognitive theorists proposed that there is a dynamic interplay between individuals and the environment. These theorists believe that thoughts come before feelings and actions, and thoughts about the world and our place in it are based on our own unique perspectives, which may or may not be based on reality. This section presents two of the most influential theorists and their therapies.

Rational-Emotive Therapy

Albert Ellis (1913–2007) developed rational-emotive therapy in 1955. The aim of rational-emotive therapy is to remove core irrational beliefs by helping people to recognize thoughts that are not accurate, sensible, or useful. These thoughts tend to take the form of *shoulds* (e.g., "I should always be polite."), *oughts* (e.g., "I ought to consistently win my tennis games."), and musts (e.g., "I must be thin."). Ellis described negative thinking as a simple A-B-C process. *A* stands for the activating event, *B* stands for beliefs about the event, and *C* stands for emotional consequence as a result of the event.

| A Activating Event | → | B Beliefs | → | C Emotional Consequence |

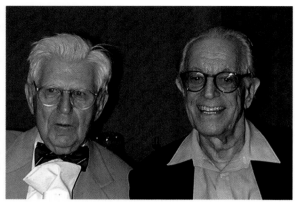

Fig. 2.5 Aaron Beck and Albert Ellis. (Courtesy of Fenichel, 2000.)

Perception influences all thoughts, which, in turn, influence our behaviors. It often boils down to the simple notion of perceiving the glass as half full or half empty. For example, imagine you have just received an invitation to a birthday party (activating event). You think, "I hate parties. Now I have to hang out with people who don't like me instead of watching my favorite television shows. They probably just invited me to get a gift" (beliefs). You will probably be miserable (emotional consequence) if you go. On the other hand, you may think, "I love parties! This will be a great chance to meet new people, and it will be fun to shop for the perfect gift" (beliefs). You could have a delightful time (emotional consequence).

Although Ellis (Fig. 2.5) recognized the role of past experiences on current beliefs, the focus of rational-emotive therapy is on present attitudes, painful feelings, and dysfunctional behaviors. If our beliefs are negative and self-deprecating, we are more susceptible to depression and anxiety. Ellis noted that, although we cannot change the past, we can change the way we are now. He was pragmatic in his approach to mental illness and colorful in his therapeutic advice. "It's too [darn] bad you panic, but you don't die from it! Get them over the panic about panic, you may find the panic disappears" (Ellis, 2000).

Cognitive Behavioral Therapy

Aaron T. Beck (see Fig. 2.5) was originally trained in psychoanalysis. He noticed that people with depression thought differently than people who were not depressed. They had stereotypical patterns of negative and self-critical thinking that seemed to distort their ability to think and process information. To challenge these negative patterns, he developed cognitive behavioral therapy (CBT), which is based on both cognitive psychology and behavioral theory.

Beck's method (Beck et al., 1979), the basis for CBT, is an active, directive, time-limited, structured approach. This evidence-based therapy is used to treat a variety of psychiatric disorders, such as depression, anxiety, phobias, and pain. It is based on the underlying theoretical principle that feelings and behaviors are largely determined by the way people think about the world and their place in it (Beck, 1967). Their cognitions (verbal or pictorial events in their streams of consciousness) are based on attitudes or assumptions developed from previous experiences. These cognitions may be fairly accurate or distorted.

According to Beck, people have *schemas*, or unique assumptions about themselves, others, and the world in general. For example, if a man has the schema, "The only person I can trust is myself," he will have expectations that everyone else has questionable motives, is dishonest, and will eventually hurt him. Other negative schemas include incompetence, abandonment, evilness, and vulnerability. People are typically not aware of such cognitive biases.

Rapid, unthinking responses based on schemas are known as automatic thoughts. These responses are particularly intense and frequent in psychiatric disorders such as depression and anxiety. Often automatic thoughts, or cognitive distortions, are irrational and lead to false assumptions and misinterpretations. For example, if a woman interprets all experiences in terms of whether she is competent and adequate, thinking may be dominated by the cognitive distortion, "Unless I do everything perfectly, I'm a failure." Consequently, the person reacts to situations in terms of adequacy, even when these situations are unrelated to whether she is personally competent. Table 2.3 describes common cognitive distortions.

Therapeutic techniques are designed to identify, reality test, and correct distorted conceptualizations and the dysfunctional beliefs underlying them. Patients are taught to challenge their own negative thinking and substitute it with positive, rational thoughts. They learn to recognize when thinking is based on distortions and misconceptions.

Homework assignments play an important role in CBT. A particularly useful technique is the use of a columned thought record. In this record, the precipitating event or situation is identified along with the accompanying negative feeling or emotion. The automatic thought is listed next. Challenges to the automatic thought through other potential interpretations are identified in the last column. The following is an application of these CBT concepts:

Event	Feeling	Automatic Thought	Other Possible Interpretations
While at a party, Cory asked me, "How is it going?" a few days after I was discharged from the hospital.	Anxious	Cory thinks I am crazy. I must really look bad for him to be concerned.	He really cares about me. He noticed that I look better than before I went into the hospital and wants to know if I feel better too.

TABLE 2.3 Common Cognitive Distortions

Distortion	Definition	Example
All-or-nothing thinking	Thinking in black and white, reducing complex outcomes into absolutes	Although Lindsey earned the second highest score in the state's cheerleading competition, she consistently referred to herself as "a loser."
Overgeneralization	Using a bad outcome (or a few bad outcomes) as evidence that nothing will ever go right again	Andrew had a minor traffic accident. He is reluctant to drive and says, "I shouldn't be allowed on the road."
Labeling	A form of generalization in which a characteristic or event becomes definitive and results in an overly harsh label for self or others	"Because I failed the advanced statistics exam, I am a failure. I might as well give up. I may as well quit and look for an easier major."
Mental filter	Focusing on a negative detail or bad event and allowing it to taint everything else	Anne's boss evaluated her work as exemplary and gave her a few suggestions for improvement. She obsessed about the suggestions and ignored the rest.
Disqualifying the positive	Maintaining a negative view by rejecting information that supports a positive view as being irrelevant, inaccurate, or accidental	"I've just been offered the job I thought I always wanted. There must have been no other applicants."
Jumping to conclusions	Making a negative interpretation despite the fact that there is little or no supporting evidence	"My fiancé, Juan, didn't call me for 3 hours, which just proves he doesn't love me anymore."
a. Mind-reading	Inferring negative thoughts, responses, and motives of others	Isabel is giving a presentation and a man in the audience is sleeping. She panics, "I must be boring."
b. Fortune-telling error	Anticipating that things will turn out badly as an established fact	"I'll ask her out, but I know she won't have a good time."
Magnification or minimization	Exaggerating the importance of something (e.g., a personal failure or the success of others) or reducing the importance of something (e.g., a personal success or the failure of others)	"I'm alone on a Saturday night because no one likes me. When other people are alone, it's because they want to be."
a. Catastrophizing	Catastrophizing is an extreme form of magnification in which the very worst is assumed to be a probable outcome	"If I don't make a good impression on the boss at the company picnic, she will fire me."
Emotional reasoning	Drawing a conclusion based on an emotional state	"I'm nervous about the exam. I must not be prepared. If I were, I wouldn't be afraid."
"Should" and "must" statements	Rigid self-directives that presume an unrealistic amount of control over external events	Renee believes that a patient with diabetes has high blood sugar today because she's not a very good nurse and that her patients should always get better.
Personalization	Assuming responsibility for an external event or situation that was likely outside personal control	"I'm sorry your party wasn't more fun. It's probably because I was there."

Modified from Burns, D. D. (1989). *The feeling good handbook*. New York, NY: William Morrow.

Table 2.4 compares and contrasts psychodynamic, interpersonal, cognitive behavioral, and behavioral therapies.

Trauma-Focused Cognitive Behavioral Therapy

A relatively new treatment approach, trauma-focused cognitive behavioral therapy (TF-CBT), was developed in the 1990s to address sexual abuse trauma in children. It was subsequently expanded to address the needs of individuals who are impacted by any severe trauma and abuse. Although patients are usually children, TF-CBT incorporates principles of family therapy and includes caregivers. This type of therapy tends to be short term and lasts from 12 to 16 sessions.

Traumatized children and adolescents often develop intense fear regarding memories of the trauma. This fear results in avoiding reminders and talking about what happened. Because they do not want to talk about the trauma, they become more isolated, numb, and anxious. TF-CBT combines trauma-sensitive interventions with CBT. It helps children and adolescents to identify feelings and how to manage them and to examine negative thoughts and replace them with more positive thoughts. Patients are supported in a nurturing environment as they develop a trauma narrative and gradually reduce the impact that the trauma once had.

Dialectical Behavioral Therapy

Psychologist Marsha Linehan (1993) developed dialectical behavioral therapy (DBT), a specific type of cognitive behavioral therapy. A dialectic is an integration of opposites—dialectical strategies help the patient (and the therapist) to give up extreme positions. This model was developed for individuals with intractable behavioral disorders involving emotional dysregulation. Linehan and colleagues (1991) found significant improvements for chronically suicidal and self-injuring women with borderline personality disorder. This emotionally

TABLE 2.4   Comparison of Psychoanalytic, Interpersonal, Cognitive Behavioral, and Behavioral Therapies

Aspects of Therapy	Psychodynamic Therapy	Interpersonal Therapy	Cognitive Behavioral Therapy	Behavioral Therapy
Treatment focus	Unresolved past relationships and core conflicts	Current interpersonal relationships and social supports	Thoughts and cognitions	Learned maladaptive behavior
Therapist role	Significant other Transference object	Problem solver	Active, directive, challenging	Active, directive teacher
Primary disorders treated	Anxiety Depression Personality disorders	Depression	Depression Anxiety/panic Eating disorders	Posttraumatic stress disorder Obsessive-compulsive disorder Panic disorder
Length of therapy	20+ sessions	Short term (12–20 sessions)	Short term (5–20 sessions)	Varies, typically fewer than 10 sessions
Technique	Therapeutic alliance Free association Understanding transference Challenging defense mechanisms	Facilitate new patterns of communication and expectations for relationships	Evaluating thoughts and behaviors Modifying dysfunctional thoughts and behaviors	Relaxation Thought stopping Self-reassurance Seeking social support

Data from Dewan, M. J., Steenbarger, B. N., & Greenberg, R. P. (2014). Brief psychotherapies. In R. E. Hales, S. C. Yudofsky, & L. W. Roberts (Eds.), *Textbook of psychiatry* (6th ed., pp. 1037–1064). Arlington, VA: American Psychiatric Publishing.

vulnerable and reactive population had been largely viewed as untreatable.

DBT is a long-term therapy (1 to 1.5 years) that uses strategies from CBT and other skills to enhance emotional regulation. They include (Behavioral Tech, n.d.):

- Mindfulness: Being aware and present in the moment.
- Distress tolerance: Tolerating pain in challenging situation, rather than frantically trying to transform the pain.
- Interpersonal effectiveness: Asking for what you want and saying no in the context of self-respect and effective relationships with others.
- Emotional regulation: Choosing and changing emotions that are problematic.

DBT is also an effective treatment for other disorders and symptoms. They include depression, suicidal thoughts, hopelessness, anger, substance use, and dissociation (Lenz et al., 2016).

Implications of Cognitive Theories for Nursing

Recognizing the interplay between events, negative thinking, and negative responses can be beneficial from both a patient-care standpoint and a personal one. As a supportive therapeutic measure, helping the patient identify negative thought patterns is a worthwhile intervention. Workbooks are available to aid in the process of identifying cognitive distortions.

The cognitive approach can also help nurses to understand their own responses to a variety of difficult situations. One example might be the anxiety that some students feel regarding the psychiatric nursing clinical rotation. Students may overgeneralize—"All psychiatric patients are dangerous"—or personalize—"My patient doesn't seem to be better. I'm probably not doing him any good"—the situation. The key to effectively using this approach in clinical situations is to challenge the negative thoughts that are not based on facts and then replace them with more realistic appraisals.

HUMANISTIC THEORIES

In the 1950s, humanistic theories arose as a protest against both the behavioral and psychoanalytic schools, which were thought to be pessimistic, deterministic, and dehumanizing. Humanistic theories focus on human potential and free will to choose life patterns supportive of personal growth. Humanistic frameworks emphasize a person's capacity for self-actualization. This approach focuses on understanding the subjective experience of the patient's perspective. Although there are a number of humanistic theorists, in this text we will explore Abraham Maslow and his theory.

Theory of Human Motivation

Abraham Maslow (1908–1970) is considered the father of humanistic psychology. He criticized other therapies for focusing too intently on humanity's frailties and not enough on its strengths. Maslow contended that the focus of psychology must go beyond experiences of hate, pain, misery, guilt, and conflict to include love, compassion, happiness, exhilaration, and well-being.

Hierarchy of Needs

Maslow believed that human beings are motivated by unmet needs. Maslow (1968) focused on human need fulfillment, which he categorized into six incremental stages, beginning with physiological survival needs and ending with self-transcendent needs (Fig. 2.6). The hierarchy of needs is conceptualized as a pyramid with the strongest, most fundamental needs placed on the lower levels. The higher levels—the more distinctly human needs—occupy the top sections of the pyramid. When lower-level needs are met, higher needs are able to emerge.

- **Physiological needs:** The most basic needs are the physiological drives—needing food, oxygen, water, sleep, sex, and a constant body temperature. If all needs were deprived, this level would take priority over the rest.

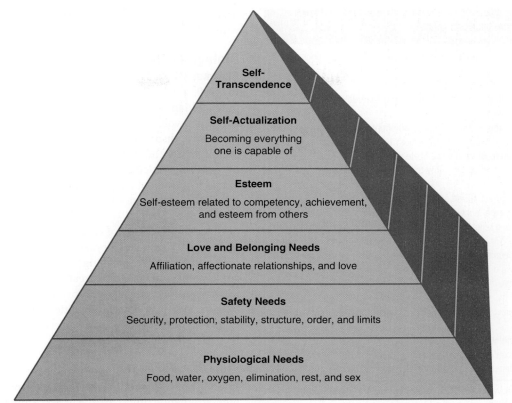

Fig. 2.6 Maslow's hierarchy of needs. (Adapted from Maslow, A. H. (1972). *The farther reaches of human nature*. New York, NY: Viking.)

- **Safety needs:** Once physiological needs are met, safety needs emerge. They include security; protection; freedom from fear, anxiety, and chaos; and the need for law, order, and limits. Adults in a stable society usually feel safe, but they may feel threatened by debt, job insecurity, or lack of insurance. It is during times of crisis, such as war, disasters, assaults, and social breakdown, when safety needs take precedence. Children, who are more vulnerable and dependent, respond far more readily and intensely to safety threats.
- **Belonging and love needs:** People have a need for intimate relationships, love, affection, and belonging and will seek to overcome feelings of loneliness and alienation. Maslow stresses the importance of having a family and a home and being part of identifiable groups.
- **Esteem needs:** People need to have a high self-regard and have it reflected to them from others. If self-esteem needs are met, they feel confident, valued, and valuable. When self-esteem is compromised, they feel inferior, worthless, and helpless.
- **Self-actualization:** Human beings are preset to strive to be everything they are capable of becoming. Maslow said, "What a man *can* be, he *must* be." What people are capable of becoming is highly individual—an artist must paint, a writer must write, and a healer must heal. The drive to satisfy this need is felt as a sort of restlessness, a sense that something is missing. It is up to each person to choose a path that will bring about inner peace and fulfillment.

Although Maslow's early work included only five levels of needs, he later took into account two additional factors: (1) cognitive needs (the desire to know and understand) and (2) aesthetic needs (Maslow, 1970). He describes the acquisition of knowledge (our first priority) and the need to understand (our second priority) as being hardwired and essential. The aesthetic need for beauty and symmetry is universal.

You may be interested to know that Maslow (1970) developed his theory by investigating people who he believed were self-actualized. Among these people were historical figures such as Abraham Lincoln, Thomas Jefferson, Harriet Tubman, Walt Whitman, Ludwig van Beethoven, William James, and Franklin D. Roosevelt. Other people he investigated were living at the time of his studies. They include Albert Einstein, Eleanor Roosevelt, and Albert Schweitzer. Box 2.1 identifies basic personality characteristics that distinguish self-actualizing people.

Implications of Motivation Theory for Nursing

The value of Maslow's model in nursing practice is twofold. First, an emphasis on human potential and the patient's strengths is key to successful nurse-patient relationships. Second, the model helps to establish what is most important in the sequencing of nursing actions. For example, to collect any but the most essential information when a patient is struggling with drug withdrawal may be dangerous. Following Maslow's model as a way of prioritizing actions, the nurse meets the patient's physiological need for stable vital

- Accurate perception of reality. Not defensive in their perceptions of the world.
- Acceptance of themselves, others, and nature.
- Spontaneity, simplicity, and naturalness. Self-actualized individuals do not live programmed lives.
- Problem-centered rather than self-centered orientation. Possibly the most important characteristic. Possibly the most important characteristic is a sense of a mission to which they dedicate their lives.
- Pleasure in being alone and in ability to reflect on events.
- Active social interest.
- People who are self-actualized don't take life for granted.
- Mystical or peak experiences. A peak experience is a moment of intense ecstasy, similar to a religious or mystical experience, during which the self is transcended.
- Self-actualized people may become so involved in what they are doing that they lose all sense of time and awareness of self *(flow experience).*
- Lighthearted sense of humor that indicates "we're in it together" and lacks sarcasm or hostility.
- Fairness and respect for people of different races, ethnicities, religions, and political views.
- Creativity, especially in managing their lives.
- Resistance to conformity (enculturation). Self-actualization results in autonomous, independent, and self-sufficient individuals.

Adapted from Maslow, A. H. (1970). *Motivation and personality.* New York, NY: Harper & Row.

signs and pain relief before collecting general information for a nursing database.

BIOLOGICAL THEORIES AND THERAPIES

Biological Model

A biological model, or medical model, of mental illness assumes that abnormal behavior is the result of a physical problem. It focuses on neurological, chemical, biological, and genetic issues. Adherents of this dominant model seek to understand how the body and brain interact to create emotions, memories, and perceptual experiences. The biological model locates the illness or disease in the body—usually in the limbic system of the brain and the synapse receptor sites of the central nervous system—and targets the site of the illness using physical interventions such as drugs, diet, or surgery.

The recognition that psychiatric illnesses are as physical in origin as diabetes and coronary artery disease serves to decrease the stigma surrounding them. Just as someone with diabetes or heart disease cannot be held responsible for being ill, patients with schizophrenia or bipolar disorder are no more to blame.

Biological Therapies

Pharmacotherapy

In 1950, a French drug firm synthesized chlorpromazine—a powerful antipsychotic medication—and psychiatry experienced a revolution. The advent of pharmacotherapy to treat psychiatric disorders presented a strong alternative to psychological approaches for mental illness. The dramatic experience of observing patients freed from the bondage of psychosis and mania by powerful drugs such as chlorpromazine and lithium left witnesses convinced of the critical role of the brain in psychiatric illness.

Since the discovery of chlorpromazine, which was later sold under the trade name Thorazine, many other medications have proven effective in controlling psychosis, mania, depression, and anxiety. These medications greatly reduce the need for hospitalization and dramatically improve the lives of people suffering from serious psychiatric difficulties. Psychotropic medications exert differential effects on a variety of neurotransmitters and help to restore brain function.

Brain Stimulation Therapies

In addition to psychotherapy and pharmacotherapy as treatment for mental illness are the brain stimulation therapies. The oldest of these therapies is electroconvulsive therapy (ECT). All of these methods involve focused electrical stimulation of the brain. In addition to treating psychiatric disorders, they also treat other neurological disorders, such as Parkinson's disease, epilepsy, and pain conditions. Table 2.5 provides a summary of FDA–approved brain stimulation treatments and their use.

Implications of the Biological Model for Nursing

Historically, psychiatric-mental health nurses have attended to the physical needs of psychiatric patients. Nurses administer medications and monitor sleep, activity, nutrition, hydration, elimination, and other functions. Nurses are responsible for preparing patients for somatic therapies such as ECT. Physical needs and physical care in psychiatric nursing are provided as part of a holistic approach to healthcare. Basic nursing strategies such as focusing on the qualities of a therapeutic relationship, understanding the patient's perspective, and communicating in a way that facilitates the patient's recovery take place alongside physical care.

TABLE 2.5   Summary of Approved Brain Stimulation Treatments and Their Use

Treatment	Convulsive?	Site	Disorders
Electroconvulsive therapy (ECT)	Yes	Cortical	Depression, mania, catatonia
Repetitive transcranial magnetic stimulation (rTMS)	No	Cortical	Depression
Vagus nerve stimulation (VNS)	No	Cervical cranial nerve	Depression
Deep brain stimulation (DBS)	No	Subcortical	Depression, obsessive-compulsive disorder

DEVELOPMENTAL THEORIES

Cognitive Development

Jean Piaget (1896–1980) was a Swiss psychologist and researcher. While working at a boys' school run by Alfred Binet, developer of the Binet Intelligence Test, Piaget helped to score these tests. He became fascinated by the fact that young children consistently gave wrong answers on intelligence tests, wrong answers that revealed a discernible pattern of cognitive processing that was different from that of older children and adults. He concluded that cognitive development was a dynamic progression from primitive awareness and simple reflexes to complex thought and responses. Our mental representations of the world, or schemata, depend on the cognitive stage we have reached.

- *Sensorimotor stage (birth to 2 years).* Begins with basic reflexes and culminates with purposeful movement, spatial abilities, and hand-eye coordination. Physical interaction with the environment provides the child with a basic understanding of the world. By approximately 9 months, object permanence is achieved, and the child can conceptualize objects that are no longer visible. This explains the delight of the game of peek-a-boo as an emerging skill, as the child begins to anticipate the face hidden behind the hands.
- *Preoperational stage (2 to 7 years).* Operations is a term used to describe thinking about objects. Children are not yet able to think abstractly or generalize qualities in the absence of specific objects, but rather think in a concrete fashion. Egocentric thinking is demonstrated through a tendency to expect others to view the world as they do. They are also unable to conserve mass, volume, or number. An example of this inability is thinking that a tall, thin glass holds more liquid than a short, wide glass.
- *Concrete operational stage (7 to 11 years).* Logical thought appears and abstract problem solving is possible. The child is able to see a situation from another's point of view and can take into account a variety of solutions to a problem. Conservation is possible. For example, two small cups hold an amount of liquid equal to a tall glass. They are able to classify based on discrete characteristics, order objects in a pattern, and understand the concept of reversibility.
- *Formal operational stage (11 years to adulthood).* Conceptual reasoning commences at approximately the same time as does puberty. At this stage, the child's basic abilities to think abstractly and problem solve mirror those of an adult.

Theory of Psychosocial Development

Erik Erikson (1902–1994), an American psychoanalyst, began as a follower of Freud. Erikson (1963) came to believe that Freudian theory was restrictive and negative in its approach. He also stressed that more than the limited mother-child-father triangle influences an individual's development. He emphasized the role of culture and society on personality development. According to Erikson, personality was not set in stone at age 5, as Freud suggested, but continued to evolve throughout the life span.

Erikson described development as occurring in eight predetermined and consecutive life stages (psychosocial crises), each of which results in a positive or negative outcome. The successful or unsuccessful completion of each stage will affect the individual's progression to the next (Table 2.6). For example, Erikson's crisis of industry versus inferiority occurs from the ages of 7 to 12. During this stage, the child's task is to gain a sense of personal abilities and competence and to expand relationships beyond the immediate family to include peers. The attainment of this task (industry) brings with it the virtue of confidence. The child who fails to navigate this stage successfully is unable to master age-appropriate tasks, cannot make a connection with peers, and will feel like a failure (inferiority).

Theory of Object Relations

The theory of object relations was developed by interpersonal theorists who emphasize past relationships in influencing a person's sense of self as well as the nature and quality of relationships in the present. The term *object* refers to another person, particularly a significant person.

Margaret Mahler (1895–1985) was a Hungarian-born child psychologist who worked with emotionally disturbed children. She developed a framework for studying how an infant transitions from complete self-absorption, with an inability to separate from its mother, to a physically and psychologically differentiated toddler. Mahler and colleagues (1975) believed that psychological problems were largely the result of a disruption of this separation.

During the first 3 years, the significant other (e.g., the mother) provides a secure base of support that promotes enough confidence for the child to separate. This is achieved by a balance of holding (emotionally and physically) a child enough for the child to feel safe while encouraging independence and natural exploration.

Problems may arise in this process. If a toddler leaves his or her mother on the park bench and wanders off to the sandbox, the child should be encouraged with smiles and reassurance, "Go on honey. It's safe to go away a little." Then the mother needs to be reliably present when the toddler returns, thereby rewarding his or her efforts. Mahler notes that raising healthy children does not require that parents never make mistakes and that "good enough parenting" will promote successful separation-individuation.

Theories of Moral Development

Stages of Moral Development

Lawrence Kohlberg (1927–1987) was an American psychologist whose work reflected and expanded on Piaget's by applying his theory to moral development, a development that coincided with cognitive development (Crain, 1985). While visiting Israel, Kohlberg became convinced that children living in a kibbutz had advanced moral development, and he believed that the atmosphere of trust, respect, and self-governance nurtured this development. In the United States, he created schools or "just communities" that were grounded on these concepts. Based on interviews with youths, Kohlberg developed a theory of how people progressively develop a sense of morality (Kohlberg & Turiel, 1971).

His theory provides a framework for understanding the progression from black-and-white thinking about right and wrong

TABLE 2.6   Erikson's Eight Stages of Development

Approximate Age	Developmental Task	Psychosocial Crisis	Successful Resolution of Crisis	Unsuccessful Resolution of Crisis
Infancy (0–1½ years)	Forming attachment to mother, which lays foundations for later trust in others	Trust versus mistrust	Sound basis for relating to other people; trust in people; faith and hope about environment and future "If he's late in picking me up, there must be a good reason."	General difficulties relating to people effectively; suspicion; trust-fear conflict; fear of future "I can't trust anyone; no one has ever been there when I needed them."
Early childhood (1½–3 years)	Gaining some basic control of self and environment (e.g., toilet training, exploration)	Autonomy versus shame and doubt	Sense of self-control and adequacy; will power "I'm sure that with the proper diet and exercise program, I can achieve my target weight."	Independence/fear conflict; severe feelings of self-doubt "I could never lose the weight they want me to, so why even try?"
Preschool (3–6 years)	Becoming purposeful and directive	Initiative versus guilt	Ability to initiate one's own activities; sense of purpose "I like to help mommy set the table for dinner."	Aggression/fear conflict; sense of inadequacy or guilt "I wanted the candy, so I took it."
School age (6–12 years)	Developing social, physical, and school skills	Industry versus inferiority	Competence; ability to work "I'm getting really good at swimming since I've been taking lessons."	Sense of inferiority; difficulty learning and working "I can't read as well as the others in my class; I'm just dumb."
Adolescence (12–20 years)	Making transition from childhood to adulthood; developing sense of identity	Identity versus role confusion	Sense of personal identity; fidelity "I'm going to go to college to be an engineer; I hope to get married before I am 30."	Confusion about who one is; weak sense of self "I belong to the gang because without them, I'm nothing."
Early adulthood (20–35 years)	Establishing intimate bonds of love and friendship	Intimacy versus isolation	Ability to love deeply and commit oneself "My husband has been my best friend for 25 years."	Emotional isolation; egocentricity "There's no one out there for me."
Middle adulthood (35–65 years)	Fulfilling life goals that involve family, career, and society; developing concerns that embrace future generations	Generativity versus self-absorption	Ability to give and to care for others "I'm joining the political action committee to help people get the healthcare they need."	Self-absorption; inability to grow as a person "After I work all day, I just want to watch television and don't want to be around people."
Later years (65 years to death)	Looking back over one's life and accepting its meaning	Integrity versus despair	Sense of integrity and fulfillment; willingness to face death; wisdom "I've led a happy, productive life, and I still have plenty to give."	Dissatisfaction with life; denial of or despair over prospect of death "What a waste my life has been; I'm going to die alone."

Data from Erikson, E. H. (1963). *Childhood and society*. New York, NY: W. W. Norton; and Altrocchi, J. (1980). *Abnormal psychology* (p. 196). New York, NY: Harcourt Brace Jovanovich.

to a complex, variable, and context-dependent decision-making process regarding the rightness or wrongness of action.

Preconventional level

Stage 1: Obedience and punishment. The hallmarks of this stage are a focus on rules and on listening to authority. People at this stage believe that obedience is the method to avoid punishment.

Stage 2: Individualism and exchange. Individuals become aware that not everyone thinks the way that they do and that different people see rules differently. If they or others decide to break the rules, they are risking punishment.

Conventional level

Stage 3: Good interpersonal relationships. Children begin to view rightness or wrongness as related to motivations, personality, or the goodness or badness of the person. In general, people should get along and have similar values.

Stage 4: Maintaining the social order. A "rules are rules" mindset returns. However, the reasoning behind it is not simply to avoid punishment; it is because the person has begun to adopt a broader view of society. Listening to authority maintains the social order; bureaucracies and big government agencies often seem to operate with this tenet.

TABLE 2.7 Gilligan's Stages of Moral Development

Stage	Goal	Action
Preconventional	Goal is individual survival—selfishness	Caring for self
Conventional	Self-sacrifice is goodness—responsibility to others	Caring for others
Postconventional	Principle of nonviolence—do not hurt others or self	Balancing caring for self with caring for others

Postconventional level

Stage 5: Social contract and individual rights. People in stage 5 still believe that the social order is important, but the social order must be *good*. For example, if the social order is corrupt, then rules should be changed and it is a duty to protect the rights of others.

Stage 6: Universal ethical principles. Actions should create justice for everyone involved. We are obliged to break unjust laws.

Ethics of Care Theory

Carol Gilligan (born 1936) is an American psychologist, ethicist, and feminist who inspired the normative ethics of care theory. She worked with Kohlberg as he developed his theory of moral development and later criticized his work for being based on a sample of boys and men. In addition, she believed that he used a scoring method that favored males' methods of reasoning, resulting in lower moral development scores for girls as compared with boys. Based on Gilligan's critique, Kohlberg later revised his scoring methods, which resulted in greater similarity between girls' and boys' scores.

Gilligan (1982) suggests that a morality of care should replace Kohlberg's "justice view" of morality, which maintains that we should do what is right no matter the personal cost or the cost to those we love. Gilligan's care view emphasizes the importance of forming relationships, banding together, and putting the needs of those for whom we care above the needs of strangers. Gilligan asserts that a female approach to ethics has always been in existence but had been trivialized. Like Kohlberg, Gilligan asserts that moral development progresses through three major divisions: preconventional, conventional, and postconventional. These transitions are not dictated by cognitive ability but rather through personal development and changes in a sense of self (Table 2.7).

CONCLUSION

This chapter introduced you to some of the historically significant theories and therapies widely used currently and the theoretical implications for nursing care. Table 2.8 lists additional theorists whose contributions influence psychiatric-mental health nursing.

TABLE 2.8 Additional Theorists Whose Contributions Influence Psychiatric-Mental Health Nursing

Theorist	School of Thought	Major Contributions	Relevance to Psychiatric Mental Health Nursing
Carl Rogers	Humanism	Developed a person-centered model of psychotherapy. Emphasized the concepts of: Congruence—authenticity of the therapist in dealings with the patient. Unconditional acceptance and positive regard—climate in the therapeutic relationship that facilitates change. Empathetic understanding—therapist's ability to apprehend the feelings and experiences of the patient as if these things were happening to the therapist.	Encourages nurses to view each patient as unique. Emphasizes attitudes of unconditional positive regard, empathetic understanding, and genuineness that are essential to the nurse-patient relationship. *Example:* The nurse asks the patient, "What can I do to help you regain control over your anxiety?"
Jean Piaget	Cognitive development	Identified stages of cognitive development, including sensorimotor (0–2 years); preoperational (2–7 years); concrete operational (7–11 years); and formal operational (11 years–adulthood). These describe how cognitive development proceeds from reflex activity to application of logical solutions to all types of problems.	Provides a broad base for cognitive interventions, especially with patients with negative self-views. *Example:* The nurse shows an 8-year-old all the equipment needed to start an IV when discussing the fact that he will need one before surgery.
Lawrence Kohlberg	Moral development	Posited a six-stage theory of moral development.	Provides nurses with a framework for evaluating moral decisions.
Albert Ellis	Existentialism	Developed approach of rational emotive behavioral therapy that is active and cognitively oriented; confrontation used to force patients to assume responsibility for behavior; patients are encouraged to accept themselves as they are and are taught to take risks and try out new behaviors.	Encourages nurses to focus on "here-and-now" issues and to help the patient live fully in the present and look forward to the future. *Example:* The nurse encourages the patient to vacation with her family even though she will be wheelchair-bound until her leg fracture heals.

Continued

TABLE 2.8   Additional Theorists Whose Contributions Influence Psychiatric-Mental Health Nursing—cont'd

Theorist	School of Thought	Major Contributions	Relevance to Psychiatric Mental Health Nursing
Albert Bandura	Social learning theory	Responsible for concepts of modeling and self-efficacy: person's belief or expectation that he or she has the capacity to affect a desired outcome through his or her own efforts.	Includes cognitive functioning with environmental factors, which provides nurses with a comprehensive view of how people learn. *Example:* The nurse helps the teenage patient to identify three negative outcomes of tobacco use.
Viktor Frankl	Existentialism	Developed "logotherapy," a form of support offered to help people find their sense of self-respect. Logotherapy is a future-oriented therapy focused on one's need to find meaning and value in living as one's most important life task.	Focuses nurse beyond mere behaviors to understanding the meaning of these behaviors to the patient's sense of life meaning. *Example:* The nurse listens attentively as the patient describes what it's been like since her daughter died.

Data from Bandura, A. (1977). *Social learning theory.* Englewood Cliffs, NJ: Prentice-Hall; Bernard, M. E., & Wolfe, J. L. (Eds.). (1993). *The RET resource book for practitioners.* New York, NY: Institute for Rational-Emotive Therapy; Ellis, A. (1989). *Inside rational emotive therapy.* San Diego, CA: Academic Press; Frankl, V. (1969). *The will to meaning.* Cleveland, OH: New American Library; Kohlberg, L. (1986). A current statement on some theoretical issues. In S. Modgil & C. Modgil (Eds.), *Lawrence Kohlberg.* Philadelphia, PA: Palmer; Rogers, C. R. (1961). *On becoming a person.* Boston, MA: Houghton Mifflin.

There are literally hundreds of therapies currently in use. The Substance Abuse and Mental Health Services Administration (SAMHSA) maintains an Evidence-Based Practice and Resource Center. New therapies are entered into the database all the time. The registry may be accessed at https://www.samhsa.gov/ebp-resource-center.

You will be introduced to other therapeutic approaches later in the book. Crisis intervention (see Chapter 26) is an approach you will find useful not only in psychiatric-mental health nursing but also in other nursing specialties. This book will also discuss group therapy (see Chapter 34) and family interventions (see Chapter 35), which are appropriate for the basic level practitioner.

KEY POINTS TO REMEMBER

- Freud articulated levels of awareness (unconscious, preconscious, conscious) and demonstrated the influence of our unconscious behavior on everyday life as evidenced by the use of defense mechanisms.
- Freud identified three psychological processes of personality (id, ego, and superego) and described how they operate and develop.
- Freud articulated one of the first modern developmental theories of personality based on five psychosexual stages.
- Various psychoanalytical therapies have been used over the years. Currently, a short-term, time-limited version of psychotherapy is common.
- Harry Stack Sullivan proposed the interpersonal theory of personality development, which focuses on interpersonal processes that can be observed in a social framework.
- Interpersonal therapy seeks to improve interpersonal relationships and improve communication patterns.
- Hildegard Peplau, a nursing theorist, developed an interpersonal theoretical framework that has become the foundation of psychiatric-mental health nursing practice.
- Behavioral theorists argue that changing a behavior changes a personality.

- Pavlov focused on classical conditioning (in which an involuntary reaction is caused by a stimulus), while Skinner experimented with operant conditioning (in which voluntary behavior is learned through reinforcement).
- Common behavioral treatments include modeling, operant conditioning, exposure therapy, aversion therapy, and biofeedback.
- Cognitive theory is based on the belief that thoughts come before feelings and actions. Thoughts may not be a clear representation of reality and may be distorted.
- Cognitive behavioral therapy is the most commonly used, accepted, and empirically validated psychotherapeutic approach. It focuses on identifying, understanding, and changing distorted thought patterns.
- Abraham Maslow, the founder of humanistic psychology, offered the theory of self-actualization and human motivation that is basic to all nursing education. He argued that humans are motivated by unmet needs. Basic needs must be met before higher-level needs.
- A biological model of mental illness and treatment dominates care for psychiatric disorders. Current biological treatments include pharmacotherapy and brain stimulation therapy.

- Erik Erikson expanded on Freud's developmental stages to include middle age through old age. Erikson called his stages psychosocial stages and emphasized the social aspect of personality development.
- Lawrence Kohlberg provides us with a framework to understand the progression of moral development from black-and-white thinking to a complex decision-making process that coincides with intellectual development.
- Carol Gilligan expanded on Kohlberg's moral theory of development to emphasize relationships and tending to the needs of others.

CRITICAL THINKING

1. Consider how the theorists and theories discussed in this chapter have had an effect on your practice of nursing:
   a. How do Freud's concepts of the conscious, preconscious, and unconscious affect your understanding of patients' behaviors?
   b. Do you believe Erikson's psychosocial stages represent a sound basis for identifying disruptions in stages of development in your patients? Support your position with a clinical example.
   c. What are the implications of Sullivan's focus on the importance of interpersonal relationships for your interactions with patients?
   d. Peplau believed that nurses must exercise self-awareness within the nurse-patient relationship. Describe situations in your student experience in which this self-awareness played a vital role in your relationships with patients.
   e. Identify someone you believe to be self-actualized. What characteristics does this person have that support your assessment? How do you make use of Maslow's hierarchy of needs in your nursing practice?
   f. What do you think about the behaviorist point of view that to change behaviors is to change personality?
2. Which of the therapies described in this chapter do you think can be the most helpful to you in your nursing practice? What are your reasons for this choice?

CHAPTER REVIEW

1. A male patient reports to the nurse, "I'm told I have memories of childhood abuse stored in my unconscious mind. I want to work on this." Based on this statement, what information should the nurse provide the patient?
   a. To seek the help of a trained therapist to help uncover and deal with the trauma associated with those memories.
   b. How to use a defense mechanism such as suppression so that the memories will be less threatening.
   c. Psychodynamic therapy will allow the surfacing of those unconscious memories to occur in just a few sessions.
   d. Group sessions are valuable to identify underlying themes of the memories being suppressed.
2. Which question should the nurse ask when assessing for what Sullivan's Interpersonal Theory identifies as the most painful human condition?
   a. "Is self-esteem important to you?"
   b. "Do you think of yourself as being lonely?"
   c. "What do you do to manage your anxiety?"
   d. "Have you ever been diagnosed with depression?"
3. When discussing therapy options, the nurse should provide information about interpersonal therapy to which patient? *Select all that apply.*
   a. The teenager who is the focus of bullying at school
   b. The older woman who has just lost her life partner to cancer
   c. The young adult who has begun demonstrating hoarding tendencies
   d. The adolescent demonstrating aggressive verbal and physical tendencies
   e. The middle-aged adult who recently discovered her partner has been unfaithful
4. When considering the suggestions of Hildegard Peplau, which activity should the nurse regularly engage in to ensure that the patient stays the focus of all therapeutic conversations?
   a. Assessing the patient for unexpressed concerns and fears
   b. Evaluating the possible need for additional training and education
   c. Reflecting on personal behaviors and personal needs
   d. Avoiding power struggles with the manipulative patient
5. Which action reflects therapeutic practices associated with operant conditioning?
   a. Encouraging a parent to read to their children to foster a love for learning
   b. Encouraging a patient to make daily journal entries describing their feelings
   c. Suggesting to a new mother that she spend time cuddling her newborn often during the day
   d. Acknowledging a patient who is often verbally aggressive for complimenting a picture another patient drew
6. A nurse is assessing a patient who graduated at the top of his class but now obsesses about being incompetent in his new job. The nurse recognizes that this patient may benefit from the following type of psychotherapy:
   a. Interpersonal
   b. Operant conditioning
   c. Behavioral
   d. Cognitive behavioral
7. According to Maslow's hierarchy of needs, the most basic needs category for nurses to address is:
   a. Physiological
   b. Safety
   c. Love and belonging
   d. Self-actualization

8. In an outpatient psychiatric clinic, a nurse notices that a newly admitted young male patient smiles when he sees her. One day the young man tells the nurse, "You are pretty like my mother." The nurse recognizes that the male is exhibiting:
   a. Transference
   b. Id expression
   c. Countertransference
   d. A cognitive distortion

9. Linda is terrified of spiders and cannot explain why. Because she lives in a wooded area, she would like to overcome this overwhelming fear. Her nurse practitioner suggests which therapy?
   a. Behavioral
   b. Biofeedback
   c. Aversion
   d. Exposure and response prevention therapy

10. A patient is telling a tearful story. The nurse listens empathically and responds therapeutically with:
    a. "The next time you find yourself in a similar situation, please call me."
    b. "I am sorry this situation made you feel so badly. Would you like some tea?"
    c. "Let's devise a plan on how you will react next time in a similar situation."
    d. "I am sorry that your friend was so thoughtless. You should be treated better."

1. **a;** 2. **b;** 3. **a, b, e;** 4. **c;** 5. **d;** 6. **d;** 7. **a;** 8. **a;** 9. **d;** 10. **c.**

🌐 Visit the Evolve website for a posttest on the content in this chapter: http://evolve.elsevier.com/Varcarolis

---

REFERENCES

Bandura, A., Blanchard, A. B., & Ritter, B. (1969). The relative efficacy of desensitization and modeling approaches for inducing behavioral, affective, and attitudinal changes. *Journal of Personality and Social Psychology, 13,* 173–179.

Beck, A. T. (1967). *Depression: clinical, experimental and theoretical aspects.* New York, NY: Harper & Row.

Beck, A. T., Rush, A. J., Shaw, B. F., & Emery, G. (1979). *Cognitive therapy of depression.* New York, NY: Guilford Press.

Behavioral Tech. (n.d.). Skills training. Retrieved from https://behavioraltech.org/resources/faqs/dialectical-behavior-therapy-dbt/skills-training/

Crain, W. C. (1985). *Theories of development.* New York, NY: Prentice-Hall.

Ellis, A. (2000). *On therapy: A dialogue with Aaron T. Beck and Albert Ellis.* Discussion at the American Psychological Association's 108th Convention, Washington, DC.

Erikson, E. H. (1963). *Childhood and society.* New York, NY: W. W. Norton.

Freud, S. (1960). *The ego and the id* (J. Strachey, trans.). New York, NY: W. W. Norton (original work published in 1923).

Freud, S. (1969). *An outline of psychoanalysis* (J. Strachey, trans.). New York, NY: W. W. Norton (original work published in 1940).

Gilligan, C. (1982). *In a different voice.* Boston, MA: Harvard University Press.

Kohlberg, L., & Turiel, E. (1971). Moral development and moral education. In G. S. Lesser (Ed.), *Psychology and educational practice* (pp. 410–465). Glenview, IL: Scott, Foresman, & Company.

Lenz, A. S., Del Conte, G., Hollenbaugh, K. M., & Callendar, K. (2016). Emotional regulation and interpersonal effectiveness as mechanisms of change for treatment outcomes within a DBT program for adolescents. *Counseling Outcome Research, 7*(2), 73–85.

Linehan, M. M., Armstrong, H. E., Suarez, A., Allmon, D., & Heard, H. L. (1991). Cognitive-behavioral treatment of chronically parasuicidal borderline patients. *Archives of General Psychiatry, 48*(12), 1060–1064.

Linehan, M. M. (1993). *Cognitive behavioral treatment of border personalit disorder.* New York: Guilford Press.

Mahler, M. S., Pine, F., & Bergman, A. (1975). *The psychological birth of the human infant.* New York: Basic Books.

Maslow, A. H. (1968). *Toward a psychology of being.* Princeton, NJ: Van Nostrand.

Maslow, A. H. (1970). *Motivation and personality* (2nd ed.). New York, NY: Harper & Row.

Pavlov, I. (1928). *Lectures on conditioned reflexes* (W. H. Grant, trans.). New York, NY: International Publishers.

Peplau, H. E. (1952). *Interpersonal relations in nursing: A conceptual frame of reference for psychodynamic nursing.* New York, NY: Putnam.

Skinner, B. F. (1987). Whatever happened to psychology as the science of behavior? *American Psychologist, 42,* 780–786.

Sullivan, H. S. (1953). *The interpersonal theory of psychiatry.* New York, NY: W. W. Norton.

Watson, J. B. (1919). *Psychology from the standpoint of a behaviorist.* Philadelphia, PA: Lippincott.

Weissman, M. M., Markowitz, J. W., & Klerman, G. L. (2007). *Clinician's quick guide to interpersonal psychotherapy.* Oxford, United Kingdom: Oxford University Press.

3

Neurobiology and Pharmacotherapy

Chris Paxos and Jessica B. Emshoff

🌐 Visit the Evolve website for a pretest on the content in this chapter: http://evolve.elsevier.com/Varcarolis

OBJECTIVES

1. Discuss the structure and major functions of the brain and how psychotropic medications can alter these functions.
2. Identify how specific brain functions are altered in certain psychiatric disorders (e.g., major depressive disorder, anxiety, schizophrenia).
3. Describe how a neurotransmitter functions as a chemical messenger.
4. Describe how the use of imaging techniques can be helpful for understanding mental illness.
5. Differentiate pharmacodynamics and pharmacokinetics.
6. Identify the main neurotransmitters that are affected by the following psychotropic medications and their subgroups:
   Antianxiety and hypnotic medications
   Antidepressant medications
   Mood stabilizers
   Antipsychotic medications
   Psychostimulants
   Cholinesterase inhibitors
7. Identify cautions you might incorporate into your medication teaching plan with regard to herbal treatments.

KEY TERMS AND CONCEPTS

antagonists
antianxiety (anxiolytic) medications
cholinesterase inhibitors
circadian rhythms
first-generation antipsychotics
hypnotic
limbic system
lithium
monoamine oxidase inhibitors (MAOIs)

mood stabilizers
neurons
neurotransmitters
norepinephrine and serotonin specific antidepressants (NaSSAs)
pharmacodynamics
pharmacogenetics
pharmacokinetics
psychotropic medication
receptors

reuptake
second-generation antipsychotics
selective serotonin reuptake inhibitors (SSRIs)
serotonin norepinephrine reuptake inhibitors (SNRIs)
synapse
therapeutic index
tricyclic antidepressants (TCAs)

Genetics, neurodevelopmental factors, substances, infections, and traumatic experiences can interact and produce a psychiatric disorder. No matter the cause, physical changes in the brain can result in disturbances in the patient's mood and behavior. These physiological alterations are the targets of psychotropic (Greek for *psyche,* or mind, + *trepein,* to turn) medications used to treat psychiatric disorders.

Despite the availability of psychotropic medications for more than half a century, the actions of some of these medications to improve psychiatric symptoms are poorly understood. Early biological theories associated a single neurotransmitter with a specific disorder: for example, a dopamine theory to explain schizophrenia, or a serotonin theory to explain depression. Experts view these theories as overly simplistic. Other neurotransmitters, hormones, and coregulators play important and complex roles. Recent discoveries have influenced the direction of research and treatment.

Before examining specific medications, this chapter will provide an overview of normal brain function and how these functions operate. Theories of the neurobiological basis of various types of emotional and physiological dysfunctions are presented next. Finally, the chapter reviews the major classifications of medications used to treat psychiatric disorders, explains how they work, and identifies both their beneficial and problematic effects. Additionally, detailed information regarding adverse and toxic effects, nursing implications, and teaching tools are presented in the appropriate clinical chapters (Chapters 11 to 24).

STRUCTURE AND FUNCTION OF THE BRAIN

Functions and Activities of the Brain

Regulating behavior and carrying out mental processes are important responsibilities of the brain, but certainly not the

BOX 3.1   Functions of the Brain

- Monitor changes in the external world
- Monitor the composition of body fluids
- Regulate the contractions of skeletal muscles
- Regulate the internal organs
- Control basic drives: hunger, thirst, sex, aggressive self-protection
- Mediate conscious sensation
- Store and retrieve memories
- Regulate mood (affect) and emotions
- Think and perform intellectual functions
- Regulate sleep cycle
- Produce and interpret language
- Process visual and auditory data

only ones. Box 3.1 summarizes some of the major functions and activities of the brain.

Maintenance of Homeostasis

The brain directs and coordinates the body's response to both internal and external changes. Appropriate responses require a constant surveillance of the environment, interpretation and integration of the incoming information, and control over the appropriate organs of response. The goal of these responses is to maintain homeostasis (an organism's process for maintaining a stable internal environment) and, therefore, to maintain life.

Various sensory organs relay information about the external world to the brain by the peripheral nerves. Stimuli such as light, sound, or touch must ultimately be interpreted as, say, a lamp, doorbell, or a tap on the back. These sensations can be altered, particularly in psychotic disorders such as schizophrenia, where an individual may register sensory information, such as an audible voice, that does not originate in the external world.

To respond to the external world, the brain controls skeletal muscles. This control includes the ability to initiate contraction. It also fine-tunes and coordinates contraction so that a person can, for example, guide the fingers to the correct keys on a piano. Unfortunately, disturbances in movement may result from either psychiatric disorders or psychotropic medications. For example, antipsychotic medications can cause tremor or muscle rigidity.

It is important to remember that the skeletal muscles controlled by the brain include the diaphragm, which is essential for breathing, and the muscles of the throat, tongue, and mouth, which are essential for speech. Therefore, medications that affect brain function can stimulate or depress respiration or lead to slurred speech.

In addition to surveying the outside world, the brain also monitors internal functions. It continuously receives information about blood pressure, body temperature, blood gases, and the chemical composition of body fluids so that it can direct the appropriate responses required to maintain homeostasis. For example, if blood pressure drops, the brain must direct the heart to pump more blood and the smooth muscles of the arterioles to constrict. These compensatory mechanisms allow the body to return blood pressure to its normal level.

Regulation of the Autonomic Nervous System and Hormones

The autonomic nervous system and the endocrine system serve as links between the brain and cardiac muscle, smooth muscle, and glands of which the internal organs are composed (Fig. 3.1). To stimulate the heart, the brain must activate sympathetic nerves that innervate the sinoatrial node and the ventricular myocardium. Activation of parasympathetic nerves innervating the gastrointestinal tract increases gut motility and facilitates digestion.

The homeostatic linkage between the brain and the internal organs explains why psychiatric disturbances, such as anxiety, alter internal function. Anxiety activates the sympathetic nervous system, leading to symptoms such as increased heart rate, shortness of breath, facial blushing, and sweaty palms (Jameson et al., 2018).

The brain also influences internal organs by regulating hormonal secretions of the pituitary gland, which, in turn, regulates other glands. A specific area of the brain, the hypothalamus, secretes hormones called releasing factors. These hormones act on the pituitary gland to stimulate or inhibit the synthesis and release of pituitary hormones. Once in the general circulation, they influence various internal activities.

An example of this linkage is the release of thyroid-releasing hormone by the hypothalamus. This hormone stimulates the anterior pituitary gland to release thyroid-stimulating hormone into the bloodstream. Thyroid-stimulating hormone then binds to the thyroid gland, which stimulates the production of thyroxine (T4) and triiodothyronine (T3). An overactive thyroid, resulting in hyperthyroidism, is associated with symptoms of anxiety. Conversely, an underactive thyroid, or hypothyroidism, is associated with depressive symptoms.

The relationship between the brain, pituitary gland, and adrenal glands is particularly important in normal and abnormal mental function. The steps in this system are:

1. The hypothalamus secretes corticotropin-releasing hormone (CRH).
2. CRH stimulates the pituitary to release adrenocorticotropic hormone.
3. Adrenocorticotropin stimulates the cortex of each adrenal gland (located on top of the kidneys) to secrete the stress hormone, cortisol.

This system is referred to as the hypothalamic-pituitary-adrenal axis, or HPA axis. It is part of the normal response to a variety of mental and physical stressors (Fig. 3.2). All three hormones—CRH, adrenocorticotropin, and cortisol—influence the functions of the nerve cells of the brain. There is considerable evidence that this system influences psychiatric disturbances. For example, elevated cortisol levels are found in patients with major depressive disorder. Elevated cortisol levels suppress the immune response and make patients with depression more vulnerable to infection. Patients with posttraumatic stress disorder (PTSD) appear to have lower than normal circulating cortisol. Lower cortisol levels are associated with more severe PTSD symptoms in particular patients (Stahl, 2013).

Control of Biological Drives and Behavior

To understand the basis of psychiatric disorders, it is helpful to distinguish between the various types of brain activity.

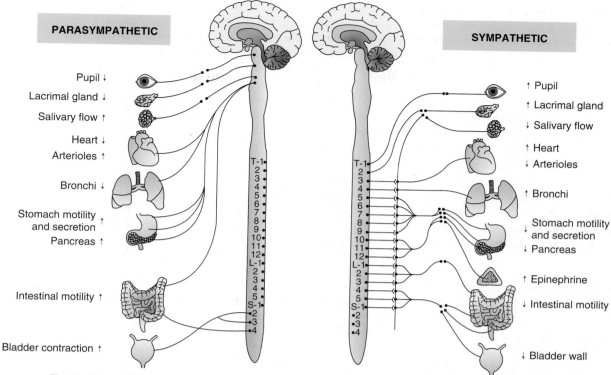

PARASYMPATHETIC

Pupil ↓
Lacrimal gland ↓
Salivary flow ↑
Heart ↓
Arterioles ↑
Bronchi ↓
Stomach motility and secretion ↑
Pancreas ↑
Intestinal motility ↑
Bladder contraction ↑

SYMPATHETIC

↑ Pupil
↑ Lacrimal gland
↓ Salivary flow
↑ Heart
↓ Arterioles
↑ Bronchi
↓ Stomach motility and secretion
↓ Pancreas
↑ Epinephrine
↓ Intestinal motility
↓ Bladder wall

Fig. 3.1 The autonomic nervous system has two divisions: sympathetic and parasympathetic. The sympathetic division is dominant in stress situations, such as fear and anger (described as fight-or-flight). The parasympathetic division conserves and restores energy (described as rest-and-digest).

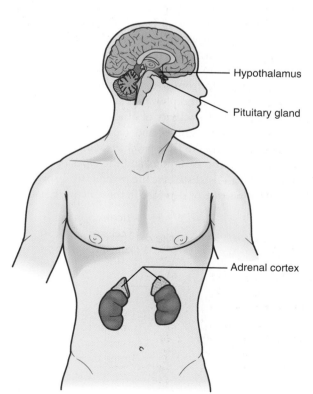

Hypothalamus

Pituitary gland

Adrenal cortex

Fig. 3.2 The hypothalamic-pituitary-adrenal axis.

An understanding of these activities shows where to look for disturbed function and what to expect with treatment. The brain is responsible for such basic drives as sex and hunger. Disturbances of these drives (e.g., loss of sexual interest, overeating or undereating) can be an indication of an underlying psychiatric disorder such as depression.

Cycle of sleep and wakefulness. Various regions of the brain regulate and coordinate the entire cycle of sleep and wakefulness, as well as the intensity of alertness while awake. Sleep is essential for both physiological and psychological well-being. Sleep pattern disturbances occur in virtually every psychiatric disorder. Improvement in sleep is often an important marker in determining response and tracking recovery from these illnesses.

Psychotropic medications may interfere with the normal regulation of sleep and alertness. Sedative-hypnotic medications will reduce alertness and can cause drowsiness. These medications require caution while engaging in activities requiring mental alertness, such as driving or operating machinery. One way of minimizing the danger is to take sedating medications at night just before bedtime. Psychostimulants, on the other hand, promote wakefulness and may cause insomnia if taken near bedtime. Therefore, they should be taken early in the day.

Circadian Rhythms

Circadian rhythms are the fluctuation of various physiological and behavioral patterns over a 24-hour cycle. Changes in sleep, body temperature, secretion of hormones such as corticotropin and cortisol, and secretion of neurotransmitters such as norepinephrine and serotonin are influenced by these rhythms. Both norepinephrine and serotonin are thought to be involved in mood. There is evidence that the circadian rhythm of neurotransmitter secretion is altered in psychiatric disorders, particularly in those that involve mood.

Conscious Mental Activity

All aspects of conscious mental experience and sense of self originate from the activity of the brain. Conscious mental activity can be a basic, meandering stream of consciousness that flows from thoughts of future responsibilities, memories, fantasies, and so on. Conscious mental activity can also be much more complex when it is applied to problem solving or interpretation of the external world. Unfortunately, conscious mental experiences can become distorted in psychiatric disorders. A patient with schizophrenia may have chaotic and incoherent speech and thought patterns (e.g., unconnected phrases and topics) and delusional interpretations of personal interactions such as beliefs about people or events that are not supported by data or reality.

Memory

An extremely important component of mental activity is memory. It is the ability to retain and recall past experiences. From both an anatomical and a physiological perspective, there is a major difference in the processing of short- and long-term memory. Alzheimer's disease provides a stark example. A patient with Alzheimer's disease may have no recall of the events of the previous few minutes but may have vivid recall of events that occurred decades earlier.

Social Skills

An important, and often neglected, aspect of brain functioning involves social skills that make interpersonal relationships possible. In almost all psychiatric disorders, from social anxiety disorder to schizoaffective disorder, difficulties in interpersonal relationships are an important aspect of the disorders. As with sleep, improvements in these relationships help gauge progress toward goals and recovery.

Cellular Composition of the Brain

The brain is composed of approximately 100 billion **neurons**, nerve cells that conduct electrical impulses. Most functions of

the brain, from regulation of blood pressure to the conscious sense of self, result from the actions of individual neurons and the interconnections between them. Although neurons come in a great variety of shapes and sizes, all carry out the same three types of physiological actions:

1. Responding to stimuli
2. Conducting electrical impulses
3. Releasing chemicals called neurotransmitters

Neurons have the ability to communicate by conducting an electrical impulse, also called an action potential, from one end of the cell to the other. All cellular membranes are electrically charged due to ions inside and outside the cell. Communication between neurons occurs mainly through sodium (Na^+) and potassium (K^+) ions. In a resting state, there is an unequal distribution of these two ions on either side of the cell membrane. When the neuron is at rest, potassium ions are located inside the membrane and sodium ions (along with some potassium ions) are on the outside. This distribution of ions results in intracellular space that is more negatively charged when compared with the extracellular space.

Stimulation of the nerve cell membrane changes this resting state within milliseconds. First, the stimulus causes sodium gates to open. Sodium ions flow into the neuron and potassium ions flow out. The entry of positively charged ions into the cell actually reverses the electrical potential from a negative one to a positive one. The current at one end of the cell is conducted along the membrane until it reaches the opposite end (Fig. 3.3).

Once an electrical impulse reaches the end of a neuron, a neurotransmitter is released. A **neurotransmitters** is a chemical substance that functions as a neuromessenger. Neurotransmitters are released from the axon terminal of the presynaptic neuron on excitation. The neurotransmitter then crosses the space, or **synapse**, to an adjacent postsynaptic neuron where it attaches to **receptors** on the neuron's surface.

It is this interaction from one neuron to another, by way of a neurotransmitter and receptor, that allows the activity of one neuron to influence the activity of other neurons. The interaction between neurotransmitter and receptor is a major target of the medications used to treat psychiatric disorders. Table 3.1 lists important neurotransmitters and the types of receptors to which they attach. Also listed are the psychiatric disorders associated with an increase or decrease in these neurotransmitters.

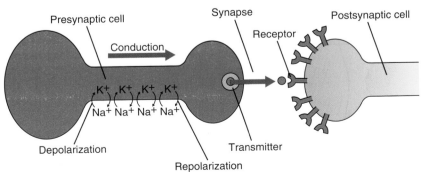

Fig. 3.3 Activities of neurons. Conduction along a neuron involves the inward movement of sodium ions (Na^+) followed by the outward movement of potassium ions (K^+). When the current reaches the end of the cell, the neurotransmitter is released. The neurotransmitter crosses the synapse and attaches to a receptor on the postsynaptic cell. Neurotransmitter attachment to a receptor either stimulates or inhibits the postsynaptic cell.

TABLE 3.1   Neurotransmitters and Receptors

Neurotransmitters	Receptors	Effects/Comments	Association with Mental Health
Monoamines			
Dopamine (DA)	D_1, D_2, D_3, D_4, D_5	Involved in fine motor movement Involved in integration of emotions and thoughts Involved in decision making Stimulates hypothalamus to release hormones	*Decrease:* Parkinson's disease Depression *Increase:* Schizophrenia Mania
Norepinephrine (NE) (noradrenaline)	α_1, α_2, β_1, β_2, β_3	Level in brain affects mood Attention and arousal Stimulates sympathetic branch of autonomic nervous system for "fight or flight" in response to stress	*Decrease:* Depression *Increase:* Mania Anxiety states Schizophrenia
Serotonin (5-HT)	5-HT_1, 5-HT_2, 5-HT_3, 5-HT_4, others	Plays a role in sleep regulation, hunger, mood states, and pain perception Hormonal activity Plays a role in aggression and sexual behavior	*Decrease:* Depression
Histamine (H)	H_1, H_2	Involved in alertness Involved in inflammatory response Stimulates gastric secretion	*Decrease:* Sedation Weight gain
Amino Acids			
γ-aminobutyric acid (GABA)	GABA_A, GABA_B	Plays a role in inhibition; reduces aggression, excitation, and anxiety May play a role in pain perception Has anticonvulsant and muscle-relaxing properties May impair cognition and psychomotor functioning	*Decrease:* Anxiety Schizophrenia Mania Huntington's disease *Increase:* Reduction of anxiety
Glutamate	NMDA, AMPA	Excitatory AMPA plays a role in learning and memory	*Decrease (NMDA):* Psychosis *Increase (NMDA):* Prolonged increased state can be neurotoxic Neurodegeneration in Alzheimer's disease *Increase (AMPA):* Improvement of cognitive performance in behavioral tasks
Cholinergics			
Acetylcholine (ACh)	Nicotinic ($\alpha_4\beta_2$, others), muscarinic (M_1, M_2, M_3)	Plays a role in learning and memory Stimulates parasympathetic branch of autonomic nervous system for "resting and digesting" actions Affects sexual and aggressive behavior	*Decrease:* Alzheimer's disease Huntington's disease Parkinson's disease *Increase:* Depression
Peptides			
Substance P	NK1	Facilitates the transmission of pain signals along the spinal cord Antagonists of NK1 have shown antidepressant effects	Involved in regulation of pain and possibly mood and anxiety
Hypocretin/Orexin	OX1R, OX2R	Promotes and sustains wakefulness	*Decrease:* Narcolepsy

Continued

TABLE 3.1   Transmitters and Receptors—cont'd

Neurotransmitters	Receptors	Effects/Comments	Association with Mental Health
Neurotensin	NTR_1, NTR_2, NTR_3	Endogenous antipsychotic-like properties	Possibly involved in disorders involving dopamine, such as schizophrenia and Parkinson's disease

AMPA, α-Amino-3-hydroxy-5-methyl-4-isoxazolepropionic acid; *GABA*, γ-aminobutyric acid; *NMDA*, N-methyl-D-aspartate.

After attaching to a receptor and exerting its influence on the postsynaptic cell, the neurotransmitter separates from the receptor and is destroyed. Box 3.2 describes the process of neurotransmitter destruction. Neurotransmitters can be destroyed in one of two ways. Some enzymes (identified by the suffix -ase) destroy neurotransmitters at the postsynaptic cell. For example,

acetylcholine is destroyed by the enzyme acetylcholinesterase (referred to as cholinesterase from here on) at the postsynaptic cell. Other neurotransmitters are taken back into the presynaptic cell from which they were originally released by a process called cellular reuptake. These neurotransmitters are either reused or destroyed by intracellular enzymes. For example, monoamine

BOX 3.2   Destruction of Neurotransmitters

A full explanation of the various ways in which psychotropic medications alter neuronal activity requires a brief review of the manner in which neurotransmitters are destroyed after attaching to the receptors. To avoid continuous and prolonged action on the postsynaptic cell, the neurotransmitter is released shortly after attaching to the postsynaptic receptor. Once released, the neurotransmitter is destroyed in one of two ways.

One way is the immediate inactivation of the neurotransmitter at the postsynaptic membrane. An example of this method of destruction is the action of the enzyme cholinesterase. Cholinesterase is present at the postsynaptic membrane and destroys the neurotransmitter, acetylcholine, shortly after it attaches to nicotinic or muscarinic receptors on the postsynaptic cell.

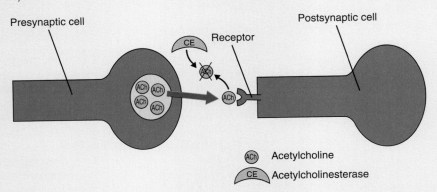

ACh   Acetylcholine

CE   Acetylcholinesterase

A second method of neurotransmitter inactivation is more complex. After interacting with the postsynaptic receptor, the neurotransmitter is released and taken back into the presynaptic cell, the cell from which it was released. This process, referred to as the reuptake of neurotransmitter, is a common target for medications. Once inside the presynaptic cell, an enzyme within the cell breaks down the neurotransmitter. The monoamine neurotransmitters norepinephrine, dopamine, and serotonin are all inactivated in this manner by the enzyme monoamine oxidase.

Looking at this second method, what would prevent the enzyme from destroying the neurotransmitter before its release? The answer is that before a neurotransmitter is released, it is stored within a membrane (i.e., vesicle) and is protected. After release and reuptake, the neurotransmitter is either destroyed by the enzyme or reenters the membrane to be stored and eventually used again.

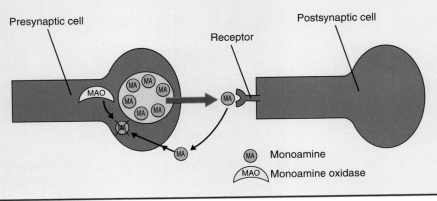

MA   Monoamine

MAO   Monoamine oxidase

neurotransmitters (e.g., norepinephrine, dopamine, serotonin) are taken back into the cell and either stored or destroyed by the intracellular enzyme, monoamine oxidase (MAO).

Organization of the Brain
Brainstem

The most primitive area of the brain is the brainstem. It connects directly to the spinal cord and is central to the survival of all animals by controlling such functions as heart rate, breathing, digestion, and sleeping.

Ascending pathways in the brainstem, referred to as mesolimbic and mesocortical pathways, seem to play a strong role in modulating the emotional value of sensory material. These pathways project to areas of the cerebrum collectively known as the limbic system. The limbic system plays a crucial role in emotional status and psychological function using norepinephrine, serotonin, and dopamine as its neurotransmitters.

The role of these pathways in normal and abnormal mental activity is significant. For example, experts believe that the release of dopamine from the mesolimbic pathway plays a role in psychological reward and substance use disorders. The neurotransmitters released by these neurons are major targets of the medications used to treat psychiatric disorders.

Hypothalamus

In a small area above the brainstem lies the hypothalamus, which plays a vital role in:

- Controlling basic drives, such as hunger, thirst, and sex
- Linking higher activities (e.g., thought and emotion) to the functioning of internal organs
- Processing sensory information that is then sent to the cerebral cortex
- Regulating the sleep and wakefulness cycle and the ability of the cerebrum to carry out conscious mental activity

Cerebellum

Located behind the brainstem where the spinal cord meets the brain, the cerebellum (Fig. 3.4) receives information from the sensory systems, the spinal cord, and other parts of the brain and then regulates voluntary motor movements. It plays a crucial role in coordinating contractions so that movement is accomplished in a smooth and directed manner. It is also involved in balance and the maintenance of equilibrium.

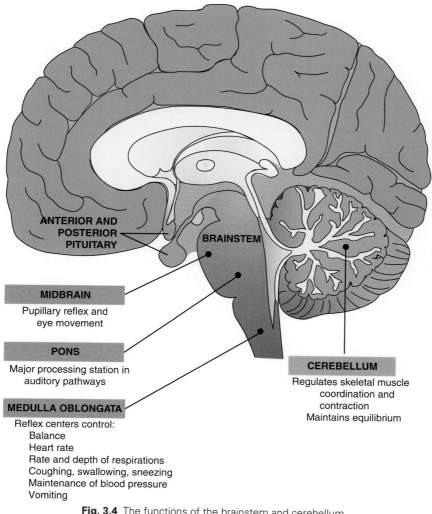

ANTERIOR AND POSTERIOR PITUITARY

BRAINSTEM

MIDBRAIN
Pupillary reflex and eye movement

PONS
Major processing station in auditory pathways

MEDULLA OBLONGATA
Reflex centers control:
Balance
Heart rate
Rate and depth of respirations
Coughing, swallowing, sneezing
Maintenance of blood pressure
Vomiting

CEREBELLUM
Regulates skeletal muscle coordination and contraction
Maintains equilibrium

Fig. 3.4 The functions of the brainstem and cerebellum.

Cerebrum

The human brainstem and cerebellum are similar in both structure and function to these same structures in other mammals. The development of a much larger and more elaborate cerebrum is what distinguishes humans from the rest of the animal kingdom.

The cerebrum, situated on top of and surrounding the brainstem, is responsible for mental activities and a conscious sense of being. This is responsible for our conscious perception of the external world and our own body, emotional status, memory, and control of skeletal muscles that allow willful direction of movement. The cerebrum is also responsible for language and the ability to communicate.

The surface of the cerebrum is called the cerebral cortex. There are four major lobes of the cortex, each responsible for specific functions. For example, conscious sensation and the initiation of movement reside in the frontal lobe, the sensation of touch resides in the parietal lobe, sounds are processed in the temporal lobe, and vision is housed in the occipital lobe. Of course, all areas of the cortex are interconnected so that you can form an appropriate picture of the world and, if necessary, link it to a proper response (Fig. 3.5).

Both sensory and motor aspects of language reside in specialized areas of the cerebral cortex. Sensory language functions include the ability to read, understand spoken language, and know the names of objects perceived by the senses. Motor functions involve the physical ability to use muscles properly for speech and writing. In both neurological and psychological dysfunction, the use of language may become compromised or distorted. The change in language ability may be a factor in determining a diagnosis.

Underneath the cerebral cortex are pockets of gray matter deep within the cerebrum. Some of these, the basal ganglia, are involved in the regulation of movement. Others, the amygdala and hippocampus in the limbic system, are involved in emotions, learning, memory, and basic drives. Significantly, these areas overlap both anatomically and in the types of neurotransmitters involved. One important consequence is that medications used to treat emotional disturbances may cause movement disorders, and medications used to treat movement disorders may cause emotional changes. In the limbic system specifically, abnormalities in the amygdala play a role in anxiety disorders, whereas changes in the hippocampus are found in Alzheimer's disease.

Visualizing the Brain

A variety of noninvasive imaging techniques are used to visualize brain structure, functions, and metabolic activity. Table 3.2 identifies some common brain imaging techniques and preliminary findings as they relate to psychiatry. There are two types of neuroimaging techniques: structural and functional. Structural imaging techniques (e.g., computed tomography [CT] and magnetic resonance imaging [MRI]) provide overall images of the brain and layers of the brain. Functional imaging techniques (e.g., functional magnetic resonance imaging [fMRI], positron emission tomography [PET], single photon emission computed tomography [SPECT] reveal physiological activity in the brain.

PET scans are particularly useful in identifying physical and chemical changes as they occur in living tissue. For scanning the brain, a radioactive atom is applied to glucose to create a radionuclide (also referred to as a tag), because the brain uses glucose for its metabolism.

In unmedicated patients with schizophrenia, PET scans may show a decreased use of glucose in the frontal lobes. Twin studies demonstrate lower brain activity in the frontal lobe of a twin diagnosed with schizophrenia compared with the twin who does not have the diagnosis. The area affected in the frontal cortex of the twin with schizophrenia is an area associated with reasoning skills, which are greatly impaired in people with schizophrenia.

PET scans of patients with depression show decreased brain activity in the prefrontal cortex. Fig. 3.6 shows a patient with depression with reduced brain activity compared with someone who does not have depression. Fig. 3.7 shows three views of a PET scan of the brain of a patient with Alzheimer's disease (Stahl, 2013).

Modern imaging techniques have become important tools in assessing molecular changes in psychiatric disorders and marking the receptor sites of medication action. From a psychiatric perspective, it is important to understand what areas of the brain are implicated in dysfunction.

CAN WE MEASURE NEUROTRANSMITTERS?: The answer is that there is no perfect or easy way to measure levels of neurotransmitters in the brain. In fact, much of what is known about neurotransmitters and brain disturbances comes from pharmacology of the medications used to treat these conditions. For example, treatments that effectively reduce the delusions and hallucinations of schizophrenia block the dopamine-2 (D_2) receptors. With this knowledge, researchers concluded that delusions and hallucinations result from overactivity of dopamine at these receptors.

Psychiatric diagnoses are based on signs and symptoms and not quantifiable, biological evidence. Advances in genetics, imaging, and behavioral sciences may help psychiatry move from broad, category-based diagnoses to more precise classifications.

National Institute of Mental Health. (n.d.). *Research domain criteria.* Retrieved from https://www.nimh.nih.gov/research-priorities/rdoc/index.shtml

---

Disturbances of Mental Function

Most origins of mental dysfunction are unknown. Some known causes include recreational drugs (e.g., lysergic acid diethylamide, also known as LSD), prescription medications (e.g., high daily doses of corticosteroids, levodopa), excess levels of hormones (e.g., thyroxine, cortisol), infection (e.g., acquired immunodeficiency syndrome, encephalitis), and trauma. Even when the cause is known, the link between the causative factor and the mental dysfunction is difficult to understand.

Genetics

There is often a genetic predisposition for psychiatric disorders. The incidence of both psychotic and mood disorders is higher in relatives of people who have these diseases than in the general population. Monozygotic (identical) twins provide us with an understanding of inheritance of a disorder through a concept known as concordance rate. Concordance refers to how often an

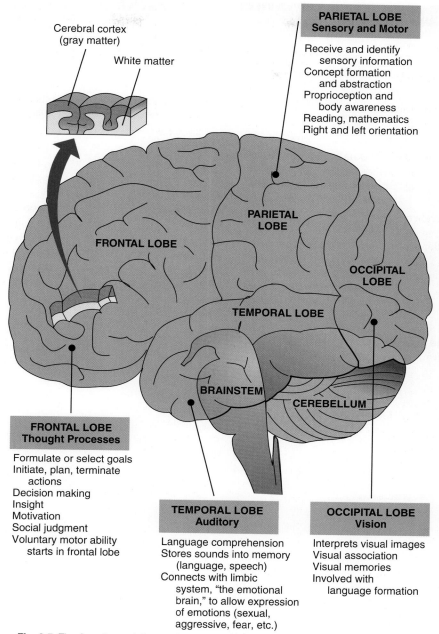

Cerebral cortex
(gray matter)

White matter

**PARIETAL LOBE
Sensory and Motor**

Receive and identify
sensory information
Concept formation
and abstraction
Proprioception and
body awareness
Reading, mathematics
Right and left orientation

PARIETAL
LOBE

FRONTAL LOBE

OCCIPITAL
LOBE

TEMPORAL LOBE

BRAINSTEM

CEREBELLUM

**FRONTAL LOBE
Thought Processes**

Formulate or select goals
Initiate, plan, terminate
actions
Decision making
Insight
Motivation
Social judgment
Voluntary motor ability
starts in frontal lobe

**TEMPORAL LOBE
Auditory**

Language comprehension
Stores sounds into memory
(language, speech)
Connects with limbic
system, "the emotional
brain," to allow expression
of emotions (sexual,
aggressive, fear, etc.)

**OCCIPITAL LOBE
Vision**

Interprets visual images
Visual association
Visual memories
Involved with
language formation

Fig. 3.5 The functions of the cerebral lobes: frontal, parietal, temporal, and occipital.

illness will affect both twins even when they are raised apart. A 100% concordance rate would mean that if one twin has a disorder, the other one would also have it. For schizophrenia, the concordance rate is 50%, meaning that inheritance is half of the equation and that other factors are involved (Jameson et al., 2018).

Neurotransmitters

Important neurotransmitters include monoamine neurotransmitters (norepinephrine, dopamine, and serotonin), the amino acid neurotransmitters (glutamate and γ-aminobutyric acid [GABA]), the neuropeptides (CRH and endorphin), and acetylcholine. Alteration of these chemicals is the basis of psychiatric disorders and is the target for pharmacological treatment. Understanding neurotransmitter abnormalities will lead to

better treatments and possibly prevent mental disorders. Research interest is focused on certain neurotransmitters and their receptors, particularly in the limbic system, which links the frontal cortex, basal ganglia, and upper brainstem.

Consider the example of major depressive disorder. It is postulated that a deficiency of norepinephrine, serotonin, dopamine, or a combination of these is the biological basis of depression. How this deficiency happens is illustrated in Fig. 3.8. Fig. 3.8A shows normal transmission of neurotransmitters. Fig. 3.8B depicts a deficiency in the amount of neurotransmitter in the presynaptic cell. Fig. 3.8C shows a deficiency or loss of the ability of postsynaptic receptors to respond to the neurotransmitters.

Changes in neurotransmitter release and receptor response can be both a cause and a consequence of intracellular changes

TABLE 3.2   Common Brain Imaging Techniques

Technique	Description	Uses	Psychiatric Relevance and Preliminary Findings
Electrical: Recording Electrical Signals From the Brain			
Electroencephalography (EEG)	A recording of electrical signals from the brain made by hooking up electrodes to the patient's scalp.	Can show the state a person is in—asleep, awake, anesthetized—because the characteristic patterns of current differ for each of these states.	Provides support from a wide range of sources that brain abnormalities exist; may lead to further testing.
Structural: Show Gross Anatomical Details of Brain Structures			
Computed tomography (CT)	A series of x-ray images is taken of the brain and a computer analysis produces "slices" providing a precise 3D-like reconstruction of each segment.	Can detect: Lesions Abrasions Areas of infarct Aneurysm	Schizophrenia Cortical atrophy Third ventricle enlargement Cognitive disorders
Magnetic resonance imaging (MRI)	A magnetic field is applied to the brain. The nuclei of hydrogen atoms absorb and emit radio waves that are analyzed by computer, which provides 3D visualization of brain structure in sectional images.	Can detect: Brain edema Ischemia Infection Neoplasm Trauma	Schizophrenia Enlarged ventricles Reduction in temporal lobe and prefrontal lobe
Functional: Show Some Activity of the Brain			
Functional magnetic resonance imaging (fMRI)	Measures brain activity indirectly by changes in blood oxygen in different parts of the brain as subjects participate in various activities.	See MRI	See MRI
Positron emission tomography (PET)	Radioactive substance (tracer) is injected, travels to the brain, and is detected as bright spots on the scan. Data collected by the detectors are relayed to a computer, which produces images of the activity and 3D visualization of the brain.	Can detect: Oxygen utilization Glucose metabolism Blood flow Neurotransmitter-receptor interaction	Schizophrenia Increased D_2, D_3 receptors in caudate nucleus Abnormalities in limbic system Mood disorder Abnormalities in temporal lobes Adult ADHD Decreased utilization of glucose
Single photon emission computed tomography (SPECT)	Similar to PET but uses radionuclides that emit gamma radiation (photons). Measures various aspects of brain functioning and provides images of multiple layers of the brain.	Can detect: Circulation of cerebrospinal fluid Similar functions to PET	See PET

3D, Three-dimensional; *ADHD,* attention-deficit/hyperactivity disorder.

in the neurons involved. Psychotic disorders, such as schizophrenia, are associated with excess transmission of dopamine from presynaptic neurons. As illustrated in Fig. 3.9, this may be caused by either excessive release of the neurotransmitter or an increase in receptor responsiveness. Aside from dopamine, the neurotransmitter glutamate may have a role in the pathology of schizophrenia. Glutamate may have a direct influence on the activity of dopamine-releasing cells. First, glutamate activity increases in the hippocampus, followed by increased metabolism in the hippocampus, and then the hippocampus atrophies or shrinks the brain's memory center. This process happens early in the disease and may become a primary tool for early diagnosis and a target for treatment (Stahl, 2013).

The neurotransmitter GABA appears to play a role in modulating neuronal excitability and anxiety. Due to the role of GABA in anxiety, many antianxiety (anxiolytic) medications act by increasing the effectiveness of this neurotransmitter. This is accomplished primarily by increasing receptor responsiveness.

It is important to keep in mind that a vast network of neurons interconnects the various areas of the brain. This network serves to integrate the activities of the brain. A limited number of neurotransmitters are used in the brain and, thus, a particular neurotransmitter is often used by different neurons to carry out quite different activities.

For example, dopamine is not only involved in thought processes but also the regulation of movement. As a result, alterations in neurotransmitter activity, resulting from a mental disturbance or medications used to treat the disturbance, can affect both thinking and movement. Basic body processes such as sleep patterns, body movement, and autonomic functions can be affected by alterations in mental status, whether arising from disease or from medication.

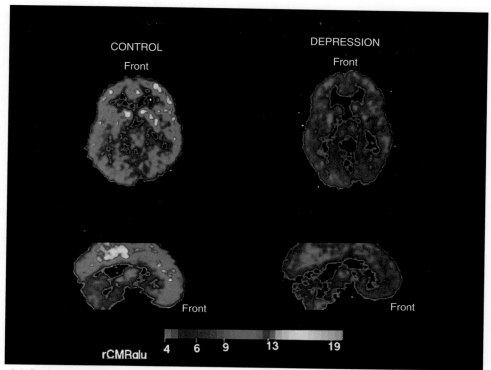

Fig. 3.6 Positron emission tomographic (PET) scans of a patient with depression *(right)* and a person without depression *(left)* reveal reduced brain activity *(darker colors)* in depression, especially in the prefrontal cortex. A form of radioactively tagged glucose was used as a tracer to visualize levels of brain activity. (From Mark George, MD, courtesy National Institute of Mental Health, Biological Psychiatry Branch.)

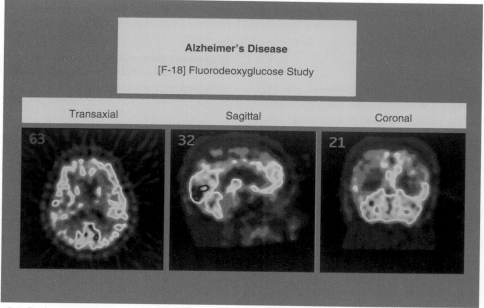

Fig. 3.7 Positron emission tomographic (PET) scan of a patient with Alzheimer's disease demonstrates a classic pattern for areas of hypometabolism in the temporal and parietal regions of the brain. Areas of reduced metabolism *(dark blue* and *black* regions) are very noticeable in the sagittal and coronal views. (Courtesy PET Imaging Center, Department of Radiology, University of Iowa Hospitals and Clinics, Iowa City.)

ACTION OF PSYCHOTROPIC MEDICATIONS

Two essential concepts to understand when studying medications are pharmacodynamics and pharmacokinetics. The term **pharmacodynamics** comes from two Greek words: *pharmakon* (drug) and *dynamikos* (power). It is the study of what a drug does to the body and how it does it. It includes drug action and responses. Both the action and responses are dose-related.

The term **pharmacokinetics** comes from the Greek words: *pharmakon* (drug) and *kinesis* (motion). As these words imply,

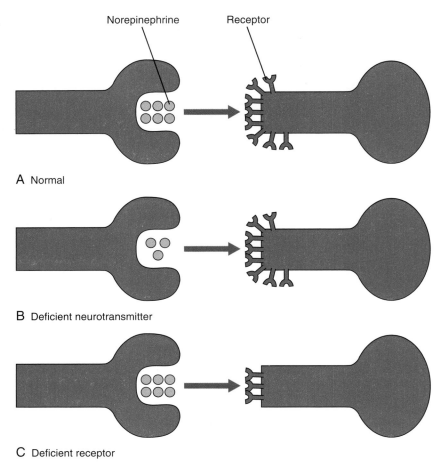

A Normal

B Deficient neurotransmitter

C Deficient receptor

Fig. 3.8 Normal transmission of neurotransmitters (A). Deficiency in transmission may be resulting from deficient release of neurotransmitter, as shown in (B), or from a reduction in receptors, as shown in (C).

pharmacokinetics is the movement of a drug through the body. The four basic processes of pharmacokinetics, which determine the concentration of a drug at its site of action, are easily remembered with the acronym ADME:

Absorption—How is the drug absorbed into the body?

Distribution—How is the drug distributed throughout the body?

Metabolism—How is the drug transformed for use and eventual excretion?

Excretion—How is the drug excreted from the body?

An understanding of pharmacokinetics maximizes the benefits and minimizes the harms of a medication. Benefits are derived by achieving a high enough level of the medication at the site of action, while minimizing harm by using the lowest dose possible. Pharmacokinetics helps guide selection of the most effective medication route, dosage, and schedule (Brunton et al., 2018). For example, knowledge of pharmacokinetics allows for the safer use of lithium. By understanding how renal function (i.e., excretion) affects lithium, healthcare providers can make more informed decisions regarding the dosing of lithium and the timing of lithium blood level monitoring.

Pharmacokinetics and pharmacodynamics are impacted by genetic factors that give rise to interindividual and cross-ethnic variations in medication response. The Considering Culture box discusses how the area of pharmacogenetics influences the way healthcare providers tailor their prescriptions for patients.

🌐 CONSIDERING CULTURE

Pharmacogenetics

Pharmacogenetics explains how genetic variations lead to differences in medication tolerability and responses in individuals and ethnic groups. The cytochrome P450 (CYP) system, enzymes responsible for metabolizing most medications, is susceptible to genetic variations.

Patients found to be poor metabolizers degrade medications more slowly. Therefore, they will experience more side effects due to higher blood levels of the medication. Conversely, patients who are rapid metabolizers will experience less response to treatment due to lower blood levels. If a patient does not respond as expected to medication treatment, consider pharmacogenetic influences as a possible cause.

About 10% of Caucasians are poor metabolizers of the enzyme CYP 2D6, which metabolizes medications such as risperidone. Approximately 20% of Asian subgroups are poor metabolizers of CYP 2C19, an enzyme involved in the metabolism of citalopram and diazepam.

Carbamazepine is an anticonvulsant mood stabilizer for bipolar disorder. Individuals of Asian ancestry with the HLA-B*1502 allele are at greater risk for developing life-threatening skin reactions such as toxic epidermal necrolysis and Stevens-Johnson syndrome. The US Food and Drug Administration (FDA) recommends testing all at-risk patients for the HLA-B*1502 allele before starting treatment. Avoid carbamazepine use in patients who test positive.

There are still many challenges to achieving the goal of personalized treatments in psychiatric medicine. As testing becomes more widespread and research clarifies the impact on clinical care, the potential for pharmacogenetics to maximize medication response and minimize side effects may be realized.

Adapted from Corponi, F., Fabbri, C., & Serretti, A. (2018). Pharmacogenetics in psychiatry. *Advances in Pharmacology, 83,* 297–331.

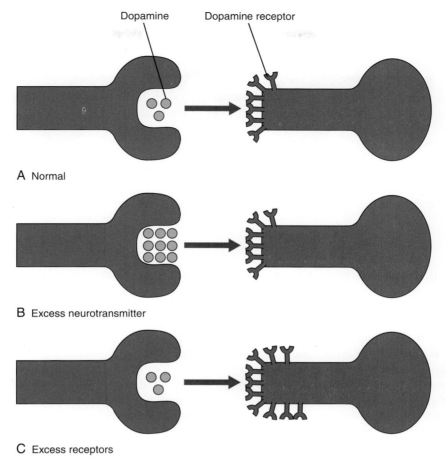

Fig. 3.9 Transmission of neurotransmitters (A). Excess transmission may be resulting from excess release of neurotransmitter, as shown in (B), or from excess responsiveness of receptors, as shown in (C).

The liver metabolizes most medications into active metabolites—chemicals that also have pharmacological actions. Researchers use this knowledge in designing new medications that make use of the body's own mechanisms to activate a chemical for pharmacological use.

An ideal medication would relieve the patient's psychological symptoms without inducing additional cerebral (mental) or somatic (physical) effects. Unfortunately, in psychopharmacology—as in most areas of pharmacology—there are no medications that are both fully effective and free of undesired side effects. Researchers work toward developing medications that target the symptoms while producing fewer side effects.

Because all activities of the brain involve actions of neurons, neurotransmitters, and receptors, these are the primary targets of pharmacological intervention. Most psychotropic medications act by either increasing or decreasing the activity of certain neurotransmitter-receptor systems.

Drug Agonism and Antagonism

Two important concepts affecting many of the psychotropic medications are **agonism** and **antagonism**. The word *agonist* comes from the Latin word *agōnista* and means contender. **Agonists** mimic the effects of a neurotransmitter naturally found in the human brain by binding to and stimulating the neurotransmitter's receptor. Partial agonists also stimulate receptors but produce a smaller response than agonists.

The word *antagonist* is derived from the Latin word *antagōnista* and means adversary or opponent. Rather than binding to and stimulating the receptor site, medications that are **antagonists** block a neurotransmitter from binding to its receptor, thereby obstructing the neurotransmitter's action.

Antianxiety and Hypnotic Medications

The major inhibitory (calming) neurotransmitter in the central nervous system (CNS) is GABA. Benzodiazepines are among the most commonly used antianxiety medications.

Benzodiazepines

Benzodiazepines promote the activity of GABA by binding to a specific site on the $GABA_A$ receptor complex. This binding results in an increased frequency of chloride channel opening, causing membrane hyperpolarization, which reduces cellular excitation. If cellular excitation is decreased, the result is a calming effect. Fig. 3.10 shows that benzodiazepines enhance the effects of GABA.

Benzodiazepines possess antianxiety, **hypnotic** (sleep-inducing), anticonvulsant, amnestic (loss of memory), and

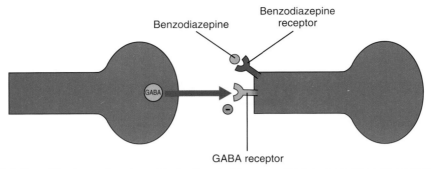

Benzodiazepine

Benzodiazepine receptor

GABA

GABA receptor

Fig. 3.10 Action of the benzodiazepines. Medications in this group attach to a specific area on receptors for the neurotransmitter γ-aminobutyric acid *(GABA)*. Attachment to these receptors results in a strengthening of the inhibitory effects of GABA. In the absence of GABA, there is no pharmacological effect of benzodiazepines.

muscle relaxant properties. Common benzodiazepines for anxiety or panic symptoms include alprazolam (Xanax), clonazepam (Klonopin), diazepam (Valium), and lorazepam (Ativan). Several benzodiazepines are FDA approved solely for treatment of insomnia, with a predominantly hypnotic effect: flurazepam (Dalmane), temazepam (Restoril), and triazolam (Halcion). Benzodiazepines reduce the neuronal overexcitation of alcohol withdrawal, and chlordiazepoxide (Librium), diazepam, or lorazepam are commonly used to prevent alcohol withdrawal seizures. The anticonvulsant properties of benzodiazepines make them the treatment of choice for status epilepticus.

Medications with CNS depressant effects will have a variety of side effects, and benzodiazepines are no exception. Sedation, ataxia, and anterograde amnesia (trouble forming new memories after taking a dose) are all possible side effects. Sedation is the most common side effect, but tolerance to sedating effects will develop over time with routine use. Ataxia occurs because of the abundance of GABA receptors in the cerebellum. When used alone, even at high dosages, benzodiazepines rarely inhibit the brain to the degree of respiratory depression and death. However, when combined with other CNS depressants, such as alcohol and opioids, life-threatening CNS depression becomes more likely. Rarely, benzodiazepines may cause paradoxical reactions, such as anxiety or agitation, especially in pediatric and geriatric patients.

Benzodiazepines are controlled substances with the potential for misuse. With routine use, physical dependence develops, and withdrawal is possible. Benzodiazepine withdrawal is characterized by symptoms that are often the opposite of their pharmacological actions: anxiety, insomnia, muscle tension, and possibly seizures. Patients receiving high dosages or an extended duration of therapy must have their doses gradually tapered to avoid benzodiazepine withdrawal symptoms. Patients with substance use disorders are often treated with alternative, noncontrolled medications.

Healthcare providers must caution patients taking benzodiazepines about engaging in activities requiring mental alertness, such as driving a car or operating machinery, secondary to sedation, ataxia, and slowed reflexes. Educate patients to avoid other CNS depressants, including alcohol, to avoid worsening these effects. In older adults, benzodiazepine use is associated with falls, bone fractures, and delirium. Elderly patients are generally best treated with alternative medications.

Short-Acting Sedative-Hypnotic Sleep Agents

Nonbenzodiazepine receptor agonists, or Z-hypnotics, include zolpidem (Ambien), zaleplon (Sonata), and eszopiclone (Lunesta). They possess hypnotic and amnestic effects without the antianxiety, anticonvulsant, or muscle relaxant effects of benzodiazepines. This is due to their selectivity for GABA$_A$ receptors containing an alpha (α)-1 subunit. Similar to benzodiazepines, nonbenzodiazepine receptor agonists can cause sedation, ataxia, and harmful effects in the elderly, including falls, bone fractures, and delirium. They are controlled substances but reportedly cause less tolerance and dependence than benzodiazepines. Nevertheless, exercise caution or consider alternatives for patients with substance use disorders. Eszopiclone can cause an unpleasant, bitter taste upon awakening in about one-third of patients.

Compared to benzodiazepines, the nonbenzodiazepines generally have shorter half-lives and no active metabolites. Zaleplon has the shortest half-life, approximately 1 hour, and helps patients to fall asleep, whereas eszopiclone has a half-life of approximately 6 hours and will also assist patients with staying asleep. Zolpidem metabolism occurs more slowly in women than men, resulting in higher blood levels in female patients. Based on this finding, the FDA lowered the starting dose for all zolpidem products for female patients.

The FDA has issued warnings on all approved hypnotic medications regarding complex sleep-related behaviors. Behaviors include sleepwalking, driving, cooking, or eating. Behaviors occur while the patient is not fully awake, and patients may have no memory of the event. While these events are rare, the use of other CNS depressants, including alcohol, may increase this risk. The FDA has strengthened warnings for nonbenzodiazepine receptor agonists and recommends that patients not take these medications if an episode of complex sleep behaviors has previously occurred (National Library of Medicine, 2019).

Melatonin Receptor Agonists

Melatonin is a naturally occurring hormone that is excreted by the pineal gland at night as part of the normal circadian rhythm. Ramelteon (Rozerem) is a melatonin (MT) receptor agonist and acts similarly to endogenous melatonin. It has high selectivity and potency at the MT_1 receptor site—which regulates sleepiness—and at the MT_2 receptor site—which regulates circadian rhythms. Ramelteon is FDA approved for insomnia characterized by difficulty falling asleep. It is not a controlled substance and lacks misuse potential. Side effects include headache and dizziness. Ramelteon may decrease testosterone and increase prolactin levels, possibly causing a decreased interest in sex or problems with fertility. Ramelteon and fluvoxamine, a selective serotonin reuptake inhibitor (SSRI), interact and are contraindicated together.

Doxepin

Doxepin (Silenor) is the low-dose formulation of a tricyclic antidepressant (TCA). Doxepin is FDA approved for insomnia characterized by difficulty staying asleep. It does not improve time to sleep onset. Histamine in the brain promotes wakefulness. Therefore, doxepin most likely produces its sedative effect by histamine-1 (H_1) receptor antagonism. Patients with severe urinary retention, glaucoma, or those taking **monoamine oxidase inhibitors (MAOIs)** should avoid this medication. Doxepin is not a controlled substance and lacks misuse potential.

Orexin Receptor Antagonists

Orexins, neuropeptides produced in the hypothalamus, promote wakefulness. Orexins naturally bind to orexin-1 and orexin-2 receptors. Suvorexant (Belsomra) and lemborexant (Dayvigo) are orexin receptor antagonists. They selectively block both orexin receptors and suppress wakefulness. They are FDA approved for insomnia characterized by difficulty falling asleep or staying asleep. Orexin-containing neurons appear to be diminished in narcolepsy. Therefore, suvorexant and lemborexant, orexin blockers, are contraindicated in patients with narcolepsy. Rare side effects of sleep paralysis, hallucinations upon waking or falling asleep, or cataplexy-like symptoms (loss of muscle tone prompted by strong emotions, such as laughter or surprise) have occurred with use. Orexin receptor antagonists are controlled substances, so use caution in patients with substance use disorders.

Buspirone

Buspirone (BuSpar) is FDA approved for the treatment of generalized anxiety disorder. Although the mechanism of action of buspirone is not clear, one possibility is illustrated in Fig. 3.11. It acts as a partial serotonin (5-HT)-1A receptor agonist. Buspirone is well tolerated. Common side effects include dizziness, headache, and nausea. There are several differences between buspirone and benzodiazepines, including:

- Buspirone is serotonergic, whereas benzodiazepines affect GABA.
- Buspirone is not a controlled substance, whereas benzodiazepines are controlled.
- Buspirone is taken every day. Benzodiazepines can be taken daily or as needed.
- Buspirone takes several weeks for antianxiety onset. Benzodiazepines work quickly.

Refer to Chapter 15 on anxiety disorders for a discussion of the adverse reactions, dosages, nursing implications, and patient and family teaching points for the antianxiety medications. Refer to Chapter 19 on sleep disorders for a more detailed discussion on medications to promote sleep.

Treating Anxiety Disorders with Antidepressants

The symptoms, neurotransmitters, and circuits associated with anxiety disorders overlap extensively with those of depressive disorders (refer to Chapters 14 and 15). Antidepressant

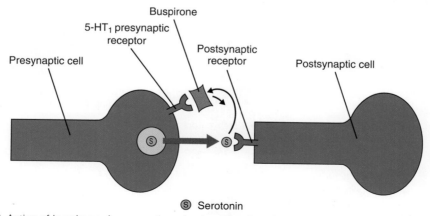

Fig. 3.11 Action of buspirone. A proposed mechanism of action of buspirone is that it blocks feedback inhibition by serotonin. This leads to increased release of serotonin by the presynaptic cell. *5-HT₁*, Serotonin.

medications possess antianxiety effects and are first-line treatment options for anxiety and anxiety-related disorders. Several antidepressants are FDA approved for generalized anxiety disorder, panic disorder, social anxiety disorder, obsessive-compulsive disorder, or PTSD. Antidepressants have several important differences from other antianxiety medications, especially benzodiazepines. Whereas benzodiazepines have a fast onset of action, antidepressants require 4 to 8 weeks for onset of antianxiety effects. Nevertheless, antidepressants are first-line and preferred for long-term treatment—unlike benzodiazepines—due to their lack of misuse potential and ability to treat co-occurring anxiety and depressive disorders.

Antidepressant Medications

While the neurophysiological basis of mood disorders is far from complete, a great deal of evidence indicates that the neurotransmitters norepinephrine and serotonin play a major role in regulating mood. A transmission deficiency of these monoamine neurotransmitters within the limbic system may underlie depression. Fig. 3.12 identifies the side effects of specific neurotransmitters being blocked or activated. Fig. 3.13 illustrates the normal release, reuptake, and destruction of the monoamine neurotransmitters. A grasp of this underlying physiology is essential for understanding how antidepressants act.

Hypotheses of antidepressant actions:

1. The *monoamine hypothesis of depression* suggests that there is a deficiency in one or more of the following neurotransmitters: serotonin, norepinephrine, and dopamine. Medications that deplete these neurotransmitters and produce depressive symptoms support this theory. The theory implies that, by increasing these neurotransmitters, depression is alleviated. The theory also suggests that low levels of neurotransmitters cause postsynaptic receptors to be up-regulated (increased in sensitivity or number). Increasing neurotransmitters by antidepressants results in down-regulation (desensitization) of key neurotransmitter receptors. Delayed length of time for down-regulation may explain why it takes 4 to 8 weeks for antidepressants to work, especially if they rapidly increase neurotransmitters (Stahl, 2013).

2. Another hypothesis for the mechanism of antidepressants suggests that with prolonged use they increase production of neurotrophic factors. These factors regulate the survival of neurons and enhance the sprouting of axons to form new synaptic connections (Stahl, 2013)

Selective Serotonin Reuptake Inhibitors

Selective serotonin reuptake inhibitors (SSRIs) block the reuptake of serotonin, thereby making more of this neurotransmitter available in the synapse. The SSRIs include fluoxetine

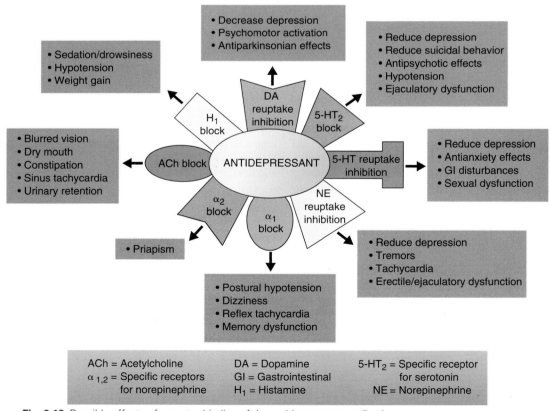

Fig. 3.12 Possible effects of receptor binding of the antidepressant medications.

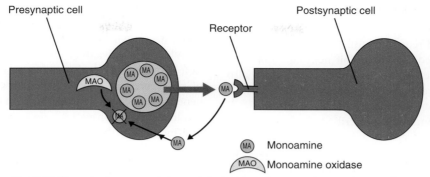

Fig. 3.13 Normal release, reuptake, and destruction of monoamine neurotransmitters.

(Prozac), sertraline (Zoloft), paroxetine (Paxil), citalopram (Celexa), escitalopram (Lexapro), and fluvoxamine (Luvox). They are first-line medications for the treatment of major depressive disorder and anxiety disorders. Common side effects include nausea, restlessness or jitteriness, sleep disturbances, and sexual dysfunction.

Side effects result from stimulation of different serotonin receptors. Stimulation of 5-HT$_{2A}$ and 5-HT$_{2C}$ receptors in the spinal cord may inhibit the spinal reflexes of orgasm, contributing to sexual dysfunction. Stimulation of 5-HT$_{2A}$ receptors in the mesocortical area may decrease dopamine activity in this area, leading to apathy and low libido. Nausea and vomiting may result from stimulation of 5-HT$_3$ receptors in the hypothalamus or brainstem, whereas other gastrointestinal side effects may be secondary to 5-HT$_3$ and/or 5-HT$_4$ receptors directly in the gastrointestinal tract (Fig. 3.14; Brunton et al., 2018).

Despite sharing many characteristics, SSRIs differ in a number of ways. Fluoxetine is the most activating agent and causes insomnia and nervousness. It has a very long half-life, enabling a once-weekly formulation. Due to its long half-life, the elderly and patients with hepatic impairment may be more susceptible to its activating effects. Sertraline appears to cause the most gastrointestinal distress (i.e., diarrhea). The most sedating agent is fluvoxamine and, unlike other SSRIs, should be started at bedtime. Paroxetine is the most anticholinergic due to muscarinic-1 (M$_1$) receptor antagonism and may not be ideal for patients with contraindications to anticholinergic agents (e.g., narrow-angle glaucoma). Citalopram prolongs the QT interval in a dose-dependent fashion. Exercise caution in patients with electrolyte disturbances (e.g., hypokalemia) or those prescribed other QT-interval-prolonging medications. Electrocardiogram (ECG) monitoring may be indicated in high-risk patients. Escitalopram is the S-enantiomer of racemic citalopram.

Norepinephrine and Serotonin Specific Antidepressant

Mirtazapine (Remeron) is known as a **norepinephrine and serotonin specific antidepressants**, or NaSSA. It enhances norepinephrine and serotonin neurotransmission by antagonizing both presynaptic α$_2$ receptors and postsynaptic 5-HT$_2$ and 5-HT$_3$ receptors. Sedation, appetite stimulation, and weight gain are common side effects. It is frequently given to patients with symptoms of insomnia or decreased appetite and weight loss. Antagonism of postsynaptic serotonin receptors results in additional benefits, including fewer gastrointestinal symptoms and less sexual dysfunction than SSRIs.

Norepinephrine and Dopamine Reuptake Inhibitor

Bupropion (Wellbutrin) is a norepinephrine and dopamine reuptake inhibitor, or NDRI. It is also FDA approved for smoking cessation (Zyban). Side effects include insomnia, tremor, anorexia, and weight loss. With no serotonergic properties, it causes less sexual dysfunction than other antidepressants and is often given for SSRI-induced sexual dysfunction. Contraindications include patients with seizure disorders, eating disorders, or those abruptly discontinuing the use of alcohol or sedatives (including benzodiazepines) secondary to seizure risk.

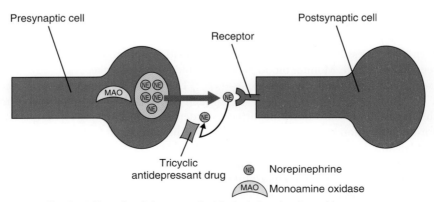

Fig. 3.14 Norepinephrine reuptake blockade by tricyclic antidepressants.

Serotonin Antagonist and Reuptake Inhibitors

Nefazodone (Serzone) and trazodone (Desyrel) belong to the serotonin antagonist and reuptake inhibitor, or SARI, class of antidepressants. Both medications inhibit neuronal uptake of serotonin and antagonize $5-HT_{2A}$ receptors. Nefazodone also inhibits norepinephrine reuptake. Common side effects include sedation, headache, nausea, dizziness, and blurred vision.

Nefazodone is not commonly prescribed. Sexual dysfunction is minimal with its use, but it is associated with rare, life-threatening liver failure. Avoid nefazodone in patients with pre-existing liver impairment. Nefazodone is also contraindicated with several medications due to its inhibition of cytochrome P450 (CYP) 3A4, a common drug metabolizing enzyme.

Trazodone is FDA approved for depression, but it is most commonly prescribed off-label as a hypnotic. Due to its sedating effects, it is prescribed at low doses (e.g., 50 mg) at bedtime for insomnia. Trazodone is a potent α_1 receptor antagonist which contributes to dizziness and orthostatic hypotension. Educate patients to rise slowly when awakening to avoid falls. Potent α_1 antagonists with little anticholinergic activity, such as trazodone, can cause priapism, a painful prolonged erection caused by the inability for detumescence (subsidence of erection).

Serotonin Modulator and Stimulator

Vortioxetine (Trintellix) has multiple pharmacological actions at serotonergic sites. Actions include $5-HT_{1A}$ receptor agonism (similar to buspirone), $5-HT_3$ receptor antagonism (similar to ondansetron), and neuronal inhibition of serotonin uptake (similar to SSRIs). Vortioxetine interacts with several other serotonin receptors, including $5-HT_{1B}$, $5-HT_{1D}$, and $5-HT_7$. Common side effects include nausea, constipation, and vomiting. Some data indicate that sexual dysfunction induced by SSRIs may improve when patients are switched to vortioxetine.

Serotonin Norepinephrine Reuptake Inhibitors

Serotonin norepinephrine reuptake inhibitors (SNRIs) increase both serotonin and norepinephrine in the synapse by inhibiting neuronal reuptake. The SNRIs include venlafaxine (Effexor), desvenlafaxine (Pristiq), duloxetine (Cymbalta), and levomilnacipran (Fetzima). All are FDA approved and first-line for the treatment of major depressive disorder, and several have indications for anxiety disorders. Another SNRI, milnacipran (Savella), is indicated only for fibromyalgia. The SNRIs have a similar side effect profile to the SSRIs, but SNRIs are more likely to cause excessive sweating. In addition, SNRIs cause dose-dependent increases in blood pressure and heart rate due to their norepinephrine reuptake blockade. Monitor blood pressure and heart rate at baseline and periodically thereafter, particularly at dose changes.

While all SNRIs inhibit serotonin and norepinephrine reuptake, the selectivity for inhibiting norepinephrine reuptake differs between agents. Venlafaxine is a serotonergic agent at lower therapeutic doses, and norepinephrine reuptake blockage only occurs at higher doses (i.e., over 150 mg/day). Duloxetine is also more selective for serotonin reuptake blockade, but it will inhibit both neurotransmitters throughout its entire dosing spectrum. Levomilnacipran is the most selective for norepinephrine reuptake of all of the SNRIs.

While a disadvantage of norepinephrine reuptake inhibition is increased blood pressure and heart rate, an advantage of noradrenergic activity is pain reduction. The SNRIs have beneficial effects on neuropathic pain. The common underlying mechanism of neuropathic pain is nerve injury or dysfunction. The mechanism by which SNRIs reduce neuropathic pain is by activation of the descending norepinephrine and serotonin pathways to the spinal cord, thereby limiting pain signals from reaching the brain.

Individual SNRIs have unique characteristics. Venlafaxine is the most likely to produce antidepressant discontinuation syndrome (i.e., flu-like symptoms, insomnia, nausea, dizziness, paresthesia, anxiety) if abruptly discontinued. Desvenlafaxine is the primary active metabolite of venlafaxine. When a patient takes venlafaxine, it will eventually be metabolized into desvenlafaxine. Duloxetine holds a number of FDA-approved indications in the realm of pain management, including diabetic peripheral neuropathy, fibromyalgia, and chronic musculoskeletal pain. Levomilnacipran, the most noradrenergic SNRI, causes urinary hesitancy in up to 6% of patients secondary to the actions of norepinephrine on the genitourinary tract.

Serotonin Partial Agonist and Reuptake Inhibitor

Vilazodone (Viibryd) enhances serotonin neurotransmission via $5-HT_{1A}$ receptor partial agonism (similar to buspirone) and neuronal inhibition of serotonin reuptake (similar to SSRIs). Side effects are similar to SSRIs and include diarrhea, nausea, vomiting, and insomnia. Instruct patients to take with food to enhance its bioavailability.

Tricyclic Antidepressants

Tricyclic antidepressants (TCAs) were widely used before the development of SSRIs. They are no longer considered first-line medications secondary to side effects and greater lethality in overdose. The TCAs are frequently used off-label for a number of indications, including migraine headaches and neuropathic pain. They act primarily by blocking the reuptake of serotonin and norepinephrine. Secondary amine TCAs (e.g., nortriptyline [Pamelor], desipramine [Norpramin]) primarily act by blocking norepinephrine reuptake. As shown in Fig. 3.15, this blockade prevents norepinephrine from coming into contact with its degrading enzyme, MAO, increasing the level of norepinephrine at the synapse. Tertiary amine TCAs (e.g., amitriptyline [Elavil], imipramine [Tofranil]) block both serotonin and norepinephrine reuptake.

The TCAs antagonize several receptors, including H_1, α_1, and M_1, and these receptor effects are responsible for several side effects. By blocking H_1 receptors in the brain, sedation and weight gain occur (see Fig. 3.12). Blockade of α_1 receptors on blood vessels results in vasodilation and the side effects of dizziness and orthostatic hypotension. The effects of acetylcholine are blunted by M_1 receptor blockade, and this leads to anticholinergic effects such as blurred vision, dry mouth, tachycardia,

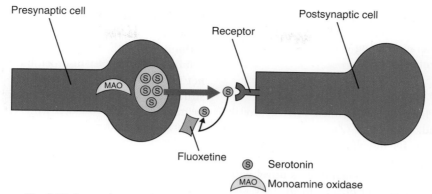

Fig. 3.15 Serotonin reuptake blockade by selective serotonin reuptake inhibitors.

urinary retention, and constipation. In elderly patients, anticholinergic activity causes memory difficulties or confusion.

The TCAs block sodium channels on the heart, and an overdose can be fatal secondary to cardiac conduction disturbances. Therefore, provide TCAs to suicidal patients only with great caution and for the smallest quantity possible to minimize overdose risk.

Monoamine Oxidase Inhibitors

Monoamine oxidase inhibitors are a class of antidepressants that are rarely used in practice today. They are considered last-line agents secondary to multiple interactions and dietary restrictions. The MAOIs consist of phenelzine (Nardil), isocarboxazid (Marplan), tranylcypromine (Parnate), and selegiline (Emsam). Selegiline offers a unique antidepressant dosage form as the only antidepressant available as a transdermal patch. MAOIs are medications that inhibit the action of MAO enzymes, thereby preventing the destruction of monoamines.

The MAO enzymes metabolize monoamines, including serotonin, norepinephrine, and dopamine. By inhibiting MAO, the MAOI antidepressants increase synaptic levels of these neurotransmitters, resulting in the antidepressant effects of these medications (Fig. 3.16). Unfortunately, MAOIs are contraindicated with a number of medications that also amplify these neurotransmitters.

Medications that enhance serotonin (e.g., SSRIs, buspirone) should be avoided with MAOIs due to the risk of serotonin syndrome. For example, paroxetine inhibits serotonin reuptake, making more serotonin available. At the same time, if MAO is inhibited and not degrading serotonin as quickly, dangerous levels of serotonin can result. Similarly, medications that enhance the sympathomimetic effects of norepinephrine or dopamine (e.g., psychostimulants) should be avoided with MAOIs due to the risk of hypertensive crisis. Instruct patients that several over-the-counter medications are serotonergic (e.g., dextromethorphan) or sympathomimetic (e.g., pseudoephedrine) and must be avoided with MAOI therapy. In order to avoid these serious reactions, washout periods are required when starting or stopping MAOIs.

MAO enzymes also degrade monoamine substances that enter the body from food. One particular monoamine, tyramine, is present in most protein-based foods. Some foods are extremely rich in tyramine, such as aged cheeses, pickled or smoked fish, and wine. If MAO cannot break down the tyramine from these food substances secondary to the MAOI antidepressant, tyramine can produce significant vasoconstriction. This vasoconstriction results in an elevation of blood pressure and may precipitate a hypertensive crisis.

Because of the dangers that result from inhibition of hepatic and intestinal MAO, patients taking MAOIs must be given a

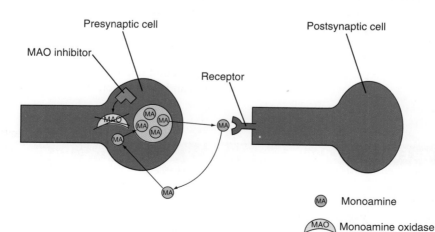

Fig. 3.16 Blocking monoamine oxidase *(MAO)* by monoamine oxidase inhibitors (MAOIs), which prevents the breakdown of monoamine neurotransmitters by MAO.

list of foods and medications to avoid. Chapter 14 discusses the treatment of depression and contains a list of foods to avoid and foods to be taken in moderation along with nursing measures and instructions for patient education.

Miscellaneous Antidepressants

Two novel medications have recently gained FDA approval: esketamine (Spravato) and brexanolone (Zulresso). They represent new possible directions for the pharmacological management of depression.

Esketamine, the s-enantiomer of ketamine, is novel with regard to mechanism of action and dosage form. Like ketamine, it is a controlled substance with the potential for misuse. Esketamine is an antagonist of the N-methyl-D-aspartate (NMDA) receptor. Glutamate stimulates NMDA receptors. Esketamine, therefore, alleviates depression by directly antagonizing the effects of glutamate. It is unknown how NMDA receptor antagonism improves depression. Esketamine is available only as an intranasal spray, and patients require education on proper administration (i.e., do not prime device, blow nose before first spray only, recline head at 45-degree angle for administration, rest 5 minutes between devices if multiple devices are required to achieve desired dose). Esketamine is FDA approved specifically for treatment-resistant depression, defined as two failed antidepressant trials. It should be used along with an oral antidepressant. Common side effects include dissociation (feeling disconnected from one's thoughts or identity) and increased blood pressure.

Esketamine is only available through a restricted program and is not intended for home use. Administration can only occur under the direct supervision of a healthcare provider, and patients must be monitored for dissociation and other side effects for at least 2 hours after every session. Monitor blood pressure before and after administration.

Brexanolone is the first medication to receive FDA approval for postpartum depression. The pharmacology of brexanolone is not fully known, but it appears to interact with GABA_A receptors. It is a neuroactive steroid and identical to a metabolite of progesterone, called allopregnanolone. Brexanolone is administered over 60 hours via continuous infusion. Monitor all patients receiving treatment for hypoxia using continuous pulse oximetry. During treatment, accompany mothers during interactions with their children as excessive sedation and sudden loss of consciousness have been reported. Brexanolone is a controlled substance.

Mood Stabilizers

Lithium

Lithium (Eskalith, Lithobid) is the gold standard among mood stabilizers for bipolar disorder, but its mechanism of action is not fully understood. As a positively charged cation, similar in structure to sodium and potassium, lithium may act by affecting neuronal electrical conductivity. Overexcitement of neurons in the brain may underlie bipolar disorder, and lithium interacts in some complex way with sodium and potassium at the cell membrane to stabilize electrical activity. Furthermore, lithium may produce an overall reduction in the activity of the excitatory neurotransmitter glutamate, exerting an antimanic effect. Inhibition of the enzyme inositol monophosphatase is another possible mechanism. Lithium enhances serotonergic neurotransmission, which may explain its antidepressant properties. Some data suggest lithium possesses antisuicidal properties (Stahl, 2013).

In addition to complex pharmacology, lithium has a number of side effects and interactions. Table 3.3 provides a list of potential lithium side effects. Medications affecting renal function or salt and water balance can alter lithium concentrations. Hydrochlorothiazide, angiotensin converting enzyme inhibitors (e.g., lisinopril), and nonsteroidal antiinflammatory drugs (e.g., ibuprofen) increase lithium levels. Conversely, caffeine decreases lithium levels.

Lithium has a narrow therapeutic index. The therapeutic index represents the ratio of the lethal dose to the effective dose. It is a measure of overall medication safety with regard to the possibility of overdose or toxicity. A narrow therapeutic index means that the blood level of a medication that can cause death is not far above the blood level required for drug effectiveness. Monitor lithium levels on a regular basis. Dehydration, medication interactions, and decreasing renal function can all increase lithium levels. Chapter 13 considers lithium treatment in more depth and discusses specific dosage-related adverse and toxic effects, nursing implications, and the patient teaching plan.

Anticonvulsant Medications

In addition to treating seizure disorders, valproate, carbamazepine, and lamotrigine are mood stabilizers that are FDA approved for bipolar disorder. Their anticonvulsant properties derive from the alteration of electrical conductivity in membranes. It is possible that this membrane-stabilizing effect accounts for the ability of these medications to reduce the mood swings that occur in patients with bipolar disorder. Other proposed mood stabilizing mechanisms include glutamate antagonism and GABA agonism.

TABLE 3.3 Adverse Effects of Lithium	
System	Adverse Effects
Dermatologic	Acne, alopecia, psoriasis
Digestive	Diarrhea, nausea, vomiting
Endocrine	Hypothyroidism, weight gain
Fluid and electrolyte	Edema, polydipsia, polyuria
Nervous and musculoskeletal	Ataxia, sedation, fine tremor

Valproate

Valproate (Depakote, Depakene) is FDA approved for manic episodes associated with bipolar disorder. It is recommended for mixed episodes and has been found to be useful for rapid cycling. Antimanic effects may result from inhibiting sodium channels on neurons or enhancing the effects of GABA, an inhibitory neurotransmitter. Common side effects include sedation, weight gain, and tremor. Serious side effects are thrombocytopenia, pancreatitis, hepatic failure, and hyperammonemia. Monitor liver function tests (LFTs) and a complete blood count (CBC) at baseline and periodically thereafter. Therapeutic blood levels are also monitored during treatment. A pregnancy test in women of childbearing age is necessary before starting treatment due to the risk of serious birth defects (e.g., spina bifida).

Carbamazepine

Carbamazepine (Equetro, Tegretol) is a second-line agent for bipolar disorder. It is FDA approved for manic or mixed episodes associated with bipolar disorder. It reduces the firing rate of overexcited neurons by reducing the activity of sodium channels. Monitor LFTs, CBC, ECG, and sodium levels at baseline and periodically thereafter. Blood levels are monitored to avoid toxicity, but there is no established therapeutic range for bipolar disorder. A pregnancy test is necessary before starting treatment due to the risk of serious birth defects.

Common side effects include dizziness, somnolence, nausea, vomiting, ataxia, and blurred vision. Hyponatremia or leukopenia may occur. Potentially life-threatening Stevens-Johnson syndrome may occur, and the FDA requires genetic testing before starting in patients of Asian descent. If the test reveals a patient is positive for the HLA-B*1502 allele, do not initiate carbamazepine.

Carbamazepine has numerous interactions. It is known to induce, or speed up, the activity of CYP metabolizing enzymes. Therefore, it commonly reduces blood levels—and diminishes the therapeutic effects—of many other medications. Oral contraceptives, antiretrovirals, and immunosuppressants may all be affected.

Lamotrigine

Lamotrigine (Lamictal) is FDA approved for maintenance therapy in bipolar disorder. It is not effective for acute mania, but it is used for bipolar depression. Lamotrigine appears to inhibit sodium channels and modulates the release of excitatory neurotransmitters, glutamate and aspartate. Lamotrigine has a gradual dose titration, because rapid dose escalations increase the risk for rash. Educate patients to promptly report any rashes, which could be a sign of Stevens-Johnson syndrome. Valproate dramatically increases lamotrigine blood levels and increases Stevens-Johnson syndrome risk. Therefore, the lamotrigine dose must be halved if valproate is initiated.

Refer to Chapter 13 for more detailed discussion on mood stabilizers.

Antipsychotic Medications

First-Generation Antipsychotics

First-generation antipsychotics, also known as typical antipsychotics, decrease dopamine activity in the CNS by antagonizing D_2 receptors. By binding to these receptors and blocking the attachment of dopamine, they reduce dopaminergic stimulation. Dopaminergic overactivity in the mesolimbic system may be responsible for some of the symptoms of schizophrenia. Fig. 3.17 illustrates the proposed mechanism of action of the first-generation antipsychotics, which include the phenothiazines, thioxanthenes, butyrophenones, and pharmacologically related agents. These medications are effective for the "positive" symptoms of schizophrenia, such as delusions (e.g., paranoid or grandiose ideas) and hallucinations (e.g., hearing or seeing things not present in reality). Refer to Chapter 12 for a more detailed discussion of schizophrenia and its symptoms.

While D_2 receptor antagonism in the mesolimbic area alleviates positive symptoms of schizophrenia, blocking dopamine receptors in other areas of the brain results in side effects.

- Nigrostriatal area, causing movement side effects known as extrapyramidal symptoms (EPSs).
- Mesocortical area, worsening cognitive and negative symptoms of schizophrenia.
- Tuberoinfundibular area, increasing the release of the hormone prolactin.

Dopamine in the basal ganglia plays a major role in the regulation of movement. Therefore, D_2 receptor blockade in the nigrostriatal pathway leads to EPS. Different types of EPS include acute dystonic reactions, akathisia, parkinsonism, and tardive dyskinesia. Acute dystonia, akathisia, and parkinsonism develop over days, weeks, or months of treatment, whereas tardive dyskinesia develops over months to years of treatment. Tardive dyskinesia may be irreversible even after antipsychotic discontinuation. Monitoring and early detection of tardive dyskinesia with the Abnormal Involuntary Movement Scale, or AIMS, is of the utmost importance.

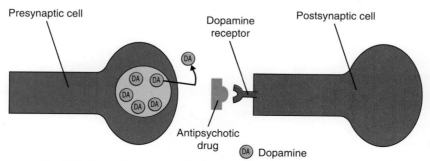

Fig. 3.17 Dopamine receptor blockade by first-generation antipsychotics.

Dopamine acts as the hypothalamic factor that inhibits the release of prolactin from the anterior pituitary gland. Therefore, blockade of dopamine transmission in the tuberoinfundibular pathway leads to increased pituitary secretion of prolactin. In women, hyperprolactinemia can result in amenorrhea (absence of the menses) or galactorrhea (excessive or inappropriate breast milk production). In men, it can lead to gynecomastia (development of the male mammary glands) or galactorrhea. In both men and women, hyperprolactinemia contributes to sexual dysfunction. Chronically high prolactin levels will decrease bone mineral density.

The acute depletion of dopamine in the CNS produced by antipsychotic medications may cause neuroleptic malignant syndrome (NMS). While rare, NMS is potentially life-threatening and requires immediate treatment. Symptoms include muscle rigidity, altered mental status, hyperthermia, and abnormalities in autonomic nervous system functioning (e.g., blood pressure and heart rate fluctuations, rapid breathing).

First-generation antipsychotics block several other receptors, resulting in a number of side effects. They are antagonists of the H_1 receptors for histamine, M_1 receptors for acetylcholine, and α_1 receptors for norepinephrine. Therefore, first-generation antipsychotics produce—to varying degrees—sedation, anticholinergic effects, and dizziness upon standing. As summarized in Fig. 3.18, many side effects are logical given their receptor-blocking activity.

By blocking H_1 receptors for histamine, sedation and weight gain occur. Sedation may be beneficial in severely agitated patients. Sedation dissipates with time, because tolerance will develop if medications are taken routinely. Both sedation and weight gain are side effects that may potentially lead to medication nonadherence.

Blockade of M_1 receptors for acetylcholine results in anticholinergic effects. Anticholinergic side effects include blurred vision, dry mouth, constipation, urinary hesitancy, and tachycardia. In the elderly, memory impairment and confusion may also occur. Tolerance to anticholinergic side effects generally does not occur with time. Taking other anticholinergic medications (e.g., diphenhydramine) at the same time will produce additive, or more pronounced, anticholinergic side effects.

First-generation antipsychotics with α_1 antagonist properties produce dizziness and orthostatic hypotension. These receptors are found on smooth muscle and constrict blood vessels in response to norepinephrine from sympathetic nerves. Vasoconstriction mediated by the sympathetic nervous system and norepinephrine is essential for maintaining normal blood pressure when the body is in the upright position. As a result, blockade of α_1 receptors results in vasodilation and a consequent drop in blood pressure.

Refer to Chapter 12 for a discussion of the clinical use of antipsychotics, side effects, specific nursing interventions, and patient teaching strategies.

Second-Generation Antipsychotics

Second-generation antipsychotics are also known as atypical antipsychotics. They are considered first-line treatments over first-generation antipsychotics due a more favorable side effect profile. They are less likely to produce EPS, including tardive dyskinesia, and target both the positive and negative symptoms of schizophrenia (see Chapter 12).

Second-generation antipsychotics are serotonin and dopamine receptor antagonists. They antagonize both D_2 and $5\text{-}HT_{2A}$ receptors. Most agents antagonize other receptors, as well. In general, second-generation antipsychotics have more $5\text{-}HT_{2A}$

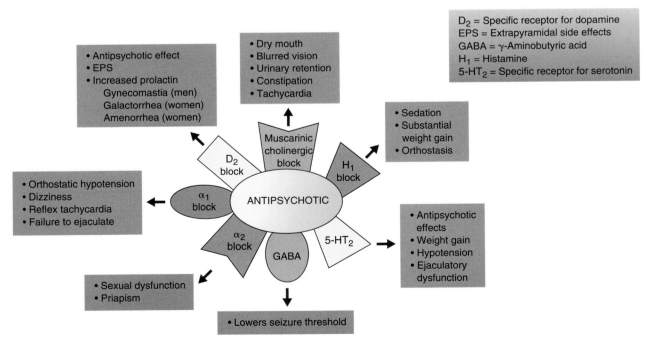

Fig. 3.18 Side effects of antipsychotic medications caused by receptor blockage. *EPS*, Extrapyramidal symptoms; *GABA*, γ-aminobutyric acid. (From Varcarolis, E. [2004]. *Manual of psychiatric nursing care plans* [2nd ed.]. St. Louis, MO: Elsevier.)

than D_2 antagonist effects. Like first-generation antipsychotics, D_2 receptor blockade in the mesolimbic pathway by second-generation antipsychotics decreases psychosis. Blocking 5-HT_{2A} receptors, however, facilitates dopamine release from neurons. This may explain why second-generation antipsychotics produce less EPS and hyperprolactinemia than first-generation antipsychotics. Pimavanserin (Nuplazid), a second-generation antipsychotic only FDA approved for Parkinson's disease psychosis, is unique in that it antagonizes only serotonin receptors.

In addition to treating psychosis and mania, several second-generation antipsychotics are FDA approved to treat depressive symptoms. Aripiprazole, brexpiprazole, and quetiapine are approved for major depressive disorder as adjuncts to antidepressant medications. Cariprazine, lurasidone, and quetiapine are approved for depression associated with bipolar disorder. Possible mechanisms explaining the antidepressant actions of antipsychotics include 5-HT_{2A} receptor antagonism (causes the release of dopamine from neurons), partial 5-HT_{1A} receptor agonism, and serotonin and norepinephrine reuptake inhibition.

Second-generation antipsychotics can increase metabolic syndrome risk. They produce weight gain, hyperglycemia, and hyperlipidemia to varying degrees. The simultaneous blockade of 5-HT_{2C} and H_1 receptors is associated with weight gain from increased appetite stimulation via the hypothalamic eating centers. Strong antimuscarinic properties at the M_3 receptor on pancreatic beta cells can cause insulin resistance leading to hyperglycemia. Rarely, second-generation antipsychotics have been associated with diabetic ketoacidosis. Clozapine and olanzapine have the highest risk for metabolic disturbances.

Clozapine. Clozapine (Clozaril) is FDA approved for treatment-resistant schizophrenia, typically defined as at least two failed antipsychotic trials. It is superior in efficacy to all other antipsychotic medications and has been shown to reduce the risk of suicidal behavior in patients with schizophrenia and schizoaffective disorder. Clozapine preferentially blocks the D_1 and D_2 receptors in the mesolimbic pathway rather than those in the nigrostriatal pathway. This allows it to exert antipsychotic action with minimal EPS risk.

Despite its many benefits, clozapine has a significant side effect profile. It is high risk for causing metabolic disturbances, including weight gain and diabetes. Sedation, orthostatic hypotension, and anticholinergic effects are all common and can be severe. Clozapine lowers seizure threshold in a dose-dependent fashion. Avoid its use in patients with uncontrolled epilepsy. Rarely, clozapine suppresses bone marrow and causes life-threatening neutropenia. This makes patients susceptible to serious infection. Therefore, clozapine is available only through a restricted program. Specific training and regular reporting of the patient's absolute neutrophil count (ANC) are program requirements. Typically, the ANC is monitored once weekly for 6 months, then once every 2 weeks for 6 months, then once every 4 weeks thereafter. The ANC values are reported directly to the clozapine program.

Clozapine is metabolized by CYP 1A2. Hydrocarbons from tobacco smoke induce CYP 1A2 enzymes. Therefore, patients who smoke will increase clozapine metabolism, lowering clozapine levels. If a patient cuts down or quits smoking, clozapine levels are expected to rise.

Risperidone. Risperidone (Risperdal) is a potent D_2 antagonist. It produces high rates of EPS compared to most second-generation antipsychotics, particularly at high dosages (>6 mg/day). As a potent D_2 antagonist, it also causes hyperprolactinemia. Risperidone also antagonizes α_1 receptors, causing orthostatic hypotension. Elderly patients are more susceptible to both EPS and orthostatic hypotension and should be monitored closely. Risperidone has a moderate risk of weight gain.

The long-acting injectable formulation (Risperdal Consta) is administered every 2 weeks, whereas a subcutaneous formulation (Perseris) is administered every 4 weeks. Consider long-acting injections for patients with frequent hospitalizations secondary to medication nonadherence or for patients who prefer not to take oral medications daily.

Quetiapine. Quetiapine (Seroquel, Seroquel XR) has very low D_2 receptor binding and rapidly dissociates (removes itself) from the D_2 receptor. Therefore, both EPS and prolactin elevation are minimal. Quetiapine is very sedating secondary to H_1 receptor antagonism, and it is often selected when sedation is desired. Combination H_1 and 5-HT_{2C} receptor blockade contribute to weight gain. Overall, quetiapine has a moderate risk for metabolic disturbances.

Olanzapine. Olanzapine (Zyprexa) is similar to clozapine in chemical structure. It possesses sedating and anticholinergic effects. Olanzapine has a high risk of causing metabolic disturbances, including weight gain and hyperglycemia. Olanzapine is available in a combination product with the SSRI fluoxetine (Symbyax).

A long-acting injectable formulation (Zyprexa Relprevv) is available. It is associated with a severe postinjection delirium/sedation syndrome caused by an unintended rapid rise in blood levels. The FDA requires patient observation for at least 3 hours after every injection to monitor for signs of excessive sedation, agitation, or disorientation.

Ziprasidone. Ziprasidone (Geodon) produces dose-dependent QT interval prolongation. Therefore, it is contraindicated in patients with uncompensated heart failure or recent myocardial infarction. Avoid use with other QT-interval-prolonging medications. Ziprasidone is low risk for metabolic disturbances. Each dose of ziprasidone must be taken with food (500 calories) to enhance absorption.

Aripiprazole. Aripiprazole (Abilify) is a partial D_2 receptor agonist. In areas of the brain with high dopamine activity, it acts as an antagonist. But in areas with low dopamine activity, it stimulates receptors by acting as an agonist. Partial D_2 receptor agonism enables aripiprazole to keep prolactin levels low, but this may be the possible mechanism responsible for rare cases of compulsive behaviors (e.g., gambling, shopping, or sex). Similar to ziprasidone, aripiprazole is low risk for metabolic disturbances. Multiple long-acting injectables (Abilify Maintena, Aristada, Aristada Initio) are available.

Paliperidone. Paliperidone (Invega), or 9-hydroxy-risperidone, is the major active metabolite of risperidone. Like risperidone, paliperidone is associated with hyperprolactinemia.

Paliperidone tablets do not fully dissolve. Avoid in patients with severe gastrointestinal narrowing, and educate patients that tablet shells may appear in stool.

Two long-acting injectable formulations are available. Paliperidone (Invega Sustenna) is administered every 4 weeks, whereas paliperidone (Invega Trinza) is administered every 12 weeks.

Iloperidone. Iloperidone (Fanapt) produces significant α_1 receptor blockade. Therefore, dizziness and orthostatic hypotension are possible. When starting iloperidone, a slow dosage titration over the first few days is necessary to minimize orthostatic hypotension. Iloperidone is associated with QT interval prolongation. Avoid use with other QT-interval-prolonging medications.

Lurasidone. Lurasidone (Latuda) antagonizes D_2 and 5-HT_{2A} receptors, similar to other second-generation antipsychotics. In addition, it is an antagonist with high affinity for the 5-HT_7 receptor. It has minimal H_1 or M_1 receptor effects. The risk of metabolic disturbances or QT interval prolongation is low. Each dose of lurasidone must be taken with food (350 calories) to enhance absorption.

Asenapine. Asenapine (Saphris, Secuado) is available as either a sublingual tablet or transdermal patch. Educate patients to place the sublingual tablet under the tongue and allow it to dissolve. Instruct patients not to eat or drink for 10 minutes. Oral hypoesthesia (numbness or tingling of the mouth) can occur after sublingual administration and usually resolves within 1 hour. If the tablet is swallowed, bioavailability is less than 2%. Asenapine antagonizes H_1 and α_1 receptors, resulting in sedation and orthostatic hypotension, respectively. It has little to no affinity for muscarinic receptors.

Brexpiprazole. Brexpiprazole (Rexulti) is the second partial D_2 receptor agonist available. Similar to aripiprazole, it is unlikely to increase prolactin levels but may rarely cause compulsive behaviors. The risk of metabolic disturbances and QT interval prolongation is low.

Cariprazine. Cariprazine (Vraylar) is the third partial D_2 receptor agonist available. Rates of EPS are high. Monitor patients for signs of movement disorders. Because cariprazine has a long half-life, response to treatment or side effect development may take several weeks to appear after starting the medication or changing the dose.

Lumateperone. Lumateperone (Caplyta) has a low overall risk for both EPS and metabolic disturbances. It is sedating, with high rates of drowsiness reported in clinical trials. Valproate may increase lumateperone serum levels and increase the risk of side effects. Educate patients to take lumateperone once daily with food.

Chapter 12 discusses the first- and second-generation antipsychotics in detail, including the indications for use, adverse reactions, nursing implications, and patient and family teaching.

Medication Treatment for Attention-Deficit/Hyperactivity Disorder

Psychostimulants are first-line pharmacological treatments for attention-deficit/hyperactivity disorder (ADHD).

Methylphenidate (Ritalin, Concerta) and amphetamines (Adderall, Vyvanse) are first-line treatment options. They are sympathomimetic amines that act by blocking the reuptake of norepinephrine and dopamine. Amphetamines also work to increase neurotransmitter release. While the mechanism of action in ADHD is not fully understood, it is thought that the monoamines may inhibit an overactive part of the limbic system. They are controlled substances with the potential for misuse. Due to their norepinephrine- and dopamine-enhancing effects, psychostimulants cause insomnia and increased blood pressure and heart rate. Agitation and growth suppression are also possible side effects. Rarely, psychostimulants may cause or exacerbate symptoms of psychosis or mania, likely due to their dopamine potentiating effects.

The FDA has approved three nonstimulants for ADHD: atomoxetine (Strattera), guanfacine (Intuniv), and clonidine (Kapvay). These medications may be preferred if a patient has a substance use disorder, psychostimulant contraindication (e.g., MAOI use), or preference for nonstimulant treatment. Nonstimulant medications are less effective for ADHD than psychostimulants.

Atomoxetine is a norepinephrine reuptake inhibitor. Common side effects include decreased appetite and weight loss, fatigue, and dizziness. Urinary hesitancy or urinary retention is less common. The noradrenergic effects of atomoxetine may cause increases in blood pressure and heart rate, and both should be monitored throughout therapy. Monitor liver function due to rare cases of liver damage. Guanfacine and clonidine are centrally acting α_2 receptor agonists. Increase the dose of both slowly to avoid hypotension and bradycardia. Avoid discontinuing these agents abruptly due to the risk of rebound hypertension.

Medication Treatment for Alzheimer's Disease

Pharmacological treatment for Alzheimer's disease has thus far been unable to prevent or slow structural degeneration. Therefore, medication treatment has centered on attempting to maintain normal brain function for as long as possible. All FDA-approved medications target the neurotransmitters glutamate or acetylcholine.

Acetylcholine is essential for learning, memory, and behavior regulation. Much of the memory loss in Alzheimer's disease has been attributed to insufficient acetylcholine. Cholinesterase inhibitors slow the rate of memory loss. Cholinesterase is the enzyme that breaks down acetylcholine. By inhibiting cholinesterase, these medications increase the amount of acetylcholine in the synapse by inhibiting its breakdown. As cholinergic neurons deteriorate with disease progression, cholinesterase inhibitors become less effective.

Three cholinesterase inhibitors are FDA approved for Alzheimer's disease: donepezil (Aricept), galantamine (Razadyne), and rivastigmine (Exelon, Exelon Patch). All are approved for mild to moderate Alzheimer's disease, but donepezil and transdermal rivastigmine are also approved for severe Alzheimer's disease. Rivastigmine is FDA approved for Parkinson's disease dementia as well. Increased cholinergic stimulation by these medications causes gastrointestinal symptoms such as nausea, vomiting, and diarrhea, as well as urinary incontinence. The increased cholinergic effect is also responsible for bradycardia, and syncopal episodes have been reported. Abrupt discontinuation of cholinesterase inhibitors can cause worsening of cognition and behavior in some patients.

Glutamate, an excitatory neurotransmitter, plays an important role in memory. However, too much glutamate can be excitotoxic (i.e., damaging from too much stimulation) to neurons. Normally, glutamate stimulates NMDA receptors, causing calcium to flow into neurons. However, pathological changes in Alzheimer's disease are associated with excess glutamate stimulation. This results in excess NMDA receptor stimulation and excess calcium in the cell, which damages neurons. Memantine (Namenda, Namenda XR) is an NMDA receptor antagonist. It fills some of the NMDA receptor sites, reduces glutamate binding, prevents excess calcium, and reduces damage. Common memantine side effects include constipation and confusion. Memantine is FDA approved for moderate to severe Alzheimer's disease, and it is often added to a cholinesterase inhibitor as the disease progresses.

A combination of memantine and donepezil (Namzaric) is available.

Refer to Chapter 23 for a more detailed discussion of these medications, as well as their nursing considerations, and patient and family teaching.

Herbal Treatments

Herbal supplement use is growing. Patients choose herbal treatments for a variety of reasons. They may believe that herbals are safer than prescription medications or have fewer side effects and interactions. If patients have experienced a lack of substantial benefit with prescription medicine, they may turn to herbal treatments. Herbals may also be less expensive. While many have been studied and some show positive results, many herbals continue to lack adequate safety and efficacy data. Lack of regulation by the FDA is also a major concern. Studies have shown that herbals may not always contain the active ingredient displayed on the label (Brown, 2017).

Chapter 36 covers complementary and integrative approaches in more detail.

KEY POINTS TO REMEMBER

- All actions of the brain—sensory, motor, and intellectual—are carried out physiologically through the interactions of nerve cells. These interactions involve impulse conduction, neurotransmitter release, and receptor response. Alterations in these basic processes can lead to mental disturbances and physical manifestations.
- In particular, it appears excess dopamine activity is involved in the thought disturbances of schizophrenia, and deficiencies of norepinephrine, serotonin, or both underlie depression and anxiety. Insufficient GABA activity may also play a role in anxiety. Excess glutamate and insufficient acetylcholine are involved in Alzheimer's disease.
- Pharmacological treatment of mental disturbances is directed at the suspected neurotransmitter-receptor problem. Thus, antipsychotics decrease dopamine, antidepressants increase serotonin and/or norepinephrine, antianxiety medications increase GABA or serotonin and/or norepinephrine,

Alzheimer's disease medications increase acetylcholine or decrease glutamate, and ADHD medications increase dopamine and/or norepinephrine.
- Psychotropic medications work in a variety of ways, and examples include receptor agonism, receptor antagonism, neurotransmitter reuptake inhibition, and enzyme inhibition. Because the immediate target activity of a medication can result in many downstream alterations in neuronal activity, medications with a variety of chemical actions may show efficacy in treating the same clinical condition.
- Unfortunately, agents used to treat psychiatric disorders can cause undesirable effects. Prominent among these are sedation, motor disturbances, anticholinergic effects, orthostatic hypotension, sexual dysfunction, and weight gain. Pharmacogenetics affects the way patients respond to and tolerate medications. It is an area of continuing research and discovery.

CRITICAL THINKING

1. Regardless of practice setting, nurses will care for many patients taking psychotropic medications. How important is it for nurses to understand normal brain structure and function as they relate to psychiatric disorders and psychotropic medications? Include the following in your answer:
   a. How nurses can use the knowledge about how normal brain function (control of peripheral nerves, skeletal muscles, the autonomic nervous system, hormones, and circadian rhythms) can be affected by either psychotropic medications or psychiatric disorders
   b. How brain imaging can help in understanding and treating people with psychiatric disorders

   c. How the understanding of neurotransmitters may affect your ability to assess a patient's response to specific medications
2. What specific information would you include in medication teaching based on your understanding of side effects that may occur when neurotransmitters are altered in the following ways?
   a. Dopamine—D_2 receptor antagonism by first- and second-generation antipsychotics
   b. Acetylcholine—M_1 receptor antagonism by first-generation antipsychotics
   c. Norepinephrine—α_1 receptor antagonism by tricyclic antidepressants

d. Histamine—H$_1$ receptor antagonism by second-generation antipsychotics

e. MAO—enzyme inhibition by monoamine oxidase inhibitors

f. GABA—increased GABA$_A$ receptor affinity by benzodiazepines

g. Serotonin—increased effects by selective serotonin reuptake inhibitors

h. Norepinephrine—increased effects by serotonin norepinephrine reuptake inhibitors

CHAPTER REVIEW

1. Which neurotransmitter is potentiated by benzodiazepines?
   a. Acetylcholine
   b. Dopamine
   c. γ-aminobutyric acid
   d. Serotonin

2. Which antidepressant is contraindicated in a patient diagnosed with a seizure disorder?
   a. Bupropion
   b. Mirtazapine
   c. Paroxetine
   d. Venlafaxine

3. Antagonism of which receptor contributes to orthostatic hypotension observed with trazodone therapy?
   a. Alpha-1
   b. Dopamine-2
   c. Histamine-1
   d. Muscarinic-1

4. Which antidepressant requires special dietary restrictions to prevent the possible development of hypertensive crisis?
   a. Amitriptyline
   b. Duloxetine
   c. Escitalopram
   d. Phenelzine

5. Which part of the brain regulates voluntary motor movements?
   a. Brainstem
   b. Cerebellum
   c. Cerebrum
   d. Hypothalamus

6. Which antidepressant is FDA approved for the treatment of postpartum depression?
   a. Brexanolone
   b. Esketamine
   c. Fluoxetine
   d. Levomilnacipran

7. Which mood stabilizer most commonly causes hypothyroidism with long-term use?
   a. Carbamazepine
   b. Lamotrigine
   c. Lithium
   d. Valproate

8. Which medication increases blood levels of lamotrigine, increasing Stevens-Johnson syndrome risk?
   a. Carbamazepine
   b. Lithium
   c. Quetiapine
   d. Valproate

9. Which pathway is involved in the development of extrapyramidal symptoms secondary to antipsychotic-induced dopamine receptor blockade?
   a. Mesocortical
   b. Mesolimbic
   c. Nigrostriatal
   d. Tuberoinfundibular

10. Which second-generation antipsychotic requires routine absolute neutrophil count monitoring?
    a. Brexpiprazole
    b. Clozapine
    c. Risperidone
    d. Ziprasidone

1. **c**; 2. **a**; 3. **a**; 4. **d**; 5. **b**; 6. **a**; 7. **c**; 8. **d**; 9. **c**; 10. **b**

Visit the Evolve website for a posttest on the content in this chapter: http://evolve.elsevier.com/Varcarolis

REFERENCES

Brown, A. C. (2017). An overview of herb and dietary supplement efficacy, safety, and government regulations in the United Sates with suggested improvements. *Food and Chemical Toxicology, 107,* 449–471.

Brunton, L. L., Hilal-Dandan, R., & Knollmann, B. C. (2018). *Goodman and Gilman's: The pharmacological basis of therapeutics* (13th ed.). New York, NY: McGraw-Hill.

Corponi, F., Fabbri, C., & Serretti, A. (2018). Pharmacogenetics in psychiatry. *Advances in Pharmacology, 83,* 297–331.

Jameson, J. L., Fauci, A. S., Kasper, D. L., Hauser, S. L., Longo, D. L., & Loscalzo, J. (2018). *Harrison's principles of internal medicine* (20th ed.). New York, NY: McGraw-Hill.

National Library of Medicine (US). (2019). *DailyMed.* Bethesda, MD: U.S. National Library of Medicine, National Institutes of Health, Health & Human Services.

Stahl, S. M. (2013). *Stahl's essential psychopharmacology* (4th ed.). New York, NY: Cambridge University Press.

4

Treatment Settings

Monica J. Halter and Christine M. Tebaldi

🌐 Visit the Evolve website for a pretest on the content in this chapter: http://evolve.elsevier.com/Varcarolis

OBJECTIVES

1. Discuss the unique challenges in accessing and navigating care for psychiatric disorders.
2. Analyze the continuum of psychiatric care and the variety of care options available.
3. Describe the role of the primary care provider and the psychiatric specialist in treating psychiatric disorders.
4. Explain the purpose of patient-centered medical homes and implications for holistically treating individuals with psychiatric disorders.
5. Identify key components and benefits of community-based care, such as psychiatric home care.
6. Discuss other community-based care providers, including assertive community treatment teams, partial

hospitalization programs, and alternate delivery of care methods such as telepsychiatry.
7. Describe the role of the nurse as it pertains to outpatient psychiatric settings.
8. Identify the main types of inpatient care and the functions of each.
9. Discuss the purpose of identifying the rights of hospitalized psychiatric patients.
10. Define the therapeutic milieu.
11. Describe the role of the nurse as it pertains to inpatient psychiatric settings.

KEY TERMS AND CONCEPTS

assertive community treatment (ACT)
clinical pathway
community mental health center
continuum of psychiatric-mental healthcare
decompensation

elopement
least restrictive environment
milieu
patient-centered medical home
prevention
psychiatric case management

recovery
stabilization
stigma
triage

Obtaining traditional healthcare is fairly straightforward. For example, if you wake up with a sore throat, you know what to do and basically what will happen. It is likely that if you feel bad enough, you will see your primary care provider to be examined, and maybe get a throat culture to diagnose the problem. If the cause is bacterial, you will probably be prescribed an antibiotic. If you do not improve in a certain length of time, your primary care provider may order more tests or recommend that you see an ear, nose, and throat specialist.

Compared with obtaining treatment for other physical disorders, entry into the healthcare system for the treatment of psychiatric problems can be a mystery. Challenges in accessing and navigating this care system exist for several reasons. One reason is that we just do not have much of a frame of reference.

We are unlikely to benefit from the experience of others because having a psychiatric illness is often concealed. This concealment is often a result of embarrassment or concern over the stigma or a sense of responsibility, shame, and being flawed associated with these disorders (refer to Chapter 1 for more on stigma). You may know that when your grandmother had heart disease, she saw a cardiac specialist and had a coronary artery bypass. However, you may be unaware that she was also treated for depression by a psychiatrist.

Seeking treatment for mental health problems is also complicated by the very nature of mental illness. At the most extreme, disorders with a psychotic component may disorganize thoughts and impede a person's ability to recognize the need for care. There is even a word for this inability: anosognosia (ah-no-sag-NOH-zee-uh). Major depressive disorder, a common psychiatric condition, may interfere with motivation to seek care because the illness often causes feelings of apathy, hopelessness, and anergia (lack of energy).

Mental health symptoms are also confused with other problems. For example, anxiety disorders often manifest in somatic symptoms such as racing heartbeat, sweaty palms, and dizziness, which could be symptoms of cardiac problems. Prudence would dictate ruling out other causes, such as physical illness, particularly because diagnosing psychiatric illness is largely based on symptoms and not on objective measurements such as electrocardiograms (ECGs) and blood counts. Unfortunately, this necessary process of ruling out other illnesses often results in a troublesome treatment delay.

Further complicating treatment for mental illness is the unique nature of the system of care, which is rooted in the public and private sectors. The purpose of this chapter is to provide an overview of this system, briefly examine the evolution of mental healthcare, and explore different venues by which people receive treatment for mental health problems. Treatment options are presented in order of acuteness, beginning with those in the least restrictive environment, which is the setting that provides the necessary care while allowing the greatest personal freedom.

BACKGROUND

Psychiatric care in the United States has its roots in asylums, which were created in most existing states before the Civil War. These asylums were created with good intentions and a belief that states had a special responsibility to care for people who were "insane." Effective treatments were not yet developed, and community care was virtually nonexistent. By the early 1950s, there were only two real options for psychiatric care—a private psychiatrist's office or a mental hospital. At that time, there were 550,000—compared to 40,000 today—patients in state hospitals (National Association of State Mental Health Program Directors, 2017). A majority of these patients had disabling conditions and became stuck in the asylums.

The number of people in state-managed psychiatric hospitals began to decrease with the creation of Medicare and Medicaid during the Great Society reform period in the 1960s. Medicaid had an especially potent effect because it paid for short-term hospitalization in general hospitals and medical centers and for long-term care in nursing homes. It did not, however, cover care for most patients in psychiatric hospitals. These incentives stimulated development of general hospital psychiatric units and also led states to transfer geriatric patients from 100% state-paid psychiatric hospitals to Medicaid-reimbursed nursing facilities.

In the 1999 Olmstead decision, the Supreme Court decreed that keeping people in psychiatric hospitals was "unjustified isolation." The opinion of the court was that mental illness is a disability, that institutionalization is in violation of the Americans with Disabilities Act, and that all people with disabilities have a right to live in the community.

These forces led to the creation of state- and county-financed community care systems to complement, and largely replace, the functions of the state hospitals. The population in state

---

BOX 4.1   Policy and Politics of the Provision of Psychiatric Care

Mental health advocates develop policies to create an ideal image of what we should be striving for in our healthcare delivery system. Organizations such as the World Health Organization (WHO) work hard to strategically plan policies that help direct government goals for healthcare. Improvements in mental health policy across the world are needed and impact how people with mental illness are treated. Policies can address various issues, including availability and accessibility of care, discrimination, and basic human rights (WHO, 2012).

Grassroots organizations such as the National Alliance on Mental Illness (NAMI) along with groups specific to each state advocate for better mental healthcare. These organizations are able to share information with legislators about special interest issues. Nurses are encouraged to contact their legislators and work collaboratively on legislation that may positively impact patient care and the profession of psychiatric-mental health nursing. This is a special advocacy role for a nurse to engage in and provides a way to be involved in policymaking.

---

hospitals dropped dramatically and many of these institutions were closed. The number of state psychiatric hospitals has been reduced from 322 in 1950 to approximately 195 in 2019 and continues to be cut (National Association of State Mental Health Program Directors, 2019).

Related to the shift from hospital to community care were the pharmacological breakthroughs in the mid-20th century that resulted in dramatic changes in the provision of psychiatric care. In the 1950s, the introduction of chlorpromazine (Thorazine)—the first antipsychotic medication—contributed to hospital discharges. Gradually, more psychopharmacological agents were added to treat psychosis, depression, anxiety, and other disorders. Treatment provision expanded beyond specialists in psychiatry as general practitioners began to feel more comfortable prescribing medication and managing symptoms.

Our current system of psychiatric care includes outpatient and inpatient settings. Decisions regarding the level of care tend to be based on the condition being treated and the acuteness of the problem. However, these are not the only criteria. Levels of care may be influenced by such factors as a concurrent psychiatric or substance use problem, medical problems, acceptance of treatment, social supports, disease chronicity, or potential for relapse (Box 4.1).

CONTINUUM OF CARE

What if you, your friend, or a family member needed psychiatric treatment or care? What would you do or recommend? Fig. 4.1 presents a continuum of psychiatric-mental healthcare that may help you to decide.

Movement along the continuum is fluid and can go in either direction. For example, patients discharged from the most acute levels of care (e.g., hospitalization) may need intensive services to maintain their initial gains. Failure to follow up with outpatient treatment increases the likelihood of rehospitalization and other adverse outcomes. Patients may also reverse direction on the treatment continuum. That is, if symptoms do not improve, professionals from a lower-intensity service may refer

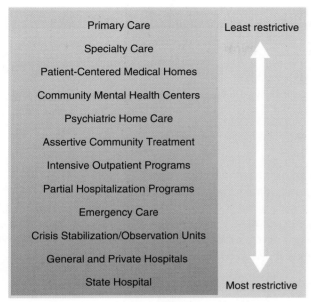

Fig. 4.1 The continuum of psychiatric-mental health treatment.

the patient to a higher level of care to prevent decompensation (deterioration of mental health) and hospitalization.

Differences in characteristics, treatment outcomes, and interventions between inpatient and outpatient settings are identified in Table 4.1.

OUTPATIENT CARE SETTINGS

Primary Care Providers

Primary care providers are the first choice for most people when they are ill, but what about psychiatric symptoms? Imagine that you are feeling depressed, so depressed in fact that you are miserable and cannot carry out your normal activities. You recall that a friend who was depressed saw a psychiatrist (or was that a psychologist?), but that seems too drastic. You do not feel *that* bad. Perhaps you are coming down with something like a cold or flu. After all, you have been tired and you do not really have an appetite. You decide to visit your primary care provider, a general healthcare provider who may be a physician, an advanced practice nurse, or a physician assistant in an office, clinic, or hospital.

This is not an unusual choice. Seeking help for mental health problems from primary care providers rather than from mental health specialists is common and similar to seeking help for other medical disorders. This is especially true because most psychiatric disorders are accompanied by unexplained physical symptoms such as headaches, backaches, and digestive problems. Many people treated for psychiatric disorders will not go beyond this level of care and may feel more comfortable being treated in a familiar setting. Being treated in primary care rather than in the mental health system may also lessen the degree of stigma, self-perceived or societally, attached to getting psychiatric care.

Disadvantages to being treated by primary care providers include time constraints because a 15-minute appointment is usually inadequate for a mental and physical assessment.

Additionally, primary care providers typically have limited training in psychiatry and may lack expertise in the diagnosis and treatment of psychiatric disorders. These professionals may refer people to mental healthcare specialists.

> **VIGNETTE:** Josh Miller is a registered nurse at a primary care office where he works with a nurse practitioner. He greets his next patient, Mr. Newton, a 56-year-old man Josh knows from previous admission and with whom he has established a solid rapport.
>
> While taking vital signs, he notices that Mr. Newton isn't his usual self. His affect is dull and his eye contact is poor. He vaguely responds with short answers. Mr. Newton reports that within the past couple of months he has been increasingly tired, doesn't enjoy anything, aches constantly, and has been eating mostly carbohydrates.
>
> After documenting his findings, Josh leans forward slightly on his stool and states in a caring tone, "Mr. Newton, I've known you for a while. The change in your behavior has me concerned. Is there anything going on in your life that you'd like to talk about?" Mr. Newton hesitates but then tells Josh that he was demoted at work last year and that he hasn't felt right since then.
>
> Josh shares his assessment with the nurse practitioner, who subsequently diagnoses Mr. Newton with major depressive disorder. The nurse practitioner prescribes escitalopram (Lexapro) 10 mg daily and educates him about his diagnosis and new medication. Josh reinforces this teaching and provides him with written educational material. He also provides him with referrals for therapy and support groups.

Specialized Psychiatric Care Providers

Most primary care providers feel comfortable in treating common psychiatric illnesses such as uncomplicated depression. However, they may feel less comfortable when suicidal ideation is present or with more severe disorders, such as schizophrenia.

Specialized psychiatric care providers have an educational background and experience in care of psychiatric problems and mental health. These providers include psychiatrists, psychiatric-mental health advanced practice registered nurses (nurse practitioners or clinical nurse specialists), psychologists, social workers, counselors, and other licensed therapists. Many primary care practices are partnering with specialty psychiatric providers who work in the same location, allowing for rapid access to care and effective triage and screening.

Specialized care providers can provide numerous services. Psychiatrists can prescribe medications. Advanced practice psychiatric nurses and physician assistants can prescribe medications as well, but the degree of prescriptive authority varies in each state. Most specialized care providers are educated to use individual psychotherapy (talk therapy) and lead group therapy. These providers may have subspecialties, such as a provider who specializes in working with veterans with posttraumatic stress disorder (PTSD).

How do you locate one of these specialized psychiatric care providers? One of the first steps is to inquire with a local care organization, such as a primary care office, hospital, clinic, or therapy practice. Other ways to find specialty care include asking peers, seeking help through support organizations, or contacting one's insurance company for a list of covered providers. Electronic searches are also good options. Reputable websites, particularly those with state or federal funding, can provide

TABLE 4.1   Characteristics, Treatment Outcomes, and Interventions by Setting

Outpatient/Community Mental Health Setting	Inpatient Setting
Characteristics	
Intermittent supervision	24-Hour supervision
Independent living environment with self-care, safety risks	Therapeutic milieu with hospital-/staff-supported healing environment
Treatment Outcomes	
Stable or improved level of functioning in community	Stabilization of symptoms and return to community
Interventions	
Establish long-term therapeutic relationship	Develop short-term therapeutic relationship
Develop comprehensive plan of care with patient and support system, with attention to sociocultural needs and maintenance of community living	Develop comprehensive plan of care, with attention to sociocultural needs of patient and focus on reintegration into the community
Encourage adherence with medication regimen	Administer medication
Teach and support adequate nutrition and self-care, with referrals as needed	Monitor nutrition and self-care, with assistance as needed
Assist patient in self-assessment, with referrals for health needs in community as needed	Provide health assessment and intervention as needed
Use creative strategies to refer patient to positive social activities	Offer structured socialization activities
Communicate regularly with family/support system to assess and improve level of functioning	Plan for discharge with family/significant other with regard to housing and follow-up treatment

a wealth of information designed to point consumers in the proper direction. Reviews of the care provider on these websites can be helpful in making your decision.

Patient-Centered Medical Homes

Patient-centered medical homes (PCMHs) or primary care medical homes received strong support from the Affordable Care Act of 2010 under President Barack Obama. These health homes were developed in response to fragmented care that resulted in some services never being delivered while others were duplicated. The focus of care is patient centered and provides access to physical health, behavioral health, and supportive community and social services. Patients are provided with a range of support for preventive care, acute care, chronic disease management, and end-of-life issues. According to the Agency for Healthcare Research and Quality (n.d.), these homes have five key characteristics:

1. Patient centered—Care is relationship based with the patient and takes into account the unique needs of the whole person. The patient is a core member of the team.
2. Comprehensive care—All levels (preventive, acute, and chronic) of mental and physical care are addressed. Physicians or advanced practice nurses lead teams that include nurses, physician assistants, pharmacists, nutritionists, social workers, educators, and care coordinators.
3. Coordination of care—Care is coordinated with the broader health system, such as hospitals, specialty care, and home health.
4. Improved access—Patients are not limited to Monday through Friday from 9 a.m. to 5 p.m. to get the care they need. In addition to extended hours of service, these homes provide e-mail and phone support. Electronic communication (e.g., follow-up e-mails and reminders)

and record keeping are viewed as essential aspects of this process.
5. Systems approach—Evidence-based care is provided with a continuous feedback loop of evaluation and quality improvement.

Community Mental Health Centers

Beginning in the 1960s, patients with severe mental illness were diverted from state psychiatric hospitals to community mental health centers. Since that time, these centers have become the mainstay for those who lack funding for mental healthcare. They offer free or low-cost sliding scale care.

Community mental health centers provide emergency services, community/home-based services, and outpatient services across the lifespan. Common treatments include medication prescription and administration, individual therapy, psychoeducational and therapy groups, family therapy, and dual-diagnosis (mental health and substance use) treatment. A clinic may also be aligned with a structured program that offers rehabilitation, vocational services, and residential services. Some community mental health centers have an associated intensive psychiatric case management service to assist patients in finding housing or obtaining entitlements.

Community mental health centers also utilize multidisciplinary teams. Psychiatric-mental health registered nurses are key members of these teams. Nurses provide medication administration and mental health education to help individuals continue treatment and reach an optimal level of functioning. Advanced practice psychiatric registered nurses hold a significant role in community mental health centers by conducting patient intakes, psychotherapy, and medication management.

Psychiatric Home Care

Psychiatric home care is a community-based treatment modality. Medicare requires that four elements be met in order for these services to be reimbursed: (1) homebound status of the patient, (2) presence of a psychiatric diagnosis, (3) need for the skills of a psychiatric registered nurse, and (4) development of a plan of care under orders of a physician or advanced practice registered nurse. Reimbursement and guidelines for psychiatric home care by other payers besides Medicare vary greatly.

Homebound refers to the patient's inability to leave home independently due to physical or mental conditions. Patients may be referred for psychiatric home care after an acute inpatient hospitalization episode of care or to prevent hospitalization.

Medicare allows two groups of healthcare providers to be involved in psychiatric home care. They are social workers with a master's degree and psychiatric registered nurses. Social workers provide counseling and medical social services such as linking people with necessary healthcare and services.

Psychiatric registered nurses provide evaluation, therapy, and teaching. Typically, the nurse visits the patient one to three times per week for a limited period of time. By going to the patient's home, the nurse is better able to address the concerns of access to services and adherence with treatment. Nurses working in the home have to be especially adept at assessing anxiety, agitation, and the potential for violence in this nonclinical setting.

Assertive Community Treatment

Assertive community treatment (ACT) is an intensive type of case management developed in the 1970s. This treatment was in response to the hard-to-engage, community-living needs of people with serious and persistent psychiatric symptoms. Due to the severity of their symptoms, they are often unable or unwilling to participate in traditional forms of treatment. As a result, this population has unnecessary and expensive repeat hospitalizations for services such as emergency room and inpatient care.

ACT teams work intensively with patients in their homes or in agencies, hospitals, and clinics—whatever settings patients find themselves in. Creative problem solving and interventions are hallmarks of care provided by mobile teams. The ACT concept takes into account that people need support and resources after 5 p.m. Therefore, teams are on call 24 hours a day.

ACT teams are multidisciplinary and typically composed of psychiatric-mental health registered nurses, social workers, psychologists, advanced practice registered nurses, and psychiatrists. One of these professionals (often the registered nurse) serves as the case manager and may have a caseload of patients who require visits three to five times per week. An advanced practice registered nurse or a psychiatrist usually supervises the case manager. Length of treatment may extend to years until the patient is more stabilized or ready to accept transfer to a more structured site for care.

Intensive Outpatient Programs and Partial Hospitalization Programs

Intensive outpatient programs (IOPs) and partial hospitalization programs (PHPs) function as intermediate steps between inpatient and outpatient care. The primary difference between the two groups is the amount of time that patients spend in them. PHPs meet Monday through Friday and have longer hours (about 6 hours because they are "partially hospitalized"), while IOPs meet anywhere from three to five times each week for sessions lasting around 3 hours. They provide structured activities along with nursing and medical supervision, intervention, and treatment. These programs tend to be located within general hospitals, psychiatric hospitals, or community mental health facilities.

A multidisciplinary team facilitates group therapy, individual therapy, other therapies (e.g., art and occupational), and medication management. Coping strategies learned during the program can be applied and practiced between sessions, then later explored and discussed. Patients admitted to IOPs and PHPs are closely monitored in case of a need for readmission to inpatient care.

Other Outpatient Venues for Psychiatric Care

New forms of treatment through technology are becoming increasingly popular. The COVID-19 pandemic resulted in adaptations to support social distancing that are likely to transform the delivery of mental health. Telepsychiatry, a subset of telemedicine, is providing therapy and even prescription services from a distance, usually through videoconferencing. Online counselors such as BetterHelp and Talkspace identify themselves as more

BETWEEN OUTPATIENT OR INPATIENT: RESIDENTIAL TREATMENT

Residential treatment centers house patients and provide 24-hour supervision. Observation and treatment may occur over a period of weeks to months or even years. Candidates for residential treatment typically are in acute or sub-acute crises, which makes outpatient treatment less effective. Yet, their needs are not severe enough to warrant hospitalization.

Sometimes, residential treatment is used as a step-down after hospitalization. This is especially true for individuals whose disorders include a psychotic element such as schizophrenia and bipolar disorder. Another type of patient that may benefit from this setting are individuals who have a psychiatric condition accompanied by a physical condition such as cerebral palsy.

Most commonly, patients are referred to residential treatment through outpatient providers. Patients may not be showing improvement in daily functioning and interactions even with increased frequency and intensity of outpatient therapy. Sometimes, continued observation is the best way to understand the nature of the patient's illness, as in the case of rapid bipolar cycling or when then are concerns about undisclosed alcohol or substance use.

affordable, convenient, and discrete options for consumers. These direct-to-consumer venues allow individuals to take the lead in their own care by initiating therapy and are expected to surge in popularity over the next decade (Boyce, n.d.). Despite the patient and provider not being in the same room, telepsychiatry has been found to be reliable and effective. However, in some populations, such as individuals with autism spectrum disorder, in-person interaction may still be preferred (American Psychiatric Association [APA], 2019). Benefits of telepsychiatry include:

- Treating people in remote areas
- Reducing emergency department visits
- Reducing delays in care
- Improving continuity of care and follow-up
- Reducing competing interests, such as employment or childcare
- Eliminating transportation barriers
- Reducing the barrier of stigma

Healthcare providers need to be licensed in the state in which the patient is living. Licensing boards and legislatures consider the place where care is provided as the setting. In terms of financial reimbursement, most US states have enacted legislation requiring insurance coverage similar to in-person provision of care.

Mobile mental health units have been developed in some service areas. In a growing number of communities, mental health programs are collaborating with other health or community services to provide integrated approaches to treatment. A prime example of this is the growth of dual-diagnosis programming at both mental health and substance use disorders clinics.

Emergency Care

Patients and families seeking emergency care range from the worried well to those with acute symptoms. The primary goal in emergency services is to perform triage and stabilization. Triage refers to determining the severity of the problem and the urgency of a response. Stabilization is the resolution of the immediate crisis. Emergency department (ED) care often provides a bridge from the community to more intensive psychiatric services, such as inpatient care.

Individuals may seek emergency care voluntarily. However, there are times when family, friends, treatment providers, schools, emergency medical personnel, or law enforcement may suggest or require an individual to undergo emergency evaluation. When emergency evaluation and stabilization are needed, psychiatric clinicians, including psychiatric-mental health nurses, will determine the correct interventions and level of care required. Refer to Chapter 6 for a more detailed discussion about involuntary treatment.

Emergency psychiatric care varies across the nation due to differences in state mental health system design, access to care, and workforce. Despite these differences, emergency psychiatric care can be categorized into three major models:

1. **Comprehensive emergency service model** is often affiliated with a full-service ED in a hospital or medical center setting. Typically, there is dedicated clinical space with specialty staffing. Psychiatric-mental health nurses, psychiatric technicians, mental health specialists, social workers, mental health counselors, and psychiatrists generally make up the multidisciplinary workforce. The concepts of triage and stabilization are incorporated into the individualized care plan for each patient.
2. **Hospital-based consultant model** utilizes the concepts of the comprehensive model by incorporating triage and stabilization. However, there is generally no dedicated clinical space or comprehensive separate staffing. Psychiatric clinical staff members are assigned to a specific hospital and are on-site or on-call, serving as part of the ED staff. Psychiatric clinicians manage emergency psychiatric evaluations as requested. Clinicians complete a "level of care" assessment, attempt to stabilize patients, and arrange for discharge or transfer. The ED staff is responsible for all immediate care needs.
3. **Mobile crisis team model** is considered for stabilization in the field. The team meets face to face with the person in crisis to assess and de-escalate the situation. While the composition of teams can vary, they often include psychiatric-mental health nurses, social workers, and counselors in collaboration with a psychiatrist and/or an advanced practice nurse.

PREVENTION IN OUTPATIENT CARE

A distinct concept in the healthcare literature is that of treatment based on a public health model that takes a community approach to prevention. Primary, secondary, and tertiary prevention are levels at which interventions are directed.

Primary Prevention

Primary prevention occurs before any problem manifests and seeks to reduce the incidence or rate of new cases. Primary prevention may prevent or delay the onset of symptoms in genetically or otherwise predisposed individuals. Coping strategies and psychosocial support for vulnerable young people are effective interventions in preventing mood and anxiety disorders.

Secondary Prevention

Secondary prevention is also aimed at reducing the prevalence of psychiatric disorders. Early identification of problems,

Role	Basic Practice (Diploma, AD, BS)	Advanced Practice (MS, DNP, PHD)
Practice	Provide nursing care; assist with medication management as prescribed, under direct supervision	Nurse practitioner or clinical nurse specialist; manage consumer care and prescribe or recommend interventions independently
Consultation	Consult with staff about care planning and work with nurse practitioner or physician to promote health and mental healthcare; collaborate with staff from other agencies	Consultant to staff about plan of care, to consumer and family about options for care; collaborate with community agencies about service coordination and planning processes
Administration	Take leadership role within mental health treatment team	Administrative or contract consultant role within mental health agencies or mental health authority
Research and education	Participate in research at agency or mental health authority; serve as preceptor to undergraduate nursing students	Role as educator or researcher within agency or mental health authority

TABLE 4.2 Roles Relevant to Educational Preparation in Outpatient and Community Settings

screening, and prompt and effective treatment are hallmarks of this level. While it does not stop the actual disorder from beginning, it is intended to delay or avert progression.

Tertiary Prevention

Tertiary prevention is the treatment of disease with a focus on preventing the progression to a severe course, disability, or even death. Tertiary prevention is closely related to rehabilitation, which aims to preserve or restore functional ability. In the case of treating major depressive disorder, the aim is to avoid loss of employment, reduce disruption of family processes, and prevent suicide.

OUTPATIENT PSYCHIATRIC NURSING CARE

Psychiatric-mental health nursing in the outpatient or community setting requires strong problem-solving and clinical skills, cultural competence, flexibility, solid knowledge of community resources, and comfort in functioning more autonomously than acute care nurses. Patients need assistance with problems related to individual psychiatric symptoms, family and support systems, and basic living needs, such as housing and financial support.

Psychiatric-mental health nurses can be leaders in transforming an illness-driven and dependency-oriented system into a system that emphasizes recovery and empowerment. Nurses are adept at understanding the system and coordinating care. Further, nurses are respected members of the interdisciplinary team. They serve not only in lead clinical roles but also as advocates for the inclusion of patient-centered and trauma-informed care models.

The role of the outpatient or community psychiatric-mental health registered nurse ideally includes service provision in a variety of these treatment settings. For example, psychiatric needs are well known in the criminal justice system and the homeless population. Individuals suffering from a mental illness tend to cycle through the correctional systems and generally comprise 50% of the incarcerated population, and from that number, 20% have a serious mental illness (American Psychological Association, 2014). The nurse's role is not only to provide care to individuals as they leave the criminal justice system and reenter the community but also to educate police officers and justice staff in how to work with individuals entering the criminal system.

Table 4.2 describes the educational preparation for a variety of outpatient and community roles.

Promoting Recovery and Continuation of Treatment

In the not-too-distant past, treatment for mental illness consisted of patients being told what medications to take and what treatments to accept. Good patients were those who were compliant. A newer model of recovery promotes self-involvement in care. **Recovery** is "a process of change through which individuals improve their health and wellness, live self-directed lives, and strive to reach their full potential" (Substance Abuse Mental Health Services Administration [SAMHSA], 2019).

Nurses are real assets in supporting patients in the recovery process, especially with medication management. Nurses are in a position to help the patient recognize side effects and be aware of interactions among medications prescribed for both physical illness and mental illness. This knowledge increases the individual's ability to self-advocate. Patient-family education and behavioral strategies, in the context of a therapeutic relationship with the nurse, promote adherence with a medication regimen.

Patient-centered care, also referred to as person-centered care, supports values in the recovery model. It is respectful and responsive care that incorporates patients' preferences, needs, and values. This concept is essential for ensuring that the patient's wishes and values are the guiding principle for care management and shared decision making.

INPATIENT CARE SETTINGS

Hospitalization is available for the treatment of acute symptoms or safety concerns for patients with mental disorders and emotional crises. In fact, in 2014, 2.4 million adult patients with a mental illness were treated in hospitals (SAMHSA, 2019). The top five mental health diagnoses treated were mood disorders, substance use disorders, neurocognitive disorders, anxiety disorders, and schizophrenia. Admission is commonly reserved for those people who are suicidal, homicidal, or extremely disabled and in need of acute care.

Crisis Stabilization/Observation Units

Care models that prioritize rapid stabilization and short length of stay have become more prevalent in medical and psychiatric settings. Overnight short-term observation, often 1 to 3 days, is designed for individuals who have symptoms that are expected to remit in 72 hours or less. This observation is also helpful for individuals who have a psychosocial stressor that can be addressed in that timeframe, maximizing their stability and allowing them to rapidly return to a community treatment setting.

General Hospitals and Private Hospitals

Acute care hospital psychiatric units tend to be housed on a floor or floors of a general hospital. Private psychiatric hospitals are freestanding facilities. As noted, the dramatic growth of acute care psychiatric hospitals and hospital units is the result of a shift away from institutionalization in state-managed hospitals. Since that time, reduced reimbursement, increased managed care, enhanced outpatient options, and expanded availability of outpatient and PHPs have resulted in the steady decline of these facilities.

State Psychiatric Hospitals

Although the quality of care in state hospitals has improved dramatically, today's state-operated psychiatric hospitals are an extension of what remains of the old system. The clinical role of state hospitals is to serve the most seriously ill patients. However, this role varies widely, depending on available levels of community care and on payments by state Medicaid programs. In some states, these hospitals primarily provide intermediate treatment for patients unable to be stabilized in short-term general hospital units and long-term care for individuals judged too ill for community care. In other states, the emphasis is on acute care that is reflective of gaps in the private sector, especially for the uninsured or for those who have exhausted limited insurance benefits.

In most states, state hospitals provide forensic (court-related) care and monitoring as part of their function. The state or county system also advises the courts as to a defendant's sanity. In some criminal cases, defendants may be judged to have been so ill when they committed the criminal act that they cannot be held responsible but instead require treatment. These judgments are termed "not guilty by reason of insanity" (NGRI). One tragic example is that of Andrea Yates, the Texas woman who, in 2001, drowned her five young children under the delusional belief she was saving them from their sinfulness. She was found NGRI and was committed to a Texas state psychiatric facility.

CONSIDERATIONS FOR INPATIENT CARE

Entry to Acute Inpatient Care

Some patients are admitted directly to inpatient care based on a specialized care provider or primary care provider referral. However, the majority of patients receiving inpatient acute psychiatric care are admitted through an ED or crisis intervention service. In the United States, mental health conditions are second only to abdominal pain as the most common reason to visit the ED (Hooker et al., 2019).

Patients may be admitted voluntarily or involuntarily (see Chapter 6). Units may be unlocked or locked. Locked units provide privacy and prevent elopement—leaving before being

discharged (also referred to as being away without leave or AWOL). There may also be psychiatric intensive care units (PICUs) within the general psychiatric units to provide better monitoring of those who pose an increased risk for danger to themselves or others.

VIGNETTE: Mr. Reese is a 22-year-old who was brought to the emergency department by police after expressing thoughts of suicide. He is restless and irritable. When approached, he becomes agitated and threatening to the nurses and physicians. He states that his mother and brother, who are only trying to have him admitted so they can take his money, tricked him. He is exhibiting poor judgment, insight, and impulse control. He stopped taking his antipsychotic medication 3 weeks ago because of side effects.

The psychiatric nurse, Morgan, in the ED approaches Mr. Reese in a non-threatening manner. She calmly asks him if he'd be more comfortable sitting while they speak with one another. Mr. Reese chooses to sit on the gurney, and the nurse sits on a chair near the door. Mr. Reese already appears calmer after accepting a cold drink and nods as the nurse observes that he seems anxious. When asked if any medication ever helps him with feeling anxious, he responds that he has taken lorazepam (Ativan) before and it helps. Morgan obtains an order for the medication and provides Mr. Reese with education about lorazepam.

BOX 4.2 Typical Items Included in Hospital Statements of Patients' Rights

- Right to be treated with dignity
- Right to be involved in treatment planning and decisions
- Right to refuse treatment, including medications
- Right to request to leave the hospital, even against medical advice
- Right to be protected against harming oneself or others
- Right to a timely evaluation in the event of involuntary hospitalization
- Right to legal counsel
- Right to vote
- Right to communicate privately by telephone and in person
- Right to informed consent
- Right to confidentiality regarding one's disorder and treatment
- Right to choose or refuse visitors
- Right to be informed of research and to refuse to participate
- Right to the least restrictive means of treatment
- Right to send and receive mail and to be present during any inspection of packages received
- Right to keep personal belongings unless they are dangerous
- Right to lodge a complaint through a plainly publicized procedure
- Right to participate in religious worship

Rights of the Hospitalized Patient

Patients admitted to any psychiatric unit retain rights as citizens, which vary from state to state, and are entitled to certain privileges. Laws and regulatory standards require that patients' rights be provided in a timely fashion after an individual has been admitted to the hospital, and that the treatment team must always be aware of these rights. Any infringement by the team during the patient's hospitalization—such as a failure to protect patient safety—must be documented and actions must be justifiable. All mental health facilities must provide a written statement of patients' rights often with copies of applicable state laws attached. Box 4.2 provides a sample list of patients' rights.

BOX 4.3   Members of the Multidisciplinary Treatment Team

Psychiatric-mental health registered nurses: Licensed registered nurses whose focus is on mental health and mental illness and who may or may not be certified in psychiatric-mental health nursing. The registered nurse is typically the only 24-hour-a-day, 7-days-a-week professional working in acute care. Among the responsibilities of the registered nurse are diagnosing and treating responses to psychiatric disorders, coordinating care, counseling, giving medication and evaluating responses, and providing education.

Psychiatric-mental health advanced practice registered nurses: Licensed registered nurses who are prepared at the master's or doctoral level and hold specialty certification as either clinical nurse specialists or nurse practitioners. These nurses are qualified for clinical functions such as diagnosing psychiatric conditions, prescribing psychotropic medications and integrative therapy, and conducting psychotherapy. They are also involved in case management, consulting, education, and research.

Psychiatrists: Psychiatrists prescribe medication for psychiatric symptoms. They may also provide psychotherapy. As physicians, psychiatrists may be employed by the hospital or may hold practice privileges in the facility.

Psychologists: In keeping with their doctoral or doctorate degree preparation, psychologists conduct psychological testing, provide consultation for the team, and offer direct services such as specialized individual, family, or marital therapies.

Social workers: Basic level social workers help the patient prepare a support system that will promote mental health on discharge from the hospital. This includes contacts with day treatment centers, employers, sources of financial aid, and landlords. Licensed clinical social workers undergo training in individual, family, and group therapies.

Counselors: Counselors prepared in disciplines such as psychology, rehabilitation counseling, and addiction counseling may augment the treatment plan by co-leading groups, providing basic supportive counseling, or assisting in psychoeducational and recreational activities.

Occupational, recreational, art, music, and dance therapists: Based on their specialist preparation, these therapists assist patients in gaining skills that help them cope more effectively, gain or retain employment, use leisure time to the benefit of their mental health, and express themselves in healthy ways.

Medical advanced practice nurses, medical doctors, and physician assistants: Medical professionals provide diagnoses and treatments on a consultation basis. Occasionally, a medical professional who is trained as an addiction specialist may play a more direct role on a unit that offers treatment for addictive disease.

Mental health workers (mental health specialists/psychiatric technicians): Mental health workers, including nursing assistants, function under the direction and supervision of registered nurses. They provide assistance to patients in meeting basic needs and also help the community to remain supportive, safe, and healthy.

Pharmacists: In view of the intricacies of prescribing, coordinating, and administering combinations of psychotropic and other medications, the consulting pharmacist can offer a valuable safeguard. Physicians and nurses collaborate with the pharmacist regarding new medications, which are proliferating at a steady rate.

Teamwork and Collaboration

Psychiatric-mental health nurses are core members of a team of professionals and nonprofessionals who work together to provide care (Box 4.3). The team (including the patient) generally formulates a full treatment plan. The nurse's role in this process is often to lead the planning meeting. This nursing leadership reflects the holistic nature of nursing as well as the fact that nursing is the discipline that is represented on the unit at all times. Nurses are in a unique position to contribute valuable information, such as continuous assessment findings, the patient's adjustment to the unit, any health concerns, psychoeducational needs, and deficits in the patient's self-care. Additionally, nurses have an integral function to facilitate a patient's achievement of therapeutic goals by offering education and support in an individual or group format.

Ultimately, the treatment plan will be the guide for the patient's care during the hospital stay. It is based on goals for the hospitalization and defines how achievement of the goals will be measured. Input from the patient and family (if available and desirable) is critical in formulating goals. Incorporating the patient's feedback in developing the treatment plan goals increases the likelihood of the success of the outcomes.

Members of each discipline are responsible for gathering data and participating in the planning of care. Newly admitted patients may find multiple professionals asking them similar questions to be extremely stressful or threatening. The urgency of the need for data should be weighed against the patient's ability to tolerate assessment. Often, assessments made by the intake team and the nurse provide the basis for care. In most settings, the psychiatrist or advanced practice nurse evaluates the patient and provides orders within a limited timeframe. Medical problems are usually referred to a medical consultant service often consisting of physicians and advanced practice nurses who assess the patient and consult with the unit clinical team.

To provide standardization in treatment and improve outcomes, inpatient units use **care pathways**, also known as **clinical pathways** and **integrated care pathways**. These task-oriented plans detail the essential steps in the care of patients with specific clinical problems based on the usual and expected clinical course. These tools provide an essential link between evidence-based knowledge and clinical practice. The treatment plan is revised if the patient's progress differs from the expected outcomes. Care pathways result in decreased costs, lengths of stay, and complications while improving outcomes.

Fig. 4.2 shows a clinical pathway for pediatric patients in the ED.

Therapeutic Milieu

Milieu (meel-yoo) is a word of French origin (mi "middle" + lieu "place") and refers to surroundings and physical environment. In a therapeutic context, it refers to the overall environment and interactions within that environment. Peplau (1989) referred to this as the therapeutic milieu. It is an all-inclusive term that recognizes the people (patients and staff), the setting, the structure, and the emotional climate as important to healing. Regardless of whether the setting involves treatment of psychotic children, adult patients in a psychiatric hospital, substance users in a residential treatment center, or psychiatric patients in a day treatment program, a well-managed milieu offers patients a sense of security and promotes healing. Structured aspects of the

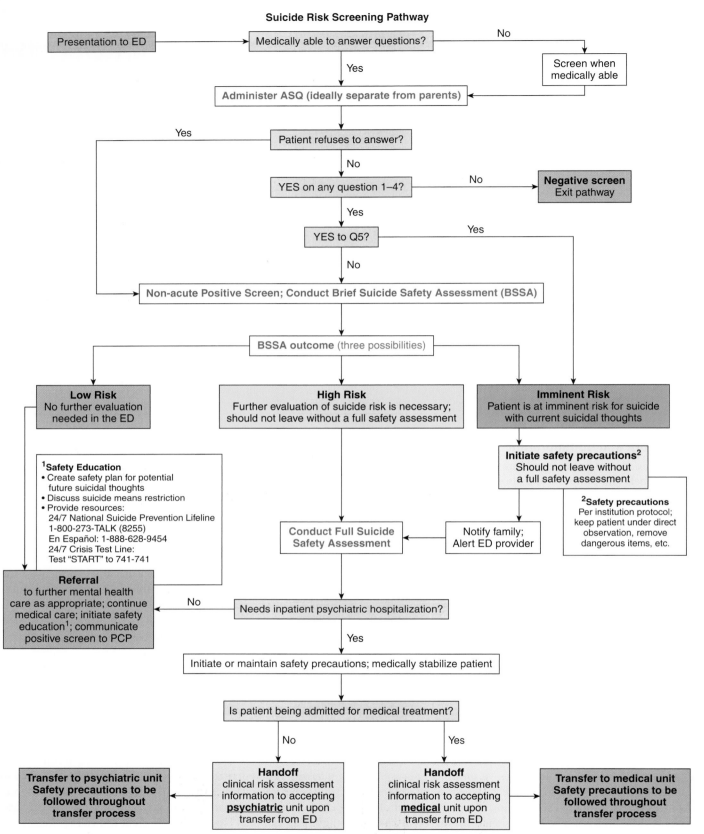

Fig. 4.2 Pediatric Emergency Room Clinical Pathway. *ASQ*, Ask Suicide-Screening Questions tool, a four-item suicide-risk questionnaire; *BSSA*, Brief Suicide Safety Assessment, another tool used to screen for suicidality; *ED*, emergency department; *PCP*, primary care provider. (From Brahmbhatt, K., Kurtz, B. P., Afzal, K. I., Giles, L. L., Kowal, E. D., Johnson, K. P. ... PaCC Workgroup. (2019). Suicide risk screening in pediatric hospitals: Clinical pathways to address a global health crisis. *Psychosomatics, 60*(1), 1–9; National Institute of Mental Health. (2019). ASQ toolkit. Retrieved from https://www.nimh.nih.gov/research/research-conducted-at-nimh/asq-toolkit-materials/emergencydepartment/emergency-department-clinical-pathway.shtml.)

TABLE 4.3 National Patient Safety Goals in Behavioral Healthcare

Goal	Process	Example
Identify patients correctly	Use at least two identifiers when providing care, treatment, or services.	Use the patient's name *and* date of birth for identification before drawing blood.
Use medicines safely	Maintain and communicate accurate medication information for the individual served.	Find out what medications the patient is taking and compare them to newly ordered medications.
Prevent infection	Use the hand-cleaning guidelines from either the Centers for Disease Control and Prevention or the World Health Organization.	Wet hands first; apply an amount of product recommended by the manufacturer to hands, and rub hands together for at least 15 s, covering all surfaces of the hands and fingers. Rinse with water and dry thoroughly with a disposable towel. Use towel to turn off the faucet.
Identify patient safety risk	Determine which patients are most likely to attempt suicide.	Routinely administer a screening tool such as the Beck Scale for Suicidal Ideation, a 21-item tool that takes 5–10 min to complete.

From The Joint Commission. (2020). *Behavioral health care: 2020 National Patient Safety Goals.* Retrieved from https://www.jointcommission.org/assets/1/6/NPSG_Chapter_BHC_Jan2020.pdf.

milieu include activities, rules, reality orientation practices, and environment.

Managing Behavioral Crises

Behavioral crises can lead to patient violence toward self or others and usually, but not always, escalate through fairly predictable stages. Staff members in most mental health facilities practice crisis prevention and management techniques. Training generally consists of a full-day course learning the skills to recognize and avoid crisis and de-escalate behavioral emergencies. Hands-on techniques, which are only used as a last resort, are also taught. At minimum, annual training is recommended to maintain competency.

Some facilities have special teams of nurses, psychiatric technicians, mental health specialists, and other professionals who respond to psychiatric emergencies called codes. Each member of the team takes part in the team effort to defuse a crisis in its early stages. If preventive measures fail and imminent risk of harm to self or others persists, each member of the team participates in a rapid, organized plan to safely manage the situation. The nurse is most often this team's leader not only in organizing the plan but also in timing the actions and managing the concurrent administration of medications.

Seclusion, restraint, and emergency medication are actions of last resort. The trend is to reduce or completely eliminate these practices whenever safely possible. The nurse can initiate such an intervention in the absence of a physician in most places but must secure a physician's order for restraint or seclusion within a specified time. Refer to Chapters 6 and 27 for further discussions and protocols for use of restraints and seclusion. The concept of trauma-informed care is a guiding principle for clinical interventions and unit philosophy and is addressed more comprehensively in Chapter 16.

Safety

A safe environment is an essential component of any inpatient setting. Protecting the patient is essential, but equally important is the safety of the staff and other patients. Safety needs are identified, and individualized interventions begin on admission. Staff members check all personal property and clothing to prevent any potentially harmful items (e.g., medication, alcohol, or sharp objects) from being taken onto the unit or left in their immediate possession. Some patients are at greater risk for suicide than others, and psychiatric-mental health nurses are skillful in evaluating this risk through questions and observations.

The Joint Commission, an agency that accredits hospitals, developed National Patient Safety Goals (2019) specific to specialty areas within hospitals to promote patient safety. Table 4.3 lists safety goals specific to behavioral healthcare. Centers for Medicare and Medicaid Services also emphasize safety and have identified several preventable hospital-acquired injuries for which they will not provide reimbursement. For example, they will not compensate healthcare organizations when a patient falls and fractures a hip, as nearly all falls are preventable. It is likely that other health insurance providers will also begin to limit payment for preventable injuries under the regulatory concept of pay for performance.

Tracking patients' whereabouts and activities is done periodically or continuously depending upon patients' risk for harming themselves or others. For patients with active suicidal thoughts, continuous in-person observation is essential because even checking on a patient every 15 minutes may not prevent a suicide that takes only several minutes.

Monitoring visitation is an important aspect of patient well-being and safety. Although visitors can contribute to patients' healing, visits may be overwhelming or distressing. Also, visitors may unwittingly or purposefully provide patients with unsafe items. Staff should inspect bags and packages. Sometimes, the unsafe items take the form of comfort foods from home or a favorite restaurant and should be monitored because they may be incompatible with diets or medications.

Intimate relationships between patients are prohibited. There are risks for sexually transmitted diseases, pregnancy, and emotional distress at a time when patients are vulnerable and may lack the capacity for consent.

Unit Design

The goal in designing psychiatric units is to provide a therapeutic and aesthetically pleasing environment while balancing the need for safety since patients on inpatient psychiatric units may be at risk for suicide or violence. Full compliance

TABLE 4.4   Sample Nursing Diagnoses Outcomes and Interventions for Patients in Acute Care Settings

Nursing Diagnoses	Outcomes	Interventions
Risk for suicide: Demonstrating behaviors indicating the potential for suicide	*Decreased suicide risk:* Personal actions to refrain from gestures and attempts at killing self	*Suicide prevention:* Reducing the risk for self-inflicted harm with intent to end life
Risk for violence against others: Vulnerable to behaviors in which an individual demonstrates that he or she can be physically, emotionally, and/or sexually harmful to others	*Decreased violence risk:* Personal actions to refrain from assaultive, combative, or destructive behaviors toward others	*Violence prevention:* Monitoring and manipulation of the physical environment to decrease the potential for violent behavior directed toward self, others, or environment
Mood disequilibrium: A mental state characterized by shifts in mood or affect … [with] affective, cognitive, somatic, and/or physiological manifestations…	*Mood equilibrium:* Appropriate adjustment of prevailing emotional tone in response to circumstances	*Mood management:* Providing for safety, stabilization, recovery, and maintenance of a patient who is experiencing dysfunctionally depressed or elevated mood

Data from International Council of Nurses. (2013). *Hospitalized adult mental health client.* Retrieved from https://www.icn.ch/what-we-do/projects/ehealth-icnp/about-icnp/icnp-catalogues.

with regulatory and accrediting bodies should be required for each clinical setting. Promoting an environment of safety and empowering patients to partner with clinical staff and take ownership of their own health and safety is critical.

Safety precautions are considered for all areas of the unit. For example, closets may be equipped with breakaway bars or hooks designed to hold a minimal amount of weight to prevent strangulation by hanging. Windows are locked and are made of safety glass, and safety mirrors are typically used. Showers may have non-weight-bearing or non-looping designed showerheads. Beds are often platforms rather than mechanical hospital beds, which can be dangerous because of their crushing potential, looping hazard, and cords. However, standard hospital beds may be indicated, depending on patient physical health needs. Other important design elements on inpatient psychiatric units include:

- Doors that open out instead of in to prevent patients from barricading themselves in their rooms.
- Continuous hinges on doors rather than three butt hinges to prevent hanging risk.
- Furniture that is anchored in place with the exception of a desk chair to prevent their use as a weapon or barricade.
- Drapes that are mounted on a track firmly anchored to the ceiling rather than curtain rods.
- Mini blinds contained within window glass provide significantly more safety than those whose mountings are accessible.
- Plumbing fixtures that are boxed in.

INPATIENT PSYCHIATRIC NURSING CARE

Management of these acute care units, ideally, is by nurses who have backgrounds in psychiatric-mental health nursing, preferably with advanced practice degrees. Staff nurses tend to be nurse generalists, that is, nurses who have basic training as registered nurses. Some registered nurses achieve national certification in psychiatric-mental health nursing through the American Nurses Credentialing Center. The staff psychiatric registered nurse carries out the following nursing responsibilities:

- Completing comprehensive data collection that includes the patient, family, and other healthcare workers
- Developing, implementing, and evaluating plans of care
- Assisting or supervising mental healthcare workers (e.g., nursing assistants with or without additional training in working with people who have mental illnesses)
- Maintaining a safe and therapeutic environment
- Facilitating health promotion through teaching
- Monitoring behavior, affect, and mood
- Maintaining oversight of restraint and seclusion
- Coordinating care by the treatment team

Medication management is an essential skill for psychiatric nurses. In this specialty area, nurses often influence medication decisions. This influence is based on frequent observation of and interaction with the patient to assess therapeutic effects and adverse effects of medications. For example, feedback about a patient's excessive sedation or increased agitation may lead to a decision to decrease or increase the dosage of an antipsychotic medication.

A common misperception regarding psychiatric nurses is that because they "just talk," they lose their skills for physical tasks such as starting and maintaining intravenous (IV) lines and changing dressings. In fact, most psychiatric nurses provide some degree of physical care. Patients on psychiatric units are not limited to psychiatric disorders and often have complex healthcare needs. For example, an older adult male with brittle diabetes and a recent foot amputation may become actively suicidal. In this case, it is likely he will be transferred to the psychiatric unit, where his blood glucose level will be monitored and wound care provided.

Table 4.4 provides sample nursing diagnoses, outcomes, and interventions for patients during admission to the acute care setting.

SPECIALTY TREATMENT SETTINGS

Treatment options are available that provide specialized care for specific groups of people. These options include inpatient, outpatient, and residential care.

Pediatric Psychiatric Care

Children with mental illnesses have the same range of treatment options as do adults but receive them in pediatric settings apart from adults. Inpatient care may be necessary if the child's symptoms become severe. Parental or guardian—including the Department of Children and Families—involvement in the plan of care is integral so that they understand the illness, treatment, and the family's role in supporting the child. Additionally, hospitalized children, if able, attend school several hours a day.

Geriatric Psychiatric Care

The older adult population may be treated in specialized mental health settings that consider the effects of aging on psychiatric symptoms. Physical illness and loss of independence can be strong precipitants in the development of depression and anxiety. Dementia is a particularly common problem encountered in geriatric psychiatry. Treatment is aimed at careful evaluation of the interaction of mind and body and provision of care that optimizes strengths, promotes independence, and focuses on safety.

Veterans Administration Centers

Active military personnel and veterans who were honorably discharged may receive federally funded inpatient or outpatient care and medication for psychiatric and alcohol or substance use disorders. One of the challenges veterans face is dealing with the aftereffects of the traumas of active combat. During Civil War times, these late effects were termed "soldier's heart." After World War I, soldiers had "shell shock," and after World War II, it was termed "battle fatigue." Currently, the mental health services available for people suffering from PTSD are laden with the demand for care. The prevalence of PTSD in the general population is about 7% and nearly 14% for veterans of the wars in Iraq and Afghanistan. This creates a tremendous need for strong psychiatric services for this population (Gradus, 2019). The Evidence-Based Practice box describes the use of telepsychiatry with veterans.

EVIDENCE-BASED PRACTICE

Veterans and Telepsychiatry

Problem
Military service members and veterans have an increased risk for psychiatric conditions after active service. Telepsychiatry has become a popular delivery method and can provide a potential solution to issues related to access to healthcare. What is less clear is whether veterans are open to using telepsychiatry.

Purpose of Study
The purpose of this study was to examine veterans' attitudes about using telepsychiatry for treatment.

Methods
Psychiatric symptoms were assessed in 253 veteran outpatients. Veterans also provided information regarding attitudes and level of comfort with receiving treatment through telehealth at home or at a clinic. Researchers developed and used a Telehealth Attitudes Questionnaire.

Key Findings
- Most of the veterans screened positive for posttraumatic stress disorder (82.9%), followed by major depressive disorder (42.9%) and traumatic brain injury (32.3%).
- A minority of veterans expressed feeling "extremely comfortable" using telehealth from home (13.4%) and clinic (8.3%) settings.
- About one third of veterans (32.8%) reported they preferred telehealth to in-person mental health visits.
- Veterans who considered geographic distance from the clinic to be a barrier to treatment did not have higher preferences for telehealth.
- Comfort with telepsychiatry was not correlated with symptom severity or age.

Implications for Nursing Practice
Despite societal acceptance of technology as a part of daily life, a minority of these veterans expressed comfort in using telepsychiatry. Nurses can provide opportunities for patients to increase comfort with these modalities through education and support. As patient advocates, nurses can also help in exploring alternatives for using healthcare.

Although not stated in the article, other factors may influence uncomfortable responses to telehealth. One of the most compelling factors is that the veterans may find clinic visits and interaction with providers as one of their main social outlets and connections. Future studies could examine the socialization variable for its influence on patients' perception.

From Goetter, E. M., Blackburn, A. M., Bui, E., Laifer, L. M., & Simon, N. (2019). Veterans' prospective attitudes about mental health treatment using telehealth. *Journal of Psychosocial Nursing, 57*, 9, 38–43.

Forensic Psychiatric Care

Incarcerated populations, both adult and juvenile, have higher than average incidences of mental disorders or substance use disorders. About 20% of jail inmates and 15% of prison inmates have a serious mental illness (Torrey et al., 2014). These statistics reflect the approximately 356,000 incarcerated individuals with serious mental illness. This is 10 times more than the 35,000 individuals with serious mental illness who remain in state hospitals.

Treatment may be provided within the prison system, where inmates are often separated from the general prison population. State hospitals also treat forensic patients. Most facilities provide psychotherapy, group counseling, medication management, and assistance with transition to the community. See Chapter 33 for more information on forensic psychiatric care and forensic nursing.

Alcohol and Drug Use Disorder Treatment

All the mental health settings that were previously described may provide treatment for alcohol and substance use disorders, although specialized treatment centers exist apart from the mental healthcare system. More than 20 million individuals aged 12 or older needed treatment in 2018 for illicit drug or alcohol use problems. Only 3.7 million received specialized care (Substance Abuse and Mental Health Services Administration [SAMHSA], 2019). This treatment is typically outpatient and includes counseling, education, medication management, and 12-step programs. Because alcohol detoxification and other substance withdrawal can be life-threatening, inpatient care may be required for medical management.

Self-Help Options

Obtaining sufficient sleep, meditating, eating right, exercising, abstaining from smoking, and limiting the use of alcohol are healthy responses to a variety of illnesses, such as diabetes and hypertension. As with other medical conditions, lifestyle choices and self-help responses can have a profound influence on the quality of life and the course, progression, and outcome of psychiatric disorders.

If we accept the notion that psychiatric disorders are usually a combination of biochemical interactions, genetics, and environment, then it stands to reason that by providing a healthy living situation, we are likely to fare better. If, for example, a person has a family history of anxiety and has demonstrated symptoms of anxiety, then a good first step (or an adjunct to psychiatric treatment) could be to learn yoga and balance the amounts of life's obligations with relaxation.

A voluntary network of self-help groups operates outside the formal mental healthcare system to provide education, contacts, and support. Since the introduction of Alcoholics Anonymous in the early 20th century, self-help groups have multiplied and have proven to be effective in the treatment and support of psychiatric problems. Groups specific to anxiety, depression, loss, caretakers' issues, bipolar disorder, PTSD, and almost every other psychiatric issue are widely available in most communities.

Consumers, people who use mental health services, and their family members have successfully united to shape the delivery of mental healthcare. Nonprofit organizations such as the National Alliance on Mental Illness (NAMI) encourage self-help and promote the concept of recovery from or self-management of mental illness. These grassroots groups also confront social stigma, influence policies, and support the rights of people experiencing mental illness.

▌ KEY POINTS TO REMEMBER

- Entry into the mental health system can be a bewildering process due to people's reluctance to share their own experiences, cognitive changes from the disorders themselves, and confusion over physical versus mental symptoms.
- Treatment options should be based on the least restrictive environment, that is, the setting that provides the necessary care while allowing the greatest personal freedom.
- Psychiatric care settings evolved during the 20th century from mass institutionalization to a variety of outpatient and inpatient settings.
- A continuum of care model helps differentiate between levels of acuity within treatment settings.
- Primary care providers have an increasingly important role in identifying and treating mental disorders. This treatment choice may feel familiar and reduce stigma. Time limitations may impact a complete mental assessment and training limitations may make some providers uncomfortable.
- Specialty care providers possess an educational and experiential background in psychiatric and mental health.
- Patient-centered medical homes with multiple services and an array of providers are becoming increasingly popular as a way to integrate mental and other physical care.
- Community mental health centers provide a wide range of mental health services for individuals who lack funding for care.

- Registered nurses and social workers provide psychiatric home care for individuals who are homebound.
- Assertive community treatment (ACT) is an intensive case management for people who are unable or unwilling to participate in traditional treatment. ACT teams are composed of a variety of professionals who provide 24-hour, 7-days-a-week support.
- Intensive outpatient and partial hospitalization programs are available as a step-down from inpatient care or as a step-up from other less restrictive treatment settings.
- Emergency psychiatric care and crisis stabilization is available in emergency rooms and from emergency teams.
- Primary, secondary, and tertiary prevention are aimed at reducing the effects of mental illness by preventing its occurrence, preventing its progression, or by restoring functional ability.
- Inpatient settings include crisis stabilization units, general hospital and private hospital acute care, and a state-funded acute care system.
- Inpatient psychiatric-mental health nursing requires strong skills in management, communication, and collaboration.
- Basic level inpatient nursing interventions include admission, providing a safe environment, psychiatric and physical assessments, milieu management, documentation, medication administration, and preparation for discharge to the community.

▌ CRITICAL THINKING

1. You are a nurse working at a local community mental health center and doing an assessment of Dion, a 45-year-old single patient. Dion reports that he has not been sleeping and that his thoughts seem to be "all tangled up." Although Dion does not admit directly to being suicidal, he remarks, "I hope that this helps today because I don't know how much longer I can go on like this."

Dion is disheveled and has been sleeping in homeless shelters. He has little contact with his family and becomes agitated when you suggest that it might be helpful to contact them. He reports a recent hospitalization at the local

veterans' hospital and previous treatment at a dual-diagnosis facility, yet he denies substance use. When asked about his physical condition, he says that he has tested positive for hepatitis C and is "supposed to take" multiple medications that he cannot name.

   a. List your concerns about this patient in order of priority.
   b. Which of these concerns must be addressed before he leaves the clinic today?
   c. Do you feel there is an immediate need to consult with any other members of the interprofessional team today about this patient?

d. Keeping in mind the concept of patient-centered care, how will you start to develop trust with the patient to increase his involvement with the treatment plan?

2. Imagine that you were asked for your opinion with regard to your patient's ability to make everyday decisions independently. What sorts of things would you consider as you weighed safety versus autonomy and personal rights?

3. If nurses function as equal members of the interprofessional mental health team, what differentiates the nurse from the other members of the team?

CHAPTER REVIEW

1. A patient needs supportive care for the maintenance treatment of bipolar disorder. The new nurse demonstrates an understanding of the services provided by the various members of the patient's mental healthcare team when he makes which statement:
   a "Your social worker will help you learn to budget your money effectively."
   b "Your counselor asked me to remind you of the group session on critical thinking at 2:00 today."
   c "The mental health technician on staff today will administer the medication that you require."
   d "Remember to ask the occupational therapist about sources of financial help that you are qualified for."

2. A patient has been voluntarily admitted to a mental health facility after an unsuccessful attempt to harm himself. Which statement demonstrates a need to better educate the patient on his patient's rights?
   a. "I understand why I was restrained when I was out of control."
   b. "You can't tell my boss about the suicide attempt without my permission."
   c. "I have a right to know what all of you are planning to do to me."
   d. "I can hurt myself if I want to. It's none of your business."

3. Which intervention demonstrates an attempt by nursing staff to meet the goals identified by The Joint Commission as National Patient Safety Goals? *Select all that apply.*
   a. Identifying patients using both name and date of birth before drawing blood.
   b. Sitting with the patient diagnosed with an eating disorder during meals.
   c. Administering the Beck Scale on each patient at the time of admission.
   d. Performing a medication history assessment on each new patient.
   e. Using appropriate hand washing technique at all times.

4. The mental health team is determining treatment options for a male patient who is experiencing psychotic symptoms. Which question(s) should the team answer to determine whether a community outpatient or inpatient setting is most appropriate? *Select all that apply.*
   a. "Is the patient expressing suicidal thoughts?"
   b. "Does the patient have intact judgment and insight into his situation?"
   c. "Does the patient have experiences with either community or inpatient mental healthcare facilities?"
   d. "Does the patient require a therapeutic environment to support the management of psychotic symptoms?"
   e. "Does the patient require the regular involvement of their family/significant other in planning and executing the plan of care?"

5. The nurse frequently includes daily sessions involving relaxation techniques. Which assessment data would most indicate a need for this intervention to be included in the initial plan of care for a patient?
   a. Family history of anxiety and symptoms of anxiety
   b. Significant other has a chronic health issue
   c. Hopes to retire in 6 months
   d. Recently adopted infant twins

6. A newly divorced 36-year-old mother of three has difficulty sleeping. When she shares this information to her gynecologist, she suggests which of the following services as appropriate for her patient's needs?
   a. Assertive community treatment
   b. Patient-centered medical home
   c. Psychiatric home care
   d. Primary care provider

7. An Afghanistan Conflict veteran has been homeless since being discharged from military service. He is now diagnosed with schizophrenia. The nurse practitioner recognizes that assertive community treatment (ACT) is a good option for this patient since ACT provides:
   a. Psychiatric home care
   b. Care for hard-to-engage, seriously ill patients
   c. Outpatient community mental health center care
   d. A comprehensive emergency service model

8. An adolescent female is readmitted for inpatient care after a suicide attempt. What is the most important nursing intervention to accomplish upon admission?
   a. Allowing the patient to return to her previous room so that she will feel safe
   b. Orienting the patient to the unit and introducing her to patients and staff
   c. Building trust through therapeutic communication
   d. Checking the patient's belongings for dangerous items

9. Emma is a 40-year-old married female who has found it increasingly difficult to leave her home due to agoraphobia. Emma's family is appropriately concerned and suggests that she seek psychiatric care. After investigating her options, Emma decides to try:
   a. Telepsychiatry
   b. Assertive community treatment
   c. Psychiatric home care
   d. Outpatient psychiatric care

10. Pablo is a homeless adult who has no family connection. Pablo passed out on the street and emergency medical

services took him to the hospital, where he expresses a wish to die. The physician recognizes evidence of substance use problems and mental health issues and recommends inpatient treatment for Pablo. What is the rationale for this treatment choice? *Select all that apply.*

   a. Intermittent supervision is available in inpatient settings.
   b. He requires stabilization of multiple symptoms.
   c. He has nutritional and self-care needs.
   d. Medication adherence will be mandated.
   e. He is in imminent danger of harming himself.

1. **b**; 2. **d**; 3. **a, c, d, e**; 4. **a, b, d, e**; 5. **a**; 6. **d**; 7. **b**; 8. **d**; 9. **a**; 10. **b, c, e**

⊕ Visit the Evolve website for a posttest on the content in this chapter: http://evolve.elsevier.com/Varcarolis

REFERENCES

Agency for Healthcare Research and Quality. (n.d.). *Defining the PCMH*. Retrieved from http://www.pcmh.ahrq.gov/page/defining-pcmh.

American Psychiatric Association. (2019). *The evidence base in telepsychiatry*. Retrieved from https://www.psychiatry.org/psychiatrists/practice/telepsychiatry/toolkit/evidence-base.

American Psychological Association. (2014). Incarceration nation. *Monitor on Psychology, 45*(9). Retrieved from http://www.apa.org/monitor/2014/10/incarceration.aspx.

Boyce, G. (n.d.). Telepsychiatry: What to look for in 2018. Retrieved from https://arraybc.com/news-media/telepsychiatry-what-to-look-for-in-2018.

Gradus, J. L. (2019). Epidemiology of PTSD. United States Department of Veterans Affairs. Retrieved from https://www.ptsd.va.gov/professional/treat/essentials/epidemiology.asp.

Hooker, E. A., Mallow, P. J., & Oglesby, M. M. (2019). Characteristics and trends of emergency department visits in the United States (2010-2014). *Journal of Emergency Medicine, 56*(3), 344–3451.

National Association of State Mental Health Directors. (2017). *Trends in total psychiatric inpatient and other 24-hour residential treatment capacity*. Retrieved from https://www.nri-inc.org/media/1302/t-lutterman-and-r-manderscheid-distribution-of-psychiatric-inpatient-capacity-united-states.pdf.

National Association of State Mental Health Directors. (2019). State hospital organizations. Retrieved from https://www.nasmhpd.org/content/state-hospital-organizations.

Peplau, H. E. (1989). Interpersonal constructs for nursing practice. In A. W. O'Toole, & S. R. Welt (Eds.), *Interpersonal theory in nursing practice: Selected works of Hildegard E. Peplau* (pp. 42–55). New York, NY: Putnam.

Substance Abuse and Mental Health Services Administration (SAMHSA). (2019). *Key substance use and mental health indicators in the United States: Results from the 2018 National Survey on Drug Use and Health*. Retrieved from https://www.samhsa.gov/data/.

Substance Abuse and Mental Health Services Administration (SAMHSA). (2019). *Recovery and recovery support*. Retrieved from http://www.samhsa.gov/recovery.

Torrey, E. G., Zdanowicz, M. T., Kennard, A. D., Lamb, H. R., Eslinger, D. F., Biasotti, M. I., & Fuller, D. A. (2014). *The treatment of persons with mental illness in prisons and jails: A state survey*. Retrieved from https://nicic.gov/treatment-persons-mental-illness-prisons-and-jails-state-survey.

World Health Organization. (2012). *Mental health policy, planning and service development*. Retrieved from http://www.who.int/mental_health/policy/services/en/index.html.

5

Cultural Implications

Rick Zoucha and Kimberly M. Wolf

Visit the Evolve website for a pretest on the content in this chapter: http://evolve.elsevier.com/Varcarolis

OBJECTIVES

1. Define key cultural terms, including minority, race, ethnicity, and culture.
2. Explain the importance of culturally relevant care in psychiatric–mental health nursing practice.
3. Discuss potential problems in applying Western methods of care to patients of other cultures.
4. Compare and contrast Western nursing beliefs, values, and practices with the beliefs, values, and practices of patients from diverse cultures.
5. Identify cultural barriers to accessing and providing mental health services.
6. Discuss special at-risk populations, including immigrants, refugees, and cultural minorities.
7. Perform culturally sensitive assessments that include risk factors and barriers to quality mental healthcare that culturally diverse patients frequently encounter.
8. Develop culturally congruent nursing care plans for all patients.

KEY TERMS AND CONCEPTS

acculturation
assimilation
cultural competence
cultural concepts of distress
cultural encounters
cultural explanations
cultural idioms of distress
culturally congruent practice
cultural norms

cultural syndromes
culture
Eastern tradition
enculturation
ethnicity
ethnocentrism
Indigenous culture
minority
multiple heritage

pharmacogenetics
race
refugee
somatization
stereotyping
stigma
Western tradition
worldview

How a society views psychiatric conditions and disorders has an impact on how mental health resources are allocated and how mental healthcare is funded. Societal attitudes also affect whether individuals are access mental healthcare and the type of treatments in which they engage. Stigma—negative attitudes toward mental illness and its treatment—is a phenomenon found across cultures globally.

What constitutes a psychiatric disorder or mental health condition and its subsequent treatment are culturally influenced or based. Not all racial/ethnic/cultural groups in the United States have the same beliefs about mental health and illness. According to a Substance Abuse and Mental Health Services Administration report (SAMHSA, 2015), discrepancies in the use of mental health services among racial/ethnic groups are a national problem.

Psychiatric–mental health nurses can help to address discrepancies by promoting culturally relevant and congruent nursing care that meets the needs of a diverse patient population. All mental health providers should strive to promote care as congruent as possible with patients' cultural beliefs, values, and practices.

MINORITY, RACE, ETHNICITY, AND CULTURE

Before examining broader issues in terms of culturally relevant care, we will review words and terms associated with culture. These terms include *minority, race, ethnicity, culture,* and *cultural norms.*

Minority

The term minority refers to groups characterized by their own cultural, ethnic, religious, or religious identity, which differs from that of the majority population. Sometimes, groups with a numerical majority may also find themselves in a minority-like position, lacking in in political or social power. For example, although the numbers of men and women in the world are roughly equal, women experience social inequalities relative to men in most societies. Other minority groups include disabled individuals, gender and sexuality minorities, and political minorities.

Race

In the United States and other countries, race has traditionally reflected social definitions based on biology, anthropology, and, more recently, genetics. Race categories are now recognized as including racial and national origins and sociocultural groups. Furthermore, many people identify themselves as biracial or multiracial. Recent US census forms (United Census Bureau, 2018a) included a check-box list for race along with a write-in area where individuals could self-identify or specify their racial identity. The races that were in the 2020 census include White, Black or African American, American Indian or Alaska Native, Asian, Native Hawaiian or Pacific Islander, or some other race.

Ethnicity

Ethnic groups have a common heritage and history, which is referred to as ethnicity. These groups may share a worldview, a system of thinking about how the world works and how people should act, especially in relation to one another. Ethnic groups may share beliefs, values, and practices that guide members of the group in how they think and act in different situations.

Increasingly, there are emerging groups of people in the United States who do not identify in terms of a single race or ethnicity. The term multiple heritage refers to biracial, multiracial, biethnic, and multiethnic individuals (Jeffreys & Zoucha, 2017).

Culture

Culture is the shared beliefs, values, and practices that guide a group's members in patterned ways of thinking and acting. Culture includes religious, geographic, socioeconomic, occupational, ability- or disability-related, and sexual orientation–related beliefs and behaviors. Each group has cultural beliefs, values, and practices that guide its members in ways of thinking and acting.

Cultural norms are attitudes and behaviors that are culturally defined and considered normal, typical, or average within a given group. Because cultural norms prescribe what is normal and abnormal, culture helps to develop concepts of mental health and illness.

For us as nurses, assessing cultural needs is paramount in providing culturally and holistically congruent care. Providing this type of care works best when planning is done in collaboration with the patient and family (when desirable and practical) and other members of the treatment team.

Measuring Race and Ethnicity in the United States

One purpose of categorizing individuals according to racial-ethnic descriptions is to help the government understand the needs of its citizens. The US Census helps to identify disparities in healthcare along racial and ethnic lines. The recording of these classifications also helps to determine when and how the healthcare needs of these populations are being met.

Despite the benefits, classifying groups of people can be confusing, confounding, and offensive. Consider the following:

- There are more than 573 federally recognized Indian Nations. About 229 of these ethnically, culturally, and linguistically diverse nations exist in Alaska (National Council for American Indians, 2019).
- The cultural norms of Blacks or African Americans whose ancestors were brought to the United States centuries ago are different from the norms of those who have recently immigrated from Africa or the Caribbean.
- Americans of European origin are a diverse group; some have been in the United States for hundreds of years, and some are new immigrants.
- Latinx (gender-neutral or nonbinary form of Latino and Latina) relates to people of Latin American origin or descent. However, all of its members are also members of a racial group or groups, such as White, Black, Native American, Mexican American, Puerto Rican, and Cuban American.
- Persons from the Middle East and the Arabian subcontinent are considered White in the US Census Bureau's classification system.

The difficulty of classifying minority groups continues to be an issue. As previously discussed, the 2020 census used two separate questions for capturing race and ethnicity (US Census Bureau, 2018a). The Census collected data regarding multiple Hispanic ethnicities, adding a write-in area for the racial category, and adding examples of a few of the racial categories, including White, Black, American Indian, and Alaska Native.

DEMOGRAPHIC SHIFTS IN THE UNITED STATES

In 2045, the United States is projected for the first time to become a majority-minority nation. This change means that no one group will make up the majority or make up 51% of the population (US Census Bureau, 2018b). However, non-Hispanic Whites will continue to remain the largest single group. The Hispanic and Asian populations are growing at the fastest rates. A comparison of population composition in 2016 and the projected population for 2060 is shown in Table 5.1.

TABLE 5.1 Year 2060 Population Projections (Percentage of Total Population)		
	2016	**2060**
White, non-Hispanic	61.3	44.3
Black, non-Hispanic	13.3	15
Hispanic (of any race)	17.8	27.5
Asian	5.7	9.1
Two or more races	2.6	6.2
American Indian and Alaska Native	1.3	1.4
Native Hawaiian or Other Pacific Islander	0.2	0.3

Population percentages are rounded to the nearest 0.1%.
Data from US Census Bureau. (2017). *Percentage distribution of population in the US in 2016 and 2060, by race and Hispanic origin.* Retrieved from https://www.statista.com/statistics/270272/percentage-of-us-population-by-ethnicities/.

BASIC WORLDVIEWS

Western Tradition

Nursing theories, psychological theories, and the understanding of mental health and illness used by nurses in the United States derive from a Western philosophical and scientific framework based on Western cultural ideals, beliefs, and values. Because psychiatric–mental health nursing is grounded in Western culture, nurses should be aware of how their assumptions regarding personality development, emotional expression, ego boundaries, culture, cultural expressions of mental illness, and interpersonal relationships affect their care of any patient.

A long history of Western science and European-American norms of mental health has shaped present-day American beliefs and values regarding people. Our understanding of how a person relates to the world and to others is based on Greek, Roman, and Judeo-Christian thought.

In the Western tradition, a person finds identity in individuality. Individuality is accompanied by the values of autonomy, independence, and self-reliance. Mind and body are two separate entities. Because they are seen as separate, different practitioners treat disorders of the mind versus those of the body. Disease has a specific, measurable, and observable cause, and care providers focus treatment on eliminating the cause. Time is seen as linear, always moving forward, and waiting for no one. Success in life is achieved by preparing for the future.

Eastern Tradition

The Eastern tradition is based on Chinese and Indian philosophers and the spiritual traditions of Confucianism, Taoism, Buddhism, and Hinduism. Native Americans, African tribes, Australian and New Zealand aborigines, and tribal peoples on other continents frequently include rich cultural traditions based on deep personal connections to the natural world and the tribe.

Eastern tradition and some Western collective cultures see the family as the basis for a person's identity; family interdependence and group decision making are the norm. Time is circular and recurring and consistent with a belief in reincarnation. One is born into an unchangeable fate based on one's past life; therefore, having a child that is mentally ill may be viewed as a punishment for one's behavior in a past life (Camann & Wilson, 2017).

Indigenous Culture

The term Indigenous culture refers to the culture of people who have inhabited a country or a geographical region at the time when people of different cultures or ethnic origins arrived. Indigenous cultures include such groups as the New Zealand Maoris, indigenous Australians, Native Americans, and Native Hawaiians. These groups may place special significance on the place of humans within the natural world. There may be less of a concept of person; instead, a person is an entity in relation to others. The holistic view of body-mind-spirit may be so complete that there may be no adequate words in the language to describe them as separate entities. Disease may be considered to be caused by a lack of harmony with others or the environment.

Worldview shapes how cultures perceive reality, the person, and the person in relation to the world and to others. Worldview also shapes perceptions about time, health and illness, and rights and obligations in society. Table 5.2 provides an overview of core differences among Western, Eastern, and Indigenous culture. The three worldviews compared here are broad categories and generalizations created to contrast some of the themes found in diverse world cultures. We are speaking in general terms in the description of these differences and are in no way indicating that individuals or individual cultures share the same worldviews.

TABLE 5.2 **Worldviews**		
Western	**Eastern**	**Indigenous**
Roman, Greek, Judeo-Christian; the Enlightenment; Descartes	Chinese and Indian philosophers: Buddha, Confucius, Lao-tse	Deep relationship with nature
The "real" has form and essence; reality tends to be stable	The "real" is a force or energy; reality is always changing	The "real" is multidimensional; reality transcends time and space
Cartesian dualism: body and mind-spirit	Mind-body-spirit unity	Mind, body, and spirit are united; there may not be words to indicate them as distinct entities
Self is the starting point of identity	Family is the starting point of identity	Community is the starting point of identity; a person is only an entity in relation to others; there may be no concept of person or personal ownership
Time is linear	Time is circular, flexible	Time is focused on the present
Wisdom: preparation for the future	Wisdom: acceptance of what is	Wisdom: knowledge of nature
Disease has a cause (e.g., pathogen, toxin) that creates the effect; disease can be observed and measured	Disease is caused by a lack of balance in energy forces (e.g., yin-yang, hot-cold); imbalance between daily routine, diet, and constitutional type	Disease is caused by a lack of personal, interpersonal, environmental, or spiritual harmony; thoughts and words can shape reality; evil spirits exist

IMPACT OF CULTURE

Cultures develop norms consistent with their worldviews and adapted to their own historical experiences and the influences of the outside world. Cultures are evolutionary; they change and adjust.

Nonverbal communication. Each culture has different patterns of nonverbal communication (Table 5.3). For instance, in the American culture, eye contact is a sign of respectful attention, but in many other cultures, it is considered arrogant and intrusive. In Western culture, emotional expressiveness is valued, but in other cultures, it may be a sign of immaturity.

Etiquette. People tend to feel offended when their rules for polite behavior are violated. However, the rules for polite behavior vary greatly from one culture to another. Unless we are aware of cultural differences in etiquette norms, we could infer rudeness on the part of patients. In reality, they are operating from a different set of cultural norms and believe their behavior to be respectful. Box 5.1 identifies norms for etiquette that may be different based on the prevailing culture.

Beliefs and values. Cultural beliefs and values that are dominant in the United States are often in contrast with those that are common in other cultures. Beliefs and values and health and illness are contrasted in Table 5.4.

A culture's worldview, beliefs, values, and practices are transmitted to its members. This enculturation occurs as children learn from parents which behaviors, beliefs, values, and actions are right and which are wrong in the context of their culture. The individual is free to make choices, but the culture expects these choices to be made from its acceptable range of options.

BOX 5.1   Norms of Etiquette

Norms of etiquette that vary across cultures include the following:
- Whether promptness is expected and how important it is to be on time
- How formal one should be in addressing others
- Which people deserve recognition and honor and how respect is shown
- Whether shaking hands and other forms of social touch are appropriate
- Whether or not shoes can be worn in the home
- How much clothing should be worn to be modest
- What it means to accept or reject offers of food or drink and other gestures of hospitality
- What importance is given to small talk and how long it should continue before getting down to business
- Whether communication should be direct or subtle
- What the tone of voice and pace of the conversation should be
- Which topics are considered taboo
- The degree of attention that children receive

Deviance from cultural expectations may be defined by the cultural group as illness. Mental health is often considered to be the degree to which a person fulfills the expectations of the culture. The culture defines which differences are still within the range of normal (mentally healthy) and which are outside that range (mentally ill). The same thoughts and behaviors considered mentally healthy in one culture can indicate mental illness in another.

People are raised to view the world through their own cultural lens, and nurses are no exception. We are products of our own culture and that of professional socialization. Nurses may think that the only good care is the care they have learned to believe in, value, and practice. This sort of thinking can lead to

---

TABLE 5.3   Selected Nonverbal Communication Patterns

Nonverbal Communication	Patterns in the United States	Patterns in Other Cultures
Eye contact	Eye contact is associated with attentiveness, politeness, respect, honesty, and self-confidence.	Eye contact may be avoided as a sign of rudeness, arrogance, challenge, or sexual interest.
Personal space	*Intimate space:* 0–1.5 ft *Personal space:* 1.5–4 ft In a personal conversation, if a person enters into the intimate space of the other, the person is perceived as aggressive, overbearing, and offensive. If a person stays more distant than expected, the person is perceived as aloof.	Personal space is closer or more distant than in US culture. When closer is the norm, standing very close may indicates acceptance of the other.
Touch	Moderate touch indicates personal warmth and conveys caring	Touch norms vary. *Low-touch cultures*—Touch may be considered a sexual gesture or taboo between men and women *High-touch cultures*—People touch one another frequently and may link arms or hold hands
Facial expressions and gestures	A nod means "yes." Smiling and nodding means "I agree." Thumbs up means "good job." Rolling one's eyes while another is talking is an insult.	Raising eyebrows or rolling the head from side to side means "yes." Smiling and nodding means "I respect you." Thumbs up may be a negative gesture. Pointing one's foot at another may be an insult.

TABLE 5.4 Cultural Beliefs and Values About Health and Illness

	Western Perspective	Potential Perspectives of Other Cultures
Health	Absence of disease Ability to function at a high level	Being in a state of balance Being in a state of harmony Ability to perform family roles
Disease causation	Measurable, observable cause that leads to measurable, observable effect Pathogens, mutant cells, toxins, or poor diet	Frequently intangible, immeasurable cause Lack of balance (yin and yang) Lack of harmony with the environment
Location of disorder	Dualism of body and mind	Whole entity (mind, body, and spirit) are impacted. Disorder causing disease in the person may be in the family or environment.
Decisions about care	Made by patient or holder of power of attorney Goals are autonomy and confidentiality. Patient should have information to make decisions.	Made by the whole family or family head Goals are protection and support of the patient. Patient should be protected from knowledge of the prognosis.
Sick role	Sick people should be as independent and self-reliant as possible. Self-care is encouraged; one gets better by getting up and getting going.	Family members should take care of and care for the sick person. Passivity promotes recovery.
Best treatments	Provider-prescribed medications and treatments Medical technology	Counteracting negative forces with positive ones and vice versa Treatment by traditional healers and remedies
Pain	Quantitative scales tend to be useful. Able to pinpoint location of pain Pain may not be expressed openly.	Quantitative scales may be less useful. Pain may be experienced globally. Pain may be expressed openly.
Ethics Patient protection from painful knowledge	Based on bioethical principles of autonomy, beneficence, justice, and confidentiality. Informed consent requires truthfulness.	Based on virtue or community needs Hope should be preserved and painful truth hidden. Support and care should be provided. Utilitarian emphasis is on greatest good for the greatest number.

Copyright © 2002, 2004 by Mary Curry Narayan.

ethnocentrism, which is the universal tendency of humans to think that their way of thinking and behaving is the only correct and natural way (Purnell, 2018).

CULTURAL BARRIERS TO MENTAL HEALTH SERVICES

US healthcare providers are increasingly aware of the importance of engaging in culturally appropriate care. Yet barriers continue to prevent culturally nondominant persons from seeking the care they need as well as preventing psychiatric nurses from providing the care they want to give (Wolf, Umland, & Lo, 2019). The following sections describe issues that nurses are likely to encounter when they are providing care to culturally diverse patients. Suggestions to overcome these barriers are provided.

Communication Barriers

Communication is a key aspect of caring for patients. However, a major obstacle exists when providers and patients do not speak the same language or when the patient is hard of hearing or deaf. The US Department of Health and Human Services

(HHS) Office of Minority Health (2018) states that healthcare organizations should provide language assistance services at all points of contact and in a timely manner during all hours of operation. These services should be provided at no cost to patients with limited English proficiency or who have reduced hearing ability or no ability to hear.

One essential language service is that of a professional interpreter. Interpreters should match the patient as closely as possible in terms of gender, age, and social status. This close match allows the interpreter to help not only with the language but also to act as a cultural broker, bridging one culture to the other.

Especially important in psychiatric settings, interpreters should not be relatives or friends of the patient. Embarrassing topics may not be shared with healthcare providers. The gender of the patient, the interpreter, and the provider may also impact the flow of information depending upon the gender hierarchy. Relatives and friends may not have the language skills necessary to meet the demands of interpretation, which is a complex task, particularly with medical terms and medications. Additionally, literal translations of words in one language can carry many different connotations in the other language. Certain concepts are so culturally linked that an adequate translation is difficult.

For instance, the terms *feeling blue* or *feeling down* may have no meaning at all in the patient's literal understanding of English.

In addition to interpreters for the spoken word, translators provide patients with written materials in the language that they understand. The use of a professional translator can be critically important in healthcare settings where a serious translation error could be a matter of life or death.

Stigma of Mental Illness

Mental illnesses are commonly stigmatized in the United States. This stigma presents significant barriers that delay or prevent individuals from seeking treatment. People often associate mental illness with weakness or dangerousness. However, in some cultural groups, the stigma of mental illness may be more severe and prevalent.

In cultural groups that emphasize the interdependence and harmony of the family, mental illness may be perceived as a failure of the family. The pressures on both the individual with the mental illness and the family are increased as attempts at concealment of the problem are made. In this view, the individual and family are both tainted by the illness, which reflects badly on the character of the family. Stigma and shame can lead to reluctance to seek help, so members of these cultural groups may delay or prevent entry into the mental healthcare system.

Misdiagnosis

Another barrier to mental healthcare is misdiagnosis. One reason for misdiagnosis is the use of culturally inaccurate assessment tools, because most of the available tools are validated using subjects of European origin.

In cultures where the body and mind are considered one entity or in those where a high degree of stigma is associated with mental health problems, individuals frequently somatize their feelings of psychological distress. In somatization, psychological distress is experienced as physical problems. For example, a woman may describe feelings of back pain, fatigue, and dizziness and say nothing about her feelings of sadness or hopelessness.

Somatization is just one example of how psychological distress is manifested in a way that seems different. Psychiatric diagnostic criteria that were developed based on studies with predominantly White U.S. participants are often invalid when they are applied to individuals from other cultures.

The impact of cultural concepts on a psychiatric diagnosis is reflected in the diagnostic criteria of the American Psychiatric Association's (APA, 2013a) fifth edition of the *Diagnostic and Statistical Manual of Mental Disorders* (*DSM-5*). The *DSM-5* also includes a standardized tool for taking into account cultural variations during the assessment phase of patient care. The Cultural Formulation Interview (APA, 2013a) is a 16-question inventory that helps clinicians plan for care based on orientation, values, and assumptions that originate from particular cultures. It takes into consideration the meaning of the illness for the patient, the role of family and others as support, the patient's attempts to cope with previous illness, and expectations of current care. The Cultural Formulation Interview is available online and can be reproduced without permission by clinicians and researchers.

Cultural Concepts of Distress

All forms of distress are local constructs and locally shaped. That is, distress is defined and descriptions are developed within the context of the culture. Even commonly diagnosed US disorders included in the *DSM-5* probably originated as cultural syndromes that eventually gained wide acceptance with the support of research.

In the previous edition of the *DSM*, a list of 25 "culture-bound syndromes" was included. These syndromes were defined as a combination of psychiatric and somatic symptoms that were considered to be recognizable diseases within a specific society or culture. The *DSM-5* (2013) eliminated the term *culture-bound syndromes* and replaced it with cultural concepts of distress. This term takes into account the way in which groups experience, understand, and communicate problematic behaviors, suffering, or troubling emotions and thoughts (APA, 2013a). The three main types of cultural concepts are cultural idioms of distress, cultural explanations or perceived causes, and cultural syndromes.

When the dominant culture encounters people with different cultural concepts of distress, the stage is set for miscommunication and a further barrier to care. One way in which people communicate emotional suffering is through cultural idioms of distress. These are specific ways of expressing distress that people in particular cultures understand. In the United States, saying, "I was as sick as a dog" or "I'm a nervous wreck" may refer to a variety of problems and not a specific disorder. Imagine how people from other cultures might literally interpret those comments.

Cultural explanations or **perceived causes** refer to explanations for symptoms, illness, or distress understood within the context of a particular culture. These explanations may be important features of folk classifications for disease that may be used by laypeople or healers. For example, it was once common to explain obsessive-compulsive symptoms or seizures as being the result of demonic possession.

Cultural syndromes exist when clusters of symptoms occur in specific groups and are recognized by these groups as a known pattern of experience. Cultural syndromes may seem exotic or irrational to nurses who have been trained within a Western medical framework. The symptoms may be shocking, and other-culture explanations regarding causation and treatment may be mystifying. These illnesses, however, are usually well understood by the people within the cultural group. They know the name of the problem, its etiology (i.e., cause), its course, and the way it should be treated. Frequently, when these illnesses are treated in culturally prescribed ways, the remedies are quite effective.

There are many cultural syndromes. Some syndromes seem to be mental health problems manifested in somatic ways. These syndromes are typically given a distinct name. *Hwa-byung* and *neurasthenia* have many similarities to depression and do not carry the degree of stigma associated with a mental disorder.

Because the somatic complaints are so prominent and patients frequently deny feelings of sadness or depression, they may not fit the *DSM-5* diagnostic criteria for depression.

Ataque de nervios and *ghost sickness* belong to another group of culture-based illnesses characterized by a variety of behaviors. These illnesses seem to be culturally acceptable ways for patients to express that they can no longer endure the stressors in their lives. People in the culture understand the patient is ill and provide support using culturally prescribed treatments, which often relieve the symptoms. A list of some of the syndromes that psychiatric nurses may see is provided in Box 5.2.

When we consider culture in diagnosis and treatment, we are more likely to see culturally different behavior as normal. For example, in some Christian demoninations, it may be common to refer to spiritual experiences in terms such as "I was talking to Jesus this morning." Rather than considering the speaker to be delusional, the care provider should understand that the person was praying. If a Vietnamese father says he tried to take the wind illness out of his child by vigorously rubbing a coin down her back, the care provider may understand that the father is not a potential threat to the child.

Genetic Variation in Pharmacodynamics

Another clinical practice issue that presents a barrier to quality mental health services for some groups is genetic variation in drug responses. There is a growing realization that many drugs vary in their actions and effects along genetic and psychosocial lines (Burchum & Rosenthal, 2018). In most clinical trials a high percentage of participants are White, while other racial subgroups are underrepresented.

The field of pharmacogenetics focuses on how genes affect individual responses to medicines (National Institutes of Health, 2020). Genes carry "recipes" for making specific protein molecules. Medications interact with thousands of proteins, and the smallest difference in the quantities or composition of these molecules can make a big difference in how they work. By understanding how genes influence drug responses, we hope one day to be able to prescribe drugs that are uniquely suited for each patient.

Genetic variations in drug metabolism have been documented for several classifications of drugs, including antidepressants and antipsychotics. An important variation that affects the ability to metabolize drugs relates to the more than 20 cytochrome P-450 (CYP) enzymes present in human beings (Chen et al., 2018). Genetic variations in these enzymes may alter drug metabolism, and these variations tend to be propagated through racial/ethnic populations.

CYP enzymes metabolize most antidepressants and antipsychotics. Some genetic variations result in rapid metabolism, and if the body metabolizes medications too quickly, serum levels become too low, thus minimizing therapeutic effects. Other variations may result in poor metabolism. If the body metabolizes medications too slowly, serum levels become too high, thus increasing the risk of intolerable side effects.

Although genetic testing to support prescribing practices has gained widespread attention and support rapidly, some

---

BOX 5.2   Examples of Cultural Syndromes and Explanations

There are many cultural syndromes; however, they cannot all be described in this chapter. The following list includes some of the syndromes that might be encountered by the psychiatric–mental health nurse.

Ataque de nervios: Latin American. Characterized by a sudden attack of trembling, palpitations, dyspnea, dizziness, and loss of consciousness. Thought to be caused by an evil spirit and related to intolerable stress. Treated by an espiritista (spiritual healer) and by the support of the family and community who provide aid to the patient.

Ghost sickness: Navajo. Characterized by "being out of one's mind," dyspnea, weakness, and bad dreams. Thought to be caused by an evil spirit. Treated by overcoming the evil spirit with a stronger spiritual force the healer, a "singer," calls forth through a powerful healing ritual.

Hwa-byung: Korean. Characterized by epigastric pain, anorexia, palpitations, dyspnea, and muscle aches and pains. Thought to be caused by a lack of harmony in the body or in interpersonal relationships. Treated by reestablishing harmony. Some feel that it is closely related to depression.

"Jin" possession: Somalian. Symptoms of psychological distress and anxiety. Thought to be caused by possession by a Jin, an invisible being that is angry with the human. Intermittent, involuntary, abnormal body movements occur along with the psychological distress. Treatment consists of an exorcism by a religious leader, such as an Imam, who will ask the Jin what the person has done to anger it so that the person can apologize and make amends. (Somali inpatient psychiatric nurse, personal communication, March 8, 2012.)

Neurasthenia: Chinese. Characterized by somatic symptoms of depression such as anorexia, weight loss, fatigue, weakness, trouble concentrating, and insomnia. Feelings of sadness or depression are denied. Thought to be related to a lack of yin-yang balance. Traditional treatment includes eating healthier, exercise, massage, rest, and lifestyle adjustment. Antidepressant therapy is now common.

Susto: Latin American. Characterized by a broad range of somatic and psychological symptoms similar to posttraumatic stress disorder. Precipitated by a traumatic incident or fright that caused the patient's soul to leave the body. Treated by an espiritista (spiritual healer).

Wind illness: Chinese, Vietnamese. Characterized by a fear of cold, wind, or drafts. Derived from the belief that yin-yang and hot-cold elements must be in balance in the body or illness occurs. Treated by keeping warm and avoiding foods, drinks, and herbs that are cold or considered to have a cold quality as well as cold colors, emotions, and activities. Also treated by pulling the "cold wind" out of the patient by coining (vigorously rubbing a coin over the body) or cupping (applying a heated cup to the skin, creating a vacuum).

---

individuals and groups are not so enthusiastic. One high authority, the US Food and Drug Administration (FDA, 2019), has issued strong warnings about misleading the public as to the evidence behind genetic testing. It contends that patients are being put at risk with false promises of positive responses to certain drugs. These reports may keep patients from using medications that could actually help them.

SPECIAL AT-RISK POPULATIONS

Many people of the nondominant cultures in the United States are subject to experiences that challenge their mental health in ways that members of the majority group do not have to face. Among these challenges are issues related to the experience of being an immigrant, a refugee, or living in poverty.

Immigrants

Immigrants face many unknowns. Upon arriving in the United States, they may not speak English, yet they must learn how to navigate their new country's economic, political, legal, educational, transportation, and healthcare systems. Many who had status and skills in their homelands—having been teachers, physicians, or other professionals—find that, because of licensing and certification requirements or their own limited language skills, only unskilled jobs are open to them.

After immigration, traditional family roles may be challenged by women finding jobs more easily than men. Immigrant families may find the struggle to live successfully in the United States arduous and wearisome. Long-honored cultural values and traditions, which once provided stability, are challenged by new cultural norms. During the period of adjustment, many immigrants find that the hope that led them to immigrate quickly turns into anxiety and depression.

Immigrants and their families embark on a process of **acculturation**—learning the beliefs, values, and practices of their new cultural setting—that sometimes takes several generations to complete. Some immigrants adapt to the new culture quickly, absorbing the new worldview, beliefs, values, and practices rapidly, until they are more natural than the ones with which they arrived. This process of adaptation is called **assimilation**. Others attempt to maintain their traditional cultural ways. Some may become bicultural—able to move in and out of their traditional culture and their new culture. Some immigrants may suffer culture shock, finding the new norms disconcerting or offensive because they contrast so deeply with their traditional beliefs, values, and practices.

Children tend to assimilate the new culture at a rapid pace, whereas older adults are more likely to maintain their traditional cultural beliefs, values, and practices. This sets the stage for intergenerational conflict. Children who are assimilating different values about family may challenge the traditional status of elders in a hierarchical family. Some children may feel lost between two cultures and unsure of where to place their cultural identity.

Refugees

A **refugee** is a special kind of immigrant. In general, immigrants seek to move to a new location, value the new culture, and hope to benefit by a change in life circumstances. In comparison, refugees leave their homeland to escape intolerable conditions; they have been forced to flee and may have preferred to remain within their native country. Refugees do not perceive entry into the new culture as an active choice and may experience the stress of adjusting as being imposed on them. In addition, both refugees and immigrants may not always feel welcome in the United States, depending on location, and this may add to their stress and anxiety.

Refugees from the Middle East, Southeast Asia, Central America, and Africa may have been traumatized by such events as war, genocide, torture, and starvation. Many have lost family members, a way of life, and a homeland to which they can never return. The degree of trauma and loss they have experienced may make them particularly vulnerable to a variety of psychiatric disorders, including major depressive disorder and posttraumatic stress disorder.

Poverty

Individuals who are considered minorities (non-Whites or Whites of non-European heritage) may be vulnerable to a variety of disadvantages, including poverty and limited opportunities for education and jobs. Cultural minority groups are frequent victims of bias, discrimination, and racism—subtle but pervasive forms of rejection that diminish self-esteem and self-efficacy and leave victims feeling excluded and marginalized.

In the United States, the prevalence of psychiatric disorders among cultural and racial minority groups is similar to that among Whites *if* you exclude the poor and other vulnerable populations (e.g., homeless, institutionalized, children in foster care, and victims of trauma) within the minority groups. The higher incidence of mental health problems is related to poverty, not race and ethnicity.

People who live in poverty are two to three times more likely to develop mental illness than those who live above the poverty line. In 2017, about 9% of non-Hispanic Whites, 10% of Asians, 19% of Latino-Hispanics, and 22% of Blacks in the United States lived below the poverty line (US Census Bureau, 2017). Poverty is associated with other disadvantages, such as scarce educational and economic opportunities, which, in turn, may be associated with substance use and violent crime. People who are poor are often subjected to a daily struggle for survival, which takes its toll on mental health.

CULTURALLY CONGRUENT CARE AND ASSOCIATED COMPETENCIES

So far, this chapter has explained why the nursing needs of culturally diverse patient populations are so varied. The remainder of this chapter suggests techniques that address the promotion of culturally congruent care and associated competencies.

Although the terms *cultural congruence* and *cultural competence* are often used interchangeably, there is a nuanced difference between the two. According to the American Nurses Association (ANA), **culturally congruent practice (care)** is *applying* evidence-based nursing care that corresponds with patients' values, beliefs, practices, and worldview. **Cultural competence** is the *process* of demonstrating culturally congruent practice. Box 5.3 identifies culturally congruent practice and the associated competencies.

Campinha-Bacote developed a model that psychiatric–mental health nurses can use to support culturally effective care. It is called the Process of Cultural Competence in the Delivery of Healthcare Services (Campinha-Bacote, 2015; Sagar & Sagar, 2019). In this model, nurses view themselves as *becoming* culturally competent rather than *being* culturally competent. This

BOX 5.3 Culturally Congruent Practice and Associated Competencies

The registered nurse practices in a manner that is congruent with cultural diversity and inclusion principles.

Competencies for the registered nurse:

1. Demonstrates respect, equity, and empathy in actions and interactions with all healthcare consumers.
2. Participates in lifelong learning to understand cultural preferences, worldview, choices, and decision-making processes of diverse consumers.
3. Creates an inventory of personal values, beliefs, and cultural heritage.
4. Applies knowledge of variations in health beliefs, practices, and communication patterns in all nursing practice activities.
5. Identifies the stage of the consumer's acculturation and accompanying patterns of needs and engagement.
6. Considers the effects and impact of discrimination and oppression on practice within and among vulnerable cultural groups.
7. Uses skills and tools that are appropriately vetted for the culture, literacy, and language of the population served.
8. Communicates with appropriate language and behaviors, including the use of medical interpreters and translators in accordance with consumer preferences.
9. Identifies the culture-specific meaning of interactions, terms, and content.
10. Respects consumers' decisions based on age, tradition, belief and family influence, and stage of acculturation.
11. Advocates for policies that promote health and prevent harm among culturally diverse, underserved, or underrepresented consumers.
12. Promotes equal access to services, tests, interventions, health promotion programs, enrollment in research, education, and other opportunities.
13. Educates nurse colleagues and other professionals about cultural similarities and differences of healthcare consumers, families, groups, communities, and populations.

Data from American Nurses Association. (2015). *Nursing: Scope and standards of practice* (3rd ed.). Silver Spring, MD: Nursesbooks.org.

model suggests that nurses should constantly see themselves as learners throughout their careers—always open to the immense cultural diversity they will see among their patients and learning from it. The model consists of five constructs:

1. Cultural awareness
2. Cultural knowledge
3. Cultural encounters
4. Cultural skill
5. Cultural desire

Cultural Awareness

Through cultural awareness, the nurse recognizes the enormous impact that culture has on patients' health values and practices. Culture also affects how and when patients decide that they are ill and need care and what treatments they will seek when illness arises.

Cultural awareness allows nurses to acknowledge themselves as cultural beings. Through cultural awareness, nurses often discover that many of their norms are cultural, few are universal, and that they have an obligation to be open and respectful of patients' cultural norms.

By practicing cultural awareness, nurses also examine their cultural assumptions and expectations about what constitutes mental health, a healthy self-concept, a healthy family, and the way to behave in society. They also examine assumptions and expectations about how people manifest psychological distress. The culturally aware nurse understands that evidence-based practice guidelines may not be applicable to all people, since they are derived from studies involving people of primarily European origin.

A culturally aware nurse recognizes that three cultures may be intersecting during any encounter with a patient: the culture of the patient, the culture of the nurse, and the culture of the setting (e.g., agency, clinic, hospital). As patient advocates, our job is to negotiate and support the patient's cultural needs and preferences.

Cultural Knowledge

Nurses can enhance their cultural knowledge in various ways. They can attend cultural events and programs, develop friendships with members of diverse cultural groups, and participate in in-service programs about diversity and inclusion. In addition, they may take advantage of formal and informal classes and resources designed for healthcare providers.

Cultural knowledge can help us to understand behaviors that might otherwise be misinterpreted. It helps nurses to establish rapport, ask appropriate questions, avoid misunderstandings, and identify the cultural variables that should be considered in the planning of nursing care. A summary of cultural knowledge, some of which we have already discussed, includes the following:

- Worldview, beliefs, and values that permeate the culture
- Nonverbal communication patterns, such as the meaning of eye contact, facial expressions, gestures, and touch
- Etiquette norms, such as the importance of punctuality, the pace of conversation, and the way respect and hospitality are shown
- Family roles and psychosocial norms, such as the way in which decisions are made and the degree of independence versus interdependence of family members
- Cultural views about mental health and illness, such as the degree of stigma and the nature of the "sick role"
- Patterns related to health and illness, including cultural syndromes, pharmacogenetic variations, and folk and herbal treatments used within a given culture

Cultural Encounters

Although obtaining cultural knowledge sets a foundation, an understanding of cultural concepts cannot tell us fully about a particular patient. **Cultural encounters** occur when we directly engage in interactions with patients from culturally diverse backgrounds. According to Campinha-Bacote (2011), multiple cultural encounters with patients of diverse backgrounds will decrease the likelihood of stereotyping. **Stereotyping** is the tendency to believe that every member of a group is like all other members. After several cultural encounters, we recognize that, although there are patterns that characterize a culture, individual members of the culture exhibit the culture's norms in individual ways.

Cultural encounters help nurses to develop confidence in their interactions. All nurses are likely to make cultural mistakes, no matter how well intentioned they may be. Cultural encounters help us to develop the skill of recognizing, avoiding, and reducing cultural pain caused by an insensitivity to cultural norms. Nurses can learn to recognize signs of cultural pain and take measures to regain trust and rapport by asking about the offense, apologizing for lack of sensitivity, and expressing willingness to learn from the patient.

Cultural Skill

Cultural skill is the ability to perform a cultural assessment in a sensitive way (Campinha-Bacote, 2011). The first step is to ensure meaningful communication. If the patient is not proficient in English, a professional medical interpreter should be engaged.

Many cultural assessment tools are available (Andrews & Boyle, 2016; Giger, 2016; Leininger, 2002; Purnell, 2019; Spector, 2012). An appendix in the *DSM-5* (APA, 2013b), "Outline for Cultural Formulation," recommends cultural assessment areas. A useful mental health assessment tool is the classic set of questions proposed by Kleinman and colleagues (1978):

- What do you call this illness? (*diagnosis*)
- When did it start? Why then? (*onset*)
- What do you think caused it? (*etiology*)
- How does the illness work? What does it do to you? (*course*)
- How long will it last? Is it serious? (*prognosis*)
- How have you treated the illness? How do you think it should be treated? (*treatment*)

These questions allow the patient to feel heard and understood. They also help in understanding cultural syndromes. You can expand on this list to include questions such as

- What kind of problems has this illness caused you?
- What do you fear most about this illness? Do you think it is curable?
- Do you know others who have had this problem? What happened to them? Do you think this will happen to you?

Approaching these questions conversationally is generally more effective than using a direct, formal approach. One indirect technique is to ask the patient what another family member thinks is causing the problem. The nurse can ask, "What does your family think is wrong? Why do they think it started? What do they think you should do about it?" After the patient describes what the family thinks, the nurse can simply ask if the patient agrees. For instance, before asking about cultural treatments the patient has tried, the nurse can first say, "People have remedies they find helpful when they are ill. Are there any special healers or treatments you have used or that you think might be helpful to you?"

The following are some areas that deserve special attention during an assessment interview:

- Ethnicity, religious affiliation, and degree of acculturation to Western medical culture
- Spiritual practices that are important to preserving or regaining health
- Proficiency in speaking and reading English

- Dietary patterns, including foods prescribed for sick people
- Attitudes about pain and experiences with pain in a Western medical setting
- Attitudes about and experience with Western medications
- Cultural remedies, such as healers, herbs, and practices the patient may find helpful
- Who is considered family, who should receive health information, and how decisions are made in the family
- Cultural customs the patient feels are essential to preserve and is fearful will be violated in the mental health setting

The purpose of a culturally sensitive assessment is to develop a therapeutic plan that is mutually agreeable, culturally acceptable, and that carries potentially positive outcomes. While gathering assessment data, you should identify cultural patterns that may support or interfere with the patient's health and recovery process. You can use your professional knowledge to categorize the patient's cultural norms into three different groups, such as these:

1. Those that facilitate the patient's health and recovery from the Western medical perspective
2. Those that are neither helpful nor harmful from the Western medical perspective
3. Those that are harmful to the patient's health and well-being from the Western medical perspective

Wehbe-Alamah (2019) suggest a preservation/maintenance, accommodate/negotiate, repatterning/restructuring framework for care planning as part of their Culture Care Theory. Using this framework, effective nursing care preserves the aspects of the patient's culture that, from a Western perspective, promote health and well-being—such as a strong family support system and traditional values such as cooperation and emphasis on relationships.

You can accommodate for cultural values and practices that are neither helpful nor harmful or negotiate as needed. You may encourage the patient's use of neutral values and practices, such as folk remedies and healers. Including these culture-specific interventions in nursing care builds on the patient's own coping and healing systems. For example, Native Americans with substance abuse problems may find tribal healing ceremonies helpful as a complement to the therapeutic program.

Finally, when you have determined that cultural patterns are harmful, make attempts to repattern and restructure them. For instance, if a patient is taking an herb that interferes with the prescription medication regimen, educate and negotiate with the patient until you have developed a mutually agreeable therapeutic program.

Cultural Desire

The final construct in Campinha-Bacote's model is cultural desire. Cultural desire indicates that the nurse is not acting from a sincere and genuine concern for patients' welfare. This concern ideally leads to truly understand each patient's viewpoint. Nurses exhibit cultural desire through patience, consideration, and empathy. Giving the impression that you are willing to learn from the patient is the hallmark of cultural desire as opposed to behaving as if you know what is best.

Cultural desire inspires openness and flexibility in applying nursing principles to meet the patient's cultural needs. Cultural desire enables the nurse to achieve good outcomes with culturally diverse patients.

KEY POINTS TO REMEMBER

- As the diversity of the world and the United States increases, psychiatric–mental health nurses will be caring for more and more people from diverse cultural groups.
- Nurses should learn to promote culturally competent and congruent care.
- *Culture* is the shared beliefs, values, and practices of a group. It shapes the group's thinking and behavior in patterned ways. Cultural groups share these norms with new members of the group through enculturation.
- A group's culture influences its members' worldview, nonverbal communication patterns, etiquette norms, and ways of viewing the person, the family, and the right way to think and behave in society.
- The concept of mental health is formed within a culture, and other members of the group may define deviance from cultural expectations as illness.
- Psychiatric–mental health nursing is based on personality and developmental theories advanced by Europeans and Americans and grounded in Western cultural ideals and values.
- Nurses are as influenced by their own professional and ethnic cultures as patients are by theirs. Monitoring and modifying ethnocentric tendencies helps nurses to provide culturally congruent care.
- Cultural barriers to quality mental health care include communication problems, mental illness stigma, misdiagnosis, differences in cultural concepts of distress, and genetic variations in psychotropic drug metabolism.

- Immigrants (especially refugees) and minority groups, who may suffer from the effects of low socioeconomic status, including poverty and discrimination, are at particular risk for mental illness.
- Cultural competence consists of five constructs: cultural awareness, cultural knowledge, cultural encounters, cultural skill, and cultural desire.
- Through cultural awareness, nurses recognize that they as well as patients have cultural beliefs, values, and practices.
- Nurses obtain cultural knowledge by seeking cultural information from friends, participating in in-service programs, immersing themselves in the culture, or consulting print and online sources (transcultural nursing theories, models, and approaches).
- Nurses experience intraethnic diversity through multiple cultural encounters, which can prevent nurses from stereotyping their patients.
- Nurses demonstrate cultural skill by performing culturally sensitive assessment interviews and adapting care to meet patients' cultural needs and preferences.
- Cultural desire is a genuine interest in the patient's unique perspective; it enables nurses to provide considerate, flexible, and respectful care to patients of all cultures.

CRITICAL THINKING

1. Describe the cultural factors that have influenced the development of Western psychiatric–mental health nursing practice. Contrast these Western influences with the cultural factors that influence patients who come from Eastern, Indigenous, or collective cultures.
2. What do you think about the claim that mental illness is a cultural phenomenon and that individuals are judged to be mentally ill if they do not fit within the social definition of normal? What implications (good or bad) does a diagnosis of a mental illness have?

3. Analyze the effects cultural competence can have on psychiatric–mental health nurses and their patients.
4. How can barriers such as communication problems, stigma, and misdiagnosis impede the promotion of competent psychiatric–mental health care? What can the members of the healthcare team do to overcome such barriers?

CHAPTER REVIEW

1. Which intervention demonstrates the nurse's understanding of what guides effective nursing care with a diverse patient population?
   a. Treating all patients the same to avoid prejudicial actions.
   b. Identifying the cultural norms of the population being served.
   c. Recognizing that race and ethnicity result in specific illness management views.
   d. Addressing the physical and emotional needs that originate from genetic factors.

2. Which statement indicates the beliefs and values that tend to be representative of a member of an Indigenous culture? *Select all that apply.*
   a. "I've reinforced the importance of taking medications at the time they are prescribed."
   b. "The patient believes that illness is a result of being out of harmony with nature."
   c. "Spending money on medicine for his diabetes is not a comfortable concept for my patient."
   d. "The patient refuses treatment."
   e. "We discussed the patient's needs regarding warding off evil spirits before her surgery."

3. Which assessment questions will support effective communication with a patient who recently emigrated from an Asian country? *Select all that apply.*
   a. "What do you call this kind of pain?"
   b. "What do you think is causing your pain?"
   c. "How do you think your pain should be treated?"
   d. "Do you consider this kind of pain a serious problem?"
   e. "Do you think American medicine will help your pain?"

4. When one is considering culturally competent care for a Muslim patient diagnosed with cardiac problems, which intervention is particularly important initially when a low-fat diet is prescribed?
   a. Requesting a dietary consult
   b. Identifying dietary considerations
   c. Explaining the importance of a low-fat diet
   d. Including the family in conversation about food preparation

5. Which statement by the nurse demonstrates ethnocentrism toward the Latinx patient?
   a. "What do you want us to do to help your symptoms?"
   b. "Tell me more about what you think is causing these symptoms."
   c. "I'm sure we can do something to make your symptoms more manageable."
   d. "How much have these symptoms made it more difficult for you to go to work?"

6. Ling has a nursing diagnosis of risk for violence. Ling's Eastern culture family is having difficulty coping with the illness because of their beliefs. A favorable therapeutic modality for this patient might include
   a. outpatient therapy.
   b. family therapy.
   c. long-term inpatient care.
   d. assimilation therapy.

7. A nurse practitioner is interviewing a female patient from Southeast Asia. She complains of stomach pain and chest discomfort. Knowing that the patient's adult son died in a car accident a month earlier, the nurse suspects
   a. vulnerability.
   b. acid reflux.
   c. somatization.
   d. transference.

8. Which nursing intervention can help a Hindu patient to maintain his religious practice?
   a. Helping the patient to choose his own food from the menu
   b. Contacting the hospital pastor for a visit
   c. Showing him which side of the room faces east
   d. Offering him a Torah

9. Intergenerational conflict may arise in immigrant families because the process of acculturation may be
   a. ignored due to cultural beliefs.
   b. filled with traumatic experiences.
   c. easier for children.
   d. a function of assimilation.

10. Which nursing actions demonstrate cultural competence? *Select all that apply.*
    a. Planning mealtime around the patient's prayer schedule
    b. Helping a patient to visit with the hospital chaplain
    c. Researching foods that a lacto-ovo-vegetarian patient will eat
    d. Providing time for a patient's spiritual healer to visit
    e. Ordering standard meal trays to be delivered three times daily

1. **b**; 2. **a, b, c, e**; 3. **a, b, c, d**; 4. **b**; 5. **c**; 6. **b**; 7. **c**; 8. **a**; 9. **c**; 10. **a, b, c, d**

Visit the Evolve website for a posttest on the content in this chapter: http://evolve.elsevier.com/Varcarolis

REFERENCES

American Nurses Association. (2015). *Nursing: Scope and standards of practice.* Spring, MD: Nursesbooks.org: Silver.

American Psychiatric Association. (2013a). *Diagnostic and statistical manual of mental disorders* (5th ed.). Washington, DC: Author.

American Psychiatric Association. (2013b). *DSM-5 cultural formulation interview.* Retrieved from http://www.dsm5.org/proposedrevision/Pages/Cult.aspx.

Andrews, M., & Boyle, J. (2016). *Transcultural concepts in nursing care* (8th ed.). Philadelphia, PA: Wolters Kluwer.

Burchum, J., & Rosenthal, R. (2018). Individual variation in drug responses. In *Lehne's pharmacology for nursing care* (pp. 74–81). St. Louis, MO: Elsevier.

Camann, M. A., & Wilson, A. H. (2017). Global perspectives in mental health. In C. Holtz (Ed.), *Global health care: Issues and policies* (3rd ed.) (pp. 173–196). Burlington, MA: Jones and Bartlett.

Campinha-Bacote, J. (2011). Delivering patient-centered care in the midst of a cultural conflict: The role of cultural competence. *Online Journal of Issues in Nursing, 16*(2).

Campinha-Bacote, J. (2015). *The process of cultural competence in the delivery of healthcare services.* Retrieved from http://transcultural-care.net/the-process-of-cultural-competence-in-the-delivery-of-healthcare-services/.

Chen, J. A., Durham, M. P., Madu, A., Trinh, N., Fricchione, G. L., & Henderson, D. C. (2018). Culture and psychiatry. In T. A. Stern, O. Freudenreich, F. A. Smith, G. L. Fricchione, & J. F. Rosenbaum (Eds.), *Massachusetts General Hospital comprehensive clinical psychiatry* (pp. 559–568). St. Louis, MO: Elsevier.

Giger, J. N. (2016). *Transcultural nursing: Assessment and intervention* (7th ed.). St. Louis, MO: Elsevier.

Jeffreys, M., & Zoucha, R. (2017). The indivisible culture of the multicultural, multiethnic individual: A transcultural imperative (reprint from 2001). *Journal of Cultural Diversity, 1*, 6–10.

Kleinman, A., Eisenberg, L., & Good, B. (1978). Culture, illness and care: Clinical lessons from anthropologic and cross-cultural research. *Annals of Internal Medicine, 88*, 251–258.

Leininger, M. (2002). *Culture care assessments for congruent competency practices.*

National Council for American Indians. (2019). *Tribaons and the United States: An introduction.* Retrieved from http://www.ncai.org/about-tribes.

National Institute of Health. (2020). *Pharmacogenetics.* Retrieved from https://www.nih.gov/about-nih/what-we-do/nih-turning-discovery-into-health/pharmacogenomics.

Purnell, L. D. (2018). Knowledge of cultures. In M. M. Douglas, D. Pacquiao, & L. D. Purnell (Eds.), *Global applications of culturally competent health care: Guidelines for practice* (pp. 31–42). New York, NY: Springer.

Purnell, L. D. (2019). Update: The Purnell Theory and Model for Culturally Competent Health Care. *Journal of Transcultural Nursing, 30*(2), 98–105.

Sagar, P.L., & Sagar, D.Y. (2019). Current state of transcultural nursing theories, models, and approaches. In C. Kasper, & R. Zoucha (Eds.), *Annual review of nursing research, transcultural and social research,* 37(1), 25-41. New York, NY: Springer.

Spector, R. E. (2012). *Cultural diversity in health and illness* (8th ed.). Upper Saddle River, NJ: Prentice-Hall.

Substance Abuse and Mental Health Services Administration. (2015). *Racial/ethnic differences in mental health service use among adults.* HHS Publication No. SMA-15-4906. Rockville, MD: Author. Retrieved from http://www.samhsa.gov/data/sites/default/files/MHServicesUseAmongAdults/MHServicesUseAmongAdults.pdf.

US Census Bureau. (2017). *Income, poverty and health insurance coverage in the US, 2017.* Retrieved from https://www.census.gov/library/publications/2018/demo/p60-263.html.

US Census Bureau. (2018a). *Census Bureau statement on 2020 census race and ethnicity questions.* Retrieved from https://www.census.gov/newsroom/press-releases/2018/2020-race-questions.html.

US Census Bureau. (2018b). *Older people projected to outnumber children for the first time in US history.* Retrieved from https://www.census.gov/newsroom/press-releases/2018/cb18-41-population-projections.html.

US Department of Health and Human Services Office of Minority Health. (2018). *The national CLAS standards.* Retrieved from https://minorityhealth.hhs.gov/omh/browse.aspx?lvl=2&lvlid=53.

US Food and Drug Administration. (2019). *The FDA warns against the use of many genetic tests with unapproved claims to predict patient response to specific medications.* Retrieved from https://www.fda.gov/medical-devices/safety-communications/fda-warns-against-use-many-genetic-tests-unapproved-claims-predict-patient-response-specific.

Wehbe-Alamah, H. (2019). Leininger's Culture Care Diversity and Universality Theory. In C. C. Kasper, & R. Zoucha (Eds.), *Annual review of nursing research, transcultural and social research,* 37(1), 1-23. New York, NY: Springer.

Wolf, K.M., Umland, K.N., & Lo, C. (2019). The current state of transcultural mental health nursing: A synthesis of the literature. In C. Kasper, & R. Zoucha (Eds.), *Annual review of nursing research, transcultural and social research,* 37(1), 209-222. New York, NY: Springer.

6

Legal and Ethical Considerations

Margaret Jordan Halter

🌐 Visit the Evolve website for a pretest on the content in this chapter: http://evolve.elsevier.com/Varcarolis

OBJECTIVES

1. Differentiate the terms ethics and bioethics.
2. Describe six ethical principles central to bioethics.
3. Describe the legal process for admissions and discharges.
4. Discuss patients' rights, including the right to treatment, the right to refuse treatment, and informed consent.
5. Describe patients' rights and legal concerns with regard to restraint and seclusion.
6. Explain the concept and legal issues regarding confidentiality in psychiatric care.
7. Identify situations in which healthcare professionals have a duty to break patient confidentiality.

8. Define laws, including torts, negligence, and malpractice, as they pertain to psychiatric nursing.
9. Discuss the basic standards by which nurses are held, including nurse practice acts, professional associations, institutional policies and procedures, and customary practice.
10. Identify the steps nurses are advised to take if they suspect negligence or illegal activity in the provision of healthcare.
11. Discuss the importance of clear and thorough documentation.
12. Identify healthcare workers' legal protection from violence in the healthcare setting.

KEY TERMS AND CONCEPTS

assault
assisted outpatient treatment
battery
bioethics
competency
conditional release
confidentiality
duty to protect
duty to warn
emergency commitment
ethical dilemma

ethics
false imprisonment
Health Insurance Portability and
    Accountability Act (HIPAA)
implied consent
informed consent
intentional torts
involuntary commitment
least restrictive alternative doctrine
malpractice
negligence

parity
right to privacy
right to refuse treatment
right to treatment
tort
unconditional release
unintentional torts
voluntary admission
writ of habeas corpus

While a basic understanding of ethical and legal issues is important in every healthcare setting, the type of problems encountered in psychiatric care elevates the significance of these issues. Patients in this population experience alterations in thought, mood, and/or behavior that impact decision making regarding their care. For example, paranoia may cause a patient to be suspicious of medications, profound depression may result in apathy to help-seeking, and hyperactivity puts people in physical danger. Additionally, individuals with mental illness are often vulnerable and may need their rights protected through the legal system. This chapter introduces ethical concepts that will

inform decision making and legal issues that will protect the rights of patients in psychiatric settings.

ETHICAL CONCEPTS

Psychiatric nurses often encounter complex situations when caring for patients and dealing with their significant others. Some decision making when working with patients is fairly simple based on **morals**, which are beliefs about what is right or wrong. Basic morality generally condemns murder, lying, and stealing. Our moral code would prevent a nurse from engaging in euthanasia, misrepresenting facts about medications, or the diversion of pain medication for personal use.

Ethics is the branch of knowledge and philosophical beliefs about what is right or wrong in a society. It describes what ought to be rather than what is. The term **bioethics** is the study of specific ethical questions that arise in healthcare.

Ethical principles help practitioners to make decisions for care and also help to evaluate care that has been given. Important ethical principles are:

1. **Autonomy**: Respecting the rights of others to make their own decisions (e.g., acknowledging the patient's right to refuse medication supports autonomy).
2. **Beneficence**: The duty to act to benefit or promote the health and well-being of others (e.g., spending extra time to help calm an anxious patient).
3. **Nonmaleficence:** Doing no harm to the patient (e.g., protecting confidential information about a patient).
4. **Justice:** The duty to distribute resources or care equally, regardless of personal attributes (e.g., an intensive care unit [ICU] nurse devotes equal attention to someone who has attempted suicide as to someone who suffered a brain aneurysm).
5. **Fidelity**: Maintaining loyalty and commitment to the patient and doing no wrong to the patient (e.g., maintaining expertise in nursing skill through continuing nurse education).
6. **Veracity**: The duty to communicate truthfully (e.g., describing the purpose and side effects of psychotropic medications in a truthful and non-misleading way).

An **ethical dilemma** results when there is a conflict between two or more courses of action, each carrying favorable and unfavorable consequences. The response to these dilemmas is based partly on morals and values. Suppose you are caring for a pregnant woman with schizophrenia who wants to have the baby but whose family insists she get an abortion. To promote fetal safety, her antipsychotic medication would need to be reduced, putting her at risk of exacerbating (worsening) the psychiatric illness. Furthermore, there is a question as to whether she can safely care for the baby. If you rely on the ethical principle of autonomy, you may conclude that she has the right to decide. Beneficence, or doing good, could be continuing medications for the sake of the mother or discontinuing medications for the sake of the child.

At times, your values may be in conflict with the value system of the organization where you work. This situation further complicates the decision-making process and requires careful consideration of the patient's desires and rights. For example, you may experience a conflict of values in a setting where older adults are routinely sedated to a degree to which you do not feel comfortable. When your value system is challenged, this increases stress. Some nurses respond proactively by working to change the system or even advocate for legislation related to some particular issue.

An ethical nursing practice has a profound impact on patient safety and quality of care. In recognition of that impact, the American Nurses Association (ANA, 2015a) designated 2015 as the "Year of Ethics" and released a revised *Code of Ethics for Nurses* for the profession. The revision was driven by the

BOX 6.1 Code of Ethics for Nurses

1. The nurse, in all professional relationships, practices with compassion and respect for the inherent dignity, worth, and uniqueness of every individual, unrestricted by considerations of social or economic status, personal attributes, or the nature of health problems.
2. The nurse's primary commitment is to the patient, whether an individual, family, group, or community.
3. The nurse promotes, advocates for, and strives to protect the rights, health, and safety of the patient.
4. The nurse has authority, accountability, and responsibility for nursing practice; makes decisions; and takes action consistent with the obligation to promote health and provide optimal care.
5. The nurse owes the same duties to self as to others, including the responsibility to promote health and safety, preserve wholeness of character and integrity, maintain competence, and continue personal and professional growth.
6. The nurse, through individual and collective effort, establishes, maintains, and improves the ethical environment of the work setting and conditions of employment that are conducive to safe, quality care.
7. The nurse, in all roles and settings, advances the profession through research and scholarly inquiry, professional standards development, and the generation of both nursing and health policy.
8. The nurse collaborates with other health professionals and the public to protect human rights, promote health diplomacy, and reduce health disparities.
9. The profession of nursing, collectively through its professional organizations, must articulate nursing values, maintain the integrity of the profession, and integrate principles of social justice into nursing and health policy.

From American Nurses Association. (2015). *Code of ethics for nurses with interpretive statements*. Washington, DC: American Nurses Publishing.

changing dynamics in healthcare and issues facing contemporary nursing. The code provides the professional ethical foundation for registered nurses in the United States (Box 6.1).

EVOLVING ETHICAL ISSUES IN PSYCHIATRIC CARE

Pharmacogenetic Testing

For over a decade, clinicians have used **pharmacogenetic testing** to help identify which antidepressant to use on specific patients based on a DNA profile. The goal of this testing is to eliminate the trial-and-error approach to prescribing antidepressants and improve recovery time. Companies offering this service have sprung up overnight and many prescribers routinely order these panels. Some insurance companies provide reimbursement for genetic testing for predictive pharmacy.

Zeier and colleagues (2018) reviewed the literature and concluded that there is insufficient data to support the widespread use of genetic testing, although they may be helpful in predicting side effects. The US Food and Drug Administration (FDA, 2018) has also taken a position. The FDA does not support the use of genetic testing since there has not been adequate research and clinical evidence. They contend the tests may influence providers and patients to select or change drugs or doses, thereby exposing the patient to harm. In 2019, the FDA issued a letter to one genetic testing company, Inova Genomics, for illegally marketing tests that have not been reviewed or approved by the FDA.

Based on the FDA's claims, pharmacogenetic testing raises several ethical issues. The first is based on the principle of nonmaleficence. If these tests are not useful, then patients are potentially being harmed as previously discussed. Further, the lack of an evidence base may raise questions as to the ethics of prescribing these panels and justifying the cost.

Predictive Psychiatry

Although genetic testing for psychiatric disorders has not become routine, it is likely that developing technology will bring about more ethical issues (Roberts & Dunn, 2019). For example, would early genetic testing for schizophrenia benefit an adolescent in the absence of preventative treatment?

There are potential consequences for insurance, employment, and general discrimination and stigmatization should the results of genetic testing be known. Anecdotally, people have been known to lose their jobs because their employer found out that they had first-degree relatives with schizophrenia. Imagine how much more is at stake with personal genetic information.

Autonomy may also be an issue. Consider the adult whose grandmother died from Alzheimer's disease. If he wants to know if he carries at-risk genes and his father does not want to know, whose autonomy should be supported?

Right now, for a small fee, anyone can mail a saliva sample and receive results of a genome scan within weeks. The companies are able to reveal risk for a variety of conditions, including Parkinson's disease, Alzheimer's disease, certain rare blood disorders, and breast, ovarian, and prostate cancers.

Genome scans carry many ethical concerns. Before these commercially manufactured tests were available, people generally learned of their health risks in the presence of a care provider who could provide support. Now, people view the, at times, devastating test results alone. Are we causing emotional distress by testing for the genetic variant for Alzheimer's disease if little or nothing can be done to prevent its onset? Research indicates that just knowing you have a genetic risk can alter your physiology (Turnwald et al., 2019). In this study, participants were tested for exercise capacity and for appetite satiety genes. After receiving genetic results, which might or might not be true, there were changes in exercise tests and feeling of fullness after food consumption. These results point to added concerns over genome scans actually influencing feelings, thoughts, and behaviors.

MENTAL HEALTH LAWS

Federal and state legislatures have enacted laws to regulate the care and treatment of people with mental illness. At the state level, mental health laws—or statutes—vary from state to state. Therefore, you are encouraged to review your state's code to better understand the legal climate in which you will be practicing. You can accomplish this by visiting the web page of your state's mental health department or by doing an internet search using the keywords "mental + health + statutes + (your state)."

Many of the state laws underwent substantial revision after the landmark Community Mental Health Centers Act of 1963 enacted under President John F. Kennedy that promoted deinstitutionalization of people with mental illness. The changes reflect a shift in emphasis from institutional care to community-based care. There was an increasing awareness of the need to provide people who have psychiatric disorders with humane care that respects their civil rights. Widespread, progressive use of psychotropic drugs in the treatment of mental illness enabled many patients to integrate more readily into the larger community.

Additionally, the legal system has adopted a more therapeutic approach to persons with substance use disorders and mental health disorders. There are now drug courts where the emphasis is more on rehabilitation than punishment. Similarly, mental health courts handle criminal charges against people with mental illness by diverting them to community resources to prevent reoffending by, among other things, monitoring medication adherence.

Federal legislation providing equality for the people with mental illness with other patients in terms of payments for services from health insurance plans also improves access to treatment. This equal payment is called parity. The Paul Wellstone and Pete Domenici Mental Health Parity and Addiction Equity Act, which went into effect in July 2010, and the Affordable Care Act, also enacted in 2010, provide for insurance funding for mental illness (Bazelton Center for Mental Health Law, 2012).

HOSPITALIZATION

While most people can be treated on an outpatient basis, some individuals experience such severe symptoms that they require hospitalization for evaluation and close monitoring. Hospitalization may occur when a person decides to seek treatment at the insistence of a family member or professional or as the result of an encounter with law enforcement personnel.

Admission Procedures

All admissions are based on several fundamental guidelines:
- Neither voluntary admission nor involuntary commitment determines a patient's ability to make informed decisions about personal healthcare.
- Care providers establish that a well-defined psychiatric problem exists based on current illness classifications in the *Diagnostic and Statistical Manual of Mental Disorders, Fifth Edition* (*DSM-5*; American Psychiatric Association [APA], 2013).
- The illness and its symptoms should result in an immediate crisis situation and other less-restrictive alternatives (i.e., outpatient care) are inadequate or unavailable.
- There is a reasonable expectation that the hospitalization and treatment will improve the presenting problems.

You are encouraged to become familiar with the laws in your state and provisions for admissions, discharges, patients' rights, and informed consent. The admissions described in the following paragraphs provide a general overview of the standards and process.

Voluntary Admissions

Voluntary admissions occur when patients apply in writing for admission to the facility. The person should understand the need for treatment and be willing to be admitted. If the individual is under 16, the parent, legal guardian, custodian, or next of kin may have authority to apply on the person's behalf. Adolescents between 16 and 18 may seek admission independently or on the application by an authorized individual or agency.

Voluntarily admitted patients have the right to request and obtain release. Before being released, reevaluation may be necessary. Reevaluation can result in a decision on the part of the care provider to initiate an involuntary commitment according to criteria established by state law.

Involuntary Commitment

Involuntary commitment, also known as assisted inpatient psychiatric treatment, is a court-ordered admission to a facility without the patient's approval. State laws vary, but they address both the criteria for commitment and the process for commitment. The criteria for commitment are the legal standards under which the court decides whether admission is necessary. These standards include a person who is:

1. Diagnosed with mental illness
2. Posing a danger to self or others
3. Gravely disabled (unable to provide for basic necessities such as food, clothing, and shelter)
4. In need of treatment and the mental illness itself prevents voluntary help-seeking

The process for commitment has evolved. Many years ago, it was fairly easy to have someone committed. For example, a common problem in 1930s Maine was husbands ridding themselves of wives through psychiatric commitment (Curtis, 2001). Legislation was enacted to penalize husbands who brought false testimony. One startling chief complaint listed on an actual admitting record was, "Patient does not do her housework." Forced hospitalization was also considered appropriate for "treating" homosexuality.

In reaction to abusive practices of the past, the pendulum has swung the other way and forced hospitalization is far less common. The US has a complex system for involuntary commitment. Generally, involuntary commitment begins with someone who is familiar with the individual and believes that treatment is necessary. Often, when things become unbearable, a call is made to a primary care provider, police, or a local mental health facility: "I can't take it anymore. He's making threats and hearing voices. Can you help us get him into treatment?" The person making the call might be a family member, legal guardian, custodian, or someone who lives with the individual. It could also be a healthcare professional. At this point, a formal application for admission is initiated. To support the application, a specified number of physicians (usually two) or a combination of other mental health professionals certify that a person's mental health status justifies detention and treatment.

Patients have the right to access legal counsel and the right to take their case before a judge, who may order a release. If they are not released, patients can be kept involuntarily for a state-specified number of days with interim court appearances. In most states,

psychiatric commitment cannot extend beyond 72 hours with a formal hearing. During this 3-day period, patients can receive basic care and hopefully understand the need for treatment. After that time, a panel of professionals that includes psychiatrists, medical doctors, lawyers, and private citizens reviews their cases.

Patients who believe they are being held without just cause can file a petition for a **writ of habeas corpus**, which means a "formal written order" to "free the person." The writ of habeas corpus is the procedural mechanism used to challenge unlawful detention by the government. The hospital must immediately submit the document to the court. The court will then decide if the patient has been denied due process of law.

Patients can also challenge the hospitalization based on the **least restrictive alternative doctrine**. The least restrictive alternative doctrine mandates that care providers take the least drastic action to achieve a specific purpose. For example, if you can treat someone safely for depression on an outpatient basis, hospitalization would be too restrictive and unnecessarily disruptive.

> **VIGNETTE:** Elizabeth is a 50-year-old with a long history of admissions to psychiatric hospitals. During previous hospitalizations, she was diagnosed with paranoid schizophrenia. She has refused visits from her caseworker, quit taking medication, and her young-adult children have become increasingly concerned about her behavior. When they stop to visit, she is typically unkempt and smells bad and her apartment is filthy and filled with cats. There is no food in the refrigerator except for ketchup and an old container of yogurt, and she is not paying her bills.
>
> Elizabeth accuses her children of spying on her. She believes they are in collusion with the government to get secrets of mind control and oil-rationing plans. She is making vague threats to the local officials, claiming that people who have caused the problems need to be "taken care of." Her daughter contacts her psychiatrist with this information, and they decide to begin emergency involuntary commitment proceedings.

Emergency Commitment

Emergency commitment is also known as a temporary admission or emergency hospitalization. Emergency commitment is used (1) for people who are so confused they cannot make decisions on their own or (2) for people who are so ill they need emergency admission. In some states, anyone can initiate these proceedings through the court system. Other states require that care providers—such as a physician, an advanced practice psychiatric nurse, a social worker, or an officer of the law—initiate a temporary admission. Generally, a psychiatrist employed by the facility needs to confirm the need for hospitalization.

The primary purpose of this type of hospitalization is observation, diagnosis, and treatment of patients who have mental illness or pose a danger to themselves or others. The length of time that patients can be held in a temporary admission ranges from 24 to 96 hours depending on the state. A court hearing is held and a decision is made for discharge, voluntary admission, or involuntary commitment.

Discharge Procedures

Release from hospitalization depends on the patient's admission status. As previously discussed, voluntarily admitted patients have the right to request and receive release. Some states, however, do provide for conditional release of voluntary patients, which enables the treating physician or administrator to order continued treatment on an outpatient basis if the patient needs further care.

Unconditional Release

The most common type of release from a hospital after admission is an unconditional release, which is the termination of the legal patient-institution relationship. This release may be ordered by the attending psychiatrist or other advanced practice mental health professional (e.g., psychiatric registered nurse practitioner or physician assistant) or it may be court ordered.

Sometimes, patients wish to be released due to issues such as being unsatisfied with care, lack of insurance coverage, or the need to return to work. When the patient requests a discharge, the care provider may agree with the request. If the clinician has doubts as to the safety of a discharge, a patient may be held for similar to an involuntary admission. As previously discussed, nearly every state allows a 72-hour holding period for professional evaluation.

Release Against Medical Advice

In some cases, there is a disagreement between the mental healthcare providers and the patient as to whether continued hospitalization is necessary. In cases where treatment seems beneficial but there is no compelling reason (e.g., danger to self or others) to seek an involuntary continuance of stay, patients may be released against medical advice (AMA). Patients are required to sign a form indicating that they are leaving AMA. This form becomes part of the patient's permanent record.

An AMA discharge may present an ethical dilemma for clinicians. On the one hand, patient autonomy and the right to refuse treatment support the patient's wishes for discharge. On the other, the clinician beneficence would support benefiting and promoting good, which includes protecting the patient.

Conditional Release

A conditional release usually requires outpatient treatment for a specified period of time. During this time, the individual is evaluated for follow-through with the medication regimen, ability to meet basic needs, and the ability to reintegrate into the community. Generally, a voluntarily admitted patient who is conditionally released can only be involuntarily admitted through the usual methods described earlier. However, an involuntarily admitted patient who is conditionally released may be readmitted based on the original commitment order.

Assisted outpatient treatment is similar to a conditional release. The main difference is in legal implications since, unlike conditional release, this is a court-ordered outpatient treatment. While patients are often discharged into this care, they may also be committed directly from the community. This type of involuntary outpatient commitment arose in the 1990s when states began to pass legislation that permitted court-ordered outpatient treatment as an alternative to forced inpatient treatment. As of 2019, only three states—Connecticut, Massachusetts, and Maryland—had not adopted this model of less restrictive care.

The order for involuntary outpatient care is usually tied to receipt of goods and services provided by social welfare agencies, including disability benefits and housing. To access these goods and services, the patient participates in treatment and may face inpatient admission for failing to participate in treatment.

While assisted outpatient treatment is often used to reduce length of hospital stay, it can also be a preventive measure. For example, a patient successfully discharged after acute care can avoid rehospitalization by maintaining treatment.

Specific procedures vary by state, but typically a candidate for this type of treatment will have a history of repeated hospitalizations or arrests caused by treatment nonadherence. These individuals would be thought unlikely to voluntarily participate in outpatient treatment, need treatment to prevent relapse, and would pose a threat to self or others if they did relapse.

PATIENTS' RIGHTS UNDER THE LAW

Psychiatric facilities usually provide patients with a written list of basic rights derived from a variety of sources, especially legislation that came out of the 1960s. Since that time, rights have been modified to some degree, but most lists share commonalities described in the following sections.

Right to Treatment

One of the most fundamental rights of a patient admitted for psychiatric care is the right to quality care. We refer to this as the right to treatment. Particularly in the case of involuntary commitment, how can we deny a person's liberty and then not provide treatment?

Based on the decisions of a number of early court cases, patients have specific rights to treatment. They include:
- The right to be free from excessive or unnecessary medication
- The right to privacy and dignity
- The right to the least restrictive environment
- The right to an attorney, clergy, and private care providers
- The right to not be subjected to lobotomies, electroconvulsive treatments, and other treatments without fully informed consent

Right to Refuse Treatment

Just as patients have the right to receive treatment, they also have the right to refuse it. Patients may withhold consent or withdraw consent at any time, even if they are involuntarily committed. Patients can also retract consent previously given, and care providers must respect this whether it is a verbal or written retraction. However, the patient's right to refuse treatment with psychopharmacological drugs has been debated in the courts. This debate is based partly on the issue of patients' mental ability to give or withhold consent to treatment and their status under the civil commitment statutes.

Early court cases—initiated by patients in state psychiatric hospitals—considered medical, legal, and ethical issues such as basic treatment problems, the doctrine of informed consent, and the bioethical principle of autonomy. Tables 6.1 and 6.2

TABLE 6.1 Right to Refuse Treatment: Evolution from Massachusetts Case Law to Present Law

Case	Court	Decision
Rogers v. Okin, 478 F. Supp. 1342 (D. Mass. 1979)	Federal district court	Ruled that involuntarily hospitalized patients with mental illness are competent and have the right to make treatment decisions. Forcible administration of medication is justified in an emergency if needed to prevent violence and if other alternatives have been ruled out. A guardian may make treatment decisions for an incompetent patient.
Rogers v. Okin, 634 F.2nd 650 (1st Cir. 1980)	Federal court of appeals	Affirmed that involuntarily hospitalized patients with mental illness are competent and have the right to make treatment decisions. The staff has substantial discretion in an emergency. Forcible medication is also justified to prevent the patient's deterioration. A patient's rights must be protected by judicial determination of competency or incompetency.
Mills v. Rogers, 457 U.S. 291 (1982)	US Supreme Court	Set aside the judgment of the court of appeals with instructions to consider the effect of an intervening state court case.
Rogers v. Commissioner of the Department of Mental Health, 458 N.E.2d 308 (Mass. 1983)	Massachusetts Supreme Judicial Court answering questions certified by federal court of appeals	Ruled that involuntarily hospitalized patients are competent and have the right to make treatment decisions unless they are judicially determined to be incompetent.

TABLE 6.2 Right to Refuse Treatment: Evolution from New Jersey Case Law to Present Law

Case	Court	Decision
Rennie v. Klein, 476 F. Supp. 1292 (D. N.J. 1979)	Federal district court	Ruled that involuntarily hospitalized patients with mental illness have a qualified constitutional right to refuse treatment with antipsychotic drugs. Voluntarily hospitalized patients have an absolute right to refuse treatment with antipsychotic drugs under New Jersey law.
Rennie v. Klein, 653 F.2d 836 (3d Cir. 1981)	Federal court of appeals	Ruled that involuntarily hospitalized patients with mental illness have a constitutional right to refuse antipsychotic drug treatment. The state may override a patient's right when the patient poses a danger to self or others. Due process protections must be complied with before forcible medication of patients in nonemergency situations.
Rennie v. Klein, 454 U.S. 1078 (1982)	US Supreme Court	Set aside the judgment of the court of appeals, with instructions to consider the case in light of the US Supreme Court decision in *Youngberg v. Romeo*.
Rennie v. Klein, 720 F.2d 266 (3d Cir. 1983)	Federal court of appeals	Ruled that involuntarily hospitalized patients with mental illness have the right to refuse treatment with antipsychotic medications. Decisions to forcibly medicate must be based on accepted professional judgment and must comply with due process requirements of the New Jersey regulations.

summarize the evolution of two landmark sets of cases regarding the patient's right to refuse treatment.

In an emergency situation where a person may cause serious and imminent harm to self or others, institutions can medicate a person without a court hearing. Beyond emergency situations, after a court hearing, a person can be medicated if all of the following criteria are met:
1. The person has a serious mental illness
2. The person's functioning is deteriorating and if the person is suffering or exhibiting threatening behavior
3. The benefits of treatment outweigh the harm
4. The person lacks the capacity to make a reasoned decision about the treatment
5. Less-restrictive services have been found inadequate

Right to Informed Consent

Informed consent is a legal term that means the patient has been provided with basic information regarding risks and benefits,

and alternatives to treatment. The person must be voluntarily accepting the treatments. While registered nurses routinely provide education about treatment, typically it is the prescriber who is legally responsible for securing informed consent.

The principle of informed consent is based on a person's right to self-determination as described in the landmark case of *Canterbury v. Spence* (1972):

> *The root premise is the concept, fundamental in American jurisprudence, that every human being of adult years and sound mind has a right to determine what shall be done with his own body ... True consent to what happens to one's self is the informed exercise of choice, and that entails an opportunity to evaluate knowledgeably the options available and the risks attendant on each. (p. 780)*

Consent is secured for surgery, electroconvulsive treatment, or the use of experimental drugs or procedures. Patients have the right to refuse participation in experimental treatments or research and the right to voice grievances and recommend changes in policies or services offered by the facility, without fear of punishment or reprisal.

Patients are informed of the following elements:

- The nature of the problem or condition
- The nature and purpose of a proposed treatment
- The risks and benefits of that treatment
- The alternative treatment options
- The probability that the proposed treatment will be successful
- The risks of not consenting to treatment

Implied Consent

Many procedures nurses perform carry an element of **implied consent**. For example, if you approach the patient with a medication in hand, and the patient indicates a willingness to receive the medication, implied consent has occurred. Many institutions—particularly state psychiatric hospitals—have a requirement to obtain signed informed consent documents for every medication given. This consent can be retracted by the patient at any time.

A general rule for you to consider is that the more intrusive or risky the procedure, the greater the need for you to obtain informed consent. While you may not have a legal duty to inform the patient of the associated risks and benefits of a particular medical procedure, morally and ethically you are bound to clarify the procedure to the patient and ensure expressed or implied consent. If after attempting to clarify with the patient you believe he really does not understand what is happening, the next step is to notify the prescriber of your concerns.

Capacity and Competency

For individuals to provide informed consent, as previously mentioned, they should have the capacity to understand. **Capacity** is a person's ability to make an informed decision. Capacity is a fluid concept and individuals may possess capacity one minute and lack capacity in another. Mental health providers may provide opinions about capacity. For example, "Does the patient have the capacity to provide consent for electroconvulsive therapy (ECT)?"

Competency is a different but closely related term to capacity. **Competency** is a legal term related to the degree of mental soundness a person has to make decisions or to carry out specific acts. Like the phrase "innocent until proven guilty," patients are considered competent until they have been declared incompetent. If found incompetent through a formal legal proceeding, the patient may be appointed a legal guardian or representative who is responsible for giving or refusing consent for the patient while always considering the patient's wishes.

Guardians are typically selected from among family members. The order of selection is usually (1) spouse or partner, (2) adult children or grandchildren, (3) parents, (4) adult siblings, and (5) adult nieces and nephews. In the event a family member is either unavailable or unwilling to serve in this role, the court may also appoint a court-trained volunteer guardian.

Rights Regarding Psychiatric Advance Directives

Patients who have experienced an episode of severe mental illness have the opportunity to express their treatment preferences in a psychiatric advance directive. This document is prepared when the individuals are well and identifies, in detail, their wishes and treatment choices.

These directives vary somewhat from state to state, but generally cover the same basic areas. The following choices are addressed in Ohio's Declaration for Mental Health Treatment:

- Designation of preferred physician and therapists
- Appointment of someone to make mental health treatment decisions
- Preferences regarding medications to take or not take
- Consent or lack of consent for ECT
- Consent or lack of consent for admission to a psychiatric facility
- Preferred facilities and unacceptable facilities
- Individuals who should not visit

Rights Regarding Restraint and Seclusion

The history of restraint and seclusion is marked by abuse, overuse, and even a tendency to use restraint as punishment. This was especially true before the 1950s when there were no effective medications to calm agitation, hyperactivity, and psychosis. In the book *The Shame of the States*, Deutsch (1949) wrote that in 1948 one out of every four patients was restrained during the day. The practice of restraining patients rose to one in three patients at night.

Legislation and accreditation requirements have dramatically reduced this problem by mandating strict guidelines. In fact, the pendulum has swung so far from the days of rampant use of restraint and seclusion that these methods have been referred to disparagingly as therapeutic assault.

The American Psychiatric Nurses Association (APNA) promotes a culture that minimizes and eventually eliminates the use of seclusion and restraint (APNA, 2018). As previously mentioned, the use of the least restrictive means of restraint for the shortest duration is always the general rule. According to the Centers for Medicare and Medicaid Services (CMS, 2008), in emergency situations, less-restrictive measures do not necessarily have to be tried; they only need to be considered ineffective in the staff's professional judgment.

Sometimes agitation, confusion, and combative behavior can have physical origins. Drug interaction, drug side effects, temperature elevation, hypoglycemia, hypoxia, and electrolyte imbalances can all result in behavioral disturbances. Addressing these problems can reduce or eliminate the need for restraint or seclusion. Nurses should consider the following before using seclusion and restraint:

- Verbally intervening (e.g., asking the patient for cooperation)
- Reducing stimulation
- Actively listening
- Providing diversion
- Offering as needed (PRN) medications

While we tend to think of classical restraining devices, a restraint can actually be any mechanical or physical device, equipment, or material that prevents or reduces movement of the patient's legs, arms, body, or head. Even side rails are a restraint if you use them to prevent the patient from exiting the bed.

Restricting a person's movement by holding is also a restraint. This controversial and dangerous method of behavior management is often referred to as "therapeutic holding" or "physical management." These so-called therapeutic holds have resulted in the deaths of many young people. A 16-year-old boy in a residential treatment center for disturbed youth in New York died after being placed in a therapeutic hold by several staff members (Bernstein, 2012). According to witnesses, the boy had complained he could not breathe, then became unresponsive. As of 2019, 23 states had enacted legislation to limit restraint of children to threats of physical danger (Butler, 2019).

A restraint may be chemical. Chemical restraints are medications or doses of medication that are not being used for the patient's condition. Chemical interventions are usually less restrictive than physical or mechanical interventions. However, they can have a greater impact on the patient's ability to relate to the environment due to their effect on levels of awareness and their side effects. Still, when used for symptom management, medication can be extremely effective and helpful as an alternative to physical methods of restraint.

Seclusion is confining patients alone in an area or a room and preventing them from leaving. Seclusion is limited to patients who are demonstrating violent or self-destructive behavior that jeopardizes the safety of others or themselves. Even if the door is not locked, making threats if the patient tries to leave the room is still considered secluding. However, a person who is physically restrained in an open room is not considered to be in seclusion.

Seclusion should be distinguished from timeout. Timeout is when a patient chooses to or accepts a suggestion to spend time alone in a specific area for a certain amount of time. The patient can leave the timeout area at any point.

Orders and Documentation with Restraint and Seclusion

In an emergency, a nurse may place a patient in seclusion or restraint but obtains a written or verbal order as soon as possible thereafter. Orders for restraint or seclusion are never written as an as needed or as a standing order. These orders to manage self-destructive or violent behavior may be renewed for a total of 24 hours with limits depending upon the patient's age (CMS, 2008). Adults 18 years or older are limited to 4 hours, children and adolescents 9 to 17 years old are limited to 2 hours, and children under 9 years old have a 1-hour limit. After 24 hours, a physician or an advanced practice professional responsible for the patient's care will personally assess the patient. Restraint or seclusion is discontinued as soon as safer and calmer behavior begins. Once a patient is removed from restraints or seclusion, a new order is required to reinstitute the intervention.

The nurse should carefully document restraint or seclusion in the treatment plan or plan of care. The documentation should include the specific behaviors leading to restraint

or seclusion, and the time the patient is placed in and released from restraint. The patient is monitored through continuous observation. Patients in restraints are assessed at regular and frequent intervals, such as every 15 to 30 minutes for physical needs (e.g., food, hydration, and toileting), safety, and comfort. Each of these assessments requires documentation. While in restraints, patients require protection from harm since they are in a vulnerable state.

Rights Regarding Confidentiality

Confidentiality is an ethical responsibility of healthcare professionals that prohibits the disclosure of privileged information without the patient's consent. Confidentiality of care and treatment remains an important right for all patients, particularly psychiatric patients. Only the patient can waive the legal privilege of confidentiality.

Discussions about a patient in public places such as elevators and the cafeteria should be completely avoided. Even if the patient's name is not mentioned, such discussions can lead to disclosures of confidential information and liability for you and the facility. Your clinical paperwork for school should never contain full patient identifiers.

VIGNETTE: During the psychiatric rotation in her senior year, Lori learned that her mother's best friend, Sandy, was a patient. In the report the nurse shared that Sandy was diagnosed with major depressive disorder, is going through a painful divorce, and that she has breast cancer.

Though she was uncomfortable and uncertain, Lori approached Sandy on the unit, gave her a hug, and asked how she's doing. To Lori's relief, Sandy seemed to take comfort in having a familiar person around and openly shared what was happening.

When Lori suggests that Sandy call her mom so that she can visit, Sandy's eyes widen, she shakes her head, and adamantly says, "I don't want anyone to know I'm here. I'm so ashamed." As a friend, Lori believes that her mom would be hurt if she didn't know, and, more importantly, she could also provide strong social support. As a future nurse, Lori knows that she will maintain confidentiality and never mentions the encounter to her mother.

Health Insurance Portability and Accountability Act

The Health Insurance Portability and Accountability Act (HIPAA), enacted in 1996, legally protects the psychiatric patient's right to receive treatment and to have medical records kept confidential. Generally, your legal duty to maintain confidentiality is to protect the patient's right to privacy.

According to the 2003 HIPAA Privacy Rule, you may not, without the patient's consent, disclose information obtained from the patient or the medical record to anyone except those persons for whom it is necessary for implementation of the patient's treatment plan. HIPAA also gives special protection to notes taken during psychotherapy that are kept separate from the patient's health information.

Confidentiality and Social Media

It is essential that people working in mental health understand the legal implications of social media and the internet. The internet is not confidential and is open to legal subpoenas. Some mental health workers have blogged about patients, thinking that they had disguised the identity. People in these posts have been identified and lawsuits have followed.

Even what seems to be a fairly innocent electronic transmission can be disastrous. Consider the nursing students in Kansas who posted a picture of a placenta on social media. Standing next to the placenta were four smiling nursing students wearing lab coats and surgical gloves. What they considered to be victimless fun resulted in these students being expelled from nursing school. Fortunately for them, a federal judge ruled for reinstatement of one of the students. Subsequently, the other three were also allowed back in school.

Confidentiality After Death

A person's reputation can be damaged even after death. It is important that you do not divulge information after a person's death that you could not legally share before the death. In the courtroom setting, the Dead Man's Statute protects confidential information about individuals when they are not alive to speak for themselves. About half the states have such a law; again, these laws vary from state to state.

Confidentiality of Professional Communications

A legal privilege exists as a result of specific laws to protect the confidentiality of certain professional communications (e.g., physician-patient, attorney-patient). The theory behind providing a privilege is to ensure that patients will speak frankly and be willing to disclose personal information because they know that care providers will not repeat or distribute confidential conversations.

In 12 states, the legal privilege of confidentiality has been extended to advanced practice registered nurses (Pierce, 2014). In nine states, privileged communication is also provided for registered nurses who work in mental health. In the remaining states, nurses must answer a court's questions regarding the patient, even if this information implicates the patient in a crime. In these states, the confidentiality of communications cannot be guaranteed.

Exceptions to the Rule

Duty to warn and protect third parties. The California Supreme Court in its 1974 landmark decision *Tarasoff v. Regents of University of California* ruled that a therapist has a duty to warn a patient's potential victim of potential harm. This **duty to warn** is an obligation to warn third parties when they may be in danger from a patient.

This ruling came about as a result of a tragic case. Prosenjit Poddar, a university student who was being counseled at the University of California, was despondent over a rejection by Tatiana Tarasoff, whom he had once kissed. The psychologist notified police verbally and in writing that the young man might pose a danger to Tarasoff. The police questioned the student, found him to be rational, and he promised to stay away from his love interest. Subsequently, he stalked and fatally stabbed Tarasoff 2 months later.

This case created much controversy and confusion in the psychiatric and medical communities over issues concerning (1) breach of patient confidentiality and its impact on the

therapeutic relationship in psychiatric care and (2) the ability of the therapist to predict when a patient is truly dangerous. The court found the patient-therapist relationship sufficient to create a duty of the therapist to warn the victim.

When a therapist determines that a patient presents a serious danger of violence to another, the therapist has the **duty to protect** that other person. In fulfilling this duty, the therapist may be required to call and warn the intended victim, the victim's family, or the police or to take whatever steps are reasonably necessary under the circumstances.

Most states have similar laws regarding the duty to protect third parties of potential life threats. The duty to protect usually includes the following:

- Assessing and predicting the patient's danger of violence toward another
- Identifying the specific persons being threatened
- Taking appropriate action to protect the identified victims
  Implications for psychiatric-mental health nursing. Staff nurses are obligated to report a patient's threats of harm against specified victims or classes of victims to other members of the treatment team. Advanced practice psychiatric-mental health nurses in private practice who provide individual therapy are obligated to warn the endangered party themselves.

Statutes for reporting child and older adult abuse. All 50 states and the District of Columbia have child abuse reporting statutes. Although these statutes differ from state to state, they generally include a definition of child abuse, a list of persons required or encouraged to report abuse, and the governmental agency designated to receive and investigate the reports. Most statutes include civil penalties for failure to report. Many states specifically require nurses to report cases of suspected abuse.

There is a conflict between federal and state laws with respect to child abuse reporting. This conflict occurs when the health-care professional discovers child abuse or neglect during the suspected abuser's alcohol or substance use treatment. Federal laws and regulations governing confidentiality of patient records, which apply to almost all drug abuse and alcohol treatment providers, prohibit any disclosure without a court order. In this case, federal law supersedes state reporting laws, although compliance with the state law may be maintained under the following circumstances:

- If a court order is obtained
- If a report can be made without identifying the abuser as a patient in an alcohol or drug treatment program
- If the report is made anonymously, although some states, to protect the rights of the accused, do not allow anonymous reporting

States may require health professionals to report other kinds of abuse. Most states have enacted older adult abuse reporting statutes, which require registered nurses and others to report cases of abuse of adults 65 and older. Agencies that receive federal funding (e.g., Medicare or Medicaid) are required to follow strict guidelines for reporting and preventing this type of abuse.

These laws also apply to dependent or disabled adults. These are adults between the ages of 18 and 64 whose physical or mental limitations restrict their ability to carry out normal activities or to protect themselves. Under most state laws, failure to report suspected abuse, neglect, or exploitation of a disabled adult may result in a misdemeanor crime. Most state statutes protect individuals who make a report in good faith by providing immunity from civil liability. Because state laws vary, students should become familiar with the requirements of their states.

Failure to Protect Patients

A common legal issue in psychiatric-mental health nursing concerns the failure to protect the safety of patients. For example, if a suicidal patient is left alone with the means of self-harm, the nurse who has a duty to protect the patient will be held responsible for any resultant injuries. Leaving a suicidal patient alone in a room on the sixth floor with an open window is an example of unreasonable judgment on the part of a nurse.

Miscommunications and medication errors are common in all areas of nursing, including psychiatric care. Because most psychiatric patients are ambulatory, carefully checking identification before medicating is essential.

Another area of liability in psychiatry arises from the abuse of the therapist-patient relationship. Issues of sexual misconduct during the therapeutic relationship have been a source of concern in the psychiatric community. This is particularly significant given the connection that exists between care providers and patients and the power differential between them.

As previously discussed, the nurse also takes precautions to prevent harm whenever a patient is restrained, as there is a risk of strangulation from the restraints. They may even be at risk from other patients given the vulnerable state of being restrained. For example, incidents of rape by other patients while restrained have occurred.

Even without restraints, you need to protect patients from other patients. One patient sued a hospital when she was beaten unconscious by another patient who entered her room looking for a fight. Her lawsuit alleged that there was inadequate staffing to monitor and supervise the patients under the hospital's care.

Potential threats from the patient's family or friends present another source of concern for patient safety. Patients may come from families where domestic violence is common. The nurse may witness controlling behavior by these family members that is based in fear, anxiety, and possibly guilt. The nurse can promote safety by remaining calm, listening carefully, and assuring family members of the importance of their contributions to the patient's welfare. If a patient reports domestic violence to the nurse or the nurse witnesses it, objective documentation of the information or event is also necessary and for reporting to authorities.

LAWS RELEVANT TO PSYCHIATRIC NURSING

Tort Law

The term *tort* originates from a French word meaning twisted and is synonymous with wrong. A **tort** is defined as any wrongful act, intentional or accidental, that results in an injury to another. Tort law is one of the major areas of law (others are contract, real property, and criminal) and results in more civil litigation than the other areas. When a person wrongfully harms another, the injured party (the plaintiff) can seek money for damages from the responsible party (the defendant). The injury can be to person, property, or reputation.

> ### BOX 6.2 Workplace Bullying: *Raess v. Doescher*
>
> Daniel Raess was a cardiovascular surgeon at a hospital near Indianapolis. According to testimony, Raess got into a verbal confrontation with Joseph Doescher, an operating room perfusionist (a professional who manages the heart-lung machine during surgeries). According to the testimony of Doescher, Raess was angry because he had complained to the hospital's administration about the surgeon's treatment of perfusionists. There was evidence, some of it inadmissible, that Raess had a history of hostile acts toward the hospital staff.
>
> On the day in question, Raess approached Doescher outside the operating room. He was described as having clenched fists, piercing eyes, a red face, and popping veins. As Raess screamed and cursed at him, Doescher backed up against a wall and raised his hands in a defensive stance, believing he was going to be struck.
>
> Doescher (the plaintiff) filed a lawsuit against Raess (the defendant). A jury found in his favor and awarded a judgment of $325,000 against the surgeon. The Indiana Supreme Court reviewed the traditional legal components of assault and determined that there was sufficient evidence to support the jury's conclusion that an assault had occurred, that the defendant acted with intent, and that the plaintiff acted reasonably under the circumstances.

Intentional Torts

Nurses in psychiatric settings should understand **intentional torts**, which are willful or intentional acts that violate another person's rights or property. Examples of intentional torts include assault, battery, and false imprisonment.

Assault is the intentional threat designed to make another person fearful that you will cause that person harm. Verbal threats such as "You'll never get out of here" or pretending to hit a patient are both examples of assault that can occur in a healthcare setting. Assault can even occur in the context of workplace bullying, as shown in Box 6.2.

Battery, on the other hand, is the actual harmful or offensive touching of another person. Shoving a patient from behind to hurry the patient up is an example of battery. Often, assault and battery occur together when a threat is made and then carried out.

False imprisonment occurs when a person is confined in a limited area or within an institution. A charge of false imprisonment may be made after a person is placed in restraints or seclusion. Medications that result in chemical restraint may also fit in this category of tort.

Other types of intentional torts may hurt a person's sense of self. **Invasion of privacy** in healthcare has to do with breaking a person's confidences or taking photographs without explicit permission. An interesting example of invasion of privacy occurred when a psychology firm in New Jersey attempted to collect on past due bills by suing 24 former patients (Ornstein, 2015). These publicly available lawsuits included patient names, diagnoses, and listings of their treatments. Philip, a lawyer and patient of the psychology firm, believed that his professional life could be negatively impacted and countersued for invasion of privacy.

In the context of healthcare, defamation of character occurs when a provider makes a false statement that causes some degree of harm, usually to the reputation of the patient. Defamation includes slander (verbal), such as talking about patients in the lunchroom with others around, and libel (printed), where written information about the patient is shared, intentionally or unintentionally, with people outside the professional setting.

Unintentional Torts

Unintentional torts are unintended acts against another person that produce injury or harm. Negligence is the most common unintentional tort. It is defined as the failure to use ordinary care in any professional or personal situation when there is a duty to do so. Failure to question a physician's order, failure to protect a patient from self-harm, and failure to provide patient teaching are all examples of negligence.

Malpractice is a special type of professional negligence. The five elements required to prove negligence are:

1. Duty
2. Breach of duty
3. Cause in fact
4. Proximate cause
5. Damages

Duty. When nurses represent themselves as being capable of caring for psychiatric patients and accept employment, a duty of care has been assumed. As a nurse working in the psychiatric setting, you have the duty to understand the principles of care and medications used in this specialty. The staff nurse assigned to a psychiatric unit should be knowledgeable enough to assume a reasonable duty of care for the patients. Persons who represent themselves as possessing superior knowledge and skill, such as advanced practice psychiatric registered nurses, are held to a higher standard of care in the practice of their profession.

Breach of duty. If you do not meet the standard of care that other nurses would be expected to supply under similar circumstances, you have breached the duty of care. A breach of duty occurs if the nursing performance falls below the standard of care and exposes the patient to an unreasonable risk of harm. This breach of duty includes doing something that results in harm (an act of *commission*) or failing to do something that results in harm (an act of *omission*).

Cause in fact and proximate cause. One of the issues in a negligence claim is causation, which involves two different issues—cause in fact and proximate cause. Both must be present for a lawsuit to be successful. Cause in fact is sometimes known as actual cause and may be evaluated by asking the question, "If it were not for what this nurse did (or failed to do), would this injury have occurred?" Proximate cause, or legal cause, is determined by whether the event was foreseeable. For example, a nurse who is misusing substances at work recognizes that she could harm a patient. Sometimes an indirect sequence of events occurs in which a patient is injured.

Damages. These include actual damages (e.g., loss of earnings, medical expenses, and property damage) as well as pain and suffering. They also include incidental or consequential damages. For example, giving a patient the wrong medication increased sleepiness. It may also result in permanent disability, requiring such things as special education needs and special accommodations in the home. Furthermore, incidental damages may deprive others of the benefits of the injured person, such as losing a normal relationship with a spouse or parent.

Foreseeability of harm evaluates the likelihood of the outcome under the circumstances. If the average reasonable nurse could foresee that injury would result from the action or inaction, then the injury was foreseeable.

TABLE 6.3 Common Liability Issues

Issue	Examples
Patient safety	Failure to notice or take action on suicide risks Failure to use restraints properly or monitor the patient Miscommunication Medication errors Violation of boundaries (e.g., sexual misconduct) Misdiagnosis
Intentional torts May carry criminal penalties Punitive damages may be awarded Not covered by malpractice insurance	Voluntary acts intended to bring a physical or mental consequence Purposeful acts Recklessness Not obtaining patient consent *Note:* Self-defense or protection of others may serve as a defense to charges of an intentional tort.
Negligence/malpractice	Carelessness Foreseeability of harm
Assault and battery	Person apprehensive (assault) of harmful/offensive touching (battery) Threat to use force (words alone are not enough) with opportunity and ability Treatment without patient's consent
False imprisonment	Intent to confine to a specific area Indefensible use of seclusion or restraints Detention of voluntarily admitted patient, with no agency or legal policies to support detaining
Invasion of privacy	Notifying parents of a 21-year-old that she is being treated on a psychiatric unit
Defamation of character Slander Libel	Telling friends that your patient is a local mayor Telling your Facebook friends that your patient is a local mayor
Unintentional torts	Unintended acts against another person that produce injury or harm
Negligence	Leaving an unlocked car running in front of a high school
Malpractice	Failure to follow up with patient teaching after finding orthostatic hypotension

Table 6.3 summarizes laws relevant to psychiatric nursing and provides examples of each. Box 6.3 describes of a case of false imprisonment, negligence, and malpractice.

STANDARDS FOR NURSING CARE

Nurses are held to a basic standard of care. This standard is based on what other nurses who possess the same degree of skill or knowledge in the same or similar circumstances would do.

State boards of nursing, professional associations, policies and procedures from various institutions, and even historical customs influence how nurses practice. They contribute standards by which nurses are measured and are important in determining legal responsibility and liability.

State Boards of Nursing

Nursing boards are state governmental agencies that regulate nursing practice and whose primary goal is to protect the health

BOX 6.3 False Imprisonment, Negligence, and Malpractice: *Plumadore v. State of New York* (1980)

Delilah Plumadore was admitted to Saranac Lake General Hospital for a gallbladder condition. During her medical workup, she confessed that marital problems had resulted in suicide attempts several years before her admission. After a series of consultations and tests, the attending surgeon scheduled gallbladder surgery for later that day. After the surgeon's visit, a consulting psychiatrist who examined Mrs. Plumadore told her to dress and pack her belongings because she was going to be admitted to a state hospital at Ogdensburg.

Subsequently, two uniformed state troopers handcuffed Mrs. Plumadore and strapped her into the back seat of a patrol car and transported her to the state hospital. On arrival, the admitting psychiatrist realized that the referring psychiatrist lacked the authority to order this involuntary commitment. He therefore requested that Mrs. Plumadore sign a voluntary admission form, which she refused to do.

Despite Mrs. Plumadore's protests regarding her admission to the state hospital, the psychiatrist assigned her to a ward without physical or psychiatric examination. She did not even have the opportunity to contact her family or her medical doctor and remained in the hospital for the weekend.

The court awarded $40,000 to Mrs. Plumadore for malpractice and false imprisonment on the part of healthcare professionals and negligence on the part of the troopers. This settlement was greatly influenced by the fact that she had an acute medical illness that was left untreated for days due to being locked in a psychiatric ward.

a nurse met or failed to meet them. A weakness of this method is that the hospital's policy may be substandard. For example, an institution may determine that patients can be kept in seclusion for up to 6 hours based on the original physician's order, but state licensing laws for institutions might set a limit of 4 hours. Substandard institutional policies may put nurses at risk of liability, so be sure to follow laws and professional standards of nursing care. As advocates for patients and the profession, nurses should address questionable policies and advocate for positive change.

Custom as a Standard of Care

Custom can also be used as evidence of a standard of care. In the absence of a written policy on the use of restraint, testimony might be offered regarding the customary use of restraint in emergency situations in which the combative, violent, or confused patient poses a threat of harm to self or others.

Using custom to establish a standard of care may have the same weakness as in using hospital policies and procedures. After all, customs may not comply with the laws, recommendations of the accrediting body, or other recognized standards of care. Custom should be carefully and regularly evaluated to ensure that substandard routines have not developed. Substandard customs do not protect you when a psychiatric patient charges that a right has been violated or that harm has been caused by the staff's common practices.

ACTING ON QUESTIONABLE PRACTICE

Negligence, Irresponsibility, or Impairment

In your professional life, you may suspect negligence on the part of a peer. In most states, you have a legal duty to intervene and to report such risks of harm to the patient. It is important to document the evidence clearly and accurately before making serious accusations against a peer.

Imagine that you are working with Doreen, a nurse on the night shift on a busy medical floor. She shows up for work disheveled, angry, and uncommunicative. As the shift progresses, her mood lightens. You notice that she keeps a bottle of soda close by and regularly drinks from it. You realize with horror that she is slurring a bit. Thinking back on previous shifts, you realize that this behavior is not new.

How should you respond? In less dangerous situations, the first step might be to communicate directly with your colleague. However, in this case you have an obligation to immediately communicate your concerns to a supervisor. The supervisor should then intervene to protect the patient's rights and wellbeing. If the supervisor is unavailable or unresponsive, you have no choice but to act to protect the patient's life. If you do not intervene, the patient may be injured, and you may be liable for these injuries.

Some problems are not life-threatening but are troubling—*maybe* something bad could happen. Whom do you tell? The answer is, "It depends." It depends on which state you live in. State laws vary in the following ways:

- Some states require that nurses report incompetence or impairment to the state board of nursing but not to the institution.

of the public by overseeing the safe practice of nursing. They have the authority to license nurses who meet a minimum competency score on board examinations, and also have the power to revoke licenses. Each state has its own Nurse Practice Act that identifies the qualifications for registered nurses, identifies the titles that registered nurses will use, defines what nurses are legally allowed to do (scope of practice), and describes the actions that are followed if nurses do not follow the nursing law.

Professional Associations

As a profession, nursing also self-regulates through professional associations. A professional association's primary focus is to elevate the practice of its members by setting standards of excellence.

Two of the main nursing associations that influence psychiatric nursing are the ANA and the APNA, each with individual state chapters. The ANA fosters high standards of nursing practice. The ANA's *Nursing: Scope and Standards of Practice* (2015b) provides parameters for nursing practice through 16 standards and outlines the role of nurses regardless of level, setting, or specialty area.

The APNA is a professional association that is organized to advance the science and education of psychiatric-mental health nursing. More specific guidelines for psychiatric nursing practice are provided in *Psychiatric-Mental Health Nursing: Scope and Standards of Practice* (2014). This publication is a joint effort of the ANA, APNA, and the International Society of Psychiatric-Mental Health Nurses.

Institutional Policies and Procedures

Institutional policies and procedures define criteria for care, and these criteria can be used during legal proceedings to prove that

- Some states require that nurses report *themselves* for incompetence, negligence, unethical or unprofessional conduct, or physical, mental, or chemical impairment.
- Some states require that nurses treating patients who are also nurses report them for problems that constitute a public danger.
- Some states allow a nurse to report a colleague to a peer assistance program rather than the state board of nursing.
- Most states do not require a nurse to report an impaired member of a different profession.

The problem of reporting impaired colleagues causes deep concerns, especially if you have not observed direct harm to a patient. Nurses may feel protective of other nurses due to concerns for professional reputations and personal privacy. The ANA (2015a, p. 12) identifies "acting on questionable practice" as being part of a nurse's professional responsibility. As a patient advocate, the nurse should be alert and take proper actions in cases of impaired colleagues.

The issues are less complex when a professional colleague's conduct (including that of a student nurse) is criminally unlawful. Specific examples include the diversion of drugs from the hospital and sexual misconduct with patients. These are criminal behaviors and must be immediately reported.

VIGNETTE: Amanda recently completed the hospital and unit orientations and has begun to care for patients independently. As she prepares to give the 5 p.m. medications, Amanda notices that Greg Thorn, a 55-year-old admitted after a suicide attempt, has been ordered the antidepressant sertraline (Zoloft). Amanda remembers that Mr. Thorn had been taking another antidepressant, phenelzine (Nardil), before his admission. She seems to recall something dangerous about mixing these two classifications of medications.

She looks the antidepressants up in her drug guide. She relearns that Nardil is a monoamine oxidase inhibitor (MAOI) and the other is a selective serotonin reuptake inhibitor (SSRI) antidepressant. Beginning the new medication within 2 weeks of discontinuing the Nardil could result in severe side effects and a potentially lethal response.

After clarifying with Mr. Thorn that he had been on Nardil and discussing the issue with another nurse, Amanda puts the Zoloft on hold and contacts Mr. Thorn's psychiatrist, Dr. Cruz, by phone. Amanda begins by saying, "I see that Mr. Thorn has been ordered Zoloft. His nursing admission assessment says that he had been taking Nardil up until a few days ago. However, I don't see it listed on the assessment that was done by the medical resident."

First Possible Outcome
Dr. Cruz responds, "Really? Wow, thanks for calling that to my attention. When I make rounds in the morning, I'll decide what to do with his medications. For now, I definitely agree that we hold the Zoloft." Amanda clarifies what Dr. Cruz has said, writes the order, and documents what happened in the nurses notes.

Second Possible Outcome
Dr. Cruz responds, "It sounds like you must have earned a medical degree. Listen, if the medication wasn't listed on my resident's assessment, then he wasn't taking it. Probably another nursing error. I wrote an order for Zoloft. Give it to him." The doctor hangs up on Amanda, who then documents the exchange. She determines that the safest and most appropriate response is to continue to hold the medication and contact her nursing supervisor. The supervisor supports her decision and follows up with the chief of psychiatry.

When the nurse is given an assignment to care for a patient, the nurse provides the care or ensures that the patient is safely reassigned to another nurse. Abandonment, a legal concept, occurs if a nurse does not deliver a patient safely to another health professional before discontinuing treatment. Abandonment is also when a nurse does not provide accurate, timely, and thorough reporting or when follow-through of patient care, on which the patient is relying, has not occurred.

The same principles apply for the psychiatric-mental health nurse working in a community setting. For example, if a suicidal patient refuses to come to the hospital for treatment, you take the necessary steps to ensure the patient's safety. These actions may include enlisting the assistance of the law in involuntarily admitting the patient on a temporary basis.

DOCUMENTATION OF CARE

The purposes of the medical record are to provide accurate and complete information about the care and treatment of patients. It also gives healthcare personnel a means of communicating with one another, allowing for continuity of care. A record's usefulness is determined by how accurately and completely it portrays the patient's behavioral status at the time it was written. The patient has the right to see the medical record, but it belongs to the institution. The patient is instructed on the facility's protocol to view personal records.

For example, if a psychiatric patient describes intent to harm himself or another person and the nurse fails to document the information—including the need to protect the patient or the identified victim—the information will be lost when the nurse leaves work. If the patient's plan is carried out, the harm caused could be linked directly to the nurse's failure to communicate the patient's intent. Even though documentation takes time away from patient care, its importance in communicating and preserving the nurse's assessment and memory cannot be overemphasized.

Medical Records and Quality Improvement

The medical record has many other uses aside from providing information on the course of the patient's care and treatment by healthcare professionals. According to the Institute of Medicine (2011), quality improvement is a key goal for the future of nursing and healthcare. A retrospective medical record review provides valuable information to the facility on the quality of care provided and on ways to improve that care.

A facility may also conduct reviews for risk management purposes. These reviews help to determine areas of potential liability for the facility and to evaluate methods used to reduce the facility's exposure to liability. For example, risk managers often review documentation of the use of restraints and seclusion for psychiatric patients. Accordingly, risk managers may use the medical record to evaluate care for quality assurance or peer review. Utilization review analysts evaluate the medical record to determine appropriate use of hospital and staff resources consistent with reimbursement schedules. Insurance companies and other reimbursement agencies rely on the medical record in determining which payments they will make on the patient's behalf.

Medical Records as Evidence

From a legal perspective, the medical record is a recording of data and opinions made in the normal course of the patient's hospital care. Courts consider it good evidence because it is presumed to be true, honest, and untainted by memory lapses. Accordingly, the medical record finds its way into a variety of legal cases for a variety of reasons.

Medical records help to determine:

1. The extent of the patient's damages and pain and suffering in personal injury cases, such as when a psychiatric patient attempts suicide while under the protective care of a hospital.
2. The nature and extent of injuries in child abuse or older adult abuse cases.
3. The nature and extent of physical or mental disability in disability cases.
4. The nature and extent of injury and rehabilitative potential in workers' compensation cases.

Medical records may also be used in police investigations, civil conservatorship proceedings, competency hearings, and involuntary commitment procedures. In states that mandate mental health legal services or a patients' rights advocacy program, audits may be performed to determine the facility's compliance with state laws or violation of patients' rights. Finally, medical records may be used in professional and hospital negligence cases.

Guidelines for Electronic Documentation

Informatics provides the healthcare system with essential technology to manage knowledge, communicate, reduce error, and facilitate decision making (Quality and Safety Education for Nurses, 2012). However, electronic record keeping creates challenges for protecting the confidentiality of the records of psychiatric patients. Sensitive information regarding treatment for mental illness can adversely impact patients seeking employment, insurance, and credit.

Federal laws address concerns for the privacy of patients' records and provide guidelines for agencies that use electronic documentation. Only staff members who have a legitimate need to know about the patient are authorized to access a patient's electronic medical record. There are penalties, including termination of employment, if a staff member enters a record without authorization.

You are responsible for all entries into records using your password. As a result, your password should remain private and should be changed periodically. In the event a documentation error is made, the various systems allow specific time frames to make medical record corrections.

Institutions should encourage documentation methods that improve communication between care providers. Courts assume that nurses and physicians read each other's notes on patient progress. They also assume that if care is not documented, it did not occur. Your notes may serve as a valuable memory refresher if the patient sues years after the care is provided.

FORENSIC NURSING

The evolving specialty of forensic nursing includes the application of nursing principles in a court of law to assist in reaching a decision on a contested issue. The nurse often educates the court about the science of nursing. The witness applies nursing knowledge to the facts in the lawsuit and may provide opinions using appropriate nursing standards.

Some situations in which a psychiatric-mental health nurse may be helpful include testimony related to patient competency, fitness to stand trial, involuntary commitment, or responsibility for a crime. Forensic nurses may also focus on victims and perpetrators of crime and violence, the collection of evidence, and the provision of healthcare in prison settings. Refer to Chapter 33 for a complete discussion of forensic nursing.

VIOLENCE IN THE PSYCHIATRIC SETTING

Registered nurses can get hurt in a variety of ways, such as heavy lifting, exposure to chemicals, and needle pricks. Violent events are only about 12% of all injuries to registered nurses (U.S. Department of Labor, 2018), yet the incidence rate of 12.7 cases per 10,000 full-time workers is about three times greater than the rate of violence in other occupations (3.8 cases per 10,000 workers). Injuries from acts of violence require workers to take time off work for treatment and recovery. Although emergency department nurses are more likely to be assaulted, psychiatric nurses also have fairly high rates.

In a survey of 3765 nurses and nursing students, 21% reported being physically assaulted during a 1-year period (ANA, 2015c). Over 50% of this sample reported being verbally abused.

Nurses, as citizens, have the same rights as patients not to be threatened or harmed. In recent years, nurses have actively sought workplace violence legislation. New laws enhance criminal charges and penalties for striking nurses and other healthcare workers in the course of duty. Usually, a prosecutor will not bring charges against disoriented, delirious, psychotic, or otherwise mentally impaired patients. However, violent patients, friends of patients, and family members who are aware of their actions can be charged with serious crimes.

▋ KEY POINTS TO REMEMBER

- Psychiatric-mental health nurses frequently encounter problems requiring ethical choices. Understanding ethical principles and applying them to ethical dilemmas can help in making choices.
- Mental health laws protect both patients and caregivers.
- Psychiatric admissions are either voluntary or involuntary.

- State laws vary in how involuntary commitments are handled. In general, a significant mental health problem exists that interferes with a person's safe functioning. Psychiatric professionals confirm this problem and courts are responsible for determining competency and continuing involuntary treatment.

- Patients have the right to quality treatment, the right to refuse treatment, and the right to informed consent (i.e., knowing their treatment options and voluntarily accepting treatment).
- Restraint and seclusion abuses in the past have resulted in strict laws concerning their use and documentation of their use.
- Confidentiality is one of the most important legal concepts in psychiatry. Only patients can waive the right to confidentiality.
- Exceptions to the confidentiality rule include warning third parties of threats by patients and in cases of suspected child and older adult abuse.

- The nurse's privilege to practice carries with it the responsibility to practice safely, competently, and in a manner consistent with state and federal laws.
- Important laws for psychiatric nurses include intentional torts such as assault, battery, false imprisonment, invasion of privacy, and defamation of character.
- Unintentional torts are a type of negligence called malpractice where professionals fail to act in accordance with professional standards. They fail to foresee consequences of their action or inaction at the level that would be expected of someone with similar training and experience.
- Knowledge of the law, professional association standards, organizational policies and procedures, and customs are essential for providing safe, effective nursing care.

CRITICAL THINKING

1. As Joe, a registered nurse, prepares the medication for the evening shift, he notices that two of his patients' medications are missing. Both are bedtime Ativan (lorazepam). When he phones the pharmacy to send up the missing medications, the pharmacist responds, "You people need to watch your carts more carefully because this has become a pattern."
Shortly after, another patient complains to Joe that he did not receive his 5 p.m. Xanax (alprazolam). On the medication administration record, Beth has recorded that she has given the drugs. Joe suspects that Beth may be diverting the drugs.
   a. What actions can Joe take regarding his suspicions of Beth?
   b. If Beth admits that she has been diverting the drugs, should Joe's next step be to report Beth to the supervisor or to the board of nursing?
   c. When Joe talks to the nursing supervisor, should he identify Beth or should he state his suspicions in general terms?
2. One day, Linda arrives at work on the behavioral care unit. She is informed that the staffing office has requested that a nurse from the psychiatric unit report to the ICU. They need help in caring for an agitated car accident victim with a history of schizophrenia.
Linda goes to the ICU and joins a nurse named Corey in providing care for the patient. Eventually, the patient is stabilized and goes to sleep, and Corey leaves the unit for a break. Because Linda is unfamiliar with the telemetry equipment, she fails to recognize that the patient is having an arrhythmia, and the patient experiences a cardiopulmonary arrest. Although he is successfully resuscitated, he suffers permanent brain damage.

   a. Can Linda legally practice in this situation? (That is, does her registered nurse license permit her to practice in the ICU?)
   b. Does the ability to practice legally in an area differ from the ability to practice competently in that area?
   c. Did Linda have any legal or ethical grounds to refuse the assignment to the ICU?
   d. What are the risks in accepting an assignment in an area of specialty in which you are professionally unprepared to practice?
   e. Would there have been any way for Linda to minimize the risk of retaliation by the employer had she refused the assignment?
   f. If Linda is negligent, is the hospital liable for any harm to the patient caused by her?
3. A 40-year-old man is admitted to the emergency department for a severe nosebleed and has both of his nostrils packed. Because of a history of alcoholism and the possibility for developing withdrawal symptoms, the patient is transferred to the psychiatric unit. His physician orders a private room, restraints, continuous monitoring, and 15-minute checks of vital signs and other indicators. At the next 15-minute check, the nurse discovers that the patient does not have a pulse or respiration. The patient had apparently inhaled the nasal packing and suffocated.
   a. Does it sound as if the nurse was responsible for the patient's death?
   b. Was the order for the restraint appropriate for this type of patient?
   c. What factors did you consider in making your determination?

CHAPTER REVIEW

1. Which statement made by the nurse concerning ethics demonstrates the best understanding of the concept?
   a. "It isn't right to deny someone healthcare because they can't pay for it."
   b. "I never discuss my patient's refusal of treatment."
   c. "The hospital needs to buy more respirators so we always have one available."
   d. "Not all ICU patients have the right to unbiased attention from the staff."

2. Which nursing intervention demonstrates the ethical principle of beneficence?
   a. Refusing to administer a placebo to a patient.
   b. Attending an in-service on the operation of the new IV infusion pumps
   c. Providing frequent updates to the family of a patient currently in surgery
   d. Respecting the right of the patient to make decisions about whether or not to have electroconvulsive therapy

3. How can a newly hired nurse best attain information concerning the state's mental health laws and statutes?
   a. Discuss the issue with the facility's compliance officer
   b. Conduct an internet search using the keywords "mental + health + statutes + (your state)"
   c. Consult the ANA's *Code of Ethics for Nurses*
   d. Review the facility's latest edition of the policies manual

4. When considering facility admissions for mental health-care, what characteristic is unique to a voluntary admission?
   a. The patient poses no substantial threat to themselves or to others
   b. The patient has the right to seek legal counsel
   c. A request in writing is required before admission
   d. A mental illness has been previously diagnosed

5. Which situations demonstrate liable behavior on the part of the staff? *Select all that apply.*
   a. Forgetting to obtain consent for electroconvulsive therapy for a cognitively impaired patient
   b. Leaving a patient with suicidal thoughts alone in the bathroom to shower
   c. Promising to restrain a patient who stole from another patient on the unit
   d. Reassuring a patient with paranoia that his antipsychotic medication was not tampered with
   e. Placing a patient who has repeatedly threatened to assault staff in seclusion

6. A nurse makes a post on a social media page about his peer taking care of a patient with a crime-related gunshot wound in the emergency department. He does not use the name of the patient. The nurse:
   a. Has not violated confidentiality laws because he did not use the patient's name.
   b. Cannot be held liable for violating confidentiality laws because he was not the primary nurse for the patient.
   c. Has violated confidentiality laws and can be held liable.

   d. Cannot be held liable because postings on a social media site are excluded from confidentiality laws.

7. In providing care for patients of a mental health unit, Li recognizes the importance of standards of care. When Li notices that some policies fall short of the state licensing laws, which of the following statements represents the most appropriate standard of care pathway?
   a. Professional association, customary care, facility policy
   b. State board of nursing, facility policy, customary care
   c. Facility policy, professional associations, state board of nursing
   d. State board of nursing, professional association, facility policy

8. Lucas has completed his inpatient psychiatric treatment, which was ordered by the court system. Which statement reveals that Lucas does not understand the concept of conditional release?
   a. "I will continue treatment in an outpatient treatment center."
   b. "My nurse practitioner has recommended group therapy."
   c. "I am finally free, no more therapy."
   d. "Attending therapy and taking my meds are a part of this conditional release."

9. Implied consent occurs when no verbal or written agreement takes place prior to a caregiver delivering treatment. Which of the following examples represents implied consent?
   a. The mother of an unconscious patient saying okay to surgery
   b. Care given to a heroin overdose victim
   c. Immobilizing a patient who has refused to take medication
   d. Signing general intake paperwork with specific parameters

10. Based on Maslow's hierarchy of needs, physiological needs for a restrained patient include: *Select all that apply.*
   a. Private toileting, oral hydration
   b. Checking the tightness of the restraints
   c. Therapeutic communication
   d. Maintaining a patent airway

1. a; 2. c; 3. b; 4. c; 5. a, b, c; 6. c; 7. d; 8. c; 9. b; 10. a, b, d

Visit the Evolve website for a posttest on the content in this chapter: http://evolve.elsevier.com/Varcarolis

REFERENCES

American Nurses Association. (2015a). *Code of ethics for nurses with interpretive statements.* Washington, DC: American Nurses Publishing.

American Nurses Association. (2015b). *Health risk appraisal.* Retrieved from http://www.nursingworld.org/HRA-Executive-Summary.

American Nurses Association. (2015c). *Nursing: Scope and standards of practice* (3rd ed.). Silver Spring, MD: NursesBooks.org.

American Nurses Association, American Psychiatric-Mental Health Nurses Association, & International Society of Psychiatric-Mental Health Nurses. (2014). *Psychiatric-mental health nursing: Scope and standards of practice.* Silver Spring, MD: American Nurses Association.

American Psychiatric Association. (2013). *Diagnostic and statistical manual of mental disorders (DSM-5)* (5th ed.). Washington, DC: Author.

American Psychiatric Nurses Association. (2018). *APNA position statement on the use of seclusion and restraint.* Retrieved from https://www.apna.org/m/pages.cfm?pageid=3728.

Bazelton Center for Mental Health Law. (2012). *Where we stand: Mental health parity.* Retrieved from http://www.bazelton.org/Where-We-Stand?Access-to-Services/Mental-Health-Parity.aspx.

Bernstein, N. (2012). Restrained youth's death in Yonkers is investigated. *New York Times*. Retrieved from http://www.nytimes.com/2012/04/21/nyregion/death-of-youth-at-leake-watts-center-in-yonkers-is-investigated.html?_r=0.

Butler, J. (2019). How safe is the schoolhouse? Retrieved from https://www.autcom.org/pdf/HowSafeSchoolhouse.pdf.

Canterbury v. Spence, 464 F.2d 722 (D.C. Cir. 1972), quoting Schloendorf v. Society of N.Y. Hosp., 211 N.Y. 125 105 N.E.2d 92, 93 (1914).

Centers for Medicare and Medicaid Services. (2008). *Hospitals—Restraint/seclusion interpretive guidelines and updated state operations manual*. Retrieved from http://www.cms.gov/Medicare/Provider-Enrollment-and-Certification/SurveyCertificationGenInfo/downloads/SCLetter08-18.pdf.

Curtis, A. (2001). *Involuntary commitment*. Retrieved from http://psychrights.org/states/Maine/InvoluntaryCommitmentbyAliciaCurtis.htm.

Deutsch, A. (1949). *The shame of the states*. New York, NY: Harcourt Brace.

Health Insurance Portability and Accountability Act, U.S.C.45C.F.R § 164.501 (2003).

Institute of Medicine (IOM). (2011). *The future of nursing: Focus on education*. Retrieved from http://www.iom.edu/Reports/2010/The-Future-of-Nursing-Leading-Change-Advancing-Health/Report-Brief-Education.aspx.

Ornstein, C. (2015). A patient is sued, and his mental health diagnosis becomes public. *New York Times*. Retrieved from http://www.nytimes.com/2015/12/24/nyregion/a-patient-is-sued-and-his-mental-health-diagnosis-becomes-public.html.

Pierce, R. (2014). *Statutory solutions for a common law defect: Advancing the nurse practitioner-patient privilege*. Retrieved from http://repository.jmls.edu/cgi/viewcontent.cgi?article=1961&context=lawreview.

Plumadore v. State of New York. (1980). 427 N.Y.S.2d 90.

Quality and Safety Education for Nurses. (2012). *Competency knowledge, skills, and attitudes*. Retrieved from http://www.qsen.org/ksas_prelicensure.php#informatics.

Raess v. Doescher, 883 N.E.2d 790 (Indiana 2008)

Roberts, L. W., & Dunn, L. B. (2019). Ethical considerations in psychiatry. In L. W. Roberts (Ed.), *The American Psychiatric Association Publishing textbook of psychiatry* (7th ed.) (pp. 177–199). American Psychiatric Association Publishing.

Tarasoff v. Regents of University of California (1974). 529 P.2d 553, 118 Cal Rptr 129.

Turnwald, B. P., Goyer, J. P., Boles, D. Z., Silder, A., Delp, S. L., & Crum, A. J. (2019). Learning one's genetic risk changes physiology independent of actual genetic risk. *Nature Human Behaviour, 3*, 48–56.

United States Department of Labor. (2018). *Occupational injuries and illnesses among registered nurses*. Retrieved from https://www.bls.gov/opub/mlr/2018/article/occupational-injuries-and-illnesses-among-registered-nurses.htm.

United States Food and Drug Administration. (2018). *The FDA warns against the use of many genetic tests*. Retrieved from https://www.fda.gov/medical-devices/safety-communications/fda-warns-against-use-many-genetic-tests-unapproved-claims-predict-patient-response-specific.

United States Food and Drug Administration. (2019). *FDA issues warning letter to genomics lab*. Retrieved from https://www.fda.gov/news-events/press-announcements/fda-issues-warning-letter-genomics-lab-illegally-marketing-genetic-test-claims-predict-patients.

Zeier, Z., Carpenter, L. L., Kalin, N. H., Rodriguez, C. I., McDonald, W. M., Widge, A. S., & Nemeroff, C. B. (2018, April). Clinical implementation of pharmacogenetic decision support tools for antidepressant drug prescribe. *American Journal of Psychiatry*. Retrieved from https://ajp.psychiatryonline.org/doi/10.1176/appi.ajp.2018.17111282.

7

The Nursing Process and Standards of Care

Margaret Jordan Halter and Elizabeth M. Varcarolis

🌐 Visit the Evolve website for a pretest on the content in this chapter: http://evolve.elsevier.com/Varcarolis

OBJECTIVES

1. Identify the steps in the nursing process.
2. Describe the purpose of the *Psychiatric–Mental Health Nursing: Scope and Standards of Practice* publication.
3. Compare the different approaches you would consider when you are performing an assessment of a child, an adolescent, and an older adult.
4. Differentiate between the use of an interpreter and a translator during an assessment of a non–English-speaking patient.
5. Conduct a mental status examination (MSE).
6. Perform a psychosocial assessment, including brief cultural and spiritual components.
7. Explain three principles a nurse should follow in planning actions to reach agreed-upon outcome criteria.
8. Construct a plan of care for a patient with a psychiatric disorder or mental health condition.
9. Describe three advanced practice psychiatric–mental health nursing interventions.
10. Discuss the evaluation of care based on professional standards of practice.

KEY TERMS AND CONCEPTS

evidence-based practice (EBP)
health teaching
mental status examination (MSE)

milieu therapy
objective data
outcome criteria

psychosocial assessment
self-care activities
subjective data

The term *nursing process* was first used in a speech by Lydia Hall, a nursing theorist (de la Cuesta, 1983). She used it to describe the care given by nurses and suggested a three-stage process of observation, ministration of care, and validation. Other nurse leaders and theorists, including Dorothy Johnson (1959) and Ida Orlando (1961), later began using the term. Interest in a systematic method for guiding nursing actions culminated in the American Nurses Association (ANA) 1965 publication of a position paper calling for a change in nursing education and use of the nursing process to support patient care. Further support for this movement arose during the 1970s, when the Joint Commission on Accreditation of Hospitals required the use of the nursing process as a condition for accreditation (de la Cuesta, 1983).

The steps of the nursing process evolved over time. In 1967, Yura and Walsh identified those four steps:

- Assessing
- Planning
- Implementing
- Evaluating

In 1973, the ANA published the forerunner of future standards publications, *Standard for Nursing Practice*. In this publication a separate step in the nursing process, nursing diagnosis, was included. In 1991, the ANA added outcome identification as a distinct step of the planning process. These changes resulted in a six-step problem-solving approach, including

- Assessment
- Diagnosis
- Outcomes identification
- Planning
- Implementation
- Evaluation

The nursing process is intended to facilitate and identify appropriate, safe, culturally competent, developmentally relevant quality care for individuals, families, groups, or communities. Psychiatric–mental health nurses base judgments and behaviors on this accepted theoretical framework (Fig. 7.1). Whenever possible, we support our interventions with scientific

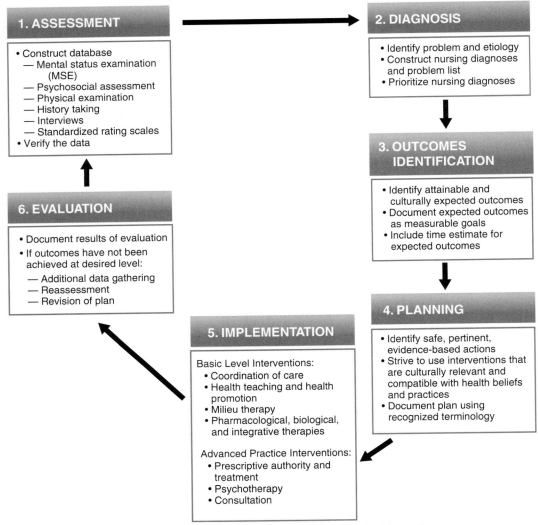

NURSING ASSESSMENT

The assessment interview requires culturally effective communication skills and encompasses a large database (e.g., significant support system; family; cultural and community system; spiritual and philosophical values, strengths, and health beliefs and practices; as well as many other factors).

1. ASSESSMENT

- Construct database
  — Mental status examination (MSE)
  — Psychosocial assessment
  — Physical examination
  — History taking
  — Interviews
  — Standardized rating scales
- Verify the data

2. DIAGNOSIS

- Identify problem and etiology
- Construct nursing diagnoses and problem list
- Prioritize nursing diagnoses

3. OUTCOMES IDENTIFICATION

- Identify attainable and culturally expected outcomes
- Document expected outcomes as measurable goals
- Include time estimate for expected outcomes

6. EVALUATION

- Document results of evaluation
- If outcomes have not been achieved at desired level:
  — Additional data gathering
  — Reassessment
  — Revision of plan

5. IMPLEMENTATION

Basic Level Interventions:
- Coordination of care
- Health teaching and health promotion
- Milieu therapy
- Pharmacological, biological, and integrative therapies

Advanced Practice Interventions:
- Prescriptive authority and treatment
- Psychotherapy
- Consultation

4. PLANNING

- Identify safe, pertinent, evidence-based actions
- Strive to use interventions that are culturally relevant and compatible with health beliefs and practices
- Document plan using recognized terminology

Fig. 7.1 The nursing process in psychiatric-mental health nursing.

documentation as we apply evidence-based research to our nursing plans and actions of care.

The nursing process is also the foundation of the standards of practice as presented in *Psychiatric-Mental Health Nursing: Scope and Standards of Practice,* second edition (ANA et al., 2014). The word *scope* in the book's title answers the following questions about psychiatric nursing: What do they do? Where do they do it? When do they do it? Why do they do it? and How do they do it? The book also provides a historical description of psychiatric nursing, current issues and trends, and levels of practice (i.e., registered nurses and advanced practice registered nurses).

The standards of practice are statements that identify the duties and obligations for which psychiatric–mental health nurses are held accountable. These standards provide the basis for

- Certification criteria
- A legal definition of psychiatric–mental health nursing
- National Council of State Boards of Nursing Licensure Examination (NCLEX-RN) questions

Quality and Safety Education in Nursing

Safety and quality care for patients is an essential focus for nursing education. In the late 1990s, the Institute of Medicine (IOM)[a] and other organizations sought to improve the quality of patient care and safety. The competencies mandated by the National Academy of Sciences require a change in the way

---

[a]Now known as the Health and Medicine Division of the National Academy of Medicine.

BOX 7.1 Quality and Safety Education for Nurses Competencies

Patient-centered care: Recognize the patient or designee as the source of control and full partner in providing compassionate and coordinated care based on respect for the patient's preferences, values, and needs.

Quality improvement: Use data to monitor the outcomes of care processes and use improvement methods to design and test changes to continuously improve the quality and safety of healthcare systems.

Safety: Minimize risk of harm to patients and provide optimal healthcare through both system effectiveness and individual performance.

Informatics: Use information and technology to communicate, manage knowledge, mitigate error, and support decision making.

Teamwork and collaboration: Function effectively within nursing and interprofessional teams, fostering open communication, mutual respect, and shared decision making to achieve quality patient care.

Evidence-based practice (EBP): Integrate best current evidence with clinical expertise and patient/family preferences and values for delivery of optimal healthcare.

From Cronenwett, L., Sherwood, G., Barnsteiner, J., et al. (2007). Quality and safety education for nurses. *Nursing Outlook, 55*(3), 122–131.

that all healthcare professionals are educated. According to the IOM (2003), healthcare workers in the 21st century should be able to

1. Provide patient-centered care
2. Work in interdisciplinary teams
3. Employ evidence-based practice
4. Apply quality improvement
5. Utilize informatics

A group of faculty adapted these competencies for nursing students in an initiative known as *Quality and Safety Education in Nursing (QSEN)*. They developed definitions that describe essential features of a competent and respected nurse. These competency definitions provide the basis for statements regarding the knowledge, skills, and attitudes (KSAs) that should be developed in nursing education (Cronenwett et al., 2007). The six QSEN competencies reflect the IOM's competencies with the addition of safety as a separate competency. These competencies are integrated into this chapter and throughout this textbook (Box 7.1).

Suggestions for the use of QSEN competencies in nursing education can be found in "Competency Knowledge, Skills, Attitudes (KSAs) (Pre-Licensure)" at the website www.qsen.org/competencies/pre-licensure-ksas/.

Standards of Practice in Psychiatric–Mental Health Nursing

The following sections describe the standards of practice for psychiatric–mental health nursing. These standards describe the care provided by a competent psychiatric–mental health nurse.

STANDARDS OF PRACTICE FOR PSYCHIATRIC–MENTAL HEALTH NURSING: STANDARD 1: ASSESSMENT

The psychiatric–mental health registered nurse collects and synthesizes comprehensive health data pertinent to the healthcare consumer's health and/or situation (ANA et al., 2014, p. 44).

A view of the individual as a complex blend of many parts is consistent with nurses' holistic approach to care. Nurses who work in psychiatric–mental health must assess or have access to the past and present medical history, a recent physical examination, and knowledge of physical complaints. Psychiatric nurses also document observable physical conditions or behaviors, such as an unsteady gait, abnormal breathing patterns, wincing as if in pain, and doubling over to relieve discomfort.

The assessment process begins with the initial patient encounter and continues throughout the patient stay. To develop a basis for the plan of care and in preparation for discharge, every patient should have a thorough formal nursing assessment upon entering treatment.

Subsequent to the formal assessment, the nurse collects data continually and systematically as the patient's condition changes and—hopefully—improves. Perhaps the patient came into treatment with active suicidal thoughts, and the initial focus of care was on protection from injury. Through regular assessment, the nurse may determine that although suicidal ideation has diminished, negative thinking may still be a problem.

A variety of professionals conduct assessments, including nurses, psychiatrists, social workers, dietitians, and other therapists. Virtually all facilities have standardized nursing assessment forms to aid in organization and consistency among reviewers. These forms may be paper or electronic versions according to the resources and preferences of the institution.

The time required for the nursing assessment varies depending on the assessment form. Longer interviews may be required based on the patient's response pattern. For example, such responses may be long or rambling, patients may have tangential thoughts or memory disturbances, or they may provide profoundly slowed responses. Refer to Chapter 9 for guidelines for setting up and conducting a clinical interview.

In all situations, the patient is provided with a copy of the Health Insurance Portability and Accountability Act (HIPAA) guidelines. Essentially, the purpose of the HIPAA privacy rule is to ensure that an individual's health information is protected while at the same time allowing healthcare providers to obtain health information for the purpose of giving and promoting high-quality healthcare (US Department of Health and Human Services, 2003). Chapter 6 has a more detailed discussion of HIPAA.

In patient-centered care, the nurse's primary source of data is the patient. However, there may be times when it is necessary to supplement or rely completely on other sources for the assessment information. These secondary sources are essential when the nurse is caring for a patient who is silent or is experiencing psychosis, agitation, or catatonia. Such secondary sources include members of the family, friends, neighbors, police, healthcare workers, and medical records.

Age Considerations

Assessment of Children

Although the child is the best source for understanding the child's inner feelings and emotions, the caregivers (parents or guardians) can often best describe the child's behavior, performance, and conduct. Caregivers are also helpful in interpreting the child's words and responses, but a separate interview is advisable when a child is reluctant to share information, especially in cases of suspected abuse by the parents or guardians.

Consider developmental levels in the evaluation of children. One of the hallmarks of psychiatric disorders in children is the tendency to regress (i.e., return to a previous level of development). For example, although it is developmentally appropriate for toddlers to suck their thumbs, such a gesture is unusual in an older child.

Children are assessed through a combination of interview and observation. Watching children at play provides important clues to their functioning. Play is a safe area for children to act out thoughts and emotions. Asking the child to tell a story, draw a picture, or engage in specific therapeutic games can be useful, particularly when the child is having difficulty with verbal expression.

Assessment of Adolescents

Adolescents are especially concerned with confidentiality and may fear that you will repeat what they say to their parents. This may be a difficult area to navigate. In the eyes of the law, parents give consent for treatment and therefore have a right to know how their child will be treated. Clinically and ethically, nurses should understand that certain zones of privacy exist even for adolescents. In such situations, it is is appropriate to use your best judgment. When in doubt, you may have to consult with your clinical instructor or supervisor.

The adolescent and the adolescent's family should be given an overview of how information sharing will work, what information will be shared, with whom, and when. Adolescents should receive an explanation of the role of the treatment team in providing care and the need to share certain information. Threats of suicide, homicide, sexual abuse, or behaviors that put the patient or others at risk for harm are shared with other professionals as well as with the parents.

One of the key objectives in the assessment of adolescents is the identification of risk factors. It is helpful to use a brief structured interview technique such as the HEADSSS interview (Box 7.2).

Assessment of Older Adults

As we get older, our five senses (taste, touch, sight, hearing, and smell) and brain function begin to diminish. The extent to which this affects each person varies. Your patient may be a spry and alert 80-year-old or a frail and confused 60-year-old. Therefore it is important not to stereotype older adults and expect them to be physically and mentally deficient.

On the other hand, many older adults need special attention. The nurse evaluates physical limitations, which may be sensory (difficulty seeing or hearing), motor (difficulty walking or maintaining balance), or medical (back pain, cardiac or pulmonary deficits). All of these problems can increase anxiety, embarrassment, or physical discomfort.

It is wise to identify physical deficits at the onset of the assessment and to make accommodations for them. Sometimes healthcare providers will speak loudly to an older adult, regardless of the patient's hearing ability. You can usually gauge the amount, if any, of hearing loss after a few sentences. If the patient is hard of hearing, speak a little more slowly in clear, louder tones (but not too loud). Without invading personal space, seat the patient close to you. Often, a voice that is lower in pitch is easier for older adults to hear. Refer to Chapter 31 for more on assessing and communicating with the older adult.

Language Barriers

Psychiatric–mental health nurses can best care for their patients if they understand the complex cultural and social factors that influence health and illness. Awareness of individual cultural beliefs and healthcare practices can help nurses minimize stereotypical assumptions that can lead to ineffective care. There are many opportunities for misunderstandings when you are assessing a patient from a different cultural or social background from your own. This is particularly problematic when the patient does not speak the same language as the caregiver.

Often healthcare professionals require an interpreter or translator to understand the patient's history and healthcare needs. An interpreter is someone who interprets the spoken words of a foreign language speaking person or someone who uses American Sign Language (ASL). A translator is an individual who speaks one or more languages in addition to English who translates the written word. Healthcare providers who receive federal funding are required by law to provide interpreters and translators to limited English proficient patients free of charge. Typically, interpreters are on staff, although they may be telephone based, particularly with less common languages.

The use of untrained interpreters such as family members, friends, and neighbors may be tempting, especially because they are convenient and there is no fee involved. However, the cost of even one malpractice lawsuit brought on by incorrect interpretations can be devastating to organizations, not to mention the

---

BOX 7.2   The HEADSSS Psychosocial Interview Technique

H Home environment (e.g., relations with parents and siblings)
E Education and employment (e.g., school performance)
A Activities (e.g., sports participation, after-school activities, peer relations)
D Drug, alcohol, or tobacco use
S Sexuality (e.g., whether the patient is sexually active, practices safe sex, or uses contraception)
S Suicide risk or symptoms of depression or other mental disorder
S Safety (e.g., how safe does the patient feel at home and school, wear a safety belt, or engage in dangerous or risky activities)

From Reif, C. J., & Elster, A. B. (1998). Adolescent preventive services. *Primary Care: Clinics in Office Practice, 25*(1), 1–21.

consequences to the patient. Unpaid nonprofessionals may censor or omit certain content (e.g., profanity, psychotic thoughts, and sexual topics) owing to a desire to protect the patient. They can also make subjective interpretations based on their own feelings, share confidential details with others, or leave out traumatic topics because the subject matter is too familiar or painful for them.

Psychiatric–Mental Health Nursing Assessment

The purpose of the psychiatric–mental health nursing assessment is to

- Establish rapport
- Obtain an understanding of the current problem or chief complaint
- Review the patient's physical status and obtain baseline vital signs
- Assess for risk factors affecting the safety of the patient or others
- Perform a mental status examination
- Assess psychosocial status
- Identify mutual goals for treatment
- Formulate a plan of care
- Document data in a retrievable format

Gathering Data

Review of systems. The mind-body connection is significant in the understanding and treatment of psychiatric disorders. An advanced care provider such as an advanced practice psychiatric registered nurse (i.e., nurse practitioner, clinical nurse specialist), a physician, or a physician assistant typically conducts a physical examination on patients who are admitted for treatment of psychiatric disorders and conditions. A complete physical examination may be deferred depending on the setting or the condition of the patient. Registered nurses gather a baseline set of vital signs, a historical and current review of body systems, and a documentation of allergies and responses.

Psychiatric symptoms such as depression, anxiety, and psychosis are often associated with certain physical conditions (Box 7.3). Therefore it important to rule out or address physical causes of symptoms. Conversely, psychiatric disorders can lead to physical or somatic symptoms such as abdominal discomfort, headaches, lethargy, insomnia, intense fatigue, and even pain.

Laboratory data. Hypothyroidism may have the clinical appearance of major depressive disorder. Hyperthyroidism may share symptoms (e.g., anxiety, weight loss, insomnia) with a hypomanic or manic phase of bipolar disorder. A simple blood test can usually differentiate between a mood disorder and thyroid problems, although a person could certainly have both. Abnormal liver enzyme levels can explain irritability, depression, and lethargy. People who have chronic renal disease often suffer from the same symptoms when their blood urea nitrogen and electrolyte levels are abnormal. Results of a toxicology screen for the presence of either prescription or illicit drugs also may provide explanations for unusual psychiatric signs and symptoms.

Mental status examination. Fundamental to the psychiatric–mental health nursing assessment is a **mental status examination (MSE)**. In fact, an MSE is part of the assessment in all areas of medicine. The MSE in psychiatry is analogous to the physical examination in general medicine, and the purpose is to evaluate an individual's current cognitive processes. Box 7.4 is an example of a basic MSE.

The MSE aids in collecting and organizing objective information. **Objective data** refers to all things that nurses observe or are verified through tests. Examples of objective data include heart rate, blood pressure, body temperature, oxygen saturation, height, weight, and levels of consciousness based on a rating scale.

Other sources of data made through observing the patient's appearance and nonverbals help us to make inferences. The nurse observes the patient's physical behavior, nonverbal communication, appearance, speech patterns, mood and affect, thought content, perceptions, cognitive ability, and insight and judgment.

Psychosocial assessment. A **psychosocial assessment** provides additional information from which to develop a plan of care. This type of assessment always begins by asking the patient to describe how treatment became necessary. This is known as the chief complaint and should be documented verbatim, that is, in the patient's own words; for example, "I have been completely miserable and alone since my husband died."

The patient's psychosocial history is the subjective part of the assessment. **Subjective data** refers to all information that you gather from a patient and from people who may accompany the patient. The focus of the history is the *patient's perceptions and recollections* of current lifestyle and life in general. Support, such as family and friends, education, work experience, coping styles, and spiritual and cultural beliefs, is typically discussed during a psychosocial history.

To conduct such an assessment, the nurse should have fundamental knowledge of growth and development, pathophysiology, psychopathology, and pharmacology as well as a basic understanding of various cultural and religious practices. Box 7.5 identifies items that are usually included in a basic psychosocial assessment tool.

Spiritual/religious assessment. Spirituality and religious beliefs have the potential to exert an influence on how people understand meaning and purpose in their lives and how they use critical judgment to solve problems (e.g., crises of illness). The terms *spirituality* and *religion* are different but not mutually exclusive. Spirituality refers to how we find meaning, hope, purpose, and a sense of peace in our lives. It is more of an inner phenomenon centering on universal personal questions and needs. It is the part of us that seeks to understand life. A person's spiritual beliefs may or may not be connected with the community or with religious rituals.

In contrast, **religion** is an external system that includes beliefs, patterns of worship, and symbols. An individual connects personal and spiritual beliefs with a larger organized group or institution. Belonging to a religious community can provide support during difficult times. Although religion is often concerned with spirituality, religious groups are social entities and

BOX 7.3   Psychiatric Symptoms Associated With Medical Conditions

Depression
Neurological disorders
- Cerebrovascular accident (stroke)
- Alzheimer's disease
- Brain tumor
- Huntington's disease
- Epilepsy
- Multiple sclerosis
- Parkinson's disease

Infections
- Mononucleosis
- Encephalitis
- Hepatitis
- Neurosyphilis
- Human immunodeficiency virus (HIV)

Endocrine Disorders
- Hypothyroidism and hyperthyroidism
- Cushing's syndrome
- Addison's disease
- Parathyroid disease

Gastrointestinal Disorders
- Liver cirrhosis
- Pancreatitis

Cardiovascular Disorders
- Hypoxia
- Congestive heart failure

Respiratory Disorders
- Sleep apnea

Nutritional Disorders
- Thiamine deficiency
- Protein deficiency
- B_{12} deficiency
- B_6 deficiency
- Folate deficiency

Collagen Vascular Disorders
- Lupus erythematosus
- Rheumatoid arthritis

Cancer

Anxiety
Neurological Disorders
- Alzheimer's disease
- Brain tumor
- Stroke
- Huntington's disease

Infections
- Encephalitis
- Meningitis
- Neurosyphilis
- Septicemia

Endocrine Disorders
- Hypothyroidism and hyperthyroidism
- Hypoparathyroidism
- Hypoglycemia
- Pheochromocytoma
- Carcinoid

Metabolic Disorders
- Low calcium
- Low potassium
- Acute intermittent porphyria
- Liver failure

Cardiovascular Disorders
- Angina
- Congestive heart failure
- Pulmonary embolus

Respiratory Disorders
- Pneumothorax
- Acute asthma
- Emphysema

Drug Effects
- Stimulants
- Sedatives (withdrawal)
- Lead, mercury poisoning

Psychosis
Medical Conditions
- Temporal lobe epilepsy
- Migraine headaches
- Temporal arteritis
- Occipital tumors
- Narcolepsy
- Encephalitis
- Hypothyroidism
- Addison's disease
- Human immunodeficiency virus (HIV)

Drug Effects
- Hallucinogens (e.g., LSD)
- Phencyclidine
- Alcohol withdrawal
- Stimulants
- Cocaine
- Corticosteroids

are also characterized by cultural, economic, political, social, and nonspiritual goals.

Spiritual and religious practices typically enhance healthy behaviors. For example, many major religions place a taboo on unhealthy practices such as smoking and drinking, thereby reducing these behaviors. Spirituality and religiosity also provide social support and a sense of meaning in people's lives. These behaviors, support, and meaning are linked to decreased mental and physical stress. This, in turn, relates to a decreased incidence of illness in many people. In rare but significant instances, a church doctrine may lead to unhealthy responses such as discouraging or forbidding the use of psychotropic medications. Religious leaders may even deny the existence of a psychiatric disorder in favor

BOX 7.4   Mental Status Examination

Appearance
- Grooming and dress
- Level of hygiene
- Pupil dilation or constriction
- Facial expression
- Height, weight, nutritional status
- Presence of body piercing or tattoos, scars, etc.
- Relationship between appearance and age

Behavior
- Excessive or reduced body movements
- Peculiar body movements (e.g., scanning of the environment, odd or repetitive gestures, level of consciousness, balance, and gait)
- Abnormal movements (e.g., tardive dyskinesia, tremors)
- Level of eye contact (keep cultural differences in mind)

Speech
- Rate: slow, rapid, normal
- Volume: loud, soft, normal
- Disturbances (e.g., articulation problems, slurring, stuttering, mumbling)

Mood
- Affect: flat, bland, animated, angry, withdrawn, appropriate to context
- Mood: sad, labile, euphoric

Disorders of the Form of Thought
- Thought process (e.g., disorganized, coherent, flight of ideas, neologisms, thought blocking, circumstantiality)
- Thought content (e.g., delusions, obsessions)

Perceptual Disturbances
- Hallucinations (e.g., auditory, visual)
- Illusions

Cognition
- Orientation: time, place, person
- Level of consciousness (e.g., alert, confused, clouded, stuporous, unconscious, comatose)
- Memory: remote, recent, immediate
- Fund of knowledge
- Attention: performance on serial sevens, digit span tests
- Abstraction: performance on tests involving similarities, proverbs
- Insight
- Judgment

Ideas of Harming Self or Others
- Suicidal or homicidal history and current thoughts
- Presence of a plan
- Means to carry out the plan
- Opportunity to carry out the plan

BOX 7.5   Psychosocial Assessment

Previous hospitalizations
Educational background
Occupational background
  Employed? Where? What length of time?
  Special skills
Social patterns
  Describe family
  Describe friends
  Household members
  Support system
  Describe a typical day
Sexual patterns
  Sexually active? Practices safe sex? Practices birth control?
  Sexual orientation
  Sexual difficulties
Interests
  How does the patient spend spare time?
  Interest in sports, hobbies, or leisure activities
  What gives the patient pleasure?
Substance use
  What prescribed medications does the patient take? How often? How much?
  What herbal or over-the-counter drugs does the patient take (e.g., St. John's wort, cold medicines)? How often? How much?
  What types of alcoholic beverages and how many drinks does the patient consume per day? Per week?
  What recreational drugs does the patient use (e.g., marijuana, psychedelics, cocaine)? How often? How much?
  Does the patient misuse prescription drugs (e.g., benzodiazepines, pain medications)?
  Does the patient identify the use of drugs as a problem?
Coping abilities
  What does the patient do when upset?
  To whom can the patient talk?
  What usually helps relieve stress?
  What coping mechanisms did the patient try prior to being admitted or seeking healthcare?
Spiritual assessment
  What importance does religion or spirituality have in the patient's life?
  Do the patient's religious or spiritual beliefs relate to self-care practices? How?
  Does the patient's faith help in stressful situations?
Health behaviors
  Whom does the patient see when medically ill?
  Are there special healthcare practices within the patient's culture that address particular mental problems?

of explanations of spiritual weakness or even demonic involvement.

The following types of questions are included in a spiritual or religious assessment:
- Do you have a religious affiliation?
- Do you practice any spiritual activities (e.g., yoga, meditation, spending time in nature)?
- Do you participate in any religious activities?
- What role does religion or spiritual practice play in your life?
- Does your faith help you in stressful situations?
- Do you pray or meditate?
- Has your illness affected your religious/spiritual practices?
- Would you like to have someone from your church/synagogue/temple or from our facility visit you?

Cultural and social assessment. Nursing assessments, diagnoses, and subsequent care should be planned around the unique cultural healthcare beliefs, values, and practices of each patient. Chapter 5 provides a detailed discussion of the cultural implications for psychiatric–mental health nursing and how to conduct a cultural and social assessment.

Questions we can ask to help with a cultural and social assessment include the following:
- What is your primary language? Would you like an interpreter?
- How would you describe your cultural background?

- Who are you close to?
- Who do you live with?
- How is your family responding to your treatment?
- Where do you go when you are physically ill? Emotionally upset or concerned?
- What do you do to get better when you have physical problems?
- What are the attitudes toward mental illness in your culture?
- How is your current problem viewed by your culture? Is it seen as a problem that can be fixed? A disease? A taboo? A fault or curse?
- Are there special foods that you eat or cannot eat?
- Are there special healthcare practices within your culture that address your particular mental or emotional health problem?
- Are there any special cultural beliefs about your illness that might help me give you better care?

After the cultural and social assessment, it is useful to summarize and review the data with the patient. This summary provides patients with reassurance that they have been heard and gives them the opportunity to clarify misinformation. The patient should be told what will happen next. For example, if the initial assessment takes place in the hospital, you should tell the patient who else will require a meeting. Tell patients when and how often they will meet with the nurse. If you believe a referral—such as talking with a dietician—is necessary, discuss this with the patient.

Validating the Assessment

To gain a clearer understanding of your patient, it is helpful to look to outside sources. Ideally, patients will have electronic medical records where all healthcare information is available. Emergency department records can be a valuable resource in understanding an individual's presenting problems. Police reports may be available in cases in which legal interactions occurred. Prior medical records, most accessible electronically, are a great help in validating information you already have or in adding new information to your database. If the patient has been admitted to a psychiatric unit in the past, information about the patient's previous level of functioning and behavior gives you a baseline for making clinical judgments. Consent forms usually have to be signed by the patient or family member/guardian to obtain access to records.

Using Rating Scales

Standardized rating scales are useful for psychiatric evaluation and monitoring. A clinician often administers rating scales, but many are self-administered. These rating scales highlight important areas in psychiatric assessment. Because many of the answers are subjective, experienced clinicians use these tools as a guide when planning care and also draw on their knowledge of their patients.

The American Psychiatric Association provides online measures that are available to clinicians and students at https://www.psychiatry.org/psychiatrists/practice/dsm/dsm-5/online-assessment-measures. Table 7.1 lists some of the common tools

TABLE 7.1   Standardized Rating Scales

USE	Scale
Major depressive disorder	Beck Inventory
	Brief Patient Health Questionnaire (Brief PHQ)
	Geriatric Depression Scale (GDS)
	Hamilton Depression Scale
	Zung Self-Report Inventory
	Patient Health Questionnaire-9 (PHQ-9)
	Patient Health Questionnaire for Adolescents (PHQ-A)
Anxiety	Brief Patient Health Questionnaire (Brief PHQ)
	Generalized Anxiety Disorder-7 (GAD-7)
	Modified Spielberger State Anxiety Scale
	Hamilton Anxiety Scale
	Severity Measure for Generalized Anxiety Disorder Child (11–17)
Trauma	Adverse Childhood Experiences Questionnaire
	Brief Trauma Questionnaire
	PTSD Scale for DSM-5 (CAPS-5)
	PTSD Symptom Scale Interview (PSS-I and PSS-I-5)
Substance use disorders	Addiction Severity Index (ASI)
	Recovery Attitude and Treatment Evaluator (RAATE)
	Brief Drug Abuse Screen Test (B-DAST)
Obsessive-compulsive behavior	Yale-Brown Obsessive-Compulsive Scale (Y-BOCS)
Mania	Mania Rating Scale
Schizophrenia	Scale for Assessment of Negative Symptoms (SANS)
	Brief Psychiatric Rating Scale (BPRS)
Abnormal movements	Abnormal Involuntary Movement Scale (AIMS)
	Simpson Neurological Rating Scale
General psychiatric assessment	Brief Psychiatric Rating Scale (BPRS)
	Global Assessment of Functioning Scale (GAF)
Cognitive function	Mini-Mental State Examination (MMSE)
	St. Louis University Mental Status Examination (SLUMS)
	Cognitive Capacity Screening Examination (CCSE)
	Alzheimer's Disease Rating Scale (ADRS)
	Memory and Behavior Problem Checklist
	Functional Assessment Screening Tool (FAST)
	Global Deterioration Scale (GDS)
Family assessment	McMaster Family Assessment Device
Eating disorders	Eating Disorders Inventory (EDI)
	Body Attitude Test
	Diagnostic Survey for Eating Disorders

These rating scales highlight important areas in psychiatric assessment. Because many of the answers are subjective, experienced clinicians use these tools as a guide when planning care and also draw on their knowledge of their patients.

in use. Many of the clinical chapters in this book provide rating scales to help you identify symptoms and symptom severity.

STANDARDS OF PRACTICE FOR PSYCHIATRIC–MENTAL HEALTH NURSING: STANDARD 2: DIAGNOSIS

The psychiatric–mental health registered nurse analyzes the assessment data to determine diagnoses, problems, and areas of focus for care and treatment, including level of risk (ANA et al., 2014, p. 46).

In 1953, Dr. Vera Fry coined the term *nursing diagnosis* in an article called "The Creative Approach to Nursing." Twenty years later, in 1973, diagnosis became an official component of the nursing process in the ANA's *Standards of Practice*. A nursing diagnosis is a clinical judgment about a patient's response to actual and potential problems (ANA, n.d.).

An accurate, clear, standardized nursing diagnosis is the basis for selecting therapeutic outcomes and interventions. NANDA International (NANDA-I, 2018) is group of professionals who have developed, researched, and refined a taxonomy of nursing diagnoses. Eleven editions of Herdman and Kamitsuru's (2018) *Nursing Diagnoses: Definitions and Classification* have been used by American nursing students.

Like NANDA-I, the International Classification for Nursing Practice (ICNP) provides a classification of nursing diagnoses. In addition to these diagnoses, the INCP also provides nursing interventions and nursing outcomes. The ICNP is published by the International Council of Nurses (ICN, 2017) as part of the World Health Organization (WHO) family of classifications. The WHO publishes the International Classification of Disease (ICD), a widely used system for diagnosing all types of diseases and disorders. Both the ICNP and ICD were developed for global use.

The ICNP supports nursing care in general settings and specialty areas through publication subsets that focus on areas such as dementia care, disaster nursing, and adult mental health. The wording for the diagnoses, outcomes, and interventions is both logical and intuitive. The ICNP is easily integrated with other healthcare classification systems, such as the ICD. It can be used to create multidisciplinary health vocabularies within information systems. The continued development of the ICNP is structured to support eHealth and statistical reporting practices across healthcare disciplines.

The ICNP is increasingly popular in US education settings and at the point of care. This system can also be used for healthcare decision making and policy development to improve delivery systems. The ICNP has international recognition and has been translated into 19 languages (ICN, 2019). This classification system will be used to support the nursing process throughout the clinical chapters in this textbook.

Diagnostic Statements

Nursing diagnostic statements are made up of the following structural components:
1. Problem/potential problem
2. Probable cause
3. Supporting data

The **problem**, or unmet need, describes the state of the patient at present. Problems that are within the nurse's domain to treat are termed *nursing diagnoses*. The nursing diagnostic label indicates what should change.

Probable cause is linked to the diagnostic label with the words *related to*. Probable causes usually indicate what needs to be addressed to bring about change through nursing interventions. In the case of *hopelessness related to long-term*

stress, the nurse would work with the patient to reduce or prevent the negative impacts of stress. However, in the case of *hopelessness related to abandonment,* there may be nothing the nurse can do to change the abandonment. In that case, the focus would be on symptom management by addressing the supporting data.

Supporting data include signs (objective and measurable) and symptoms (subjective and reported by the patient). All types of nursing diagnoses use supporting data. They may be linked to the diagnosis with the words *as evidenced by*. The previous example would then become "Hopelessness related to abandonment as evidenced by the statement, 'Nothing will change,' lack of involvement with family and friends, and inattention to self-care."

Types of Nursing Diagnoses

In **problem-focused diagnoses,** we make a judgment about adverse human responses to a health condition or life process. This category of nursing diagnosis is accompanied by probable cause and supporting data. An example of a problem-focused diagnosis is "Anxiety related to losing employment and financial burdens as evidenced by the statement, 'I can't concentrate,' crying, restlessness, and insomnia" (Formula: Problem + probable cause + supporting data).

Risk diagnoses pertain to vulnerability that carries a high probability of developing problematic experiences or responses. Common problems in this category include preventable occurrences such as falls, self-injury, pressure ulcers, and infection.

This category of diagnosis always begins with the phrase "risk for," followed by the problem. Because the problem has not yet happened, we do not cite causation in the form of "related to." An example of a risk diagnosis is "Risk for self-mutilation as evidenced by impulsivity, inadequate coping, isolation, and unstable self-esteem" (Formula: Problem + supporting data).

STANDARDS OF PRACTICE FOR PSYCHIATRIC–MENTAL HEALTH NURSING: STANDARD 3: OUTCOMES IDENTIFICATION

The psychiatric–mental health registered nurse identifies expected outcomes and the healthcare consumer's goals for a plan individualized to the healthcare consumer or to the situation (ANA et al., 2014, p. 48).

Outcome criteria are the hoped-for outcomes that reflect the maximum level of patient health that the patient can realistically achieve through nursing interventions. Whereas nursing diagnoses identify nursing problems, outcomes reflect the desired change. The expected outcomes provide direction for continuity of care (ANA et al., 2014).

All outcomes and goals are written in positive terms. The clinical chapters in this book include these short- and long-term outcomes. Table 7.2 shows how to state specific outcome criteria for an individual with suicidal ideation with a nursing diagnosis of "Risk for suicide related to depression and suicide attempt."

TABLE 7.2 Examples of Long- and Short-Term Goals for a Suicidal Patient

Long-Term Goals or Outcomes	Short-Term Goals or Outcomes
Patient will remain free from injury throughout the hospital stay.	Patient will identify the rationale and procedure of the unit's protocol for suicide precautions shortly after admission. Patient will seek out staff when feeling overwhelmed or self-destructive during hospitalization.
By discharge, patient will express hope and a desire to live and identify at least two people to contact if suicidal thoughts arise.	Patient will meet with social worker to find supportive resources in the community before discharge and work on trigger issues (e.g., housing, job). By discharge, patient will state the purpose of medication, time and dose, adverse effects, and whom to call for questions or concerns. Patient will have the written name and telephone numbers of at least two people to turn to if feeling overwhelmed or self-destructive. Patient will have a follow-up appointment to meet with a mental health professional by discharge.

STANDARDS OF PRACTICE FOR PSYCHIATRIC–MENTAL HEALTH NURSING: STANDARD 4: PLANNING

The psychiatric–mental health registered nurse develops a plan that prescribes strategies and alternatives to help the healthcare consumer reach his or her expected outcomes (ANA et al., 2014, p. 50).

Once you have done an assessment and formulated nursing diagnoses, it is time to prioritize them. Maslow's hierarchy of needs (see Chapter 2) provides a useful framework for doing so. Physiological needs and safety always come first because they have the potential for the most serious harm. Then the higher-order needs can be addressed, including love and belonging; self-esteem can then be the focus. For each nursing diagnosis, measurable goals are set and interventions for attaining the goals are selected.

The nurse considers the following specific principles when interventions are being planned:

- **Safe:** Interventions must be safe for the patient as well as for other patients, staff, and family.
- **Compatible and appropriate:** Interventions must be compatible with other therapies and with the patient's personal goals and cultural values and also institutional rules.
- **Realistic and individualized:** Interventions should be (1) within the patient's capabilities given the patient's age, physical strength, condition, and willingness to change; (2) based on the number of staff available; (3) reflective of the actual available community resources; and (4) within the student's or nurse's capabilities.
- **Evidence based:** Interventions should be based on scientific evidence and principles when available.

Evidence-based interventions and treatments constitute the gold standard in healthcare. **Evidence-based practice (EBP)** for nurses is a combination of clinical skill and the use of clinically relevant research in the delivery of effective patient-centered care. Using the best available research, incorporating patient preferences, and implementing sound clinical judgment and skills will provide an optimal patient-centered nurse–patient relationship. This evidence-based approach to care is consistent with QSEN standards.

STANDARDS OF PRACTICE FOR PSYCHIATRIC–MENTAL HEALTH NURSING: STANDARD 5: IMPLEMENTATION

The psychiatric–mental health registered nurse implements the identified plan (ANA et al., 2014, p. 52).

The psychiatric–mental health registered nurse accomplishes patient care through the nurse–patient partnership and the use of therapeutic intervention skills. The nurse implements the plan using evidence-based interventions whenever possible, utilizing community resources, and collaborating with colleagues. Provision of care implies that interventions are age appropriate and culturally and ethnically sensitive.

The psychiatric–mental health registered nurse has passed a state board examination to provide basic-level interventions. This level of practice may be enhanced by experience, competency, and successfully passing a psychiatric nursing certification examination resulting in a credential of registered nurse–board certified (RN-BC). The psychiatric–mental health advanced practice registered nurse (PMH-APRN) is educated at the master's or doctorate level and is prepared to function at an advanced level. A majority of states also require the PMH-APRNs to be certified through an examination and licensed by the state board of nursing. The first five intervention categories that follow apply to registered nurses with all levels of education, basic and advanced. The last three intervention categories (consultation, prescriptive authority, and psychotherapy) are relevant only to nurses functioning in the advanced practice role.

REGISTERED NURSE INTERVENTIONS

Coordination of Care

The psychiatric–mental health registered nurse coordinates care delivery (ANA et al., 2014, p. 54).

One of the most important jobs that a registered nurse does is to coordinate care. The nurse is generally in the most contact with the patient and communicates patient status, needs, and goals with the interprofessional team. Nurses also tend to be the families' advocates and help them to navigate an often bewildering healthcare system at a difficult time in their lives. Documentation of the coordination of care is an essential aspect of this standard.

Health Teaching and Health Promotion

The psychiatric–mental health registered nurse employs strategies to promote health and safe environment (ANA et al., 2014, p. 55).

Psychiatric–mental health nurses use a variety of health teaching methods adapted to the patient's special needs (age, culture, ability to learn, readiness) and recovery goals. Healthcare teaching includes coping skills, self-care activities, stress management, problem-solving skills, relapse prevention, conflict management, and interpersonal relationships. A vital part of health promotion is identifying resources for services in the community.

Pharmacological, Biological, and Integrative Therapies

The psychiatric–mental health registered nurse incorporates knowledge of pharmacological, biological, and complementary interventions with applied clinical skills to restore the healthcare consumer's health and prevent further disability (ANA et al., 2014, p. 59).

Nurses are knowledgeable regarding current research findings, intended action, therapeutic dosage, adverse reactions, and safe blood levels of medications being administered. Monitoring of the patient for any negative effects protects the patient from unnecessary harm. The nurse communicates the assessment of the patient's response to psychobiological interventions to other members of the mental health team.

Milieu Therapy

The psychiatric–mental health registered nurse provides, structures, and maintains a safe, therapeutic, recovery-oriented environment in collaboration with healthcare consumers, families, and other healthcare clinicians (ANA et al., 2014, p. 60).

Milieu refers to a physical and social environment. Milieu therapy is a psychiatric philosophy that involves a secure environment including people, settings, structure, and emotional climate to support recovery. Milieu therapy takes naturally occurring events in the environment and uses them as learning opportunities for patients. A consistent routine and structure are maintained to provide predictability and trust.

Milieu management includes the following:
- Orienting patients to their rights and responsibilities
- Providing culturally sensitive care
- Selecting activities (both individual and group) that meet the patient's physical and mental health needs
- Using the least restrictive environment

Therapeutic Relationship and Counseling

The psychiatric–mental health registered nurse uses the therapeutic relationship and counseling interventions to assist healthcare consumers in their individual recovery journeys by improving and regaining their previous coping abilities, fostering mental health, and preventing mental disorder and disability (ANA et al., 2014, p. 62).

The therapeutic relationship is the basis of interactions between the nurse and patient. Although medications and other treatments are important for recovery from a psychiatric disorder, nurses are vital in providing presence and being sounding boards. In an individual or group setting, you can reinforce healthy behavior and help the patient to recognize maladaptive behaviors, identify positive coping methods, and try out new coping methods.

ADVANCED PRACTICE REGISTERED NURSE INTERVENTIONS

Consultation

The psychiatric–mental health advanced practice registered nurse provides consultation to influence the identified plan, enhance the abilities of other clinicians to promote services for healthcare consumers, and effect change (ANA et al., 2014, p. 57).

Consultation is an advanced practice role. Consultation involves assisting other registered nurses and members of the interprofessional team in addressing complex clinical and other situations. Evidence-based information, clinical data, and theoretical frameworks provide the foundation for nurse consultants.

Prescriptive Authority and Treatment

The psychiatric–mental health advanced practice registered nurse uses prescriptive authority, procedures, referrals, treatments, and therapies in accordance with state and federal law and regulation (ANA et al., 2014, p. 58).

Prescribing—another advanced practice role—is accomplished by using evidence-based treatments, procedures, and therapies for healthcare consumers. Medication is prescribed in collaboration with the patient based on clinical symptoms and the results of diagnostic and laboratory tests. Evaluation of the therapeutic benefit and adverse effects of pharmacology is assisted by using standard symptom measurements along with the healthcare consumer's appraisal.

Psychotherapy

The psychiatric–mental health advanced practice registered nurse conducts individual, couples, group, and family psychotherapy using evidence-based psychotherapeutic frameworks and nurse–patient therapeutic relationships (ANA et al., 2014, p. 63).

The practice of psychotherapy is an advanced practice skill that builds upon principles of therapeutic communication. Evidence-based therapies are chosen in order to meet the needs of healthcare consumers who are encouraged to be active participants in treatment. When possible, standardized tools are used to evaluate effectiveness of interventions.

STANDARDS OF PRACTICE FOR PSYCHIATRIC–MENTAL HEALTH NURSING: STANDARD 6: EVALUATION

The psychiatric–mental health registered nurse evaluates progress toward the attainment of expected outcomes (ANA et al., 2014, p. 65).

TABLE 7.3   Narrative Versus Problem-Oriented Charting

	Narrative Charting	Problem-Oriented Charting: SOAPIE
Characteristics	A descriptive statement of patient status written in chronological order throughout a shift. Used to support assessment findings from a flow sheet. In charting by exception, narrative notes are used to indicate significant symptoms, behaviors, or events that are exceptions to norms identified on an assessment flow sheet.	Developed in the 1960s for physicians to reduce inefficient documentation. Intended to be accompanied by a problem list. Originally SOAP, with IE added later. The emphasis is on problem identification, process, and outcome. S: Subjective data (patient statement) O: Objective data (nurse observations) A: Assessment (nurse interprets *S* and *O* and describes either a problem or a nursing diagnosis) P: Plan (proposed intervention) I: Interventions (nurse's response to problem) E: Evaluation (patient outcome)
Example	(Date/time/discipline) Patient was agitated in the morning and pacing in the hallway. Blinked eyes, muttered to self, and looked off to the side. Reported heard voices. Verbally hostile to another patient. Offered 2 mg haloperidol (Haldol) PRN and sat with staff in quiet area for 20 min. Patient returned to community lounge and was able to sit and watch television.	(Date/time/discipline) S: "I'm so stupid. Get away, get away." "I hear the devil telling me bad things." O: Patient paced the hall, mumbling to self, and looking off to the side. Shouted insulting comments when approached by another patient. Watched walls and ceiling closely. A: Patient was having auditory hallucinations and increased agitation. P: Offered patient haloperidol PRN. Redirected patient to less stimulating environment. I: Patient received 2 mg haloperidol PO PRN. Sat with patient in quiet room for 20 min. E: Patient calmer. Returned to community lounge, sat, and watched television.
Advantages	Uses a common form of expression (narrative writing). Can address any event or behavior. Explains flow-sheet findings. Provides multidisciplinary ease of use.	Structured. Provides consistent organization of data. Facilitates retrieval of data for quality assurance and utilization management. Contains all elements of the nursing process. Minimizes inclusion of unnecessary data. Provides multidisciplinary ease of use.
Disadvantages	Unstructured. May result in different organization of information from note to note. Makes it difficult to retrieve quality assurance and utilization management data. Frequently leads to omission of elements of the nursing process. Commonly results in inclusion of unnecessary and subjective information.	Requires time and effort to structure the information. Limits entries to problems. May result in loss of data about progress. Not chronological. Carries negative connotation.

Unfortunately, nurses often neglect evaluation of patient outcomes during the nursing process. Evaluation of the individual's response to treatment should be systematic, ongoing, and based on criteria. You should include supporting data to clarify the evaluation. Ongoing assessment of data allows for revisions of nursing diagnoses, changes to more realistic outcomes, or identification of more appropriate interventions when outcomes are not met.

Documentation

Documentation has been referred to as the seventh step in the nursing process. Keep in mind that medical records are legal documents and may be used in a court of law. Besides the evaluation of stated outcomes, the medical record should include changes in patient condition, informed consents for medications and treatments, reaction to medication, documentation of symptoms (verbatim when appropriate), concerns of the patient, and adverse incidents in the healthcare setting. Documentation of patient progress is the responsibility of the entire healthcare team.

Communication among team members and coordination of services are the primary goals when choosing a system for documentation. Information is recorded in a format that is retrievable for quality improvement monitoring, utilization management, peer review, and research. Documentation—using the nursing process as a guide—may be reflected in two of the formats commonly used in healthcare settings and described in Table 7.3.

Informatics in general and electronic medical records specifically are the preferred formats in both inpatient and outpatient settings. Nurses need to be trained to use these technologies in the medical setting. We should also be prepared to provide further training for nurses in the use of terminology, progress notes relating to needs assessment, nursing interventions, and nursing diagnoses. Whatever format is used, documentation must be focused, organized, pertinent, and conform to certain legal and other generally accepted principles (Box 7.6).

Documentation of Nonadherence

When patients do not follow medication and treatment plans, they are often labeled as "noncompliant." Applied to patients, the

---

BOX 7.6   Legal Considerations for Documentation of Care

Do

- Chart in a timely manner all pertinent and factual information.
- Follow the nursing documentation policy in your facility and make your charting conform to this standard. The policy generally states the method, frequency, and assessments, interventions, and outcomes to be recorded. If your agency's policies and procedures do not encourage or allow for quality documentation, bring the need for change to the administration's attention.
- Chart facts fully, descriptively, and accurately.
- Chart what you see, hear, feel, and smell.
- Chart observations: psychosocial interactions, physical symptoms, and behaviors.
- Chart follow-up care provided when a problem has been identified in earlier documentation. For example, if a patient has fallen and injured a leg, describe how the wound is healing.
- Chart fully the facts surrounding unusual occurrences and incidents.
- Chart *all* nursing interventions, treatments, and outcomes (including teaching and patient responses) and safety and patient-protection interventions.
- Chart the patient's subjective feelings and symptoms.
- Chart each time you notify the advanced practice provider and record the reason for notification, the information that was communicated, the time, the provider's instructions or orders, and the follow-up activity.

- Chart discharge medications and instructions given for their use, as well as all discharge teaching, and note if family members included in the process.

Do Not

- Do *not* chart opinions that are not supported by facts.
- Do *not* defame patients by calling them names or making derogatory statements about them (e.g., "an unlikable patient who is demanding unnecessary attention").
- Do *not* chart before an event occurs.
- Do *not* chart generalizations, suppositions, or pat phrases (e.g., "patient in good spirits").
- Do *not* obliterate, erase, alter, or destroy a record. If an error is made, draw one line through the error, write "mistaken entry," the date, and initial. Follow your agency's guidelines for mistakes.
- Do *not* leave blank spaces for chronological notes. If you must chart out of sequence, chart "late entry." Identify the time and date of the entry and the time and date of the occurrence.
- If an incident report is filed, do not note in the chart that one was filed. This form is generally a privileged communication between the hospital and the hospital's legal team. Describing it in the chart may eliminate the privileged nature of the communication.

---

term *noncompliant* has negative connotations because compliance traditionally referred to the extent that a patient obediently and faithfully followed healthcare providers' instructions. "That patient is noncompliant" often translates into the patient being bad or lazy, subjecting the patient to blame and criticism. The term *noncompliant* is invariably judgmental. A much more useful term is nonadherent. This term encourages healthcare providers to find out what is going on in the patient's life and to explore barriers to taking medication and participating in treatment.

Furthermore, "patient did not comply" does not protect nurses, physicians, or healthcare workers from malpractice lawsuits. Meticulous records that document the reasons for interventions, clarify explanations and teaching, and include the patient's responses will support healthcare workers in the case of lawsuits. Probably the biggest problem in a malpractice lawsuit is whether the patient understood the instructions given by the healthcare provider. Even if patients are given instructions or printed information sheets, it is possible that some patients will not understand the instructions or fail to realize how important the treatment (e.g., medication, a follow-up) is to their health.

KEY POINTS TO REMEMBER

- The nursing process is a six-step, problem-solving approach to patient care.
- The Institute of Medicine (IOM) and Quality and Safety Education for Nurses (QSEN) have established mandates to prepare future nurses with the knowledge, skills, and attitudes (KSAs) necessary for achieving quality and safety as they engage in the six competencies of nursing: patient-centered care, teamwork and collaboration, evidence-based practice (EBP), quality improvement (QI), safety, and informatics.
- The primary source of assessment is the patient. Secondary sources of information include family members, neighbors, friends, police, and other members of the health team.
- A professional interpreter is required by law to prevent serious misunderstandings during the assessment, treatment, and evaluation of patients with limited English proficiency or those using ASL. Translators are used to transcribe written documents into English.

- The assessment interview includes mental or emotional status and psychosocial assessment.
- Medical examination, history, and systems review round out a complete assessment.
- Assessment tools and standardized rating scales may be used to evaluate and monitor a patient's progress.
- Determination of the nursing diagnosis defines the practice of nursing, improves communication between staff members, and supports accountability.
- Nursing diagnoses always include a problem or unmet need. Depending upon the type of diagnosis (e.g., actual or risk), probable cause and supporting data are included in the diagnostic statement.
- Outcomes are measurable and positively stated in terms that reflect a patient's actual state.
- Behavioral goals support outcomes. Goals are short, specific, and measurable; they indicate the desired patient behaviors and include a set time for achievement.

- Planning nursing actions to achieve outcomes includes the use of specific principles. The plan is (1) safe, (2) compatible with and appropriate for implementation with other therapies, (3) realistic and individualized, and (4) evidence-based whenever possible.
- Psychiatric–mental health nursing practice includes five basic-level interventions: coordination of care; health teaching and health promotion; milieu therapy; pharmacological, biological, and integrative therapies; and therapeutic relationships and counseling.
- Nurses who are educated as psychiatric–mental health advanced practice nurses (PMH-APRNs) may engage in

consultation, prescribe psychiatric medications, and practice psychotherapy.
- Evaluation of care is a continual process of determining to what extent the outcome criteria have been achieved. The plan of care may be revised based on the evaluation.
- Documentation of patient progress through evaluation of the outcome criteria is considered to be the seventh step of the nursing process. The medical record is a legal document and should accurately reflect the patient's condition, medications, treatments, tests, and responses.

CRITICAL THINKING

Pedro Gonzales, a 37-year-old Hispanic man, arrived by ambulance from a supermarket, where he had fallen. On his arrival at the emergency department (ED), his breath smelled "fruity." He appeared confused and anxious, saying that "they put the evil eye on me, they want me to die, they are drying out my body … it's draining me dry … they are yelling, they are yelling … no, no, I'm not bad … oh, God, don't let them get me!" When his mother arrived in the ED, she told the staff, through an interpreter, that Pedro has severe diabetes and a diagnosis of paranoid schizophrenia. She says with frustration, "This happens when he doesn't take his medications. In a group or in collaboration with a classmate, respond to the following:

1. A number of nursing diagnoses are possible in this scenario. Given the provided information, formulate at least two nursing diagnoses and include *related to* and *as evidenced by* as appropriate.
2. For each of your nursing diagnoses, write out one long-term outcome (the problem, what should change, etc.). Include a time frame, desired change, and three criteria that will help you evaluate whether the outcome has been met, not met, or partially met.
3. What specific needs might you consider when planning nursing care for Mr. Gonzales?
4. Using the SOAPIE format (see Table 7.3), formulate an initial nurse's note for Mr. Gonzales.

CHAPTER REVIEW

1. What is the purpose of the Health Insurance Portability and Accountability Act (HIPAA)? *Select all that apply.*
   a. Ensuring that an individual's health information is protected
   b. Providing third-party players with access to patient's medical records
   c. Facilitating the movement of a patient's medical information to the interested parties
   d. Guaranteeing that all those in need of healthcare coverage have options to obtain it
   e. Allowing healthcare providers to obtain health information to provide high-quality healthcare.
2. Which intervention demonstrates a nurse's understanding of the initial action associated with the assessment of a patient's spiritual beliefs?
   a. Offering to pray with the patient
   b. Providing a consult with the facility's chaplain
   c. Asking the patient what role spirituality plays in his daily life
   d. Arranging for care to be provided with respect to religious practices
3. Which nursing interventions best demonstrate an understanding of the Quality and Safety Education in Nursing (QSEN) competences? *Select all that apply.*

   a. Asking the patient what she expects from the treatment she is receiving
   b. Seeking recertification for cardiopulmonary resuscitation (CPR)
   c. Accessing the internet to monitor social media related to opinions on healthcare
   d. Consulting with a dietitian to discuss a patient's cultural food preferences and restrictions
   e. Reviewing the literature regarding the best way to monitor the patient for a fluid imbalance
4. Which disadvantage is inherent to the problem-oriented charting system (SOAPIE)?
   a. Does not support a universal organizational system
   b. Commonly allows for the inclusion of subjective information
   c. Documentation is not listed in chronological order
   d. Does not support the nursing process as a format
5. Which standardized rating scale will the nurse specifically include in the assessment of a newly admitted patient diagnosed with major depressive disorder?
   a. Mini-Mental State Examination (MMSE)
   b. Body Attitude Test
   c. Global Assessment of Functioning Scale (GAF)
   d. Beck Inventory

6. A 13-year-old boy is undergoing a mental health assessment. The nurse practitioner assures him that his medical records are protected and private. The nurse recognizes that this promise cannot be kept when the youth divulges:
   a. "I lost my virginity last year."
   b. "I am angry with my parents most of the time."
   c. "I have thoughts of being in love with boys."
   d. "My parents do not know that I hit my grandpa."

7. During an interview with a non–English-speaking middle-aged woman recently diagnosed with major depressive disorder, the patient's husband states, "She is happy now and doing very well." The patient, however, sits motionless, looking at the floor, and wringing her hands. A professional interpreter would provide better information due to the fact that a family member in the interpreter role may *Select all that apply.*
   a. Be too close to accurately capture the meaning of the patient's mood
   b. Censor the patient's thoughts or words
   c. Avoid interpretation
   d. Leave out unsavory details

8. A nurse identified a nursing diagnosis of *self-mutilation* for a female diagnosed with borderline personality disorder. The patient has multiple self-inflicted cuts on her forearms and inner thighs. What is the most important patient outcome for this nursing diagnosis? Patient will
   a. Identify triggers to self-mutilation
   b. Refrain from self-harm
   c. Describe strategies to increase socialization on the unit
   d. Describe two strategies to increase self-care

9. Medical records are considered legal documents. Proper documentation needs to reflect patient condition along with changes. It should also be based on professional standards designated by the state board of nursing, regulatory agencies, and reimbursement requirements. Proper documentation can be enhanced by:
   a. Only using objective data
   b. Using the nursing process as a guide
   c. Using language the specific patient can understand
   d. Avoiding legal jargon

10. Amadi is a 40-year-old African national being treated in a psychiatric outpatient setting due to a court order. Amadi's medical record is limited in scope, so where can Renata, his registered nurse, obtain more data on Amadi's condition within legal parameters? *Select all that apply.*
    a. Emergency department records
    b. Police records related to the offense resulting in the court order for treatment
    c. Calling his family in Africa for details about Amadi's mental health
    d. Past medical records in the current facility

1. **a, e**; 2. **c**; 3. **a, b, d, e**; 4. **c**; 5. **d**; 6. **d**; 7. **b**; 8. **a**; 9. **b**; 10. **a, b, d**

🌐 Visit the Evolve website for a posttest on the content in this chapter: http://evolve.elsevier.com/Varcarolis

---

REFERENCES

American Nurses Association. (1973). *Standards of nursing practice*. Kansas City, MO: American Nurses Association.

American Nurses Association.(n.d.).The nursing process. Retrieved from https://www.nursingworld.org/practice-policy/workforce/what-is-nursing/the-nursing-process/.

American Nurses Association, American Psychiatric Nurses Association, & International Society of Psychiatric–Mental Health Nurses. (2014). *Psychiatric–mental health nursing: Scope and standards of practice* (2nd ed.). Washington, DC: Nursebooks.org.

Cronenwett, L., Sherwood, G., Barnsteiner, J., Disch, J., Johnson, J., Mitchell, P., et al. (2007). Quality and safety education for nurses. *Nursing Outlook, 55*(3), 122–131.

De la Cuesta, C. (1983). The nursing process: From development to implementation. *Journal of Advanced Nursing, 8,* 365–371.

Fry, V. S. (1953). The creative approach to nursing. *American Journal of Nursing, 53*(3), 301–302.

Herdman, T. H., & Kamitsuru, S. (Eds.). (2018). *NANDA International nursing diagnoses: Definitions and classification 2018-2020.* New York, NY: Thieme.

Institute of Medicine. (2003). *Health professions education*. Washington, DC: National Academies Press.

International Council of Nurses. (2017). *ICNP download*. Retrieved from https://www.icn.ch/what-we-do/projects/ehealth/icnp-download.

International Council of Nurses. (2019). *International Council of Nurses adds new content and updates the International Classification for Nursing Practice (ICNP)*. Retrieved from https://www.icn.ch/news/international-council-nurses-adds-new-content-and-updates-international-classification-nursing.

Johnson, D. E. (1959). A philosophy of nursing. *Nursing Outlook, 7*(4), 198–200.

Orlando, I. (1961). *The dynamic nurse-patient relationship*. New York, NY: Putnam.

United States Department of Health and Human Services. (2003). *Summary of HIPAA privacy rule*. Retrieved from http://www.hhs.gov/sites/default/files/ocr/privacy/hipaa/understanding/summary/privacysummary.pdf.

Yura, H., & Walsh, M. B. (1967). *The nursing process: Assessing, planning, implementing, and evaluating*. Washington, DC: Catholic University of America.

8

Therapeutic Relationships

Margaret Jordan Halter and Elizabeth M. Varcarolis

Visit the Evolve website for a pretest on the content in this chapter: http://evolve.elsevier.com/Varcarolis

OBJECTIVES

1. Compare and contrast a personal relationship and a therapeutic relationship regarding purpose, focus, communications style, and goals.
2. Explore qualities that foster a therapeutic nurse-patient relationship.
3. Describe legal, ethical, and professional boundaries, along with boundary crossings, violations, and sexual misconduct.
4. Identify the influence of transference and countertransference on boundary blurring.
5. Discuss the influences of different values and cultural beliefs on the therapeutic relationship.
6. Explain Peplau's four phases of the nurse-patient relationship.
7. Define and discuss the roles of genuineness, empathy, and positive regard on the part of the nurse in a nurse-patient relationship.
8. Identify the use of attending behaviors such as eye contact, body language, and vocal qualities.

KEY TERMS AND CONCEPTS

beliefs
boundaries
clinical supervision
confidentiality
contract
counseling
countertransference
empathy

genuineness
orientation phase
patient-centered care
personal relationship
positive regard
preorientation phase
professional nurse-patient relationship
psychotherapy

rapport
termination phase
therapeutic encounter
therapeutic relationship
therapeutic use of self
transference
values
working phase

Psychiatric-mental health nursing is in many ways based on principles of *science*. A background in anatomy, physiology, and chemistry is the basis for providing safe and effective biological treatments. Knowledge of pharmacology—a medication's mechanism of action, indications for use, and adverse effects based on evidence-based studies and trials—is vital to nursing practice. However, it is the caring relationship and the development of the interpersonal skills needed to enhance and maintain such a relationship that make up the *art* of psychiatric nursing. A therapeutic relationship creates a space where caring and healing can occur.

CONCEPTS CENTRAL TO THE NURSE-PATIENT RELATIONSHIP

The healthcare community accepts the concept of patient-centered care as the gold standard. The core concepts of patient- and family-centered care consist of (1) dignity and respect, (2) information sharing, (3) patient and family participation, and (4) collaboration in policy and program development (Institute for Patient- and Family-Centered Care, n.d.). These concepts are consistent with and basic to the nurse-patient relationship.

The nurse-patient relationship is the basis of all psychiatric-mental health nursing treatment approaches, regardless of the specific goals. The first connections between nurse and patient are to establish an understanding that the nurse is safe, confidential, reliable, and consistent. Another essential characteristic of this relationship is that it will occur within appropriate and clear boundaries.

Virtually all psychiatric disorders, including schizophrenia, bipolar disorder, major depressive disorder, and substance use disorders, have genetic and biochemical components. However, many accompanying problems, such as poor self-image, low self-esteem, and difficulties with adherence to a treatment regimen, can be significantly improved through a therapeutic nurse-patient relationship. What makes this relationship even more important is that patients entering treatment have often taxed or exhausted their family and social resources and find themselves isolated and in need of emotional support.

We all have distinct gifts—unique personality traits and talents—that we can learn to use creatively to form positive bonds with others. The use of these gifts to promote healing in others is referred to as the therapeutic use of self. A positive therapeutic alliance, which is collaborative and respectful, is one of the best predictors of positive outcomes in therapy (Gordon & Beresin, 2016).

Importance of Talk Therapy

A formalized approach to talk therapy that is based on theoretical models is called psychotherapy. Healthcare providers with advanced degrees and specialized knowledge, including psychiatric-mental health advanced practice registered nurses, psychiatrists, and psychologists, are licensed to practice psychotherapy. Evidence suggests that psychotherapy within a therapeutic partnership actually changes brain chemistry in much the same way as medication (Malhotra & Sahoo, 2017). Thus, the best treatment for most psychiatric problems—less so with psychotic disorders—is a combination of medication and psychotherapy.

Basic-level psychiatric-mental health nurses do not practice psychotherapy because this is an advanced skill. They do, however, use counseling techniques in the context of the therapeutic relationship. Counseling is a supportive face-to-face process that helps individuals problem solve, resolve personal conflicts, and feel supported.

Goals and Functions

The nurse-patient relationship is often loosely defined, but a therapeutic nurse-patient relationship has specific goals and functions, including the following:

- Facilitating communication of distressing thoughts and feelings
- Assisting with problem solving to help facilitate activities of daily living
- Examining self-defeating thoughts and behaviors and testing alternatives
- Promoting self-care and independence
- Providing education about disorders, medications, and symptom management

An additional goal of the nurse-patient relationship is promoting recovery. Mental health and substance use recovery is a process that begins with diagnoses and the eventual management of the psychiatric condition. This process takes illness management a step further by empowering the individual to be the key player in partnerships with healthcare providers to make decisions about personal care and treatment. Increasing family and the social support of peers is another important aspect of recovery.

Personal Versus Therapeutic

A relationship is an interpersonal process that involves two or more people. Throughout life, we meet people in a variety of settings and share a variety of experiences. With some individuals, we develop long-term relationships. With others, the relationship lasts only a short time. Naturally, the kinds of relationships we enter vary from person to person and from situation to situation.

In general, relationships can be categorized as *intimate, personal,* or *therapeutic.* Intimate relationships occur between people who have an emotional commitment to each other. Within intimate relationships, mutual needs are met and intimate desires and hopes are shared. Obviously, there are moral and ethical concerns about intimate relationships with patients, and most certainly legal and professional restrictions. In this chapter, we will focus on clarifying the differences between personal and therapeutic relationships.

Personal Relationships

A personal relationship is primarily initiated for the purpose of friendship, socialization, enjoyment, or accomplishment of a task. Mutual needs are met during social interaction (e.g., participants share ideas, feelings, and experiences). Communication skills may include giving advice and sometimes meeting basic dependency needs, such as lending money and helping with jobs. Often, the content of the communication is superficial.

During social interactions, roles may shift, such as being the listener one day and being listened to the next. Within a personal relationship, there is little emphasis on the evaluation of the interaction. In the following example, notice the casual friend-like tone of the nurse:

Patient: "Oh, I just hate to be alone. It's getting me down, and sometimes it hurts so much."

Nurse: "I know how you feel. I don't like being alone either. What I do is get on Instagram and see if anyone wants to do something. Maybe you should try this?" (*In this response, the nurse is minimizing the patient's feelings and giving advice prematurely.*)

Patient: "I don't get on Instagram. Anyway, I usually don't even feel like going out. I just sit at home feeling lonely and empty."

Nurse: "Most of us feel like that at one time or another. Maybe if you took a class or joined a group, you could meet more people. I know of some great groups you could join." (*Again, the nurse is not "hearing" the patient's distress and is minimizing her pain and isolation. The nurse goes on to give the patient unwanted and unhelpful advice, thus closing off the patient's feelings and experience.*)

Therapeutic Relationships

In a therapeutic relationship, the nurse maximizes communication skills, understanding of human behaviors, and personal strengths to enhance the patient's growth. Patients more easily engage in the relationship when the clinician's interactions address their concerns, respect patients as partners in decision-making, and use straightforward language. These interactions are evidence that the focus of the relationship is on the patient's ideas, experiences, and feelings.

Inherent in a therapeutic relationship is addressing issues introduced by the patient during the initial nursing assessment or in subsequent meetings. The nurse and the patient identify areas that need exploration and periodically evaluate the degree of progress of the patient.

Although the nurse may assume a variety of roles (e.g., teacher, counselor, socializing agent, liaison), the relationship is consistently focused on the patient's problem and needs. Nurses' needs are met outside the relationship. Nurses who want the patient to "like me," "do as I suggest," or "give me recognition" devalue the needs of the patient.

Nursing students have the opportunity to develop a therapeutic relationship with patients while having the support of both clinical faculty and nursing staff. This clinical supervision is a mentoring relationship characterized by feedback and evaluation. Typically, students experience a gradual increase in autonomy and responsibility.

Communication skills and knowledge of the stages and phenomena in a therapeutic relationship are crucial tools in the formation and maintenance of that relationship. Within the context of a therapeutic relationship, the nurse will do the following:

- Identify the needs of the patient and explore them.
- Establish clear boundaries.
- Encourage alternate problem-solving approaches.
- Help the patient develop new coping skills.
- Support behavioral change.

Just like staff nurses, nursing students may struggle with the boundaries between personal and therapeutic relationships because there is a fine line between the two. In fact, students often feel more comfortable being a friend because it is a familiar role, especially with patients close to their own age. When this occurs, students need to make it clear (to themselves and the patient) that the relationship is a therapeutic one.

This does *not* mean that the nurse is not friendly toward the patient, and it does *not* mean that talking about everyday topics (e.g., television, weather, and children's pictures) is forbidden. In fact, a small amount of self-disclosure on the nurse's part may strengthen the therapeutic relationship. For example, your patient is about 24 years old (your age) and asks you about nursing school and what the hardest parts are. Briefly sharing your experience with nursing education will increase your connection with the patient. Although the focus is on the patient, can you imagine responding to the question about nursing school with, "We won't be talking about me."?

In a therapeutic relationship, the patient's problems and concerns are explored. Both patient and nurse discuss potential solutions. The patient, as in the following example, implements the solutions:

Patient: "Oh, I just hate to be alone. It's getting me down, and sometimes it hurts so much."

Nurse: "Loneliness can be painful. What is going on now that you are feeling so alone?"

Patient: "Well, my mom died 2 years ago, and last month, my— oh, I am so scared." (*Patient takes a deep breath, looks down, and looks as if she might cry.*)

Nurse: (*Sits in silence while the patient recovers.*) "Go on."

Patient: "My boyfriend is a member of the US special operations force in the Middle East. I haven't heard from him. He is my best friend, and we are supposed to get married. If he dies, I don't want to live."

Nurse: (*Leans in slightly, nodding gently.*) "That must be scary not knowing what is going on with your boyfriend."

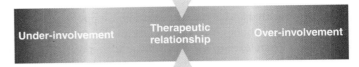

Fig. 8.1 Continuum of therapeutic involvement.

Patient: (*Nods. Is momentarily silent.*) "I think that losing my mom and now worrying about my boyfriend has just been too much."

Sometimes the relationship may be informal and not extensive, such as when the nurse and patient meet only a few times. Even though the relationship is limited, it may be substantial, useful, and important for the patient. This type of limited relationship is referred to as a therapeutic encounter. When the nurse shows genuine concern for another's circumstances, along with positive regard and empathy, even a short encounter can have a powerful effect.

At other times, sessions with patients may be longer and more formal in such places as inpatient settings, community mental health centers, crisis centers, and freestanding psychiatric facilities. This longer time span allows the therapeutic nurse-patient relationship to be more fully developed.

Relationship Boundaries and Roles
Boundaries

Boundaries can be considered the "edge" of professional behavior and exist to protect patients. Nurses, not patients, are responsible for maintaining professional boundaries. Boundaries are the expected and accepted legal, ethical, and professional standards that separate nurses from patients. This separation is essential, considering the power differential between the nurse and the patient. This differential also exists between nursing students and patients, even if you do not feel powerful. Consider that you have read the patient's chart, you are there to help the patient, you are close to becoming a registered nurse, and you are not a patient. These qualities put nursing students in a position of some authority, particularly from the patient's perspective.

Nurses and other healthcare workers should seek a level of involvement that is healthy. A well-defined therapeutic nurse-patient relationship allows for the establishment of clear boundaries. These boundaries provide a safe space in which the patient can explore feelings and treatment concerns. This safe space may be threatened by under-involvement and over-involvement on the part of the nurse. Nurses who are under-involved with patients may be at the least disinterested and neglectful and at the worst guilty of patient abandonment (National Council of State Boards of Nursing, 2018). Over-involvement may result in boundary crossings, boundary violations, and professional sexual misconduct. Fig. 8.1 illustrates a continuum of professional involvement in a therapeutic relationship.

Boundary Crossings

Boundary crossings are the least serious form of over-involvement. They tend to give the impression of "something's not quite right" but do not actually violate ethical standards. In

BOX 8.1 Nurse Behaviors Indicating Boundary Crossing

- Spending long periods of time with the patient, more than is necessary or is comparable to time spent with other patients
- Doing tasks for the patient that could be done independently
- Sharing too much personal information with the patient
- Thinking about the patient outside of the care setting
- Being defensive when others comment on the special attention the patient is receiving
- Accepting personal comments and questions made by the patient

fact, some boundary crossing may actually support the work being done by the patient.

Nurses may recognize that their behavior is crossing a line and return to established boundaries, or repeatedly cross the line. Self-awareness and supervision can often correct these types of behaviors.

Two common circumstances in which boundaries are crossed are (1) when the relationship slips into a personal context and (2) when the nurse's needs (for attention, affection, and emotional support) are met at the expense of the patient's needs. Box 8.1 provides examples of behaviors that indicate boundary crossing.

Boundary Violations

Boundary violations take advantage of the patient's vulnerability and are ethically wrong. They are harmful or potentially harmful to the patient. Boundary violations are characterized by a reversal of roles where the needs of the nurse are being met rather than the needs of the patient. Boundary violations usually start small but may become increasingly problematic.

Context is an important part of determining whether an action is considered a boundary violation. For example, a small amount of self-disclosure is useful in establishing a therapeutic relationship. If you disclose to your patient that you are not married, it may be harmless. If, however, you are disclosing your single status as an initial act of romance, you are heading into boundary violation territory.

Other examples of boundary violations include accepting gifts or cash, planning a business together, excessive touching of the patient, and trying to influence a patient's political or religious beliefs. Boundaries may even be violated indirectly. For example, if a patient's case is discussed on Facebook, it may breach confidentiality and the patient's right to privacy, also violating boundaries.

Professional Sexual Misconduct

While less common than other boundary violations, the most extreme boundary violation is professional sexual misconduct. This behavior may be physical or verbal and may include expressions of feelings and thoughts or gestures that are sexual or could reasonably be interpreted by the patient as sexual.

This breach of trust results in high levels of malpractice actions, loss of professional licensure, and damaged reputations. Consider the case of the 48-year-old psychiatric nurse who had, in his words, a "loving and sexual relationship" with a 19-year-old patient after she was discharged (BBC News, 2014). The licensing board determined that his actions could have resulted in harm due to her clear vulnerability. The board also stated that this serious misconduct was abuse due to the special position of trust he held. The nurse lost his job and his license.

Blurring of Roles

Blurring of roles in the nurse-patient relationship is often a result of unrecognized transference or countertransference.

Transference. Sigmund Freud originally identified transference as a phenomenon when he used psychoanalysis to treat patients. Transference occurs when the patient unconsciously and inappropriately displaces (transfers) onto the nurse feelings and behaviors related to significant figures in the patient's past. The patient may even say, "You remind me of my [mother, sister, father, brother, etc.]."

Patient: "Oh, you are so high and mighty. Did anyone ever tell you that you are a cold, unfeeling machine, just like others I know?"

Nurse: "Let's talk about a person who is or was cold and unfeeling toward you." (*In this example, the patient is experiencing the nurse in the same way she experienced significant other[s] during her formative years. In this case, the patient's mother was cold and distant, leaving the patient with feelings of isolation, worthlessness, and anger.*)

Although transference occurs in all relationships, it seems to be intensified in relationships where one person is in authority. This may occur because parental figures were the original figures of authority. Nurses, physicians, and social workers all are potential objects of transference.

This transference may be positive or negative. If a patient is motivated to work with you, completes assignments between sessions, and shares feelings openly, it may be that the patient is experiencing positive transference.

Negative transference may result in the patient directing painful or angry feelings toward the nurse. The nurse may need to explore negative transference that threatens the nurse-patient relationship. Also, if patients are made aware of these negative emotions, they may be able to better understand themselves.

Common forms of transference include the desire for affection or respect and the gratification of dependency needs. Other transferential feelings are hostility, jealousy, competitiveness, and love.

Sometimes patients experience positive or negative thoughts, feelings, and reactions that are realistic and appropriate and *not* a result of transference onto the healthcare worker. For example, if a nurse makes promises to the patient that are not kept, such as not showing up for a meeting, the patient may feel resentment and mistrust toward the nurse.

Countertransference. Countertransference is transference in reverse. It occurs when the nurse unconsciously displaces feelings related to significant figures in the nurse's past onto the patient. Frequently, the intense emotions of transference on the part of the patient bring out countertransference in the nurse. For example, say you remind your patient of his much-loved older sister and he works very hard to please you. In response to this idealization and caring, you experience feelings of tenderness toward the patient and spend extra time with him each day.

Countertransference often results in overinvolvement and impairs the therapeutic relationship. Patients are experienced not as individuals but rather as extensions of ourselves. For example:

Patient: "Well, I decided not to go to that dumb group. 'Hi, I'm so-and-so, and I'm an alcoholic.' Who cares?"(*Patient sits slumped in a chair chewing gum, and nonchalantly looking around.*)

Nurse: (*In an impassioned tone.*) "You seem to always sabotage your chances. You need AA to get in control of your life. Yesterday, you were going to go, and now you're letting people down." (*In this case, the patient reminds the nurse of her mother, who was an alcoholic. The nurse took it as a personal failure that her mother never sought recovery. The nurse sorts her feelings and realizes her feelings of disappointment and failure belong with her mother and not the patient. She starts out the next session with the following approach.*)

Nurse: "Look, I was thinking about yesterday, and I realize the decision to go to AA or find other help is solely up to you. Let's talk about what happened to change your mind about going to the meeting."

If the nurse feels either a strongly positive or a strongly negative reaction to a patient, the feeling most often signals countertransference. One common sign is over-identification with the patient. In this situation, the nurse may have difficulty recognizing or objectively seeing patient problems that are similar to the nurse's own. For example, a nurse who is struggling with a depressed family member may feel disinterested or disgusted with a depressed patient. Other indicators of countertransference are when the nurse gets involved in power struggles, competition, or arguments with the patient.

Identifying and working through transference and countertransference issues is crucial in accomplishing professional growth and in helping the patient meet goals. No matter how hard clinicians try to examine their responses objectively, professional support and help are extremely helpful. Supervision by peers or by the therapeutic team can help with working through transference and countertransference, as well as numerous other issues.

A FOCUS ON SELF-AWARENESS

While nurses routinely perform clinical assessments on patients, they are not usually trained to know and understand themselves. In psychiatric nursing, self-awareness is a key component to forming a therapeutic relationship. We all have likes (e.g., sweets or salty food) and areas of interest (e.g., sports and reality shows). We are usually aware of those aspects of our personality, and it is fairly simple not to let a difference in what we like interfere with our ability to provide care.

More sacred to us than likes or dislikes are our values and beliefs. These two concepts provide us with a way to conduct ourselves and give life meaning. It is easy to become threatened by others who possess different values and beliefs. It is important to develop awareness, acknowledge, and then monitor our responses to patients who possess different values and beliefs.

Values are abstract standards and represent an ideal, either positive or negative. It is your judgment of what is important in life. Examples of values are self-reliance, honesty, cleanliness, organization, justice, respect, and a healthy lifestyle. You can probably list those things that you find most personally important and valuable.

Beliefs are another area of self-awareness. They are defined in several different ways. Each of the definitions has relevance to the practice of psychiatric nursing and the therapeutic relationship.

1. An opinion or conviction, something that you hold to be true. For example, "Healthcare is a right for everyone, just like having paved roads." This type of belief may be rational ("The earth is round") or irrational or delusional ("My brain is being monitored").
2. Confidence, trust, or faith. For example, "I believe that my doctor is the best in her field."
3. Religious tenets, creed, or faith. For example, "It's fine if you celebrate birthdays, but in my religion, we don't."

When working with patients, it is important for nurses to understand that our values and beliefs are not necessarily right and certainly are not right for everyone. It is helpful to realize that our values and beliefs (1) reflect our own culture or subculture, (2) are derived from a range of choices, and (3) are those we have *chosen* for ourselves from a variety of influences and role models. These chosen values stem from religious, cultural, and societal forces. Our values guide us in making decisions and taking actions that we hope will make our lives meaningful, rewarding, and fulfilled.

Working with others whose values and beliefs are radically different from our own can be a challenge. Topics that cause controversy in society in general—including religion, gender roles, abortion, war, politics, money, drugs, alcohol, sex, and corporal punishment—also can cause conflict between nurses and patients. What happens when the nurse's values and beliefs are very different from those of a patient? Consider the following examples of possible conflicts:

- The patient is planning to have an abortion, which is against the nurse's belief that life begins at conception.
- The nurse values cleanliness while the patient believes that showering more than once a week wastes water and harms the environment.
- The nurse is a feminist and values women's rights. She resents her female patient who wears a hijab (head covering) for religious reasons.
- The patient makes disparaging remarks and uses insulting language about a certain race of people.
- The nurse has a strong religious belief system and thinks that everyone needs the support of a church, whereas the patient is agnostic.

Self-awareness requires that we understand what we value and those beliefs that guide our behavior. Being self-aware helps us accept the uniqueness and differences in others.

PEPLAU'S MODEL OF THE NURSE-PATIENT RELATIONSHIP

Hildegard Peplau introduced the concept of the nurse-patient relationship in 1952 in her groundbreaking book *Interpersonal Relations in Nursing*. This model of the nurse-patient relationship is well accepted in the United States and Canada as an important tool for all nursing practice. A professional nurse-patient relationship consists of a nurse who has skills and expertise and a patient who wants to feel better, find solutions to problems, explore different methods to improve quality of life, or find an advocate.

Peplau (1952) proposed that the nurse-patient relationship "facilitates forward movement" for both the nurse and the patient (p. 12). This interactive nurse-patient process is designed to facilitate the patient's boundary management, independent problem solving, and decision-making that promotes autonomy.

Peplau (1952, 1999) described the nurse-patient relationship as evolving through three distinct interlocking and overlapping phases. An additional preorientation phase, during which the nurse prepares for the orientation phase, is useful and is included here. The four phases are:

1. Preorientation phase
2. Orientation phase
3. Working phase
4. Termination phase

Most likely, you will not have time to develop all phases of the nurse-patient relationship in your brief psychiatric-mental health nursing rotation. However, it is important to be aware of these phases to recognize and use them later.

Preorientation Phase

The preorientation phase begins with preparing for your assignment. The chart is a rich source of information, including mental and physical evaluation, progress notes, and patient orders. You will probably be required to research your patient's condition, learn about prescribed medications, and understand laboratory results. Staff may be available to share more anecdotal information or provide you with tips on how to best interact with your patient.

Another task before meeting your patient is recognizing your own thoughts and feelings regarding this first meeting. Nursing students usually have many concerns and experience anxiety on their first clinical day. These universal concerns include being afraid of persons with psychiatric disorders, of saying "the wrong thing," and of not knowing what to do in response to certain patient behaviors. Table 8.1 identifies patient behaviors and gives examples of possible reactions and suggested responses.

Experienced faculty and staff monitor the unit atmosphere and have a sixth sense for behaviors that indicate escalating tension. They are trained in crisis interventions, and formal security is often available on-site to give support to the staff. Your instructor will set the ground rules for safety during the first clinical day. These rules may include not going into a patient's room alone, interacting with patients in an open area, and reporting signs and symptoms of escalating anxiety.

Orientation Phase

The orientation phase can last for a few meetings or extend over a longer period. It is the first time the nurse and the patient meet and is the phase in which the nurse conducts the initial interview (refer to Chapter 9). During the orientation phase, the patient may begin to express thoughts and feelings, identify problems, and discuss realistic goals. Specific tasks of the orientation phase are discussed in the following sections.

Introductions

The first task of the orientation phase is introductions. The patient needs to know about the nurse (who the nurse is and the nurse's background) and the purpose of the meetings. For example, a student might furnish the following information:

TABLE 8.1 Patient Behaviors, Possible Nurse Reactions, and Suggested Nurse Responses	
Possible Reactions	**Useful Responses**
If the Patient Threatens Suicide	
The nurse may feel overwhelmed or responsible for "talking the patient out of it."	The nurse assesses whether the patient has a plan and the lethality of the plan.
The nurse may pick up some of the patient's feelings of hopelessness.	The nurse tells the patient that this is serious, that the nurse does not want harm to come to the patient, and that this information needs to be shared with other staff:
	"This is serious, Mr. Lamb. I don't want any harm to come to you. I need to share how you're feeling with the other staff."
	The nurse can then discuss with the patient the feelings and circumstances that led up to this decision. (Refer to Chapter 25 for strategies in suicide intervention.)
If the Patient Asks the Nurse to Keep a Secret	
The nurse may feel conflict because the nurse wants the patient to share important information but is unsure about making such a promise.	The nurse *cannot* make such a promise. The information may be important to the health or safety of the patient or others:
	"I cannot make that promise. It might be important for me to share it with other staff."
	The patient then decides whether to share the information.

Continued

TABLE 8.1   Patient Behaviors, Possible Nurse Reactions, and Suggested Nurse Responses—cont'd

Possible Reactions	Useful Responses
If the Patient Asks the Nurse a Personal Question The nurse may think that it is rude not to answer the patient's question. A new nurse may feel relieved to put off having to start the interview. The nurse may feel put on the spot and want to leave the situation. New nurses are often manipulated by a patient into changing roles. This keeps the focus off the patient and prevents the building of a relationship.	The nurse may or may not answer the patient's query. If the nurse decides to answer a natural question, the answers should be short, and then refocused on the patient: **Patient:** Are you married? **Nurse:** Yes. Do you have a spouse? **Patient:** Do you have any children? **Nurse:** Yes, I have two… But, this time is for you. Tell me about yourself….
If the Patient Makes Sexual Advances The nurse feels uncomfortable but may feel conflicted about "rejecting" by making the patient feel "unattractive" or "not good enough."	The nurse sets clear limits on expected behavior: "I'm not comfortable discussing my looks. We are here to focus on your problems and concerns." Frequently restating the nurse's role throughout the relationship can help maintain boundaries. If the behavior persists, the nurse might say: "I'm going to leave for now. I'll be back at [time] to spend time with you then." Leaving gives the patient time to gain control. In some cases, reassignment to another nurse (if possible) is the best alternative.
If the Patient Cries The nurse may feel uncomfortable and experience increased anxiety or feel somehow responsible for making the person cry.	The nurse should stay with the patient and reinforce that it is all right to cry. Often it is at that time that feelings are closest to the surface and can be best identified: "You are still upset about your brother's death." "What are you thinking right now?" The nurse offers tissues when appropriate.
If the Patient Leaves Before the Session Is Over The nurse may feel rejected. The nurse may experience increased anxiety or feel abandoned by the patient.	Some patients are not able to relate for long periods without experiencing an increase in anxiety. Check back with them later.
If the Patient Does Not Want to Talk The nurse new to this situation may feel rejected or ineffective.	At first, the nurse might say something like: "It's all right. I would like to spend time with you. We don't have to talk." The nurse might spend short, frequent periods (e.g., 5 minutes) with the patient throughout the shift. This gives patients the opportunity to understand that the nurse can be relied upon. It also gives patients time between visits to assess feelings and perhaps to feel less threatened.
If the Patient Gives the Nurse a Present The nurse may feel uncomfortable when offered a gift. The meaning needs to be examined. Is the gift (1) a way of getting better care, (2) a way to maintain self-esteem, (3) a way of making the nurse feel guilty, (4) a sincere expression of thanks, or (5) a cultural expectation?	Possible guidelines: If the gift is expensive, the only policy is to graciously refuse. If it is inexpensive, then (1) if it is given at the end of hospitalization when a relationship has developed, graciously accept; (2) if it is given at the beginning of the relationship, graciously refuse and explore the meaning behind the present: "Thank you, but it is our job to care for our patients. Are you concerned that some aspect of your care will be overlooked?" If the gift is money, it is always graciously refused.
If Another Patient Interrupts During Time with Your Current Patient The nurse may feel a conflict. The nurse does not want to appear rude. Sometimes the nurse tries to engage both patients in conversation.	The time the nurse had contracted with a selected patient is that patient's time. By keeping his or her part of the contract, the nurse demonstrates that the nurse means what he or she says and views the sessions as important: "I am with Mr. Rob for the next 20 minutes. At 10:00 a.m., after our time is up, I can talk to you for 5 minutes."

Student: "Hello, Ms. Chang. I am Bob Jacobs, and I'm a registered nursing student from Fairlawn University. I am in my psychiatric rotation. We will be coming here on Thursdays and Fridays until the end of the semester. I would like to spend time with you on these days until you are discharged.

I'm here to be a support person for you as you work on your treatment goals."

Knowing what the patient would like to be called is also essential, as names and titles are meaningful to most people. In the previous example, the student began by using a formal title of Ms. Chang. After checking the patient's identification band and reading it out loud, "Dorothy Chang," ask, "What would you like to be called?"

Establishing rapport. A major emphasis during the initial encounter with the patient is on providing an atmosphere in which trust and understanding, or rapport, can grow. Rapport is a relationship characterized by understanding and harmony, which is facilitated by genuineness, empathy, and unconditional positive regard on the part of the nurse. Being consistent, aiding in problem solving, and providing support are also essential aspects of establishing and maintaining rapport.

Specifying a contract. A contract emphasizes the patient's participation and responsibility because it shows that the nurse does something *with* the patient rather than *for* the patient. The contract, either stated or written, contains the place, time, date, and duration of the meetings. You should also discuss the termination of the relationship.

Student: "Ms. Chang, we will meet at 10:00 AM on Thursdays and Fridays. We have 30 minutes to discuss how you are doing and any concerns you may have. We will also discuss your diagnosis, symptom management, and review your medications and blood work. Like I said earlier, we will be able to work together until you are discharged."

Explaining confidentiality. Confidentiality is an integral part of caring for people in the mental health field. Confidentiality refers to information being held in confidence unless an authorization is made to share this information. The patient has a right to know (1) who else will be given the information shared with the nurse and (2) that the information may be shared with specific people such as a clinical supervisor, the physician, the staff, or other students in postconference. The patient also needs to know that the information will not be shared with relatives, friends, or others outside the treatment team, except in extreme situations. Extreme situations include child or older adult abuse and threats of self-harm or harm to others.

Nurses are aware of the patient's right to confidentiality. Safeguarding the confidentiality of patients is not only an ethical obligation but a legal responsibility as well. Breach of confidentiality is a common law tort, which is a civil wrong. This wrong can lead to a lawsuit resulting in monetary damages. See Chapter 6 for more information about torts.

Working Phase

A strong working relationship allows the patient to safely experience increased levels of anxiety and recognize dysfunctional responses. New and more adaptive coping behaviors can be practiced within the context of the working phase. Specific tasks for the nurse in this phase include:

- Gathering further data
- Identifying problem-solving skills and self-esteem
- Providing education about the disorder
- Promoting symptom management
- Providing medication education
- Evaluating progress

During the working phase, the nurse and patient identify and explore areas that are causing problems in the patient's life. Often, the patient's coping methods were developed to survive in a chaotic and dysfunctional family environment. Although coping methods may have worked for the patient at an earlier age, they may now interfere with the patient's functioning and interpersonal relationships.

An essential aspect of this working relationship is patient education. In order to facilitate this education, you need to become familiar with biological factors (e.g., genetic, biochemical) and also with psychological factors (e.g., cognitive distortions, learned helplessness) that may be the basis of your patients' psychiatric disorders. Understanding psychotropic medication, laboratory tests and results, and other treatments is also essential. This knowledge prepares you to help your patients learn, which, in turn, prepares them to take an active role in their own care and eventual recovery.

Termination Phase

The termination phase is the final, integral phase of the nurse-patient relationship. You discuss termination during the first meeting and again during the working stage at appropriate times. Termination may occur when the patient is discharged or when the student's clinical rotation ends. Basically, the tasks of termination include the following:

- Summarizing the goals and objectives achieved
- Reviewing patient education and providing handouts
- Discussing ways for the patient to incorporate new coping strategies
- Reviewing situations that occurred during the nurse-patient relationship
- Exchanging memories, which can help validate the experience for both nurse and patient and facilitate closure of that relationship

Termination may be a trigger for strong feelings in both the nurse and the patient. Termination of the relationship signifies a loss for both, although the intensity and meaning of termination may be different for each. If a patient has unresolved feelings of abandonment, loneliness, or rejection, these feelings may be reawakened during the termination process. This process can be an opportunity for the patient to express these feelings—perhaps for the first time.

If a nurse has been working with a patient for a while, it is important for the nurse to recognize that separation may be difficult for the patient. A general question—such as "How do you feel about being discharged?"—may provide the opening necessary for the patient to describe feelings.

Part of the termination process is to discuss the patient's plans for the future. If the termination is the result of a discharge, some of these plans have usually been discussed with the advanced practice care provider, including follow-up care and referrals. Registered nurses generally reinforce those plans and emphasize understanding of medications and recognizing when symptoms are getting out of control. Self-help groups can also be encouraged.

FACTORS THAT PROMOTE PATIENTS' GROWTH

Rogers and Truax (1967) identified three personal characteristics of the nurse that help promote change and growth in patients—factors still valued today as vital components for establishing a therapeutic relationship. They are: (1) genuineness, (2) empathy, and (3) positive regard and are some of the intangibles that are at the heart of the art of nursing and patient-centered care.

Genuineness

Genuineness refers to the nurse's ability to be open, honest, and authentic in interactions with patients. Being genuine is a key ingredient in building trust. When a person is genuine, one gets the sense that what is displayed on the outside of the person is congruent with who the person is on the inside. Nurses convey genuineness by listening to and communicating clearly with patients. Being genuine in a therapeutic relationship implies the ability to use therapeutic communication tools in an appropriately spontaneous manner rather than rigidly or in a parrot-like fashion.

Empathy

Empathy occurs when the helping person attempts to understand the world from the patient's perspective. Simply put, it is attempting to put oneself in the other's position. It is empathy that allows us to know what sort of emotional response to use, depending on another person's mental state.

Empathy is consistent with improved patient outcomes and increased patient satisfaction with care. However, it does not seem like we are doing a great job of instilling empathy in nursing students. In a study by Ward and colleagues (2012), 214 undergraduate nursing students demonstrated a decline in empathy after a year of clinical courses. These findings are consistent with those of medical students as they progress through years of school. It may be that these once-empathetic students are following the cue of other nurses.

Empathy Versus Sympathy

You may wonder how empathy differs from sympathy. A simple way to distinguish them is that in empathy, we *understand* the feelings of others, and in sympathy, we *feel* pity or sorrow for others. Although these are considered nurturing human traits, they may not be particularly useful in a therapeutic relationship.

The following examples clarify the distinction between empathy and sympathy. A friend tells you that her mother was just diagnosed with inoperable cancer. Your friend then begins to cry and pounds the table with her fist.

Sympathetic response: "I feel so bad for you (*tearing up*). I know how close you are to your mom. She is such an amazing person. Oh, I am so sorry." (*You hug your friend.*)

Empathetic response: "This must be devastating for you (*silence*). It must seem so unfair. What thoughts and feelings are you having?" (*You stay with your patient and listen.*)

Empathy is not a technique but rather an attitude that conveys respect, acceptance, and validation of the patient's strengths. Empathy may be one of the most important qualities that a psychiatric-mental health nurse can possess.

Positive Regard

Positive regard is respecting a person and viewing another person as being worthy of caring about and as someone who has strengths and achievement potential. Positive regard is usually communicated indirectly by attitudes and actions rather than directly by words. It is not necessary to like all people or approve of what they have done, especially if they have done terrible and hurtful things.

Attitudes

One attitude that might convey positive regard, or respect, is willingness to work with the patient. That is, the nurse takes the patient and the relationship seriously. The experience is viewed not as "a job" or "part of a course," but as an opportunity to work with patients to help them develop personal resources and actualize more of their potential in living.

Actions

Some actions that manifest an attitude of respect are attending, suspending value judgments, and helping patients develop their own resources.

Attending. Attending behavior is the foundation of a therapeutic relationship. To succeed, nurses must pay attention to their patients in culturally and individually appropriate ways. *Attending* is a special kind of listening that refers to an intensity of presence or being with the patient. At times, simply being with another person during a painful time can make a difference.

Posture, eye contact, and body language are nonverbal behaviors that reflect the degree of attending and are highly culturally influenced. Refer to Chapter 9 for a more detailed discussion of the cultural implications of nonverbal communication.

Suspending value judgments. As previously discussed, we all have values and beliefs. Using our own value systems to judge patients' thoughts, feelings, or behaviors is not helpful or productive. For example, if a patient is taking drugs or is involved in risky sexual behavior, the nurse recognizes that these behaviors are unhealthy. However, labeling these activities as bad or good is not useful. Rather, the nurse should help the patient explore the thoughts and feelings that influence this behavior. Judgment on the part of the nurse will most likely interfere with further exploration.

The first steps in eliminating judgmental thinking and behaviors are to (1) recognize their presence, (2) identify how or where you learned these responses, and (3) construct alternative ways to view the patient's thinking and behavior. Denying judgmental thinking will only compound the problem.

Patient: "I guess you could consider me an addictive personality. I love to gamble when I have money and spend most of my time in the casino. It seems like I'm hooking up with a different woman every time I'm there, and it always ends in sex."

A judgmental response would be:

Nurse A: "So your compulsive gambling and promiscuous sexual behaviors really haven't brought you much happiness, have they? You're running away from your problems and could end up with a sexually transmitted disease and broke."

A more helpful response would be:

Nurse B: "So, sexual and gambling activities are part of the picture also. How do these activities impact your life?"

In this example, Nurse B focuses on the patient's behaviors and how they affect his life. Nurse B does not introduce personal value statements or apply labels to the patient's behaviors.

Helping patients develop resources. It is important that patients remain as independent as possible to develop new resources for problem solving. The nurse does not do the work that patients should be doing unless it is absolutely necessary and then only as a step toward helping them act on their own. The following are examples of helping the patient develop independence:

Patient: "This medication makes my mouth so dry. Could you get me something to drink?"

Nurse: "There is juice in the refrigerator. I'll wait here for you until you get back." *Or* "I'll walk with you while you get some juice from the refrigerator."

Patient: "Could you ask the doctor to let me have a pass for the weekend?"

Nurse: "Your doctor will be on the unit this afternoon. I'll let her know that you want to speak with her."

Consistently encouraging patients to use their own resources helps minimize patients' feelings of helplessness and dependency. It also validates their ability to bring about change.

KEY POINTS TO REMEMBER

- The nurse-patient relationship is the basis of all psychiatric-mental health nursing treatment approaches, regardless of the specific goals.
- Using unique personality traits and talents to promote healing in others is referred to as the therapeutic use of self.
- Counseling is used by psychiatric-mental health registered nurses and other entry-level psychiatric care professionals as a supportive face-to-face process that helps individuals problem solve, resolve personal conflicts, and feel supported.
- Psychotherapy refers to a group of theoretically based therapies that are used by psychiatric-mental health advanced practice registered nurses and other advanced practice psychiatric care professionals.
- A personal relationship is a relationship for the purpose of friendship, socialization, enjoyment, or accomplishment of a task. A therapeutic nurse-patient relationship focuses on the patient's needs, thoughts, feelings, and goals.
- Professional boundaries protect patients. Boundaries are the expected and accepted social, physical, and psychological boundaries that separate nurses from patients.
- Values and beliefs give our life meaning and influence our conduct. It is important to develop awareness, acknowledge, and then monitor our responses to patients who possess different values and beliefs.
- Peplau's phases of the nurse-patient relationship provide a framework to structure care. They are the preorientation, orientation, working, and termination phases.
- Factors vital for establishing a therapeutic relationship include genuineness, empathy, and positive regard.

CRITICAL THINKING

1. On your first clinical day, you are assigned to work with an older adult, Ms. Schneider, who is depressed. Your first impression is, "Oh, my, she looks like my rude Aunt Elaine. She even dresses like her." You approach her with a vague feeling of uneasiness and say, "Hello, Ms. Schneider. My name is Alisha. I am a nursing student, and I will be working with you today." She tells you that "a student" could never understand what she is going through.
   a. Identify transference and countertransference issues in this situation. What is your most important course of action?
   b. What other information will you give Ms. Schneider during this first clinical encounter? Be specific.
   c. What are some useful responses you could give Ms. Schneider regarding her concern about whether you could understand what she was going through?

2. You are interviewing Tom Stone, a 17-year-old who was admitted to a psychiatric unit after a suicide attempt. How would you best respond to each of the following patient requests and behaviors?
   a. "I would feel so much better if you would sit closer to me and hold my hand."
   b. "I will tell you if I still feel like killing myself, but you have to promise not to tell anyone else. If you do, I can't trust you, ever."
   c. "I don't want to talk to you. I have absolutely nothing to say."
   d. "I will be going home tomorrow, and you have been so helpful and good to me. I want you to have my watch to remember me by."
   e. Tom breaks down and starts sobbing.

CHAPTER REVIEW

1. Which statement made by either the nurse or the patient demonstrates an ineffective patient-nurse relationship?
   a. "I've given a lot of thought about what triggers me to be so angry."
   b. "Why do you think it's acceptable for you to be so disrespectful to staff?"
   c. "Will your spouse be available to attend tomorrow's family group session?"

d. "I wanted you to know that the medication seems to be helping me feel less anxious."

2. The patient expresses sadness at "being all alone with no one to share my life with." Which response by the nurse demonstrates the existence of a therapeutic relationship?
   a. "Loneliness can be a very painful and difficult emotion."
   b. "Let's talk and see if you and I have any interests in common."
   c. "I use Facebook to find people who share my love of cooking."
   d. "Loneliness is managed by getting involved with people."

3. Which patient outcome is directly associated with the goals of a therapeutic nurse-patient relationship?
   a. Patient will be respectful of other patients on the unit.
   b. Patient will identify suicidal feelings to staff whenever they occur.
   c. Patient will engage in at least one social interaction with the unit population daily.
   d. Patient will consume a daily diet to meet both nutritional and hydration needs.

4. What is the greatest trigger for the development of a patient's nurse-focused transference?
   a. The similarity between the nurse and someone the patient already dislikes
   b. The nature of the patient's diagnosed mental illness
   c. The history the patient has with the patient's parents
   d. The degree of authority the nurse has over the patient

5. Which patient statement demonstrates a value held regarding children?
   a. "Nothing is more important to me than the safety of my children."
   b. "I believe my spouse wants to leave both me and our children."
   c. "I don't think my child's success depends on going to college."
   d. "I know my children will help me through my hard times."

6. Mary is a 39-year-old attending a psychiatric outpatient clinic. Mary believes that her husband, sister, and son cause her problems. Listening to Mary describe the problems, the nurse displays therapeutic communication in which response?
   a. "I understand you are in a difficult situation."
   b. "Thinking about being wronged repeatedly does more harm than good."
   c. "I feel bad about your situation, and I am so sorry it is happening to you and your family."
   d. "It must be so difficult to live with uncaring people."

7. A registered nurse is caring for an older male who reports depressive symptoms since his wife of 54 years died suddenly. He cries, maintains closed body posture, and avoids eye contact. Which nursing action describes attending behavior?
   a. Reminding the patient gently that he will "feel better over time"
   b. Using a soft tone of voice for questioning
   c. Sitting with the patient and taking cues for when to talk or when to remain silent
   d. Offering medication and bereavement services

8. A male patient frequently inquires about the female student nurse's boyfriend, social activities, and school experiences. Which is the best *initial* response by the student?
   a. The student requests assignment to a patient of the same gender as the student.
   b. She limits sharing personal information and stresses the patient-centered focus of the conversation.
   c. The student shares information to make the therapeutic relationship more equal.
   d. She explains that if he persists in focusing on her, she cannot work with him.

9. Morgan is a third-year nursing student in her psychiatric clinical rotation. She is assigned to an 80-year-old widow admitted for major depressive disorder. The patient describes many losses and sadness. Morgan becomes teary and says meaningfully, "I am so sorry for you." Morgan's instructor overhears the conversation and says, "I understand that getting tearful is a human response. Yet, sympathy isn't helpful in this field." The instructor urges Morgan to focus on:
   a. "Adopting the patient's sorrow as your own"
   b. "Maintaining pure objectivity"
   c. "Using empathy to demonstrate respect and validation of the patient's feelings"
   d. "Using touch to let her know that everything is going to be alright"

10. Emily is a 28-year-old nurse who works on a psychiatric unit. She is assigned to work with Jenna, a 27-year-old who was admitted with major depressive disorder. Emily and Jenna realize that they graduated from the same high school and each has a 2-year-old daughter. Emily and Jenna discuss getting together for a play date with their daughters after Jenna is discharged. This situation reflects:
    a. Successful termination
    b. Promoting interdependence
    c. Boundary blurring
    d. A strong therapeutic relationship

1. **b**; 2. **a**; 3. **b**; 4. **d**; 5. **a**; 6. **a**; 7. **c**; 8. **b**; 9. **c**; 10. **c**

Visit the Evolve website for a posttest on the content in this chapter: http://evolve.elsevier.com/Varcarolis

REFERENCES

BBC News. (2014). Bodmin Hospital nurse struck off. *BBC News.* Retrieved from http://www.bbc.com/news/uk-england-cornwall-25596856.

Gordon, C., & Bereson, E. V. (2016). The doctor-patient relationship. In T. A. Stern, M. Fava, T. E. Wilens, & J. F. Rosenbaum (Eds.), *Massachusetts General Hospital comprehensive clinical psychiatry* (2nd ed.) (pp. 1–7). Philadelphia, PA: Saunders.

Institute for Patient- and Family-Centered Care. (n.d.). *Frequently asked questions*. Retrieved from https://www.ipfcc.org/about/pfcc.html.

Malhotra, S., & Sahoo, S. (2017). Rebuilding the brain with psychotherapy. *Indian Journal of Psychiatry, 59*(4), 411–419.

National Council of State Boards of Nursing. (2018). *A nurse's guide to professional behaviors*. Retrieved from https://www.ncsbn.org/ProfessionalBoundaries_Complete.pdf.

Peplau, H. E. (1952). *Interpersonal relations in nursing: A conceptual frame of reference for psychodynamic nursing*. New York, NY: Putnam.

Peplau, H. E. (1999). *Interpersonal relations in nursing: A conceptual frame of reference for psychodynamic nursing*. New York, NY: Springer.

Rogers, C. R., & Truax, C. B. (1967). The therapeutic conditions antecedent to change: A theoretical view. In C. R. Rogers (Ed.), *The therapeutic relationship and its impact*. Madison, WI: University of Wisconsin Press.

Ward, J., Cody, J., Schaal, M., & Hojat, M. (2012). The empathy enigma: An empirical study of decline in empathy among undergraduate nursing students. *Journal of Professional Nursing, 28*, 34–40.

9

Therapeutic Communication

Margaret Jordan Halter and Elizabeth M. Varcarolis

 Visit the Evolve website for a pretest on the content in this chapter: http://evolve.elsevier.com/Varcarolis

OBJECTIVES

1. Describe two theoretical models of communication.
2. Identify two personal, two environmental, and two relationship factors that can interfere with communication.
3. Discuss the differences between verbal and nonverbal communication.
4. Discuss verbal and nonverbal communication of different cultural groups in the areas of communication style, eye contact, and touch.
5. Identify four techniques that can enhance communication, highlighting what makes them effective.
6. Identify four types of nontherapeutic communication and what makes them ineffective.
7. Relate problems that can arise when nurses are insensitive to cultural influences on patients' communication styles.
8. Discuss the increasing role of information communication technology in the delivery of healthcare, both in terms of advantages and concerns.
9. Summarize the best pace, setting, and seating arrangement for engaging in the nurse-patient interaction.
10. Identify two attending behaviors the nurse might focus on to increase communication skills.
11. Describe the importance of clinical supervision.

KEY TERMS AND CONCEPTS

active listening
closed-ended questions
cultural filters
debriefing
double-bind messages

information communication
 technology
mobile medical applications
nontherapeutic communication
nonverbal behaviors
nonverbal communication

open-ended questions
patient-centered
telehealth technologies
therapeutic communication techniques
verbal communication

INTRODUCTION

Humans have an inherent need to relate to others. Our advanced ability to communicate with others gives substance and meaning to our lives. All our actions, words, and facial expressions convey meaning to others. It has been said that we cannot *not* communicate. Even silence can convey acceptance, anger, or thoughtfulness. Effective communication is the foundation for productive relationships and positive feelings. On the other hand, ineffective communication within a relationship often results in stress and negative feelings.

In the provision of nursing care, communication takes on a new emphasis. Just as personal relationships are different from therapeutic relationships, *basic communication* is different from patient-centered, goal-directed, and scientifically based *therapeutic communication*.

The ability to form patient-centered therapeutic relationships is fundamental and essential to effective nursing care.

Patient-centered refers to the patient as a full partner in care whose values, preferences, and needs are respected (Quality and Safety Education for Nurses, 2012). Therapeutic communication is crucial to the formation of patient-centered therapeutic relationships. Determining levels of pain in the postoperative patient, listening as parents express feelings of fear concerning their child's diagnosis, or understanding, without words, the needs of the intubated patient in the intensive care unit are essential skills in providing quality nursing care.

Ideally, therapeutic communication is a professional ability you learn and practice early in your nursing curriculum. But in psychiatric–mental health nursing, communication skills take on a new emphasis. Psychiatric disorders cause physical symptoms (e.g., fatigue, loss of appetite, or insomnia), cognitive symptoms (e.g., difficulty with concentration or memory loss), and emotional symptoms (e.g., sadness, anger, or euphoria) that affect a patient's ability to relate to others.

It is often during the psychiatric rotation that students discover the usefulness of therapeutic communication and begin to rely on techniques they may have once considered artificial. For example, restating sounds so simplistic, you may hesitate to use it:

Patient: "At the moment they told me my daughter would never be able to walk like her twin sister, I felt like I couldn't go on."

Student: *(Restates the patient's words after a short silence)* "You felt like you couldn't go on."

The technique, and the empathy it conveys, is supportive in such a situation. Developing therapeutic communication skills takes time, and with continued practice, you will find your own style and rhythm. Eventually, these techniques will become a part of the way you instinctively communicate with others in the clinical setting.

Saying the Wrong Thing

Nursing students are often concerned that they may say the wrong thing. Will you say the "wrong thing"? Yes, that may happen. Making mistakes helps us to find more useful and effective ways of helping individuals reach their goals.

Will saying the wrong thing be harmful to the patient? Consider that symptoms of psychiatric disorders—irritability, negativity, limited communication, or hyperactivity—often frustrate and alienate friends and family. It is likely that the interactions the patient had been having recently were not always pleasant. Patients tend to appreciate a well-meaning person who conveys genuine acceptance, respect, and concern for their situation. Even if you make mistakes in communication or when you say the "wrong thing," there is little chance that the comments will do actual harm.

Benefits of Therapeutic Communication

Just as personal relationships are different from therapeutic relationships, basic communication is different from the professional and goal-directed communication we call therapeutic communication. Research supports the use of this type of communication. Benefits include feeling safe and protected, being more satisfied with the care, increased recovery rates, and improved adherence to treatment (Neese, 2015).

Conversely, poor communication can create serious problems. More than 250,000 people in the United States die each year because of medical mistakes, making it the third leading cause of death after heart disease and cancer (Makary & Daniel, 2016). In 2015, communication failure caused about 30% of all malpractice claims, resulting in 1744 deaths and $1.7 billion in malpractice costs (CRICO Strategies, 2016). This impaired communication is particularly problematic during patient handoffs, such as change of shift reports.

THEORETICAL MODELS OF COMMUNICATION

The Transactional Model of Communication

Communication is an interactive process between two or more persons who interact with one another. Models provide a visual representation of communication. The transactional model of communication (Barnlund, 1970) is systematic and useful for psychiatric–mental health nurses. The following components are included in this model:

1. **Communicator:** Senders and receivers are both considered to be communicators, which makes roles fluid. Communicators are interdependent. For example, communication is not occurring if the receiver is not listening.
2. **Message:** The message is the content and the ideas that are being exchanged. Messages are also relational, which are communicated nonverbally by such elements as tone and body posture.
3. **Channel:** The method by which the communication takes place (e.g., in person or by telepsychiatry).
4. **Feedback:** The messaging takes place with a constant feedback being given by both parties. Feedback for one is the message for the other.
5. **Encoding/decoding:** While interacting, individuals encode (develop) messages and send to the other and decode (determine meaning) messages received from the other.
6. **Context:** Context frames and influences our interactions. The more contextual elements that people share in common, the easier the communication.
   - **Social context** refers to stated or unstated rules or norms (socially accepted ways of interacting) that guide communication.
   - **Relational context** includes interpersonal history and the type of relationship that is involved. Personal relationships are less highly scripted than are therapeutic relationships due to the nature of the connection.
   - **Cultural context** refers to the influence that our cultural identities have on communication. This context includes gender, race, ethnicity, nationality, sexual orientation, and socioeconomic class.
7. **Environmental noise:** Noise disturbs the message flow and serves as a barrier to interaction.
   - **Physical noise** is experienced by such conditions as loud units, background music, or overhead announcements.
   - **Physiological noise** includes biological factors (e.g., illness, headache, or fatigue) that reduce the quality of interactions.
   - **Psychological noise** refers to the factors within a person's mind such as not wanting to converse or being preoccupied about finances.

The transactional model of communication identifies communication as occurring in the context of social, relational, and cultural contexts. We do not just communicate to share information; rather, we communicate to create relationships and to shape self-concepts. This model stresses that participants are simultaneously senders and receivers. By recognizing the fluid nature of the interaction, we can adapt our message in the middle of sending it based on the communication we are receiving.

The method or medium of communication affects the reliability of what is being said. Face-to-face communication, whether in person or by teleconferencing, is more effective than phone conversations since nonverbals enrich the interaction.

Fig. 9.1 shows the transactional model of communication.

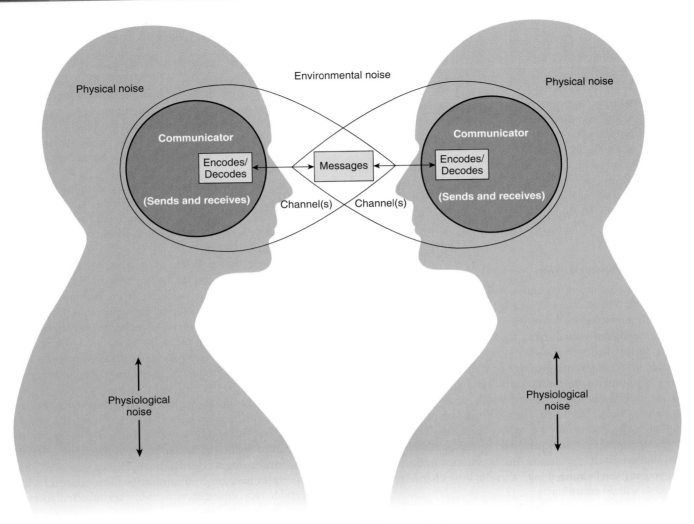

Fig. 9.1 Transactional model of communication.

Peplau's Interpersonal Theory

Hildegard Peplau (1952) was the first published nurse since Florence Nightingale. Her book, *Interpersonal Relations in Nursing*, emphasizes the nurse-patient relationship. At the heart of this relationship is a commitment to clear communication. The two main principles that guide the communication process are: (1) clarity, which ensures that the meaning of the message is accurately understood by both parties and (2) continuity, which promotes connections among ideas, feelings, events, and themes. Peplau also recommends nondirective listening. Using this form of communication allows nurses to provide reflective and nonjudgmental feedback, thereby helping patients to clarify their thoughts.

See Chapter 2 for more information about Peplau's Interpersonal Theory.

FACTORS THAT AFFECT COMMUNICATION

Personal Factors

Personal factors can impede accurate transmission or interpretation of messages. Patients may have difficulty communicating due to a psychiatric disorder. For example, depression may result in slow thinking and reduced communication, anxiety can cause lack of concentration, and mania creates an inability to focus for any length of time.

Even with an interpreter, language barriers will reduce the normal flow of communication. Cultural differences such as gender–related beliefs (i.e., the role of women in caring for male patients) can negatively impact communication.

Cognitive factors have to be considered when communicating and providing education. Problem-solving ability, knowledge level, and language use are reduced in intellectual development disability, neurocognitive disorders, and psychotic states.

Environmental Factors

Environmental factors within a healthcare setting that may affect communication include physical factors. Background noise, lack of privacy, and uncomfortable accommodations are not conducive to a smooth flow of communication. While units are not as crowded and noisy as they once were, it may still be difficult to carry on a private conversation in the day hall or other common area.

TABLE 9.1 Nonverbal Behaviors

Behavior	Possible Nonverbal Cues	Example
Body behaviors	Posture, body movements, gestures, gait	The patient is slumped in a chair, puts her face in her hands, and occasionally taps her right foot.
Facial expressions	Frowns, smiles, grimaces, raised eyebrows, pursed lips, licking of lips, tongue movements	The patient grimaces when speaking to the nurse; when alone, he smiles and giggles to himself.
Eye expression and gaze behavior	Lowering brows, intimidating gaze	The patient's eyes harden with suspicion.
Voice-related behaviors	Tone, pitch, level, intensity, inflection, stuttering, pauses, silences, fluency	The patient talks in a loud singsong voice.
Observable autonomic physiological responses	Increase in respirations, diaphoresis, pupil dilation, blushing, paleness	When the patient mentions discharge, her respirations increase and her face becomes diaphoretic.
Personal appearance	Grooming, dress, hygiene	The patient is dressed in a wrinkled shirt, his pants are stained, his socks are dirty, and he is unshaven.
Physical characteristics	Height, weight, physique, complexion	The patient is pale and emaciated.

Relationship Factors

For the purpose of this discussion, relationship factors refer to the level of equality within the relationship. When the two participants are equal, such as friends or colleagues, the relationship is symmetrical. However, when there is a difference in status or power, such as between nurse and patient or teacher and student, the relationship is characterized by inequality. One participant has more control. This is called a complementary relationship. Usually, the inequality decreases as the patient recovers and as the student progresses and graduates. Complementary relationships also exist based on social status, age or developmental differences, gender differences, and educational differences.

VERBAL AND NONVERBAL COMMUNICATION

Verbal Communication

Verbal communication consists of all the words a person speaks. We live in a society of symbols, and our main social symbols are words. Words are the symbols for emotions and mental images. Talking is our link to one another and the primary instrument of instruction. Talking is a need, an art, and one of the most personal aspects of our private lives. When we speak, we:

- Communicate our beliefs and values.
- Communicate perceptions and meanings.
- Convey interest and understanding *or* insult and judgment.
- Convey messages clearly *or* convey conflicting or implied messages.
- Convey clear, honest feelings *or* disguised, distorted feelings.

Nonverbal Communication

It is said, "It's not what you say but how you say it." In other words, it is the nonverbal behaviors that may be defining the real message. The tone of voice, emphasis on certain words, and the manner in which a person paces speech are examples of nonverbal communication. Other common examples of nonverbal communication are physical appearance, body posture,

eye contact, hand gestures, sighs, fidgeting, and yawning. Table 9.1 identifies examples of nonverbal behaviors.

Some elements of nonverbal communication, such as facial expressions, seem to be inborn and are similar across cultures. For example, some cultural groups may control their facial expressions in public while others tend to be open with facial expressions. Gender also plays a role in facial expressions. Men tend to hide surprise and fear while women control disgust, contempt, and anger.

Facial expression is extremely important in terms of nonverbal communication. The eyes and the mouth seem to hold the biggest clues into how people are feeling through emotional decoding. Eisenbarth and Alpers (2011) examined how participants looked at various parts of the face in response to different emotions. Participants focused on the eyes more frequently when looking at a sad face. They focused on the mouth more frequently when looking at a happy face. Like sadness, anger was more frequently decoded in the eyes. When presented with either a fearful or neutral expression, there was an equal amount of attention given to both the eyes and the mouth.

Some types of nonverbal behaviors, such as how close people stand to each other when speaking, depend on cultural conventions. Some nonverbal communication is formalized and has specific meanings (e.g., the military salute, the Japanese bow).

Interaction of Verbal and Nonverbal Communication

Spoken words represent our public selves and can be straightforward or used to distort, conceal, deny, or disguise true feelings. Nonverbal behaviors include a wide range of human activities, from body movements to facial expressions to physical reactions to messages from others. How a person listens and uses silence and sense of touch may also convey important information about the private self that is not available from conversation alone, especially in consideration of cultural norms.

The verbal message is sometimes referred to as the *content* of the message (what is said), and the nonverbal behavior is called the *process* of the message (nonverbal cues a person uses along with the verbal message). People usually have greater awareness of their verbal messages than what is projected nonverbally.

Typically, when verbal content is congruent with the nonverbal processes, the communication is more clearly understood and is considered healthy. For example, a student may say, "It's important that I get good grades in this class," and then proceed to purchase the required textbook, take thorough notes, and engage a study buddy; this sends a congruent message. In this case, the content and process are congruent. If, however, the verbal message is not reinforced or is contradicted by the nonverbal behavior, the message is incongruent. If a student says, "It's important that I get good grades in this class" and does not have the required textbook, skips classes, and does not study, the content and process do not match. The student's verbal and nonverbal behaviors are incongruent.

With experience in making observations, nurses become increasingly aware of the verbal and nonverbal communication of the patient. Nurses can compare patients' dialogue with their nonverbal behaviors to gain important clues about the real message.

One way a nurse can respond to verbal and nonverbal incongruity is to reflect and validate the patient's feelings. For example, the nurse could say, "You say you are upset you did not pass pathophysiology this semester, but I notice you don't look upset. What do you think about that?"

Bateson and colleagues (1956) coined the term **double-bind messages**. They are characterized by two or more mutually contradictory messages given by a person in power. Opting for either choice will result in displeasure of the person in power. Such messages may be a mix of content (what is said) and process (what is conveyed nonverbally) that has both nurturing and hurtful aspects. The following vignette gives an example.

> **VIGNETTE:** A 21-year-old female who lives at home with her chronically ill mother wants to go out for an evening with her friends. She is told by her frail but not helpless mother: "Oh, go ahead, have fun. I'll just sit here by myself, and I can always call 911 if I don't feel well. You go ahead and have fun." The mother says this with a sad expression and eyes downcast. She slumps down in her chair and lets her cane drop to the floor.
>
> The recipient of this double-bind message is caught between contradictory messages. If she goes out, she will feel guilty and selfish for leaving her sick mother alone. Yet, if she stays, her mother could say, "I told you to go have fun." As is the nature of double-bind communication, she is trapped in a no-win situation.

COMMUNICATION SKILLS FOR NURSES

Therapeutic Communication Techniques

Once you have established a therapeutic relationship, you and your patient can identify specific needs and problems. You can then begin to work with the patient on increasing problem-solving skills, learning new coping behaviors, and experiencing more appropriate and satisfying ways of relating to others. Strong communication skills will facilitate your work. These skills are called **therapeutic communication techniques** and include words and actions that help to achieve health-related goals. Some useful techniques for nurses when communicating with their patients are (1) silence, (2) active listening, (3) clarifying techniques, and (4) questions.

Using Silence

Students and practicing nurses alike may find that, when the flow of words stops, they become uncomfortable. They may rush to fill the void with questions or idle comments. This response may cut off important thoughts and feelings the patient might be taking time to think about. Silence is not the absence of communication but a specific channel for transmitting and receiving messages. Therefore, the nurse learns to appreciate that silence is a significant means of influencing and being influenced by others.

When the nurse and patient first meet, patients may be reluctant to speak because of the newness of the situation and the fact that the nurse is a stranger. Some patients may also be profoundly depressed, distrustful, self-consciousness, embarrassed, or shy. The nurse recognizes and respects individual differences in styles and tempos of responding.

Although there is no universal rule concerning how much silence is too much, silence is worthwhile only as long as it is serving some function and not frightening the patient. Knowing when to speak during interactions largely depends on the nurse's perception about what is being conveyed through the silence. For example, icy silence may be an expression of anger and hostility and may be addressed by making observations.

Silence may provide meaningful moments of reflection for both participants. It provides an opportunity to contemplate thoughtfully what has been said and felt, weigh alternatives, formulate new ideas, and gain a new perspective. If the nurse waits to speak and allows the patient to break the silence, the patient may share thoughts and feelings that would have been withheld otherwise.

It is important to note that some psychiatric disorders, such as major depressive disorder, Alzheimer's disease, and schizophrenia, along with medications may cause an overall slowing of thought processes. This slowing may be so severe that it may seem like an eternity before the patient responds. Patience and gentle prompting can help patients gather their thoughts. For example, "You were saying that you are looking forward to your husband's visit."

Conversely, silence is not always therapeutic. Prolonged and frequent silences by the nurse may hinder a communication that requires verbal articulation. This technique may make the patient feel uncomfortable. Without feedback from the nurse, patients have no way of knowing whether what they said was understood. Also, children and adolescents in particular tend to feel uncomfortable with silence, so this technique should be used sparingly, if at all, with young people.

Active Listening

People want more than just a physical presence in human communication. Most people want the other person to be there for them fully. In **active listening**, nurses focus, respond, and remember what the patient is saying verbally and nonverbally.

Active listening enhances self-esteem and encourages the patient to direct energy toward finding ways to deal with problems. This technique helps strengthen the patient's ability to solve problems. Serving as a sounding board, the nurse listens as the patient tests thoughts by voicing them aloud. This form of interpersonal interaction often enables the patient to clarify thinking, link ideas, and tentatively decide what should be done and how best to do it.

Clarifying Techniques

Understanding depends on clear communication, which is aided by verifying the nurse's interpretation of the patient's messages. The nurse can request feedback on the accuracy of the message received from verbal and nonverbal cues.

Paraphrasing. Paraphrasing occurs when you restate the basic content of a patient's message in different, usually fewer, words. Using simple, precise, and culturally relevant terms, the nurse may confirm an interpretation of the patient's message. Prefacing statements with a phrase such as "You seem to be saying…" or "I'm not sure I understand" helps the nurse sort through a bewildering amount of details. It helps the patient to feel heard and may provide greater focus. The patient may confirm or deny the perceptions nonverbally by nodding or looking uncertain, or by direct responses, "Yes, that is what I was trying to say" or "No, I meant…"

Restating. Restating is an active listening strategy that helps the nurse to understand what the patient is saying. It also lets the patient know he is being heard. Restating differs from paraphrasing in that it involves repeating the same key words the patient has just spoken. If a patient remarks, "My life is empty… it has no meaning," additional information may be gained by restating, "Your life is empty?"

While this is a valuable technique, it should be used sparingly. Patients may interpret frequent and indiscriminate use of restating as inattention or disinterest. Overuse makes restating sound mechanical. To avoid overuse of restating, the nurse can combine restatements with direct questions that encourage descriptions: "What does your life lack?" "What kind of meaning is missing?" "Describe a day in your life that seems empty to you."

Reflecting. Reflection is a means of assisting patients to better understand their own thoughts and feelings. Reflecting may take the form of a question or a simple statement that conveys the nurse's observations of the patient when discussing sensitive issues. The nurse might then describe briefly to the patient the apparent meaning of the emotional tone of the patient's verbal and nonverbal behaviors. For example, to reflect a patient's feelings about her life, a good beginning might be, "You sound as if you have had many disappointments."

When you reflect, you make the patient aware of inner feelings and encourage the patient to own them. For example, you may say to a patient, "You look sad." Perceiving your concern may allow the patient to spontaneously share feelings. The use of a question in response to the patient's question is another reflective technique. For example:

Patient: "Nurse, do you think I really need to be hospitalized?"

Nurse: "What do you think, Kelly?"

Patient: "I don't know. That's why I'm asking you."

Nurse: "I'm willing to share my impression with you. However, you've probably thought about hospitalization and have some feelings about it. Let's talk about this."

Exploring. A technique that enables the nurse to examine important ideas, experiences, or relationships more fully is exploring. For example, if a patient tells you he does not get along well with his wife, you will want to further explore this area. Possible openers include the following:

"*Tell me more* about your relationship with your wife."

"*Describe* your relationship with your wife."

"*Give me an example* of how you and your wife don't get along."

Asking for an example can greatly clarify a vague or generic statement made by a patient.

Patient: "No one likes me."

Nurse: "Give me an example of one person who doesn't like you."

or

Patient: "Everything I do is wrong."

Nurse: "Let's talk about one thing you do that you think is wrong."

Table 9.2 lists more examples of therapeutic communication techniques.

Questions

Open-ended questions. Open-ended questions encourage patients to share information about experiences, perceptions, or responses to a situation. For example:

- "What do you perceive as your biggest problem right now?"
- "What is an example of some of the stresses you are under right now?"
- "How would you describe your relationship with your wife?"

Because open-ended questions are not intrusive and do not put the patient on the defensive, they help the nurse obtain information. This technique is especially useful in the beginning of an interview or when a patient is guarded or resistant to answering questions. They are particularly useful when establishing rapport with a person.

Closed-ended questions. Nurses commonly ask open-ended questions to induce more than a "yes" or "no" response. However, closed-ended questions, when used sparingly, can give you specific and needed information. Closed-ended questions are most useful during an initial assessment or intake interview or to determine specific results such as "Are the medications helping you?" "When did you start hearing voices?" "Did you get into therapy after your first suicide attempt?"

Projective questions. Projective questions usually start with a "*what if*" to help people articulate, explore, and identify thoughts and feelings. They are surprisingly strong in their ability to facilitate a patient's thinking about problems differently and to identify priorities. Projective questions can also help people imagine thoughts, feelings, and behaviors they might have in certain situations:

- If you had three wishes, what would you wish for?
- If you could go back and change how you acted in (a situation/significant life event), what would you do differently now?
- What would you do if you were given $1 million with no strings attached?

TABLE 9.2 Therapeutic Communication Techniques

Therapeutic Technique	Description	Example
Silence	Gives the person time to collect thoughts or think through a point.	Encouraging a person to talk by waiting for the answers.
Accepting	Indicates that the person has been understood. An accepting statement does not necessarily indicate agreement but is nonjudgmental.	"Yes." "Uh-huh." "I follow what you say."
Giving recognition	Indicates awareness of change and personal efforts. Does not imply good or bad, right or wrong.	"Good morning, Mr. James." "You've combed your hair today." "I see you've eaten your whole lunch."
Offering self	Offers presence, interest, and a desire to understand. Is not offered to get the person to talk or behave in a specific way.	"I would like to spend time with you." "I'll stay here and sit with you awhile."
Offering general leads	Allows the other person to take direction in the discussion. Indicates that the nurse is interested in what comes next.	"Go on." "And then?" "Tell me about it."
Giving broad openings	Clarifies that the lead is to be taken by the patient. However, the nurse discourages pleasantries and small talk.	"Where would you like to begin?" "What are you thinking about?" "What would you like to discuss?"
Placing the events in time or sequence	Puts events and actions in better perspective. Notes cause-and-effect relationships and identifies patterns of interpersonal difficulties.	"What happened before?" "When did this happen?"
Making observations	Calls attention to the person's behavior (e.g., trembling, nail-biting, restless mannerisms). Encourages patient to notice the behavior and describe thoughts and feelings for mutual understanding. Helpful with mute and withdrawn people.	"You appear tense." "I notice you're biting your lips." "You seem nervous whenever John enters the room."
Encouraging description of perception	Increases the nurse's understanding of the patient's perceptions. Talking about feelings and difficulties can lessen the need to act them out inappropriately.	"What do these voices seem to be saying?" "What is happening now?" "Tell me when you feel anxious."
Encouraging comparison	Brings out recurring themes in experiences or interpersonal relationships. Helps the person clarify similarities and differences.	"Has this ever happened before?" "Is this how you felt …?"… "Was it something like…?"…
Restating	Repeats the main idea expressed. Gives the patient an idea of what has been communicated. If the message has been misunderstood, the patient can clarify it.	*Patient:* "I can't sleep. I stay awake all night." *Nurse:* "You have difficulty sleeping?" *or* *Patient:* "I don't know… he always has some excuse for not coming over or keeping our appointments." *Nurse:* "You think he no longer wants to see you?"
Reflecting	Directs questions, feelings, and ideas back to the patient. Encourages the patient to accept personal ideas and feelings. Acknowledges the patient's right to have opinions and make decisions and encourages the patient to think of oneself as a capable person.	*Patient:* "What should I do about my husband's affair?" *Nurse:* "What do you think you should do?" *or* *Patient:* "My brother spends all of my money and then has the nerve to ask for more." *Nurse:* "You feel angry when this happens?"
Focusing	Concentrates attention on a single point. It is especially useful when the patient jumps from topic to topic. If a person is experiencing a severe or panic level of anxiety, the nurse should not persist until the anxiety lessens.	"This point you are making about leaving school seems worth looking at more closely." "You've mentioned many things. Let's go back to your thinking of 'ending it all.'"
Exploring	Examines certain ideas, experiences, or relationships more fully. If the patient chooses not to elaborate by answering no, the nurse does not probe or pry. In such a case, the nurse respects the patient's wishes.	"Tell me more about that." "Would you describe it more fully?" "Could you talk about how it was that you learned your mom was dying of cancer?"
Giving information	Makes facts the person needs available. Supplies knowledge from which decisions can be made or conclusions drawn. For example, the patient needs to know the role of the nurse, the purpose of the nurse-patient relationship, and the time, place, and duration of the meetings.	"My purpose for being here is…"… "This medication is for…"… "The test will determine…"…
Seeking clarification	Helps patients clarify their own thoughts and maximize mutual understanding between nurse and patient.	"I am not sure I follow you." "What would you say is the main point of what you just said?" "Give an example of a time you thought everyone hated you."

TABLE 9.2 Therapeutic Communication Techniques—cont'd

Therapeutic Technique	Description	Example
Presenting reality	Indicates what is real. The nurse does not argue or try to convince the patient, just describes personal perceptions or facts in the situation.	"That was Dr. Todd, not a man from the Mafia." "That was the sound of a car backfiring." "Your mother is not here; I am a nurse."
Voicing doubt	Expressing uncertainty regarding the reality of the patient's perceptions or conclusions, especially in hallucinations and delusions.	"Isn't that unusual?" "Really?" "That's hard to believe."
Seeking consensual validation	Clarifies that both the nurse and patient share mutual understanding of communications. Helps the patient to clarify thoughts.	"Tell me whether my understanding agrees with yours."
Verbalizing the implied	Puts into concrete terms what the patient implies, making the patient's communication more explicit.	*Patient:* "I can't talk to you or anyone else. It's a waste of time." *Nurse:* "Do you feel that no one understands?"
Encouraging evaluation	Aids the patient in considering other persons and events from the perspective of the patient's own set of values.	"How do you feel about…?" "What did it mean to you when he said he couldn't stay?"
Attempting to translate into feelings	Responds to the feelings expressed, not just the content. Often termed *decoding*.	*Patient:* "I am dead inside." *Nurse:* "Are you saying that you feel lifeless? Does life seem meaningless to you?"
Suggesting collaboration	Emphasizes working with the patient, not doing things for the patient. Encourages the view that change is possible through collaboration.	"Perhaps you and I can discover what produces your anxiety." "Perhaps by working together, we can come up with some ideas that might improve your communication with your spouse."
Summarizing	Brings together important points of discussion to enhance understanding. Also allows the opportunity to clarify communications so that both nurse and patient leave the interview with the same ideas in mind.	"Have I got this straight?" "You said that…" "During the past hour, you and I have discussed…"
Encouraging formulation of a plan of action	Allows the patient to identify alternative actions for interpersonal situations the patient finds disturbing (e.g., when anger or anxiety is provoked).	"What could you do to let anger out harmlessly?" "The next time this comes up, what might you do to handle it?" "What are some other ways you can approach your boss?"

Adapted from Hays, J. S., & Larson, K. (1963). *Interacting with patients.* New York, NY: Macmillan. Copyright © 1963 by Macmillan Publishing Company.

The miracle question. The miracle question is a goal-setting question that helps patients to see what the future would look like if a particular problem were to vanish. The question should be asked deliberately and dramatically. For example:

Nurse: "We've talked about some serious topics. Now I am going to ask you an unusual question, one that might really make you think. What if while you were sleeping tonight a miracle occurred. When you wake up in the morning how will your life be different if this miracle came true?"

You can use the miracle question to identify goals that the patient may be motivated to pursue. This very basic question often gets to the source of the most important issues in a person's thinking and life. Try this question out on yourself and see if you find any surprises.

Nontherapeutic Communication

Although people may use "nontherapeutic" or ineffective communication techniques in their daily lives, using them at work can cause problems for nurses because they tend to impede or shut down nurse-patient interaction. Table 9.3 describes types of **nontherapeutic communication** and suggests more helpful responses.

Excessive Questioning

Excessive questioning—asking multiple questions (particularly closed-ended) consecutively or rapidly—casts the nurse in the role of interrogator who demands information without respect for the patient's willingness or readiness to respond. This approach conveys a lack of respect for and sensitivity to the patient's needs. Excessive questioning controls the range and nature of patient responses. It can result in decreased quality of communication or may completely shut down communication. It is better to ask open-ended questions and follow the patient's lead. For example:

Excessive questioning: "Why did you leave your husband? Did you feel angry with him? What did he do to you? Would you consider going back to him?"

More therapeutic approach: "Tell me about the situation between you and your husband."

Giving approval or disapproval. "You look great in that dress." "I'm proud of the way you controlled your temper at lunch." What could be bad about giving someone a pat on the back once in a while? Nothing, if it is done without conveying a positive or negative judgment. We often give our friends and family approval when they do something well, but giving praise and approval becomes much more complex in a nurse-patient relationship.

TABLE 9.3 Nontherapeutic Communication

Nontherapeutic Communication	Description	Example	More Helpful Response
Giving premature advice	Assumes the nurse knows best and the patient can't think for oneself. Inhibits problem solving and fosters dependency.	"Get out of this situation immediately."	**Encouraging problem solving:** "What are the pros and cons of your situation?" "What were some of the actions you thought you might take?" "What are some of the ways you have thought of to meet your goals?"
Minimizing feelings	Indicates that the nurse is unable to understand or empathize with the patient. Here the patient's feelings or experiences are being belittled, which can cause the patient to feel small or insignificant.	*Patient:* "I wish I were dead." *Nurse:* "Everyone gets down in the dumps." "I know what you mean." "You should feel happy you're getting better." "Things get worse before they get better."	**Empathizing and exploring:** "You must be feeling very upset. Are you thinking of hurting yourself?"
Falsely reassuring	Underrates a person's feelings and belittles a person's concerns. May cause the patient to stop sharing feelings if not taken seriously.	"I wouldn't worry about that." "Everything will be all right." "You will do just fine, you'll see."	**Clarifying the patient's message:** "What specifically are you worried about?" "What do you think could go wrong?" "What are you concerned might happen?"
Making value judgments	Prevents problem solving. Can make the patient feel guilty, angry, misunderstood, not supported, or anxious to leave.	"How come you still smoke when your wife has lung cancer?"	**Making observations:** "I notice you are still smoking even though your wife has lung cancer. Is this a problem?"
Asking "why" questions	Implies criticism; often has the effect of making the patient feel defensive.	"Why did you stop taking your medication?"	**Asking open-ended questions; giving a broad opening:** "Tell me some of the reasons that led up to your not taking your medications."
Asking excessive questions	Results in the patient not knowing which question to answer and possibly being confused about what is being asked.	*Nurse:* "How's your appetite? Are you losing weight? Are you eating enough?" *Patient:* "No."	**Clarifying:** "Tell me about your eating habits since you've been depressed."
Giving approval, agreeing	Implies the patient is doing the *right* thing—and that not doing it is wrong. May lead the patient to focus on pleasing the nurse or clinician; denies the patient the opportunity to change her mind.	"I'm proud of you for applying for that job." "I agree with your decision."	**Making observations:** "I noticed that you applied for that job." "What factors will lead up to your changing your mind?" **Asking open-ended questions; giving a broad opening:** "What led to that decision?"
Disapproving, disagreeing	Can make a person defensive.	"You really should have shown up for the medication group." "I disagree with that."	**Exploring:** "What was going through your mind when you decided not to come to your medication group?" "That's one point of view. How did you arrive at that conclusion?"
Changing the subject	May invalidate the patient's feelings and needs. Can leave the patient feeling alienated and isolated and increase feelings of hopelessness.	*Patient:* "I'd like to die." *Nurse:* "Did you go to Alcoholics Anonymous like we discussed?"	**Validating and exploring:** *Patient:* "I'd like to die." *Nurse:* "This sounds serious. Have you thought of harming yourself?"

Adapted from Hays, J. S., & Larson, K. (1963). *Interacting with patients.* New York, NY: Macmillan. Copyright © 1963 by Macmillan Publishing Company.

Patients may be feeling overwhelmed, experiencing low self-esteem, and feeling unsure of where their lives are going. They may be desperate for recognition, approval, and attention. Yet, when people are feeling vulnerable, a value comment might be misinterpreted. For example:

Giving approval: "You did a great job in group telling Jacob what you thought about how he treated you."

This message implies that the nurse was pleased by the manner in which the patient talked to Jacob. The patient then sees such a response as a way to please the nurse by doing the right thing. To continue to please the nurse and get approval, the patient may continue the behavior. The behavior might be useful for the patient, but when the patient is doing a behavior to please another person, it is not coming from the individual's own conviction. Also, when the other person the patient needs to please is not around, the motivation for the new behavior might not be there either. Thus, the new response really is not a change in behavior as much as it is an act to win approval and acceptance from another.

Giving approval also cuts off further communication.

More therapeutic approach: "I noticed that you spoke up to Jacob in group yesterday about his response to you. How did it feel to be more assertive?"

This opens the way for finding out if the patient was scared, was comfortable, or wants to work more on assertiveness. It also suggests that this was a self-choice the patient made. The nurse gives the patient recognition for the change in behavior and also opens the topic for further discussion.

Giving disapproval implies that the nurse has the right to judge the patient's thoughts or feelings. Again, an observation should be made instead.

Giving disapproval: "You really should not cheat on exams even if you think everyone else is doing it."

More therapeutic approach: "Let's talk about how cheating could impact your goal of graduating."

Giving advice. We ask for and give advice all the time. Yet, when a nurse gives advice to a patient, the nurse is interfering with the patient's ability to make personal decisions. When nurses offer patients solutions, patients may believe that they are not viewed as capable of making decisions. People often feel inadequate when they are given no choices over decisions in their lives. Giving advice to patients also can foster dependency ("I'll have to ask the nurse what to do about …") and undermine the patient's sense of competence and adequacy.

However, people do need information to make informed decisions. Often, you can help a patient define a problem and identify what information might be needed to come to an informed decision. A useful approach would be to ask, "What do you see as some possible actions you can take?" It is much more constructive to encourage problem solving by the patient. At times you might suggest alternatives a patient might consider (e.g., "Have you ever thought of telling your friend about the incident?"). The patient is then free to give you a yes or no answer and make a decision from among the suggestions.

Asking "why" questions. "Why" demands a justification for actions and implies wrongdoing. Think of the last time someone asked you why: "Why were you late?" "Why didn't you go to the funeral?" "Why didn't you study for the exam?" Such questions imply criticism. We may ask our friends or family such questions, and in the context of a solid relationship, the *why* may be understood more as "What happened?" With people we do not know—especially those who may be anxious or overwhelmed—a *why* question from a person in authority (e.g., nurse, physician, or teacher) can be experienced as intrusive and judgmental, which serves only to make the person defensive.

It is much more useful to ask what is happening rather than why it is happening. Questions that focus on who, what, where, and when often elicit important information that can facilitate problem solving and further the communication process. See Table 9.3 for additional types of ineffective communication and statements that would better facilitate interaction and patient comfort.

Cultural Considerations

Communicating across cultures poses many challenges for healthcare workers. We all need a frame of reference to help us function in our world. The trick is to understand that other people use many other frames of reference to help them function in their worlds. Acknowledging that others view the world quite differently and trying to understand other people's ways of experiencing and living in the world can minimize our personal distortions in listening. Building acceptance and understanding of those culturally different from ourselves is a skill, too.

The US Census Bureau (2018) reports that by 2045 the nation will become "minority white." At that time, white Americans will make up 49.7% of the population. In contrast, Hispanics will make up 24.6% of the population, blacks 13.1%, and Asians 7.9% (Fig. 9.2). Healthcare professionals need to be familiar with the cultural meaning of certain verbal and nonverbal communications. Cultural awareness in initial face-to-face encounters with a patient can lead to the formation of positive therapeutic alliances with members of a diverse society. Always assess the patient's ability to speak and understand English well and provide an interpreter when needed.

Unrecognized differences in cultural identities can result in assessment and interventions that are not optimally respectful of the patient and can be inadvertently biased or prejudiced. Healthcare workers need to have knowledge of various patients' cultures and also awareness of their own cultural identities. Nurses' attitudes and beliefs derived from their own cultural background toward those from ethnically diverse populations and subcultures (e.g., different socioeconomic groups, those with disabilities, different ethnic backgrounds, lifestyle differences, the elderly) can greatly impact their ability to be effective healers.

There is no quick and easy-to-use reference guide for culturally based behaviors, and lists of cultural dos and don'ts are ineffective. Even if it were possible to assemble a truly comprehensive list of facts for each culture, memorizing such information and keeping it straight is unrealistic. It is important to recognize that there are varying degrees of diversity among and within cultural groups. Several areas may be difficult for nurses in interpreting verbal and nonverbal messages from patients from different cultures. They are:

1. Communication style.
2. Use of eye contact.
3. Perception of touch.
4. Cultural filters.

Communication Style

Some people may consider it normal to use expressive body language when describing emotional problems, and others may perceive such behavior as being out of control or reflective of some degree of pathology. In other cultures, a calm facade may mask severe distress. For example, in some cultures, expression of positive

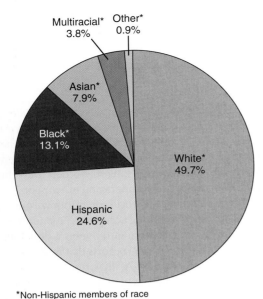

Fig. 9.2 Racial profile of the US population, 2045.

*Non-Hispanic members of race

or negative emotions is a private affair, and open expression of them is considered to be in bad taste and possibly a weakness. A quiet smile may express joy, an apology, stoicism in the face of difficulty, or even anger. German and British individuals also tend to highly value the concept of self-control and may show little facial emotion in the presence of great distress or emotional turmoil.

Eye Contact

Culture also influences the presence or absence of eye contact. Cultural norms dictate a person's comfort or lack of comfort with direct eye contact. Therefore, do not use the amount of eye contact to assess attentiveness, judge truthfulness, or make assumptions on the degree of engagement one has with a patient.

Some cultures consider direct eye contact disrespectful and improper. Individuals may have been taught to avoid eye contact with authority figures such as nurses, physicians, and other healthcare professionals. Avoidance of direct eye contact is a sign of respect to those in authority, but it could be misinterpreted as disinterest or even as a lack of respect. Some people may try to avoid eye contact. However, once it is established, they believe it is important to return and maintain eye contact. In some cultures, gender impacts eye contact. For example, a woman making direct eye contact with a man may imply a sexual interest or even promiscuity. In some cultures, direct eye contact is viewed as disrespectful or even a sign of aggression to engage in direct eye contact, especially if the speaker is younger.

On the other hand, in other cultures, direct and sustained eye contact indicates that the person listens or trusts, is somewhat aggressive, or, in some situations, is sexually interested. These cultures may interpret avoidance of eye contact by another person as being disinterested, not telling the truth, or avoiding the sharing of important information.

Touch

The therapeutic use of touch is a basic aspect of the nurse-patient relationship and is generally considered a gesture of warmth,

support, and consolation. Holding a patient's hand in response to a distressing situation or giving the patient a reassuring pat on the shoulder may be experienced as supportive and thus help facilitate openness.

However, some people perceive personal touch within the context of the nurse-patient relationship as an invasion of privacy. Touch may be experienced as patronizing, intrusive, aggressive, or sexually inviting in other cultures. Even among people from similar cultures, the use of touch has different interpretations and rules regarding gender and class.

Students are urged to find out if their facility has a "no touch" policy. This is particularly important when working with adolescents and children who have experienced inappropriate touch. They may not know how to interpret therapeutic touch from the healthcare worker.

Cultural Filters

It is important to recognize that it is impossible to listen to people in an unbiased way. In the process of socialization, we develop cultural filters through which we listen to the world around us (Egan, 2013). Cultural filters are a form of cultural bias or cultural prejudice that determines what we pay attention to and what we ignore. These cultural filters provide structure for our lives and help us interpret and interact with the world. However, these filters also unavoidably introduce various forms of bias into our communication because they are bound to influence our personal, professional, familial, and sociological values and interpretations.

We all need a frame of reference to help us function in our world; the trick is to understand that other people use many other frames of reference to help them function in their worlds. Acknowledging that everyone views the world differently and understanding that these various views impact each person's beliefs and behaviors can go a long way toward minimizing our personal distortions in listening. Building acceptance and understanding of cultural diversity is a skill that you can learn. Chapter 5 provides an in-depth discussion of cultural considerations in psychiatric nursing.

Information Communication Technologies

Telehealth is the use of electronic information and telecommunication technologies to support long-distance clinical healthcare. It is used primarily to eliminate barriers from the delivery of healthcare services. Telehealth technologies include video conferencing, the internet, phone consultation and counseling, image transmission, and interactive video sessions.

In the days of handwritten notes and records, keeping information private was fairly straightforward. However, technology creates new challenges. Issues such as confidentiality, documentation, informed consent, record maintenance, and the safety of transmitted information are all impacted by technology.

Telehealth technologies are used as a live interactive mechanism, as a way to track clinical data, and to provide access to people who otherwise might not receive good medical or psychosocial help. These people include those in rural areas and chronically ill, homebound, and underserved individuals.

Information communication technology is a valuable tool for consumers and practitioners to access current psychiatric and medical breakthroughs, diagnoses, and treatment options. As information communication technologies advance, it is possible that electronic house calls, internet support groups, and virtual health examination may well be the wave of the future, eliminating office visits altogether.

Technology is being adopted for psychiatric and mental healthcare. Telehealth can be of tremendous value for people with mental health concerns. Often, these mental health issues are not addressed due to fear of stigma, scarcity of mental health providers in remote areas, or lack of transportation. These technologies can be used for telepsychiatric appointments ranging from treating posttraumatic stress disorder and depression to providing wellness and resiliency interventions, especially in rural areas.

Mobile Applications

Mobile phones have been the most rapidly adopted consumer technology in human history. In 2019, 96% of Americans owned a cellphone of some kind and 81% of them owned smartphones (Pew Research Center, 2019). Clinicians are increasingly drawn to mobile medical applications (apps) as tools to monitor, diagnose, treat, and communicate with patients.

The Substance Abuse and Mental Health Services Administration (SAMHSA) has a line of free apps that can help address some of the toughest mental health and substance use challenges. Three of these apps are:

- **Suicide Safe** helps healthcare providers integrate suicide prevention strategies into their practice and addresses suicide risk among their patients.
- **KnowBullying** provides information and guidance on ways to prevent bullying and build resilience in children. A great tool for parents and educators, KnowBullying is for kids ages 3 to 18.
- **Talk. They Hear You** is an interactive game that can help parents and caregivers prepare for one of the more important conversations they may ever have with children—underage drinking.

Mobile apps are evolving quickly and concerns about privacy and confidentiality issues, and lack of data for efficacy and safety, as well as liability issues have been raised. Research is needed to evaluate the risks versus the benefits of these apps. Professional organizations will need to develop professional and ethical guidelines for the use of apps.

THE CLINICAL INTERVIEW

Ideally, the patient decides and leads the content and direction of the clinical interview. The nurse employs communication skills and active listening to better understand the patient's situation.

Preparing for the Interview
Pace

As previously discussed, psychiatric conditions may cause changes in the ability to process information. Major depressive disorder, for example, tends to slow thinking. Therefore, it is critical to any kind of counseling to permit the patient to set the pace of the interview, no matter how slow or halting the

progress may be. In the case of mania, which speeds up thought processes and also impairs them, counseling sessions may be shorter and more frequent.

Setting

Effective communication can take place almost anywhere. Establishing a setting that enhances feelings of security is important to the therapeutic relationship. A conference room or a quiet part of the unit that has relative privacy but is within view of others is ideal. Sometimes, patients are cared for in their home. This provides the nurse a valuable opportunity to assess the patient in the context of everyday life.

Seating

Some patients who are experiencing hyperactivity may find it difficult to sit still and are more comfortable talking while walking or even pacing. However, most of the time, nurses and patients will be sitting during counseling and education sessions. In either case, the nurse should be in the same vertical space (height) as the patient, that is, standing or sitting.

Seating arrangements can be face-to-face with a table in between, face-to-face with no table, at an angle with a table in between, or at an angle with no table. Some people believe that face-to-face with a table suggests a power differential and that the desk serves as a barrier. However, face-to-face discussion does facilitate the best reading of nonverbals.

Safety and psychological comfort in terms of exiting the room is an additional consideration. The patient should not be positioned between the nurse and the door. In cases where behavior escalation occurs, it may be necessary to exit the room. At the same time, you should position yourself in such a way that does not make the patient feel trapped in the room.

Introductions

Introductions occur during the orientation phase of the nurse-patient relationship. Refer to Chapter 8 to review the nurse's responsibilities in the orientation phase. Once you have made introductions, you can turn the interview over to the patient by using one of a number of open-ended questions or statements:

- "Where should we start?"
- "Tell me a little about what has been going on in your life."
- "What are some of the stresses you have been coping with recently?"
- You were admitted for a medication adjustment. Tell me, what has been going on with your medications?"

You can facilitate communication by appropriately offering leads (e.g., "Go on"), making statements of acceptance (e.g., "Uh-huh"), or otherwise conveying interest.

Tactics to Avoid

Certain behaviors are counterproductive and should be avoided. The following table identifies some don'ts and dos of communication during a counseling session.

Don't	Do
Argue with, minimize, or challenge the patient.	Keep focus on facts and the patient's perceptions.
Give false reassurance.	Make observations of the patient's behavior: "Change is always possible."
Interpret to the patient or speculate on the dynamics.	Listen attentively, use silence, and try to clarify the patient's problem.
Question or probe patients about sensitive areas they do not wish to discuss.	Pay attention to nonverbal communication. Strive to keep the patient's anxiety to a minimum.
Try to sell the patient on accepting treatment.	Encourage the patient to look at pros and cons.
Join in attacks patients launch on their mates, parents, friends, or associates.	Focus on facts and the patient's perceptions. Be aware of nonverbal communication.
Participate in criticism of another nurse or any other staff member.	Focus on facts and the patient's perceptions.
	Check out serious accusations with the other nurse or staff member.
	Have the patient meet with the nurse or staff member in question in the presence of a senior staff member/clinician and clarify perceptions.

Behaviors That Support Counseling

As discussed in Chapter 8, engaging in attending behaviors and actively listening are two key principles of counseling. Positive attending behaviors help to open up communication and encourage free expression, whereas negative attending behaviors are more likely to inhibit expression. All behaviors are evaluated in terms of cultural patterns and past experiences of both the interviewer and the interviewee.

Kinesic Communication

Kinesic communication is a type of nonverbal communication made by body movement. Facial expressions, body posture, and gestures are all kinesic types of communication.

In facial expressions, the eyes are particularly important. Cultural and individual variations influence a person's comfort with eye contact. For some patients and interviewers, sustained eye contact is normal and comfortable. For others, it may be more comfortable and natural to make brief eye contact and look away or down much of the time. A general rule of communication and eye contact is that it is appropriate for nurses to maintain more eye contact when the patient speaks and less constant eye contact when the nurse speaks.

The way the head tilts conveys information. For example, a slight tilt indicates interest on the part of the nurse. Eyebrows, too, convey information. Raised eyebrows indicate surprise and inwardly compressed eyebrows may indicate serious interest or anger.

Posture can provide immediate clues to what another is feeling or experiencing. A person who slumps in a chair, rolls the eyes, and sits with arms crossed in front of the chest can be perceived as resistant and unreceptive. On the other hand, a person who leans in slightly toward the speaker maintains a relaxed and attentive posture. Copying a patient's posture, where appropriate, shows agreement, trust, and acceptance.

During conversations or counseling with patients, it is wise to do a self-check on your body language. Are you crossing your arms and legs? If so, consciously uncross them. Is your index finger held to your lips? This is an unconscious move that often means that the listener wants to talk. Are you leaning away from the patient? Perhaps your seats are too close together and some adjustment is in order.

Gestures refer to communicating with the body—mainly the hands and arms. Making hand gestures that are unobtrusive and smooth while minimizing the number of other movements can be perceived as open to and respectful of the communication. Monitor the amount of gesturing you use since excessive gesturing can be distracting and even annoying.

Vocal Quality

Vocal quality, or, paralanguage, refers to qualities of speech that do not involve words. These qualities include voice volume, pitch, rate, and fluency. Vocal qualities can improve rapport, demonstrate empathy and interest, and add emphasis to words or concepts. Speaking in soft and gentle tones is likely to encourage a person to share thoughts and feelings. Conversely, speaking in a rapid, high-pitched tone may convey anxiety and create it in the patient. Consider, for example, how tonal quality can affect communication in a simple sentence like "I will see you tonight."

1. "*I* will see you tonight." (I will be the one who sees you tonight.)
2. "I *will* see you tonight." (No matter what happens, or whether you like it or not, I will see you tonight.)
3. "I will see *you* tonight." (Even though others are present, it is you I want to see.)
4. "I will see you *tonight*." (It is definite, tonight is the night we will meet.)

Proxemics

Proxemics refers to the significance of the physical distance between individuals. Central to proxemics is the concept of space, which is the area surrounding a person. Most people have a comfort zone in terms of space and feel anxious, uncomfortable, or angry when this boundary is crossed. Consider being in an elevator with one other person. Most people will stand on opposite sides of the elevator. Imagine for a moment that the other person boards the elevator and stands right next to you instead. You would likely feel discomfort or even concern for your safety because your space has been invaded.

Hall (1966) categorized distance as follows:
- **Intimate distance** in the United States is up to 18 inches and is reserved for those we trust most and with whom we feel most safe.
- **Personal distance** (18 inches to 4 feet) is for personal communications such as those with friends or colleagues.
- **Social distance** (4 to 12 feet) applies to strangers or acquaintances, often in public places or formal social gatherings.

- **Public distance** (12 feet or more) relates to public space (e.g., public speaking). In public space, one may hail another, and the parties may move about while communicating (refer to Fig. 9.3).

In general, when working with patients you will want to maintain a distance that is equal to personal or social distance. Although patients are not friends or colleagues, you are engaging in a personal conversation with them. Four feet, which is the low end of social distance, is quite far away for a nurse-patient interaction.

Some patients may require expanded distance due to anxiety or paranoia that accompanies psychotic disorders. Getting too close increases anxiety and agitation in some patients. Additionally, culture dictates what is appropriate in terms of distance. Some patients from other cultures will naturally move into a space where you may not feel comfortable. Usually, backing up into your comfort zone will be sufficient. Sometimes the issue of discomfort may need to be addressed directly: "I'm not comfortable standing so closely."

Clinical Supervision and Debriefing

Communication and interviewing techniques are acquired skills. You will learn to increase these abilities through practice and clinical supervision. In clinical supervision, the focus is on your skills within the context of the nurse-patient relationship. The student and clinical faculty have opportunities to examine and analyze the nurse's feelings and reactions to the patient and the way they affect the relationship. Clinical supervision can occur in a one-on-one conversation or as part of a group discussion in postconference.

An increasingly popular method of providing clinical supervision is through debriefing. According to the National League for Nursing (2015), debriefing is such an excellent learning method that it should be incorporated into all clinical experiences. Debriefing refers to a critical conversation and reflection regarding an experience that results in growth and learning. Debriefing supports essential learning along a continuum of "knowing what" to "knowing how" and "knowing why."

Process Recordings

A good way to increase communication and interviewing skills is to review your clinical interactions exactly as they occur. This process offers the opportunity to identify themes and patterns in both your own and your patients' communications. As students, clinical review helps you learn to deal with the variety of situations that arise in the clinical interview.

Process recordings are written records of a segment of the nurse-patient session that reflect as closely as possible the verbal and nonverbal behaviors of both patient and nurse. Process recordings have some disadvantages because they rely on memory and are subject to distortions. However, you may find them useful in identifying communication patterns.

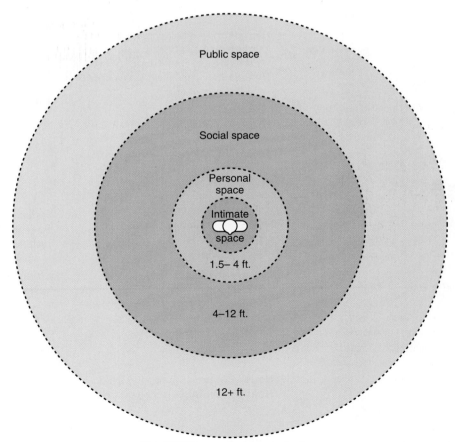

Fig. 9.3 Distance for communication.

Sometimes, an observing clinician takes notes during the interview, but this practice may be distracting for both interviewer and patient. Some patients (especially those with a paranoid disorder) may resent or misunderstand the student's intent.

Assigning process recordings is becoming less common in schools of nursing. Videotaping clinical simulations in a laboratory setting and subsequent debriefing are becoming the mainstay in nursing education. Psychiatric–mental health simulation experiences are used for students to practice therapeutic communication along with other psychiatric nursing skills such as crisis management and medication administration. A wide range of patient problems—such as alcohol and drug use problems, hallucinations, delusions, aggression, and cognitive impairment—can be simulated safely in a laboratory setting.

After the simulation, debriefing helps students realize what went right and what may have gone wrong.

Table 9.4 gives an example of a process recording.

Evaluation of Communication Skills

After you have had some introductory clinical experience, you may find the facilitative skills checklist in Fig. 9.4 useful for evaluating your progress in developing interviewing skills. Note that some of the items might not be relevant for some of your patients (e.g., numbers 11 through 13 may not be possible when a patient is experiencing psychosis [disordered thought, delusions, and/or hallucinations]). Self-evaluation of clinical skills is a way to focus on therapeutic improvement. Role-playing can help prepare you for clinical experience and to practice effective and professional communication skills.

TABLE 9.4 Example of a Process Recording

Nurse	Patient	Communication Technique	Student's Thoughts and Feelings
"Good morning, Mr. Long."		**Therapeutic.** Giving recognition. Acknowledging a patient by name can enhance self-esteem and communicates that the patient is viewed as an individual by the nurse.	I was feeling nervous. He had attempted suicide, and I didn't know if I could help him. Initially I was feeling somewhat overwhelmed.
	"Who are you, and where the devil am I?" Gazes around with a confused look on his face—quickly sits on the edge of the bed.		
"I am Ms. Rodriguez. I am a student nurse from the college, and you are at Mount Sinai Hospital. I would like to spend some time with you today."		**Therapeutic.** Giving information. Informing the patient of facts needed to make decisions or come to realistic conclusions. **Therapeutic.** Offering self. Making oneself available to the patient.	
	"What am I doing here? How did I get here?" (*Spoken in a loud, demanding voice.*)		I felt a bit intimidated when he raised his voice.
"You were brought in by your wife last night after swallowing a bottle of aspirin. You had to have your stomach pumped."		**Therapeutic.** Giving information. Giving needed facts so that the patient can orient himself and better evaluate his situation.	
	"Oh … yeah." Silence for 2 min. Shoulders slumped, Mr. Long stares at the floor and drops his head and eyes.		I was uncomfortable with the silence, but because I didn't have anything useful to say, I stayed with him in silence for the 2 min.
"You seem upset, Mr. Long. What are you thinking about?"		**Therapeutic.** Making observations. He looks sad. **Therapeutic.** Giving broad openings in an attempt to get at his feelings.	I began to feel sorry for him; he looked so sad and helpless.
	"Yeah, I just remembered … I wanted to kill myself." (*Said in a low tone almost to himself.*)		
"Oh, Mr. Long, you have so much to live for. You have such a loving family."		**Nontherapeutic.** Defending. **Nontherapeutic.** Introducing an unrelated topic.	I felt overwhelmed. I didn't know what to say—his talking about killing himself made me nervous. I could have said, "You must be very upset" (*verbalizing the implied)* or "Tell me more about this" (*exploring).*

TABLE 9.4 Example of a Process Recording—cont'd

Nurse	Patient	Communication Technique	Student's Thoughts and Feelings
	"What do you know about my life? You want to know about my family? … My wife is leaving me, that's what." (*Faces the nurse with an angry expression on his face and speaks in loud tones.*)		Again, I felt intimidated by his anger, but now I linked it with his wife's leaving him, so I didn't take it as personally as I did the first time.
"I didn't know. You must be terribly upset by her leaving."		**Therapeutic.** Reflective. Observing the angry tone and content of the patient's message and reflecting back the patient's feelings.	I really felt for him, and now I thought that encouraging him to talk more about this could be useful for him.

FACILITATIVE SKILLS CHECKLIST

Instructions: Periodically during your clinical experience, use this checklist to identify areas where growth is needed and progress has been made. Think of your clinical client experiences. Indicate the extent of your agreement with each of the following statements by marking the scale: *SA,* strongly agree; *A,* agree; *NS,* not sure; *D,* disagree; *SD,* strongly disagree.

1. I maintain good eye contact.	SA	A	NS	D	SD
2. Most of my verbal comments follow the lead of the other person.	SA	A	NS	D	SD
3. I encourage others to talk about feelings.	SA	A	NS	D	SD
4. I am able to ask open-ended questions.	SA	A	NS	D	SD
5. I can restate and clarify a person's ideas.	SA	A	NS	D	SD
6. I can summarize in a few words the basic ideas of a long statement made by a person.	SA	A	NS	D	SD
7. I can make statements that reflect the person's feelings.	SA	A	NS	D	SD
8. I can share my feelings relevant to the discussion when appropriate to do so.	SA	A	NS	D	SD
9. I am able to give feedback.	SA	A	NS	D	SD
10. At least 75% or more of my responses help enhance and facilitate communication.	SA	A	NS	D	SD
11. I can assist the person to list some alternatives available.	SA	A	NS	D	SD
12. I can assist the person to identify some goals that are specific and observable.	SA	A	NS	D	SD
13. I can assist the person to specify at least one next step that might be taken toward the goal.	SA	A	NS	D	SD

Fig. 9.4 Facilitative skills checklist. (Adapted from Myrick, D., & Erney, T. (2000). *Caring and sharing* [2nd ed., p. 168]. Minneapolis, MN. Copyright © 2000 by Educational Media Corporation.)

KEY POINTS TO REMEMBER

- Knowledge of communication and interviewing techniques is the foundation for developing any nurse-patient relationship. Goal-directed professional communication is referred to as therapeutic communication.
- Communication is a complex, interactive process. Theoretical models such as the transactional model of communication and theories such as Peplau's interpersonal theory provide frameworks for supporting therapeutic communication.
- A number of factors can minimize, enhance, or otherwise influence the communication process: culture, language, knowledge level, noise, lack of privacy, presence of others, and expectations.

- There are verbal and nonverbal elements in communication. Verbal communication consists of all the words a person speaks. Nonverbal communication consists of the behaviors displayed by an individual in addition to the actual content of speech. Nonverbal communication is particularly useful in understanding feelings and attitudes.
- Communication has two levels: the content level (verbal speech) and the process level (nonverbal behavior). When content is congruent with process, the communication is considered to be healthy. When the verbal message is incongruent with the communicator's actions, the message is ambiguous.

- There are a number of therapeutic communication techniques nurses can use to enhance their nursing practices.
- There are also nontherapeutic types of communication that nurses can learn to avoid to enhance their effectiveness with people.
- Cultural background (as well as individual differences) has a great deal to do with communication styles. The degree of eye contact and the use of touch are two nonverbal behaviors that may differ depending on culture.

- Telehealth is particularly helpful in the field of psychiatry and may eliminate barriers such as stigma, scarcity of mental healthcare providers in remote areas, and transportation problems thereby improving the delivery of mental healthcare.
- The clinical interview is a key component of psychiatric–mental health nursing. The nurse establishes a safe setting and plan for appropriate seating, introductions, and initiation of the interview.
- Attending behaviors (e.g., eye contact, body language, and vocal qualities) are key elements in effective communication.

CRITICAL THINKING

1. Keep a written log of a conversation you have with a patient. In your log, identify the therapeutic techniques and types of nontherapeutic communication you noticed yourself using. Rewrite the nontherapeutic communications and replace them with statements that would better facilitate discussion of thoughts and feelings. Share your log and discuss the changes you are working on with one classmate.
2. Role-play with a classmate at least five nonverbal communications and have your partner identify the message received.
3. With the other students in your class watching, plan and role-play a nurse-patient conversation that lasts about three minutes. Use both therapeutic and nontherapeutic commuication. When you are finished, have your other classmates try to identify the types of communication that you used.
4. Demonstrate how the nurse would use touch and eye contact when working with patients from three different cultural groups.

CHAPTER REVIEW

1. Which statement made by the nurse demonstrates the best understanding of nonverbal communication?
   a. "The patient's verbal and nonverbal communication is often different."
   b. "When my patient responds to my question, I check for congruence between verbal and nonverbal communication to help validate the response."
   c. "If a patient is slumped in the chair, I can be sure he's angry or depressed."
   d. "It's easier to interpret verbal communication than to interpret nonverbal communication."
2. Which nursing statement is an example of reflection?
   a. "I think this feeling will pass."
   b. "So you are saying that life has no meaning."
   c. "I'm not sure I understand what you mean."
   d. "You look sad."
3. When should a nurse be most alert to the possibility of communication errors resulting in harm to the patient?
   a. Change of shift report
   b. Admission interviews
   c. One-on-one conversations with patients
   d. Conversations with patients' families
4. During an admission assessment and interview, which channels of information communication should the nurse be monitoring? *Select all that apply.*
   a. Auditory
   b. Visual
   c. Written
   d. Tactile
   e. Olfactory

5. What principle about nurse-patient communication should guide a nurse's fear about "saying the wrong thing" to a patient?
   a. Patients tend to appreciate a well-meaning person who conveys genuine acceptance, respect, and concern for their situation.
   b. The patient is more interested in talking to you than listening to what you have to say and so is not likely to be offended.
   c. Considering the patient's history, there is little chance that the comment will do any actual harm.
   d. Most people with a mental illness have by necessity developed a high tolerance of forgiveness.
6. You have been working closely with a patient for the past month. Today, he tells you he is looking forward to meeting with his new psychiatrist but frowns and avoids eye contact while reporting this to you. Which of the following responses would most likely be therapeutic?
   a. "A new psychiatrist is a chance to start fresh; I'm sure it will go well for you."
   b. "You say you look forward to the meeting, but you appear anxious or unhappy."
   c. "I notice that you frowned and avoided eye contact just now. Don't you feel well?"
   d. "I get the impression you don't really want to see your psychiatrist—can you tell me why?"
7. Which student behavior is consistent with therapeutic communication?
   a. Offering your opinion when asked to convey support.
   b. Summarizing the essence of the patient's comments in your own words.

c. Interrupting periods of silence before they become awkward for the patient.

d. Telling the patient he did well when you approve of his statements or actions.

8. James is a 42-year-old patient with schizophrenia. He approaches you as you arrive for your day shift and anxiously reports, "Last night, demons came to my room and tried to rape me." Which response would be most therapeutic?

a. "There are no such things as demons. What you saw were hallucinations."

b. "It is not possible for anyone to enter your room at night. You are safe here."

c. "You seem upset. Please tell me more about what you experienced last night."

d. "That must have been frightening, but we'll check on you at night and you'll be safe."

9. Therapeutic communication is the foundation of a patient-centered interview. Which of the following techniques is not considered therapeutic?

a. Restating

b. Encouraging description of perception

c. Summarizing

d. Asking "why" questions

10. Carolina is surprised when her patient does not show up for a regularly scheduled appointment. When contacted, the patient states, "I don't need to come see you anymore. I have found a therapy app on my phone that I love." How should Carolina respond to this news?

a. "That sounds exciting, would you be willing to visit and show me the app?"

b. "At this time, there is no real evidence that the app can replace our therapy."

c. "I am not sure that is a good idea right now; we are so close to progress."

d. "Why would you think that is a better option than meeting with me?"

1. **b**; 2. **d**; 3. **a**; 4. **a, b, d, e**; 5. **a**; 6. **b**; 7. **b**; 8. **c**; 9. **d**; 10. **a**

Visit the Evolve website for a posttest on the content in this chapter: http://evolve.elsevier.com/Varcarolis

REFERENCES

Bateson, G., Jackson, D., & Haley, J. (1956). Toward a theory of schizophrenia. *Behavioral Sciences, 1*(4), 251–264.

Barnlund, D. (1970). A transactional model of communication. In K. Sereno, & C. Mortensen (Eds.), *Foundations of communication theory*. New York, NY: Harper Row.

CRICO Strategies. (2016). *Malpractice risks in communication failures: 2015 benchmarking report*. Retrieved from https://www.rmf.harvard.edu/Malpractice-Data/Annual-Benchmark-Reports/Risks-in-Communication-Failures.

Egan, G. (2013). *The skilled helper: A problem-management approach and opportunity-development approach to helping* (10th ed.). Belmont, CA: Brooks/Cole, Cengage Learning.

Eisenbarth, H., & Alpers, G. W. (2011). Happy mouth and sad eyes: Scanning emotional facial expressions. *Emotion, 11*(4), 860–865.

Hall, E. T. (1966). *The hidden dimension*. New York, NY: Anchor Books.

Makary, M. A., & Daniel, M. (2016). Medical error—The third leading cause of death. *British Medical Journal.* https://doi.org/10.1136/bmj.i2139.

National League for Nursing. (2015). *Debriefing across the curriculum*. Retrieved from http://www.nln.org/docs/default-source/about/nln-vision-series-(position-statements)/nln-vision-debriefing-across-the-curriculum.pdf?sfvrsn=0.

Neese, B. (2015). *Effective communication in nursing: Theory and best practices*. Retrieved from http://online.seu.edu/effective-communication-in-nursing/#sthash.hNHpFiV3.dpuf.

Peplau, H. E. (1952). *Interpersonal relations in nursing: A conceptual frame of reference for psychodynamic nursing*. New York, NY: Putnam.

Pew Research Center. (2019). *Mobile fact sheet*. Retrieved from https://www.pewresearch.org/internet/fact-sheet/mobile/.

Quality and Safety Education for Nurses. (2012). *Patient centered care.* Retrieved from http://www.qsen.org/definition.php?id=1.

Substance Abuse and Mental Health Services Administration. (n.d.). *Get connected with SAMHSA's free mobile apps*. Retrieved from http://www.store.samhsa.gov/apps/.

United States Census Bureau. (2018). *National population projections tables, 2017*. Retrieved from https://www.census.gov/data/tables/2017/demo/popproj/2017-summary-tables.html.

Stress Responses and Stress Management

Margaret Jordan Halter and Elizabeth M. Varcarolis

 Visit the Evolve website for a pretest on the content in this chapter: http://evolve.elsevier.com/Varcarolis

OBJECTIVES

1. Recognize the short- and long-term physiological consequences of stress.
2. Compare and contrast Cannon's (fight-or-flight) and Selye's (general adaptation syndrome) models of stress.
3. Describe how responses to stress are mediated through perception, individual temperament, social support, support groups, culture, spirituality, and religion.
4. Assess stress level using the Recent Life Changes Questionnaire.
5. Describe relaxation techniques that help to manage stress responses.
6. Teach a classmate or patient a relaxation technique to help lower stress and anxiety.
7. Explain how cognitive techniques can help increase a person's tolerance for stressful events.

KEY TERMS AND CONCEPTS

adverse childhood experiences (ACEs)
biofeedback
cognitive reframing
coping styles
deep-breathing exercises
distress
eustress

fight-or-flight response
general adaptation syndrome (GAS)
guided imagery
humor
journaling
meditation
mindfulness

physiological stressors
progressive relaxation
psychological stressors
relaxation response
stressors

Before turning our attention to the clinical disorders in the chapters that follow, we will explore the important subject of stress. According to the National Institute of Mental Health (2016), stress is simply the brain's response to any demand. Stress is natural, and humans have evolved with a capacity to respond to internal and external demands.

Stress and responses to it are central to understanding psychiatric disorders and providing mental healthcare. The interplay between stress, the development of psychiatric disorders, and the exacerbation (worsening) of psychiatric symptoms has been widely researched.

ADVERSE CHILDHOOD EXPERIENCES

The old adage "what doesn't kill you will make you stronger" does not hold true with the development of psychiatric disorders. In fact, early exposure to stressful events actually sensitizes people to stress in later life. These early exposures are referred to as **adverse childhood experiences (ACEs)** and include the following:

- Any form of psychological, physical, and sexual abuse
- Violence against a parent, particularly the mother

- Living with people who have substance use disorders, have mental illness, or were ever incarcerated

ACEs occur more frequently than many of us would imagine. In a large-scale study ($N = 9508$) by Felitti and colleagues (2019), more than half of respondents reported at least one ACE, and one-fourth reported two or more ACEs. They found a positive relationship (i.e., as one goes up, so does the other) between the number of ACEs and adult risk behaviors and diseases. A summary of these risks and diseases reporting four or more ACEs is presented in Table 10.1.

While an understanding of the connection between stress and mental illness is essential in the psychiatric setting, it is also important when caring for any patient, in any setting, with any condition. Imagine having an appendectomy and being served with an eviction notice on the same day. How well could you cope with either situation, let alone both simultaneously? The nurse's role is to intervene to reduce stress by promoting a healing environment, facilitating successful coping, and developing future coping strategies. In this chapter, we will explore how we are equipped to respond to stress, what can go wrong with the stress response, and how to care for our patients and even ourselves during times of stress.

RESPONSES TO AND EFFECTS OF STRESS

Early Stress Response Theories

Fight-or-Flight Response

The earliest research into the stress response began as a result of observations that stressors increased the incidence of physical disorders and made existing conditions worse. Stressors are any psychological or physical stimuli or events that provoke a stress response in an organism. Stressors can be acute or chronic and may be external or internal.

Walter Cannon (1871–1945) methodically investigated the sympathetic nervous system, which is a part of the autonomic nervous system. Specifically, he studied animals' responses to stressors. His work revealed a phenomenon that he referred to as an *acute stress response*, now commonly described with the words *fight* (aggression) *and flight* (withdrawal). The well-known fight-or-flight response is the body's way of preparing for a situation an individual perceives as a threat. This response results in increased blood pressure, heart rate, respirations, and cardiac output.

While groundbreaking, Cannon's theory has been criticized for being simplistic, as not all animals or people respond by fighting or fleeing. In the face of danger, some animals become frozen—think of a deer in the headlights—to avoid being noticed or to observe the environment in a state of heightened awareness. Freezing may also happen when you are not sure whether you should fight or flee.

General Adaptation Syndrome

Hans Selye (1907–1982) was another pioneer in stress research who introduced the concept of stress into both the scientific and popular literature. Selye (1936) defined stress as "a nonspecific response of the body to any demand for change." He incorporated Cannon's fight-or-flight response into an expanded theory of stress known as the general adaptation syndrome (GAS). While Cannon focused on the sympathetic nervous system, Selye included the hypothalamus-pituitary-adrenal axis in his research.

According to Selye (1974), the GAS occurs in three stages (Fig. 10.1):

1. The *alarm* stage is the initial, brief, and adaptive response (fight or flight) to the stressor. It begins with the eyes or ears sending information, such as the sight of car headlights or the sound of a fire alarm, to the brain's amygdala. If the amygdala, which processes emotional data, interprets the event as dangerous, it sounds the alarm to the hypothalamus, which responds in two ways:

   - *Sympathetic.* The hypothalamus signals through the autonomic nerves to the adrenal glands. The adrenals then pump the catecholamine epinephrine (also known as *adrenaline*) into the bloodstream, thereby activating the sympathetic nervous system. This results in a faster heart rate and increased blood pressure that pushes blood to muscles and the heart. Breathing becomes more rapid, and the lungs expand more fully. Extra oxygen is sent to the brain to aid in cognitive processing. All senses, including sight (pupils dilate for a broad view of the environment) and hearing, become sharper. Glucose is dumped in the bloodstream to supply additional energy. Blood is shunted away from the digestive tract (resulting in a dry mouth) and kidneys to more essential organs.

     All of this happens so quickly that most people are not aware of the full scope of the threat. This is why you can jump out of the way of an oncoming car before you realize what is happening.

   - *Hypothalamic-pituitary-adrenal (HPA) axis.* As the initial surge of epinephrine subsides, the HPA axis, which is composed of the hypothalamus, the pituitary, and the adrenal gland, is activated. You can conceptualize this axis as the gas pedal of the system that keeps it on high alert.

     The hypothalamus secretes a corticotropin-releasing hormone that stimulates the pituitary to release the adrenocorticotropic hormone (ACTH). ACTH travels through the bloodstream to the adrenal cortex. The adrenal cortex then produces extra cortisol to increase blood glucose and muscle endurance. At the same time, other nonessential functions (e.g., digestion) are decreased. Unfortunately, cortisol also impacts the immune system and memory.

     The alarm stage is extremely intense, and no organism can sustain this level of reactivity and excitement for long. If the threat subsides, the other part of the autonomic nervous system, the parasympathetic nervous system, slowly puts on the brakes. It allows the body to rest and digest (versus fight or flight) and dampens the stress response. However, if the threat continues, the resistance stage follows.

2. The *resistance* stage could also be called the *adaptation stage* because it is during this time that sustained and optimal resistance to the stressor occurs. Usually, stressors are successfully overcome. Recovery, repair, and renewal may occur.

TABLE 10.1 Four or More Adverse Childhood Experiences (ACEs) and Adult Health Impact	
Increase Compared to Individuals With No ACEs	**Adult Risk Behaviors and Diseases**
4- to 12-fold	Alcohol use Substance use Major depressive disorder Suicide attempts
2- to 4-fold	Smoking Poor self-reported health 50+ sexual intercourse partners Sexually transmitted disease
1.4- to 1.6-fold	Physical inactivity Obesity
↑ ACEs and ↑ diseases	Ischemic heart disease Cancer Chronic lung disease Skeletal fractures Liver disease

↑, Graded increase.

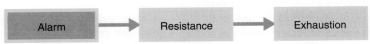

Fig. 10.1 Stages of the general adaptation syndrome.

At this point, individuals have used up valuable resources and have reduced defenses and adaptive energy. If stressors continue, the body remains in a state of arousal and may transition to the final stage of the syndrome.

3. The *exhaustion* stage occurs when attempts to resist the stressor prove futile. At this point, resources are depleted and the stress may become chronic. The impact of long-term overexposure to cortisol results in vulnerability to stress-related illnesses. These illnesses include anxiety disorders, major depressive disorder, sleep disorders, digestive problems, heart disease, and weight gain.

Bad Stress Versus Good Stress? Selye also noted that individuals become energized by both negative and positive events. These reactions are *distress* and *eustress*:

- **Distress** is a negative, draining energy that results in anxiety, depression, confusion, helplessness, hopelessness, and fatigue. Stressors such as a death in the family, financial overload, or school/work demands may cause distress.
- **Eustress** ("*eu*" is Greek for well or good) refers to the normal physiological workings of an organism. It is a positive energy that motivates individuals and results in feelings of happiness, hopefulness, and purposeful movement. Examples of eustress are a much-needed vacation, playing a favorite sport, the birth of a baby, or the challenge of a new job.

Critique of the General Adaptation Syndrome. Selye's GAS remains a popular theory, but it has been expanded and reinterpreted since the 1950s. Some researchers question the notion of "nonspecific responses" and believe that different types of stressors bring about different patterns of responses and that it is the *degree* of stress that is important (Koolhaas et al., 2011).

Furthermore, the GAS is most accurate in the description of how males respond when threatened. Females do not always respond to stress by fighting or fleeing but often by "tending and befriending," a survival strategy that emphasizes the protection of the young and a reliance on the social network for support. Also, women are more vulnerable to stress-related disorders. This may be due to females being more sensitive to even low levels of corticotropin-releasing hormone, a peptide hormone released from the hypothalamus in response to stress (Bangasser et al., 2010).

Increased understanding of the exhaustion stage of the GAS has revealed that illness results not only from the depletion of reserves but also from the stress mediators themselves. For example, people experiencing chronic distress may have wounds that heal more slowly. Table 10.2 describes some reactions to acute and prolonged (chronic) stress.

Immune System Stress Responses

Cannon and Selye focused on the physical and mental responses of the nervous and endocrine systems to acute and chronic stress. Later work revealed that there was also an interaction between the nervous system and the immune system that occurs during the alarm phase of the GAS.

In one study, rats were given saccharine, an artificial sweetener, along with a drug that reduces the immune system (Ader & Cohen, 1975). Afterward, when given *only* the saccharine, the rats continued to have decreased immune responses, contracted bacterial and viral infections, and often died. The taste of the sweetener by itself was sufficient to bring about neural signals in the rats' brains that

TABLE 10.2 Some Reactions to Acute and Prolonged (Chronic) Stress

Acute Stress Can Cause	Prolonged (Chronic) Stress Can Cause
Uneasiness and concern	Anxiety and panic attacks
Sadness	Major depressive disorder
Loss of appetite	Anorexia or overeating
Suppression of the immune system	Lowered resistance to infections, leading to an increase in opportunistic viral and bacterial infections
Increased metabolism and use of body fats	Insulin-resistant diabetes
Hypertension	
Infertility	Amenorrhea or loss of sex drive
Impotence, anovulation	
Increased energy mobilization and use	Increased fatigue and irritability
Decreased memory and learning	
Increased cardiovascular tone	Increased risk for cardiac events (e.g., heart attack, angina, and sudden heart-related death)
Increased risk of blood clots and stroke	
Increased cardiopulmonary tone	Increased respiratory problems

suppressed their immune systems. This research contradicted the notion that the immune system functioned autonomously and pointed to a brain–immune system connection.

Researchers continue to find evidence that stress, through the hypothalamic-pituitary-adrenal and sympathetic-adrenal medullary axes, can induce changes in the immune system. This model helps explain what many researchers and clinicians have believed and witnessed for centuries: There are links among stress (biopsychosocial), the immune system, and disease—a clear mind-body connection that may alter health outcomes. Stress may result in malfunctions in the immune system that are implicated in autoimmune disorders, immunodeficiency, and hypersensitivities.

Stress influences the immune system in several complex ways. It can enhance the immune system and prepare the body to initially respond to injury by fighting infections and healing wounds. Immune cells normally release cytokines, which are proteins and glycoproteins used for communication between cells when a pathogen is detected. Cytokines activate and recruit other immune cells. During times of stress, these cytokines are released and the immune system is activated. The activation is limited because the cytokines stimulate further release of corticosteroids, which inhibits the immune system.

The immune response and the resulting cytokine activity in the brain raise questions regarding their connection with psychological and cognitive states. Researchers have found significantly higher concentrations of cytokines that cause systemic inflammation in subjects with major depressive disorder compared with control subjects (Dahl et al., 2014). Recovery from depression is associated with a reduction to normal levels of most of the cytokines.

Cancer patients are often treated with cytokine molecules known as *interleukins*. Unfortunately, but understandably, these chemotherapy drugs tend to cause or increase depression (National Cancer Institute, 2019).

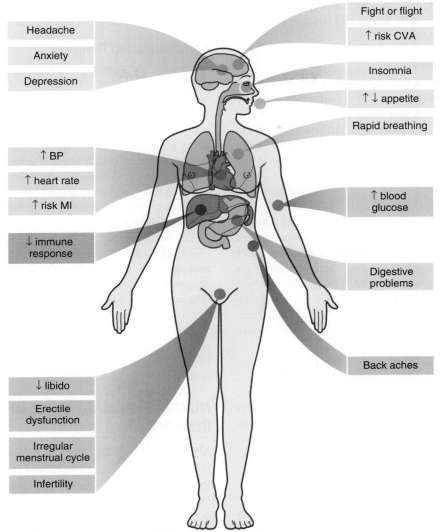

Headache
Anxiety
Depression
↑ BP
↑ heart rate
↑ risk MI
↓ immune response
↓ libido
Erectile dysfunction
Irregular menstrual cycle
Infertility

Fight or flight
↑ risk CVA
Insomnia
↑ ↓ appetite
Rapid breathing
↑ blood glucose
Digestive problems
Back aches

Fig. 10.2 Effects of stress on the body. *BP*, Blood pressure; *CVA*, Cerebrovascular accident; *MI*, Myocardial infarction.

Research in this field is promising. Investigators are examining how psychosocial factors, such as optimism and social support, moderate the stress response. They are mapping the biological and cellular mechanisms by which stress affects the immune system and are testing new theories.

Fig. 10.2 illustrates the effects of stress on the body.

MEDIATORS OF THE STRESS RESPONSE

Many situations, such as emotional arousal, fatigue, fear, humiliation, loss of blood, extreme happiness, or unexpected success, are capable of producing stress and triggering the stress response (Selye, 1993). Stressors can be divided into two broad categories: physiological and psychological.

Physiological stressors include environmental conditions such as trauma and excessive cold or heat, and physical conditions such as infection, hemorrhage, hunger, and pain. **Psychological stressors** include such events as divorce, loss of a job, unmanageable debt, the death of a loved one, retirement,

and fear of a terrorist attack. Psychological stressors also include changes we consider positive, such as marriage, the arrival of a new baby, or unexpected success. Both physiological and psychological stressors may be either buffered or bolstered by mediators specific to the individual.

Perception

Have you ever noticed that something that upsets your friend does not bother you at all? Or that your professor's habit of continuing to teach beyond the scheduled class time drives you up a wall, yet (to your annoyance) your best friend does not seem to notice? It is not always the stressor itself that determines a response but the *perception* of the stressor that determines the person's emotional and psychological reactions to it.

The way that we perceive stressors is affected by factors such as age, gender, culture, life experience, and lifestyle. All of these factors may work to either lessen or increase the degree of emotional or physical influence and the sequelae (consequence or result) of stress. For example, a man in his 40s who has a new baby, a new home, and gets laid off may feel more stress than a man in his 60s who is financially secure and is asked to take an early retirement.

Individual Temperament

As mentioned earlier, part of the response to stressors is based on our own individual perceptions. These perceptions are colored by a variety of factors, including genetic structure and vulnerability, childhood experiences, coping strategies, and personal outlook on life and the world. All these factors combine to form a unique personality with specific strengths and vulnerabilities.

Social Support

The benefit of social support cannot be emphasized enough, whether it is for you or for your patients. Humans once lived in close communities with extended families sharing the same living quarters. Essentially, neighbors were the therapists of the past. Suburban life often results in isolated living spaces where neighbors interact sporadically. In fact, you may not even know your neighbors. People in crowded cities may also live in isolation, where even eye contact and communication may be considered an invasion of privacy.

Strong social support from significant others can enhance mental and physical health and act as a substantial buffer against distress. A shared identity—whether with a family, social network, religious group, or colleagues—helps people overcome stressors more adaptively. Researchers have found a strong correlation between intact support systems and lower mortality rates (Cruces et al., 2014). People, and even animals, without social companionship have higher rates of illness and even risk early death.

Support Groups

The proliferation of self-help groups attests to the need for social supports. Many of the support groups currently available are for people going through similar stressful life events: Alcoholics Anonymous (the prototype for 12-step programs), Gamblers Anonymous, Reach for Recovery (for cancer patients), and Parents Without Partners. Online support groups provide cost-effective, anonymous, and easily accessible self-help for people with every disorder imaginable. A Google search for online + support + groups yielded more than one billion hits. There is a group out there for nearly everyone, although quality and fit are always variables to be considered. Videoconferencing software such as Zoom expanded tremendously during the coronavirus pandemic as isolated individuals came together to address stressors in their lives. It is likely that this crisis will reshape the way that support groups are offered well into the future.

Culture

Each culture not only emphasizes certain problems of living more than others but also interprets emotional problems differently. Although Western European and North American cultures tend to subscribe to a psychophysiological view of stress and somatic distress, this is not the dominant view in other cultures. An overwhelming majority of Asians, Africans, and Central Americans tend to express distress in somatic terms and actually experience it physically (Lanzara et al., 2018).

Spirituality and Religion

Spirituality and religious affiliation help people cope with stress. Studies have demonstrated that spiritual practices can even enhance the immune system and sense of well-being (Jacobson, 1938). Spiritual well-being helps people deal with health issues, primarily because spiritual beliefs help people cope with issues of living. People who include spiritual solutions to physical or mental distress often gain a sense of comfort and support that can aid in healing and lowering stress. Even prayer, in and of itself, can elicit the relaxation response (discussed later in this chapter). Prayer is known to reduce stress physically and emotionally and to reduce the impact of stress on the immune system.

For many people, religious beliefs promote hope and optimism. Organized religious groups provide structure and may promote a feeling of belonging. Beyond coming together as a congregation to listen to a sermon or take part in religious rites, religious groups are an important social outlet. As discussed earlier, social support is an essential mediator to the stress response.

Fig. 10.3 operationally defines the process of stress and the positive or negative results of attempts to relieve stress, and Box 10.1 identifies several stress busters that can be incorporated into our lives with little effort.

NURSING MANAGEMENT OF STRESS RESPONSES

Measuring Stress

In 1967, psychiatrists Holmes and Rahe developed the Social Readjustment Scale. This life-change scale measures positive or negative life events. Each life-change event is assigned a weight depending on its severity. For example, the death of a parent was rated significantly higher than attending college. The purpose of the scale is to assess a person's vulnerability to stress-related disorders.

Since the scale was developed in 1967, perceptions of stress have changed. To more accurately measure life-change events, 1306 online participants were collected and then compared with data collected in the original study (First30Days, 2008). Although some life-change events were viewed as more stressful in 1967, most events were viewed as more stressful in 2007 (Table 10.3).

Take a few minutes to assess your stress level for the past 6 or 12 months using the Recent Life Changes Questionnaire, a revised version of the Social Readjustment Scale (Table 10.4). A 6-month score of 300 or more, or a year score of 500 or more, indicates high stress. When you self-administer the questionnaire, consider the following:

- Not all events are perceived to have the same degree of intensity or disruptiveness.
- Culture may dictate whether or not an event is stressful or how stressful it is.
- Different people may have different thresholds beyond which disruptions occur.
- The questionnaire equates change with stress.

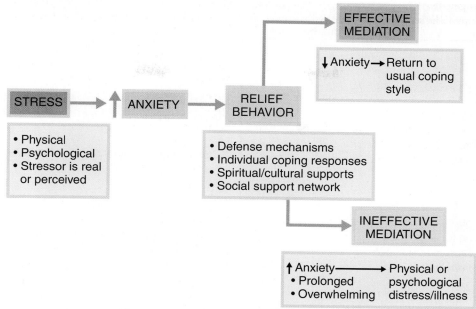

Fig. 10.3 Stress and anxiety operationally defined.

<table>
<tr><td colspan="2">

BOX 10.1   Effective Stress Busters

Sleep
- 7–9 h of sleep is recommended.
- Try going to sleep 30–60 min early each night for a few weeks.
- Sleeping later in the morning is not helpful and can disrupt body rhythms.
- Invest in a tracker that can monitor sleep and make adjustments based on the data it provides.

Exercise (Aerobic)
- 150 min a week (about 20 min a day) of moderate-intensity aerobic activity such as walking is recommended.
- Reduces chronic and acute stress
- Decreases levels of anxiety, depression, and sensitivity to stress
- Decreases muscle tension and increases endorphin levels
- Exercise at least 3 h before bedtime to prevent sleep disruption

Reduction or Cessation of Caffeine Intake
- No more than four cups of coffee or colas are recommended for anyone.
- Overuse or sensitivity may cause insomnia, nervousness, restlessness, irritability, stomach upset, rapid heartbeat, muscle tremors, and shakiness.
- Slowly wean off coffee, tea, colas, and chocolate drinks.

Music
- Listening to familiar music promotes relaxation.
- Rates of healing may be improved with music.
- Music can decrease agitation and confusion in older adults.
- Quality of life in hospice settings is enhanced by music.

Pets
- Can bring joy and reduce stress
- May provide real social support
- Alleviate medical problems aggravated by stress

Massage
- Slows the heart rate and relaxes the body
- Improves alertness by reducing anxiety

</td></tr>
</table>

TABLE 10.3   Perception of Life Stressors in 1967 and 2007

Life Change Event	1967	2007
Death of spouse	100	80
Death of family member	63	70
Divorce/separation	73/65	66
Job layoff or firing	47	62
Birth of child/pregnancy	40	60
Death of friend	50	50
Marriage	50	50
Retirement	45	49
Marital reconciliation	45	48
Change job field	36	47
Child leaves home	29	43

Data from First30Days. (2008). *Making changes today considered more difficult to handle than 40 years ago.* Retrieved from http://www.first30days.com/pages/press_changereport.html.

Other stress scales that may be useful to nursing students have been developed. You might want to try the Perceived Stress Scale, a popular scale that measures perceived stress (Fig. 10.4). Although there are no absolute scores, this scale measures how relatively uncontrollable, unpredictable, and overloaded you find your life. You might try this scale alone or suggest that it be used in a clinical postconference for comparison and discussion.

Assessing Coping Styles

People cope with life stressors in a variety of ways, and a number of factors can act as effective mediators to decrease stress in our lives. Four personal attributes, or coping styles, that people can develop to help manage stress include:

1. Health-sustaining habits (e.g., medical adherence, proper diet, relaxation, pacing one's energy)

TABLE 10.4 Recent Life Changes Questionnaire

Life-Changing Event	Life Change Unit[a]	Life-Changing Event	Life Change Unit[a]
Health		**Child Leaving Home**	
An injury or illness that:		To attend college	41
Kept you in bed a week or more or sent you to the hospital	74	Due to marriage	41
Was less serious than above	44	For other reasons	45
Major dental work	26	Change in arguments with spouse	50
Major change in eating habits	27	In-law problems	38
Major change in sleeping habits	26	**Change in the Marital Status of Your Parents**	
Major change in your usual type and/or amount of recreation	28	Divorce	59
		Remarriage	50
Work		**Separation from Spouse**	
Change to a new type of work	51	Due to work	53
Change in your work hours or conditions	35	Due to marital problems	76
		Divorce	96
Change in Your Responsibilities at Work		Birth of grandchild	43
More responsibilities	29	Death of spouse	119
Fewer responsibilities	21	**Death of Another Family Member**	
Promotion	31	Child	123
Demotion	42	Brother or sister	102
Transfer	32	Parent	100
		Personal and Social	
Troubles at Work		Change in personal habits	26
With your boss	29	Beginning or ending of school or college	38
With coworkers	35	Change of school or college	35
With persons under your supervision	35	Change in political beliefs	24
Other work troubles	28	Change in religious beliefs	29
Major business adjustment	60	Change in social activities	27
Retirement	52	Vacation	24
		New close personal relationship	37
Loss of Job		Engagement to marry	45
Laid off from work	68	Girlfriend or boyfriend problems	39
Fired from work	79	Sexual differences	44
Correspondence course to help you in your work	18	"Falling out" of a close personal relationship	47
		An accident	48
Home and Family		Minor violation of the law	20
Major change in living conditions	42	Being held in jail	75
		Death of a close friend	70
Change in Residence		Major decision regarding your immediate future	51
Move within the same town or city	25	Major personal achievement	36
Move to a different town, city, or state	47	**Financial**	
Change in family get-togethers	25	**Major Change in Finances**	
Major change in health or behavior of family member	55	Increase in income	38
Marriage	50	Decrease in income	60
Pregnancy	67	Investment and/or credit difficulties	56
Miscarriage or abortion	65	Loss or damage of personal property	43
		Moderate purchase	20
Gain of a New Family Member		Major purchase	37
Birth of a child	66	Foreclosure on a mortgage or loan	58
Adoption of a child	65		
A relative moving in with you	59		
Spouse beginning or ending work	46		

[a]One-year totals ≥500 life change units are considered indications of high recent life stress.
From Miller, M.A., & Rahe, R.H. (1997). Life changes scaling for the 1990s. *Journal of Psychosomatic Research, 43*(3), 279–292.

Perceived Stress Scale–10 Item (PSS-10)

Instructions: The questions in this scale ask you about your feelings and thoughts during the last month. In each case, please indicate with a check how often you felt or thought a certain way.

1. In the last month, how often have you been upset because of something that happened unexpectedly?
   ___0 never   ___1 almost never   ___2 sometimes   ___3 fairly often   ___4 very often

2. In the last month, how often have you felt that you were unable to control the important things in your life?
   ___0 never   ___1 almost never   ___2 sometimes   ___3 fairly often   ___4 very often

3. In the last month, how often have you felt nervous and "stressed"?
   ___0 never   ___1 almost never   ___2 sometimes   ___3 fairly often   ___4 very often

4. In the last month, how often have you felt confident about your ability to handle your personal problems?
   ___0 never   ___1 almost never   ___2 sometimes   ___3 fairly often   ___4 very often

5. In the last month, how often have you felt that things were going your way?
   ___0 never   ___1 almost never   ___2 sometimes   ___3 fairly often   ___4 very often

6. In the last month, how often have you found that you could not cope with all the things that you had to do?
   ___0 never   ___1 almost never   ___2 sometimes   ___3 fairly often   ___4 very often

7. In the last month, how often have you been able to control irritations in your life?
   ___0 never   ___1 almost never   ___2 sometimes   ___3 fairly often   ___4 very often

8. In the last month, how often have you felt that you were on top of things?
   ___0 never   ___1 almost never   ___2 sometimes   ___3 fairly often   ___4 very often

9. In the last month, how often have you been angered because of things that were outside of your control?
   ___0 never   ___1 almost never   ___2 sometimes   ___3 fairly often   ___4 very often

10. In the last month, how often have you felt difficulties were piling up so high that you could not overcome them?
   ___0 never   ___1 almost never   ___2 sometimes   ___3 fairly often   ___4 very often

Perceived stress scale scoring

Items 4, 5, 7, and 8 are the positively stated items. PSS-10 scores are obtained by reversing the scores on the positive items, e.g., 0=4, 1=3, 2=2, etc. and then adding all 10 items.

Fig. 10.4 Perceived Stress Scale–10 Item (PSS-10). (Modified from Cohen, S., & Williamson, G. 1988. Perceived stress in a probability sample of the US. In S. Spacepan & S. Oskamp (Eds.), *The social psychology of health: Claremont Symposium on applied social psychology.* Newbury Park, CA: Sage.)

2. Life satisfaction (e.g., work, family, hobbies, humor, spiritual solace, arts, nature)
3. Social support
4. Effective and healthy responses to stress

Examining these four coping categories can help nurses identify areas to target for improving their patients' responses to stress.

Managing Stress Through Relaxation Techniques

Poor management of stress has been correlated with an increased incidence of a number of physical and emotional conditions, such as cardiac disease, poor diabetes control, chronic pain, and significant emotional distress. There is considerable evidence that many mind-body therapies can be used as effective adjuncts to conventional medical treatment for a number of common clinical conditions.

Psychiatric problems that are known to benefit from relaxation techniques include anxiety, depression, insomnia, and nightmares (National Center for Complementary and Alternative Medicine, 2016). Stress- and anxiety-reduction techniques may also have benefits for some other conditions, including asthma, childbirth, epilepsy, fibromyalgia, headache, irritable bowel syndrome, cardiac disease and cardiac symptoms, menopause symptoms, menstruation, nausea, and pain. Although the results are not clear, there is some evidence to indicate that stress-reduction techniques may aid in smoking cessation and may improve temporomandibular disorder, ringing in the ears, and overactive bladder.

Because no single stress-management technique feels right for everyone, employing a mixture of techniques brings the best results. Essentially, there are stress-reducing techniques for every personality type, situation, and level of stress. Give them a try. Practicing relaxation techniques will help you to help your

---

BOX 10.2   Deep-Breathing Exercise

- Find a comfortable position.
- Relax your shoulders and chest; let your body relax.
- Shift to relaxed, abdominal breathing. Take a deep breath through your nose, expanding the abdomen. Hold it for 3 s and then exhale slowly through the mouth; exhale completely, telling yourself to relax.
- With every breath, turn attention to the muscular sensations that accompany the expansion of the belly.
- As you concentrate on your breathing, you will start to feel focused.
- Repeat this exercise for 2–5 min.

BOX 10.3   Script for Guided Imagery

- Imagine releasing all the tension in your body…letting it go.
- Now, with every breath you take, feel your body drifting down deeper and deeper into relaxation…floating down…deeper and deeper.
- Imagine a peaceful scene. You are sitting beside a clear, blue mountain stream. You are barefoot, and you feel the sun-warmed rock under your feet. You hear the sound of the stream tumbling over the rocks. The sound is hypnotic, and you relax more and more. You see the tall pine trees on the opposite shore, bending in the gentle breeze. Breathe the clean, scented air, with each breath moving you deeper and deeper into relaxation. The sun warms your face.
- You are very comfortable. There is nothing to disturb you. You are experiencing a feeling of well-being.
- Come back to this peaceful scene by taking time to relax. The positive feelings can grow stronger and stronger each time you choose to relax.
- You can return to your activities now, feeling relaxed and refreshed.

---

patients reduce their stress levels and also help you manage your own responses to stressors.

Biofeedback

Through the use of sensitive instrumentation, **biofeedback** provides immediate and exact information regarding muscle activity, brain waves, skin temperature, heart rate, blood pressure, and other bodily functions. Indicators of the particular internal physiological process are detected and amplified by a sensitive recording device. An individual can achieve greater voluntary control over phenomena once considered to be exclusively involuntary by knowing whether a somatic activity is increasing or decreasing.

The use of biofeedback was once reserved for clinicians with specialized training. Now, with increasingly sophisticated technology, most people can use some form of biofeedback themselves. Exercise trackers and smartwatches provide us with the ability to track sleep patterns and heart rates. One high-tech gadget is a clip-on device that tracks respiration changes that indicates tension. A companion application (app) suggests relaxation techniques such as meditation. One handheld device that measures electrodermal changes that indicate stress also comes with an app that teaches calming techniques.

Deep-Breathing Exercises

In a study by the US Department of Health and Human Services (2015), researchers found that the most common relaxation technique used in the United States was **deep-breathing exercises**. About a third of respondents used this technique as a mainstay or as a quick fix to calm down. Breathing exercises are simple and easy to remember, even when anxiety begins to escalate. This technique involves focusing on taking slow, deep, and even breaths.

One breathing exercise that has proved helpful for many people coping with anxiety and anxiety disorders has two parts (Box 10.2). The first part focuses on abdominal breathing, while the second part helps patients interrupt trains of thought, thereby quieting mental noise. With increasing skill, breathing becomes a tool for dampening the cognitive processes likely to induce stress and anxiety reactions.

Guided Imagery

Long before we learn to speak, our experience is based on mental images. With **guided imagery**, people are taught to focus on pleasant images to replace negative or stressful feelings. This focus diverts a person from less positive thoughts or obsessions, resulting in a refreshed outlook. Guided imagery may be self-directed, accessed online, or led by a practitioner. Specific scripts address a variety of psychiatric problems, such as anxiety or insomnia. Other scripts may be useful for different populations, such as children, incarcerated individuals, or refugees.

Imagery techniques are also useful in the management of medical conditions. One recent study found that guided imagery reduced anxiety and postoperative pain in children undergoing surgery (Vagnoli et al., 2019). During chemotherapy, cancer patients have experienced reduced fatigue, anxiety, and improved quality of life using this technique (Pattanshetty et al., 2018). Patients with cancer have successfully used guided imagery along with progressive muscle relaxation (discussed in the next section) to reduce pain-related distress (De Paolis et al., 2019).

Many sources of generic guided imagery are available to patients and healthcare workers online, especially on YouTube and TikTok. See Box 10.3 for a short sample script for guided imagery.

Progressive Relaxation

In 1938, Edmund Jacobson, a Harvard-educated physician, developed a rather simple procedure that elicits a **relaxation response**, which he coined **progressive relaxation** or progressive muscle relaxation. This technique can be done without any external gauges or feedback and can be practiced almost anywhere by anyone.

The premise behind progressive relaxation is that because anxiety results in tense muscles, one way to decrease anxiety is to relax muscle contraction. This is accomplished by deliberately tensing groups of muscles (beginning with feet and ending with face or vice versa) as tightly as possible for about 8 seconds and then releasing the tension you have created.

Considerable research supports the use of progressive relaxation as helpful for a number of medical conditions, such as tension headaches. People with major depressive disorder and posttraumatic stress disorder have been found to benefit from this relaxation technique (Bryan, 2013).

There are many free progressive relaxation scripts, audios, and videos on the internet, and some of them can be quite

BOX 10.4 Short Progressive Muscle Relaxation

Find a quiet, comfortable place to sit. A reclining chair is ideal. Take five slow, deep breaths before you begin. Now, tense and relax each area listed below. Tighten your muscles only until you feel tension, not pain.

- First, let's focus on your neck and shoulders. Raise your shoulders up toward your head...tighten the muscles there...hold...feel the tension there...and now release. Let your shoulders drop to a lower, more comfortable position.
- Now, let's move to your hands. Tighten your hands into fists. Very tight...as if you are squeezing a tennis ball tightly in each hand...hold...feel the tension in your hands and forearms...and now release. Shake your hands gently, shaking out the tension. Feel how much more relaxed your hands are now.
- Now, your forehead: Raise your eyebrows, feeling the tight muscles in your forehead. Hold that tension. Now, tightly lower your eyebrows and scrunch your eyes closed, feeling the tension in your forehead and eyes. Hold it tightly. And now, relax...let your forehead be relaxed and smooth, your eyelids gently resting.
- Your jaw is the next key area: Tightly close your mouth, clamping your jaw shut, very tightly. Your lips will also be tight and tense across the front of your teeth. Feel the tension in your jaws. Hold...and now relax. Release all of the tension. Let your mouth and jaw be loose and relaxed.
- There is only one more key area to relax, and that is your breathing: Breathe in deeply, and hold that breath. Feel the tension as you hold the air in. Hold...and now relax. Let the air be released through your mouth. Breathe out all the air.
- Once more, breathe in...and now hold the breath. Hold...and relax. Release the air, feeling your entire body relax. Breathe in...and out...in...and out...
- Continue to breathe regular breaths.
- You have relaxed some of the key areas where tension can build up. Remember to relax these areas a few times each day, using this quick progressive muscle relaxation script, to prevent stress symptoms.

lengthy. An abbreviated example of a script that focuses on key muscle tension areas is listed in Box 10.4. Many people prefer to hear their own voice reciting the script, so you may want to make a recording of yourself.

Meditation

Meditation is a discipline for training the mind to develop greater calm and then using that calm to bring penetrative insight into one's experience. Meditation can be used to help people tap into their deep inner resources for healing, calm their minds, and help them operate more efficiently in the world. It can help people develop strategies to cope with stress, make sensible adaptive choices under pressure, and feel more engaged in life.

Meditation elicits a relaxation response by creating a hypometabolic state of quieting the sympathetic nervous system. Some people meditate using a visual object or a sound to help them focus. Others may find it useful to concentrate on their breathing while meditating. Meditation is easy to practice anywhere. Some students find that meditating before an exam helps them focus and reduces test anxiety. Keep in mind that meditation, like most other techniques, becomes better with practice.

Mindfulness, a centuries-old form of meditation that dates back to Buddhist tradition, has received increased attention among healthcare professionals. Mindfulness is based on two ways our brains work. One is a default network that includes the medial prefrontal cortex and memory regions such as the hippocampus. In this state, we operate on a sort of mental autopilot or "mind wandering." You are thinking about what to make for dinner or how your hair looks and are continually compiling the narrative of your life and people you know. This type of thinking tends to be dominant.

The other network is the direct experience network that is the focus of mindfulness. Several areas of the brain are activated in this state. The insular cortex is active and makes us aware of bodily sensation and a sense of self. The anterior cingulate cortex is active and is central to attention and focuses us on what is happening around us. In this state, you are in tune with your environment, live in the moment, and take a break from planning, strategizing, and setting goals.

Being mindful includes being in the moment by paying attention to what is going on around you—what you are seeing, feeling, and hearing. Imagine how much you miss during an ordinary walk to class, staring straight ahead as your mind wanders from one concern to the next. You miss the pattern of sunlight filtered through the leaves, the warmth of the sunshine on your skin, and the sounds of birds calling out to one another. By focusing on the here and now, rather than past and future, you are practicing mindfulness.

With practice, people can gradually learn to let go of internal dialogue and reactiveness. Practicing mindfulness can be done at any time, and proponents suggest that it should become a way of life. One mindfulness technique can be found in Box 10.5.

OTHER WAYS TO RELAX

Physical Exercise

Physical exercise can lead to protection from the harmful effects of stress on both physical and mental states. Researchers have been particularly interested in the influence exercise has over major depressive disorder. Even in individuals who have a high genetic vulnerability to the disorder, physical activity is associated with a reduced incidence (Choi et al., 2019). The type of exercise does not seem to matter. Spending at least 3 hours a week participating in any activity, such as walking, running, or biking, reduces the risk for depression. Adding an additional 30 minutes of exercise reduces risk by another 17%.

Yoga, an ancient form of exercise, incorporates principles of meditation that use postures, breathing, and relaxation. There is growing evidence of yoga's neurobiological effects (Varambally et al., 2019). These effects include modulation of the HPA axis, enhancement of calming neurotransmitters, autonomic modulation, and a positive neuroendocrinological impact.

BOX 10.5   A Mindfulness Technique

Creating space to come down from the worried mind and back into the present moment has proven enormously helpful to people. When we are present, we have a firmer grasp on all our options and resources that often make us feel better. Next time you find your mind racing with stress, try the acronym STOP.

S—Stop what you are doing; put things down for a minute.

T—Take a breath. Breathe normally and naturally and follow your breath coming in and out of your nose. You can even say to yourself "in" as you're breathing in and "out" as you're breathing out, if that helps with concentration.

O—Observe your thoughts, feelings, and emotions. You can reflect about what is on your mind and also notice that thoughts are not facts and they are not permanent. If the thought arises that you are inadequate, just notice the thought, let it be, and continue on. Notice any emotions that are there and just name them. Just naming your emotions can have a calming effect. Then notice your body. Are you standing or sitting? How is your posture? Any aches and pains?

P—Proceed with something that is important to you in the moment, whether that is talking with a friend, appreciating your children, or walking while paying attention to the world.

From Goldstein, E. (2012). *The now effect.* New York, NY: Atria Books.

TABLE 10.5   Cognitive Reframing of Irrational Thoughts

Irrational Thought	Positive Statements
"I'll never be happy until I am loved by someone I really care about."	"If I do not get love from one person, I can still get it from others and find happiness that way."
	"If someone I deeply care for rejects me, that will seem unfortunate, but I will hardly die."
	"If the only person I truly care for does not return my love, I can devote more time and energy to winning someone else's love and probably find someone better for me."
	"If no one I care for ever cares for me, I can still find enjoyment in friendships, in work, in books, and in other things."
"He should treat me better after all I do for him."	"I would like him to do certain things to show that he cares. If he chooses to continue to do things that hurt me after he understands what those things are, I am free to make choices about leaving or staying in this hurtful relationship."

Adapted from Ellis, A., & Harper, R.A. (1975). *A new guide to rational living.* North Hollywood, CA: Wilshire.

Cognitive Reframing

Cognitive reframing stems from an evidenced-based practice known as cognitive-behavioral therapy. The goal of cognitive reframing (also known as *cognitive restructuring*) is to change an individual's perceptions of stress by reassessing a situation and replacing irrational beliefs. For example, the thought "I can't pass this course" is replaced with a more positive self-statement, "If I choose to study for this course, I will increase my chances of success." We can learn from most situations by asking ourselves the following:

- "What positive things came out of this situation or experience?"
- "What did I learn in this situation?"
- "What would I do differently?"

The desired result is to reframe a disturbing event or experience as less disturbing and to give the person a sense of control over the situation. When the perception of the disturbing event is changed, there is less stimulation to the sympathetic nervous system, which, in turn, reduces the secretion of cortisol and catecholamines that disrupt the balance of the immune system.

Cognitive distortions often include overgeneralizations ("He always…" or "I'll never…") and "should" statements ("I should have done better" or "He shouldn't have said that").

Table 10.5 shows some examples of cognitive reframing of anxiety-producing thoughts.

Journaling

Writing in a journal, or **journaling**, is an extremely useful and surprisingly simple method of identifying stressors. It is a technique that can ease worry and obsession, help identify hopes and fears, increase energy levels and confidence, and facilitate the grieving process. Keeping an informal diary of daily events and activities can reveal surprising information on sources of daily stress. Simply noting which activities put a strain on energy and time, which trigger anger or anxiety, and which precipitate a negative physical experience (e.g., headache, backache, fatigue) can be an important first step in stress reduction. Writing thoughts and feelings is helpful not only in dealing with stress and stressful events but also in healing both physically and emotionally.

Humor

The use of **humor** as a cognitive approach is a good example of how a stressful situation can be "turned upside down." The intensity attached to a stressful thought or situation can be dissipated when it is made to appear absurd or comical. Essentially, the bee loses its sting.

KEY POINTS TO REMEMBER

- Stress is a universal experience and an important concept when caring for any patient in any setting.
- The body responds similarly whether stressors are real or perceived and whether the stressor is negative or positive.
- Physiologically, the body reacts to anxiety and fear by arousal of the sympathetic nervous system. Specific symptoms include rapid heart rate, increased blood pressure, diaphoresis, peripheral vasoconstriction, restlessness, repetitive questioning, feelings of frustration, and difficulty concentrating.
- Cannon introduced the fight-or-flight model of stress, and Selye introduced the widely known GAS.
- Prolonged stress can lead to chronic psychological and physiological responses.

- There are basically two categories of stressors: physiological (e.g., heat, hunger, cold, noise, trauma) and psychological (e.g., death of a loved one, loss of job, schoolwork, humiliation).
- Age, gender, culture, life experience, and lifestyle all are important in identifying the degree of stress a person is experiencing.
- Lowering the effects of chronic stress can alter the course of many physical conditions; decrease the need for some medications; diminish or eliminate the urge for unhealthy and destructive behaviors such as smoking, insomnia, and drug addiction; and increase a person's cognitive functioning.
- An extremely important factor to assess is a person's support system. High-quality social and intimate supports can go a long way toward minimizing the long-term effects of stress.
- Cultural differences exist in the extent to which people perceive an event as stressful and in the behaviors they consider appropriate to deal with a stressful event.
- Spiritual practices have been found to lead to an enhanced immune system and a sense of well-being.
- A variety of relaxation techniques are available to reduce the stress response and elicit the relaxation response, which results in improved physiological and psychological functioning.

CRITICAL THINKING

1. Assess your level of stress using the Recent Life Changes Questionnaire found in Table 10.4 and evaluate your potential for illness in the coming year. Identify stress-reduction techniques you think would be useful to learn.
2. Teach a classmate the deep-breathing exercise identified in this chapter (see Box 10.2).
3. Using Fig. 10.1, explain to a classmate the short-term effects of stress on the sympathetic–adrenal medulla system, and identify three long-term effects if the stress is not relieved. How would you use this information to provide patient teaching? If your classmate were the patient, how would his or her response indicate that effective learning had taken place?
4. Using Fig. 10.1, have a classmate explain to you the short-term effects of stress on the hypothalamus–pituitary–adrenal cortex and the eventual long-term effects if the stress becomes chronic. Summarize to your classmate your understanding of what was presented. Using your knowledge of the short-term effects of stress on the hypothalamus–pituitary–adrenal cortex and the long-term effects of stress, develop and present a patient education model related to stress for your clinical group.
5. In postconference, discuss a patient you have cared for who had one of the stress-related effects identified in Fig. 10.1. See if you can identify some stressors in the patient's life and possible ways to lower chronic stress levels.

CHAPTER REVIEW

1. What assessment question is focused on identifying a long-term consequence of chronic stress on physical health?
   a. "Do you have any problems with sleeping well?"
   b. "How many infections have you experienced in the past 6 months?"
   c. "How much moderate exercise do you engage in on a regular basis?"
   d. "What management techniques do you regularly use to manage your stress?"
2. Which nursing assessments are directed at monitoring a patient's fight-or-flight response? *Select all that apply.*
   a. Blood pressure
   b. Heart rate
   c. Respiratory rate
   d. Abdominal pain
   e. Dilated pupils
3. The patient you are assigned unexpectedly suffers a cardiac arrest. During this emergency situation, your body will produce a large amount of:
   a. Carbon dioxide
   b. Growth hormone
   c. Epinephrine
   d. Aldosterone
4. Which question is focused on the assessment of an individual's personal ability to manage stress? *Select all that apply.*
   a. "Have you ever been diagnosed with cancer?"
   b. "Do you engage in any hobbies now that you have retired?"
   c. "Have you been taking your antihypertensive medication as it is prescribed?"
   d. "Who can you rely on if you need help after you're discharged from the hospital?"
   e. "What do you do to help manage the demands of parenting a 4-year-old and a newborn?"
5. When considering stress, what is the primary goal of making daily entries into a personal journal?
   a. Providing a distraction from the daily stress
   b. Expressing emotions to manage stress
   c. Identifying stress triggers
   d. Focusing on one's stress
6. Jackson has suffered from migraine headaches all of his life. Fatima, his nurse practitioner, suspects muscle tension as a trigger for his headaches. Fatima teaches him a technique that promotes relaxation by using:
   a. Biofeedback
   b. Guided imagery
   c. Deep breathing
   d. Progressive muscle relaxation

7. Hugo is 21 and diagnosed with schizophrenia. His history includes significant turmoil as a child and adolescent. Hugo reports his father was abusive and routinely beat him, all of his siblings, and his mother. Hugo's early exposure to stress most likely:
   a. Made him resilient to stressful situations
   b. Increased his future vulnerability to psychiatric disorders
   c. Developed strong survival skills
   d. Shaped his nurturing nature

8. Hugo has a fraternal twin named Franco who is unaffected by mental illness, even though they were raised in the same dysfunctional household. Franco asks the nurse, "Why Hugo and not me?" The nurse replies:
   a. "Your father was probably less abusive to you."
   b. "Hugo likely has a genetic vulnerability."
   c. "You probably ignored the situation."
   d. "Hugo responded to perceived threats by focusing on an internal world."

9. First responders and emergency department healthcare providers often use dark humor in an effort to:
   a. Reduce stress and anxiety
   b. Relive the experience
   c. Rectify moral distress
   d. Alert others to the stress

10. Your 39-year-old patient Samantha, who was admitted with anxiety, asks you what the stress-relieving technique of mindfulness is. The best response is:
    a. Mindfulness is focusing on an object and repeating a word or phrase while deep breathing.
    b. Mindfulness is progressively tensing, then relaxing, body muscles.
    c. Mindfulness is focusing on the here and now, not the past or future, and paying attention to what is going on around you.
    d. Mindfulness is a memory system to assist you in short-term memory recall.

1. **b**; 2. **a, b, c, e**; 3. **c**; 4. **b, d, e**; 5. **c**; 6. **d**; 7. **b**; 8. **b**; 9. **a**; 10. **c**

Visit the Evolve website for a posttest on the content in this chapter: http://evolve.elsevier.com/Varcarolis

REFERENCES

Ader, R., & Cohen, N. (1975). Behaviorally conditioned immunosuppression. *Psychosomatic Medicine, 37*(4), 333–340.

Bangasser, A., Curtis, A., Reyes, B. A. S., Bethea, T. T., Parastatidis, I., Ischiropoulos, H., et al. (2010). Sex differences in corticotropin-releasing factor receptor signaling and trafficking: Potential role in female vulnerability to stress-related psychopathology. *Molecular Psychiatry, 15*(9), 896–904.

Bryan, D. (2013). *Progressive muscle relaxation as a CAM.* Retrieved from http://www.camcommons.org/progressive-muscle-relaxation-as-an-evidence-based-cam-treatment.html.

Choi, K. W., Zheutlin, A. B., Karlson, R. A., Wang, M., Dunn, E. C., Stein, M. B., et al. (2019). Physical activity offsets genetic risk for incident depression assessed via electronic health records in a biobank cohort study. *Depression and Anxiety, 37*(2).

Cruces, J., Venero, C., Pereda-Perez, I., & De la Fuente, M. (2014). The effect of psychological stress and social isolation on neuroimmunoendocrine communication. *Current Pharmaceutical Design, 20*(29), 4608–4628.

Dahl, J., Ormstad, H., Aas, H. C. D., Malt, U. F., Bendz, L. T., Sandvik, L., et al. (2014). The plasma levels of various cytokines are increased during ongoing depression and are reduced to normal levels after recovery. *Psychoneuroendocrinology, 45,* 77–86.

De Paolis, G., Naccarato, A., Cibelli, F., D'Alete, A., Mastroianni, C., Surdo, L., et al. (2019). The effectiveness of progressive muscle relaxation and interactive guided imagery as a pain-reducing intervention in advanced cancer patients. *Complementary Therapies in Clinical Practice, 34,* 280–287.

Felitti, V. J., Anda, R. B., Nordenberg, D., Williamson, D. F., Spitz, A. M., Edwards, V., et al. (2019). Relationship of childhood abuse and household dysfunction to many of the leading causes of death in adults: The Adverse Childhood Experiences (ACE) Study. *American Journal of Preventive Medicine, 56*(6), 774–786.

First30Days. (2008). *First30Days' The Change Report: Making changes today considered more difficult to handle than 40 years ago.* Retrieved from http://www.first30days.com/pages/press_changereport.html.

Holmes, T. H., & Rahe, R. H. (1967). The social readjustment rating scale. *Journal of Psychosomatic Research, 11*(2), 213.

Jacobson, E. (1938). *Progressive relaxation.* Chicago, IL: University of Chicago Press.

Koenig, H. G., King, D. E., & Carson, V. B. (2012). *Handbook of religion and health* (2nd ed.). New York, NY: Oxford University Press.

Koolhaas, J. M., Bartolomucci, A., Buwalda, B., de Boer, S. F., Flugge, G., Korte, S. M., et al. (2011). Stress revisited: A critical evaluation of the stress concept. *Neuroscience & Biobehavioral Reviews, 35*(5), 1291–1301.

Lanzara, R., Scipioni, M., & Conti, C. (2018). A clinical-psychological perspective on somatization among immigrants: A systematic review. *Frontiers in Psychology, 9,* 2792.

National Cancer Institute. (2019). *Mood changes.* Retrieved from https://www.nccn.org/patients/resources/life_with_cancer/managing_symptoms/mood_changes.aspx.

National Center for Complementary and Alternative Medicine. (2016). *Mental health CAM.* Retrieved from https://www.mhanational.org/sites/default/files/MHA_CAM.pdf.

National Institute of Mental Health. (2016). *Fact sheet on stress.* Retrieved from http://www.nimh.nih.gov/health/publications/stress/index.shtml.

Pattanshetty, R., Moniz, C. C., & Patil, S. (2018). Guided imagery—Effectiveness in cancer fatigue in patients undergoing chemotherapy: A clinical trial. *International Journal of Applied Research, 4*(2), 141–145.

Selye, H. (1936). A syndrome produced by diverse nocuous agents. *Nature, 138*(32).

Selye, H. (1974). *Stress without distress*. Philadelphia, PA: Lippincott.

Selye, H. (1993). History of the stress concept. In L. Goldberger, & S. Breznitz (Eds.), *Handbook of stress: Theoretical and clinical aspects* (pp. 7–17). New York, NY: Free Press.

US Department of Health and Human Services. (2015). Trends in the use of complementary health approaches among adults: United States, 2002-2012. *National Health Statistics Reports, 79*, 1–16.

Vagnoli, L., Bettini, A., Amore, E., De Masi, S., & Messeri, A. (2019). Relaxation-guided imagery reduces perioperative anxiety and pain in children: A randomized study. *European Journal of Pediatrics, 178*(6), 913–921.

Varambally, S., George, S., & Gangadhar, B. N. (2019). Yoga for psychiatric disorders: From fad to evidence-based intervention. *British Journal of Psychiatry*. https://doi.org/10.1192/bjp.2019.249.

11

Childhood and Neurodevelopmental Disorders

Chyllia D. Fosbre and Cindy Parsons

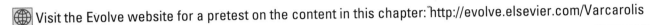 Visit the Evolve website for a pretest on the content in this chapter: http://evolve.elsevier.com/Varcarolis

OBJECTIVES

1. Identify the prevalence and significance of psychiatric disorders in children and adolescents.
2. Examine factors and influences contributing to neurodevelopmental disorders.
3. Identify characteristics of mental health and factors that promote resilience in children and adolescents.
4. Describe the specialty area of psychiatric–mental health nursing.
5. Discuss the assessment of a child or adolescent.

6. Compare and contrast at least six treatment modalities for children and adolescents with neurodevelopmental disorders.
7. Describe clinical features and behaviors of at least three childhood neurodevelopmental disorders.
8. Formulate one nursing diagnosis, state patient outcomes, and identify interventions for patients with intellectual disability, autism spectrum disorder, and attention-deficit/hyperactivity disorder.

KEY TERMS AND CONCEPTS

attention-deficit/hyperactivity disorder
autism spectrum disorder
bibliotherapy
communication disorders
early intervention programs

intellectual disability
play therapy
principle of least restrictive
  intervention
resilience

specific learning disorders
temperament
therapeutic games

We tend to think of mental illness as a phenomenon of adulthood, yet research shows that more than half of all lifetime cases began before the patient was age 14. Approximately one out of five or about 20% of children and adolescents in the United States experience a mental health disorder in any given year (Centers for Disease Control and Prevention, 2019).

Because of the timing of onset, these disorders can disrupt the normal pattern of childhood development. They may result in devastating consequences for academic, social, and psychological functioning. The symptoms of these disorders can also cause significant distress for families and disrupt family functioning. Fear of stigma can cause patients and families to attempt to conceal the conditions or even limit help seeking professional care.

Younger children are more difficult to diagnose than older children because of limited language skills and cognitive and emotional development. Additionally, children undergo more rapid psychological, neurological, and physiological changes over a briefer period than adults.

Clinicians and parents often wait to see whether symptoms are the result of a developmental lag or trauma response that will eventually correct itself. Unfortunately, this wait-and-see approach means that crucial early interventions may be delayed. Other barriers to assessment and treatment include (1) lack of consensus for screening children, (2) lack of coordination among multiple systems, (3) lack of community-based resources and long waiting lists for services, (4) lack of mental health providers, and (5) cost and inadequate reimbursement.

Fortunately, changes in the accessibility and availability of health insurance have created opportunities to improve funding, access to care, and research to understand the reasons for underutilization and early termination of services. The Substance Abuse and Mental Health Services Administration (SAMHSA, 2018) has revised and updated its 3-year strategic plan to improve the use of resources in the prevention, early detection, treatment, and recovery services for individuals with mental or substance use disorders.

The White House Conference on Mental Health in 2013 brought together community, state, and national representatives with national stakeholders. This group was charged to develop an initiative to bring about greater awareness to the mental health needs of all Americans, especially those more vulnerable populations. The "Now Is the Time" campaign followed and provided SAMHSA (2014) with increased funding for access to children's mental health services and community awareness efforts. The national budget for substance use and mental health services continues to increase, with approximately $1 trillion for 2020 (National Council for Behavioral Health, 2019).

In this chapter, we begin with an overview of the risk factors for psychiatric disorders in children and adolescents, overall assessments, and general interventions. Several neurodevelopmental disorders—communication disorder, learning disorder, and motor disorder—will be summarized. Specific disorders—intellectual disability, autism spectrum disorder, and attention-deficit/hyperactivity disorder (ADHD)—will be discussed in greater depth.

EVIDENCE-BASED PRACTICE

Functioning After Neonatal Abstinence Syndrome

Problem
Babies who are born to mothers with opioid addiction are likely to have neonatal abstinence syndrome (NAS), a drug withdrawal syndrome. There is limited longitudinal information about how these children function later in life.

Purpose of Study
The purpose of this study was to understand psychiatric outcomes for children who had NAS as infants.

Methods
According to hospital records from January 2008 through September 2010, 1046 infants were diagnosed with NAS and all other births totaled 269,726. Outcomes were mental disorders diagnosed between ages 1 and 5 years.

Key Findings
- About half of the children with NAS had a diagnosed psychiatric disorder before age 5, compared to 30% of all other births.
- Compared to other children, children born with NAS are more than twice as likely to have a conduct disturbance, ADHD, adjustment reaction, and intellectual disabilities.
- Children born with NAS were over 1.5 times more likely to have specific delays in development.

Implications for Nursing Practice
Children born to mothers with opioid addiction not only face withdrawal, but they are also at higher risk for future psychiatric conditions. Understanding the long-term consequences of opiate use supports nurses as they provide education to patients in general and pregnant mothers specifically. Recognizing the increased risk for children born with NAS helps in the long-term planning for this population.

Sherman, L. J., Ali, M. M., Mutter, R., & Larson, J. (2019). Mental disorders among children born with neonatal abstinence syndrome. *Psychiatric Services, 70*(2), 151.

RISK FACTORS

Biological Factors

Genetic

Hereditary factors are implicated in numerous childhood-onset psychiatric disorders. Because not all genetically vulnerable children develop mental disorders, researchers assume that factors such as resilience, intelligence, and a supportive environment aid in limiting the development of mental disorders.

Neurobiological

Dramatic changes occur in the brain during childhood and adolescence, including a declining number of synapses (they peak at age 5), changes in the relative volume and activity level in different brain regions, and interactions of hormones (Menzies et al., 2015). Myelination of brain fibers increases the speed of information processing, improves the conduction speed of nerve impulses, and enables faster reactions to occur.

Changes in the frontal and prefrontal cortex regions occur during the teen years. This leads to improvements in executive functions, organization and planning skills, and inhibiting responses. These changes, including cerebellum maturation and hormonal changes, reflect the emotional and behavioral fluctuations characteristic of adolescence. Early adolescence is typically characterized by low emotional regulation and intolerance for frustration. Emotional and behavioral control usually increases over the course of adolescence.

Cognitive Factors

Temperament

Temperament refers to the overall mood, attitude, and behavior that a child habitually uses to cope with the demands and expectations of the environment. These characteristics are present in infancy, are modified somewhat with maturation, and develop in the context of the social environment. All people have temperaments, and the fit between the child's and parent's temperament is critical to the child's development. If there is incongruence between parent and child temperament and the caregiver is unable to respond positively to the child, there is a risk of insecure attachment, developmental problems, and future mental disorders.

Temperament and behavioral traits can be powerful predictors of future problems. Traits such as shyness, aggressiveness, and rebelliousness, for example, may increase the risk for substance use problems. External risk factors for using illicit substances include peer or parental substance use and involvement in legal problems such as truancy or vandalism. Protective factors that shield some children from drug use include self-control, parental monitoring, academic achievement, antidrug-use policies, and strong neighborhood attachment.

Resilience

Despite risk factors for the development of psychiatric disorders, many children and adolescents develop normally. This is likely due to resilience. The phenomenon of resilience is the capacity to recover quickly from difficulties. Internal and external factors such as self-concept, future expectations, social competence, problem-solving skills, family, and school and community inter-actions all influence resilience. According to Zoloski and Bullock (2012), the *resilient child* has the following characteristics:

1. Adaptability to changes in the environment
2. Ability to form nurturing relationships with other adults when the parent is not available
3. Ability to distance self from emotional chaos
4. Social intelligence
5. Good problem-solving skills
6. Ability to perceive a long-term future

Environmental Factors
Adverse Childhood Experiences
To a far greater degree than adults, children are dependent on others. During childhood, the main context is the family. Parents model behavior and provide the child with a view of the world. If parents are abusive, rejecting, or overly controlling, the child may suffer detrimental effects at the developmental point(s) at which the trauma occurs (The National Child Traumatic Stress Network, 2019). Some familial risk factors correlate with child psychiatric disorders. These risk factors include severe marital discord, low socioeconomic status, large families and overcrowding, parental criminality, maternal psychiatric disorders, and foster-care placement.

Trauma in childhood is strongly associated with adult dysfunction. The CDC-Kaiser Permanente Adverse Childhood Experiences (ACE) study is one of the largest studies of childhood and adolescent abuse and neglect and subsequent adult health and well-being (CDC, 2019). ACEs include abuse (emotional, physical, sexual), neglect, and household challenges such as mental illness, spousal abuse, and substance use. The original study had more than 17,000 participants and was published in 1998. As the number of ACEs increase, so do the following:

- Alcohol use disorder
- Cardiac problems
- Fetal death
- Financial stress
- Intimate partner violence
- Liver disease
- Major depressive disorder
- Multiple sexual partners
- Poor academic performance
- Poor work performance
- Pregnancies (unintended)
- Sexual activity at a young age
- Sexually transmitted disease
- Smoking
- Suicide attempts

Neglect is the most prevalent form of child abuse in the United States. According to the US Department of Health and Human Services (2016), 75% of all abuse victims were neglected, 17% were physically abused, and about 8% were sexually abused.

Girls are more frequently the victims of sexual abuse. Boys are also sexually abused, but the numbers are likely underreported due to shame and stigma. Sexual abuse varies from fondling to forcing a child to observe lewd acts to sexual intercourse. All instances of sexual abuse are devastating to a child who lacks the mental capacity or emotional maturation to consent to this type of a relationship. All healthcare providers, including nurses, are required to report suspected abuse of a minor child to the local child protective services.

Witnessing violence is traumatizing and a well-documented risk factor for many mental health problems. Children who have experienced abuse are at risk for identifying with their aggressor and may act out, bully others, become abusers, or develop dysfunctional interpersonal relationships in adulthood.

Cultural Factors
Differences in cultural expectations, presence of stressors, and lack of support by the dominant culture may have profound effects on children and adolescents. Working with patients from diverse backgrounds requires an increased awareness of one's own biases and the patient's needs. Nurses should consider the social and cultural context of the patient, including factors such as age, ethnicity, gender, sexual orientation, worldview, religiosity, and socioeconomic status when assessing and planning care.

⊕ CONSIDERING CULTURE
Suicide Rates of Black Female Teens

Suicide rates among adolescents ages 15–19 have risen dramatically, with a rate of 6.7 suicides per 100,000 per year in 2007 and a rate of 11.8 per 100,000 per year in 2017. The rate increased for both boys and girls and also for white, black, and Hispanic adolescents. While black boys are experiencing an increased rate of suicide, the group with the most drastic increase was black girls: 1.2 suicides per 100,000 in 2007 and 4.0 per 100,000 per year in 2017.

This increase in suicide rates among young African American females is troubling and should influence prevention and intervention efforts. Research should be conducted to determine the reasons for the increases. If causation can be determined, strategies can be aimed at healthcare and social policy to address this problem.

Adapted from Shain, B. N. (2019). Increases in rates of suicide and suicide attempts among black adolescents. *Pediatric, 144*(5).

CHILD AND ADOLESCENT PSYCHIATRIC-MENTAL HEALTH NURSING

In 2014, the American Nurses Association (ANA), along with the American Psychiatric Nurses Association (APNA) and International Society of Psychiatric-Mental Health Nurses (ISPN) (2014), defined the functions of nurses in the *Psychiatric-Mental Health Nursing: Scope and Standards of Practice*. According to this document, psychiatric-mental health nurses utilize evidence-based psychiatric practices to provide care responsive to the patient's and family's specific problems, strengths, personality, sociocultural context, and preferences.

Nurses who work in psychiatric-mental health settings may focus on specific populations such as pediatric, adolescent, adult, and geriatric patients. All of these nurses are referred to as psychiatric-mental health registered nurses regardless of the population. Formal recognition of the role occurs through certification at either the basic or advanced practice level.

General Assessment Topics for Children
The type of data collected to assess mental health depends on the setting, the severity of the presenting problem, and the availability of resources. Box 11.1 identifies essential assessment

---

BOX 11.1 Types of Assessment Data

History of Present Illness
- Chief complaint
- Development and duration of problems
- Help sought and results
- Effect of problem on child's life at home and school
- Effect of problem on family and siblings' lives

Developmental History
- Pregnancy, birth, neonatal data
- Developmental milestones
- Description of eating, sleeping, and elimination habits and routines
- Attachment behaviors
- Types of play
- Social skills and friendships
- Sexual activity

Developmental Assessment
- Psychomotor skills
- Language skills
- Cognitive skills
- Interpersonal and social skills
- Academic achievement
- Behavior (response to stress, to changes in environment)
- Problem-solving and coping skills (impulse control, delay of gratification)
- Energy level and motivation

Neurological Assessment
- Cerebral functions
- Cerebellar functions
- Sensory functions

- Reflexes

Note: Functions can be observed during developmental assessment and while playing games involving a specific ability (e.g., "Simon says, 'Touch your nose.'")

Medical History
- Review of body systems
- Traumas, hospitalizations, operations, and child's response
- Illnesses or injuries affecting central nervous system
- Medications (past and current)
- Allergies

Family History
- Illnesses in related family members (e.g., seizures, mental disorders, intellectual disability, hyperactivity, drug and alcohol use, diabetes, cancer)
- Background of family members (occupation, education, social activities, religion)
- Family relationships (separation, divorce, deaths, contact with extended family, support system)

Mental Status Assessment
- General appearance
- Activity level
- Coordination and motor function
- Affect
- Speech
- Manner of relating
- Intellectual functions
- Thought processes and content
- Characteristics of play

---

data, including history of the present illness; medical, developmental, and family history; mental status; and neurological developmental characteristics. Local, regional, and national agencies determine which data are collected, but a nurse should be prepared to make an independent judgment about what to assess and how to assess it. In all cases, a physical examination is part of a complete assessment for children and adolescents with serious mental problems who require hospitalization.

Data Collection

Methods of collecting data include interviewing, screening, testing (neurological, psychological, intelligence), observing, and interacting with the child or adolescent. In addition to the patient, ideally, data will be taken from multiple sources, including parents, teachers, and other caregivers. Parents and teachers can complete structured questionnaires and behavior checklists. A family diagram, called a genogram, can illustrate family composition, history, and relationships (refer to Chapter 35). Numerous assessment tools and rating scales are available, and with training, nurses can use them to effectively monitor symptoms, behavioral change, and response to treatment.

The initial interview is key to observing interactions among the child, caregiver, and siblings (if available) and building trust and rapport. The observation-interaction part of a mental health assessment begins with a semi-structured interview in which the nurse asks the young person about the home environment, parents, and siblings and the school environment, teachers, and peers. In this format, the patient is encouraged to describe current problems and give information about developmental history. Nurses use play activities such as ***therapeutic games***, drawings, and puppets for younger children who have difficulty responding to a direct approach.

Mental Status Examination

Assessment of mental status of children and adolescents is similar to that of adults. The main difference is that assessment is adapted to be appropriate for the child's developmental stage, cognitive capabilities, and verbal skills. It provides information about the mental state at the time of the examination and identifies problems with thinking, feeling, and behaving. Broad categories to assess include safety, general appearance, socialization, activity level, speech, coordination and motor function, affect, manner of relating, intellectual function, thought processes and content, and characteristics of play.

Developmental Assessment

A developmental assessment will look at milestones such as the age a child starts walking, talking, or toilet training. A child or adolescent who does not have a psychiatric disorder matures with only minor regressions, coping with the stressors and developmental tasks of life. Learning and adapting to the

- Trusts others and sees his or her world as being safe and supportive
- Correctly interprets reality and makes accurate perceptions of the environment and one's ability to influence it through actions (e.g., self-determination)
- Behaves in a way that is developmentally appropriate and does not violate social norms
- Has a positive realistic self-concept and developing identity
- Adapts to and copes with anxiety and stress using age-appropriate behavior
- Can learn and master developmental tasks and new situations
- Expresses self in spontaneous and creative ways
- Develops and maintains satisfying relationships

environment and bonding with others in a mutually satisfying way are signs of mental health (Box 11.2).

The developmental assessment provides information about the child or adolescent's maturational level. These data are then reviewed in relation to the chronological age to identify developmental strengths or deficits. The Denver II Developmental Screening Test is a popular assessment tool that lists 125 items. This tool covers four areas: social/personal, fine motor function, language, and gross motor function.

Abnormal findings in the developmental and mental status assessments may be related to stress and adjustment problems or to more serious disorders. Nurses need to evaluate behaviors brought on by stress, as well as those of more serious psychopathology, and identify the need for further evaluation or referral. Stress-related behaviors or minor regressions may be managed by working with parents. Serious psychopathology requires evaluation by an advanced practice nurse in collaboration with clinicians from other specialty disciplines.

General Interventions With Children

You can use the interventions described in this section in a variety of settings: inpatient, residential, outpatient, day treatment, outreach programs in schools, and home visits. Many of the modalities can encompass activities of daily living, learning activities, multiple forms of play and recreational activities, and interactions with adults and peers.

Behavioral Interventions

Behavioral interventions reward desired behaviors to reduce maladaptive behaviors. Most child and adolescent treatment settings use a structured program that includes a behavioral program to motivate and reward age-appropriate behaviors. One popular method is the point system, in which care providers award points for desired behaviors. Specific behaviors have specific points. Privileges are awarded based on the points that are earned each day.

Play Therapy

Play is often described as the work of childhood. Through play, children develop their physical, intellectual, emotional, social,

and moral capacities. Play therapy is an intervention that allows children to express feelings such as anxiety, self-doubt, and fear through the natural use of play. It is also useful in helping young patients to access and work through painful memories. Trauma is often stuck in the nonverbal parts of the brain—amygdala, thalamus, hippocampus, or brainstem. Playing out memories helps move them to verbal frontal lobes.

> **VIGNETTE:** Seth, a 6-year-old male, was walking home from the store with his grandmother when an out of control car charged toward them on the sidewalk. Seth's grandmother was able to push him to safety, but she was struck and died at the scene. Since that time, he has become withdrawn, anxious, and has frequent nightmares. He is inconsolable when his mother goes to work or takes him to school. Seth and his mother were referred to a play therapist.
>
> During play therapy, the therapist used dolls and toy vehicles to help Seth work through his anxiety and distress related to the accident. He even reenacted the tragic event and said he was very mad at the driver. After four sessions, he begins to talk about positive memories of his grandmother and his mother reports that his anxiety is decreasing.

Bibliotherapy

Bibliotherapy involves using literature to help the child express feelings in a supportive environment, gain insight into feelings and behavior, and learn new ways to cope with difficult situations. When children listen to or read a story, they unconsciously identify with the characters and experience a catharsis of feelings. You should select stories and books that reflect the situations or feelings the child is experiencing. Also take into consideration the child's cognitive and developmental level and emotional readiness for the particular topic.

Expressive Arts Therapy

The therapeutic use of art provides a nonverbal means of expressing difficult or confusing emotions. Drawing, painting, and sculpting are commonly used mediums. Creating something may help young people express the thoughts, feelings, and tensions that they cannot express verbally, are unaware of, or are denying. Children who have experienced trauma will often show the traumatic event in their drawing when asked to draw whatever they wish.

Journaling

Another effective technique when working with younger people, particularly teenagers, is using a journal. Journaling is a tangible way of recording and viewing emotions and may be a way to begin a dialogue with others. The use of a daily journal is also effective in setting goals and evaluating progress.

Music Therapy

The healing power of music has been recognized for centuries. Music therapy is an evidence-based approach to accomplish therapeutic goals within the context of a therapeutic relationship. Music can be used to improve physical, psychological, cognitive, behavioral, and social functioning. It is a nonthreatening approach that engages multiple senses. Children and adolescents can be involved in music by listening, singing, playing, moving, and other creative activities.

Family Interventions

The family is critical to improving the functional capacity of a young person with a psychiatric illness. Family counseling is often a key component of treatment. Nurses can help family members develop specific goals, identify ways to improve, and work to achieve the goals for the family or subunits within the family (e.g., parental, sibling).

Homework assignments are often used for family members to practice new skills outside the therapeutic environment. Sometimes, families are taught in groups. Group education may be useful for (1) learning how other families solve problems and build on strengths, (2) developing insight and improved judgment about their own family, and (3) learning and sharing new information.

Teamwork and Safety

Children and adolescents with neurodevelopmental disorders may require comprehensive teamwork to promote safety in inpatient units, long-term residential care, or intensive outpatient care. Nurses collaborate with other healthcare providers in structuring and maintaining the therapeutic environment to provide physical safety, psychological security, and improve coping.

The nurse provides leadership to the nursing team in planning, implementing, and delivering safe, effective, quality care to maintain the therapeutic milieu and safety of all patients. The multidisciplinary team shares and articulates a philosophy regarding how to provide physical and psychological security, promote personal growth, and work with problematic behaviors.

Disruptive Behavior Management

To ensure the civil and legal rights of individuals are maintained, techniques are selected according to the **principle of least restrictive intervention**. This principle requires that you use more restrictive interventions *only* after attempting less restrictive interventions that have been unsuccessful to manage the behavior. Less restrictive interventions include discussion (e.g., asking if the patient would like to talk about his anger), offering medication to help him gain control, and suggesting a time-out (e.g., his room or other quiet area). Finally, as a last resort, seclusion or restraint may be considered. In general, seclusion is viewed as less restrictive than restraint, where all movement is constrained.

Time-out. Asking or directing a child or adolescent to take a time-out from an activity is an excellent intervention that promotes self-reflection and encourages self-control. It is a less restrictive alternative to seclusion and restraint. Taking a time-out may involve going to a designated room or sitting on the periphery of an activity until self-control is regained. This technique may be an integral part of the treatment plan, and the child's and family's input are considered in including this modality.

Quiet room. A unit may have an unlocked room for a child who needs an area with decreased stimulation for regaining and maintaining self-control. The types of quiet rooms include a feelings room, which can be carpeted and supplied with soft objects that can be punched and thrown, and a sensory room, which contains items for relaxation and meditation, such as music and yoga mats. The child is encouraged to express freely and work through feelings of anger or sadness in privacy and with staff support.

> **VIGNETTE:** Isabelle, a school-aged child, was admitted to the hospital from her foster home placement. She has been in foster care since her mother died from a drug overdose. Her father is incarcerated for armed robbery and drug-related offenses. Isabelle has a history of self-injurious behavior that includes biting and pinching herself and hitting her head against the wall when she is frustrated. The nurse and activity therapist have taught Isabelle to request time in the sensory room when she begins to feel upset or anxious. She has been able to identify certain triggers and to request time in the sensory room, decreasing episodes of self-injury over the past week.

Seclusion and restraint. Evidence suggests that both seclusion and restraint are psychologically harmful and can be physically dangerous. Deaths have resulted, primarily by asphyxiation, from physical holds during the use of restraints. However, a child's or adolescent's behavior may be so destructive or dangerous that physical restraint or seclusion is required for the safety of all. Members of the treatment team who use locked seclusion or physical restraint of children and adolescents must receive training to decrease the risk of injury to the young person and themselves.

The registered nurse assigned to the patient is often the one to make the decision to restrain or seclude a child. A physician, nurse practitioner, or other advanced level practitioner must authorize this action according to facility policy and state regulation. The patient's family should be notified of any incident of seclusion or restraint.

Patients in seclusion or restraints must be monitored constantly and not be left alone. Vital signs and range of motion in extremities must be monitored at a set interval. Hydration, elimination, comfort, and other psychological and physical needs should be monitored and addressed as needed. Policy and regulations should provide guidelines as to the appropriate physical monitoring and care.

Children are released as soon as they are no longer dangerous. Once the child is calm, the staff should include the child in a debriefing and discuss the events leading up to and including the restrictive interventions with the patient. Debriefings provide an opportunity for staff members to discuss the event and explore ways it may have been prevented, evaluate their emotional responses, review the plan of care, and enhance their clinical skills.

TREATMENT MODALITIES

Biological Treatments

Pharmacotherapy

The treatment of psychiatric disorders in young people requires a multimodal approach, which may include the use of medication. Medication typically works best when combined with another psychological treatment modality. Medications that target specific symptoms can improve quality of life while enhancing the child's or adolescent's potential for growth.

Psychological Therapies
Cognitive-Behavioral Therapy

Cognitive-behavioral therapy (CBT) is an evidence-based treatment approach for a number of psychiatric diagnoses. It is based on the premise that negative and self-defeating thoughts lead to psychiatric pathology. Learning to replace these thoughts with more realistic and accurate appraisals results in improved functioning.

Group Therapy

Registered nurses working in psychiatric settings may conduct education groups, teaching about a new skill, medication, or diagnosis. They may also lead task groups such as daily goal-setting groups to determine what the patients would like to accomplish during the day. A follow-up group at the end of the day provides for evaluation of the goals.

Advanced practice nurses are trained at the graduate level and qualified to conduct formal group therapy. Groups are effective when dealing with specific issues in a child's life, such as bereavement, physical abuse, or chronic illnesses such as juvenile diabetes. Group therapy for younger children uses play to introduce ideas and work through issues. For grade-school children, it combines play, learning skills, and talking about the activity. The child learns to identify feelings and improve impulse control and social skills by taking turns and sharing with peers.

For teens, this modality offers them the opportunity to see how their peers are coping with or have managed similar problems and can be a means for developing a positive source of peer support. For adolescents, group therapy involves identifying emotions, modifying responses, learning skills and talking, focusing largely on peer relationships, and addressing specific problems. Adolescent group therapy might use a popular media event or personality as the basis for a group discussion.

HEALTH POLICY

Getting Teens Mental Healthcare: Whose Choice Is It?

Washington State legislators passed an important bill in 1985 aimed at allowing adolescents older than the age of 13 to seek mental healthcare on their own. It also gave the child the choice of whether or not to include parents in their treatment. This legislation paved the way for countless young people to get the help they needed. Unfortunately, adolescents making their own mental health decisions carried the unintended consequence of them also being able to refuse care.

A parent with two children refusing psychiatric treatment approached lawmakers in 2016 to change the old law. She was joined by other parents who were concerned about their children's mental healthcare. As a result, House Bill 1874 was passed in July of 2019. The new law retained teens' ability to admit themselves for inpatient treatment, but there is also parent-initiated treatment. Parents and guardians can now request care for mental health or substance use disorders without the minors' consent. This care includes admission, evaluation, or treatment for inpatient care or outpatient counseling.

McCarty, E. (2020, January 8). It affects the entire family: Washington parents now work alongside teens in mental health recovery. *Crosscut.* Retrieved from https://crosscut.com/2020/01/it-affects-entire-family-washington-parents-now-work-alongside-teens-mental-health-recovery.

NEURODEVELOPMENTAL DISORDERS

According to the American Psychiatric Association (APA, 2013), the following disorders are considered neurodevelopmental disorders. These will be discussed through the next portion of this chapter:

- Communication disorders
- Motor disorders
- Specific learning disorder
- Intellectual disability
- Autism spectrum disorder
- ADHD

COMMUNICATION DISORDERS

Communication disorders are manifested in deficits in language, speech, and communication. These deficits result in impairments in academic achievement, socialization, or self-care. About 6% of children have some sort of communication disorder. Assessment of children must take into consideration cultural variables and language context, especially for children who grow up in bilingual families. The category of communication disorders includes language disorder, speech sound disorder, childhood-onset fluency disorder (stuttering), and social (pragmatic) communication disorder.

Children with **language disorder** have difficulties in attaining and using language due to deficits in production or comprehension of language. Children may have an *expressive* problem that results in difficulty in finding the right words, forming clear sentences, and using the right gestures and verbal signals. Other children may have *receptive* problems where they experience difficulty understanding or are unable to follow directions. Receptive impairment results in a poorer prognosis than does expressive impairment.

Language disorder may be present from birth or may occur later in life. Causes include hearing loss, neurological disorders, intellectual disabilities, drug misuse, brain injury, physical problems such as cleft palate or lip, and vocal abuse or misuse. Frequently, the cause is unknown. This disorder ranges from mild to severe and tends to show up prior to the age of 3 (American Speech, Language, and Hearing Disorders, 2019).

Speech sound disorder has to do with problems in making sounds. To have clear articulation, children must have knowledge of speech sounds and the ability to coordinate movements of speech. They may distort, add, or omit sounds. Children may have trouble making certain sounds (saying "no" for "snow" or "wabbit" for "rabbit," for example). Speech sound disorders result in problems with social participation, academic achievement, and occupational performance. Most children with this disorder respond well to treatment.

Another aspect of speech that may be disturbed is fluency. **Child-onset fluency disorder**, also known as stuttering, is manifested by hesitations and repetition. While all children may have mild and transient symptoms of stuttering, a fluency disorder significantly impacts a child's ability to communicate and participate in social, academic, and occupational activities. Most children recover from the dysfluency.

While some children have no problem with language and no problem speaking, they may have problems relating with other people. In **social communication disorder**, children have problems using verbal and nonverbal means for interacting socially with others. Impairments are also evident in written communication when the child is trying to relate to others. Prior to 2013, many children with communication problems were diagnosed with Asperger's disorder, a diagnosis which is no longer in use. Autism spectrum disorder needs to be ruled out to receive a diagnosis of social communication disorder (APA, 2013).

The Disabilities Education Act provides for early intervention services in every state for toddlers up to age 3. Service providers will meet with the family to develop a treatment plan. Special education and services are also available for individuals ages 3 to 21. Typically, the first step in the plan is a hearing test followed by involvement with a speech or language therapist.

MOTOR DISORDERS

Developmental Coordination Disorder

A key feature of growth and development is the acquisition of fine and gross motor skills and coordination. **Developmental coordination disorder** is based on (1) impairments in motor skill development, (2) coordination below the child's developmental age, and (3) problems interfering with academic achievement or activities of daily living. Symptoms include delayed sitting or walking or difficulty jumping or performing tasks such as tying shoelaces.

Serious impairments in skills development or coordination are usually obvious. Less severe impairments may be less noticeable. They may be identified by the child's avoidance of certain tasks or activities. These children typically make comments like, "I hate to draw" or "I don't want to play kickball."

Early diagnosis, treatment, and education are essential to prevent frustration and unnecessary problems in adult life. Physical therapy and occupational therapy are the treatments of choice for developmental coordination disorder.

Stereotypic Movement Disorder

Stereotypic movement disorder is manifested by repetitive purposeless movements such as hand-waving, rocking, head banging, nail biting, and teeth grinding for a period of 4 weeks or more (APA, 2013). This disorder is more common in boys than in girls. Intellectual disability is a risk factor for these repetitive movements, with up to 16% of this population affected.

Interventions for stereotypic movement disorder focus on safety and prevention of injury. Helmets may be required for children who have the potential for head injury. Behavioral therapy includes habit-reversal techniques such as folding the arms when the urge to hand-wave begins. Naltrexone, an opioid receptor antagonist, may block euphoric responses from these behaviors, thereby reducing their occurrence.

Tic Disorders

Tics are sudden, nonrhythmic, and rapid motor movements or vocalizations. Motor tics usually involve the head, torso, or limbs, and they change in location, frequency, and severity over time. Other motor tics are tongue protrusion, touching, squatting, hopping, skipping, retracing steps, and twirling when walking. Vocal tics are spontaneous production of words unrelated to conscious communication and sounds such as sniffs, barks, coughs, or grunts.

According to the APA (2013), there are three types of tic disorders. They are listed here from least to most severe:
1. Provisional tic disorder—Single or multiple motor and or vocal tics for less than 1 year.
2. Persistent motor or vocal tic disorder—Single or multiple motor or vocal tics but not both for more than 1 year.
3. Tourette's disorder—Multiple motor tics and at least one vocal tic for more than 1 year.

All of these problems occur before age 18, with the typical age of onset between 4 and 6 years. Symptoms tend to peak in early adolescence and diminish into adulthood.

The Hollywood version of Tourette's disorder is a person pouring forth a string of obscenities. In reality, coprolalia—the involuntary outburst of obscene words or socially inappropriate and derogatory remarks—occurs in fewer than 10% of cases. A child or adolescent with tics may have low self-esteem as a result of feeling ashamed, self-conscious, and rejected by peers and may severely limit public appearances for fear of displaying tics.

There is no specific gene connected to Tourette's disorder, but patterns within families indicate there may be a genetic influence. Tourette's disorder often coexists with depression, obsessive-compulsive disorder, and anxiety. Approximately 63% of those with Tourette's have also been diagnosed with ADHD (CDC, 2019). Central nervous system stimulants, like those used to treat ADHD, can increase the severity of tics, so medications must be carefully monitored in children with coexisting ADHD.

Behavioral techniques can reduce tic expression (CDC, 2019). They are referred to as habit reversal, and the most promising form is called comprehensive behavior intervention for tics (CBIT). It works by helping the patient become aware of the building up of a tic urge and then using a muscular response in competition to or incompatible with the tic.

Drugs with FDA approval for treating tics are the first-generation antipsychotics haloperidol (Haldol) and pimozide (Orap) and the second-generation antipsychotic aripiprazole (Abilify). Another second-generation drug, risperidone (Risperdal), does not have FDA approval but is commonly used for tic disorders.

Alpha 2-adrenergic agonists used to treat hypertension are also prescribed for tics. While less effective and far slower acting than the antipsychotics, they have fewer side effects. They may be appropriate as a first-line agent in many patients. Guanfacine (Tenex/Intuniv) is usually well tolerated. Side effects include somnolence, lethargy, fatigue, insomnia, nausea, dizziness, hypotension, and abdominal pain. Clonidine (Kapvay/Catapres) used for ADHD, is used to manage tics. Common side effects of clonidine are somnolence, fatigue, insomnia, nightmares, irritability, constipation, respiratory symptoms, and dry mouth.

The antianxiety drug clonazepam (Klonopin) is used as a supplement to other medications. It may work by reducing anxiety and resultant tics. Botulinum toxin type A (Botox) injections are used to calm the muscle associated with the tics.

A sort of pacemaker for the brain, deep brain stimulation (DBS), is used when more conservative treatments fail. A fine wire is threaded into affected areas of the brain and connected to a small device implanted under the collarbone that delivers electrical impulses. Users of DBS can turn the device on to control tics or shut it off when they go to sleep.

SPECIFIC LEARNING DISORDER

Children with specific learning disorders are identified during the school years. A specific learning disorder is diagnosed when a child demonstrates persistent difficulty in reading (dyslexia), mathematics (dyscalculia), and/or written expression (dysgraphia). With any of these problems, their performance is well below the expected performance of their peers. Diagnosis of a learning disorder is made through multiple assessments, including formal psychological evaluations.

Screening for learning disorders is essential so that crucial early interventions may be put in place. Most students with this type of disability are eligible for assistance at a school that is supported by the Disabilities Education Improvement Act. This assistance involves an individualized treatment plan for each child, careful monitoring of progress, special education intervention, and the establishment of an Individualized Education Program (IEP).

According to the National Center for Learning Disorders (NCLD, 2017), one in five children face a learning disability. These disabilities are associated with higher rates for those with lower family education, poverty, and male gender.

Long-term outcomes for children with learning disorders can vary. The rate of enrollment in postsecondary education has risen significantly in the past 15 years. Without educational, social, and psychiatric interventions, low self-esteem, poor social skills, higher rates of school dropout, difficulties with attaining and maintaining employment, and poorer social adjustment may result (NCLD, 2017).

INTELLECTUAL DISABILITY

Intellectual disability is characterized by deficits in three areas:

- *Intellectual functioning.* Deficits in reasoning, problem solving, planning, judgment, abstract thinking, and academic ability.
- *Social functioning.* Impaired communication and language, interpreting and acting on social cues, and regulating emotions.
- *Daily functioning.* Practical aspects of daily life are impacted by a deficit in managing age-appropriate activities of daily living, functioning at school or work, and performing self-care.

Impairments begin during childhood development, range from mild to severe, and include the consideration of the person's level of dependence on others for ongoing care and support

(American Speech, Language Hearing Association, 2019). The incidence of intellectual disability is estimated at about 1% of the population (APA, 2013).

The etiology of intellectual disability may be heredity, problems with pregnancy or perinatal development, environmental influences, or a direct result of a medical condition. Hereditary factors can include chromosomal disorders such as Fragile X, Down or Klinefelter's syndrome, inborn errors of metabolism such as phenylketonuria, or genetic abnormalities.

Approximately 10% of affected individuals are a result of problems during pregnancy or birth and include malnutrition, chronic maternal substance abuse, and maternal infection. Complications of pregnancy—such as toxemia, placenta previa, or trauma to the head during birth—are also implicated. In addition, up to 20% of cases are attributed to environmental or social neglect that does not foster the development of social or linguistic skills or a lack of a nurturing relationship. Intellectual disabilities can also be associated with other mental disorders, such as autism spectrum disorder.

APPLICATION OF THE NURSING PROCESS
ASSESSMENT

ASSESSMENT GUIDELINES
Intellectual Disability

1. Assess for delays in cognitive and physical development or lack of ability to perform tasks or achieve milestones in relation to peers. Gather information from family, caregivers, or others actively involved in the child's life.
2. Assess for delays in cognitive, social, or personal functioning, focusing on strengths and abilities.
3. Assess for areas of independent functioning and the need for support/assistance to meet requirements of daily living (examples are hygiene, dressing, or feeding).
4. Assess for physical and emotional signs of potential neglect or abuse. Be aware that children with behavioral and developmental problems are at risk for abuse.
5. Assess for need of community resources or programs that can provide resources and support the child's need for intellectual and social development and the family's need for education and emotional support.

NURSING DIAGNOSIS

The child with an intellectual disability has impairments in conceptual, social, and practical functioning, ranging from mild to severe. The severity of impairment is demonstrated in the ability to communicate effectively, meet one's self-care and safety needs, and socialize in an age-appropriate manner. Due to the increased need for supervision and assistance with daily living and the chronic nature of the disorder, families or caregivers may experience significant stress and be at risk for impaired family functioning. Table 11.1 lists potential nursing diagnoses that address intellectual disability problems.

TABLE 11.1 Signs and Symptoms and Nursing Diagnoses Neurodevelopmental Disorders

Signs and Symptoms	Nursing Diagnosis
Lack of responsiveness or interest in others, empathy, or sharing	Impaired socialization Impaired caregiver child attachment Risk for impaired parenting Risk for social isolation
Lack of cooperation or imaginative play with peers	Lack of play activity Situational low self-esteem Impaired socialization
Language delay or absence, stereotyped, or repetitive use of language	Impaired child development
Inability to feed, bathe, dress, or toilet self at age-appropriate level	Impaired child development Self-care deficit
Head banging, face slapping, hand biting	Impaired impulse control Risk for injury Self-destructive behavior
Frequent disregard for bodily needs	Risk for situational low self-esteem Self-care deficit
Failure to follow age-appropriate social norms	Impaired coping Impaired role performance Impaired socialization
Depression, inability to concentrate, withdrawal, difficulty in functioning, feeling down, change in vegetative symptoms	Risk for suicide Hopelessness Spiritual distress Impaired concentration Impaired socialization
Refusal to attend school	Impaired coping Risk for impaired school performance Readiness for enhanced parenting
Family reports insufficient knowledge about child's disorder, overprotectiveness interferes with child's autonomy, parental anxiety	Impaired family coping Impaired family process Risk for impaired caregiver child attachment

International Council of Nursing Practice. (2019). *ICNP browser*. Retrieved from https://www.icn.ch/what-we-do/projects/ehealth/icnp-browser. ICNP® is owned and copyrighted by the International Council of Nurses (ICN). Reproduced with permission of the copyright holder.

OUTCOMES IDENTIFICATION

There are a number of outcomes appropriate for the child with an intellectual disability:

- Uses spoken language to make or respond to requests.
- Engages in simple social interactions and accepts assistance or feedback regarding behavior without frustration.
- Tolerates social interaction for short periods of time without becoming disruptive or frustrated.
- Refrains from acting impulsively toward self or others when frustrated.

Additionally, the family may be in denial over the diagnosis. An outcome would be for the family to acknowledge the existence of impairment and its potential to alter family routines.

IMPLEMENTATION

Nurses provide services to children with intellectual disabilities in a variety of settings. Children with intellectual disabilities are cared for in the community through early intervention programs or public-school programs as they reach school age. Federal legislation, the Individuals with Disabilities in Education Act (IDEA), requires that public schools provide services to assist children with emotional or developmental disorders to participate in school (APA, 2015). Individuals may also require short-term hospitalization related to socially impaired behaviors such as aggression, self-harm, or severe self-care deficits.

Treatment plans should be individualized and realistic. Although the care plan is developed for the child, family members or caregivers and school personnel should be included in the process. Supportive education should be ongoing regarding the scope and nature of the illness; conceptual, social, and practical deficits; and realistic assessment of the child's potential. Long-term planning should include consideration of continuing care needs as the child ages and matures into adulthood.

EVALUATION

In evaluating the child and family with an intellectual disability, it is important for nurses to use a strength-based perspective. In the assessment, we identify the areas of need and capabilities, focusing on how to maximize the family resources and link to services where need exists. Specific areas to evaluate relate to making a connection with service providers. Are the child and family receiving timely and efficient services? Is the care patient- and family-centered, allowing for the family to take a lead role in directing the plan of care?

While the individual may be the direct recipient of care, the family system is also disrupted. Families may require a great deal of education and ongoing reinforcement to accept realistic expectations for the child. Families and individuals with intellectual disabilities require lifelong support, so evaluations will focus on both short- and long-term goals. Long-term planning should include a goal of transitioning the child to a level of supervised or assisted care as he or she ages into adulthood.

AUTISM SPECTRUM DISORDER

Autism spectrum disorder is a complex neurobiological and developmental disability that typically appears during a child's first 3 years of life. Autism spectrum disorder affects the normal development of social interaction and communication skills. It ranges in severity from mild to moderate to severe.

Symptoms associated with autism spectrum disorder include deficits in social relatedness, which are manifested in disturbances in developing and maintaining relationships. Other behaviors include stereotypical repetitive speech, obsessive focus on specific objects, over adherence to routines or rituals, hyperreactivity or hyporeactivity to sensory input, and resistance to change. The symptoms will first occur in childhood and cause impairments in everyday functioning. The *DSM-5* box provides diagnostic criteria for autism spectrum disorder.

DSM-5 CRITERIA FOR AUTISM SPECTRUM DISORDER

A. Persistent deficits in social communication and social interaction across multiple contexts, as manifested by the following, currently or by history (examples are illustrative, not exhaustive):

1. Deficits in social-emotional reciprocity, ranging, for example, from abnormal social approach and failure of normal back-and-forth conversation to reduced sharing of interests, emotions, or affect to failure to initiate or respond to social interactions.
2. Deficits in nonverbal communicative behaviors used for social interaction, ranging, for example, from poorly integrated verbal and nonverbal communication to abnormalities in eye contact and body language or deficits in understanding and use of gestures to total lack of facial expressions or nonverbal communication.
3. Deficits in developing, maintaining, and understanding relationships, ranging, for example, from difficulties adjusting behavior to suit various social contexts to difficulties in sharing imaginative play or in making friends to an absence of interest in peers.

Specify current severity:

Severity is based on social communication impairments and restricted repetitive patterns of behavior.

B. Restricted, repetitive patterns of behavior, interests, or activities as manifested by at least two of the following, currently or by history (examples are illustrative, not exhaustive):

1. Stereotyped or repetitive motor movements, use of objects, or speech (e.g., simple motor stereotypies, lining up toys or flipping objects, echolalia, idiosyncratic phrases).
2. Insistence on sameness, excessive adherence to routines, or ritualized patterns of verbal or nonverbal behavior (e.g., extreme distress at small changes, difficulties with transitions, rigid thinking patterns, greeting rituals, need to take the same route or eat the same food every day).

3. Highly restricted, fixated interests that are abnormal in intensity or focus (e.g., strong attachment to or preoccupation with unusual objects, excessively circumscribed or perseverative interests).
4. Hyperreactivity or hyporeactivity to sensory input or unusual interest in sensory aspects of the environment (e.g., apparent indifference to pain/temperature, adverse response to specific sounds or textures, excessive smelling or touching of objects, visual fascination with lights or movement).

Specify current severity:

Severity is based on social communication impairments and restricted repetitive patterns of behavior.

C. Symptoms must be present in the early developmental period (but may not fully manifest until social demands exceed limited capacities, or may be masked by learned strategies in later life).
D. Symptoms together limit and impair everyday functioning.
E. These disturbances are not better explained by intellectual disability (intellectual developmental disorder) or global developmental delay. Intellectual disability and autism spectrum disorder frequently co-occur; in comorbid diagnoses of autism spectrum disorder and intellectual disability, social communication should be below that expected for general developmental level.

Specify if:

With or without accompanying intellectual impairment

With or without accompanying language impairment

Associated with a known medical or genetic condition or environmental factor

Associated with another neurodevelopmental, mental, or behavioral disorder

With catatonia

From American Psychiatric Association. (2013). *Diagnostic and statistical manual of mental disorders* (5th ed.). Washington, DC: Author.

There is a genetic component to autism spectrum disorder. The concordance rate for monozygotic (identical) twins is 70% to 90%, meaning that most of the time if one twin is affected so is the other. Autism spectrum disorder is four times more common in boys than girls (Autism Speaks, 2019). Autism spectrum disorder has no racial, ethnic, or social boundaries and is not influenced by family income, educational levels, or lifestyles.

Without intensive intervention, individuals with severe autism spectrum disorder may not be able to live and work independently. Only about one-third achieve partial independence, with restricted interests and activities. Early intervention for children with autism spectrum disorder can greatly enhance their potential for a full, productive life. Unfortunately, many families with a child with an autism spectrum disorder may not seek or have access to early interventions.

Often, symptoms are first noticed when the infant fails to be interested in others or to be socially responsive through eye contact and facial expressions. Some children show improvement during development, but puberty can be a turning point toward either improvement or deterioration.

Some individuals with autism spectrum disorder may have low IQs yet are brilliant in specific areas. These areas include musical, visual-spatial, or intellectual abilities such as photographic memory recall or the ability to complete complex mathematical calculations. This is a condition known as savant syndrome.

APPLICATION OF THE NURSING PROCESS

ASSESSMENT

ASSESSMENT GUIDELINES

Autism Spectrum Disorder

1. Assess for developmental delays, uneven development, or loss of acquired abilities. Use baby books and diaries, photographs, videotapes, or anecdotal reports from nonfamily caregivers.
2. Assess the child's communication skills (verbal and nonverbal), sensory, social, and behavioral skills (including presence of any aggressive or self-injurious behaviors).
3. Assess the parent-child relationship for evidence of bonding, anxiety, tension, and fit of temperaments.
4. Assess for physical and emotional signs of possible abuse. Be aware that children with behavioral and developmental problems are at risk for abuse.
5. Ensure that screening for comorbid intellectual disability has been completed.
6. Assess the need for community programs with support services for parents and children, including parent education, counseling, and after-school programs.

NURSING DIAGNOSIS

The child with autism spectrum disorder has severe impairments in social interactions and communication skills, often accompanied by stereotypical behavior, interests, and activities. At least half of those diagnosed with autism spectrum disorder will have some intellectual disability (IQ <85), which will impact their academic performance as well. The stress on the family can be severe due to the chronic nature of the disease. The severity of the impairment is evident in the degree of responsiveness to or interest in others, the presence of associated behavioral problems (e.g., head banging), and the ability to bond with peers. Refer to Table 11.1 for a list of potential nursing diagnoses.

OUTCOME IDENTIFICATION

A variety of outcomes are appropriate for the child with autism spectrum disorder and the family. Outcomes for social interaction skills include cooperating with others, exhibiting consideration, and exhibiting sensitivity to others. Communication skills outcomes include accurately interpreting messages and accurately exchanging messages. Family normalization is associated with adapting to the challenges of a child with autism spectrum disorder and using community support.

IMPLEMENTATION

Children with autism spectrum disorder should be referred to **early intervention programs** once communication and behavioral symptoms are identified, typically in the second or third year of life. Through case management and coordination of care, they may be treated in therapeutic nursery schools, day treatment programs, and special education classes in public or specialized private schools. Their education and treatment with therapeutic modalities are mandated under the Children with Disabilities Act.

Treatment plans include behavior management with a reward system, teaching parents to provide structure, rewards, consistency in rules, and expectations at home to shape and modify behavior and foster the development of socially appropriate skills. Children with autism spectrum disorder may receive physical, occupational, and speech therapy as part of the plan of care.

It is important that the nurse recognize and capitalize on the individual's and family's strengths. Also, the family's goals and priorities should influence the plan of care. The multidisciplinary team serves to guide and support the family in making realistic goals for their child.

EVALUATION

Autism spectrum disorder causes deficits in communication and social skills in the individual with a range of individual severity. The *DSM-5* (APA, 2013) classifies autism spectrum disorder in three levels depending on the degree of assistance and support the individual requires:

- Level 1 requires support
- Level 2 requires substantial support
- Level 3 requires very substantial support

For children with milder forms of autism spectrum disorder, it is reasonable to expect greater participation and input from the child with supports in place to help with transitions, changes in routine, and difficulties with social and emotional reciprocity. Individuals with level 2 or 3 require increasingly more support and have increasingly more profound impairments. Children with level 3 are nonverbal and need support with activities of daily living (ADLs). For individuals with more severe impairments, there will be greater reliance on the family. Family members must have clear and realistic expectations of the long-term needs of their child and be linked with the appropriate resources to assist with care and long-term planning.

Evaluation should target the family's awareness of how to advocate for appropriate service provision. Has the early intervention program been accessed? How are the child and family coordinating appointments? For the school-aged child, is the early intervention plan reflective of realistic educational goals?

The nurse should monitor both the individual and the family for the effects of stress. Increased stress may interfere with the family's ability to utilize resources, or family members may find the coordination and integration of services to be overwhelming.

TREATMENT MODALITIES

Biological Treatments

Pharmacotherapy

Pharmacological agents target specific symptoms and may be used to improve relatedness and decrease anxiety, compulsive behaviors, or agitation. The second-generation antipsychotics risperidone (Risperdal) and aripiprazole (Abilify) have FDA approval for treating children with autism-associated agitation. These drugs improve irritability that is expressed in severe temper tantrums, aggression, and compulsive behavior. By reducing irritability, they may also improve relatedness. Side effects are significant and include extrapyramidal side effects, somnolence, and weight gain.

Other medications may be used off-label. Selective serotonin reuptake inhibitors (SSRIs) may improve mood and reduce anxiety, which provides the patient with a higher degree of tolerance for new situations and social interactions. Stimulant medications may be used to target hyperactivity, impulsivity, or inattention. Naltrexone, a drug used for addictive disorders, may reduce disability repetitive and self-injurious behaviors.

Psychological Therapies

Applied Behavior Analysis (ABA) encourages positive behaviors and discourages negative behaviors. The child's progress is tracked and measured. The Early Intensive Behavioral Intervention (EIBI) has the strongest evidence for improving language and cognitive skills in children with autism spectrum disorder (Hong et al., 2019). This long-term (several years), intensive (up to 40 hours a week) approach combines operant conditioning (reinforcement and negative consequences) and ABA. The Early Start Denver Model (ESDM) is also evidence based. Developmental considerations focusing on one-on-one interactions, joint play, and activity routines with the adult and child are used as teaching opportunities.

ATTENTION-DEFICIT/HYPERACTIVITY DISORDER

Individuals with **attention-deficit/hyperactivity disorder** show an inappropriate degree of inattention, impulsiveness, and hyperactivity. Some children are inattentive but not hyperactive. In this case, the diagnosis is still ADHD and is then further classified as primarily inattentive type (previously known as ADD).

To diagnose a child with ADHD, symptoms must be present in at least two settings (e.g., at home and school) and occur before age 12. The disorder is most often detected when the child has difficulty adjusting to elementary school. Attention problems and hyperactivity contribute to low frustration tolerance, temper outbursts, labile moods, poor school performance, peer rejection, and low self-esteem.

The behaviors and symptoms associated with ADHD can include hyperactivity and impulsivity. Peer relationships are strained due to difficulty taking turns, poor social boundaries, intrusive behaviors, and interrupting others. Those with the inattentive type of ADHD may exhibit high degrees of distractibility and disorganization. They may be unable to complete challenging or tedious tasks, become easily bored, lose things frequently, or require frequent prompts to complete tasks. The *DSM-5* box provides diagnostic criteria for ADHD.

DSM-5 CRITERIA FOR ATTENTION-DEFICIT/HYPERACTIVITY DISORDER

A. A persistent pattern of inattention and/or hyperactivity-impulsivity that interferes with functioning or development, as characterized by (1) and/or (2):

1. **Inattention**: Six (or more) of the following symptoms have persisted for at least 6 months to a degree inconsistent with developmental level and that negatively impacts directly on social and academic/occupational activities:

   Note: The symptoms are not solely a manifestation of oppositional behavior, defiance, hostility, or failure to understand tasks or instructions. For older adolescents and adults (age 17 and older), at least five symptoms are required.

   a. Often fails to give close attention to details or makes careless mistakes in schoolwork, at work, or during other activities (e.g., overlooks or misses details, work is inaccurate).

   b. Often has difficulty sustaining attention in tasks or play activities (e.g., has difficulty remaining focused during lectures, conversations, or lengthy reading).

   c. Often does not seem to listen when spoken to directly (e.g., mind seems elsewhere, even in the absence of any obvious distraction).

   d. Often does not follow through on instructions and fails to finish schoolwork, chores, or duties in the workplace (e.g., starts task but quickly loses focus and is easily sidetracked).

   e. Often has difficulty organizing tasks and activities (e.g., difficulty managing sequential tasks, difficulty keeping materials and belongings in order, messy disorganized work, has poor time management, fails to meet deadlines).

   f. Often avoids, dislikes, or is reluctant to engage in tasks that require sustained mental effort (e.g., schoolwork or homework; for older adolescents and adults, preparing reports, completing forms, reviewing lengthy papers).

   g. Often loses things necessary for tasks or activities (e.g., school materials, pencils, books, tools, wallets, keys, paperwork, eyeglasses, mobile telephones).

   h. Is often easily distracted by extraneous stimuli (for older adolescents and adults, may include unrelated thoughts).

   i. Is often forgetful in daily activities (e.g., doing chores, running errands; for older adolescents and adults, returning calls, paying bills, keeping appointments).

2. **Hyperactivity and impulsivity**: Six (or more) of the following symptoms have persisted for at least 6 months to a degree inconsistent with development level and that negatively impacts directly on social and academic/occupational activities:

   Note: The symptoms are not solely a manifestation of oppositional behavior, defiance, hostility, or a failure to understand tasks or instructions. For older adolescents and adults (age 17 and older), at least five symptoms are required.

   a. Often fidgets with or taps hands or feet or squirms in seat.

   b. Often leaves seat in situations when remaining seated is expected (e.g., leaves his or her place in the classroom, in the office or other workplace, or in situations that require remaining in place).

   c. Often runs about or climbs in situations where it is inappropriate. (**Note**: In adolescents or adults, may be limited to feeling restless.)

   d. Often unable to play or engage in leisure activities quietly.

   e. Is often "on the go," acting as if "driven by a motor" (e.g., is unable to be or uncomfortable being still for extended time, as in restaurants, meetings; may be experienced by others as being restless or difficult to keep up with).

   f. Often talks excessively.

   g. Often blurts out an answer before a question has been completed (e.g., completes people's sentences; cannot wait for turn in conversation).

   h. Often has difficulty waiting for his or her turn (e.g., while waiting in line).

   i. Often interrupts or intrudes on others (e.g., butts into conversations, games, or activities; may start using other people's things without asking or receiving permission; for adolescents and adults, may intrude into or take over what others are doing).

B. Several inattentive or hyperactive-impulsive symptoms were present before age 12.

C. Several inattentive or hyperactive-impulsive symptoms are present in two or more settings (e.g., at home, school, or work; with friends or relatives; in other activities).

D. There is clear evidence that the symptoms interfere with, or reduce the quality of, social, academic, or occupational functioning.

E. The symptoms do not occur exclusively during the course of schizophrenia or another psychotic disorder and are not better explained by another mental disorder (e.g., mood disorder, anxiety disorder, dissociative disorder, personality disorder, substance intoxication or withdrawal).

Specify if: **In partial remission**: When full criteria were previously met, fewer than the full criteria have been met for the past 6 months, and the symptoms still result in impairment in social, academic, or occupational functioning.

From American Psychiatric Association. (2013). *Diagnostic and statistical manual of mental disorders* (5th ed.). Washington, DC: Author.

About 10% of children and adolescents between the ages of 5 and 17 have ADHD. It affects about 14% of boys and about 6% of girls in that same age range (CDC, 2016). Children in poor health are more than twice as likely to have ADHD (21% versus 8%). The median age of onset is 7 years old. However, some people may go undiagnosed until functional impairments become noticeable in adulthood.

Children with ADHD are often diagnosed with comorbid disorders such as oppositional defiant disorder or conduct disorder. Other comorbid disorders include conduct disorder, disruptive mood dysregulation disorder, and specific learning disorder.

APPLICATION OF THE NURSING PROCESS
ASSESSMENT

ASSESSMENT GUIDELINES
Attention-Deficit/Hyperactivity Disorder

1. Gather data from parents, caregivers, teachers, or other adults involved with the child. Ask about level of physical activity, span, talkativeness, frustration tolerance, impulse control, and the ability to follow directions and complete tasks. Also, assess these areas through your own observations and note any developmental variance in these behaviors.
2. Assess social skills, friendship history, problem-solving skills, and school performance. Gather this data from the family or caregiver and one or two additional sources.
3. Assess for comorbidities such as anxiety and depression.
4. Assess for any indicators of learning disorders, autism spectrum disorder, or intellectual disabilities.
5. Gather data on eating and sleeping patterns and monitor these regularly for the child treated with stimulants.

NURSING DIAGNOSIS

Children and adolescents with ADHD can be overactive and may display disruptive behaviors that are impulsive, angry, aggressive, and often dangerous. They may have difficulty with maintaining attention in situations that require sustained attention. In addition, their behaviors negatively impact their ability to develop fulfilling peer and family relationships. They are often in conflict with others, are noncompliant, do not follow age-appropriate social norms, and may use inappropriate ways to meet their needs. Refer to Table 11.1 for potential nursing diagnoses.

OUTCOMES IDENTIFICATION

Outcomes appropriate for the child with ADHD target hyperactivity, impulse self-control, freedom from injury, improved social relationships, the development of self-identity and self-esteem, positive coping skills, and family functioning.

IMPLEMENTATION

Interventions for patients with ADHD focus on recognizing ineffective coping mechanisms, such as blaming others and denial of responsibility for their actions. Children and adolescents can be helped to adopt adaptive coping mechanisms and pro-social goals.

Treatment may include hospitalization for those who are an imminent danger to self or others. Typically, treatment is provided on an outpatient basis, using individual, group, and family therapy, with an emphasis on parenting issues. Children whose behavior requires longer-term intensive treatment may be referred to intensive outpatient programs and specialized charter schools. Residential treatment or group home placement may even be an option.

Families are actively engaged in therapy and given support in using parenting skills to provide nurturance and set consistent limits. They are taught techniques for modifying behavior; monitoring medication for effects; collaborating with teachers to foster academic success; and setting up a home environment that is consistent, structured, and nurturing and that promotes achievement of normal developmental milestones. If families are abusive, drug dependent, or highly disorganized, the child may require out-of-home placement.

Box 11.3 lists techniques for managing disruptive behaviors.

EVALUATION

For the family and child with ADHD, evaluation will focus on the symptom patterns and severity. For those with ADHD, inattentive type, the focus of evaluation will be academic performance, activities of daily living, social relationships, and personal perception. For those with ADHD, hyperactive-impulsive type, or combined type, the focus will be on academic performance, social skills and relationships, impulse control, and behavioral responses.

For all children with neurobiological disorders, safety is a major emphasis and an important subject of evaluation. Young people who have ADHD can have difficulties in assessing the environment or realistically assessing risks of danger. When aggressive or disruptive behaviors are present, there is always the potential for harm.

At the family system level, the nurse will assess the degree of understanding of symptoms and symptom management by family members. Unrealistic expectations can result in frustration for both the individual and family and yield unfulfilling or negative interpersonal relationships. What is the family's perception of the problem? What types of services do they need to support their attempts in implementing effective behavioral plans? Has the family system stabilized?

Finally, long-term planning and goal setting should be a core evaluation measure. ADHD is chronic and unremitting, and symptoms frequently persist into adulthood. Are the patient and family setting realistic expectations as the child prepares to transition to postsecondary education or a vocation? Has the patient assumed primary responsibility for treatment planning and symptom management? Supporting the patient and family in the decision-making process and linking them with any additional resources can assist in a smooth transition.

BOX 11.3   Techniques for Managing Disruptive Behaviors

Behavioral contract: A verbal or written agreement between the patient and nurse or other parties (e.g., family, treatment team, teacher) about behaviors, expectations, and needs. The contract is periodically evaluated and reviewed and typically coupled with rewards and other contingencies, positive and negative.

Collaborative and proactive solutions: A therapeutic intervention used with parents and children designed to help both identify and define problematic behaviors, specific triggers, and develop a collaborative method for creating mutually agreeable solutions to the specific situation or trigger.

Counseling: Verbal interactions, role-playing, and modeling to teach, coach, or maintain adaptive behavior and provide positive reinforcement. Best used with motivated youth and those with well-developed communication and self-reflective skills.

Modeling: A method of learning behaviors or skills by observation and imitation that can be used in a wide variety of situations. It is enhanced when the modeler is perceived to be similar (e.g., age, interests) and attending to the task is required.

Role-playing: A counseling technique in which the nurse, the patient, or a group of youngsters acts out a specified script or role to enhance their understanding of that role, learn and practice new behaviors or skills, and practice specific situations. It requires well-developed expressive and receptive language skills.

Planned ignoring: When behaviors are determined by staff to be attention seeking and not dangerous, they may be ignored. Additional interventions may be used in conjunction (e.g., positive reinforcement for on-task actions).

Use of signals or gestures: Use a word, a gesture, or eye contact to remind the child to use self-control. To help promote behavioral change, this may be used in conjunction with a behavioral contract and a reward system. An example is placing your finger to your lips and making eye contact with a child who is talking during a quiet drawing activity.

Physical distance and touch control: Moving closer to the child for a calming effect, perhaps putting an arm around the child (with permission). Evaluate the effect of this because some children may find this more agitating and may need more space and less physical closeness. It also may involve putting the nurse or a staff member between certain children who have a history of conflict.

Redirection: A technique used after an undesirable or inappropriate behavior to engage or re-engage an individual in an appropriate activity. It may involve the use of verbal directives (e.g., setting firm limits), gestures, or physical prompts.

Additional affection: Involves giving a child planned emotional support for a specific problem or engaging in an enjoyable activity. It can be used to redirect a child away from an undesirable activity as well. This shows acceptance of the child while ignoring the behavior and can increase rapport in the nurse-patient relationship.

Use of humor: Use well-timed appropriate kidding about some external non-personal (to the child) event as a diversion to help the child save face and relieve feelings of guilt or fear.

Clarification as intervention: Breaking down a problem situation that a child experiences can help the child understand the situation, the roles of others, and his or her own motivation for the behavior. This can be done verbally and using worksheets depending on the age and functional level of the child.

Restructuring: Changing an activity in a way that will decrease the stimulation or frustration (e.g., shorten a story or change to a physical activity). This requires flexibility and planning and an alternative if the activity is not going well.

Limit setting: Involves giving direction, stating an expectation, or telling a child what to do or where to go. Caregivers should do this firmly, calmly, without judgment or anger, preferably in advance of any problem behavior occurring, and all staff should do this consistently in a treatment setting. An example would be, "I would like for you to stop turning the light on and off."

Simple restitution: Refers to a procedure in which an individual is required or expected to correct the adverse environmental or relational effects of his or her misbehavior by restoring the environment to its prior state, making a plan to correct his or her actions with the nurse, and implementing the plan (e.g., apologizing to the people harmed, fixing the chairs that are upturned).

Physical restraint: Using mechanical means to control and protect the child from impulses to act out and hurt self or others.

TREATMENT MODALITIES

Biological Treatments

Pharmacotherapy

Paradoxically, we treat the symptoms of ADHD with stimulant drugs. Responses to these drugs are often dramatic and can quickly increase attention and task-directed behavior while reducing impulsivity, restlessness, and distractibility (Lehne, 2016). Methylphenidate (Ritalin and others) and the mixed amphetamine salts (Adderall) are the most widely used stimulants because of their relative safety and simplicity of use. As with any controlled substance, however, there is a risk of misuse, such as the sale of the medication on the street or the use by people for whom the medication was not intended.

Not surprisingly, insomnia is a common side effect while taking stimulant medications. Treating with the minimum effective dose is essential. Administering medications no later than 4:00 in the afternoon or lowering the last dose of the day helps. The extended-release formulations of these medications have improved dosing and scheduling. The long-acting versions allow for a morning administration with sustained release of the medication over the course of the day and with a decreased incidence of insomnia. Other common side effects include appetite suppression, headache, abdominal pain, and lethargy.

A nonstimulant selective norepinephrine reuptake inhibitor, atomoxetine (Strattera), is approved for childhood and adult ADHD. Therapeutic responses develop slowly, and it may take up to 6 weeks for full improvement. This medication is preferable for individuals whose anxiety is increased with stimulants. It is also useful for those with comorbid anxiety, active substance use disorders, or tics.

The most common side effects of atomoxetine are gastrointestinal disturbances, urinary retention, dizziness, fatigue, and insomnia. It may also cause liver injury in some patients and a small increase in blood pressure and heart rate. Ongoing monitoring of vital signs and regular screening of liver function are key aspects of assessment. Rarely, serious allergic reactions occur. Patients and their families should be clearly educated on the risks and benefits of treatment before starting this medication. Atomoxetine should be used with extreme caution in those patients with comorbid depression since its use has been associated with an increased suicidal ideation. See Table 11.2 for a summary of the FDA approved medications used to treat ADHD.

Two centrally acting alpha-2 adrenergic agonists, clonidine (Kapvay/Catapres) and guanfacine (Intuniv/Tenex), are FDA approved for the treatment of ADHD. They may be used alone or in conjunction with other ADHD medications. Of the two

TABLE 11.2   FDA Approved Drugs for Attention-Deficit/Hyperactivity Disorder

Generic Name	Trade Name	Indications	Duration	Schedule
Stimulants				
Amphetamine	Adzenys XR-ODT	Ages 6 and older	12 h	Once a day
	Dyanavel XR	Ages 6 and older	12 h	Once a day
	Evekeo	Ages 3 and older	4–6 h	Two or three times a day
Dexmethylphenidate	Focalin	Ages 6 and older	4–5 h	Two times a day
	Focalin XR	Ages 6 and older	8–12 h	Once a day
Dextroamphetamine	Dexedrine	Ages 3–16	4–6 h	Two or three times a day
	ProCentra	Ages 3–16	4–6 h	Two or three times a day
	Zenzedi	Ages 3–16	4–6 h	Two or three times a day
Lisdexamfetamine dimesylate	Vyvanse	Ages 6 and older	10–12 h	Once a day
Methamphetamine	Desoxyn	Ages 6 and older	6–8 h	One or two times a day
Methylphenidate HCL	Adhansia XR	Ages 6 and older	10–12 h	Once a day
	Aptensio XR	Ages 6 and older	10–12 h	Once a day
	Concerta, Relexxii	Ages 6–65	10–12 h	Once a day
	Cotempla XR-ODT	Ages 6–17	10–12 h	Once a day
	Daytrana (transdermal patch)	Ages 6–17	10–12 h (up to 3 h after removal)	Once a day
	Jornay PM	Ages 6 and older	10–12 h	Once a day in the evening
	Metadate ER	Ages 6–15	6–8 h	One or two times a day
	Metadate CD	Ages 6–15	6–8 h	Once a day
	Methylin ER	Ages 6 and older	6–8 h	Once a day
	Mydayis	Ages 13 and older	Up to 16 h	Once a day
	Quillichew ER	Ages 6 and older	12 h	Once a day
	Quillivant XR	Ages 6–17	12 h	Once a day
	Ritalin	Ages 6–12	6–8 h	One or two times a day
	Ritalin LA	Ages 6–12	7–9 h	Once a day
	Ritalin SR	Ages 6–12	6–8 h	One or two times a day
Mixed salts of a single-entity amphetamine product	Adderall	Ages 6 and older	4–6 h	Two times a day
	Adderall–XR	Ages 6 and older	10–12 h	One or two times a day
Nonstimulants				
Atomoxetine	Strattera	Ages 6–65	24 h	One or two times a day
Clonidine	Kapvay/Catapres	Ages 6–17	24 h	Two times a day
Guanfacine	Intuniv/Tenex	Ages 6–17	24 h	Once a day

ADHD, Attention-deficit/hyperactivity disorder; *FDA,* Food and Drug Administration.
Food and Drug Administration. (2019). *FDA online label repository.* Retrieved from http://labels.fda.gov.

drugs, clonidine carries more side effects: somnolence, fatigue, insomnia, nightmares, irritability, constipation, respiratory symptoms, and dry mouth. The most common side effects of guanfacine are somnolence, lethargy, fatigue, insomnia, nausea, dizziness, hypotension, and abdominal pain.

Medication for aggressive behaviors. To control aggressive behaviors, pharmacological agents—including stimulants, mood stabilizers, alpha-adrenergic agonists, and antipsychotics—are used. Stimulants have a dose-dependent effect. Low doses stimulate aggressive behaviors while moderate to high doses suppress aggression. Mood stabilizers such as lithium and anticonvulsants reduce aggressive behavior and are recommended for impulsivity, explosive temper, and mood lability.

Due to the side effects of fatigue and somnolence, clonidine and guanfacine are helpful in reducing agitation and rage and in increasing frustration tolerance. Antipsychotic medications have reduced violent behavior, hyperactivity, and social unresponsiveness. Due to the risk of tardive dyskinesia and metabolic problems associated with long-term use, antipsychotic medications are only recommended for severely aggressive behavior.

Psychological Therapies

In patients younger than 6 years of age, parent training in behavior therapy is the first line of treatment before medication is prescribed. For children older than 6, parental training in behavior therapy along with medication is indicated. Behavior therapy teaches parents skills and strategies to help their child with ADHD succeed at home, school, and socially.

CBT is used to change the pattern of misconduct by fostering the development of internal controls and working with the family to improve coping and support. Development of problem solving, conflict resolution, empathy, and social skills is an important component of the treatment program.

■ KEY POINTS TO REMEMBER

- One in five children and adolescents in the United States suffers from a major mental illness that causes significant impairments at home, at school, with peers, and in the community.
- Factors known to affect the development of mental and emotional problems in children and adolescents include genetic influences, biochemical (prenatal and postnatal) factors, temperament, psychosocial developmental factors, social and environmental factors, and cultural influences.
- The characteristics of a resilient child include an adaptable temperament, the ability to form nurturing relationships with surrogate parental figures, the ability to distance the self from emotional chaos in parents and family, good social intelligence, the ability to perceive a future, and problem-solving skills.
- Use seclusion and restraint as last resorts after less restrictive interventions have failed and only in the case of dangerous behavior toward self or others. Seclusion and restraint require continuous monitoring by trained staff and must not be used as a punishment. Notify parents/guardians if such measures are used.
- Communication disorders are a deficit in language skills acquisition that creates impairments in academic achievement, socialization, or getting self-care.
- Motor disorders are manifested by impairments in gross and fine motor skill acquisition. They can range from mild to profound in severity. Purposeless, repetitive movements that interfere with daily living activities characterize stereotypic movement disorders.

- Tics are sudden, nonrhythmic, and rapid motor movements or vocalizations. Tic disorders vary in severity and degree of interference with the child's social and academic functioning.
- Learning disorders may be in the areas of reading, mathematics, or written expression, with performance in those areas below the level expected for the age and cognitive level. Interventions are designated in an IEP and provided through special education in public schools.
- Autism spectrum disorder typically occurs within the first 3 years of life, yielding deficits in social interaction and communication skills. Children with autism spectrum disorder are referred to early intervention programs and continue to receive school-based services as they enter the public education system.
- ADHD is evidenced by symptoms of inattentiveness and/or hyperactivity and impulsivity that are developmentally inappropriate. These disorders cause the child problems in a number of settings, such as home, school, and community. ADHD is treated primarily with stimulant medications and behavioral therapies.
- Treatment of childhood and adolescent disorders requires a multimodal approach in almost all instances, and family involvement is seen as critical to improvement in outcomes.
- Nurses can be important advocates for children with severe emotional and behavioral disorders.

■ CRITICAL THINKING

1. Bettina, a 12-year-old girl, has been diagnosed with autism spectrum disorder, moderate severity. She has an Individualized Education Program (IEP) that includes remedial reading; occupational therapy to assist with her skills in feeding, dressing, and safety; and a weekly social skills group to improve relational and communication skills.
   a. Describe the specific behavioral data you would find on assessment in terms of (1) communication, (2) social interactions, and (3) behaviors and activities.
   b. Name a minimum of three specific measurable and behavioral nursing outcomes for a child with autism spectrum disorder.

   c. Which nursing and behavioral interventions do you think are the most important for a preadolescent with autism spectrum disorder? Identify at least six.
   d. List three types of community-based resources to which the family should be referred.
2. Carlos is a 6-year-old boy in first grade diagnosed with attention-deficit/hyperactivity disorder (ADHD), combined type.
   a. Describe behaviors he might be exhibiting at home and in the classroom. Identify specific behavioral examples of his (1) inattention, (2) hyperactivity, and (3) impulsivity and the correlated neurotransmitter involved.

b. Develop a nursing care plan with two priority nursing diagnoses.

c. Identify at least six intervention strategies one might use for him, including a discussion of the use of medication management. Identify at least two different medications that could be used, and identify their intended effect, potential side effects, and key patient teaching information.

d. Describe the concept of redirecting and planned ignoring and how it could be used therapeutically with Carlos.

CHAPTER REVIEW

1. Which statement demonstrates a well-structured attempt at limit setting?
   a. "Hitting me when you are angry is unacceptable."
   b. "I expect you to behave yourself during dinner."
   c. "Come here, right now!"
   d. "Good boys don't bite."

2. Which activity is most appropriate for a child with ADHD?
   a. Reading an adventure novel
   b. Monopoly
   c. Checkers
   d. Tennis

3. Cognitive-behavioral therapy is going well when a 12-year-old patient in therapy reports to the nurse practitioner:
   a. "I was so mad I wanted to hit my mother."
   b. "I thought that everyone at school hated me. That's not true. Most people like me and I have a friend named Todd."
   c. "I forgot that you told me to breathe when I become angry."
   d. "I scream as loud as I can when the train goes by the house."

4. What assessment question should the nurse ask when attempting to determine a teenager's mental health resilience? *Select all that apply.*
   a. "How did you cope when your father deployed with the Army for a year in Iraq?"
   b. "Who did you go to for advice while your father was away for a year in Iraq?"
   c. "How do you feel about talking to a mental health counselor?"
   d. "Where do you see yourself in 10 years?"
   e. "Do you like the school you go to?"

5. Which factors tend to increase the difficulty of diagnosing young children who demonstrate behaviors associated with mental illness? *Select all that apply.*
   a. Limited language skills
   b. Level of cognitive development
   c. Level of emotional development
   d. Parental denial that a problem exists
   e. Severity of the typical mental illnesses observed in young children

6. Pam, the nurse educator, is teaching a new nurse about seclusion and restraint. Order the following interventions from least (1) to most (5) restrictive:
   a. With the patient, identify the behaviors that are unacceptable and consequences associated with harmful behaviors
   b. Placing the patient in physical restraints

   c. Allowing the patient to take a time-out and sit in his or her room
   d. Offering a PRN medication by mouth
   e. Placing the patient in a locked seclusion room

7. In pediatric mental health, there is a lack of sufficient numbers of community-based resources and providers, and there are long waiting lists for services. This has resulted in: *Select all that apply.*
   a. Children of color and poor economic conditions being underserved
   b. Increased stress in the family unit
   c. Markedly increased funding
   d. Premature termination of services

8. Child protective services have removed 10-year-old Christopher from his parents' home due to neglect. Christopher reveals to the nurse that he considers the woman next door his "nice" mom, that he loves school, and gets above average grades. The strongest explanation of this response is:
   a. Temperament
   b. Genetic factors
   c. Resilience
   d. Paradoxical effects of neglect

9. April, a 10-year-old admitted to inpatient pediatric care, has been getting more and more wound up and is losing self-control in the day room. Time-out does not appear to be an effective tool for April to engage in self-reflection. April's mother admits to putting her in time-out up to 20 times a day. The nurse recognizes that:
   a. Time-out is an important part of April's baseline discipline.
   b. Time-out is no longer an effective therapeutic measure.
   c. April enjoys time-out and acts out to get some alone time.
   d. Time-out will need to be replaced with seclusion and restraint.

10. Adolescents often display fluctuations in mood along with undeveloped emotional regulation and poor tolerance for frustration. Emotional and behavioral control usually increases over the course of adolescence due to:
    a. Limited executive function
    b. Cerebellum maturation
    c. Cerebral stasis and hormonal changes
    d. A slight reduction in brain volume

1. **a**; 2. **d**; 3. **b**; 4. **a, b, d**; 5. **a, b, c**; 6. **a-1, b-5, c-3, d-2, e-4**; 7. **a, b, d**; 8. **c**; 9. **b**; 10. **b**

NGN CASE STUDY AND QUESTIONS

PHASE 1

Ming is a 12-year-old boy with autism spectrum disorder. He is ambulatory but is nonverbal. In the morning, Ming prefers the following schedule: His dad gets him out of bed and takes him to the bathroom while his mom plays his favorite YouTube clip from *Mister Rogers' Neighborhood*. They do this to encourage him to urinate, but his use of the toilet is inconsistent and he needs daily diapering. His parents know not to flush the toilet around him because the sound is disturbing to Ming. He does not really participate in dressing himself, but he does like the sound of the Velcro that his parents use on all of his clothing. Once he is dressed, his dad walks him to the kitchen, where his mom has made oatmeal with raisins, sliced banana, and cinnamon. If the bananas are not ripe, he becomes upset, so they have learned to freeze ripe banana slices ahead of time. After breakfast, Ming sits on the floor continuously spinning a beach ball.

1. Which of Ming's specific behaviors are consistent with the criteria for autism spectrum disorder? *Select all that apply.*
   a. Extreme distress at small changes
   b. Insistence on sameness
   c. Picky eating
   d. Deficits in mathematics
   e. Repetitive motor movements
   f. Hyperreactivity to sensory input
   g. Highly restricted, fixated interests
   h. Inability to learn to play a musical instrument

2. Choose the *most likely* options to complete the following statement.
   Based on his basic needs both at home and at school, this individual is *most likely* on _____1_____ of the autism spectrum disorder, particularly because he _____2_____ and _____3_____.

Options for 1	Options for 2	Options for 3
a. Level 1	a. Requires the most assistance with personal care and support	a. Can be expected to participate and provide input in activities

Options for 1	Options for 2	Options for 3
b. Level 2	b. Requires substantial assistance and support	b. Is nonverbal
c. Level 3	c. Requires the least support and can be independent	c. Can verbally negotiate and express his needs and wants and respond in kind

PHASE 2

Ming has been attending an extended-day school for 3 weeks. When Ming's parents arrive after school, the mother states, "This isn't getting easier. Working full-time, we are both overwhelmed. Sometimes we don't have a clue whether we are doing things right." His father states, "When he gets upset, Ming bites toys and even furniture. He hits himself and us. What should we be doing?" The nurse welcomes this opportunity to provide support and decides she will start with discussing Ming's priority needs.

3. Identify needs that are a priority for Ming at this time. *Select all that apply.*

Nursing Diagnoses	Priority Concerns
a. Risk for suicide	
b. Risk for injury	
c. Impaired caregiver child attachment	
d. Self-care deficit	
e. Risk for caregiver stress	
f. Risk for nutritional deficit	

4. Identify the nursing actions as 1. indicated (appropriate or necessary), 2. contraindicated (could be harmful), or 3. nonessential (not necessary) for the patient's care at this time. *Only one selection can be made for each nursing action.*

Nursing Action	1. Indicated	2. Contraindicated	3. Nonessential
a. Assess family stress levels, and teach coping mechanisms			
b. Implement behavior management strategies to help him adjust to new situations			
c. Establish a written behavioral contract between the child, music therapist, family, and treatment team regarding his expectations and needs			
d. Engage child in role playing, with the child acting out a specified script to enhance his understanding of his role			

Nursing Action	1. Indicated	2. Contraindicated	3. Nonessential
e. Redirect undesirable behavior with verbal directives that set firm limits			
f. Provide a substantial snack before the activity of interest			
g. Implement a reward system to recognize behaviors that demonstrate adaptation to new circumstances (e.g., sitting in the music class, engaging by playing the maraca)			
h. Review home plan—including structure, consistencies, and expectations—with the parents, focusing on any additional needs for support			

PHASE 3

The school's intervention team, including his parents, agree that Ming might adjust to his new school better with the introduction of two specific treatments. The first is pharmacotherapy that will relieve some of his anxiety while he adjusts to this new environment. Options are presented to the parents along with expected therapeutic responses and side effects.

The second treatment is a behavioral intervention used to gradually improve tolerance and participation through a series of small steps. At first, the music therapist sits with Ming and listens to his music from *The Jungle Book*. After several sessions, the therapist invites another student to listen as well. Both children respond independently, with Ming spinning a beach ball and the other student rocking. After adding several more students, the music therapist sits next to Ming with a hand cymbal on the floor between them. The therapist moves a soft brush over the cymbal, then leaves this at the side. Ming smiled slightly at the sound it made. The parents do the same at home with the brush and cymbal. One day during class, he briefly picks up the brush, touches it to the cymbal, runs his hand across the cymbal, sets it down, and spins the ball.

5. For each drug characteristic, indicate the corresponding drug classification. *Only one selection can be made.*

Drug Characteristic	1. Second-Generation Antipsychotics	2. Selective Serotonin Reuptake Inhibitors	3. Stimulants
a. Addresses autism-associated agitation			
b. Treats comorbid attention-deficit/hyperactivity disorder (ADHD) symptoms			
c. Treats mood and anxiety symptoms associated with autism spectrum disorder			
d. Side effects include extrapyramidal side effects			
e. Intended to target hyperactivity, impulsivity, or inattention			

6. The following are the nurse's own notes on today's observations. Identify the findings that indicate that the plan of care is effective. *Select all that apply.*
   a. Listens to music with others
   b. Others in class enjoy the student's music
   c. Sits near or alongside others
   d. Touches brush and cymbal at home
   e. Smiles slightly at the sound of the brush
   f. Runs his hand across the cymbal
   g. Spins beach ball and continues to rock

NGN case study answers are on Evolve.

Visit the Evolve website for a posttest on the content in this chapter: http://evolve.elsevier.com/Varcarolis

REFERENCES

American Nurses Association (ANA), American Psychiatric-Mental Health Nurses Association (APNA), & International Society of Psychiatric-Mental Health Nurses (ISPN). (2014). *Psychiatric mental health nursing: Scope and standards of practice*. Silver Spring, MD: American Nurses Association.

American Psychiatric Association. (2013). *Diagnostic and statistical manual of mental disorders* (5th ed.). Washington, DC: Author.

American Psychiatric Association. (2015). *Individuals with Disabilities in Education Act*. Retrieved from http://www.apa.org/about/gr/issues/disability/idea.aspx.

American Speech, Language, & Hearing Association. (2019). *Early identification of speech, language and hearing disorders*. Retrieved from https://www.asha.org/public/Early-Identification-of-Speech-Language-and-Hearing-Disorders/.

American Speech, Language, & Hearing Association. (2019). *Intellectual disability*. Retrieved from https://www.asha.org/PRPSpecificTopic.aspx?folderid=8589942540&section=Incidence_and_Prevalence.

Autism Speaks. (2019). *Autism facts and figures*. Retrieved from https://www.autismspeaks.org/autism-facts-and-figures.

Centers for Disease Control and Prevention. (2019). *Adverse childhood experiences (ACEs)*. Retrieved from https://www.cdc.gov/violenceprevention/childabuseandneglect/acestudy/index.html.

Centers for Disease Control and Prevention. (2019). *Tourette syndrome*. Retrieved from https://www.cdc.gov/features/tourettesyndromeawareness/index.html.

Hong, D. S., Fung, L. K., & Hardan, A. (2019). Neurodevelopmental disorders. In L. W. Roberts (Ed.), *Textbook of psychiatry* (7th ed.) (pp. 225–255). Washington, DC: American Psychiatric Association.

Lehne, R. A. (2016). *Pharmacology for nursing care* (9th ed.). Philadelphia, PA: Saunders.

Menzies, L., Goddings, A., Whitaker, K. J., Blakemore, S. J., & Viner, R. M. (2015). The effects of puberty on white matter development in boys. *Developmental Cognitive Neuroscience, 11*, 116–128.

National Center for Learning Disorders. (2017). *The state of LD: Understanding 1 in 5*. Retrieved from https://www.ncld.org/news/newsroom/the-state-of-ld-understanding-the-1-in-5/#:~:text=One%20in%20five%20children%20in,difficulties%2C%20and%2033%20percent%20of.

National Child Traumatic Stress Network. (2019). *Childhood trauma*. Retrieved from https://www.nctsn.org/what-is-child-trauma/trauma-types.

National Council for Behavioral Health. (2019). *FY2020 health spending package passes house*. Retrieved from https://www.thenationalcouncil.org/capitol-connector/2019/06/fy-2020-health-spending-package-passes-house/.

Substance Abuse Mental Health Administration. (2018). *SAMHSA strategic plan FY2019-FY2023*. Retrieved from https://www.samhsa.gov/about-us/strategic-plan.

US Department of Health & Human Services. (2016). *Child maltreatment 2014*. Retrieved from http://www.acf.hhs.gov/sites/default/files/cb/cm2014.pdf.

Zoloski, S., & Bullock, l (2012). Resilience in children and youth: A review. *Children and Youth Services Review, 4*(12), 2295–2303.

Schizophrenia Spectrum Disorders

Edward A. Herzog

🌐 Visit the Evolve website for a pretest on the content in this chapter: http://evolve.elsevier.com/Varcarolis

OBJECTIVES

1. Differentiate among the schizophrenia spectrum disorders.
2. Discuss at least three of the neurobiological findings indicating that schizophrenia is a brain disorder.
3. Differentiate the positive and negative symptoms of schizophrenia in terms of treatment and effect on quality of life.
4. Discuss how to deal with common reactions the nurse may experience in working with a patient with schizophrenia.
5. Create a nursing care plan incorporating evidence-based intervention for symptoms of psychosis, including hallucinations, delusions, paranoia, cognitive disorganization, anosognosia, and impaired self-care.
6. Demonstrate or role-play interventions for a patient who is experiencing hallucinations, delusions, and disorganized thinking.
7. Discuss pharmacotherapy in the treatment of schizophrenia.
8. Identify the role of both short- and long-acting injectable antipsychotic medications.
9. Compare and contrast therapeutic responses from first- and second-generation antipsychotics.
10. Identify antipsychotic side effects, including metabolic syndrome, extrapyramidal side effects, anticholinergic responses, neuromalignant syndrome, and severe neutropenia.
11. Discuss how antipsychotic side effects can be managed or reduced.
12. Identify psychological therapies such as cognitive behavioral therapy, family therapy, and support groups for individuals and families with schizophrenia.

KEY TERMS AND CONCEPTS

acute dystonia
affective symptoms
akathisia
anosognosia
anticholinergic toxicity
antipsychotic medication
associative looseness
clang association
command hallucination
concrete thinking

delusions
echopraxia
executive functioning
extrapyramidal side effects
hallucinations
illusions
long-acting injectable
metabolic syndrome
negative symptoms
neologism

neuroleptic malignant syndrome
paranoia
positive symptoms
prodromal phase
pseudoparkinsonism
psychosis
reality testing
recovery model
severe neutropenia
tardive dyskinesia

Schizophrenia spectrum disorders are disorders that share features with schizophrenia. They are characterized by **psychosis**, which refers to altered cognition, altered perception, and/or an impaired ability to determine what is or is not real. This chapter begins with an overview of schizophrenia spectrum disorders and then focuses on schizophrenia and associated nursing care.

DELUSIONAL DISORDER

Delusional disorder is characterized by delusions (i.e., false thoughts or beliefs) that have lasted 1 month or longer. The delusions include grandiose, persecutory, somatic, and referential themes. They are usually not severe enough to impair functioning. Individuals with this disorder do not tend to behave strangely or bizarrely. The lifetime prevalence of delusional disorder is about 0.2%.

BRIEF PSYCHOTIC DISORDER

Brief psychotic disorder involves the sudden onset of at least one of the following: delusions, hallucinations, disorganized speech, and disorganized or catatonic (severely decreased motor activity) behavior. The symptoms must last longer than 1 day, but no longer than 1 month, with the expectation of a return to normal functioning. Brief psychotic disorder accounts for about 9% of all first-time psychoses and is twice as common in females.

SCHIZOPHRENIFORM DISORDER

The essential features of this disorder are exactly like those of schizophrenia except that symptoms have thus far lasted less than 6 months. Also, impaired social or occupational functioning may not be apparent. Some people with schizophreniform disorder return to their previous level of functioning, whereas others develop a persistent or recurrent psychosis.

SCHIZOAFFECTIVE DISORDER

This disorder involves a major depressive, manic, or mixed episode concurrent with symptoms that meet the criteria for schizophrenia. The symptoms must not be caused by any substance use or general medical condition. It has a lifetime prevalence of 0.3%.

SUBSTANCE-INDUCED PSYCHOTIC DISORDER AND PSYCHOTIC DISORDER DUE TO ANOTHER MEDICAL CONDITION

Illicit drugs, alcohol, medications, or toxins can induce delusions and/or hallucinations. Hallucinations or delusions can also be caused by a general medical condition, such as delirium, neurological disease, hepatic or renal disease, and many more. Substance use and medical conditions should always be ruled out before a primary diagnosis of schizophrenia spectrum disorder is made.

SCHIZOPHRENIA

Clinical Picture

Schizophrenia develops gradually and insidiously, usually beginning between 15 and 25 years of age. However, there are also child-onset (before 15 years) and late-onset (after 40 years) forms. Schizophrenia is often preceded by a prodromal phase during which milder symptoms of the disorder occur, often months or years before the full disorder becomes manifest. During the prodromal phase, people may experience diminished school performance and cognitive ability. They may become less socially engaged or adept. They may also demonstrate attenuated (mild) psychotic symptoms, such as suspiciousness and/or eccentric or disorganized speech or thought (Guccione et al., 2019).

All people diagnosed with schizophrenia have at least one psychotic symptom, such as hallucinations, delusions, and/or disorganized speech or thought. These symptoms are severe enough to disrupt normal activities, such as school, work, family and social interaction, and self-care; in children and young adults, they often delay or stop the achievement of developmental milestones. Basic needs such as hygiene, nutrition, and healthcare are often neglected and socialization and relationships often disrupted. The full criteria for schizophrenia are listed in the DSM-5 box. About 1% of people develop schizophrenia.

Epidemiology

The prevalence of childhood-onset schizophrenia is about 1 in 40,000 children. It affects individuals of all races and cultures equally. It is diagnosed more frequently in males (1.4:1) and among individuals growing up in urban areas (Haddad et al., 2015). Onset in males is usually between the ages of 15 and 25 years and is associated with poorer functioning and more structural abnormality in the brain. The onset tends to be somewhat later in women (ages 25 to 35 years), who tend to have a better prognosis and experience less structural changes in the brain.

Comorbidity

Substance use disorders, particularly alcohol and marijuana, occur in nearly half of affected individuals. Substance use may be a form of self-treatment for certain symptoms (e.g., social discomfort) or side effects (e.g., sedation). It is associated with poorer treatment adherence and prognosis and with increased relapse, incarceration, homelessness, violence, and suicide (Jorgensen, Nordentoft, & Hjorthoj, 2018). About 60% of individuals with schizophrenia use nicotine, possibly owing to genetic factors or as a form of coping with cognitive impairment or anxiety (Mallet et al., 2019). Smoking doubles the risk of cancer and contributes to cardiovascular and respiratory disorders.

Anxiety, depression, and **suicide** co-occur frequently in schizophrenia. At least 20% of people with schizophrenia attempt suicide, whereas 5% to 10% die by suicide, a rate five times that of the general population. Suicide attempts are more common within 3 years of diagnosis and especially upon discharge after the first episode of schizophrenia (American Psychiatric Association, 2013).

Physical illnesses are more common among people with schizophrenia. They face a risk of premature death that is 3.5 times greater than the risk in the general population; on average, moreover, patients with schizophrenia die more than 20 years prematurely with cardiovascular disease and metabolic syndrome (Seeman, 2019).

Individuals with psychotic disorders are at greater risk for poor health maintenance behaviors (e.g., reduced physical activity), poor nutrition, substance use, poverty, limited access to healthcare, victimization, trauma, and reduced ability to recognize or respond to signs of illness. They may also receive poorer-quality healthcare owing to poverty, stigma, impaired

DSM-5 CRITERIA FOR SCHIZOPHRENIA

A. Two or more of the following, each present for a significant portion of time during a 1-month period (or less if successfully treated). At least one must be item 1, 2, or 3:
  1. Delusions
  2. Hallucinations
  3. Disorganized speech (e.g., frequent derailment or incoherence)
  4. Grossly disorganized or catatonic behavior
  5. Negative symptoms (i.e., diminished emotional expression or avolition)
B. For a significant portion of the time since the onset of the disturbance, level of functioning in one or more major areas—such as work, interpersonal relations, or self-care—is markedly below the level achieved before the onset (or when the onset is in childhood or adolescence, there is failure to achieve the expected level of interpersonal, academic, or occupational functioning).
C. Continuous signs of the disturbance persist for at least 6 months. This 6-month period must include at least 1 month of symptoms (or less if successfully treated) that meet Criterion A (i.e., active-phase symptoms) and may include periods of prodromal or residual symptoms. During these prodromal or residual periods, the signs of the disturbance may be manifested by only negative symptoms or by two or more symptoms listed in Criterion A present in an attenuated form (e.g., odd beliefs, unusual perceptual experiences).
D. Schizoaffective disorder and depressive or bipolar disorder with psychotic features have been ruled out because either (1) no major depressive or manic episodes have occurred concurrently with the active-phase symptoms or (2) if mood episodes have occurred during active-phase symptoms, they have been present for a minority of the total duration of the active and residual periods of the illness.
E. The disturbance is not attributable to the physiological effects of a substance (e.g., a drug of abuse, a medication) or another medical condition.
F. If there is a history of autism spectrum disorder or a communication disorder of childhood onset, the additional diagnosis of schizophrenia is made only if prominent delusions or hallucinations, in addition to the other required symptoms of schizophrenia, are also present for at least 1 month (or less if successfully treated).

Specify if: The following course specifiers are to be used only after a 1-year duration of the disorder and if they are not in contradiction to the diagnostic course criteria.

First episode, currently an acute episode: First manifestation of the disorder meeting the defining diagnostic symptom and time criteria. An *acute episode* is a time period in which the symptom criteria are fulfilled.

First episode, currently in partial remission: *Partial remission* is a period of time during which an improvement after a previous episode is maintained and in which the defining criteria of the disorder are only partially fulfilled.

First episode, currently in full remission: *Full remission* is a period of time after a previous episode during which no disorder-specific symptoms are present.

Multiple episodes, currently in acute episode: Multiple episodes may be determined after a minimum of two episodes (i.e., after a first episode, a remission, and a minimum of one relapse).

Multiple episodes, currently in partial remission
Multiple episodes, currently in full remission

Continuous: Symptoms fulfilling the diagnostic symptom criteria of the disorder are remaining for the majority of the illness course with subthreshold symptom periods being very brief relative to the overall course.

Unspecified
Specify if: With catatonia
Specify current severity: Severity is rated by a quantitative assessment of the primary symptoms of psychosis, including delusions, hallucinations, disorganized speech, abnormal psychomotor behavior, and negative symptoms. Each of these symptoms may be rated for its current severity (most severe in the last 7 days) on a 5-point scale ranging from 0 (not present) to 4 (present and severe).

From American Psychiatric Association. (2013). *Diagnostic and statistical manual of mental disorders* (5th ed.). Washington, DC: Author.

ability to express their needs, or stereotyping (e.g., emergency department staff assuming that chest pain complaints are imaginary or not serious).

Polydipsia is compulsive drinking of fluids; it occurs in about 20% of individuals with schizophrenia. The excess fluid reduces sodium levels, which results in hyponatremia (also known as water intoxication) in up to 5% of those affected. Symptoms of hyponatremia include confusion, delirium, hallucinations, worsening of psychotic symptoms, dilute urine, polyuria, and ultimately coma. Contributing factors include antipsychotic medications that cause dry mouth, compulsive behavior (associated with schizophrenia), and neuroendocrine abnormalities (Yang & Cheng, 2017). Hyponatremia should be considered when there is a sudden increase in psychotic symptoms, particularly if symptoms of delirium such as disorientation, restlessness, and fluctuating vital signs are also present.

Risk Factors

Schizophrenia is believed to occur when multiple inherited genetic abnormalities combine with other factors. Such other factors include viral infections, birth injuries, environmental stressors, prenatal malnutrition, trauma, and abnormal neural pruning that alters brain development or function and/or injures the brain directly.

Biological Factors

Genetic. About 80% of the risk of schizophrenia is genetic. Over 100 loci in the human genome are associated with an increased risk of schizophrenia (Ota et al., 2019). Concordance rates—that is, the percentage of twins each having the disorder—are about 50% for identical twins and about 15% for fraternal twins. Evidence suggests that multiple genes on different chromosomes interact with one another in complex ways to create vulnerability for schizophrenia.

Epigenetic factors include toxins and psychological trauma that affects the expression of genes. Even psychological trauma in a parent or grandparent may cause epigenetic changes that increase vulnerability, and this increased risk can be passed on to one's descendants.

Neurobiological.

Neurotransmission. The first antipsychotic drugs blocked the activity of dopamine-2 (D_2) receptors in the brain and reduced symptoms such as hallucinations and delusions. Symptom reduction suggested that dopamine plays a significant role in psychosis. However, because medications that reduce dopamine activity do not alleviate all the symptoms of schizophrenia, it seems likely that other neurotransmitters or other factors are involved as well.

Amphetamines and cocaine enhance dopamine activity and can induce psychosis or precipitate schizophrenia. Almost any drug of abuse, particularly marijuana, can increase the risk of schizophrenia in biologically vulnerable individuals (Renard et al., 2017).

Newer antipsychotics block serotonin (5-hydroxytryptamine 2A, or 5-HT$_{2A}$) and dopamine, which suggests that serotonin may play a role in schizophrenia as well.

Phencyclidine (PCP) induces a state that resembles schizophrenia, suggesting a possible role of glutamate in the pathophysiology of schizophrenia. Glutamate, dopamine, and serotonin act synergistically in neurotransmission; thus, glutamate may also play a role in causing psychosis. Neurotransmission by gamma-aminobutyric acid (GABA), another calming neurotransmitter, is also altered in schizophrenia (Zhand et al., 2019). Acetylcholine, active in the muscarinic system, may also play a role in psychosis (Potasiewicz, Golebioska, Popik, & Nikiforuk, 2019).

Brain Structure Abnormalities

Structural abnormalities such as atrophy cause disruption in communication within the brain. Structural differences may be neurodevelopmental errors or errors in the normal pruning of neuronal tissue, as happens in late adolescence and early adulthood. Inflammation or neurotoxic effects from factors such as oxidative stress, infection, or autoimmune dysfunction may also alter the brain's structure (Sekar et al., 2016; Miller, 2019).

Using brain imaging techniques—computed tomography (CT), magnetic resonance imaging (MRI), functional MRI (fMRI), and positron emission tomography (PET)—researchers (Zhao et al., 2018) have demonstrated structural brain abnormalities, including the following:

- Reduced volume in the right anterior insula (may contribute to negative symptoms)
- Reduced volume and changes in the shape of the hippocampus
- Accelerated age-related decline in cortical thickness
- Gray matter deficits in the dorsolateral prefrontal cortex area, thalamus, and anterior cingulate cortex as well as in the frontotemporal, thalamocortical, and subcortical-limbic circuits
- Reduced connectivity among various brain regions
- Neuronal overgrowth in some areas, possibly due to inflammation or inadequate neural pruning
- Widespread white matter abnormalities (e.g., in the corpus callosum)

PET scans also show a lowered rate of blood flow and glucose metabolism in the prefrontal cortex. This part of the brain governs executive functional skills such as planning, abstract thinking, social adjustment, and decision making. Fig. 3.5 in Chapter 3 shows a PET scan demonstrating reduced brain activity in the frontal lobe of a patient with schizophrenia. Such structural and functional changes may worsen as the disorder continues. Postmortem studies of schizophrenic individuals show a reduced volume of gray matter, especially in the temporal and frontal lobes, and people with the most tissue loss had the worst symptoms.

Prenatal Stressors

Infection during or after pregnancy increases the risk of mental illness (Allswede & Cannon, 2018). Other factors associated with an increased risk of schizophrenia include a father above 35 years of age at the child's conception and being born during late winter or early spring.

Environmental Factors

Stress increases cortisol levels, impairing hypothalamic development and causing other changes that may precipitate schizophrenia in vulnerable individuals. Schizophrenia often manifests at times of developmental and family stress, such as when a person is beginning college or moving away from home. Social, psychological, and physical stressors may play a significant role in both the severity and course of the disorder and the person's quality of life.

Toxins such tetrachloroethylene, used in dry cleaning and to line water pipes and sometimes found in drinking water, are also believed to contribute to the development of schizophrenia in vulnerable people (Aschengrau et al., 2012). Other risk factors include childhood sexual abuse, exposure to social adversity (e.g., crime or chronic poverty), migration to or growing up in a foreign culture, and exposure to psychological trauma or social defeat (Kilian et al., 2018). These factors may cause structural changes in the brain due to epigenetic changes in the genome.

Prognostic Variables

Symptoms typically improve with medications and psychosocial interventions. In many cases, however, schizophrenia does not respond fully to treatment, leaving mild to severe residual symptoms and varying degrees of dysfunction or disability. A minority of individuals require repeated or lengthy inpatient care or institutionalization. Factors associated with a less positive prognosis include a slow onset (e.g., more than 2 years), younger age at onset, longer duration between symptom onset and first treatment, longer periods of untreated illness, and more negative symptoms (described later). Reducing the frequency, intensity, and duration of *relapse* (when previously controlled symptoms return) is believed to improve the prognosis.

Phases of Schizophrenia

Schizophrenia usually progresses through predictable phases, although the presenting symptoms during a given phase and the length of the phase can vary widely. These phases are as follows:

- **Prodromal**—Before acute symptoms of schizophrenia occur, people may experience mild changes in thinking, reality testing, and mood. Speech and thoughts may be odd, and anxiety, obsessive thoughts, and compulsive behaviors may present. Concentration, school or job performance, and social functioning can deteriorate. The person may feel "not right" or that "something strange" is happening. Symptoms typically appear 1 to 12 months before the first full episode of schizophrenia.
- **Acute**—Acute symptoms vary, from few and mild to many and disabling. Symptoms such as hallucinations, delusions, apathy, social withdrawal, diminished affect, anhedonia, disorganized behavior, and impaired judgment and cognition

▶ Neurobiology of Schizophrenia and the Effects of Antipsychotics

The antipsychotics affect a number of neurotransmitters including dopamine, noradrenaline/norepinephrine, serotonin, and GABA. An excess of serotonin may contribute to both the positive and negative symptoms of schizophrenia. GABA regulates dopamine activity and in some people with schizophrenia, there is a loss of GABAergic neurons in the hippocampus, potentially causing hyperactivity of dopamine. Since dopamine is the most studied and most prominent of the neurotransmitters (D_1, D_2, D_3, D_4, and D_5) in schizophrenia, the role of dopamine is presented here.

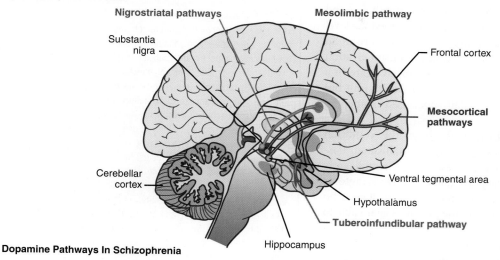

Dopamine Pathways In Schizophrenia

Mesolimbic pathway is involved in reward motivation, emotions, and positive symptoms of schizophrenia.

Mesocortical pathways are relevant to cognitive function, executive function, and negative symptoms of schizophrenia.

Nigrostriatal pathways are normally responsible for purposeful movement.

Tuberoinfundibular pathway is normally responsible for regulation of prolactin.

Pharmacotherapy

First-generation antipsychotic (FGA) drugs are potent antagonists/blockers of D_2.

Second-generation antipsychotic (SGA) drugs have less affinity for D_2 receptors, and tend to bind with D_3 and D_4 receptors. Since the expression of D_3 and D_4 is limited to the neurons of the limbic system and cerebral cortex, the action of these drugs are limited to areas involved in the pathology of schizophrenia. Second-generation drugs also inhibit the serotonin (5HT) receptors. Since serotonin inhibits the release of dopamine, the dopaminergic transmission is affected.

The potential serious effects of the SGAs (metabolic effects: weight gain, diabetes, and dyslipidemia) come from the blockade of noradrenaline/norepinephrine (alpha-1), histamine, and acetylcholine.

Dopamine Pathways and Antipsychotic Responses

Dopamine Pathway	Abnormality in Schizophrenia	Responses to Antipsychotic Drugs
Mesolimbic pathway connects the ventral tegmental area (VTA) to the nucleus accumbens Associated with reward, motivation, and emotion	Hyperactive in schizophrenia Associated with positive symptoms (hallucinations, delusions, disorganized thought)	**FGA** - D_2 blockage results in reduction in positive symptoms **SGA** - D_2, D_3, and D_4 antagonism results in reduction of positive symptoms
Mesocortical pathway made up of dopaminergic neurons that project from the VTA to the prefrontal cortex Relevant to cognition, executive function, emotions, and affect	Hypofunction in schizophrenia results in cognitive impairment and negative symptoms (apathy, anhedonia, lack of motivation)	**FGA** - D_2 blockage may result in a worsening of these symptoms **SGA** - Since there are more serotonin (5HT) receptors than D_2 receptors in this area, blockage of 5HT is more profound. Blockage of 5HT may help improve negative symptoms
Nigrostriatal pathway-substantia nigra to basal ganglia Responsible for purposeful movement	Unaffected	**FGA** (to a lesser degree SGA) - Long-term blockade of D_2 receptors can cause upregulation (increase response to a stimulus) to those receptors, which may lead to extrapyramidal side effects e.g., tardive dyskinesia (TD)
Tuberoinfundibular pathway consists of dopaminergic projections from the hypothalamus to the pituitary gland Inhibits prolactin release	Unaffected	**FGA** (to a lesser degree SGA) - Blockade of D_2 receptors increases prolactin levels resulting in hyperprolactinemia and lactation

result in functional impairment. The person can have difficulty coping, and symptoms become apparent to others. This phase can last several months, even with treatment. Increased support and additional treatment or hospitalization may be required.

- **Stabilization**—In this phase, symptoms are stabilizing and diminishing, and there is movement toward a previous level of functioning. This phase can last for months. Care in an outpatient mental health center or a partial hospitalization program may be needed. The person may receive care in a residential crisis center (similar to a mental health unit but based in the community) or a staff-supervised residential group home or apartment.

- **Maintenance or Residual**—In this phase, the condition has stabilized and a new baseline may be established. Positive symptoms (described later) are usually significantly diminished or absent, but negative and cognitive symptoms continue to be a concern. Ideally, recovery with few or no residual symptoms will occur, and the patient is again able to live independently or with family.

A pattern of recurrent exacerbations (relapses) separated by periods of reduced or dormant symptoms is common. Some people have one or several episodes and none thereafter. For most patients, however, schizophrenia is a chronic or relapsing disorder that, like diabetes or heart disease, is managed with ongoing treatment.

BOX 12.1   Can Schizophrenia Be Prevented?

Malnutrition, infection, and tobacco use during pregnancy and marijuana and drug use in biologically vulnerable people increase the risk of developing schizophrenia. Primary prevention aims at avoiding these factors. However, not all risks can be avoided. Avoiding triggers, such as environmental stressors, and interventions to promote resiliency and coping in children and families, are helpful. Two additional options are (1) early treatment with antipsychotic medications and (2) supplemental essential fatty acids.

In the future, genetic screening may help to identify those at risk. Providers now identify prodromal (early) symptoms (e.g., eccentric or magical thinking, cognitive disorganization, or quasi-hallucinations) and can consider prophylactic use of antipsychotic medications. However, only one-third of those at risk for schizophrenia actually develop it, and the prophylactic use of antipsychotics can unnecessarily expose those people to significant side effects.

Omega-3 and omega-6 fatty acids, found in fish oils and oily fish such as tuna, salmon, and sardines, are structural contributors to brain development. They also reduce inflammation and free radicals in the brain and contribute to acetylcholine and serotonin stability. They are abnormally low in the brains of people with schizophrenia, and omega-3 supplementation appears to reduce rates of conversion (from "at risk" to actually having schizophrenia) significantly.

Radic, K., Curkokvic, M., Bagaric, D., Vilibic, M., Tomic, A., & Zivkovic, M. (2018). Ethical approach to prevention of schizophrenia–concepts and challenges. *Psychiatria Danubina, 30*(1), 35–40. Rog, J., & Karakula-Juchnowicz, H. (2016). Omega-3 fatty acids in schizophrenia—part 1: Importance in the pathophysiology of schizophrenia. *Current Problems in Psychiatry, 17*(3), 198–213.

APPLICATION OF THE NURSING PROCESS

ASSESSMENT

Assessment involves interviewing the patient and observing behavior and other manifestations of the disorder. Information from people who know the patient is also important, since patients may conceal or minimize their symptoms. Assessment includes a mental status examination (MSE) along with a review of spiritual, cultural, biological, psychological, social, and environmental elements that might be affecting the presentation (e.g., impaired sleep, spiritual distress, despair).

Prodromal Phase

Early assessment is key to improving the prognosis for individuals with schizophrenia. Reducing risk factors (such as high levels of stress or substance abuse), coupled with enhancing social and coping skills, can reduce the risk of developing schizophrenia in biologically vulnerable people. Box 12.1 identifies other prevention strategies.

General Assessment

Symptoms of schizophrenia vary from person to person and from episode to episode, and some of them are also found in other disorders. Fig. 12.1 describes the four main symptom categories in schizophrenia:

1. **Positive symptoms**: The presence of symptoms that should not be present. Positive symptoms include hallucinations, delusions, paranoia, or disorganized or bizarre thoughts, behavior, or speech.
2. **Negative symptoms**: The absence of qualities that should be present. Negative symptoms include the inability to enjoy activities (anhedonia), social discomfort, or lack of goal-directed behavior.
3. *Cognitive symptoms*: Subtle or obvious impairment in memory, attention, thinking (e.g., disorganized or irrational thoughts); impaired executive functioning (e.g., impaired judgment, impulse control, prioritization, and problem solving).
4. **Affective symptoms**: Symptoms involving emotions and their expression.

Positive Symptoms

Positive symptoms usually appear early. They can be dramatic and are often what precipitates treatment. Positive symptoms are what most individuals associate with mental illness, often making schizophrenia what people imagine "mental illness" to be.

One positive symptom is alterations in reality testing. **Reality testing** is the automatic and unconscious process by which we determine what is and is not real. We all experience thoughts that are irrational or distorted, yet we usually catch and correct them via reality testing. You might think you hear a voice, but you see that no one is present, so you conclude you are mistaken—it wasn't real. With impaired reality testing, the person experiences hallucinations or delusions as real.

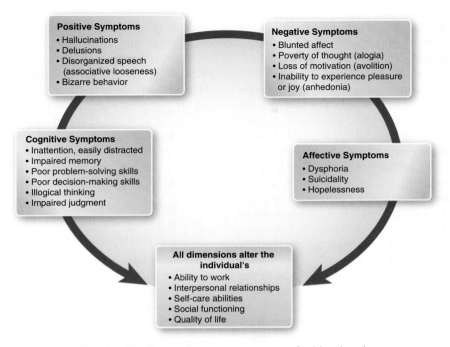

Fig. 12.1 The four main symptom groups of schizophrenia.

Delusions are false beliefs that are held despite a lack of evidence to support them. The most common delusions involve persecutory, grandiose, or religious ideas. Table 12.1 provides definitions and examples of delusions, which can reflect underlying issues or needs. For example, a person with poor self-esteem may believe that he is Beethoven or God, possibly driven by a need to feel important or powerful.

Just because someone has a mental illness does not mean that every improbable belief is delusional. One patient repeatedly told staff that criminals were out to kill him. Staff later learned that he had been selling drugs, had not paid his suppliers, and that drug dealers *were* trying to harm him.

Alterations in speech. Unusual speech patterns are common in schizophrenia. One, **associative looseness**, or looseness of association, results from haphazard and illogical thinking where concentration is poor and thoughts are only loosely connected. For example: "My friends talk about French fries but how can you trust the French?" **Word salad**, the most extreme form of associative looseness, is a jumble of words that is meaningless to the listener (e.g., "agents want strength of policy on a boat reigning supreme").

Clang association is choosing words based on their sound rather than their meaning and often involves words that rhyme or have a similar beginning sound ("On the track ... have a Big Mac" or "Click, clack, clutch, close").

Neologisms are words that have meaning for the patient but a different or nonexistent meaning for others. A patient may use a known word differently than others or create a completely new word that others do not understand (e.g., "His *mannerologies* are poor").

TABLE 12.1   Types of Delusions[a]

Delusion	Definition	Example
Persecutory	Believing that one is being singled out for harm or prevented from making progress by others	Shannon believes that her food is poisoned; therefore, she eats only prepackaged food. John believes that his coworkers are plotting to prevent his promotion.
Referential	A belief that events or circumstances that have no connection to you are somehow related to you	Christopher believes that the birds sing songs to cheer him up. Sarah believes that songs on the radio are chosen to send her a message.
Grandiose	Believing that one is a powerful or important person	Brianna believes that she is a famous playwright.
Erotomanic	Believing that another person desires you romantically	Although he barely knows her, Patty insists that Eric would marry her if only his current wife would stop interfering.
Nihilistic	The conviction that a major catastrophe will occur	Deepesh is giving away all his belongings since they won't be of any use when the comet hits.
Somatic	Believing that the body is changing in unusual ways	Chris says that her heart is dead and rotting away.
Control	Believing that another person, group, or external force controls your thoughts, feelings, impulses, or behavior	Brian covered his apartment walls with aluminum foil to block aliens' efforts to control his thoughts.

[a]A false belief held regardless of evidence to the contrary. Note that unusual beliefs that stem from one's culture or subculture are not considered delusions.

Echolalia is the pathological repetition of another's words, occurring perhaps because the patient's thought processes are so impaired that she is unable to generate speech of her own.

Nurse: Mary, come get your medication.

Mary: Come get your medication.

Note that alterations in speech often reflect altered cognitive abilities and thus can reflect cognitive deficits. The following are other pathological speech patterns:

- **Circumstantiality:** Including unnecessary and often tedious details in conversation but eventually reaching the point.
- **Tangentiality:** Wandering off topic or going off on tangents and never reaching the point.
- **Cognitive retardation:** Generalized slowing of thinking, which is represented by delays in responding to questions or difficulty finishing thoughts.
- **Pressured speech:** Urgent or intense speech; reluctance to allow comments from others.
- **Flight of ideas:** Moving rapidly from one thought to the next, often making it difficult for others to follow the conversation.
- **Symbolic speech:** Using words based on what they symbolize, not what they mean. For example, a patient reports "demons are sticking needles in me" when what he means is that he is experiencing a sharp pain (symbolized by *needles*).
- **Thought blocking:** A reduction or stoppage of thought. Cognitive disorganization or interruption of thought by hallucinations can cause this.
- **Thought insertion:** The often uncomfortable belief that someone else has inserted thoughts into the patient's brain.
- **Thought deletion:** A belief that thoughts have been taken or are missing.

Other positive symptoms manifested in disorders of thought include these:

- **Magical thinking:** Believing that reality can be changed simply by thoughts or unrelated actions. This thinking is common in children (e.g., "Because I was mad at him, he fell down").
- Paranoia: An irrational fear, ranging from mild (being suspicious, wary, guarded) to profound (believing irrationally that another person intends to kill you). Fear may result in dangerous defensive actions, such as harming another person before that person can harm the patient.

Alterations in perception. Alterations in perception involve errors in how one interprets perceptions or perceives reality. The most common perceptual errors are hallucinations. Hallucinations occur when a person perceives a sensory experience for which no external source exists (e.g., hearing a voice when no one is speaking). Types of hallucination include the following.

- **Auditory:** Hearing voices or sounds
- **Visual:** Seeing people or things
- **Olfactory:** Smelling odors
- **Gustatory:** Experiencing tastes
- **Tactile:** Feeling bodily sensations (e.g., feeling an insect crawling on one's skin)

Psychosis often involves auditory hallucinations, but they can also occur in individuals who are not psychotic. They are the most common form in psychosis, being experienced by about 70% of people with schizophrenia (Capizzi et al., 2019). They may be vague sounds or indistinct or clear voices. Hallucinations seem to come from outside the person's head and are perceived similarly to real voices. Auditory processing areas of the brain are activated during these hallucinations, just as they are when a genuine sound is heard.

John Nash, the world-renowned mathematician with schizophrenia portrayed in the film *A Beautiful Mind* (Howard, 2001), described his hallucinations this way:

I thought of the voices as … something a little different from aliens. I thought of them more like angels…. It's really my subconscious talking; it was really that, I know that now.

Hallucinatory voices may be single or multiple, distinct or indistinct, and may be attributed to specific sources (e.g., God, a family member) or unrecognized. They may be supportive and pleasant or derogatory and frightening. They can be subtle and unobtrusive or intrusive and disruptive. Hallucinations commenting on the person's behavior or conversing with the person are common. Indications that a person is hallucinating include tracking motions (turning one's head in the direction of the perceived sound), lips moving silently, talking as if to another when no one is present, and otherwise unexplained changes in affect (e.g., suddenly laughing with no apparent reason).

A person who hears voices struggles to understand the experience, sometimes developing related delusions to explain the voices. For example, a person may believe that the voices are from God or from a device implanted by the Central Intelligence Agency. Patients may try to cope by drowning out auditory hallucinations with loud music or by talking loudly, humming, or singing. Such competing auditory stimuli may, in fact, reduce hallucinations and serve as a recommended intervention.

A command hallucination is a particularly concerning symptom wherein the person is directed to take an action. Command hallucinations may be dangerous and must be evaluated carefully. For example, they may be telling a patient to "jump out the window" or to "hit that nurse." Command hallucinations are often frightening and may be a flag warning of a psychiatric emergency. It is essential to assess what the patient hears, the source to which it is attributed, the patient's ability to recognize the hallucination as "not real" and resist commands.

Visual hallucinations are the second most common form in schizophrenia. They may involve the distortion of visual stimuli or may be formed and realistic images. Seeing individuals and animals that do not exist is the most common type of visual hallucination.

Olfactory, tactile, or gustatory hallucinations are unusual in mental illness. When they are present, other possible causes should be investigated.

Other alterations in perception include the following.

- Illusions: Misinterpretations of a real experience. For example, a man sees a coat on a shadowy coat rack and believes it to be a bear.

- **Depersonalization:** A feeling of being unreal or having lost an element of one's person or identity. For example, body parts do not belong, or the body has drastically changed (e.g., a patient may see her fingers as being smaller than they actually are or not as hers).
- **Derealization:** A feeling that the environment has changed (e.g., that one is detached from the environment, that everything seems bigger or smaller, or that familiar surroundings seem somehow strange and unfamiliar).

Alterations in behavior. Alterations in behavior involve changes in the speed of movement and behaviors that are illogical or inappropriate. Behavioral alterations include the following.

- **Catatonia:** A pronounced increase or decrease in the rate and amount of movement. Excessive motor activity is purposeless. The most common form of catatonia is when the person moves little or not at all. Muscular rigidity, or **catalepsy**, may be so severe that the limbs remain in whatever position they are placed. Persistent catatonia may contribute to exhaustion, pneumonia, blood clotting, malnutrition, or dehydration.
- **Motor retardation:** A pronounced slowing of movement.
- **Motor agitation:** Excited behavior, such as running or pacing rapidly, often in response to internal or external stimuli. It can put the patient at risk (e.g., from exhaustion, by running into traffic) or put others at risk (e.g., by being knocked down).
- **Stereotyped behaviors:** Repetitive behaviors that do not serve a logical purpose.
- **Echopraxia:** The mimicking of movements of another.
- **Negativism:** A tendency to resist or oppose the requests or wishes of others.
- **Impaired impulse control:** A reduced ability to resist one's impulses. Examples include interrupting others or throwing unwanted food on the floor. It can increase the risk of assault.
- **Gesturing or posturing:** Assuming unusual and illogical expressions (often grimaces), posture, or positions.
- **Boundary impairment:** An impaired ability to sense where one's body or influence ends and another's begins. For example, a patient might stand too close to others or might drink another person's beverage, believing that because the beverage is near, it is the patient's.

Negative Symptoms

Positive symptoms are obvious to others and can make treatment seem more urgent than negative symptoms do. Yet negative symptoms are a serious problem for people with schizophrenia because they amount to the absence of essential human qualities. Treating negative symptoms is more difficult than treating positive symptoms.

Negative symptoms include the following six, which all start with the letter A:

- **Anhedonia** (*an* = without + *hedonia* = pleasure): A reduced ability or the inability to experience pleasure.
- **Avolition** (*a* = without + *volition* = initiating an action): reduced motivation or goal-directed behavior; difficulty beginning and sustaining goal-directed activities.

- **Asociality:** Decreased desire for social interaction or discomfort during it; social withdrawal.
- **Affective blunting:** Reduced or constricted affect.
- **Apathy:** Decreased interest in activities or beliefs that would otherwise be interesting or important or little attention to them.
- **Alogia:** Reduction in speech, sometimes called *poverty of speech.*

These symptoms can contribute to poor social functioning and social withdrawal. They can impair a person's ability to initiate and maintain conversations and relationships or to succeed in school or work. Apathy and avolition result in deficits in basic activities, such as maintaining adequate hygiene, grooming, and other activities of daily living.

Affect, an additional "A" word, is the external expression of a person's emotional state. In schizophrenia, affect may be diminished or may not coincide with the person's inner emotions. Some antipsychotic medications can also cause diminished affect. Affect in schizophrenia can usually be categorized in one of four ways:

- **Flat:** Immobile or blank facial expression
- **Blunted:** Reduced or minimal emotional response
- **Constricted:** Reduced in range or intensity (e.g., shows sadness or anger but no other moods)
- **Inappropriate:** Incongruent with the actual emotional state or situation (e.g., laughing in response to a tragedy)
- **Bizarre:** Odd, illogical, inappropriate, or unfounded; includes grimacing

Cognitive Symptoms

Cognitive symptoms represent the third symptom group and are evident in most patients with schizophrenia. These impairments can lead to poor judgment and leave the person less able to cope, learn, manage health, or succeed in school or work. Medication is of limited value, but other treatments such as cognitive remediation (discussed later) can be helpful. Cognitive symptoms include the following.

Concrete thinking is an impaired ability to think abstractly, resulting in interpreting or perceiving things in a literal manner. For example, a nurse might ask what brought the patient to the hospital, and the patient answers "a cab" rather than "a suicide attempt." The meanings of proverbs can be used to assess abstract thought. An abstract interpretation of "The grass is always greener on the other side of the fence" is that we feel that we might be happier given other circumstances. A concrete interpretation could be "That side gets more sun, so it's greener there." Concreteness reduces one's ability to understand and respond to concepts requiring abstract reasoning, such as love or humor. Nurses can assist by communicating in more concrete terms that do not require abstract reasoning.

Concreteness, especially when combined with an impaired ability to recognize variations in affect or tone of voice, can also make it difficult to recognize social cues, such as sarcasm. A patient who had forgotten his wallet asked a store clerk if he could pay later for a bag of chips. When the clerk sarcastically replied, "Oh sure, you can pay whenever you want," the patient took this literally. The patient was distressed when police later arrested him for theft despite his protests that he had permission not to pay.

Memory impairment primarily affects short-term memory and the ability to learn. Repetition and verbal or visual reminders (cues) may help the patient to learn and recall information. For example, a picture of a toothbrush in the bathroom may serve as a reminder to brush teeth.

Impaired information processing can lead to problems such as delayed responses, misperceptions, or difficulty understanding others. Patients may lose the ability to screen out insignificant stimuli such as background sounds or objects in their peripheral vision, leading to overstimulation. Reducing stimulation can be helpful.

Impaired *executive functioning* includes difficulty with reasoning, setting priorities, comparing options, placing things in logical order or groups, anticipating and planning, and inhibiting undesirable impulses or actions. Impaired executive functioning interferes with problem solving and can contribute to inappropriateness in social situations.

Anosognosia (ah-no-sag-NO-zsuh) is the inability to realize one is ill—an inability caused by the illness itself. It is common in severe mental illness. Anosognosia may lead the patient to resist or stop treatment, making care more challenging and frustrating to others. Anosognosia can interfere with requesting or accepting help.

Affective Symptoms

Affective symptoms involve an altered experience and expression of emotions. Mood may be unstable, erratic, labile (changing rapidly and easily), or incongruent (not what would be expected for the circumstances).

A serious affective change often seen in schizophrenia is comorbid major depressive disorder. Depression may occur as part of a shared inflammatory reaction affecting the brain, or it may simply be a reaction to the stress and despair that can come from living with a chronic illness. Depression may signal an impending relapse, further impair functioning, and increase risk of substance use disorders. Most importantly, depression puts people at increased suicide risk.

Self-Assessment

Working with individuals who have schizophrenia can prompt anxiety or fear in the caretakers. One may also have biases or stereotypical images of the illness that interfere with patient care. Reflecting on your experiences, beliefs, and feelings and discussing them with staff, faculty, and peers may help.

NURSING DIAGNOSIS

Patients with schizophrenia have multiple distressing and often disabling symptoms. They require a multifaceted approach to care and treatment for both themselves and their significant others. Table 12.2 lists signs and symptoms and potential nursing diagnoses for a person with schizophrenia.

📄 ASSESSMENT GUIDELINES

Schizophrenia and Other Psychotic Disorders

1. Ensure that the patient has had a medical workup. Concurrent medical disorders are common. Patients may have experienced trauma or illness that is affecting their mental status (e.g., dehydration, alcohol withdrawal).
2. Assess for indications of medical problems that might mimic psychosis (e.g., digitalis or anticholinergic toxicity, brain trauma, drug intoxication, delirium, fever).
3. Assess for substance use disorders.
4. Complete an MSE, including insight, reality testing, judgment, cognitive abilities, knowledge of the illness, relationships and support systems, other coping resources, role functioning, physiological functioning, and strengths and needs.
5. Assess for hallucinations:
   - Do not imply that the perceptions are real (e.g., ask: "What do you hear?" not "What are the voices saying?").
   - Assess when the hallucinations began, their content, how the patient experiences them (e.g., supportive or distressing, in the background or intrusive), what makes them worse or better, how the patient is responding (e.g., acting on commands), and what the patient does to cope.
   - Questions should include "Are you hearing a voice that is telling you to do something?" "Do you believe what you hear is real?" (a "yes" suggests an increased risk that the patient will act on the commands).
6. Assess for delusions:
   - If present, are they firmly held? Is the patient capable of reality testing (questioning his thoughts, determining what is real)?
   - Does the patient believe that there is danger? Does the patient believe that acting against a person or organization will provide protection or vengeance?
7. Assess for suicide risk (refer to Chapter 25). Depression, anhedonia, impaired cognition, and isolation can create or worsen risk.
8. Assess activities of daily living. Does the patient
   - Maintain adequate food and fluid intake?
   - Achieve adequate sleep and rest?
   - Complete hygiene and self-care?
   - Move about safely? (e.g., fall risk, distractibility that leads to walking into traffic)
   - Control impulses and make sound, safe decisions?
   - Dress safely for weather conditions? (e.g., perceive heat or cold accurately and thus able to avoid temperature-related emergencies)
   - Meet health needs? (e.g., recognize onset or worsening of medical illnesses, adhere to treatment for medical conditions)
9. Assess medication regimen: whether medications are taken, their effectiveness and side effects, and barriers to treatment, such as cost, stigma, mistrust of healthcare providers.
10. Assess the family's knowledge of and response to the illness and its symptoms. Are they overprotective, frustrated, or anxious? Are they familiar with and using family support groups, respite, and other resources?

OUTCOMES IDENTIFICATION

Outcomes should focus on illness knowledge, management, coping, and quality of life. Outcomes should be consistent with the *recovery model* (refer to Chapter 32), which stresses hope, living a full and productive life, and eventual recovery rather than focusing on controlling symptoms and adapting to disability. Desired outcomes vary with the phase of the illness.

🌐 CONSIDERING CULTURE

Stigma of Schizophrenia in Chinese Families

Mrs. Chou, a young Chinese American woman, learned that her mother died from pneumonia. Mrs. Chou commented that her mother would not have become ill if she had been a better daughter and that she brought evil upon her family.

After the funeral, Mrs. Chou became increasingly lethargic, staring into space and mumbling to herself. Her husband asked who she was talking to. She answered, "My mother." Mrs. Chou told him that her organs had died and that she was dying. Mr. Chou knew something was wrong but was reluctant to seek help. In their culture, there is strong stigma against mental illness; it is often perceived as punishment and causes shame.

When Mrs. Chou quit eating and taking care of herself, her husband took her to an herbalist, who convinced him to take her to a hospital. During her admission, the unkempt and dehydrated Mrs. Chou sat motionless and mute.

Mr. Chou apologized for burdening others with his wife's care and asked that her treatment be kept secret. Staff helped him to recognize that Mrs. Chou had a physical illness of her brain that affected her thinking, emotions, and behavior and that treatment was comparable to treatment for heart disease or diabetes. They also stressed that seeking help for brain illness is accepted in the American culture.

Mr. Chou calmed down when he realized that he did not need to feel shame and that others would help. As his wife improved, she and Mr. Chou came to attribute the illness to grief, reducing their guilt. They met with a Chinese healer who helped them to integrate their beliefs with the beliefs and resources of their adopted culture.

TABLE 12.2 Signs and Symptoms and Nursing Diagnoses for Schizophrenia

Signs and Symptoms	Nursing Diagnoses
Auditory hallucinations	*Hallucinations*
Hears voices telling him or her to hurt self or others *(command hallucinations)*	*Hallucinations* *Risk for violence*
Delusions	*Delusions*
Looseness of association, cognitive impairment, impaired concentration, memory, judgment	*Distorted thinking process* *Impaired abstract thinking* *Impaired concentration* *Impaired verbal communication*
Anosognosia	*Lack of knowledge of disease*
Poor self-esteem, internalized stigma	*Negative self-image* *Risk for loneliness*
Despair, helplessness, hopelessness, sadness, thoughts of suicide	*Risk for powerlessness* *Risk for suicide*
Lack of energy (anergia) Lack of motivation (avolition) Impaired self-care	*Impaired ability to perform hygiene* *Impaired health maintenance* *Impaired ability to perform leisure activity* *Impaired volition*
Mistrust of others, paranoia	*Lack of trust in healthcare provider* *Withdrawn behavior* *Suspicion* *Risk for violence*

ICNP is owned and copyrighted by the International Council of Nurses (ICN). Reproduced with permission of the copyright holder. International Council of Nursing Practice. (2019). ICNP browser. Retrieved from https://www.icn.ch/what-we-do/projects/ehealth/icnp-browser

Phase I: Acute

For the acute phase of schizophrenia, the overall goal is **patient safety and stabilization**. If the patient poses a risk to self or others, initial outcome criteria address such safety issues (e.g., patient refrains from self-injury, hyponatremia is prevented). Another desired outcome is that the patient consistently labels hallucinations as "not real—a symptom of an illness."

Phase II: Stabilization

Outcome criteria during phase II focus on understanding of the illness and treatment, achieving an optimal medication and psychosocial treatment regimen, and controlling and/or coping with symptoms and side effects. Outcomes target the negative and cognitive symptoms in particular, as these tend to respond less well to initial treatment than do positive symptoms, possibly reducing treatment success.

Phase III: Maintenance

Outcome criteria for phase III focus on maintaining and increasing symptom control and optimal functioning. Factors measured during the maintenance phase include treatment adherence, absence of relapse, increasing independence, and a satisfactory quality of life.

PLANNING

Again, the planning of appropriate interventions is guided by the phase of the illness and the strengths and needs of the patient. Cultural considerations, available resources, and patient preferences influence planning.

Phase I: Acute

Hospitalization is indicated if the patient is considered a danger to self (e.g., refuses to eat or is too disorganized to function safely in the community) or others (e.g., behaving in a threatening manner). It may also be needed to rapidly clarify the diagnosis and initiate treatment. Planning focuses on selecting the best strategies to ensure patient safety and control symptoms.

Phase II: Stabilization and Phase III: Maintenance

Planning during the stabilization and maintenance phases focuses on education, support, and skills training for the patient and family. Planning incorporates interpersonal, functional, coping, healthcare, shelter, educational, and vocational strengths and needs; it also addresses how and where these needs can best be met within the community.

Relapse prevention efforts are vital. Each relapse may increase residual dysfunction and deterioration and can contribute to despair, hopelessness, and suicide risk. Recognizing early warning signs of relapse—such as reduced sleep, social withdrawal, and worsening concentration—followed by close monitoring and intensification of treatment as needed is essential to minimize the duration and severity of psychotic episodes and resulting disruption of the patient's life.

IMPLEMENTATION

Phase I: Acute

Settings

In general, during the acute phase of schizophrenia, 24-hour support is required to prevent harm to self or others. Hospitalization provides external structure and support (e.g., others guiding the patient's activities). As previously discussed, anosognosia may impair a person's ability to recognize the illness. In this case, court-ordered hospitalization might be required.

Although a minority of patients require extended inpatient care (more than 1 month), the length of hospitalization or other intensive treatment during the acute phase is typically short (days to weeks), ending when acute symptoms have been stabilized. However, additional time is needed for full recovery from any serious mental illness, making continued engagement and care in the community important after discharge.

Structure within the therapeutic milieu provides a feeling of safety and security for patients who have been experiencing severe anxiety. Staff monitor patients for suicide risk and intervene promptly to address risk factors such as despair or hopelessness while providing for the patient's safety (see Chapter 25).

Nurses provide support and guidance regarding the nature of the illness and its treatment. Medication education is an essential focus of nursing care. Psychoeducation promotes patient-centered care by helping the patient to recognize and self-manage symptoms.

Working With an Aggressive Patient

A small percentage of patients with schizophrenia, especially during the acute phase, may have the potential for physical violence. Violence may be in response to hallucinations, delusions, paranoia, impaired judgment, or limited impulse control. Interpersonal conflict, fear, desperation, and disagreements (e.g., about unit rules) increase the risk of aggression.

Assessment and monitoring for risk of violence are essential. Interventions to protect the patient and others become a priority. Refer to Table 12.3 and also Chapter 27 for more information on caring for the aggressive or potentially violent patient.

Phase II: Stabilization and Phase III: Maintenance

Postdischarge care is often provided through community mental health centers. They provide medication support, monitoring, structured therapeutic activities, case management, and 24/7 crisis and psychiatric emergency services. They can also provide housing support, allied physical health services, and employment programs. Peer-led services are available in most communities, including peer support and drop-in centers, also known as clubhouses, that offer socialization, activities, and sometimes employment opportunities.

Hospital staff can connect patients and families with outpatient resources before discharge. Support groups and educational resources are also helpful. The National Alliance on Mental Illness [NAMI, http://www.nami.org] is the best-known and strongest consumer and family support organization. The Best Practices in Schizophrenia Treatment Center is also a rich source of consumer and family support available online.

Nurses provide essential family education about the illness and how best to help the patient. Education can be provided even if the patient does not consent *if* the family initiates the request *and* the information is provided without divulging confidential health information. Alternately, the family can be connected to other resources for information. NAMI's "Family-to-Family" program educates families about severe mental illnesses and their treatment. Support and respite for caregivers are also important.

A sample care plan can be found in the Case Study and Nursing Care Plan. Additional nursing interventions that are often helpful in caring for individuals with schizophrenia are provided in Table 12.3

TABLE 12.3	Additional Nursing Interventions for the Person Experiencing Psychosis	
Problem	**Considerations**	**Nursing Care**
Poor hygiene	Contributing factors include apathy, avolition, negativism, disorganized thinking, impaired memory, distractibility, reduced awareness of social expectations, reduced recognition of own appearance/odor (due to altered sensory perception/processing, internal preoccupation).	1. Concisely and explicitly identify expected hygiene. Have patient try out each hygiene action while observing, assisting when needed. 2. Break tasks into smaller, more manageable steps. 3. Use visual cues to prompt attention to hygiene tasks, such as putting a toothbrush and towels in the bathroom and clean clothes on the bed. 4. Suggest ways in which improved hygiene will benefit the patient (e.g., perhaps by receiving greater acceptance from peers). 5. Guide patient to use napkin or towel around neck when eating or if experiencing drooling. 6. Periodically remind patient and refocus to hygiene tasks as needed. 7. Reinforce progress with verbal praise or concrete rewards (e.g., more privileges).
Resistance to treatment, nonadherence	Anosognosia causes treatment to seem illogical (why accept medication for an illness one does not have?). Side effects, stigma, inconvenience, a belief that the treatment will not help, expense, impaired memory, and mistrust of staff also discourage adherence.	1. Meet the patient where he is, acknowledging his views and preferences without judgment. 2. Treat the patient with respect and actively convey empathy, caring, and support. 3. Establish trust by behaving in a consistent and reliable manner. 4. Involve the patient collaboratively in planning treatment. 5. Explore concerns about treatment and suggest solutions (e.g., perhaps medications that cause fatigue can be taken at bedtime).

TABLE 12.3 Additional Nursing Interventions for the Person Experiencing Psychosis—cont'd

Problem	Considerations	Nursing Care
		6. Convey in a clear, concrete, and confident manner your belief that the patient will benefit from the treatment. 7. Tie the treatment to the patient's own goals. For example, the patient may not agree to take the medication *for an illness*, but if he believes that it will quiet the voices or help him keep his job (his goals), he may see more value to treatment.
Cheeking or palming medications	See "Resistance to Treatment."	1. Address underlying reasons for wanting to avoid medications. 2. Seek to switch medication to a more difficult-to-conceal form, such as a liquid or fast-dissolving tablet. 3. Long-acting injectable forms need to be taken only every 2–4 weeks or even months, thus reducing episodes of medication-related conflict.
Anosognosia	Anosognosia is common in severe mental illness. It is not denial or resistance—the patient quite literally is unable to see the illness.	1. Establish trust and rapport. Even a simple act such as offering the patient gum each day can increase patient comfort with staff. 2. Seek areas of commonality: What can both the patient and others agree upon? 3. Agree to disagree about whether these issues do or don't indicate an illness but seek agreement that they are a problem. 4. The patient may be aware of illness in others. If so, suggest that, just as another patient is unaware of being ill, something similar might be happening in him or her as well. 5. Involve the patient in activities including peers who have gained insight despite once having had anosognosia (e.g., National Alliance on Mental Illness meetings). A patient may find the reports of the peer to be more valid than similar information originating with staff.
Avoids interaction with peers	Contributing factors include asociality, impaired social skills, preoccupation with hallucinatory or other internal experiences, actual or potential rejection by peers, stigma or fear of embarrassment.	1. Actively convey acceptance and *meet the patient where the patient is now,* building from there. 2. Regularly engage with the patient. Connect at intervals and initially interact briefly about low-anxiety topics like the weather. Gradually increase the duration and/or frequency as interaction becomes more comfortable. 3. Offer encouragement to participate in unit activities without pressure, such as "We would love to see you at the morning meeting" or "How about going for a walk with me?" 4. Assure the patient that he generally has control over his choices. For example, if he becomes uncomfortable in a group, he can leave and try another day. 5. Reinforce each step toward greater interaction. "It was nice to see you in the morning meeting today." 6. Pet therapy may help patients increase comfort level with people.
Depression, hopelessness, and despair	The person may be dealing with loss and may recognize that the illness has affected her life negatively; if disabled, she may grieve for the dreams that have been taken from her.	1. Engage regularly with the patient. 2. Actively convey empathy and support. "Sometimes having a mental illness can feel very discouraging … I wonder how you are feeling?" 3. If he cannot identify his feelings, suggest those that may apply. "Sometimes it's hard to say what you're feeling. Do you feel sad, frustrated, or lost?" 4. Validate the patient's feelings as understandable and assure him that he is not alone. Identify options for coping with those feelings, such as keeping a journal or using a support group. 5. Teach activities that reduce depression or use cognitive interventions, physical activity, self-nurturing (such as taking a relaxing bath or listening to uplifting music), getting support from others, and spending more time on the outside if possible.
Poor self-esteem	Contributing factors include inability to achieve personal goals due to illness, stigma, isolation, depression.	1. Actively convey unconditional acceptance. 2. Engage regularly and supportively with the patient, guiding him to identify and express feelings. 3. Help the patient to recognize her or his own positive traits, potential, or accomplishments. 4. Educate the patient about how the illness may distort one's self-view. Guide the patient to question distorted beliefs and to replace these with a more realistic self-appraisal. 5. Arrange for interaction with individuals who also once experienced poor self-esteem but who have since improved.
Fall risk	Contributing factors include impaired balance, bradykinesia, and orthostatic hypotension.	1. Walk with all patients to assess their gait, providing physical support as needed. 2. Assess for orthostatic hypotension with lying and standing blood pressure checks. 3. With orthostatic hypotension, ensure that the patient is well hydrated and teach him to slowly change position stepwise from lying to sitting to standing. 4. Encourage the use of handrails or seeking assistance when unsteady. 5. People who fear falling tend to look at their feet when they walk. Guide the patient to look ahead instead of down. 6. Locate the patient's room close to the nurses' station so that help will be readily available.

Continued

TABLE 12.3   Additional Nursing Interventions for the Person Experiencing Psychosis—cont'd

Problem	Considerations	Nursing Care
Choking risk	Contributing factors include difficulty swallowing (dysphagia) due to muscle stiffness or dry mouth, failing to chew food thoroughly, taking bites that are too large (all of these routine functions can be disrupted in schizophrenia).	1. Assess all patients for difficulty swallowing and identify the causes if possible. 2. Address causes that can be corrected. With dry mouth, taking a sip of a beverage with each bite and avoiding dry foods can make swallowing much easier. 3. Encourage smaller bites that are then thoroughly chewed. 4. Ensure that patients are not rushed to complete their meals and encourage fast eaters to eat more slowly. 5. Be available at mealtime to monitor and assist if needed. This can give patients greater confidence, reducing anxiety and improving swallowing.
Restlessness, agitation	Contributing factors include akathisia, anxiety, interpersonal conflict, sensory overload, paranoia, hallucinations, anxiety, unrealistic expectations by others, concerns about the future.	1. Reduce excess stimulation—dim the lights, lower TV volume, redirect patient to less stimulating areas or activities. 2. Assess for and treat akathisia with medications that can reduce **extrapyramidal side effects (EPSs)** and anxiety. 3. Explore the patient's feelings and perceptions that may be contributing to akathisia and address these as indicated. 4. Promote verbal expression of negative emotions to reduce desperation or distress. 5. Provide safe outlets for physical energy (e.g., walk with patient, allow pacing, provide access to safe exercise equipment). 6. Administer calming medications as needed if agitation is unresponsive to nonpharmacological interventions.
Risk for other-directed violence	Aggression may stem from paranoia (assault may be self-defense in the patient's mind), command hallucinations, conflicts with staff about treatment or limit setting, conflicts with peers (who may be frustrated by intrusive or other patient behaviors, or may tease, speak disparagingly of, or even intentionally provoke distress in the patient).	1. Assess for paranoid thoughts, command hallucinations, interpersonal conflict, irritability, impaired impulse control, increasing tension and desperation, and other factors that may increase the risk of violence. 2. Engaging regularly with the patient increases the opportunity for assessment and communication about concerns that may contribute to risk. 3. Engender goodwill via supportive activities and a strong therapeutic relationship. 4. Provide increased supervision when risk is present. Placing the patient in a room near the nurses' station facilitates monitoring. 5. Make sure that the patient is taking ordered medications (see the section "Cheeking or Palming Medications"). 6. Monitor for and promptly de-escalate increasing tension. 7. Take action to help the patient feel safe and secure (e.g., if patient fears harm from outside the unit, note the locked doors and constant presence of staff). 8. Promote communication and venting in a safe manner to reduce the patient's level of anxiety or desperation. 9. Teach and guide the patient to practice coping skills so as to reduce stress and desperation. 10. Provide constructive diversion and outlets for physical energy. 11. If the patient, due to paranoia or other factors, targets specific peers, it may be necessary to relocate the patient or the targeted peer (whichever can best tolerate the relocation). Similar action may be needed if identifiable staff are targeted. 12. Only when truly necessary: use seclusion and/or chemical (medication) or physical restraint. 13. Search thoroughly on admission and repeat the search anytime circumstances suggest that the patient may have had an opportunity to make or acquire a weapon. 14. Refer to Chapter 27 for more information on caring for an aggressive patient.
Risk for self-directed violence	People with schizophrenia have a 10% lifetime suicide rate. They may experience depression, loss, impaired impulse control, impaired problem-solving, impaired coping, social isolation, and other risk factors.	1. Assess for risk to self. Warning signs include a sudden brightening or worsening of mood, termination activities (e.g., saying goodbye or giving away possessions), increased suicidal ideation, increased withdrawal, an increased sense of calm, increased restlessness, or taking action to acquire a means of suicide. Repeat risk assessment regularly, particularly if the patient's situation changes. 2. Increase supervision when risk is present. Placing the patient in a room near the nurses' station can facilitate monitoring. 3. Make rounds at unpredictable intervals and adjust frequency based on risk. Checks at predictable intervals (e.g., every 15 min) provide the patient with a window of predictable opportunity. 4. Ensure that the patient is receiving ordered medications (see the section "Cheeking or Palming Medications"). Some medications may help to reduce suicidality in schizophrenia (e.g., clozapine). 5. Extra precautions should be taken to make sure that the patient has not acquired a weapon. See intervention 13 in the section "Risk for Self-Directed Violence." 6. Implement interventions from the sections "Depression," "Hopelessness/Despair," and "Poor Self-Esteem."

CASE STUDY AND NURSING CARE PLAN

Schizophrenia

Don, age 42, has been in and out of hospitals for 13 years. His auditory hallucinations began at age 19 while he was serving as a marine in Afghanistan. He subsequently received a medical discharge. He has been separated from his wife and four children for 3 years and reports not sleeping much "because the voices get worse at night." Don uses cocaine because "It makes me feel good, and not much else does."

This hospitalization was precipitated by auditory hallucinations and paranoia worsened by drug abuse. "I thought people were following me. The voices say people hate me and I should die. People say that it happens because I don't take my medications ... they make me tired and I can't have sex."

He had a previous episode of suicidal ideation where voices were telling him to jump off a building. During a previous admission he assaulted a peer who he thought was planning to kill him.

Sarah is Don's nurse. Initially, Don rarely made eye contact and spoke in a soft monotone. He glanced around the room as if distracted, mumbled to himself, and appeared upset.

Nurse: Don, my name is Sarah. I will be your nurse while you're in the hospital. If it's okay with you, we will meet daily to talk about anything that concerns you.

Don: Well ... don't believe what they say about me. I want to start ... Are you married?

Nurse: This time is for *you* to talk about *your* concerns.

Don: (scans the room, then lowers his eyes) I think someone is trying to kill me ...

Nurse: You seem to be focusing on something other than our conversation.

Don: Voices tell me things ... I should die ...

Nurse: That must be frightening. Tell me what is happening, and I will try to help you.

After acknowledging his distress, Sarah focuses on the here and now and on Don's security. As Don gradually engages more in the conversation, his thoughts become more connected and he appears less distracted.

Self-Assessment

In a previous admission, Don assaulted peers he thought wanted to kill him. He reports that "God told me it was me or them." This frightens Sarah. An experienced nurse suggests that Sarah meet with Don in public areas on the unit with other staff nearby until he is more stable. Sarah feels more secure knowing that other staff are nearby. After 5 days, Don is calmer and relates well with Sarah.

Assessment

Subjective Data (Patient)

- "I don't sleep much because the voices get worse at night."
- "Someone is trying to kill me."
- "I hear voices ... telling me I don't deserve to live."
- "Medications make me tired and I can't have sex."
- "[Drugs] make me feel good ... not much else does."

Subjective Data (Other Sources)

- Separated from wife and children
- History of drug abuse (cocaine, marijuana)
- First hospitalized at age 19; has not worked since leaving military
- Has had suicidal impulses twice, both associated with command hallucinations
- Assaulted a peer in the hospital and attributed the assault to paranoid ideation

Objective Data

1. Speaks in soft monotone
2. Poor eye contact
3. Impaired reality testing
4. Distracted and looks around the room during conversation
5. Thoughts disorganized when anxious

Nursing Diagnosis 1

- Hallucinations and delusions related to neurological dysfunction as evidenced by persecutory hallucinations and paranoid delusions that he perceives as real:
- "The voices get worse at night, and I can't sleep."
- "Voices" have told him "You should die" and "Someone is trying to kill you."
- Although they increase his paranoia, he abuses cocaine and marijuana. "They make me feel good."

Outcomes Identification

1. Don recognizes that his hallucinations and delusions are not real and refrains from acting on them.
2. Don and others remain safe.

Short-Term Goal	Intervention	Rationale	Evaluation
1. By (date), Don reports when he has hallucinations and identifies one or more contributing factors (e.g., telling his nurse what preceded the hallucinations).	1a. Engage regularly and supportively to establish trust and rapport. 1b. Explore times when voices are worse or become disturbing, noting and teaching how to reduce the circumstances that preceded them (triggers). 1c. Encourage use of competing auditory stimulation, such as humming or music.	1a. Regular engagement helps decrease anxiety and establish trust. 1b. Identifies events that increase anxiety and trigger hallucinations; by learning to avoid or manage triggers, Don can reduce his hallucinations. 1c. A competing reality-based auditory stimulus can reduce Don's distress from hallucinations.	**GOAL MET** By the end of the first week, Don tells the nurse when he is experiencing hallucinations and reports that "music helps."
2. By (date), Don recognizes that the hallucinations are "not real" and sees them as part of his illness.	2a. Explore content of hallucinations to identify command hallucinations. 2b. Educate Don about the nature of hallucinations and ways to determine if they are real (e.g., encourage Don to compare his experiences with those of others to determine if his are real).	2a. Identifies risks (e.g., suicidal or aggressive themes or commands). 2b. Improves reality testing so that Don can distinguish hallucinations from reality; helps him realize that any commands can safely be ignored. Gives options for controlling the experience of hallucinations.	**GOAL MET** Don notes that others do not seem to hear what he hears and that he can ignore commands.

Continued

CASE STUDY AND NURSING CARE PLAN—cont'd

Short-Term Goal	Intervention	Rationale	Evaluation
3. By discharge, Don consistently reports a decrease in hallucinations, knows they are not real, and does not act on any commands he hears.	3a. Explore with Don actions that can minimize anxiety and/or reduce hallucinations (e.g., relaxation exercises and engaging in reality-based activities). 3b. Guide Don to recognize that hallucinations are helped by medication and other techniques that he has mastered.	3a. Offers means to lower anxiety level. 3b. Helps Don recognize that he can control his hallucinations, thus reducing feelings of powerlessness.	**GOAL MET** Don states that since stopping marijuana and cocaine use and beginning his medications, he hears fewer threatening voices. He notes that if he whistles or sings, he stays calm and can control the voices. Don has not assaulted others even when command hallucinations have occurred.

Note: Additional interventions for hallucinations are found in Box 12.2.

Nursing Diagnosis 2

- *Nonadherence to medications* related to side effects as evidenced by history of nonadherence and persistence of symptoms.
- Attributes nonadherence to "They make me tired and I can't have sex."
- Pattern of relapses.

Outcome Identification

1. Don consistently adheres to treatment.

1. By the end of week 1, Don discusses his concerns about side effects with staff.	1a. Evaluate medication response and side effects. 1b. Convey empathy and support while educating Don about the management of side effects. 1c. Discuss possible medication change with the medication prescriber.	1a. Identify drugs and dosages that have increased therapeutic value and decreased side effects. 1b. Reduces patient distress and resulting resistance caused by side effects, increasing Don's sense of control. 1c. Olanzapine causes no known sexual impairment.	**GOAL MET** Don identifies the reasons for stopping his medication. He agrees to try olanzapine (Zyprexa) because he trusts staff's assurances that the side effects will improve. Don states that he sleeps better at night but is still tired during the day.
2. By the end of week 2, Don identifies advantages of taking medications.	2a. Connect Don with the local National Alliance of Mentally Ill (NAMI) support group. 2b. Explore areas where medications help Don to meet his goals (e.g., reduce tormenting hallucinations).	2a. Provides peer support and a chance to hear from others further along in recovery how medications helped them and shows that side effects can be managed. National Alliance of Mentally Ill members can also offer suggestions for dealing with loneliness and other concerns. 2b. Seeing that medication helps him achieve his goals increases Don's motivation for treatment.	**GOAL MET** Week 1: Don attends a NAMI meeting. Week 2: He speaks in the group about "not feeling good." Several peers say they understand, responding supportively and helpfully. Don describes how taking medication has helped his peers.

At discharge, Don reports that the medicines have reduced his voices and helped him to feel better and think more clearly. He voices an understanding of his medications and how to cope with side effects, also noting how they can help him to meet his goals. He knows that marijuana and cocaine make his symptoms worse and explains that when he feels down, he now knows three constructive ways to help himself feel better.

Note: Additional nursing interventions for patients with schizophrenia can be found in Table 12.3.

Counseling and Communication Techniques

Therapeutic communication techniques for patients with schizophrenia aim to build trust and reduce anxiety. Staff should remember that people with schizophrenia may have memory and attentional impairment and that repetition and visual and verbal reminders promote learning and task completion. People who think concretely also benefit from concrete examples during education (e.g., counting out the equivalent number of sugar cubes found in a bottle of cola to show its sugar content). Shorter (less than 30 minutes) but more frequent interactions may be less stimulating and better tolerated than fewer, longer interactions.

Intervening With Hallucinations

Hallucinations are real to the person who is experiencing them and may be distracting during interactions. They can be supportive or terrifying, faint or loud, episodic or constant. They can be sounds or voices and are sometimes attributed to specific sources (e.g., a parent or God).

When a patient is hallucinating, the nurse focuses on understanding the patient's experiences and responses. Suicidal or homicidal themes or commands require safety measures. For example, if voices tell a patient that a peer plans to assault him, the patient may act aggressively against that person. In this case, close monitoring, helping the patient to feel safe, and

BOX 12.2   Helping Patients Who Are Experiencing Hallucinations

Nursing Care

1. Watch the patient for hallucination indicators, such as eyes tracking an unheard speaker, muttering or talking to self, appearing distracted, suddenly stopping conversing as if interrupted, or intently watching a vacant area of the room.
2. Ask about the content of the hallucinations and how the patient is reacting to them. Assess for command hallucinations, and assess for resulting fear or distress.
3. Avoid referring to hallucinations as if they were real. Do not ask, "What are the voices saying to you?" Ask, "What are you hearing?"
4. Be alert to signs of anxiety, which may indicate that hallucinations are intensifying or that they are of a command type.
5. Do not negate the patient's experience but offer your own perceptions and convey empathy. "I don't hear angry voices that you hear, but that must be very frightening for you."
6. Focus on reality-based "here and now" activities, such as conversations or simple projects.
7. Address any underlying emotion, need, or theme that seems to be indicated by the hallucination, such as fear with menacing voices or guilt with accusing voices.
8. Promote and guide reality testing. If the patient has frightening hallucinations, guide her or him to scan the area to see if others appear frightened; if they are not, encourage the patient to consider that these might be hallucinations. Teach the patient to compare such beliefs and perceptions to those of trusted others.
9. As the patient begins to develop insight and reality testing improves, guide him or her to interpret the hallucinations as symptoms of illness. "The voice you hear is part of your illness, and it cannot hurt you. Try to listen to me and the others you can see around you."
10. Cognitive interventions, such as teaching the patient to question perceptions if they are unusual or unlikely, can help him or her to cope with hallucinations by altering how the experience is perceived (see Chapter 2).
11. Transcranial magnetic stimulation may enhance relief from auditory hallucinations.

Teach the Patient to:

1. Manage stress and stimulation
   - Avoid overly loud or stressful places or activities.
   - Avoid negative or critical people and seek out supportive people.
   - Learn assertive communication skills so you can tell others "no" if they pressure or upset you.
   - When stressed, slow and deepen your breathing. Count slowly from one to four as you inhale, hold the breath, and exhale.
   - Gently tense and then relax your muscles, one area of the body at a time, starting at your head (e.g., closing your eyes then opening them, clenching your teeth then relaxing your jaw) and working your way down to your hands and feet.
   - Discover other ways that help manage your stress (e.g., going for a walk, meditation, taking a hot bath, reading or listening to music, imagining yourself in a less stressful situation [sometimes called a *mental vacation*]).
2. Use other sounds that compete with the hallucinations (sometimes called *competing auditory stimuli*).
   - Talk with others.
   - Listen to music or television (but not too loud).
   - Read aloud.
   - Sing, whistle, or hum.
3. Find out what is and isn't real (called *promoting reality testing*).
   - Look at others; do they seem to be hearing/seeing what you are?
   - Ask trusted others if they are experiencing what you are.
   - If the answers to these questions are "no" then, although it seems very real to you, it is most likely not real, and you can safely ignore the voices/images.
4. Engage in activities that can take your mind off what you hear.
   - Walk.
   - Clean.
   - Take a relaxing bath or shower.
   - Play music or an instrument or sing.
   - Go to any place where you enjoy being where others will be present, such as a coffee shop, mall, or library.
5. Talk (if others are nearby, quietly or silently to self).
   - Tell the voices or thoughts to go away.
   - Tell yourself that the voices and thoughts are a symptom and aren't real.
   - Tell yourself that no matter what you hear, you will be safe and you can ignore what you hear.
6. Make contact with others.
   - Talk with a trusted friend, relative, or staff member.
   - Call a help line or go to a drop-in center.
   - Visit a public place where you are comfortable.
7. Develop a plan for how to cope with hallucinations; options include
   - Any of the activities already mentioned that work for you
   - Taking extra medication when ordered (call your prescriber)
   - Using breathing exercises and other relaxation methods

From Capizzi, R., Ramsay, I., & Vinogradov, S. (2019). The efficacy of transcranial direct current stimulation for the treatment of persistent auditory hallucinations in schizophrenia: a meta-analysis. *Schizophrenia Bulletin Supplement 45*, S343; and Herzog, E. (2014). Caring for the hallucinating patient: Non-pharmacological interventions. Presentation at the American Psychiatric Nurses Association 28th Annual Conference, October 22, 2014.

maintaining separation of the patient and potential victim would be indicated.

Nursing care also includes calling the patient by name, speaking simply and loudly enough to be understood during hallucinations, conveying support, maintaining eye contact, and redirecting the patient's focus to the conversation with the nurse as needed (see Box 12.2 regarding helping patients who are experiencing hallucinations).

Intervening With Delusions

Impaired reality testing prevents self-correction of irrational thoughts that normally would be disregarded. When the nurse attempts to see the world through the patient's eyes, it becomes easier to understand the patient's delusion. For example:

Patient: You people are all alike ... all part of the FBI plot to destroy me.

Nurse: It seems to you that people want to hurt you. That must be very frightening. I will not hurt you, and we can work together to help you feel safer.

Here, the nurse acknowledges and accepts the patient's experience and feelings, conveys empathy about the patient's fearfulness, provides reassurance about her intentions, avoids questioning the delusion itself, and focuses on helping the patient feel safer (addressing the underlying theme of fear).

BOX 12.3 Helping Patients Who Are Experiencing Delusions

- Build trust by being open, honest, genuine, and reliable.
- Respond to suspicion in a matter-of-fact, empathic, supportive, and calm manner.
- Ask the patient to describe beliefs. "Tell me more about someone trying to hurt you."
- Never debate the delusional content.
- As the patient's reality testing improves, supportively convey doubt as tolerated. "Although it is frightening for you, it seems as if it would be hard for a girl that small to hurt you."
- Validate if part of the delusion is real. "Yes, there was a man at the nurse's station, but I did not hear him talk about you."
- Focus on the feelings or themes within the delusion. If a patient believes that he is a famous leader, comment: "It would feel good to be more powerful." If the patient believes that others intend to hurt him, comment: "It must feel frightening to believe others want to hurt you."
- Use reality-based interventions that help meet underlying needs. If the patient believes that he is powerful, it may represent a sense of powerlessness. Increase the patient's control, such as asking the patient when he would like to take his medications.
- Acknowledge that although the belief seems real to the patient, illnesses can make things *seem* true even though they aren't. Introducing this indirectly can make it less confrontational: "I wonder if that might be what is happening here, because what seems true to you does not seem true to others."
- Do not dwell excessively on the delusion. Instead, refocus onto reality-based topics.
- Help the patient to identify triggers of delusions and find ways to avoid them.
- Promote reality testing by questioning beliefs: "I wonder if there might be any other explanation why others might be avoiding you? Instead of hating you, mightn't they simply be busy?"

Focusing on the delusion itself, the beliefs about the FBI, would not be helpful. Focusing on fear, its causes, and what can help the patient to feel more secure is therapeutic.

Until the patient's testing of reality improves, it is *never* useful to try to prove that the delusion is incorrect. This can instead intensify the delusion and cause the patient to view staff as people who cannot be trusted. However, it *is* helpful to clarify misinterpretations of the environment and gently suggest, as tolerated, a more reality-based perspective. For example:

Patient: I see the doctor is here. He wants to kill me.

Nurse: It is true the doctor wants to see you, as he talks with all patients about their treatment. Would you feel more comfortable if I stayed with you during your meeting?

Focusing on reality-based activities and events occurring in the present keeps the focus on reality and provides opportunities to distinguish what is real. The nurse works with the patient to find and promote helpful coping strategies. Box 12.3 provides strategies for working with patients experiencing delusions.

Intervening With Associative Looseness

Associative looseness is part of disorganized thinking. Increased anxiety or overstimulation worsens cognitive disorganization.

Guidelines for helping those with disorganized thinking include the following:

- Do not pretend or allow the patient to think that you understand when you don't.
- Place the difficulty in understanding on yourself, *not* on the patient. Example: "I'm having trouble following what you are saying," *not* "You're not making any sense."
- Tell the patient what you *do* understand, and reinforce clear communication of needs, feelings, and thoughts when it occurs.
- Look for recurring issues and themes in the patient's communications, and tie these to possible triggers. Example: "You've mentioned trouble with your brother several times, usually after your family has visited. Tell me about your brother and your visits with him."
- Summarize or paraphrase the patient's communications to role-model clearer communication and to give the patient a chance to correct anything you may have misunderstood.
- Speak concisely, clearly, and concretely, in sentences rather than paragraphs.

Teamwork and Safety

A therapeutic milieu provides structure and external boundaries that create a sense of security. It is a physical and social environment that maximizes safety, opportunities for learning and practicing skills (such as conflict resolution, stress reduction, and symptom management techniques), and engaging in therapeutic activities (e.g., games that promote socialization, therapy groups that help patients to develop insight or coping abilities). Hospital alternatives such as crisis centers and partial hospitalization programs also provide a therapeutic milieu in a less restrictive setting.

Activities and Groups

Participation in activities and groups appropriate to the patient's needs and abilities may decrease withdrawal, enhance motivation, modify unacceptable behaviors, improve understanding of the illness, and increase social competence and other skills. Drawing, writing poetry, journaling, and listening to music promote the expression of feelings and coping with them. Task completion and participation in activities for which there is a high likelihood of success enhance self-esteem.

Recreational activities such as games and outings to stores or restaurants are not simply diversions. They teach and provide practice opportunities that improve cognition and constructive leisure skills, increase social comfort, build interactional skills, promote independence, and improve boundaries. Outpatient programs can provide structure after discharge.

Health Teaching and Promotion

Education should include the causes, nature, and symptoms of the illness, what to expect, and how it is treated. Patients should be taught ways to cope and control the illness and its symptoms. They should also be taught about medications and side effects, helpful resources, and relapse prevention. This knowledge will help them to become actively involved in the course of their recovery.

BOX 12.4 **Patient and Family Teaching: Schizophrenia**

1. Have regular contact with supportive individuals.
2. Taking care of one's diet, health, and hygiene keeps you healthy.
3. Minimize tobacco and caffeine, as they may make your medicines less effective and hurt your health.
4. Maintain a stable weight; if you are overweight, work to lose weight.
5. Maintain a regular sleep pattern.
6. Keep active (hobbies, friends, groups, sports, job, special interests).
7. Nurture yourself and practice stress-reduction activities daily.
8. Join support groups such as the National Alliance on Mental Illness (NAMI.org) and attend local meetings where available.
9. Learn all you can about the illness (e.g., through NAMI's Family-to-Family program).
10. Read books about severe mental illness, such as the following:
    - *Surviving Schizophrenia (7th Edition): A Family Manual* by E. Fuller Torrey (2019, New York, NY: HarperCollins. ISBN-13: 978-0062880802)
    - *I Am Not Sick, I Don't Need Help! How to Help Someone with Mental Illness Accept Treatment (10th anniversary edition)* by Xavier Amador (2012, Peconic, NY: Vida Press. ISBN-13: 2940014075459). A free excerpt is available at NAMI.org
11. Access reliable websites and online videos, including these:

- *Living with Schizophrenia* (X. Amador and others, LEAP Institute). Provides basic information and hope for recovery via interviews with people living with schizophrenia, as well as mental healthcare professionals.
- *National Alliance on Mental Illness*: About schizophrenia.
- *Schizophrenia.com*, a source of online support and information about schizophrenia.
- *National Institute of Mental Health*: Provides information about schizophrenia and other mental health disorders, including research and treatment.
- *Fred Frese* was a psychologist who lived with schizophrenia. He was an advocate for others with the disorder and offers helpful suggestions for coping with the illness.
- *Minds on the Edge*, a panel discussion on issues often experienced by those seeking to obtain help for a mental illness.
- *Out of the Shadow* captures the issues that can occur when families have a loved one with severe mental illness. It also documents the obstacles to treatment created by an underfunded mental health system.
- *Schizophrenia and Related Disorders Alliance of America*, a support and advocacy organization for those who live with mental illness and those who care about them.

Ideally, significant others and caregivers are included in teaching. Often, relationships have been stressed by the illness. Significant others may have become critical, controlling, or intrusive. Lack of understanding of the disease and its symptoms can lead others to mistake symptoms such as apathy and poor hygiene as intentionally bad behavior. Teaching significant others how to recognize and respond helpfully to symptoms and how to negotiate and help the patient to achieve needed changes is important. Box 12.4 identifies patient and family teaching about schizophrenia.

Additional nursing interventions for patients with schizophrenia are listed in Table 12.3.

EVALUATION

Progress should be reevaluated regularly and treatment adjusted when needed. Staff, patients, and significant others should remember that gains may be small and difficult to see at first. Even when it seems to others that symptoms have improved considerably, the patient may still be recovering. As with other serious illnesses, full recovery can take months. Setting small goals makes it easier to identify progress that may occur in small increments.

Conveying interest in the patient's progress communicates concern and caring. This promotes recovery and treatment adherence and reduces feelings of helplessness. Involving the patient collaboratively as a true partner in care is central to the Recovery Model and increases patient trust, motivation, and buy-in.

TREATMENT MODALITIES
Biological Treatments
Pharmacotherapy
Antipsychotic medications are used to treat psychotic disorders such as schizophrenia. The first of these medications became available in the 1950s. Until the late 1960s, patients with

schizophrenia usually spent months or years in state or private hospitals, resulting in great emotional and financial costs to patients, families, and society. Antipsychotic drugs at last provided symptom control and allowed most patients to live and be treated in the community.

Drugs used to treat psychotic disorders include the following:
1. **First-generation antipsychotics**, also known as typical antipsychotics or neuroleptics, comprise the oldest and hence first generation of antipsychotics. They are dopamine (D_2 receptor) antagonists. Examples include haloperidol (Haldol) and chlorpromazine (Thorazine).
2. **Second-generation antipsychotics**, also referred to as atypical antipsychotics, are serotonin (5-HT_{2A} receptor) and dopamine (D_2 receptor) antagonists. Examples of this classification include clozapine (Clozaril) and risperidone (Risperdal).

The first-generation antipsychotics work primarily by reducing positive symptoms (e.g., hallucinations and delusions) but have little effect on negative symptoms. Second-generation antipsychotics treat positive symptoms and can also help negative symptoms (e.g., asociality, blunted affect), although improvement in negative and cognitive symptoms is usually less. Second-generation antipsychotic drugs also tend to produce fewer and better-tolerated side effects.

It usually takes 2 to 6 weeks for antipsychotic drugs to become effective. Patient-specific dosage adjustment is required to obtain an optimal balance between effectiveness and side effects. Monotherapy, the use of a single antipsychotic medication, is recommended. After the failure of two monotherapy trials, a clozapine (Clozaril) trial is justified. If clozapine treatment fails or is not tolerated, a second antipsychotic may be used to improve the response of another.

Antipsychotics are not addictive but should be discontinued gradually to minimize a discontinuation syndrome, whose symptoms include dizziness, nausea, tremors, insomnia, electric shock–like pains, and anxiety. Antipsychotic agents are unlikely to be lethal in overdose. A lesser-known risk of all antipsychotic medications, due to dopamine blockade or sedation, is impaired swallowing. This may cause drooling and the risk of choking (Funayama, Takata, & Koreki, 2019). Also, patients taking these medications are at increased fall risk due to orthostatic (postural) hypotension, sedation, and gait impairment.

Liquid or fast-dissolving forms, available for selected antipsychotics, can make it difficult for a person to cheek or palm his medicine (hide it in his cheek or palm and later dispose of it). See Table 12.3 for interventions to prevent cheeking and palming.

Some antipsychotics are available in short-acting injectable form, used primarily for the treatment of agitation and emergencies, such as assaultive behavior or when a patient refuses court-mandated oral antipsychotics. Side effects can be intensified and less easily managed when medication is administered intramuscularly.

Antipsychotics are also available in long-acting injectable (LAI) formulations that need to be administered only every 2 to 4 weeks or even months. Some require special administration protocols (Table 12.4). By requiring less frequent administration, conflict about taking medications is reduced and adherence is improved. However, patients may not like injections or can feel like they have less control over their treatment.

Additional information on antipsychotic medications can be found in Table 12.5.

First-generation antipsychotics. First-generation antipsychotics are used less often because of their minimal impact on negative symptoms and their generally higher level of challenging side effects. However, they are as effective in treating positive symptoms as newer antipsychotics and are much less expensive than some second-generation antipsychotics. For patients untroubled by their side effects, first-generation antipsychotics can remain an appropriate choice, especially when cost or the risk of a metabolic syndrome, which is more common with the newer drugs (described later in this chapter), is a concern.

Side effects of first-generation antipsychotics. First-generation antipsychotics are dopamine (D_2) antagonists in both limbic and motor centers. Blockage of D_2 receptors in motor areas causes **extrapyramidal side effects (EPSs),** including the following:

1. Acute dystonia—A sudden, sustained contraction of one or several muscle groups, usually of the head and neck. Acute dystonias can be frightening and uncomfortable, but unless they involve muscles affecting the airway, which is rare, they are not dangerous. However, they cause significant anxiety and should be treated promptly.
2. Akathisia—A motor restlessness that causes pacing and/or an inability to stay still or remain in one place. It can be severe and distressing to patients and can be mistaken for anxiety or agitation. These symptoms may lead to mistakenly administering more of the drug that originally caused the akathisia, making it worse. A tardive form can persist despite treatment.
3. Pseudoparkinsonism—A temporary group of symptoms that resemble Parkinson disease: tremor, reduced accessory movements (e.g., arms swinging when walking), gait impairment, reduced facial expressiveness (mask facies), and slowing of motor behavior (bradykinesia).

EPSs can be minimized by lowering doses of the drug, and they can be prevented by using antipsychotics less liable to cause EPSs. These unusual side effects may diminish over time. Oral **antiparkinsonian drugs** are also useful, either prophylactically or when EPSs develop. However, antiparkinsonian drugs have their own side effects (e.g., most are anticholinergic). Abuse of some antiparkinsonian drugs, particularly trihexyphenidyl (Artane) but also benztropine (Cogentin) and diphenhydramine (Benadryl), may occur.

Tardive dyskinesia is a persistent EPS involving involuntary rhythmic movements. It develops in about 25% of patients on antipsychotics. Tardive dyskinesia is more common with first-generation antipsychotics, usually after prolonged treatment, and usually persists even after the medication has been discontinued. Smoking, alcohol, and stimulant use may increase the risk of this form of EPS. It usually begins in oral and facial muscles and progresses to include the fingers, toes, neck, trunk, or pelvis. More common in women, tardive dyskinesia varies from mild to severe, and can be disfiguring or incapacitating (Margolius & Fernandez, 2019).

The National Institute of Mental Health (NIMH) developed the *Abnormal Involuntary Movement Scale* (AIMS) (Fig. 12.2) to identify and monitor involuntary movements. Assessing patients using the AIMS is a key nursing role in treating this population.

Tardive dyskinesia in adults can be treated with two drugs (U.S. Food and Drug Administration, 2017): valbenazine (Ingrezza) and deutetrabenazine (Austedo). These drugs are selective vesicular monoamine transporter inhibitors and reduce the severity of abnormal movements in tardive dyskinesia. Adverse effects include sleepiness and QT prolongation. They are contraindicated with congenital or acquired long-QT syndrome or related dysrhythmias. They should be used with caution in people who drive or operate heavy machinery or do other dangerous activities until how the drug affects them is known. Switching to a second-generation antipsychotic or reducing or (paradoxically) increasing the first-generation antipsychotic dosage can be helpful (Margolius & Fernandez, 2019).

The first-generation and some second-generation antipsychotics cause anticholinergic side effects by blocking muscarinic cholinergic receptors. Anticholinergic side effects include urinary retention, dilated pupils, constipation, reduced visual accommodation (blurred near vision), tachycardia, dry mucous membranes, reduced peristalsis (rarely leading to paralytic ileus and risk of bowel obstruction), and cognitive impairment. Taking multiple medications with anticholinergic side effects increases the risk of anticholinergic toxicity, covered later in this chapter. In general, first-generation antipsychotics have either a strong EPS potential or strong anticholinergic potential; that is, when one side effect is prominent, the other is not.

TABLE 12.4 Antipsychotic Drugs: Classification and Relative Side-Effect Profiles

Drug	Trade Name	INCIDENCE OF SIDE EFFECTS							
		Extrapyramidal Effects[a]	Sedation	Orthostatic Hypotension	Anticholinergic Effects	Metabolic Effects: Weight Gain, Diabetes Risk, Dyslipidemia	Significant QT Prolongation	Prolactin Elevation	Metabolized by CYP3A4
First-Generation (Conventional) Antipsychotics									
Low Potency									
Chlorpromazine	Generic only	Moderate	High	High	Moderate	Moderate	Yes	Low	—
Thioridazine	Generic only	Low	High	High	High	Moderate	Yes	Low	—
Medium Potency									
Loxapine	Loxitane	Moderate	Moderate	Low	Low	Low	No	Moderate	—
Perphenazine	Generic only	Moderate	Moderate	Low	Low	—	No	Low	—
High Potency									
Fluphenazine	Generic only	Very high	Low	Low	Low	—	No	Moderate	—
Haloperidol	Haldol	Very high	Low	Low	Low	Moderate	Yes	Moderate	—
Pimozide	Orap	High	Moderate	Low	Moderate	—	Yes	Moderate	—
Thiothixene	Navane	High	Low	Moderate	Low	Moderate	No	Moderate	—
Trifluoperazine	Generic only	High	Low	Low	Low	—	No	Moderate	—
Second-Generation (Atypical) Antipsychotics									
Aripiprazole[b]	Abilify	Very low	Low	Low	None	None/low	No	Low	Yes
Asenapine	Saphris	Moderate	Moderate	Moderate	Low	Low	Yes	Low	Slightly
Brexpiprazole[b]	Rexulti	Very low	Low	Low	None	Low	No	Low	Yes
Cariprazine[b]	Vraylar	Moderate	Moderate	Low	Low	Moderate	No	No	Yes
Clozapine	Clozaril, FazaClo, Versacloz	Very low	High	Moderate	High	High	No	Low	Yes
Iloperidone	Fanapt	Very low	Moderate	Moderate	Moderate	Moderate	Yes	Low	Yes
Lumateperone	Caplyta	Low	Moderate	Low	Low	Low	No	Low	Yes
Lurasidone	Latuda	Moderate	Moderate	Low	None	None/low	No	Low	Yes
Olanzapine	Zyprexa	Low	Moderate	Moderate	Moderate	High	No	Low	No
Paliperidone	Invega	Moderate	Low	Low	None	Moderate	No	High	Slightly
Quetiapine	Seroquel	Very low	Moderate	Moderate	None	Moderate/high	Yes	High	Yes
Risperidone	Risperdal	Moderate	Low	Low	None	Moderate	Yes	High	No
Ziprasidone	Geodon	Low	Moderate	Moderate	None	None/low	Yes	Low	Yes

[a]Incidence here refers to *early* extrapyramidal reactions (acute dystonia, parkinsonism, akathisia). The incidence of *late* reactions (tardive dyskinesia) is the same for all traditional antipsychotics.
[b]These are considered to be third generation antipsychotics by some sources.
Data from Burchum, J., & Rosenthal, L. (2019). *Lehne's pharmacology for nursing care* (10th ed.). St. Louis, MO: Elsevier.

Other first-generation antipsychotic side effects include sedation, orthostatic (postural) hypotension, lowered seizure threshold (which can lead to seizures in seizure-vulnerable individuals), and photosensitivity, cataracts, or other visual changes (with chlorpromazine [Thorazine] and thioridazine [Mellaril]). Neuroendocrine abnormalities, such as increased release of prolactin (hyperprolactinemia), may result in sexual dysfunction (impotence, anorgasmia, impaired ejaculation). Galactorrhea (a milky nipple discharge), amenorrhea, and gynecomastia are also side effects of first-generation antipsychotics. Weight gain can be more than 50 lb per year, causing significant psychological distress and increasing the risk of cardiovascular disorders and diabetes.

ABNORMAL INVOLUNTARY MOVEMENT SCALE (AIMS)

Public Health Service
Alcohol, Drug Abuse, and Mental Health Administration
National Institute of Mental Health

Name: _____
Date: _____
Prescribing Practitioner: _____

Code: 0 = None
1 = Minimal, may be extreme normal
2 = Mild
3 = Moderate
4 = Severe

Instructions: Complete Examination Procedure before making ratings.

Movement ratings: Rate highest severity observed. Rate movements that occur upon activation one *less* than those observed spontaneously. Circle movement as well as code number that applies.		Rater Date	Rater Date	Rater Date	Rater Date
Facial and Oral Movements	**1. Muscles of facial expression** (e.g., movements of forehead, eyebrows, periorbital area, cheeks, including frowning, blinking, smiling, grimacing)	0 1 2 3 4	0 1 2 3 4	0 1 2 3 4	0 1 2 3 4
	2. Lips and perioral area (e.g., puckering, pouting, smacking)	0 1 2 3 4	0 1 2 3 4	0 1 2 3 4	0 1 2 3 4
	3. Jaw (e.g., biting, clenching, chewing, mouth opening, lateral movement)	0 1 2 3 4	0 1 2 3 4	0 1 2 3 4	0 1 2 3 4
	4. Tongue: Rate only increases in movement both in and out of mouth — *not* inability to sustain movement. Darting in and out of mouth.	0 1 2 3 4	0 1 2 3 4	0 1 2 3 4	0 1 2 3 4
Extremity Movements	**5. Upper (arms, wrists, hands, fingers):** Include choreic movements (i.e., rapid, objectively purposeless, irregular, spontaneous) and athetoid movements (i.e., slow, irregular, complex, serpentine). *Do not include tremor* (i.e., repetitive, regular, rhythmic).	0 1 2 3 4	0 1 2 3 4	0 1 2 3 4	0 1 2 3 4
	6. Lower (legs, knees, ankles, toes) (e.g., lateral knee movement, foot tapping, heel dropping, foot squirming, inversion and eversion of foot)	0 1 2 3 4	0 1 2 3 4	0 1 2 3 4	0 1 2 3 4
Trunk Movements	**7. Neck, shoulder, hips** (e.g., rocking, twisting, squirming, pelvic gyrations)	0 1 2 3 4	0 1 2 3 4	0 1 2 3 4	0 1 2 3 4
Global Judgments	**8. Severity of abnormal movements overall**	0 1 2 3 4	0 1 2 3 4	0 1 2 3 4	0 1 2 3 4
	9. Incapacitation due to abnormal movements	0 1 2 3 4	0 1 2 3 4	0 1 2 3 4	0 1 2 3 4
	10. Patient's awareness of abnormal movements: Rate only patient's report. No awareness 0; Aware, no distress 1; Aware, mild distress 2; Aware, moderate distress 3; Aware, severe distress 4	0 1 2 3 4	0 1 2 3 4	0 1 2 3 4	0 1 2 3 4
Dental Status	**11. Current problems with teeth and/or dentures**	No Yes	No Yes	No Yes	No Yes
	12. Are dentures usually worn?	No Yes	No Yes	No Yes	No Yes
	13. Edentia	No Yes	No Yes	No Yes	No Yes
	14. Do movements disappear in sleep?	No Yes	No Yes	No Yes	No Yes

Fig. 12.2 Abnormal Involuntary Movement Scale (AIMS).

AIMS Examination Procedure
Either before or after completing the Examination Procedure, observe the patient unobtrusively, at rest (e.g., in waiting room).

The chair to be used in this examination should be a hard, firm one without arms.

1. Ask patient to remove shoes and socks.
2. Ask patient whether there is anything in his or her mouth (e.g., gum, candy) and, if there is, to remove it.
3. Ask patient about the *current* condition of his or her teeth. Ask patient if he or she wears dentures. Do teeth or dentures bother the patient *now?*
4. Ask patient whether he or she notices any movements in mouth, face, hands, or feet. If yes, ask to describe and to what extent they *currently* bother patient or interfere with his or her activities.
5. Have patient sit in chair with hands on knees, legs slightly apart, and feet flat on floor. Look at entire body movements while in this position.
6. Ask patient to sit with hands hanging unsupported: if male, between legs; if female and wearing a dress, hanging over knees. Observe hands and other body areas.
7. Ask patient to open mouth. Observe tongue at rest within mouth. Do this twice.
8. Ask patient to protrude tongue. Observe abnormalities of tongue movement. Do this twice.
9. Ask patient to tap thumb, with each finger, as rapidly as possible for 10 to 15 seconds, separately with right hand, then with left hand. Observe each facial and leg movement.
10. Flex and extend patient's left and right arms (one at a time). Note any rigidity.
11. Ask patient to stand up. Observe in profile. Observe all body areas again, hips included.
12. Ask patient to extend both arms outstretched in front with palms down. Observe trunk, legs, and mouth.
13. Have patient walk a few paces, turn, and walk back to chair. Observe hands and gait. Do this twice.

Fig. 12.2, Cont'd

Some side effects, such as sedation, occur initially but improve thereafter. Potentially dangerous side effects are infrequent but include anticholinergic toxicity, neuroleptic malignant syndrome, and prolongation of the QT interval, all discussed later in this section. Side effects that are not addressed by healthcare professionals increase the risk of treatment nonadherence. See Table 12.6 for nursing care for common or potentially dangerous side effects.

Second-generation antipsychotics. Second-generation antipsychotics include drugs such as clozapine (Clozaril), risperidone (Risperdal), olanzapine (Zyprexa), quetiapine (Seroquel), and ziprasidone (Geodon). They are D_2 receptor antagonists, as are first-generation antipsychotics, but they bind to serotonin receptors as well. Second-generation antipsychotics are often chosen as first-line antipsychotics because they are equally effective for positive symptoms and may also help negative symptoms.

Side effects of second-generation antipsychotics. As is the case with first-generation antipsychotics, second-generation antipsychotics can cause sedation, sexual dysfunction, seizures, and increased mortality in older adults with dementia. However, most drugs in this classification are less likely to cause tardive dyskinesia or significant EPSs. Although they have the same potential side effects as the first-generation antipsychotics, second-generation antipsychotic side effects are usually fewer, milder, and better tolerated.

When the first second-generation antipsychotic clozapine (Clozaril) was approved in the United States in 1989, it produced dramatic improvement in some patients whose disorder had been resistant to first-generation antipsychotics. Clozapine

helped improve negative symptoms as well. Unfortunately, clozapine causes severe neutropenia in 0.5% to 1% of those who take it. As a result, patients taking clozapine are routinely monitored for absolute neutrophil counts (ANCs) (discussed later).

Clozaril can also cause myocarditis and in rare cases can contribute to life-threatening bowel emergencies and new-onset diabetes as well as, rarely, ketoacidosis. Owing to these serious concerns, clozapine use in the United States has declined. However, it is one of the few drugs that have FDA approval for the treatment of suicidality in schizophrenia and is the drug of choice for individuals who are unresponsive to other antipsychotics. One wide-scale study of more than 62,000 people found that taking antipsychotics was associated with a substantially reduced mortality, especially among patients treated with clozapine.

All second-generation antipsychotics carry a risk of metabolic syndrome, which includes weight gain (especially in the abdominal area), dyslipidemia, increased blood glucose, and insulin resistance. Metabolic syndrome is a significant concern and increases the risk of diabetes, certain cancers, hypertension, and cardiovascular disease, making its prevention an important role for nurses (see Table 12.6). Metformin (Glucophage), an anti-diabetic medication, has shown promise in reducing antipsychotic weight gain in children, adolescents, and adults (Ellul et al., 2018; Luo et al., 2019).

Some second-generation antipsychotics also have antidepressant properties and are FDA approved for adjunctive use in the treatment of major depressive disorder as well bipolar disorder. As with all antidepressants, they carry a theoretical risk of increased suicidality, particularly in adolescents. Other potentially dangerous second-generation antipsychotic side effects include anticholinergic toxicity, neuroleptic malignant syndrome, and prolongation of the QT interval, all discussed later in this section.

Other second-generation antipsychotics. A subset of the second-generation antipsychotics—aripiprazole (Abilify), brexpiprazole (Rexulti), and cariprazine (Vraylar)—are sometimes referred to as third-generation antipsychotics. They are described as dopamine system stabilizers that reduce dopamine activity in some brain regions while increasing it in others. Aripiprazole and brexpiprazole act as D_2 partial agonists. They attach to the D_2 receptor without fully activating it, reducing the effective level of dopamine activity. Cariprazine acts as a partial agonist more on D_3 than D_2 receptors, which may help to improve cognitive symptoms.

Additional information about antipsychotics can be found in Tables 12.4 and 12.5. Table 12.6 describes common antipsychotic side effects and related nursing care.

Serious side effects of antipsychotic medications. Nurses need to know about some rare but serious and potentially fatal effects of antipsychotics, including anticholinergic toxicity, neuroleptic malignant syndrome, and severe neutropenia. Nurses in psychiatry, primary care, and emergency services in particular need to be familiar with and to monitor for the early signs of these side effects. Patients and families should be taught to recognize and respond immediately to dangerous side effects. More information and nursing care for these side effects is included in Table 12.6.

Anticholinergic toxicity is a potentially life-threatening medical emergency caused by antipsychotics or other anticholinergic medications, including many antiparkinsonian drugs and over-the-counter cold/allergy medicines. Older adults and those on multiple anticholinergic drugs are at greatest risk. Symptoms include autonomic nervous system instability, dilated pupils, urinary retention, and delirium with altered mental status. Mental status changes can include hallucinations and may be mistaken for a worsening of the patient's psychosis, so people whose psychosis is inexplicably worsening should immediately be evaluated for possible anticholinergic toxicity.

Neuroleptic malignant syndrome (NMS), caused by excessive dopamine receptor blockade, occurs in about 0.2% to 1% of patients who have taken first-generation antipsychotics. It is characterized by reduced consciousness and responsiveness, increased muscle tone (generalized muscular rigidity), and autonomic dysfunction. Although less likely, NMS can also occur with second-generation antipsychotics.

NMS is a life-threatening medical emergency that is fatal in about 6% of cases (Modi et al., 2016). Complications of this

TABLE 12.5   Long-Acting Injectable Antipsychotics

Generic (Trade)	Usual Frequency	Nursing Considerations
First-Generation Antipsychotics		
Haloperidol decanoate (Haldol Decanoate)	Every 4 weeks	Viscous, deltoid or gluteal site Z-track method
Fluphenazine decanoate (generic only)	Every 2–3 weeks	Viscous, deltoid or gluteal site Z-track method
Second-Generation Antipsychotics		
Olanzapine pamoate (Zyprexa Relprevv)	Every 2–4 weeks	Must monitor patient for excess sedation for 3 h postinjection Gluteal site only Shake vigorously just before administering
Paliperidone palmitate (Invega Sustenna)	Every 4 weeks	When initiating, the first two injections must be given deltoid on days 1 and 8. Deltoid or gluteal site afterward. Shake vigorously just before administering
Paliperidone palmitate (Invega Trinza)	Every 12 weeks	Must be treated with once-monthly paliperidone for at least 4 months before transitioning to this preparation Deltoid or gluteal site
Risperidone microspheres (Risperidal Consta)	Every 2 weeks	Deltoid or gluteal site Shake vigorously just before administering
Risperidone (Perseris)	Every 4 weeks	Subcutaneous in abdomen only Lump on abdomen will decrease in size over time; do not rub or massage injection site
Aripiprazole (Abilify Maintena)	Every 4 weeks	Deltoid or gluteal site Shake vigorously just before administering
Aripiprazole lauroxil (Aristada)	Every 4, 6, or 8 weeks depending on strength	Deltoid for lowest strength or gluteal site Shake vigorously just before administering
Aripiprazole lauroxil (Aristada Initio)	One-time injection	Deltoid or gluteal site One-time injection given with Aristada to initiate Aristada without the need for 3 weeks of oral tablet overlap, or given to catch a patient up following missed Aristada injections

Data from Burchum, J., & Rosenthal, L. (2019). *Lehne's pharmacology for nursing care* (10th ed.). St. Louis, MO: Elsevier.

TABLE 12.6 Side Effects of Antipsychotic Medication

Side Effect	Nursing Care and Considerations
Dry mouth	Encourage ingestion of ice chips or frequent sips of water. Sugarless candy or gum stimulates salivation. Xylitol-containing moisture supplements or other saliva substitutes can be helpful.
Urinary retention and hesitancy	Check for distended bladder. Try running water and a warm moist towel on abdomen. Consider catheterization if no results.
Constipation	Ensure adequate fluid and fiber intake. Promote physical activity. Consider stool softeners, laxatives, or dietary laxatives (e.g., prune juice).
Blurred vision	May improve in 1–2 weeks. Use reading or magnifying glasses. If intolerable, consult prescriber regarding medication change.
Dry eyes	Use artificial tears. Minimize wind exposure. Humidifier may help at home.
Sexual dysfunction	Consult prescriber—patient may need alternative medication. Artificial lubricants for vaginal dryness.
Anticholinergic toxicity Reduced or absent peristalsis (can lead to bowel obstruction); urinary retention; mydriasis; hyperpyrexia without diaphoresis (hot dry skin); delirium with tachycardia, unstable vital signs, agitation, disorientation, hallucinations, reduced responsiveness; worsening of psychotic symptoms; seizure; repetitive motor movements	***Potentially life-threatening medical emergency*** Hold all medications. Consult prescriber immediately. Implement emergency cooling measures as ordered (cooling blanket, alcohol, or ice bath). Urinary catheterization as needed. Administer a benzodiazepine or other sedation as ordered. Physostigmine may reverse the anticholinergic toxicity. Evaluate for anticholinergic toxicity any time psychosis appears to be worsening.
Pseudoparkinsonism Masklike face, stiff and stooped posture, shuffling gait, bradykinesia, drooling, tremor, "pill-rolling" finger movements, dysphagia or reduction in spontaneous swallowing	Administer antiparkinsonian agent such as trihexyphenidyl (Artane) or benztropine (Cogentin). If intolerable, consult prescriber regarding dose reduction or medication change. Provide towel or handkerchief to wipe excess saliva. Teach how to reduce fall risk.
Acute dystonic reactions Acute painful contractions of limited muscle groups (e.g., tongue, face, neck, and back; usually tongue and jaw first) Spasm of the muscles causing backward arching of the head, neck (torticollis), and spine Eyes roll back (oculogyric crisis) Laryngeal dystonia: could threaten airway (rare)	Monitor and assure open airway. Reassure patient that although frightening, dystonias are not dangerous except for rare airway complications. Administer antiparkinsonian agent as above (IM for faster response). Relief usually occurs in 5–15 min. Also consider diphenhydramine (Benadryl) 25–50 mg IM/IV. Stay with the patient to provide comfort and support. Consider prophylaxis with an oral antiparkinsonian agent. Assist patient to understand the event and avert mistrust of medications.
Akathisia Motor restlessness (e.g., pacing, patient unable to stand still or stay in one location, rocking while seated or shifting from one foot to other while standing)	Take care to distinguish akathisia (inability to sit still, generalized muscle restlessness) from simple anxious repetitive movement (which usually involves only the extremities). Consult prescriber regarding possible medication change. Give antiparkinsonian agent as ordered. Propranolol (Inderal), lorazepam (Ativan), or diazepam (Valium) may be used. Relaxation exercises may be helpful. In severe cases, may cause great distress and contribute to suicidality. Usually subsides when antipsychotic is discontinued (exception: tardive form of akathisia).
Tardive dyskinesia *Face:* protruding or writhing tongue; blowing, smacking, licking; facial distortion Limbs: Chorea: rapid, purposeless, and irregular movements Athetoid: slow, complex, and serpentine movements *Trunk:* neck and shoulder movements, hip jerks and rocking, or twisting pelvic thrusts	Some 20% of patients taking these drugs for more than 2 years may develop tardive dyskinesia. Screening for abnormal movements should be done at least every 3 months. Purposeful muscle contraction overrides and masks involuntary tardive movements. Administer valbenazine (Ingrezza) or deutetrabenazine (Austedo) as ordered. Discontinuing the drug rarely relieves symptoms, but onset may merit reconsideration of medication. Movements associated with tardive dyskinesia may contribute to stigmatizing response by others. Provide support. Teach the patient ways to conceal involuntary movements, such as holding one hand with the other.
Hypotension and orthostatic (postural) hypotension Upon standing, systolic pressure rises, diastolic pressure decreases, and pulse increases.	Monitor lying or sitting and standing blood pressure. Hold dose and consult prescriber if systolic pressure is below 80 mm Hg when standing. Advise patient to rise slowly to prevent dizziness and to hold onto railings/furniture while arising to reduce falls. If lying down, patient should first move slowly to sitting position and pause before standing until any dizziness passes. Effect usually subsides in 1–2 weeks. Ensure adequate hydration.

Continued

TABLE 12.6   Side Effects of Antipsychotic Medication—cont'd

Side Effect	Nursing Care and Considerations
Tachycardia, irregular pulse	Patients, especially those with existing cardiac problems, should always be evaluated by ECG before antipsychotic drugs are administered. Monitor pulse for tachycardia and irregularities. Abnormal QT interval can be a contraindication for certain antipsychotics.
Severe neutropenia Symptoms include reduced neutrophil counts and increased frequency and severity of infections. Any symptoms suggesting infection (e.g., sore throat, fever, malaise, body aches) should be carefully evaluated.	**Potentially fatal blood dyscrasia** Monitor for neutropenia weekly for 6 months, then twice monthly for 6 more months, then monthly. If neutropenia develops, hold drug and consult prescriber. Moderate neutropenia (ANC 500–999 µL) and severe neutropenia (ANC <500 µL) should result in treatment interruption (Clozapine REMS, 2015). In some cases, clozapine may be reinstituted once the ANC returns to normal. If severe, reverse isolation may be initiated temporarily. Teach patient to observe for signs of infection and to report these promptly to prescriber.
Cholestatic jaundice Rare, reversible, and usually benign if caught in time; early symptoms are fever, malaise, nausea, and abdominal pain; jaundice appears 1 week later.	Consult prescriber regarding possible medication change. Bed rest and high-protein, high-carbohydrate diet if ordered. Liver function tests should be performed every 6 months.
Neuroleptic malignant syndrome (NMS) Rare but dangerous. Severe muscle rigidity, dysphasia, flexor-extensor posturing, reduced or absent speech and movement, decreased responsiveness. *Hyperpyrexia is the main feature:* temperature over 103°F Autonomic dysfunction: hypertension, tachycardia, diaphoresis, incontinence Delirium, stupor, coma	***Acute, life-threatening medical emergency*** Early detection increases patient's chance of survival. If suspected, hold all antipsychotics and contact prescriber stat. Transfer to a critical care unit (if in community, 911 transport to ER; notify ER of referral and reason). Bromocriptine (Parlodel) and dantrolene (Dantrium, Ryanodex) can relieve muscle rigidity and reduce the heat (fever) generated by muscle contractions. Cool body to reduce fever (cooling blankets; alcohol bath, cool water or ice bath as ordered). Maintain hydration with oral or intravenous fluids; correct electrolyte imbalance. Treat dysrhythmias. Small doses of heparin may decrease risk of pulmonary emboli.
Metabolic syndrome Weight gain, dyslipidemia (abnormal lipid levels), and increased insulin resistance leading to increased risk of cardiovascular disease, diabetes, and other serious medical conditions	Teach the patient how to minimize weight gain through proper nutrition and physical activity (e.g., help the patient to identify low-calorie snacks that he enjoys, engage the patient in regular physical activity, and help the patient to identify and pursue enjoyable physical activities, such as walking or cycling. Teach the patient and family about the importance of regular medical evaluation and care to identify and correct possible changes that could lead to this syndrome, which can increase the risk of premature illness and death. Metformin has been used off label to reduce diabetes in patients with metabolic syndrome.

Data from Burchum, J., & Rosenthal, L. (2019) *Lehne's pharmacology for nursing care* (10th ed.). St. Louis, MO: Elsevier.

condition include rhabdomyolysis (protein in the blood from muscle breakdown), which can cause organ failure (30%), acute respiratory failure (16%), acute kidney injury (18%), sepsis (6%), and other systemic infections. Respiratory failure is the strongest predictor of mortality.

NMS usually occurs early in therapy but has also occurred 20 years into treatment. Prompt detection, discontinuation of the antipsychotic agent, management of fluid balance, temperature reduction, and monitoring for complications are essential.

Severe neutropenia, though most often associated with clozapine (Clozaril), is also possible with most other antipsychotics. Severe neutropenia is an acute condition involving a dangerously low white blood cell count (neutropenia), which increases the risk of a serious infection. Neutropenia is defined by an ANC of less than 500/µL. Left untreated, this life-threatening condition leads to death, most commonly through bacterial infection of the blood, or septicemia. Monitoring for neutropenia is done as part of the complete blood count through an ANC. Symptoms of severe neutropenia include signs of infection (e.g., fever, chills, and sore throat) or increased susceptibility to infection.

Some individuals have naturally lower levels of ANC. This is referred to as benign ethnic neutropenia. It is most common in those of African descent (about 25% to 50%), some Middle Eastern groups, and other non-Caucasians with darker skin. They are not at greater risk for developing severe neutropenia but should have a baseline ANC before starting clozapine. The Clozapine Risk Evaluation and Mitigation Strategies (REMS) is a mandatory FDA program for prescribers and pharmacies. It calls for the enrollment, education, and certification of prescribers and dispensers who are authorized to administer periodic ANC checks.

Prolongation of the QT interval is a delay of ventricular repolarization. This condition may result in tachycardia, fainting, seizures, and even sudden death. The first-generation antipsychotic drugs that can prolong the QT interval include chlorpromazine (Thorazine), haloperidol (Haldol), and thioridazine (Mellaril); the second-generation antipsychotic drugs quetiapine (Seroquel), risperidone (Risperdal), and ziprasidone (Geodon) can do so as well. Before being started on any antipsychotic agent, a patient should receive an electrocardiogram to detect preexisting QT prolongation, which magnifies the risk from medication-related prolongation.

Liver impairment may also occur during antipsychotic therapy, particularly with first-generation agents. Second-generation drugs also lead to serum enzyme elevations but rarely to injury or jaundice. Liver impairment usually occurs in the first weeks of therapy. Monitoring of liver function values is essential. Signs of liver problems include jaundice, abdominal pain, ascites, vomiting, lower extremity edema, dark urine, pale or tar-colored stool, and easy bruising. The patient may complain of itchy skin, chronic fatigue, nausea, and decreased appetite.

Disorders co-occurring with schizophrenia should be actively treated. Major depressive disorder is common in schizophrenia and is typically treated with antidepressants and other interventions (see Chapter 14). Antidepressants and mood-stabilizing agents may be needed for mood symptoms in schizoaffective disorder. Benzodiazepines such as lorazepam (Ativan) can reduce agitation and anxiety (which can worsen other symptoms and is quite common in schizophrenia) and can help lessen both positive and negative symptoms.

Psychological Therapies

Advanced practice registered nurses may provide diagnostic evaluations, individual and group psychotherapy (e.g., cognitive behavioral therapy [CBT]), psychoeducation, medication prescription and monitoring, health assessment, and family therapy. Cognitive deficits can be addressed with cognitive remediation or enhancement therapy, which enhances recall, attentional, and other skills to reduce cognitive impairment, improving functioning and quality of life. Although these are advance practice roles, components of some, such as helping patients to identify and correct distortions in thinking, can also be implemented by any nurse.

Family therapy is an important advanced practice role. Families often endure considerable distress related to living with individuals who have acute or residual symptoms of schizophrenia, particularly if they are the direct caregivers or the patient becomes abusive. They may not know how to help their loved ones and can feel powerless. Families can become isolated from their peers, communities, and support systems owing to the stigma of mental illness and shame they may feel. In family therapy sessions, fears, faulty communication patterns, and distortions are identified; communication, symptom management, and problem-solving skills are taught; healthier alternatives to conflict are explored; and guilt and anxiety can be lessened.

Family therapy and groups such as NAMI and the Schizophrenia and Related Disorders Alliance of America provide support, education, and opportunities to vent frustrations. This helps to make families partners in the treatment process, helps them to solve problems and reduce conflict better, and improves the quality of life for both patient and family.

This example shows how one family came to understand schizophrenia and better help their loved one:

I went to the group session. We all shared what dealing with the illness was like for us. Then my daughter and others there with schizophrenia talked about what it was like for them, how it made it hard for them to take a shower, or to listen and focus when you are hearing voices or having upsetting thoughts. I really didn't understand it before—I used to think my daughter was just being lazy... I didn't know it was her illness. I thought she could make the symptoms stop if she tried hard enough... I felt so bad for those times I yelled at her or pressured her to get a job before she was ready. We all had a good cry, and everyone agreed to talk more and to try harder to understand the other person.

EVIDENCE-BASED PRACTICE

Improving Attention With Nicotine?

Problem
People with schizophrenia smoke at much higher rates than the general population: 70% versus 22%. Individuals with schizophrenia also smoke more cigarettes, inhale harder, and obtain more nicotine from each cigarette. Smoking is a significant risk factor for cancers, respiratory disorders, and cardiovascular disease, adding significantly to the already high mortality rates associated with schizophrenia.

Purpose of Study
One hypothesis to explain these much higher rates of nicotine consumption is that the nicotine is a form of self-medication for the cognitive deficits seen in schizophrenia. This study sought to test this hypothesis by evaluating nicotine's effect on the ability to maintain attention.

Methods
Seventeen patients with schizophrenia and 20 controls without a severe mental illness took part. They were randomly assigned to receive either nicotine (through nicotine patches) or no nicotine (through a placebo). Researchers assessed their ability to attend to a task despite a distracting recording of urban environmental noises. fMRI was used to determine brain regions affected by the nicotine.

Key Findings
- Without nicotine, people with schizophrenia showed a lower capacity to focus.
- Nicotine appeared to enhance the ability of people with schizophrenia to maintain their attention despite the distracting sounds.

Implications for Nursing Practice
Because of the health consequences of smoking, nurses cannot support smoking to address impaired concentration. Therefore, nicotine agents with safer delivery systems—such as patches, lozenges, and gums—may be useful adjuncts for treating cognitive impairment. However, nicotine also interferes with the effectiveness of some antipsychotic medications (e.g., clozapine), requiring a dosage adjustment if nicotinic drugs (or smoking) are initiated or discontinued while patients are on those medications.

Smucny, J., Olincy, A., Rojas, D., & Tregellas, J. (2016). Neuronal effects of nicotine during auditory selective attention in schizophrenia. *Human Brain Mapping, 37*, 410–421.

KEY POINTS TO REMEMBER

- Schizophrenia spectrum disorders are a group of related biological disorders of the brain with overlapping symptoms and treatments but varying etiologies.
- Neurochemical, genetic, and neuroanatomical findings help explain the symptoms of schizophrenia. No one theory accounts fully for schizophrenia's complexities.
- Schizophrenia varies from person to person in terms of which symptoms dominate, their severity, and the degree of impairment in affect, cognition, and functioning.
- Psychotic symptoms are often more pronounced and obvious than symptoms of other disorders, making schizophrenia more apparent to others and increasing stigmatization.
- Positive symptoms of schizophrenia (e.g., hallucinations, delusions, associative looseness) are easier to recognize and respond best to antipsychotic drug therapy. Cognitive interventions are also helpful.
- Cognitive symptoms (e.g., impaired memory, concentration, and decision making) and negative symptoms (e.g., reduction in affect, social withdrawal and dysfunction, lack of motivation, inability to experience pleasure) respond less well to antipsychotic therapy and can be more debilitating.
- Psychosocial interventions such as support groups improve negative symptoms, and cognitive remediation treatment enhances cognition.
- Comorbid anxiety and depression must be identified and treated to reduce the potential for suicide, substance abuse, nonadherence, and relapse. It is essential to help patients learn to regulate their emotions (e.g., through stress management techniques, self-nurturance, instilling hope, and participating in rewarding activities).
- Substance use disorders affect the majority of people with schizophrenia and can intensify symptoms and cause relapse. Prevention, screening, and treatment of substance use disorders is important.
- Outcomes are chosen based on the phase of the disorder and the patient's symptoms, needs, strengths, values, and level of functioning. Short-term and intermediate indicators have been developed to better track the incremental progress typical of schizophrenia.
- It is important for nurses to assess and support functions such as hygiene, self-care, nutrition, and rest and to ensure a therapeutic milieu (e.g., reducing undue stimuli on the unit).
- Antipsychotic medications are essential in treating patients with schizophrenia. Nurses must understand the properties and desired and undesired effects of antipsychotics and adjunctive medications.
- Side effects can be distressing to patients and contribute to nonadherence.
- Side effects such as neuroleptic malignant syndrome, severe neutropenia, paralytic ileus, bowel obstruction, metabolic syndrome, and anticholinergic toxicity are potentially fatal.

CRITICAL THINKING

1. Andrea, 24, diagnosed with schizophrenia, was hospitalized after accusing colleagues of trying to poison her. She is being discharged to her mother's care. Andrea's mother is overwhelmed and asks how she is going to cope: "I can hardly talk to Andrea without upsetting her. She is still mad at me because I had her admitted. She says there is nothing wrong with her, and I'm worried she'll stop her medication once she is home. What am I going to do?"

   a. Explain Andrea's behavior and symptoms to a classmate as you would to Andrea's mother.
   b. How would you respond to the mother's immediate concerns?
   c. What priority concerns should the nurse address before Andrea's discharge?
   d. What community resources could help support this family, and how?
   e. How might this situation affect Andrea's prognosis?

CHAPTER REVIEW

1. Which characteristics suggest a man is experiencing the prodromal phase of schizophrenia? *Select all that apply.*
   a. Always afraid that others will steal his belongings.
   b. Displays unusual interest in numbers and specific topics.
   c. Has increasingly unusual thoughts and uses words oddly.
   d. Demonstrates increasing difficulty with concentration.

2. Which nursing interventions are particularly well chosen for addressing a population at high risk for developing schizophrenia? *Select all that apply.*
   a. Screening 15- to 25-year-olds for early symptoms.
   b. Forming a support group for females aged 25 to 35 who are diagnosed with substance use disorders.
   c. Teaching ways to cope and build resiliency.
   d. Educating about the risk of psychosis with marijuana use.

3. To provide effective care for the patient who is taking a second-generation antipsychotic, the nurse should frequently assess for
   a. Alcohol use disorder
   b. Major depressive disorder
   c. Stomach cancer
   d. Polydipsia
   e. Metabolic syndrome

4. A female patient diagnosed with schizophrenia has been prescribed a first-generation antipsychotic medication. What information should the nurse provide to the patient regarding her signs and symptoms?
   a. Her memory problems will likely decrease.
   b. Depressive episodes should be less severe.

c. She will probably enjoy social interactions more.

d. She should experience a reduction in hallucinations.

5. Which characteristic presents the greatest risk for injury to others by the patient diagnosed with schizophrenia?
   a. Depersonalization
   b. Pressured speech
   c. Negative symptoms
   d. Paranoia

6. Which therapeutic communication statement might a psychiatric–mental health registered nurse use when a patient's nursing diagnosis is hallucinations? *Select all that apply.*
   a. "I know you say you hear voices, but I cannot hear them."
   b. "Stop listening to the voices, they are NOT real."
   c. "Tell me more about what you hear."
   d. "Please tell the voices to leave you alone for now."

7. When patients diagnosed with schizophrenia suffer from anosognosia, they often refuse medication, believing that
   a. The medications provided are ineffective.
   b. Nurses are trying to control their minds.
   c. The medications will make them sick.
   d. They are not actually ill.

8. Kyle, a patient with schizophrenia, began to take the first-generation antipsychotic haloperidol (Haldol) a week ago. You find him sitting stiffly and not moving. He is diaphoretic, and when you ask if he is okay, he seems unable to respond verbally. His vital signs are: BP 170/100, P 110, T 104.2°F. What is the priority nursing intervention? *Select all that apply.*
   a. Hold his medication and contact his prescriber stat.
   b. Wipe him with a washcloth that has been wetted with cold water or alcohol.
   c. Administer an "as needed" medication such as benztropine intramuscularly to correct his dystonic reaction.
   d. Reassure him that no treatment is needed and that this reaction will pass.
   e. Hold his medication for now and consult his prescriber when he comes to the unit later today.

9. Tomas is a 21-year-old male with a recent diagnosis of schizophrenia. Tomas's nurse recognizes that self-medicating with excessive alcohol is common in this disorder and can be an effort to: *Select all that apply.*
   a. Self-medicate for social discomfort.
   b. Cope with anxiety.
   c. Enhance mood.
   d. Enable Tomas to better express himself.

10. A patient reports that "the voices are really bad today." Helpful nursing responses would include
    a. Giving an additional "as needed" dosage of his antipsychotic medication.
    b. Telling him that the voices are not real and that he should ignore them.
    c. Directing him to return to his room and try not to think about the voices.
    d. Encouraging the patient to use competing auditory stimuli, such as humming or listening to music.

1. **a, b, c, d;** 2. **a, c, d;** 3. **e;** 4. **d;** 5. **d;** 6. **a, c;** 7. **d;** 8. **a, b;** 9. **a, b, c;** 10. **d**

NGN CASE STUDY AND QUESTIONS

Shannon, 47 years old, is brought to the emergency department after striking her case manager at a homeless shelter. Due to the potential for danger to others and a need for care, she is admitted to the psychiatric unit. Prior documentation identifies a history of schizophrenia, which has not been consistently treated since she became homeless.

On the unit Shannon shows no interest in—and resists—all food, self-care, and social activities. She wears a sweater upside down. Her mood is labile, ranging from tearfulness, laughter, and withdrawal. She stands by the window, studying the sky "for signs," saying that messages appear in cloud formations. When a staff member asks her about the messages, she shouts, "Stay out of my head!" and pushes him away. On her way to lunch she knocks objects off the table that irritate her—a puzzle box, a small stack of magazines, and a container of buttons, saying "Clutter clutter, flutter flutter."

1. This patient is most likely experiencing which types of delusion? *Select all that apply:*
   a. Persecutory
   b. Referential
   c. Somatic
   d. Erotomanic
   e. Control
   f. Nihilistic

2. Indicate which assessment finding is associated with each of the following symptom categories. *Each item may fit more than one category.*

Symptom	Positive	Negative	Cognitive	Affective
a. Mood swings from weeping to laughing to withdrawal				
b. Shows no interest in food, self-care, and socialization				
c. Appears to hear and respond to voices				
d. Clang association in speech patterns				
e. Knocks objects that irritate her off the table				
f. Difficulty putting on an item of clothing				
g. Exhibits anhedonia				
h. Lashes out in unexpected anger				

NGN case study answers are on Evolve.

🌐 Visit the Evolve website for a posttest on the content in this chapter: http://evolve.elsevier.com/Varcarolis

REFERENCES

Allswede, D., & Cannon, T. (2018). Prenatal inflammation and risk for schizophrenia: A role for immune proteins in neurodevelopment. *Development and Psychopathology, 30*(3), 1157–1178.

American Psychiatric Association. (2013). *Diagnostic and statistical manual of mental disorders* (5th ed.). Washington, DC: Author.

Aschengrau, A., Weinberg, J., Janulewicz, P., Romano, M., Gallagher, L., Winter, M., et al. (2012). Occurrence of mental illness following prenatal and early childhood exposure to tetrachloroethylene (PCE)-contaminated drinking water: A retrospective cohort study. *Environmental Health: A Global Access Science Source, 11*(1), 1–12.

Capizzi, R., Ramsey, I., & Vinogradov, S. (2019). The efficacy of transcranial magnetic stimulation for the treatment of persistent auditory hallucinations in schizophrenia: A meta-analysis. *Schizophrenia Bulletin, 45*(Suppl. 2), S343. Retrieved from https://academic.oup.com/schizophreniabulletin/article/45/Supplement_2/S343/5434404.

Clozapine, R. E. M. S. (2015). *Clozapine and the risk of neutropenia: A guide for healthcare providers.* Retrieved from https://www.clozapinerems.com/CpmgClozapineUI/rems/pdf/resources/Clozapine_REMS_HCP_Guide.pdf.

Ellul, P., Delorme, R., & Cortese, S. (2018). Metformin for weight gain associated with second-generation antipsychotics in children and adolescents. *CNS Drugs, 32*, 1103–1112.

Funayama, M., Takata, T., & Koreki, A. (2019). Choking incidents among patients with schizophrenia may be associated with severe illness and higher-dosage antipsychotics. *General Hospital Psychiatry, 59*, 73–75.

Guccione, C., di Scalea, G. L., Ambrosecchia, M., Teronne, G., Di Cesare, G., Ducci, G., et al. (2019). Early signs of schizophrenia and autonomic nervous system dysregulation: A literature review. *Clinical Neuropsychiatry, 16*(2), 86–97.

Haddad, L., Schäfer, A., Streit, F., Lederbogen, F., Grimm, O., Wüst, S., et al. (2015). Brain structure correlates of urban upbringing, an environmental risk factor. *Schizophrenia Bulletin, 41*(1), 115–122.

Howard, R. (2001). *A beautiful mind* [film]. Universal Pictures.

Jorgensen, K., Nordentoft, M., & Hjorthoj, C. (2018). Association between alcohol and substance use disorders and psychiatric service use in patients with severe mental illness: A nationwide Danish register-based cohort study. *Psychological Medicine, 48*(15), 2592–2600.

Kilian, S., Asmal, L., Chiliza, B., Olivier, M. R., Phahladira, L., Scheffler, F., et al. (2018). Childhood adversity and cognitive function in schizophrenia spectrum disorders and healthy controls: Evidence for an association between neglect and social cognition. *Psychological Medicine, 48*(13), 2186–2193.

Luo, C., Wang, X., Huang, H., Xiaoyuan, M., Zhou, H., & Liu, Z. (2019). Effect of metformin on antipsychotic-induced metabolic dysfunction. *Frontiers in Pharmacology, 10*, 371.

Mallet, J., Strat, Y., Schuroff, F., Mazer, N., Portalier, C., Andrianarisoa, M., et al. (2019). Tobacco smoking is associated with antipsychotic medication, physical aggressiveness, and alcohol use disorder in schizophrenia: Results from the FACE-SZ national cohort. *European Archives of Psychiatry and Clinical Neuroscience, 269*(4), 449–457.

Margolius, A., & Fernandez, H. (2019). Current treatment of tardive dyskinesia. *Parkinsonism and Related Disorders, 59*, 155–160.

Miller, B. (2019). Immunotherapy as personalized medicine for schizophrenia? *Psychiatric Times, 36*(2), 1–4.

Modi, S., Dharaiya, D., Schultz, L., & Varelas, P. (2016). Neuroleptic malignant syndrome: Complications, outcomes, and mortality. *Neurocritical Care, 24*(1), 97–103.

Ota, V., Moretti, P., Santoro, M., Talarico, F., Spindola, L. M., Xavier, G., et al. (2019). Gene expression over the course of schizophrenia: From clinical high-risk for psychosis to chronic stages. *Schizophrenia, 5*, 1–6.

Potasiewicz, A., Golebioska, J., Popik, P., & Nikiforuk, A. (2019). Procognitive effects of varenicline in the animal model of schizophrenia depend on alpha4beta2 and alpha7-nicotinic acetylcholine receptors. *Journal of Psychopharmacology, 33*(1), 62–73.

Renard, J., Rosen, L., Loureiro, M., De Oliveira, C., Schmid, S., Rushlow, W. J., et al. (2017). Adolescent cannabinoid exposure induces a persistent sub-cortical hyper-dopaminergic state and associated molecular adaptations in the prefrontal cortex. *Cerebral Cortex, 27*(2), 1297–1310.

Seeman, M. (2019). Schizophrenia mortality: Barriers to progress. *Psychiatric Quarterly, 90*(3), 553–563.

Sekar, A., Bialas, A., de Rivera, H., Davis, A., Hammond, T., Kamitaki, N., et al. (2016). Schizophrenia risk from complex variation of complement component 4. *Nature, 530*, 177–183.

US Food and Drug Administration. (2017). *Ingrezza (valbenazine) capsules label.* Retrieved from https://www.accessdata.fda.gov/drugsatfda_docs/label/2017/209241lbl.pdf.

Yang, H.-J., & Cheng, W. J. (2017). Antipsychotic use is a risk factor for hyponatremia in patients with schizophrenia: A 15-year follow-up study. *Psychopharmacology, 234*(5), 869–876.

Zhand, N., Attwood, D., & Harvey, P. (2019). Glutamate modulators for treatment of schizophrenia. *Personalized Medicine in Psychiatry, 15-16*, 1–12.

Zhao, C., Zhu, J., Liu, X., Pu, C., Lai, Y., Chen, L., et al. (2018). Structural and functional brain abnormalities in schizophrenia: A cross-sectional study at different stages of the disease. *Progress in Neuropsychopharmacology & Biological Psychiatry, 83*, 27–32.

13

Bipolar and Related Disorders

Margaret Jordan Halter

🌐 Visit the Evolve website for a pretest on the content in this chapter: http://evolve.elsevier.com/Varcarolis

OBJECTIVES

1. Describe the symptoms of bipolar I, bipolar II, and cyclothymic disorder.
2. Distinguish between mania and hypomania.
3. Identify the epidemiology of bipolar disorders.
4. Discuss the biological, environmental, and cognitive risk factors for the development of bipolar disorders.
5. Formulate three nursing diagnoses that support care for a patient with mania.
6. Describe the differences in care for the acute phase versus the maintenance phase of mania and hypomania.
7. Evaluate specific indications for the use of seclusion with a patient experiencing mania.
8. Identify medications used for mood stabilization, including lithium, anticonvulsant drugs, and second-generation antipsychotics.
9. Distinguish between signs of early and severe lithium toxicity.
10. Identify five areas of patient and family teaching regarding lithium carbonate.
11. Discuss the role of brain stimulation therapies, such as electroconvulsive therapy (ECT) and repetitive transcranial magnetic stimulation (rTMS) in treating bipolar disorders.
12. Identify psychological therapies that are used in treating the patient and family with bipolar disorder.

KEY TERMS AND CONCEPTS

anticonvulsant drugs
bipolar I disorder
bipolar II disorder
circumstantial speech
clang association
cyclothymic disorder

delusions
electroconvulsive therapy (ECT)
flight of ideas
hypomania
lithium
loose associations

mania
mood stabilizers
pressured speech
rapid cycling
tangential speech

Formerly known as *manic depression*, the bipolar disorders are chronic recurrent illnesses that require careful management throughout a person's life. The distinguishing symptoms of these disorder include unusual shifts from highs (mania and hypomania) to lows (depressive symptoms). Bipolar disorder frequently goes unrecognized, and people suffer for an average of 6 years before receiving a proper diagnosis and treatment (Dagani et al., 2016).

The placement of the bipolar and related disorders chapter between the schizophrenia spectrum disorder chapter and the depressive disorder chapter was intentional in the *Diagnostic and Statistical Manual of Mental Disorders, 5th edition (DSM-5)* (American Psychiatric Association, 2013). This positioning reflects the overlap of the psychotic disorders on one side of the spectrum and the depressive disorders on the other (Miller, Ostacher, & Suppes, 2019). While genetic, neurobiological, and symptom similarities exist between the disorders, the bipolar disorders are biologically distinct from schizophrenia and depressive disorders.

CLINICAL PICTURE

While the *DSM-5* describes additional bipolar disorders, in this chapter we will focus on the three disorders: bipolar I, bipolar II, and cyclothymic disorder.

Bipolar I Disorder

Bipolar I disorder is the most severe bipolar disorder. It is marked by shifts in mood, energy, and ability to function. Periods of normal functioning may alternate with periods of illness (highs, lows, or a combination of both). Many individuals continue to experience chronic interpersonal or occupational difficulties even during remission.

The mortality rate for bipolar disorder is severe. Suicide accounts for 5% of deaths among women and 10% of deaths among men with bipolar disorder, compared with 1% and 2% in the general population (Crump et al., 2013). Factors related to completed suicide include early onset of disease, history of suicide among first-degree relatives, and previous suicide attempts (Plans et al., 2019).

Individuals with bipolar I disorder have experienced at least one manic episode. Mania is a period of intense mood disturbance with persistent elevation, expansiveness, irritability, and extreme goal-directed activity or energy. These periods last at least 1 week for most of the day, every day. Symptoms of mania are so severe that this state is a psychiatric emergency. Manic episodes usually alternate with depression or a mixed state of anxiety and depression (refer to Chapter 14 for a full discussion of depression).

Initially, individuals experiencing a manic episode are the happiest, most excited, and most optimistic people you could meet. They feel euphoric and energized. They eat and sleep little, if at all, and are in perpetual motion. Because they feel so important and powerful, they take horrific chances and engage in hazardous activities. Unfortunately, the person with mania does not recognize the behaviors as being problematic and resists treatment. As discussed in Chapter 12, this inability to recognize the illness is due to the illness itself and is referred to as anosognosia (ah-no-sag-NO-zsuh).

As the mania intensifies, individuals may become psychotic. Psychosis refers to symptoms such as hallucinations, delusions, and dramatically disturbed thoughts. Hallucinations tend to be auditory and individuals may begin to hear voices, sometimes the voice of God. Delusions commonly center around self-importance and grandeur, such as being famous or being able to end wars. Thought disturbance takes the form of distractibility and decreased concentration.

The initial euphoria of mania gives way to agitation and irritability. Utter exhaustion eventually happens and many people ultimately collapse into depression. Depression and the agitated state of mania is a dangerous combination that can lead to extreme behaviors, such as violence or attempted suicide.

People may be at equal risk for developing anxiety as depression after an episode of mania (Olfson et al., 2016). They may even experience a major depressive disorder and generalized anxiety disorder simultaneously after a manic event. If clinicians adopted a broader definition of bipolar disorder that includes anxiety as an alternating symptom, we may identify bipolar disorder earlier and develop different treatment approaches. Individuals whose main symptom is anxiety should be assessed for a history of mania before being treated for anxiety.

The *DSM-5* box contains the full criteria for bipolar I disorder.

DSM-5 CRITERIA FOR BIPOLAR I DISORDER

For a diagnosis of bipolar I disorder, it is necessary to meet the following criteria for a manic episode. The manic episode may have been preceded by and may be followed by hypomanic or major depressive episodes.

Manic Episode

A. A distinct period of abnormally and persistently elevated, expansive, or irritable mood and abnormally and persistently increased goal-directed activity or energy, lasting at least 1 week and present most of the day, nearly every day (or any duration if hospitalization is necessary).

B. During the period of mood disturbance and increased energy or activity, three (or more) of the following symptoms (four if the mood is only irritable) are present to a significant degree and represent a noticeable change from usual behavior:

1. Inflated self-esteem or grandiosity
2. Decreased need for sleep (e.g., feels rested after only 3 hours of sleep)
3. More talkative than usual or pressure to keep talking
4. Flight of ideas or subjective experience that thoughts are racing
5. Distractibility (i.e., attention too easily drawn to unimportant or irrelevant external stimuli), as reported or observed
6. Increase in goal-directed activity (either socially, at work or school, or sexually) or psychomotor agitation (i.e., purposeless non–goal-directed activity)
7. Excessive involvement in activities that have a high potential for painful consequences (e.g., engaging in unrestrained buying sprees, sexual indiscretions, or foolish business investments)

C. The mood disturbance is sufficiently severe to cause marked impairment in social or occupational functioning or to necessitate hospitalization to prevent harm to self or others, or there are psychotic features.

D. The episode is not attributable to the physiological effects of a substance (e.g., a drug of abuse, a medication, other treatment) or to another medical condition.

Note: A full manic episode that emerges during antidepressant treatment (e.g., medication, electroconvulsive therapy) but persists at a fully syndromal level beyond the physiological effect of that treatment is sufficient evidence for a manic episode and, therefore, a bipolar I diagnosis.

Note: Criteria A through D constitute a manic episode. At least one lifetime manic episode is required for the diagnosis of bipolar I disorder.

From American Psychiatric Association. (2013). *Diagnostic and statistical manual of mental disorders* (5th ed.). Washington, DC: Author.

Bipolar II Disorder

Individuals with bipolar II disorder have experienced at least one hypomanic episode and at least one major depressive episode. Hypomania refers to a low-level and less dramatic mania. The hypomania of bipolar II disorder tends to be euphoric and often increases functioning. Like mania, hypomania is accompanied by excessive activity and energy for at least 4 days and involves at least three of the behaviors listed under Criterion B in the *DSM-5*. Unlike mania, psychosis is never present with hypomania. Psychotic symptoms may, however, accompany the depressive side of the disorder.

A hypomanic episode does impact functioning in a way that is noticeable to others. For example, an individual may be much more talkative and distractible than usual. However, hypomania is not usually severe enough to cause serious impairment in occupational or social functioning. Hospitalization for hypomania is rare. However, the depressive symptoms can be quite profound and may put those who suffer from it at a particular risk for suicide.

Among adults, bipolar II disorder is believed to be underdiagnosed and is often mistaken for major depressive disorder or personality disorders when it actually may be the most common form of bipolar disorder. Clinicians may downplay bipolar II and consider it to simply be the milder version of bipolar disorders. However, it is a source of significant morbidity and mortality, particularly due to the occurrence of severe depression. Anyone with major depressive disorder should be assessed for symptoms of hypomania because these symptoms are frequently associated with a progression to bipolar disorder.

Cyclothymic Disorder

In cyclothymic disorder, symptoms of hypomania alternate with symptoms of mild to moderate depression for at least 2 years in adults and 1 year in children. Hypomanic and depressive

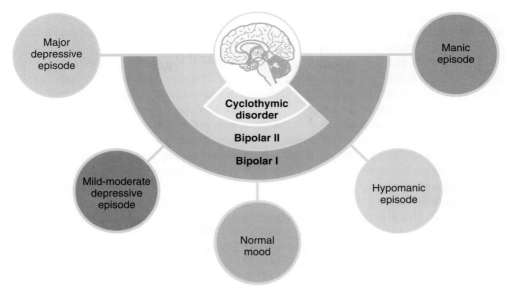

Fig. 13.1 Continuum of bipolar symptoms.

symptoms do not meet the criteria for either bipolar II or major depressive disorder, yet the symptoms are disturbing enough to cause social and occupational impairment.

As part of the spectrum of bipolar disorders (Fig. 13.1), cyclothymic disorder may be difficult to distinguish from bipolar II disorder. Individuals with cyclothymic disorder tend to have irritable hypomanic episodes. Children with cyclothymic disorder experience irritability and sleep disturbance. There is a 15% to 50% risk of this disorder progressing to bipolar I or bipolar II (APA, 2013).

Rapid Cycling

Some people with bipolar I or II will experience **rapid cycling** and may have at least four mood episodes in a 12-month period. These mood episodes can be major depressive, manic, or hypomanic. Cycling can also occur within the course of a month or even a 24-hour period. Rapid cycling is associated with more severe symptoms, such as poorer global functioning, high recurrence risk, and resistance to conventional somatic treatments.

Other Bipolar Disorders

Several other bipolar and related disorders are included in the *DSM-5*. They include:
- Substance/Medication-Induced Bipolar and Related Disorder: The disturbance of mood is directly related to a specific substance. The diagnosis is further specified by whether the onset occurred with intoxication or with withdrawal. Symptoms include elevated, expansive, or irritable mood or depressed mood, which causes clinically significant distress and impacts functioning.
- Bipolar and Related Disorder Due to Another Medical Condition: Mania or hypomania that may be mixed with depression that is directly related to a specific condition. This condition can be verified through history, physical examination, or laboratory findings. Symptoms include elevated, expansive, or irritable mood or depressed mood, which causes clinically significant distress and impacts functioning.

TABLE 13.1 Statistics Related to Bipolar I and II Disorders in Adults and Adolescents		
	Bipolar I	**Bipolar II**
Lifetime prevalence: adult	1.0%	1.1%
Lifetime prevalence: adolescent	2.5%	
12-month prevalence: adult	0.6%	0.8%
12-month prevalence: adolescent	2.2%	
Mean age of onset	18 years	20 years

From American Psychiatric Association. (2013). *Diagnostic and statistical manual of mental disorders* (5th ed.). Washington, DC: Author.

EPIDEMIOLOGY

Bipolar I and Bipolar II Disorders

The lifetime risk, or the percentage of the population that will ever have a bipolar I or bipolar II disorder, is nearly 4% (Merikangas et al., 2012). Table 13.1 provides a snapshot of statistics regarding bipolar disorders in adults and adolescents ages 13 to 18.

Men and women have nearly equal rates of bipolar disorders, yet they respond somewhat differently to their condition. Men with a bipolar disorder are more likely to have legal problems and commit acts of violence. Women with a bipolar disorder are more likely to misuse alcohol, commit suicide, and develop thyroid disease.

Women who experience a severe postpartum psychosis within 2 weeks of giving birth have a four times greater chance of subsequent conversion to bipolar disorder (Munk-Olsen et al., 2011). Giving birth may act as a trigger for the first symptoms of bipolar disorder. The precipitant may be hormonal changes and sleep deprivation. In addition, sleep loss after childbirth may trigger mania and psychosis in women with pre-existing bipolar disorder (Lewis et al., 2018).

Children and Adolescents

The existence of bipolar disorder in nonadults has been a hotly contested subject of controversy. At the beginning of the 21st century, there was an alarming increase in the number of children and adolescents being diagnosed with bipolar disorder. This diagnosis was given to young people who had chronic irritability and anger along with frequent verbal or behavioral outbursts that were an overreaction to the situation. A bipolar diagnosis for this troubled population provided for financial reimbursement from insurance companies, an answer for bewildered parents, and an established treatment pathway.

However, clinicians and parents alike had concerns over the trend of bipolar disorder in children. The most fundamental issue was that these children and adolescents did not usually go on to have bipolar disorder as adults. More commonly, they would eventually be diagnosed with major depressive disorder. Unfortunately, a bipolar diagnosis is a lifelong label—one that is stigmatized more than depression. This diagnosis also results in exposure to powerful medications during crucial growth periods. In 2013, a new diagnosis—disruptive mood dysregulation disorder—was developed to reverse this troubling diagnostic problem. Chapter 14 discusses this disorder in more detail.

Bipolar disorder in adolescence, particularly late adolescence, is a serious problem. Prevalence rates in this age group mirror that of adults (Merikangas et al., 2012). Early-onset bipolar is associated with high rates of suicide attempts. One study found that 18% of youths with bipolar made at least one suicide attempt within a 5-year study period, with girls making more attempts than boys (Goldstein, Ha, & Axelson, 2012).

Also, these young people with bipolar disorder experience role—familial, social, and academic—impairment. This impairment has significant implications for individuals who are positioning themselves for a lifetime and a career, as well as developing relationship patterns.

Cyclothymic Disorder

Cyclothymic disorder usually begins in adolescence or early adulthood. There is a 15% to 50% risk that an individual with this disorder will subsequently develop bipolar I or bipolar II disorder. A major risk factor for developing cyclothymic disorder is having a first-degree relative—parent, sibling, or child—with bipolar I.

COMORBIDITY

Bipolar I Disorder

Nearly all the anxiety disorders are associated with bipolar I, affecting about 75% of people with this disorder. Individuals may experience panic attacks, social anxiety disorder, and specific phobias.

Other challenging disorders may complicate the clinical presentation and management of the often-dramatic bipolar I. They include attention-deficit/hyperactivity disorder and all the disruptive, impulse-control, or conduct disorders. A substance use disorder is present in more than half of individuals with bipolar I, perhaps in an attempt to self-medicate. More than 50% of individuals have an alcohol use disorder—a problem associated with an increased risk for suicide.

Further complicating the picture is a higher-than-normal rate of serious medical conditions. Migraines are more common. Metabolic syndrome—a cluster of problems such as high blood pressure, high blood glucose, excess body fat around the waist, and abnormal cholesterol levels—may lead to premature death due to heart disease, stroke, and diabetes.

Bipolar II Disorder

As with bipolar I, about 75% of individuals with bipolar II disorder have comorbid anxiety disorders. Typically, the anxiety disorders come about before the hypomania and depressive symptoms. Eating disorders, particularly binge-eating disorder, affects about 14% of this population. Substance use disorders are also common and impact about 37% of people with bipolar I. Anxiety and eating disorders seem to be associated with the depressive side of bipolar II, while substance use disorder symptoms arise along with hypomanic symptoms.

Cyclothymic Disorder

Substance use disorders are also common with cyclothymic disorder. This may be due to efforts to self-medicate and subdue the symptoms. Sleep disorders where people have difficulty going to sleep and staying asleep are often present in this disorder. Attention-deficit/hyperactivity disorder is more common among children with cyclothymic disorder than with other mental health conditions.

RISK FACTORS

Biological Factors

Genetic

The lifetime prevalence for bipolar disorder is 3.9% (Kessler et al., 2005). However, for individuals with affected family members, the risk is far greater. The concordance rate among identical twins is estimated at about 60% (Johansson, Halkola, Cannon, Hultman, & Hedman, 2019). This means that if one twin has the disorder, 60% of the time the other one will too.

Some evidence suggests that bipolar disorders are more prevalent in adults who had high intelligence quotients (IQs), particularly verbally, as children (Smith et al., 2015). People with bipolar disorders appear to achieve higher levels of education and higher occupational status than individuals with unipolar depression. Also, the proportion of patients with bipolar disorders among creative writers, artists, highly educated men and women, and professionals is higher than in the general population.

Genetic relationships between psychiatric disorders are being found. Stahl and colleagues (2019) conducted a large-scale ($N > 50,000$) genetic study to identify genes involved in bipolar disorder. They found 30 loci that were genome significant containing genes for encoding ion channels, neurotransmitter transporters, and synaptic components. Based on genetic similarity, they concluded that bipolar I is strongly genetically correlated with schizophrenia with its psychotic features, while bipolar II was more strongly correlated with major depressive disorder. Another study found a genetic overlap between bipolar disorder, schizophrenia, and autism (Goes et al., 2016).

Neurobiological

Neurotransmitters such as norepinephrine, dopamine, and serotonin were the early focus for researchers who studied mania and depression. A simple explanation is that too few of these chemical messengers will result in depression, and an overabundance will bring about mania. However, proportions of neurotransmitters in relation to one another may be more important. Receptor site insensitivity could also be at the root of the problem; even if there is enough of a certain neurotransmitter, it is not getting to where it needs to go.

Brain structure and function. Structural neuroimaging techniques (e.g., computed tomography [CT] and magnetic resonance imaging [MRI]) provide still pictures of the scalp, skull, and brain. Structural imaging is useful in viewing bones, tissues, blood vessels, tumors, infection, damage, or bleeding. Functional neuroimaging techniques (e.g., positron emission tomography [PET], functional MRI [fMRI], and magnetoencephalography [MEG]) provide measures related to brain activity. Functional imaging reveals activity and chemistry by measuring the rate of blood flow, chemical activity, and electrical impulses in the brain during specific tasks.

With bipolar disorder, functional imaging techniques reveal dysfunction in the prefrontal cortical region, the region associated with executive decision making, personality expression, and social behavior (Phillips & Schwartz, 2014). Dysfunction is also evident in the hippocampus, which is primarily associated with memory, and the amygdala, which is associated with memory, decision making, and emotion. Dysregulation in these areas results in the characteristic emotional lability, heightened reward sensitivity, and emotional dysregulation of bipolar disorder. These abnormalities may be due to gray matter loss in these areas.

Neuroendicrine

In terms of the neuroendocrine system, the hypothalamic-pituitary-thyroid-adrenal (HPTA) axis has been the object of significant research in bipolar disorder. In fact, hypothyroidism is one of the most common physical abnormalities associated with bipolar disorder. Typically, the thyroid dysfunction is not dramatic and the problem is often undetected.

Peripheral Inflammation

In both manic and depressive states, peripheral inflammation is increased. This inflammation tends to decrease in between episodes (Maletic & Raison, 2014). These findings are consistent with changes in the HPTA axis, which are known to drive inflammatory activation. Systemic inflammation is associated with a broad cognitive dysfunction in people with bipolar disorder (Millett et al., 2019).

Cognitive Factors

With the advent of improved neuroimaging techniques and treatment advances, psychological theories are largely dismissed. Mania was once thought to be a defense against underlying anxiety and depression. Mania was also thought to help individuals tolerate loss or tragedy, such as the death of a loved one. Psychodynamic theorists believed that a faulty ego uses mania when it is overwhelmed by pleasurable impulses such as sex or feared impulses such as aggression. An overactive and critical superego is replaced with the euphoria of mania and has also been suggested as the cause.

Environmental Factors

Children who have a genetic and biological risk of developing bipolar disorder are most vulnerable in bad environments. Stressful family life and adverse life events may result in a more severe course of illness in these individuals. Stress is also a common trigger for mania and depression in adults.

Childhood adversity in the form of physical, sexual, and emotional abuse and emotional neglect are significantly associated with bipolar disorder (Palmier-Claus, Berry, Bucci, Mansell, & Varese, 2016). Emotional abuse has the largest association and is four times more likely to have occurred in bipolar patients than in controls. Childhood mistreatment is also associated with poorer clinical outcomes with more frequent and severe episodes, earlier onset, risk of suicide, and substance misuse (Rowland & Marwaha, 2018).

APPLICATION OF THE NURSING PROCESS

ASSESSMENT

Individuals with bipolar disorder are often misdiagnosed or underdiagnosed. Early diagnosis and proper treatment can help people avoid:

- Suicide attempts
- Alcohol or substance use problems and disorders
- Marital or work problems
- Development of medical comorbidity

Fig. 13.2 presents Altman's Self-Rating Mania Scale. The items in this scale are useful in capturing a picture of the patient's placement on the depression to mania continuum. Scores of 6 or higher suggest mania or hypomania and the need for further assessment and/or treatment.

General Assessment

Individuals with bipolar disorder tend to spend more time in a depressed state than in a manic state. For a complete discussion of nursing care for the depressive aspects of bipolar, refer to Chapter 14. In this chapter, we will focus on nursing care for individuals experiencing mania. The characteristics of mania discussed in the following sections are (1) mood, (2) behavior, (3) thought processes and speech patterns, thought content, and (4) cognitive function.

Mood

The euphoric mood associated with mania is unstable. During this euphoric period, patients may experience intense feelings of well-being, being "cheerful in a beautiful world," or are becoming "one with God." The overly joyous mood may seem out of proportion to what is going on, and cheerfulness may be inappropriate for the circumstances, considering that patients are full of energy with little or no sleep.

People experiencing a manic state may laugh, joke, and talk in a continuous stream with uninhibited familiarity. They often demonstrate boundless enthusiasm, treat others with confidential friendliness, and incorporate everyone into their plans and activities. They know no strangers, and energy and self-confidence seem boundless.

The euphoric mood associated with mania is unstable because this mood may change quickly to irritation and anger

Level 2—Mania—Adult
Altman Self-Rating Mania Scale (ASRM)

1. Please read each group of statements/question carefully.
2. Choose the one statement in each group that best describes the way you have been feeling for the past week.
3. Check the box next to the number/statement selected.
4. Please note: The word "occasionally" when used here means once or twice, "often" means several times or more, and "frequently" means most of the time.

Question 1		Score
1	I do not feel happier or more cheerful than usual.	
2	I occasionally feel happier or more cheerful than usual.	
3	I often feel happier or more cheerful than usual.	
4	I feel happier or more cheerful than usual most of the time.	
5	I feel happier or more cheerful than usual all of the time.	
Question 2		
1	I do not feel more self-confident than usual.	
2	I occasionally feel more self-confident than usual.	
3	I often feel more self-confident than usual.	
4	I frequently feel more self-confident than usual.	
5	I feel extremely self-confident all of the time.	
Question 3		
1	I do not need less sleep than usual.	
2	I occasionally need less sleep than usual.	
3	I often need less sleep than usual.	
4	I frequently need less sleep than usual.	
5	I can go all day and all night without any sleep and still not feel tired.	
Question 4		
1	I do not talk more than usual.	
2	I occasionally talk more than usual.	
3	I often talk more than usual.	
4	I frequently talk more than usual.	
5	I talk constantly and cannot be interrupted.	
Question 5		
1	I have not been more active (either socially, sexually, at work, home, or school) than usual.	
2	I have occasionally been more active than usual.	
3	I have often been more active than usual.	
4	I have frequently been more active than usual.	
5	I am constantly more active or on the go all the time.	
	TOTAL SCORE:	

Fig. 13.2 Altman Self-Rating Mania Scale (ASRM). (Reprinted by permission of Elsevier from The Altman Self-Rating Mania Scale, by Altman, E. G., Hedeker, D., Peterson, J. L., Davis, J. M. *Biological Psychiatry, 42*, 948–955, 1997 by the Society of Biological Psychiatry.)

when the person is frustrated. The irritability and belligerence may be short-lived, or it may become the prominent feature of the manic phase of bipolar disorder.

The following is a patient's description of the painful transition from hypomania to mania:

In the beginning, I'm high as a kite, it's tremendous. My thoughts are clear and my ideas are fast ... one great idea follows the last. I feel happy, I am not shy around anyone, I know just what to say. People and activities that seemed boring before become intensely interesting ... I don't want to eat, I'm not hungry ... I think about sex and consider having sex with people who I would never have before. Your whole being is super-charged ... you can do anything ... but at some point, this state of mind changes.

The thoughts start streaming in at such a speed and such an amount that clear thinking is impossible ... Your wonderful, interesting personality devolves into one that is irritable, impatient, uncontrolled ... friends and family are afraid of you ... you are trapped in the madness of your own mind.

Behavior

When people experience hypomania, they have voracious appetites for social engagement, spending, and activity, even indiscriminate sex. Constant activity and a reduced need for sleep prevent proper rest. Although short periods of sleep are possible, some patients may not sleep for several days in a row. This nonstop physical activity and the lack of sleep and food can lead to physical exhaustion and worsening of mania.

Individuals may pursue elaborate schemes to get rich, famous, and powerful despite objections and realistic constraints. Sometimes the person will make excessive phone calls and e-mails, often to well-known and influential people. Being manic means being busy during all hours of the day and night, furthering grandiose plans and wild schemes. To the person experiencing mania, no aspirations are too high and no distances are too far.

In the manic state, people often give away money, prized possessions, and expensive gifts. The person experiencing mania may throw extravagant parties and visit expensive nightclubs and restaurants. While out, they may spend money freely on friends and strangers alike—"I'll buy the next round for everyone!" This excessive spending, use of credit cards, and high living continue even in the face of seriously depleted resources. The individual often needs intervention to prevent financial ruin.

EVIDENCE-BASED PRACTICE

Symptoms Before and After a Suicide Attempt in Bipolar Disorder

Problem
Suicide rates among individuals with bipolar disorder are quite high, particularly during major depressive episodes.

Purpose of Study
The researchers were attempting to understand symptoms before and after suicide attempts in order to aid in prevention efforts.

Methods
Researchers used existing data from the Systematic Treatment Enhancement Program for Bipolar Disorder (STEP-BD) funded by the National Institute of Mental Health. The analysis focused on change in suicidal ideation and depressive symptoms in 120 days before and after the attempt. The sample included 216 who attempted suicide compared to data from a matched sample of non-attempters.

Findings
- Suicidal ideation worsened in the 120 days pre-attempt, but improved afterward, reaching non-attempter levels by 90 days post-attempt.
- Depressed mood, loss of interest, guilt, and low self-esteem followed a similar pattern of worsening prior to the attempt and improving by 90 days.

Why Should Nurses Be Interested in This Study?
Monitoring individuals with bipolar disorder for worsening suicidal ideation and depressive symptoms is essential. Also, monitoring for improvement and supporting individuals after a suicide attempt is absolutely indicated. Ninety days is a significant period of time to regain the will to live and to be free of depressive symptoms. Nurses can be advocates for follow-up care and support in the community.

Ballard, E. D., Farmer, C. A., Shovestul, B., VandeVoort, J., Machado-Vieira, R., & Park, L. (2019). Symptom trajectories in the months before and after a suicide attempt in individuals with bipolar disorder. *Bipolar Disorders, 22*(3), 245–254.

Distractibility is a hallmark symptom of mania. People with mania lose their focus and go from one activity or place to another. Many projects are started, but few, if any, are completed. Inactivity is impossible, even for the shortest period of time. Hyperactivity may range from mild constant motion to frenetic wild activity.

Individuals experiencing mania may be manipulative, profane, faultfinding, and skilled at detecting and then exploiting others' vulnerabilities. They constantly push limits. These behaviors often alienate family, friends, employers, healthcare providers, and others.

Choices of clothing often reflect the person's grandiose, yet tenuous, grasp of reality. Dress may be unusual, bizarre, colorful, and noticeably inappropriate. Makeup may be gaudy and overdone.

People often emerge from a manic state startled and confused by the shambles of their lives. The following description conveys one patient's experience:

> Now I can only go by what others said that I did. I am humiliated by their memories … I suppose if there is one saving grace to having mania, it is not remembering the details. I can tell by the way people are responding to me—being too kind maybe? Or, backing away when I walk in the room. I think that this episode is over, but I have to make sure it doesn't happen again. Pay off my credit cards, talk to my boss, make apologies, salvage some friendships. Yet … it's a slippery slope when I stay awake too late at night and begin feeling high again. The medication gives me peace, but it takes away the high and the brilliant colors.

Thought Processes and Speech Patterns

When people are thinking clearly, they are able to communicate clearly and get to the point. Mania causes a person to experience disorganized thoughts and speech patterns. This disorganization is evident in several specific ways:

- **Pressured speech** is fast, ranging from rapid to frenetic, conveying an inappropriate sense of urgency. As the name implies, the speech is pressured—if normal speech is analogous to the flow of a garden hose, then pressured speech is like the stream from a fire hose. This type of speech tends to be loud, rapid, and incoherent. Individuals may talk nonstop and usually have no interest in feedback or conversation.

- **Circumstantial speech** is adding unnecessary details when communicating with others. Unlike some of the other verbal derailments, the person eventually gets to the point:

> I planned to have my oil changed today. When I got in my car, I noticed that the leather on the seat was dirty. The dog. We got a brown and white beagle because Jim insisted upon it. He's a barker. That's how things have gone since we got married in 1986 at a lovely church. I'll never forget the minister wore a green suit and dirty shoes … After I cleaned the seat, I drove to the garage and four guys swarmed around the car and changed the oil.

- **Tangential speech** is similar to circumstantial speech with one key difference. When people think tangentially, they lose the point that they were trying to make and never find it again. Awareness of losing the point indicates less thought disturbance: "Sorry I'm so scattered; I've got a lot on my mind" indicates insight. The degree of tangentiality also helps identify how serious the thought disturbance is. Often, a common word connects sentences:

I had to do my laundry that day because it was Saturday. On Saturday, I always watch Ninja Turtles on television. Have you seen those 60-inch televisions? Giants. I used to think of giants as I fell asleep, and I thought that sleep activated them.

- **Loose associations** represent the disordered way that a person is processing information. Thoughts are only loosely connected to each other in the person's conversation. For example, a patient may say, "The sky's the limit now that I have money. I took a flight, you know, from Kennedy. Drinking beer is a belly full of bags."
- **Flight of ideas** is a continuous flow of *accelerated* speech with abrupt changes from topic to topic. The speech is usually based on understandable associations or plays on words. At times, the attentive listener can keep up with the flow of words, even though direction changes from moment to moment. Speech is rapid, verbose, and circumstantial. When the condition is severe, speech may be disorganized and incoherent. The incessant talking often includes joking, puns, and teasing:

How are you doing, kid, no kidding around, I'm going home … home sweet home … home is where the heart is, the heart of the matter is I want out and that ain't hay … hey, Doc … get me out of this place.

Speech is not only profuse but also loud or even screaming. You can hear the force and energy behind the rapid words. As mania escalates, the flight of ideas may give way to clang associations. **Clang associations** are the stringing together of words because of their rhyming sounds, without regard to their meaning:

Cinema I and II, last row. Row, row, row your boat. Don't be a cutthroat. Cut your throat. Get your goat. Go out and vote. And so I wrote.

Thought Content

The content of speech is often sexually explicit and ranges from inappropriate to vulgar. Themes in the communication of the individual with mania may revolve around extraordinary sexual skill, brilliant business ability, or unparalleled artistic talents (e.g., writing, painting, and dancing). The person may actually have only average ability in these areas.

Mania brings about disturbing ways of viewing others and the world. These distorted and generally false thoughts are called **delusions**.

- **Grandiose delusions** are manifested by a highly inflated self-regard. It is apparent in both the ideas expressed and the person's behavior. People with mania may exaggerate their achievements or importance, state that they know famous people, or believe they have great powers. Religious ("I am the Messiah"), science fiction ("I was abducted"), and supernatural ("I am possessed by my dead father") themes are common in grandiose delusions. Sometimes it is difficult to distinguish fact from fiction ("I made an absolute fortune during the real estate crash of 2008").
- **Persecutory delusions** are also disturbingly common. For example, people may think that God is punishing them, that the FBI is spying on them, or that the mayor is harassing them. Sensory perceptions may become altered as the mania escalates, and hallucinations may occur. Rarely, patients may resort to violence in retaliation for this imagined persecution.

Cognitive Function

The onset of bipolar disorder is often preceded by comparatively high cognitive function. However, a substantial portion of individuals with bipolar disorder have significant and persistent cognitive problems even when they are not experiencing acute symptoms of mania or depression (Cullen et al., 2016). These cognitive deficits in bipolar disorder are milder but similar to those in patients with schizophrenia. Bipolar I results in more severe deficits, but cognitive alterations are known to exist in bipolar II.

The potential cognitive dysfunction among many people with bipolar disorder has specific clinical implications:

- Cognitive function affects overall function.
- Cognitive deficits correlate with a greater number of manic episodes, history of psychosis, chronicity of illness, and poor functional outcome.
- Early diagnosis and treatment are crucial to prevent illness progression, cognitive deficits, and poor outcome.
- Medication selection should consider not only the efficacy of the drug in reducing mood symptoms but also the cognitive impact of the drug on the patient.

Self-Assessment

If you are around someone experiencing mania, you will probably feel uncomfortable. This discomfort may be brought on, in part, by the patient's decreased personal space and intrusive comments. You may find yourself feeling afraid, inadequate, or even angry. Understanding, acknowledging, and sharing these responses will enhance your professional ability to care for the patient. Collaborating with staff, your nursing faculty member, and sharing your experience with peers in postconference may be helpful.

📄 ASSESSMENT GUIDELINES

Bipolar Disorder

1. Assess whether the patient is a danger to self and others:
   - Patients may not eat or sleep, often for days at a time.
   - Poor impulse control may result in harm to others or self.
2. Assess the need for protection from uninhibited behaviors. External control may be needed to protect the patient from such consequences as bankruptcy.
3. Assess the need for hospitalization to safeguard and stabilize the patient.
4. Assess medical status. A thorough medical examination helps determine whether mania is primary (a mood disorder—bipolar disorder or cyclothymic disorder) or secondary to another condition.
   - Mania may be secondary to a general medical condition.
   - Mania may be substance-induced (caused by misuse of a drug or substance or by toxin exposure).
5. Assess the patient's and family's understanding of bipolar disorder, knowledge of medications, and knowledge of support groups and organizations that provide information on bipolar disorder.

TABLE 13.2 Signs and Symptoms, Nursing Diagnoses, and Outcomes for Mania

Signs and Symptoms	Nursing Diagnoses	Outcomes
Auditory hallucinations, agitation, impulsivity, poor judgment	*Risk for injury*	No injury: Delusional content reduced or eliminated, hallucinations reduced or eliminated, thinking is objectively clearer, redirectable
Alteration in cognitive functioning, impulsiveness, sexual advances, threatening violence, agitation	*Risk for violence*	No aggressive behavior: Refrains from harming others, controls impulses, respects others' space
Agitation, anxiety, confusion, perceptual disorders, restlessness	*Sleep deprivation*	Adequate sleep: Sleeps 4–6 h a night, reports feeling refreshed after sleep
Deficits in verbal communication, working memory, executive functioning, reasoning, problem solving	*Impaired cognition* *Impaired concentration*	Improved cognition: Demonstrates increase in concentration, improved memory, and hallucinations are absent
Minimal calorie intake, poor hygiene, clothing unclean	*Self-care deficit (feeding, bathing, dressing)*	Able to self-care: Completes meals, tends to hygiene, clean and appropriate clothing
Dysfunctional interaction with others, pressured speech, flight of ideas, annoyance or taunting of others, loud and crass speech	*Impaired socialization*	Improved socialization: Initiates and maintains goal-directed and mutually satisfying verbal exchanges

International Council of Nursing Practice. (2019). *ICNP browser.* Retrieved from https://www.icn.ch/what-we-do/projects/ehealth/icnp-browser. ICNP is owned and copyrighted by the International Council of Nurses (ICN). Reproduced with permission of the copyright holder.

NURSING DIAGNOSIS

Nursing diagnoses vary among people who are experiencing mania. A primary consideration for a patient in acute mania is the prevention of exhaustion. Because of the patient's poor judgment, excessive and constant motor activity, probable dehydration, and difficulty evaluating reality, *risk for injury* is a likely and appropriate diagnosis. Table 13.2 lists signs, symptoms, potential nursing diagnoses, and outcomes for bipolar disorders.

OUTCOMES IDENTIFICATION

Outcome criteria will be based on which of the three phases of the illness that the patient is experiencing. The three phases are acute, continuation, and maintenance.

Acute Phase

The acute phase begins with the onset of a new manic and hypomanic episode. The goals are symptom reduction and achieving remission from the episode. Nursing care centers around supporting these goals while supporting injury prevention and physiological integrity. For example, the patient will:

- Be well hydrated.
- Maintain stable cardiac status.
- Maintain/obtain tissue integrity.
- Get sufficient sleep and rest.
- Demonstrate thought self-control with the aid of staff or medication.
- Make no attempt at self-harm.

Manic Episodes

Maintenance Phase

During this stage, the most acute symptoms have been controlled. The longer-term maintenance phase begins after the resolution of an acute episode. The goal is now on preventing future exacerbation of the mania or hypomania. Education (e.g., knowledge of disease process, symptom management, and medication), support (e.g., individual, family, peer, and community), and problem-solving skills are areas that should be supported during this phase. For example, the patient will:

- Identify three risk factors for the development of acute mania.
- Attend group therapy on a daily basis.
- Identify new coping skills

PLANNING

Acute Phase

During an acute manic phase, planning focuses on medically stabilizing the patient while maintaining safety. Therefore, the hospital is usually the safest environment for accomplishing this stabilization (see the Case Study and Nursing Care Plan). Nursing care is geared toward managing medications, decreasing physical activity, increasing food and fluid intake, ensuring at least 4 to 6 hours of sleep per night, and intervening so that self-care needs are met. Seclusion, restraint, or electroconvulsive therapy (ECT) may be considered during the acute phase.

Maintenance Phase

During the maintenance phase, planning focuses on preventing relapse and limiting the severity and duration of future episodes. Patients with bipolar disorders require medications over long periods of time or even an entire lifetime.

During this period of time, people with bipolar disorders often face the interpersonal, familial, occupational, educational, and financial hardships that came out of the acute phase of the illness. Often, residual problems resulting from reckless, violent, or bizarre behavior leaves lives shattered and family and friends hurt and distant. Patients will need support as they not only recover from acute illness but also address repairing their lives.

IMPLEMENTATION

Patients with bipolar disorders are often ambivalent about treatment. On average, people wait almost 10 years between the onset of symptoms and receiving treatment (Conus, MacNeil, & McGorry, 2014). Self-medicating through alcohol or substances complicates the clinical picture and contributes to treatment delay. Patients may minimize the destructive consequences of their behaviors or deny the seriousness of the disease, and some are reluctant to give up the increased energy, euphoria, and heightened sense of self-esteem of hypomania.

Unfortunately, lack of adherence to mood-stabilizing medication is a major cause of relapse. Establishing a therapeutic alliance with the individual with bipolar disorder is crucial to support continued treatment.

Depressive Episodes

Depressive episodes of bipolar disorder have the same symptoms and risks as major depressive disorder (refer to Chapter 14), although they are often more intense. Hospitalization may be required if suicidal ideation, psychosis, or catatonia is present. Pharmacological treatment is impacted by concerns of bringing on a manic phase. A discussion of medication therapy is included in this chapter.

Manic Episodes

Acute Phase

Hospitalization provides safety for a person experiencing acute mania in bipolar I disorder, imposes external control on destructive behaviors, and provides medication for stabilization. Staff members continually set limits in a firm, nonthreatening, and neutral manner to prevent escalation of behavior and safe boundaries.

There are unique approaches to communicating with and maintaining the safety of the person during the hospitalization. Table 13.3 provides interventions for patients who are experiencing acute mania.

Maintenance Phase

During this phase, interventions are geared toward the prevention of relapse. Medication adherence is essential, as is regular and adequate hours of sleep, healthy nutrition, and community support. Individuals at this stage will likely be engaged with community resources and be using outpatient facilities such as community mental health centers, outpatient clinics, and

TABLE 13.3   Interventions for Mania

Intervention	Rationale
Communication	
Use firm and calm approach: "John, come with me. Eat this sandwich."	Structure and control are provided for a patient who is out of control. Believing that someone is in control may improve feelings of security.
Use short and concise explanations or statements.	Short attention span limits comprehension to small bits of information.
Be consistent in approach and expectations.	Consistent limits and expectations minimize potential for patient's manipulation of staff.
Identify expectations in simple, concrete terms with consequences. Example: "John, do not yell at or hit Peter. If you cannot control yourself, we will help you." Or "The seclusion room will help you feel less out of control and prevent harm to yourself and others."	Clear expectations help the patient experience outside controls as well as understand reasons for medication, seclusion, or restraints (if he or she is not able to control behaviors).
Hear and act on legitimate complaints.	Underlying feelings of helplessness are reduced, and acting-out behaviors are minimized.
Firmly redirect energy into more appropriate and constructive channels.	Distractibility is the most effective tool with the patient experiencing mania.
Structure in a Safe Milieu	
Maintain low level of stimuli in patient's environment (e.g., away from bright lights, loud noises, and people).	Escalation of anxiety can be decreased.
Provide structured solitary activities with nurse or aide.	Structure provides security and focus.
Provide frequent high-calorie fluids.	Serious nutritional deficiencies and dehydration are addressed.
Encourage frequent rest periods.	Exhaustion is prevented.
Redirect aggressive behavior.	Physical exercise can decrease tension and provide focus.
In acute mania, use as needed medication, seclusion, and/or restraint to minimize physical harm.	Exhaustion can result from dehydration, lack of sleep, and constant physical activity.
Observe for signs of lithium toxicity.	There is a small margin of safety between therapeutic and toxic doses.
Store valuables in hospital safe until rational judgment returns.	Patient is protected from giving away money and possessions.
Physiological Safety: Self-Care Needs	
Nutrition	
Monitor intake, output, and vital signs.	Adequate fluid and calorie intake are ensured; development of dehydration and cardiac collapse is minimized.
Offer frequent, high-calorie protein drinks and finger foods (e.g., sandwiches, fruit, milkshakes).	Fluid and calorie replacement are needed. Finger foods allow for "eating on the run."
Frequently remind patient to eat. "Tom, finish your milkshake." "Taylor, eat this banana."	The patient experiencing mania is unaware of bodily needs and is easily distracted. Needs supervision to eat.

TABLE 13.3 Interventions for Mania— cont'd

Intervention	Rationale
Sleep	
Encourage frequent rest periods during the day.	Lack of sleep can lead to exhaustion and increase mania.
Keep patient in areas of low stimulation.	Relaxation is promoted, and manic behavior is minimized.
At night, provide warm baths, soothing music, and medication when indicated. Avoid caffeine.	Relaxation, rest, and sleep are promoted.
Hygiene	
Encourage appropriate clothing choices.	The potential is decreased for ridicule, which lowers self-esteem and increases the need for manic defense. The patient is helped to maintain dignity.
Give step-by-step reminders for hygiene and dress. "Here is your razor. Shave the left side … now the right side. Here is your toothbrush. Put the toothpaste on the brush."…	Distractibility and poor concentration are countered through simple, concrete instructions.
Elimination	
Offer fluids and foods that are high in fiber. Evaluate need for laxative. Encourage patient to go to the bathroom.	Fecal impaction resulting from dehydration and decreased peristalsis is prevented.

CASE STUDY AND NURSING CARE PLAN

Mania

The police report that when they pulled over Jasmine's weaving car, she told them she was "driving to fame and fortune." She had an open bottle of bourbon on the seat next to her. She proceeded to talk rapidly and make light of the situation. Dressed provocatively, she flirted with the police officers while chanting, "Boys in blue are fun to do…"

When the police explained that they wanted to take her to the hospital for evaluation, her mood turned to anger and rage. Minutes after getting into the police car, she was singing, "You Need to Calm Down."

In the emergency department, a psychiatric nurse practitioner saw Jasmine, who loudly says, "I'm here because I was driving to fame and fortune." Jasmine then begins to pace.

Her sister arrived and reported that Jasmine stopped taking her lithium about 5 weeks ago. Her behavior had deteriorated rapidly. Apparently, Jasmine had not eaten in days, stayed up all night calling friends and strangers, and finally fled the house when the sister called an ambulance to take her to the hospital. The nurse practitioner receives her old charts, with history and medical management. Jasmine is hospitalized, and lithium therapy is restarted.

Self-Assessment

Jeff has worked as a registered nurse on the psychiatric unit for 3 years. He has learned to deal with many of the challenging behaviors associated with mania.

Yet Jeff is uncomfortable with Jasmine's sexual comments, such as "Let me be…set me free, lover." He discusses his concerns with the unit coordinator. They decide that two nurses should care for Jasmine. A female nurse will spend time with her in her room, and Jeff will provide care for her on the unit. They agree that neither Jeff nor any male staff member should be alone with Jasmine in her room.

Assessment

Subjective Data

- "I'm here because I was driving myself to fame and fortune."
- "Let me be…set me free, lover."
- Told the police, "Boys in blue are fun to do…"
- Quit lithium 5 weeks ago
- Behavior deteriorated rapidly
- Limited nutritional intake for days
- Limited sleep for days

Objective Data

- Impaired concentration
- Poor judgment
- Constant physical activity
- Loud voice
- Flight of ideas
- Seductive clothing

Priority Diagnosis

Risk for injury as evidenced by the inability to meet physiological needs and set limits on behavior.

Outcomes Identification

Physical status will remain stable during the manic phase.

Planning

The nurse plans interventions that will help de-escalate Jasmine's activity to minimize potential physical injury (e.g., dehydration, cardiac instability) through the use of medication and providing a nonstimulating environment.

Implementation

Jeff makes the following nursing care plan.

Continued

CASE STUDY AND NURSING CARE PLAN—cont'd

Short-Term Goal	Intervention	Rationale	Evaluation
1. Patient will be well hydrated, as evidenced by good skin turgor and normal urinary output and specific gravity, within 24 h.	1a. Offer high-calorie, high-protein drink (8 oz) every hour in quiet area. 1b. Frequently remind patient to drink: "Take two more sips." 1c. Offer finger food frequently in a quiet area. 1d. Maintain record of intake and output. 1e. Weigh patient daily.	1a. Proper hydration is mandatory for maintenance of cardiac status. 1b. Patient is easily distracted; reminders and small goals are useful 1c. Patient is unable to sit and snacks can be eaten while pacing 1d. A record allows staff to make accurate nutritional assessment for patient's safety. 1e. Monitoring of nutritional status is necessary.	**GOAL MET** After 3 h, patient takes small amounts of fluid (2–4 oz per hour). After 5 h, patient starts taking 8 oz per hour with encouragement. After 24 h, urine specific gravity is within normal limits.
2. Patient will sleep or rest 3 h during the first night in the hospital with aid of medication and nursing interventions.	2a. Give programmed and PRN medication as ordered. 2b. Direct patient to unit areas with minimal activity. 2c. Encourage short rest periods throughout the day (e.g., 3–5 min every hour) when possible. 2d. Patient should drink decaffeinated drinks only—decaffeinated coffee, tea, or colas. 2e. Provide nursing measures at bedtime that promote sleep: warm milk, soft music.	2a. Antipsychotic and mood stabilizers will reduce physical activity. 2b. Lower levels of stimulation can decrease excitability. 2c. Patient may be unaware of feelings of fatigue. Can collapse from exhaustion if hyperactivity continues without periods of rest. 2d. Caffeine is a central nervous system stimulant that inhibits needed rest or sleep. 2e. Such measures promote nonstimulating and relaxing mood.	**GOAL NOT MET** Patient is awake most of the first night. Slept for 2 h from 4 to 6 a.m. Patient is able to rest on the second day for short periods and engage in quiet activities for short periods (5–10 min).
3. Patient's blood pressure (BP) and pulse (P) will be within normal limits within 24 h with the aid of medication and nursing interventions.	3a. Monitor BP and P frequently throughout the day (every 30 min). 3b. Keep staff informed by verbal and written reports of baseline vital signs and patient progress.	3a. Overactivity is a great strain on the patient's heart. 3b. Alerting staff regarding patient's status can increase medical intervention if a change in status occurs.	**GOAL MET** Medical records indicate that baseline BP is 130/90 mm Hg and baseline P is 88 beats/min. BP at the end of 24 h is 130/70 mm Hg; P is 80 beats/min.

Evaluation

After 2 days, Jasmine's vital signs are within normal limits, she is consuming sufficient fluids, and her urinary output is normal. She slept 4 h during the second night. As the effect of the medications progresses, Jasmine's activity level decreases. Eventually, she sleeps 6 h. By discharge, she is able to discuss concerns with Jeff and make some decisions about her future. Follow-up care will be provided at the community center. She and her sister will attend a family psychoeducational group for patients with bipolar disorder.

psychiatric home care. In addition to medication management, outpatient services provide structure, a decrease in social isolation, and a channel for their time and energy.

Health Teaching and Health Promotion

Patients and families need information about bipolar illness, with particular emphasis on its chronic and highly recurrent nature. In addition, patients and families need to learn the warning signs and symptoms of impending episodes. For example, changes in sleep patterns are especially important because they usually precede, accompany, or precipitate mania. Even a single night of unexplainable sleep loss can be taken as an early warning of impending mania. Health teaching stresses the importance of establishing regularity in sleep patterns, meals, exercise, and other activities. Box 13.1 lists health-teaching guidelines for patients with bipolar disorder and their families.

Most of the medications used to treat bipolar disorder may cause weight gain and other metabolic disturbances, such as altered metabolism of lipids and glucose. These alterations increase the risk for diabetes, high blood pressure, dyslipidemia, cardiac problems, or all of these in combination (metabolic syndrome). Not only do these disturbances impair quality of life and shorten life span, but they are also a major reason for nonadherence. Teaching aimed at weight reduction and management is essential to keeping patients physically healthy and emotionally stable.

Recovery concepts are particularly important for patients with bipolar disorder who often have issues with adherence to treatment. The best method of addressing this problem is to follow a collaborative-care model in which responsibilities for treatment adherence are shared. In this model, patients are responsible for making it to appointments and openly communicating information, and the healthcare provider is responsible for keeping current on treatment methods and listening carefully as the patient shares perceptions. Through this sharing, treatment adherence becomes a self-managed responsibility.

The National Institute of Mental Health (2015) provides two colorful, downloadable brochures about bipolar disorder in

BOX 13.1 Patient and Family Teaching: Bipolar Disorder

1. Patients with bipolar disorder and their families need to know:
   - The chronic and episodic nature of bipolar disorder
   - The fact that bipolar disorder is long term. Treatment will require that one or more mood-stabilizing agents be taken for a long time.
   - The expected side effects and toxic effects of the prescribed medication, as well as whom to call and where to go in case of an adverse reaction
   - The signs and symptoms of relapse that may "come out of the blue"
   - The role of family members and others in preventing a full relapse
   - The phone numbers of emergency contact people, which should be kept in an easily accessed place
2. The use of alcohol, drugs, caffeine (particularly in energy drinks), and over-the-counter medications can cause a relapse.
3. Good sleep hygiene is critical to stability. Frequently, the early symptom of a manic episode is lack of sleep. In some cases, mania may be averted by the use of sleep medications.
4. Coping strategies are important for dealing with work, interpersonal, and family problems for lowering stress; for enhancing a sense of personal control; and for increasing community functioning.
5. Group and individual therapy are valuable for gaining insight and skills in relapse prevention, providing social support, increasing coping skills in interpersonal relations, improving adherence to the medication regimen, reducing functional morbidity, and decreasing the need for hospitalization.

adults and children and adolescents. They are available in both English and Spanish for you to provide to your patient. The link is: http://www.nimh.nih.gov/health/publications/bipolar-disorder-listing.shtml.

Teamwork and Safety

Interprofessional staff work together to create a climate of teamwork and safety. This is essential for patients who are at risk of self-harm during a depressive phase or at risk for self-harm or other harm during the acute phase. The whole treatment team is trained to recognize changes that may lead to unsafe behavior.

Frequent team meetings to plan strategies for dealing with challenging patient behaviors are essential. These meetings help to minimize staff splitting and may reduce feelings of anger, fear, and isolation. Limit setting (e.g., lights out after 11:00 p.m.) is the main theme in treating a person in a manic state.

Seclusion and Restraint

Control of hyperactivity during the acute phase almost always includes immediate treatment with an antipsychotic drug. When a patient is dangerously out of control, however, use of the seclusion room or restraints may be necessary. The use of seclusion or restraints is associated with complex therapeutic, ethical, and legal issues. Most state laws prohibit the use of unnecessary physical restraint or isolation. Unless it is an emergency, the use of seclusion and restraints requires the patient's consent.

Seclusion and restraint may be warranted when documented data collected by the nursing and medical staff reflect the following points:

- Substantial risk of harm to others or self is clear.
- The patient is unable to control actions.
- Other measures have failed (e.g., setting limits beginning with verbal de-escalation or using chemical restraints).

Most facilities have well-defined practices for treatment with seclusion and restraint, including a proper reporting procedure through the chain of command when a patient is to be secluded. For example, the use of seclusion and restraint is permitted only on the written order of an authorized care provider (e.g., physician, advanced practice nurse, or a physician assistant), which must be reviewed and rewritten every 24 hours. The order must include the type of restraint to be used. Only in an emergency may the charge nurse place a patient in seclusion or restraint; under these circumstances, a written order must be obtained within a specified period of time (15 to 30 minutes).

Protocols identify specific nursing responsibilities, such as how often to observe and document the patient's behavior (e.g., every 15 minutes), how often to offer the patient food and fluids (e.g., every 30 to 60 minutes), and how often the patient can use the restroom (e.g., every 1 to 2 hours). Caregivers should measure vital signs frequently (e.g., every 1 to 2 hours).

Communication with a patient in seclusion is concrete, direct, and empathetic. Patients need reassurance that seclusion is only a temporary measure and that they will be returned to the unit when they demonstrate the ability to safely be around others.

Restraints and seclusion are never for punishment or for the convenience of the staff. Refer to Chapter 6 for a more detailed discussion of the legal implications of seclusion and restraints.

Support Groups

Patients with bipolar disorder, as well as their friends and families, benefit from support groups such as those sponsored by the Depression and Bipolar Support Alliance (DBSA), the National Alliance on Mental Illness (NAMI), and Mental Health America. Prior to 2020, support groups were moving toward virtual offerings. Due to the coronavirus pandemic, there was tremendous growth in video teleconferencing and, anecdotally, this resulted in improved attendance. It is likely that many of these groups will not return to an in-person format. An online search will provide information about bipolar support groups that will fit a variety of demographics, including specific age ranges, gender identity, and sexuality.

EVALUATION

Outcome criteria often dictate the frequency of evaluation of short-term and intermediate indicators. Are the patient's vital signs stable? Is he or she well hydrated? Is the patient able to control personal behavior or respond to external controls? Is the patient able to sleep for 4 or 5 hours a night or take frequent short rest periods during the day? Does the family have a clear understanding of the patient's disease and need for medication? Do the patient and family know which community agencies may help them?

After reassessing the outcomes and care plan, the plan is revised, if indicated. Longer-term outcomes include:

- Adherence to the medication regimen
- Resumption of functioning in the community
- Achievement of stability in family, work, and social relationships and in mood
- Improved coping skills for reducing stress

TREATMENT MODALITIES

Biological Treatments

Pharmacotherapy

Agitation. Individuals with bipolar disorder may be on multiple medications. For severe agitation, lithium (Eskalith, Lithobid) or divalproex (Depakote) and a second-generation antipsychotic such as olanzapine (Zyprexa) or risperidone (Risperdal) are recommended. Individuals experiencing less severe symptoms may be given only one of these.

There may be times when a benzodiazepine antianxiety agent can help reduce agitation or anxiety. Due to concern of dependency, use of benzodiazepines is usually short term until the mania subsides. The high-potency antianxiety benzodiazepines clonazepam (Klonopin) and lorazepam (Ativan) are useful in the treatment of acute mania. They may calm agitation and reduce insomnia, aggression, and panic.

Mood stabilization. Mood stabilizers refer to classes of drugs used to treat symptoms associated with bipolar disorder. The original intent of the term "mood stabilizers" was to indicate that these drugs were effective in the treatment of both mania and depression. While all of the medications in this category are effective in treating mania, not all of them do well in treating depression.

Lithium. The chemical name for lithium carbonate is $LiCO_3$, although you may see it abbreviated as Li^+. Lithium (Eskalith, Lithobid) has US Food and Drug Administration (FDA) approval for both acute mania and maintenance treatment. Onset of action is usually within 10 to 21 days. Because the onset of action is so slow, it is usually supplemented in the early phases of treatment by second-generation antipsychotics, anticonvulsants, or antianxiety medications.

The clinical benefits of lithium can be incredible. However, newer drugs have been introduced and approved that carry lower toxicity, have more favorable side effects, and require less frequent laboratory testing. The use of these newer drugs has resulted in a decline in lithium use.

Lithium is particularly effective in reducing the following:
- Elation, grandiosity, and expansiveness
- Flight of ideas
- Irritability and manipulation
- Anxiety
- Self-injurious behavior
To a lesser extent, lithium controls the following:
- Insomnia
- Psychomotor agitation
- Threatening or assaultive behavior
- Distractibility
- Hypersexuality
- Paranoia

Actress Patty Duke describes her response to lithium after years of alternating depression, elation, and bad choices (Moore, 2008):

Lithium saved my life. After just a few weeks on the drug, death-based thoughts were no longer the first I had when I
got up and last when I went to bed. The nightmare that had spanned 30 years was over. I'm not a Stepford wife; I still feel the exultation and sadness that any person feels. I'm just not required to feel them 10 times as long or as intensively as I used to.

Therapeutic and toxic levels. There is a small window between the therapeutic and toxic levels of lithium. Lithium must reach therapeutic blood levels to be effective. This usually takes 7 to 14 days, or longer for some patients. In the acute manic phase, lithium is usually started at 600 to 1200 mg a day in two or three divided doses. It is then increased every few days by 300 mg a day with a maximum dose of 1800 mg a day. A target range for a 12-hour serum trough level is 0.8–1.2 mEq/L. A greater clinical benefit for acute mania may be found in a level of 1.0–1.2 mEq/L (Miller, Ostacher, & Suppes, 2019).

During the maintenance phase, lithium doses can be cut back to doses ranging from 900 to 1200 mg a day. The target serum lithium level for maintenance is 0.6 to 0.8 mEq/L. Even lower levels of lithium—0.4 to 0.6 mEq/L—may be considered in some cases, such as adjunctive treatment for bipolar I patients or monotherapy for bipolar II patients. Table 13.4 details the expected side effects of lithium, signs of lithium toxicity, and interventions for both.

The first lithium level should be drawn every 2 to 3 days after beginning lithium therapy and after any dosage change until the therapeutic level has been reached. Blood levels are then checked every 3 to 6 months. For older adult patients, the principle of start low and go slow applies.

Before administering lithium, complete a baseline assessment of renal function and thyroid status, including levels of thyroxine and thyroid-stimulating hormone. Perform other clinical and laboratory assessments, including an electrocardiogram as needed, depending on the individual's physical condition.

Box 13.2 outlines patient and family teaching for lithium therapy.

Contraindications. Lithium therapy is generally contraindicated in patients with cardiovascular disease, brain damage, renal disease, thyroid disease, or myasthenia gravis. Whenever possible, lithium is not given to women who are pregnant because it may harm the fetus. Lithium use is also contraindicated in mothers who are breast-feeding and in children younger than 12 years of age.

Anticonvulsant drugs. Anticonvulsant drugs (also known as antiepileptics) were developed to treat seizures associated with epilepsy. The FDA approves them for use in acute mania, acute bipolar depression, and/or bipolar maintenance. They are generally:
- Superior for continuously cycling patients
- More effective when there is no family history of bipolar disease
- Effective at diminishing impulsive and aggressive behavior in some nonpsychotic patients
- Helpful in cases of alcohol and benzodiazepine withdrawal
- Beneficial in controlling mania (within 2 weeks) and depression (within 3 weeks or longer)

TABLE 13.4 Lithium Side Effects and Signs of Lithium Toxicity

Plasma Level	Signs	Interventions
Signs of Toxicity <1.5 mEq/L	Nausea, vomiting, diarrhea, thirst, polyuria (producing too much urine), lethargy, sedation, and fine hand tremor Renal toxicity, goiter, and hypothyroidism may occur with long-term use	Symptoms often subside during treatment. Doses should be kept low. Kidney function and thyroid levels should be assessed before treatment and then on an annual basis.
Early Signs of Toxicity 1.5–2.0 mEq/L	Gastrointestinal upset, coarse hand tremor, confusion, hyperirritability of muscles, electroencephalographic changes, sedation, incoordination	Medication should be withheld, blood lithium levels measured, and dosage reevaluated.
Advanced Signs of Toxicity 2.0–2.5 mEq/L	Ataxia, giddiness, serious electroencephalographic changes, blurred vision, clonic movements, large output of dilute urine, seizures, stupor, severe hypotension, coma. Death is usually secondary to pulmonary complications.	Hospitalization is indicated. The drug is stopped, and excretion is hastened. Whole bowel irrigation may be done to prevent further absorption of lithium.
Severe Toxicity >2.5 mEq/L	Convulsions, oliguria (producing none or small amounts of urine), and death can occur.	In addition to the interventions above, hemodialysis may be used in severe cases.

Data from Burchum, J. R., & Rosenthal, L. D. (2019). *Lehne's pharmacology for nursing care* (10th ed.). St. Louis, MO: Elsevier Saunders.

Valproate. Valproate, available as divalproex (Depakote) and valproic acid, has FDA approval for treating acute mania. Valproate is also helpful in preventing future manic episodes. Common side effects include nausea, weakness, somnolence, indigestion, diarrhea, dizziness, and vomiting.

The FDA has a black box warning for several adverse responses. Although hepatotoxicity is rare, it is important to monitor liver function. Low platelets (thrombocytopenia) may also occur, so platelet counts and coagulation studies should also be monitored. Pancreatitis, including fatal hemorrhagic cases, have been reported. These conditions may be dose related, so the lowest beneficial dosages should be used.

The FDA has a black box warning against valproate use in pregnancy due to teratogenicity. Patients should be screened for pregnancy and use birth control during therapy with this drug. These risks may apply to other anticonvulsants as well but are higher with valproate. Valproate can affect how the baby develops and may result in birth defects. Defects associated with this drug include malformations such as small fingers and toes, and major malformations such as spina bifida or cleft palate. Autism is more common after use during pregnancy. As the child grows, a condition sometimes known as fetal anticonvulsant syndrome may become evident. This syndrome is characterized by developmental and learning problems, such as delayed walking and talking, poor speech and language skills, memory deficits, and decreased intelligence.

Carbamazepine. Carbamazepine (Equetro) is indicated for acute mania and mixed states. Due to complex drug interactions and adverse effects, carbamazepine is considered a second-line treatment. It is an inducer of cytochrome P450 3A4, of which many psychotropics are substrates. Thus, carbamazepine causes the rapid metabolism of these other drugs, making them less effective.

Common side effects include dizziness, somnolence, nausea, vomiting, ataxia, constipation, pruritis, dry mouth, weakness, blurred vision, and speech problems. Liver enzymes should be monitored at least weekly for the first 8 weeks of treatment because the drug can increase levels of liver enzymes that can speed its own metabolism. In some instances, this can cause bone-marrow suppression and liver inflammation. Complete blood counts should also be drawn prior to beginning treatment and periodically thereafter since carbamazepine is known to cause leukopenia and aplastic anemia.

Carbamazepine carries a black box warning for serious dermatologic reactions. These include toxic epidermal necrolysis and Stevens-Johnson syndrome. Patients of Asian ancestry have a 10 times greater risk for toxic epidermal necrolysis and should be genetically tested prior to using this drug.

Lamotrigine. Lamotrigine (Lamictal) is an FDA-approved maintenance therapy medication approved for people 18 years and older. Patients usually tolerate lamotrigine well. Common adverse reactions include dizziness, headache, diplopia (double vision), ataxia, blurred vision, nausea, somnolence, rhinitis, and pharyngitis.

In about 10% of people taking lamotrigine, a rash appears within 8 weeks of starting treatment. However, about 1% of people progress to toxic epidermal necrolysis or Stevens-Johnson syndrome. The risk is greater in children aged 2 to 16 years. These skin conditions are more common with co-administration of valproate, rapid dose increases, and doses exceeding the recommended upper limit. Since it is impossible to tell if a benign rash will become dangerous, it is essential to discontinue this drug if a rash appears.

The patient and the patient's family should receive the following information, be encouraged to ask questions, and be given the material in written form as well.

- Lithium is a mood stabilizer and helps prevent relapse. It is important to continue taking the drug even after the current episode subsides.
- Lithium is not addictive.
- It is important to monitor lithium blood levels closely until a therapeutic level is reached. After this level is reached, continued monitoring will be required to prevent toxicity. You will need more frequent blood level monitoring at first, then once every several months after that.
- It is important to maintain a consistent fluid intake (1500–3000 mL/day or six 12-oz glasses of fluid).
- Sodium intake can affect lithium levels. High sodium intake leads to lower levels of lithium and less therapeutic effect. Low sodium intake leads to higher lithium levels, which could produce toxicity. Aim for consistency in sodium intake.
- You should stop taking lithium if you have excessive diarrhea, vomiting, or sweating. All of these symptoms can lead to dehydration and increase blood lithium to toxic levels. Inform your care provider if you have any of these problems.
- Let your prescriber know if you take diuretics (water pills).
- Talk to your prescriber about having your thyroid, parathyroid, and renal function checked periodically due to risk for hypothyroidism, hyperthyroidism, hyperparathyroidism, and decreased kidney function.
- Don't take over-the-counter medicines without checking with your prescriber. Even non-steroidal anti-inflammatory drugs (e.g., ibuprofen, naproxen) may influence lithium levels.
- Take lithium with meals to avoid stomach irritation.
- In the first week, you may gain up to 5 pounds of water weight. Additional weight gain may occur, particularly with females. Discuss how much weight gain is acceptable with your prescriber.
- Groups are available to provide support for people with bipolar disorder and their families. A local self-help group is [provide a name and telephone number].
- You can find out more information by calling [provide a name and telephone number].
- Keep a list of side effects and toxic effects handy, along with the name and number of a contact person (see Table 13.4).
- If lithium is to be discontinued, the dosage will be tapered gradually to minimize the risk of relapse.

Second-generation antipsychotics. Many of the second-generation antipsychotics are approved for acute mania. In addition to showing sedative properties during the early phase of treatment (help with insomnia, anxiety, agitation), the second-generation antipsychotics seem to have mood-stabilizing properties. Evidence supports the use of olanzapine (Zyprexa), risperidone (Risperdal), quetiapine (Seroquel), ziprasidone (Geodon), aripiprazole (Abilify), asenapine (Saphris), and cariprazine (Vraylar).

This classification of drugs may cause serious side effects. These serious side effects stem from a tendency toward weight gain that may lead to insulin resistance, diabetes, dyslipidemia, and cardiovascular impairment.

Bipolar depression. Treatment of bipolar with a common antidepressant alone increases the risk of bringing on a manic episode (Viktorin et al., 2014). This risk vanishes when combining the antidepressant with a mood stabilizer.

Specific medications are indicated for bipolar depression. The second-generation antipsychotics lurasidone (Latuda), quetiapine (Seroquel), and cariprazine (Vraylar) have FDA approval for the treatment of bipolar depression. Symbyax is another drug with approval for this type of depression. It is made up of the second-generation antipsychotic olanzapine (Zyprexa) and the selective serotonin reuptake inhibitor antidepressant fluoxetine (Prozac).

Table 13.5 identifies drugs with FDA approval for bipolar disorder. You may notice that your patient is taking a drug without specific FDA approval. This is called using the medication *off-label*, meaning that it is not officially approved, but practitioners often prescribe it.

Integrative Therapy

A few generations ago, children resisted a nightly dose of cod liver oil that mothers swore by as constipation prevention. While the foul-tasting evil-smelling liquid undoubtedly helped win that particular battle, it may have had other benefits as well. Cod liver oil is rich in omega-3 fatty acids, which have drawn increasing attention as being important in mood regulation. Fish oil is the target of this attention. It contains two omega-3 fatty acids, eicosapentaenoic acid (EPA) and docosahexaenoic acid (DHA), which are important in CNS functioning.

The interest in these particular fatty acids developed as research began to suggest that people who live in areas with low seafood consumption, especially cold-water seafood, exhibited higher rates of depression and bipolar disorder. This led researchers to explore the influence of omega-3 fatty acids as protective for bipolar disorder.

In 2012 Sarris and colleagues reviewed published research about omega-3 and its influence on mania and depression. They concluded that there is no evidence to support the use of omega-3 in treating mania. However, they found strong evidence that increasing the use of this fatty acid may improve bipolar depressive symptoms.

Brain Stimulation Therapies

Electroconvulsive therapy. Electroconvulsive therapy (ECT) is the oldest, most known, and most studied brain stimulation therapy. It works by passing an electric current through the brain. One major advantage of ECT is that it works more quickly than medication in improving depressive symptoms—usually within a week. See Chapter 14 for a description of the procedure.

ECT is most commonly used with patients who have bipolar disorder with severe levels of depression. ECT has been shown to be effective in about 80% of patients, particularly in older adults (Popiolek et al., 2019). ECT has been used effectively in mania, mixed, and depressed states of bipolar disorder as well as maintenance phases of treatment (Medda et al., 2014). One study demonstrated an overall cognitive improvement with ECT for patients with bipolar disorder (Wong et al., 2019).

Repetitive transcranial magnetic stimulation. Repetitive transcranial magnetic stimulation (rTMS) is a fairly new, noninvasive neuromodulation technique with FDA approval for treatment-resistant major depressive disorder. It has not been approved for

TABLE 13.5 FDA-Approved Drugs for Bipolar Disorder

Generic (Trade) Name	Bipolar Depression	Acute Mania	Bipolar Maintenance
Mood Stabilizer			
Lithium (Eskalith, Eskalith CR, Lithobid)	—	FDA approved	FDA approved
Anticonvulsant Mood Stabilizers			
Divalproex sodium delayed release (Depakote),	—	FDA approved	—
divalproex sodium extended release (Depakote ER)	—	FDA approved	—
Valproic acid delayed release			
Carbamazepine (Equetro)	—	FDA approved	—
Lamotrigine (Lamictal)	—	—	FDA approved
First-Generation Antipsychotics			
Chlorpromazine (Thorazine)	—	FDA approved	—
Loxapine (Adasuve) inhaled	—	FDA approved bipolar I agitation	—
Second-Generation Antipsychotics			
Aripiprazole (Abilify)	—	FDA approved	FDA approved
Asenapine (Saphris)	—	FDA approved	FDA approved
Cariprazine (Vraylar)	FDA approved	FDA approved	—
Lurasidone (Latuda)	FDA approved	—	—
Olanzapine (Zyprexa)	—	FDA approved	FDA approved
Quetiapine (Seroquel, Seroquel XR)	FDA approved	FDA approved	FDA approved
Risperidone (Risperdal)	—	FDA approved	—
(Risperdal Consta)	—	—	FDA approved
Ziprasidone (Geodon)	—	FDA approved	FDA approved
Combination Second-Generation Antipsychotic and Antidepressant			
Olanzapine (Zyprexa) + fluoxetine (Prozac) = Symbyax	FDA approved	—	—

Food and Drug Administration. (2016). FDA online label repository. Retrieved from http://labels.fda.gov/; and Howland, R. H. (2015). Drugs to treat bipolar disorder. *Journal of Psychosocial Nursing, 53*(6), 17–18.

bipolar depression. It works through the daily application of repeated magnetic pulses on hypoactive or hyperactive cortical brain areas. See Chapter 14 for more information on rTMS.

Research has been conducted that provides support for rTMS in patients with bipolar disorder. Jodoin, Miron, & Lesperance (2019) found that older adults with bipolar depression responded well to this alternate treatment. rTMS has been found to improve cognitive function in patients with bipolar disorder (Yang et al., 2019)

Psychological Therapies

Like other advanced practice psychiatric professionals, psychiatric-mental health advanced practice registered nurses (PMH-APRNs) are usually able to diagnose and prescribe medications for treating bipolar disorder. In addition, they may use psychotherapy to help the patient cope more adaptively to stresses in the environment and decrease the risk of relapse. Specific approaches to psychotherapy include cognitive behavioral therapy (CBT), interpersonal and social rhythm therapy, and family-focused therapy.

Many patients have strained interpersonal relationships, marriage and family problems, academic and occupational problems, and legal or other social difficulties. Psychotherapy can help them work through these difficulties, decrease some of the psychic distress, and increase self-esteem. Psychotherapeutic treatments can also help patients improve their functioning between episodes and attempt to decrease the frequency of future episodes.

Cognitive Behavioral Therapy

CBT is typically used as an adjunct to pharmacotherapy in many psychiatric disorders. It involves identifying maladaptive thoughts ("I am always going to be a loser") and behaviors ("I might as well drink") that may be barriers to a person's recovery and ongoing mood stability.

CBT focuses on adherence to the medication regimen, early detection and intervention for manic or depressive episodes, stress and lifestyle management, and the treatment of depression and comorbid conditions. Some research demonstrates that patients treated with cognitive therapy are more likely to take their medications as prescribed than are patients who do not participate in therapy, and psychotherapy results in greater adherence to the lithium regimen.

Interpersonal and Social Rhythm Therapy

Depression and manic-type states impair a person's ability to interact with others. Even in between episodes, relationships have been so damaged it may seem impossible to correct the problems. The APRN can use a specialized approach, interpersonal and social rhythm therapy. This approach aims to regulate social routines and stabilize interpersonal relationships to improve depression and prevent relapse. Psychoeducation is a major component of this therapy and includes symptom recognition, adherence with medication and sleep routines, stress management, and maintenance of social supports.

Family-Focused Therapy

Family-focused therapy helps improve communication among family members. During depressive and manic episodes, family life can become a challenge or even intolerable. Negative patterns of communicating develop and become part of the fabric of the family. APRNs can help people recognize and reduce negative expressed emotion and stressors that provoke episodes.

KEY POINTS TO REMEMBER

- Bipolar I disorder is characterized by the presence of a history of at least one manic episode, whereas bipolar II is characterized by the presence or history of at least one hypomanic episode.
- Cyclothymia is a bipolar-related disorder with symptoms of hypomania and symptoms of mild-moderate depression.
- Genetics play a strong role in the risk for bipolar disorders.
- Early detection of bipolar disorder can help diminish comorbid substance use problems or disorders, suicide, and decline in social and personal relationships and may help promote more positive outcomes.
- Nurses assess the patient's mood (i.e., mania, hypomania, and depression), behavior, and thought processes and are alert to cognitive dysfunction.
- During the acute phase of mania, physical needs often take priority and demand nursing interventions.
- Support groups, psychoeducation, and guidance for the family can greatly affect the patient's adherence to the medication regimen.
- Patients experiencing mania can be demanding and manipulative. Nurses set limits in a firm, neutral manner and tailor communication techniques and interventions to maintain the patient's safety.
- Healthcare workers, family, and friends often feel angry and frustrated by the patient's disruptive behaviors. When these

feelings are not examined and shared with others, the therapeutic potential of the staff is reduced, and feelings of confusion and helplessness remain.
- Mood stabilizers are usually the first line of defense for bipolar disorder and include lithium and several anticonvulsants.
- Lithium is approved for treating acute mania and maintenance. Blood levels, kidney function, and thyroid function should be assessed regularly.
- Most anticonvulsant drugs are approved for acute mania. Lamotrigine (Lamictal) is approved for maintenance.
- Antipsychotic agents, particularly the second-generation antipsychotics, are used for their sedating and mood-stabilizing properties. Screening for metabolic problems (e.g., diabetes) is essential in this population.
- For some patients, ECT and rTMS may be appropriate medical treatments.
- Patient and family teaching takes many forms and is most important in encouraging adherence to the medication regimen and reducing the risk of relapse.
- Evaluation includes examining the effectiveness of the nursing interventions, changing the outcomes as needed, and reassessing the nursing diagnoses. Evaluation is an ongoing process and is part of each of the other steps in the nursing process.

CRITICAL THINKING

1. Donald has a history of bipolar disorder and has been taking lithium for 4 months. During his clinic visit, he tells you that he does not think he will be taking his lithium anymore because he feels great and is able to function well at his job and at home with his family. He tells you his wife agrees that he "has this thing licked."
   a. What are Donald's needs in terms of teaching?
   b. What are the needs of the family?
   c. Write a teaching plan or use an already constructed plan. Include the following issues with sound rationales for these teaching topics:

- Use of alcohol, drugs, caffeine, over-the-counter medications
- Need for sleep hygiene
- Types of community resources available
- Signs and symptoms of relapse
   d. Role-play with a classmate how you can teach this family about bipolar illness and approach effective medication management, stressing the need for adherence and emphasizing those things that may threaten adherence.
   e. What referral information (websites, associations) can you give Donald and his family where they can access further information regarding this disease?

CHAPTER REVIEW

1. Which nursing response demonstrates accurate information that should be discussed with the female patient diagnosed with bipolar disorder and her support system? *Select all that apply.*

   a. "Remember that alcohol and caffeine can trigger a relapse of your symptoms."
   b. "Due to the risk of a manic episode, antidepressant therapy is never used with bipolar disorder."

c. "It's critical to let your healthcare provider know immediately if you aren't sleeping well."

d. "It will be helpful for your family to understand the management of this disorder."

e. "The symptoms tend to come and go and so you need to be able to recognize the early signs."

2. Which statement made by the patient demonstrates an understanding of the effective use of newly prescribed lithium to manage bipolar mania? *Select all that apply.*

a. "I have to keep reminding myself to consistently drink six 12-ounce glasses of fluid every day."

b. "I discussed the diuretic my cardiologist prescribed with my psychiatric care provider."

c. "Lithium may help me lose the few extra pounds I tend to carry around."

d. "I take my lithium on an empty stomach to help with absorption."

e. "I've already made arrangements for outpatient lithium level monitoring."

3. The nurse is providing medication education to a patient who has been prescribed lithium to stabilize mood. Which early signs and symptoms of toxicity should the nurse stress to the patient? *Select all that apply.*

a. Increased attentiveness

b. Getting up at night to urinate

c. Improved vision

d. An upset stomach for no apparent reason

e. Shaky hands that make holding a cup difficult

4. A male patient calls to tell the nurse that his monthly lithium level is 1.7 mEq/L. Which nursing intervention will the nurse implement initially?

a. Reinforce that the level is considered therapeutic.

b. Instruct the patient to hold the next dose of medication and contact the prescriber.

c. Have the patient go to the hospital emergency department immediately.

d. Alert the patient to the possibility of seizures and appropriate precautions.

5. Which intervention should the nurse implement when caring for a patient demonstrating manic behavior? *Select all that apply.*

a. Monitor the patient's vital signs frequently.

b. Keep the patient distracted with group-oriented activities.

c. Provide the patient with frequent milkshakes and protein drinks.

d. Reduce the volume on the television and dim bright lights in the environment.

e. Use a firm but calm voice to give specific concise directions to the patient.

6. Substance use problems or disorders are often present in people diagnosed with bipolar disorder. Laura, a 28-year-old with a diagnosis of bipolar disorder, drinks alcohol instead of taking her prescribed medications. The nurse caring for this patient recognizes that:

a. Anxiety may be present.

b. Alcohol ingestion is a form of self-medication.

c. The patient is lacking a sufficient number of neurotransmitters.

d. The patient is using alcohol because she is depressed.

7. Ted, a former executive, is now unemployed due to manic episodes at work. He was diagnosed with bipolar I disorder 8 years ago. Ted has a history of IV drug use, which resulted in hepatitis C. He is taking his lithium exactly as scheduled, a fact that both Ted's wife and his blood tests confirm. To reduce Ted's mania, the psychiatric nurse practitioner recommends:

a. Clonazepam (Klonopin)

b. Fluoxetine (Prozac)

c. Electroconvulsive therapy (ECT)

d. Lurasidone (Latuda)

8. A 33-year-old female diagnosed with bipolar I disorder has been functioning well on lithium for 11 months. At her most recent checkup, the psychiatric nurse practitioner states, "You are ready to enter the maintenance therapy stage, so at this time I am going to adjust your dosage by prescribing _____":

a. A higher dosage

b. Once a week dosing

c. A lower dosage

d. A different drug

9. Tatiana has been hospitalized for an acute manic episode. On admission, the nurse suspects lithium toxicity. What assessment findings would indicate the nurse's suspicion as correct?

a. Shortness of breath, gastrointestinal distress, chronic cough

b. Ataxia, severe hypotension, large volume of dilute urine

c. Gastrointestinal distress, thirst, nystagmus

d. Electroencephalographic changes, chest pain, dizziness

10. Luc's family comes home one evening to find him extremely agitated and they suspect in a full manic episode. The family calls emergency medical services. While one medic is talking with Luc and his family, the other medic is counting something on his desk. What is the medic most likely counting?

a. Hypodermic needles

b. Fast food wrappers

c. Empty soda cans

d. Energy drink containers

1. a, c, d, e; 2. a, b, e; 3. d, e; 4. b; 5. a, c, d, e; 6. b; 7. c; 8. c; 9. b; 10. d

NGN CASE STUDY AND QUESTIONS

Darnell is a 20-year-old male being admitted to a state psychiatric hospital accompanied by his brother. His clothing is rumpled, and his overall hygiene is poor. He reports hearing voices. Darnell states, "I do not have time for this. I make and sell rare guitars. You've got to get out there and sell yourself, day and night, and that's what I do." The intake nurse notices that the patient talks rapidly and with few breaks. "I don't need sleep. I need investors, people who believe in art, real art, you know? But you have to watch your back. There are people who hate genius, and there are people who know what I've got and want to take it away from me. You have to fight for this." He eyes his brother angrily.

1. Choose the *most likely* options to complete the following statement.

This patient's symptoms are most indicative of a(n) _____1_____ episode because his symptoms include ____2_____, and ___3_____.

Options for 1	Options for 2	Options for 3
a. Hypomanic	**a.** Delusions	**a.** Withdrawal from others
b. Depressive	**b.** Loss of interest in activities of life	**b.** Persistent lowered or decreased mood
c. Manic	**c.** Alternations of elation and sadness	**c.** Euphoria
d. Cyclothymic	**d.** Increased functioning	**d.** Hallucinations

2. The patient is not progressing as well as the treatment team has hoped. Identify the assessment findings that require immediate follow-up by the nurse. *Select all that apply.*
   a. Averaging 2 to 3 hours of sleep per night.
   b. Attention to hygiene is performed every 2 days.
   c. Prefers solitary to group activities.
   d. Eats finger foods while reading as opposed to dining with others in the dining area.
   e. Is calmer but not able to concentrate on all tasks at hand.

NGN case study answers are on Evolve.

🌐 Visit the Evolve website for a posttest on the content in this chapter: http://evolve.elsevier.com/Varcarolis

REFERENCES

American Psychiatric Association. (2013). *Diagnostic and statistical manual of mental disorders* (5th ed.). Washington, DC: Author.

Conus, P., MacNeil, C., & McGorry, P. D. (2014). Public health significance of bipolar disorder: Implications for early intervention and prevention. *Bipolar Disorders, 16*(5), 548–556.

Crump, C., Sundquist, K., Winkleby, M. A., & Sundquist, J. (2013). Comorbidities and mortality in bipolar disorder: A Swedish national cohort study. *JAMA Psychiatry, 70*(9), 931–939.

Cullen, B., Ward, J., Graham, N. A., Deary, I. J., Pell, J. P., Smith, D. J., & Evans, J. J. (2016). Prevalence and correlates of cognitive impairment in euthymic adults with bipolar disorder: A systematic review. *Journal of Affective Disorders, 205*, 165–181.

Dagani, J., Signorini, G., Nielssen, O., Bani, M., Pastore, A., de Girolamo, G., & Large, M. (2016). Meta-analysis of the interval between the onset and management of bipolar disorder. *Canadian Journal of Psychiatry, 62*(4), 247–258.

Goes, F. S., Pierooznia, M., Parla, J. S., Kramer, M., Ghiban, E., Mavruk, S., & Potash, J. B. (2016). Exome sequencing of familial bipolar disorder. *Journal of the American Medical Association Psychiatry, 73*(6), 590–597.

Goldstein, T. R., Ha, W., & Axelson, D. A. (2012). Predictors of prospectively examined suicide attempts among youth with bipolar disorder. *Archives of General Psychiatry, 69*(11), 1113–1122.

Jodoin, V. D., Miron, J. P., & Lesperance, P. (2019). Safety and efficacy of accelerated repetitive transcranial magnetic stimulation protocol in elderly depressed unipolar and bipolar patients. *The American Journal of Geriatric Psychiatry, 27*(50), 548–558.

Johansson, V., Halkola, R., Cannon, T. D., Hultman, C. M., & Hedman, A. M. (2019). A population-based heritability estimate of bipolar disorder—In a Swedish twin sample. *Psychiatry Research, 278*, 180–187.

Kessler, R. C., Berglund, P. A., Demler, O., Jin, R., & Walters, E. E. (2005). Lifetime prevalence and age-of-onset distributions of DSM-IV disorders in the National Comorbidity Survey Replication. *Archives of General Psychiatry, 62*(6), 593–602.

Lewis, K. J. S., DiFlorio, A. D., Forty, L., Gordon-Smith, K., Perry, A., Craddock, N., & Jones, I. (2018). Mania triggered by sleep loss

and risk of postpartum psychosis in women with bipolar disorder. *Journal of Affective Disorders, 225*(1), 624–629.

Maletic, V., & Raison, C. (2014). Integrated neurobiology of bipolar disorder. *Frontiers in Psychiatry, 5*(98). Retrieved from http://www.ncbi.nlm.nih.gov/pmc/articles/PMC4142322/.

Medda, P., Toni, C., & Perugi, G. (2014). The mood-stabilizing effects of electroconvulsive therapy. *Journal of ECT, 30*(4), 275–282.

Merikangas, K., Cui, L., Kattan, G., Carlson, G., Youngstrom, E., & Angst, J. (2012). Mania with and without depression in a community sample of U.S. adolescents. *Archives of General Psychiatry, 69*(9), 943–951.

Miller, S., Ostacher, M., & Suppes, T. (2019). Bipolar and related disorders. In L. W. Roberts (Ed.), *The American Psychiatric Association Publishing Textbook of Psychiatry*. Washington, D.C.: American Psychiatric Association.

Millett, C. E., Perez-Rodriguez, M., Shanahan, M., Larsen, E., Yamamoto, H. S., Bukowski, C., & Burdick, K. E. (2019). C-reactive protein is associated with cognitive performance in a large cohort of euthymic patients with bipolar disorder. *Molecular Psychiatry*.

Moore, M. (2008). *Patty Duke puts celebrity face on bipolar disorder. Missoulian*. Retrieved from http://missoulian.com/articles/2008/10/11/news/local/news05.txt.

National Institute of Mental Health. (2015). *Publications about bipolar disorder*. Retrieved from https://www.nimh.nih.gov/health/publications/bipolar-disorder-listing.shtml.

Palmier-Claus, J. E., Berry, K., Bucci, S., Mansell, W., & Varese, F. (2016). Relationship between childhood adversity and bipolar affective disorder: systematic review and meta-analysis. *British Journal of Psychiatry, 209*(6), 454–459.

Plans, L., Barrot, C., Nieto, E., Rios, J., Schulze, T. G., Papiol, S., & Benabarre, A. (2019). Association between completed suicide and bipolar disorder: A systematic review of the literature. *Journal of Affective Disorders, 242*(2), 111–122.

Phillips, M. L., & Swartz, H. A. (2014). A critical appraisal of neuroimaging studies of bipolar disorder: Toward a new conceptualization of underlying neural circuitry and roadmap for future research. *American Journal of Psychiatry, 171*(8), 829–843.

Popiolek, K., Bejerot, S., Brus, O., Hammar, A., Landen, M., Lundberg, J., & Nordenskjöld, A. (2019). Electroconvulsive therapy in bipolar depression—Effectiveness and prognostic indicators. *Acta Psychiatrica Scandinavica, 140*(3), 196–204.

Rowland, T. A., & Marwaha, S. (2018). Epidemiology and risk factors for biplar disorder. *Therapeutic Advances in Psychopharmacology, 8*(9), 251–269.

Sarris, J., Mischoulon, D., & Schweitzer, I. (2012). Omega-3 for bipolar disorder: Meta-analyses of use in mania and bipolar depression. *Journal of Clinical Psychiatry, 73*(1), 81–86.

Smith, D. J., Anderson, J., Zammit, S., Meyeter, T. D., Pell, J. P., & Mackay, D. (2015). Childhood IQ and risk of bipolar disorder in adulthood: Prospective birth cohort study. *British Journal of Psychiatry Open, 1,* 74–80.

Stahl, E. A., Breen, G., Forstner, A. J., McQuillin, A., Ripke, S., Trubetskoy, V., & Sklar, P. (2019). Genome-wide association study identifies 30 loci associated with bipolar disorder. *Nature Genetics, 51,* 793–803.

Viktorin, A., Lichtenstein, P., Thase, M. E., Larson, H., Lundholm, C., Magnusson, P. K. E., & Landen, M. (2014). The risk of switch to mania in patients with bipolar disorder during treatment with an antidepressant alone and in combination with a mood stabilizer. *American Journal of Psychiatry, 171*(10), 1067–1073.

Wong, V. K. H., Tor, P. C., Martin, D. M., Mok, Y. M., & Loo, C. (2019). Effectiveness and cognitive changes with ultrabrief right unilateral and other forms of electroconvulsive therapy in the treatment of mania. *Journal of ECT, 35*(1), 40–43.

Yang, L., Dong, Z., Kong, L. L., Sun, Y. Q., Wang, Z. Y., Gao, Y. Y., & Wang, Y. M. (2019). High-frequency repetitive transcranial magnetic stimulation (rTMS) improves neurocognitive function in bipolar disorder. *Journal of Affective Disorders, 246*(1), 851–856.

14

Depressive Disorders

Margaret Jordan Halter

 Visit the Evolve website for a pretest on the content in this chapter: http://evolve.elsevier.com/Varcarolis

OBJECTIVES

1. Identify symptoms of disruptive mood dysregulation disorder, persistent depressive disorder (dysthymia), and premenstrual dysphoric disorder.
2. Discuss the epidemiology of major depressive disorder.
3. Discuss the biological and cognitive risk factors for the development of major depressive disorders.
4. Assess behaviors in a patient with depression in regard to each of the following areas: (a) behavior, (b) mood, (c) feelings and emotions, (d) thought processes, and (e) thought content and perception.
5. Formulate five nursing diagnoses for a patient with major depressive disorder and include outcome criteria.
6. Name unrealistic expectations a nurse may have while working with a patient with depression and compare them to your own personal thoughts.
7. Role-play six principles of communication that are useful in working with patients with depression.
8. Identify the major classifications of antidepressants and general advantages and disadvantages of each.
9. Discuss brain therapies for major depressive disorder, such as electroconvulsive therapy (ECT) and vagus nerve stimulation.

KEY TERMS AND CONCEPTS

affect
anergia
anhedonia
bereavement exclusion
deep brain stimulation

electroconvulsive therapy (ECT)
light therapy
repetitive transcranial magnetic stimulation (rTMS)
serotonin syndrome

suicidal ideation
vagus nerve stimulation
vegetative signs of depression

One of the most important aspects of studying psychiatric nursing is to learn about the depressive disorders. In this chapter we will focus on disorders that share symptoms of sadness, emptiness, irritability, somatic (body) concerns, and impairment of thinking. All of the disorders impact a person's ability to function adequately. While the focus in this chapter will be on the classic condition of major depressive disorder, we will begin with a discussion of the other depressive disorders:

- Disruptive mood dysregulation disorder
- Persistent depressive disorder (formerly called dysthymia)
- Premenstrual dysphoric disorder
- Substance/medication-induced depressive disorder
- Depressive disorder due to another medical condition

DISRUPTIVE MOOD DYSREGULATION DISORDER

Disruptive mood dysregulation disorder was introduced in 2013 in response to an alarming number of children and adolescents

being diagnosed with bipolar disorder. A bipolar diagnosis resulted in exposure to powerful medications that probably were not helping, along with a lifelong label of serious mental illness. Perhaps the most compelling reason to change this diagnostic practice was that most of the young people who received a diagnosis of bipolar did not go on to have bipolar symptoms as adults. In fact, most children and adolescents once diagnosed with bipolar disorder actually converted to major depressive disorder or an anxiety disorder in adulthood.

Symptoms of disruptive mood dysregulation disorder are constant and severe irritability and anger. Diagnosis is made in individuals between the ages of 6 and 18 with an onset before age 10. Temper tantrums with verbal or behavioral outbursts out of proportion to the situation occur at least 3 times a week. Sometimes children and adolescents with this problem can maintain control in certain settings, such as school. To be diagnosed with disruptive mood dysregulation disorder, individuals need to exhibit symptoms in at least two of the following settings—home, school, and with peers.

Disruptive mood dysregulation disorder prevalence is believed to fall in the range of 0.8% to 3.3% (Copeland et al., 2013). It is more common in males than females, and it is more common in children than adolescents.

There is little information available on the treatment of disruptive mood dysregulation disorder. Management of this disorder is symptomatic and problem focused (Parikh et al., 2019). If symptoms resemble major depressive disorder, antidepressants may be considered. If a manic episode occurs during antidepressant therapy, bipolar disorder may be a strong possibility. If the disorder is accompanied by attention-deficit/hyperactivity disorder (ADHD), medications for that condition could be tried. Antidepressants may be used to address irritability. The second-generation antipsychotics risperidone (Risperdal) and aripiprazole (Abilify) have US Food and Drug Administration (FDA) approval for irritability in autism and are sometimes used for disruptive mood dysregulation disorder.

Psychosocial interventions such as cognitive behavioral therapy (CBT) are essential considering the degree of turmoil this disorder brings about. Parent training helps parents to interact with a child in such a way as to predict and reduce aggression and irritability through consistency and rewarding appropriate behavior. There is some evidence that these young people may be misperceiving others' facial expressions as angry. Computer-based training can help them become more aware of the meaning of facial expressions.

PERSISTENT DEPRESSIVE DISORDER

Persistent depressive disorder, formerly known as dysthymia (dys – bad + thymia – mood), is diagnosed when low-level depression occurs most of the day, for the majority of days. These depressive feelings last at least 2 years in adults and 1 year in children and adolescents. In addition to depressed mood, individuals with this disorder have at least two of the following: decreased appetite or overeating, insomnia or hypersomnia, low energy, poor self-esteem, difficulty thinking, and hopelessness.

The symptoms are difficult for the patient to live with and bring about social and occupational distress, but they are usually not severe enough to require hospitalization. Because the onset of persistent depressive disorder is usually in the teenage years, patients will frequently express that they have "always felt this way" and that being depressed seems like normal functioning. It is not uncommon for people with this low-level depression to also have periods of full-blown major depressive episodes.

The prevalence of persistent depressive disorder ranges from 1.5% to 3.3% (Vandeleur et al., 2017). The problem tends to have an early onset and, as the name suggests, it is a chronic illness. It is more common among women. Up to 50% of people with this disorder go undiagnosed and seek care for physical symptoms.

Treatment for this disorder is similar to that of major depressive disorder, which we will discuss in more depth later in this chapter. Psychotherapy, particularly CBT, is quite useful in managing the symptoms. Antidepressants such as selective serotonin reuptake inhibitors (SSRIs), serotonin and norepinephrine reuptake inhibitors (SNRIs), and tricyclics (TCAs) are the other main treatments.

PREMENSTRUAL DYSPHORIC DISORDER

Premenstrual dysphoric disorder is a relatively new addition to the diagnostic system for psychiatry. It refers to a cluster of symptoms that occur in the last week before the onset of a woman's period. Premenstrual dysphoric disorder causes problems severe enough to interfere with the ability to work or interact with others. Symptoms include mood swings, irritability, depression, anxiety, feeling overwhelmed, and difficulty concentrating. Other physical manifestations include lack of energy, overeating, hypersomnia or insomnia, breast tenderness, aching, bloating, and weight gain. Symptoms decrease significantly or disappear with the onset of menstruation.

The prevalence of premenstrual dysphoric disorder is about 2% to 6% of menstruating women. Symptoms cease after menopause, although they may return with hormone replacement therapy.

Treatment for this disorder includes regular exercise, particularly aerobic exercise. Other recommendations include eating food rich in complex carbohydrates and getting sufficient sleep. Acupuncture, light therapy, and relaxation therapy have also been used to reduce symptoms.

Several drugs have FDA approval for treatment of this disorder. A drospirenone and ethinyl estradiol combination (Yaz, Gianvi) is a contraceptive that improves symptoms. SSRIs have been used successfully and three have FDA approval. They are fluoxetine (Prozac, Sarafem), sertraline (Zoloft), and controlled-release paroxetine (Paxil CR). Diuretics may be useful in reducing bloating and weight gain brought on by water retention.

SUBSTANCE/MEDICATION-INDUCED DEPRESSIVE DISORDER

Substance/medication-induced depressive disorder is a result of prolonged use of or withdrawal from drugs and alcohol. The depressive symptoms last longer than the expected length of physiological effects, intoxication, or withdrawal of the substance. The person with this diagnosis would not experience depressive symptoms in the absence of drug or alcohol use or withdrawal. Symptoms appear within 1 month of use. Once the substance is removed, depressive symptoms usually remit within a few days to several weeks.

The lifetime prevalence rate is fairly low—about 0.25%. Medications associated with depressive symptoms include antiviral agents, cardiovascular drugs, retinoic acid derivatives, antidepressants, anticonvulsants, antimigraine agents, antipsychotics, hormonal agents, smoking cessation agents, and immunological agents.

DEPRESSIVE DISORDER DUE TO ANOTHER MEDICAL CONDITION

Depressive disorder due to another medical condition may be caused by disorders that affect the body's systems or from long-term illnesses that cause ongoing pain. The symptoms are the

TABLE 14.1 Medical Conditions and Substances/Medications Associated With Major Depressive Disorder

Substances/Medication

Central nervous system depressants	Alcohol, barbiturates, benzodiazepines, clonidine
Central nervous system medications	Amantadine, bromocriptine, levodopa, phenothiazines, phenytoin
Psychostimulants	Amphetamines
Systemic medications	Corticosteroids, digoxin, diltiazem, enalapril, ethionamide, isotretinoin, mefloquine, methyldopa, metoclopramide, quinolones, reserpine, statins, thiazides, vincristine

Medical Conditions

Neurological	Epilepsy, Parkinson disease, multiple sclerosis, Alzheimer disease, Huntington disease, traumatic brain injury, cerebrovascular accident
Infectious or inflammatory	Neurosyphilis, HIV
Cardiac disorders	Ischemic heart disease, cardiac failure, cardiomyopathies
Endocrine	Hypothyroidism, diabetes mellitus, vitamin deficiencies, parathyroid disorders
Inflammatory disorders	Collagen-vascular diseases, irritable bowel syndrome, chronic liver disorders
Neoplastic disorders	Central nervous system tumors, paraneoplastic syndromes

same as the diagnostic criteria for the depressive disorders. It is important to review medications being used for the medical condition to rule them out as being the causative agents.

There are clear associations, along with neuroanatomical changes, with some disease states. The prevalence rate of depression in people who have suffered a cerebrovascular accident (stroke) is high—30% to 50% in the first year (Flaster et al., 2013). Parkinson disease, Huntington disease, Alzheimer disease, and traumatic brain injury are also clearly associated with depressive disorders. Neuroendocrine conditions such as Cushing disease and hypothyroidism are also commonly accompanied by depression. Arthritis, back pain, metabolic conditions (e.g., vitamin B_{12} deficiency), HIV, diabetes, infection, cancer, and autoimmune problems may also contribute to depression.

Table 14.1 summarizes the medical problems and substances that are associated with major depression.

MAJOR DEPRESSIVE DISORDER

Clinical Picture

Major depressive disorder is one of the most common psychiatric disorders. In 2017, it affected approximately 17 million adults in the United States or about 7% of the population (Substance Abuse and Mental Health Services Administration, 2018). Major depressive disorder, or major depression, is characterized by a persistently depressed mood lasting for a minimum of 2 weeks.

The length of a depressive episode may be 5 to 6 months (Parikh et al., 2019). About 20% of cases become chronic (i.e., lasting more than 2 years). While depression begins with a single occurrence, most people experience recurrent episodes. People experience a recurrence within the first year about 50% of the time and within a lifetime up to 85% of the time. The full criteria for major depressive disorder are listed in the *DSM-5* box.

DSM-5 CRITERIA FOR MAJOR DEPRESSIVE DISORDER

A. Five (or more) of the following symptoms have been present during the same 2-week period and represent a change from previous functioning; at least one of the symptoms is either (1) depressed mood or (2) loss of interest or pleasure.

B. **Note:** Do not include symptoms that are clearly attributable to another medical condition.
  1. Depressed mood most of the day, nearly every day, as indicated by either subjective report (e.g., feels sad, empty, hopeless) or observation made by others (e.g., appears tearful). (**Note:** In children and adolescents, it can be irritable mood.)
  2. Markedly diminished interest or pleasure in all, or almost all, activities most of the day, nearly every day (as indicated by either subjective account or observation).
  3. Significant weight loss when not dieting or weight gain (e.g., a change of more than 5% of body weight in a month) or decrease or increase in appetite nearly every day. (**Note:** In children, consider failure to make expected weight gain.)
  4. Insomnia or hypersomnia nearly every day.
  5. Psychomotor agitation or retardation nearly every day (observable by others, not merely subjective feelings of restlessness or being slowed down).
  6. Fatigue or loss of energy nearly every day.
  7. Feelings of worthlessness or excessive or inappropriate guilt (which may be delusional) nearly every day (not merely self-reproach or guilt about being sick).
  8. Diminished ability to think or concentrate or indecisiveness nearly every day (either by subjective account or as observed by others).
  9. Recurrent thoughts of death (not just fear of dying), recurrent **suicidal ideation** without a specific plan, or a suicide attempt or a specific plan for committing suicide.

C. The symptoms cause clinically significant distress or impairment in social, occupational, or other important areas of functioning.

D. The episode is not attributable to the physiological effects of a substance or to another medical condition.

E. **Note:** Criteria A through C represent a major depressive episode.

Continued

DSM-5 CRITERIA FOR MAJOR DEPRESSIVE DISORDER—cont'd

F. **Note:** Responses to a significant loss (bereavement, financial ruin, losses from a natural disaster, a serious medical illness or disability) may include the feelings of intense sadness, rumination about the loss, insomnia, poor appetite, and weight loss as noted in Criterion A, which may resemble a depressive episode. Although such symptoms may be understandable or considered appropriate to the loss, the presence of a major depressive episode in addition to the normal response to a significant loss should also be carefully considered. This decision inevitably requires the exercise of clinical judgment based on the individual's history and the cultural norms for the expression of distress in the context of loss.

G. The occurrence of the major depressive episode is not better explained by schizoaffective disorder, schizophrenia, schizophreniform disorder, delusional disorder, or other specified and unspecified schizophrenia spectrum and other psychotic disorders.

H. There has never been a manic or a hypomanic episode.

I. **Note:** This exclusion does not apply to all of the manic-like or hypomanic-like episodes that are substance-induced or are attributable to the physiological effects of another medical condition.

American Psychiatric Association. (2013). *Diagnostic and statistical manual of mental disorders* (5th ed.). Washington, DC: Author.

The exact diagnostic terminology identifies this disorder as major depressive disorder. However, for the sake of flow and common use, this diagnosis will be discussed using the terms major depressive disorder, major depression (the former diagnostic label), and depression interchangeably throughout this chapter.

Depression and the Seasons

Sometimes there is a regular relationship between the seasons and depressive symptoms. Commonly known as seasonal affective disorder (SAD), the exact diagnosis used in the *DSM-5* is major depressive disorder with seasonal pattern. Typically, individuals with this variation experience depressive symptoms in the fall and winter and then gain a full remission in the spring. While not as common, a subset of people will have summer depressive episodes. People with this diagnosis experience two seasonal depressive episodes within 2 years in the absence of a nonseasonal major depressive episode during the same time period.

Symptoms of the seasonal variety of depression are similar to what you would expect with hibernation: hypersomnia, overeating, weight gain, and craving carbohydrates. This disorder is more common in women and typically begins between the ages of 18 to 30. Populations that lie farthest from the equator are most affected. Treatment is similar to that of major depressive disorder, with the addition of light boxes to mimic natural outdoor light.

Depression and Grieving

People who experience a significant loss can exhibit feelings and behaviors similar to depression. They may cry, feel hopeless about the future, have disruptions in eating and sleeping, and lose pleasure in everyday activities. They may even experience a lack of interest in caring for themselves and neglect normal hygiene. At what point does grief become pathological? This is a controversial question and one that is not easily answered.

Clinicians were once advised against diagnosing a person with depression in the first 2 months following a significant loss. This was called the **bereavement exclusion**. The rationale for the bereavement exclusion follows:

1. Normal mourning could be labeled pathological.
2. A psychiatric diagnosis could result in a lifelong label.
3. Unnecessary medications might be prescribed.

Although controversial, according to the *DSM-5*, a diagnosis of major depressive disorder can now be given in the first 2 months following death of a loved one or other loss. The reason for the change is that grief, like other stressors, can result in depression. For some people, waiting 2 months for an official diagnosis of major depression may delay treatment and adversely affect prognosis. Further research about grief may clarify diagnostic categories and prevent overdiagnosis of depression in the presence of grief.

Epidemiology

Depression is a leading cause of disability worldwide (World Health Organization [WHO], 2019). In the United States, about 17 million adults had at least one major depressive episode in 2017 (Substance Abuse and Mental Health Services Administration [SAMHSA], 2018). This number represents about 7% of all US adults. The prevalence of depression was higher among adult females (8.7%) compared to males (5.3%). Young adults (18 to 25) seem to be affected the most, with a rate of 13.1%. Having two or more races or being white results in higher rates of depression. Fig. 14.1 provides a snapshot of prevalence details.

Children and Adolescents

Because symptoms vary by age and circumstance, depression in children, until recently, has been underrecognized. We now know that even infants can display symptoms of depression. With this understanding, we are just beginning to get a realistic view of the epidemiology of depression in children. We have more information about adolescents. In 2017, about 3 million adolescents aged 12 to 17 in the United States had at least one major depressive episode (SAMHSA, 2018). This number represents about 13% of all adolescents. This prevalence rate is higher than of adults, which is especially troubling since a youth onset carries a high recurrence rate, setting the stage for lifelong periods of depression. Fig. 14.2 provides a summary of prevalence statistics in adolescents.

Older Adults

Although depression in older adults is common, it is *not* a normal result of aging. The risk of depression increases as health deteriorates. About 1% to 5% of older adults who live in the community have depression. This statistic rises to 11.5% of hospitalized older adults and 13.5% for those requiring home care (National Institute of Mental Health [NIMH], 2012). A disproportionate number of older adults with depression are likely to die by suicide.

Many older adults suffer from subsyndromal depression in which they experience many, but not all, of the symptoms of a major depressive episode. These individuals have an increased risk of eventually developing major depression. Sometimes the psychomotor and cognitive slowing of depression may resemble a neurocognitive disorder, such as Alzheimer disease. This condition

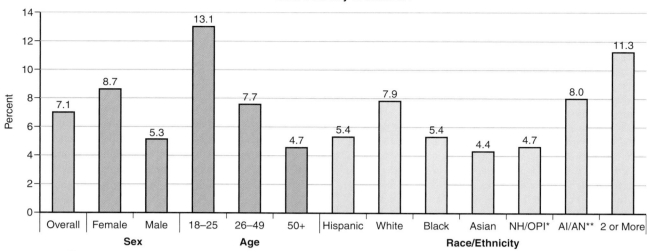

Fig. 14.1 Past year prevalence of major depressive episode among U.S. adults (2017). *Native Hawaiian/Other Pacific Islander; **American Indian/Alaskan Native. (Data from SAMHSA. [2018]. National survey on drug use and health. Retrieved from https://www.samhsa.gov/data/release/2018-national-survey-drug-use-and-health-nsduh-releases.)

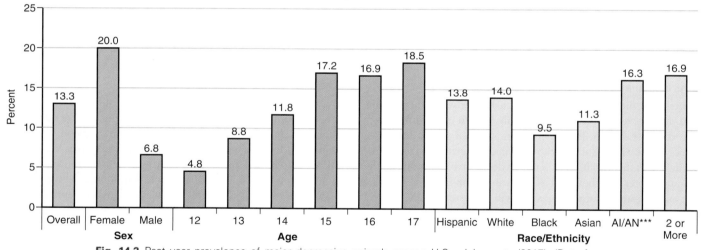

Fig. 14.2 Past year prevalence of major depressive episode among U.S. adolescents (2017). (Data from SAMHSA. [2018]. National survey on drug use and health. Retrieved from https://www.samhsa.gov/data/release/2018-national-survey-drug-use-and-health-nsduh-releases.)

is referred to as pseudodementia, a problem that can be reversed when the underlying depression is treated and eliminated.

Comorbidity

A depressive syndrome frequently accompanies other psychiatric problems such as schizophrenia, substance use, eating disorders, schizoaffective disorder, and borderline personality disorder. The combination of anxiety and depression is perhaps one of the most common psychiatric presentations. Symptoms of anxiety occur in about 70% of cases of major depressive disorder. Some clinicians believe that mixed anxiety and depression should be a stand-alone diagnosis and be treated as a distinct entity (Möller et al., 2016).

Risk Factors

Although many theories attempt to explain the cause of depression, the combination of psychological, biological, and cultural variables make identification of any one cause difficult. Furthermore, it is unlikely there is a single cause for depression. The high variability in symptom manifestation, response to treatment, and course of the illness supports the supposition that depression may result from a complex interaction of causes. For example, genetic predisposition to the illness combined with childhood stress may lead to significant changes in the central nervous system (CNS) that result in depression. However, there seem to be several common risk factors for depression, as listed in Box 14.1.

BOX 14.1 Primary Risk Factors for Depression

- Female gender
- Adverse childhood experiences
- Stressful life events
- First-degree family members with major depressive disorder
- Neuroticism (a negative personality trait characterized by anxiety, fear, moodiness, worry, envy, frustration, jealousy, and loneliness)
- Other disorders, such as substance use, anxiety, and personality disorders
- Chronic or disabling medical conditions

From American Psychiatric Association. (2013). *Diagnostic and statistical manual of mental disorders* (5th ed.). Washington, DC: Author.

Biological Factors

Genetic. Twin studies consistently show that genetic factors play a role in the development of depressive disorders. The concordance rate for major depressive disorder among monozygotic (identical) twins is nearly 50%. That is, if one twin is affected, the second has about a 50% chance of being affected as well. It is likely that multiple genes are involved, each one having a small but substantial role in the development and severity of depression. For instance, certain genetic markers seem to be related to depression when accompanied by early childhood maltreatment or a history of stressful life events. In this case, there is no gene directly related to the development of the mood disorder. There is a genetic marker associated with depression in the context of stressful life events.

EVIDENCE-BASED PRACTICE

Can Magic Mushrooms Improve Symptoms of Major Depressive Disorder?

Problem
Individuals seeking treatment for major depressive disorder may not respond to traditional antidepressant therapy. Furthermore, emotional unresponsiveness may be a long-term problem with major depression.

Purpose of Study
The purpose of this study was to determine if psilocybin, the active ingredient in magic mushrooms, would impact amygdala responses. (Note: The amygdala is one of two almond-shaped structures in the temporal lobes of the brain responsible for processing emotional responses.)

Methods
Nineteen individuals diagnosed with moderate-severe treatment-resistant depression were given two separate doses of psilocybin. Psychological support was given during and after the treatment. Functional magnetic resonance imaging (fMRI) was conducted 1 week prior to and 1 day after treatment. During the fMRI, participants were presented with neutral, happy, and angry faces.

Key Findings
- Depressive symptoms were reduced rapidly and lastingly after psilocybin.
- Increased responses to fearful and happy faces occurred in the right amygdala.
- Right amygdala increases to fearful rather than neutral faces were predictive of improvement.

- Psilocybin along with psychological support resulted in increased amygdala responses to emotional stimuli, which is opposite to previous research with SSRIs.

Implications for Nursing Practice
This study supports continuing reviews of literature and new findings. Psilocybin could end up being part of a legitimate therapeutic protocol for individuals with major depressive disorder. The FDA is supporting research on this therapy with a Breakthrough Status, meaning that clinical trials will be accelerated. Furthermore, they have increased potential participants to anyone with major depression, not just the treatment-resistant type.

Roseman, L., Demetriou, L., Wall, M. B., Nutt, D. J., & Carhart-Harris, R. L. (2018). Increased amygdala responses to emotional faces after psilocybin for treatment-resistant depression. *Neuropharmacology, 142*, 263–269.

One of the more important aspects of understanding the role of genetics in relation to mental illness such as major depression may be in pharmacological treatments. Understanding genetic influences on the role of the transport of certain neurotransmitters, such as serotonin, across synapses will make it much easier to prescribe effective medical treatment of depression based on individual genetic patterns.

Biochemical. The brain is a highly complex organ that contains billions of neurons. There is evidence to support the concept that many CNS neurotransmitter abnormalities may cause clinical depression. These neurotransmitter abnormalities may be the result of genetic or environmental factors or other medical conditions, such as cerebral infarction, Parkinson disease, hypothyroidism, acquired immunodeficiency syndrome (AIDS), or drug use.

Two of the main neurotransmitters involved in mood are serotonin (5-hydroxytryptamine [5-HT]) and norepinephrine. Serotonin is an important regulator of sleep, appetite, and libido. Therefore, serotonin-circuit dysfunction can result in sleep disturbances, decreased appetite, low sex drive, poor impulse control, and irritability. Norepinephrine modulates attention and behavior. It is stimulated by stressful situations, which may result in overuse and a deficiency of norepinephrine. A deficiency, an imbalance as compared with other neurotransmitters, or an impaired ability to use available norepinephrine can result in apathy, reduced responsiveness, or slowed psychomotor activity.

Research suggests that depression results from the dysregulation of a number of neurotransmitter systems beyond serotonin and norepinephrine. For example, glutamate is a common neurotransmitter that increases the ability of a nerve fiber to transmit information. A deficit in glutamate can interfere with normal neuron transmission in the areas of the brain that affect mood, attention, and cognition.

Stressful life events, especially losses, seem to be a significant factor in the development of depression. Norepinephrine, serotonin, and acetylcholine play a role in stress regulation. When these neurotransmitters become overtaxed through stressful events, neurotransmitter depletion may occur. In addition, research indicates that stress is associated with a reduction in neurogenesis, which is the ability of the brain to produce new brain cells.

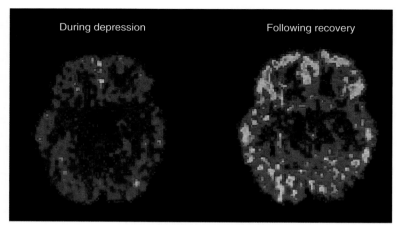

During depression   Following recovery

Fig. 14.3 Positron emission tomographic scans of a 45-year-old woman with recurrent depression. The scan on the left was taken when the patient was on no medication and very depressed. The scan on the right was taken several months later when the patient was well after she had been treated with an antidepressant. Note that her entire brain, particularly the left prefrontal cortex, is more active when she is well. (Courtesy Mark George, MD, Biological Psychiatry Branch, National Institute of Mental Health.)

No single mechanism of depressant action has been found. The relationships among the serotonin, norepinephrine, dopamine, acetylcholine, gamma-aminobutyric acid (GABA), and glutamate systems are complex and need further assessment and study. However, treatment with medication that helps regulate these neurotransmitters has proved empirically successful in the treatment of many patients. Fig. 14.3 shows a positron emission tomographic (PET) scan of the brain of a woman with depression before and after taking medication. Refer to Chapter 3 for further discussion of brain imaging and depression.

Hormonal. Neurotransmitters and hormones have the same receptors and pathways in the mood area of the brain. The most widely studied neuroendocrine area in relation to major depressive disorder has been hyperactivity of the hypothalamic-pituitary-adrenal cortical axis. People with depression have increased urine cortisol levels and elevated corticotrophin-releasing hormone.

Depression rates are almost equal for males and females in the years preceding puberty and in older adults. This has led to more research into the effect of hormones on depression in women (Ryan et al., 2012). Recent studies have found that estradiol, a form of estrogen, affects receptors sensitive to serotonin in the areas of the brain responsible for mood in rats. As the relationships between sex hormones such as estrogen in women and testosterone in males are better understood, more effective therapies may be developed.

Inflammation. Inflammation is the body's natural defense to physical injury. There is growing evidence that inflammation may be the result of psychological injury as well. Researchers have focused in on two important blood components related to inflammation, C-reactive protein and interleukin-6. In young females with a history of adversity, depression is accompanied by elevations in these blood components but not in children without a history of adversity (Miller & Cole, 2012). Adversity in life may compromise resilience and place children at risk for depression and other disorders.

While we do not believe that inflammation causes depression, research indicates that it does play a role (Krishnadas & Cavanagh, 2012). Support for this belief includes that about a third of people with major depression have elevated inflammatory biomarkers in the absence of a physical illness. Also, people who have inflammatory diseases have an increased risk of major depression. Finally, people treated with cytokines to enhance immunity during cancer treatment develop major depression at a high rate. There is some evidence to suggest that antiinflammatory agents can improve therapeutic effects of antidepressants (Köhler–Forsberg et al., 2019).

Diathesis-stress model. The diathesis-stress model of depression considers the interplay between genetic and biological predisposition toward depression and life events. The physiological vulnerabilities, such as genetic predispositions, biochemical makeup, and personality structure, are referred to as a diathesis. The stress part of this model refers to the life events that impact individual vulnerabilities. This explains why two persons exposed to relatively similar events may respond differently. One person may demonstrate resilience, and another may develop depression.

Biochemically, the diathesis-stress model of depression is believed to work this way. Psychosocial stressors and interpersonal events trigger neurophysical and neurochemical changes in the brain. Early life trauma may result in long-term hyperactivity of the CNS corticotropin-releasing factor (CRF) and norepinephrine systems with a consequent neurotoxic effect on the hippocampus, which leads to overall neuronal loss. These changes could cause sensitization of the CRF circuits to even mild stress in adulthood, leading to an exaggerated stress response (Gillespie & Nemeroff, 2005).

Cognitive Factors

Cognitive theory. In cognitive theory, the underlying assumption is that a person's thoughts will result in emotions. If a person looks at life in a positive way, the person will experience positive emotions, but negative interpretation of life events can result in sorrow, anger, and hopelessness. Cognitive theorists believe that people may acquire a psychological predisposition to depression due to early life experiences. These experiences contribute to negative, illogical, and irrational thought processes that may remain dormant until they are activated during times of stress (Beck & Rush, 1995).

Beck found that people with depression process information in negative ways and tend to ignore positive aspects of their lives. He believed that automatic, negative, repetitive, unintended, and not-readily-controllable thoughts perpetuate depression. Three assumptions constitute Beck's cognitive triad:

1. A negative, self-deprecating view of self
2. A pessimistic view of the world
3. The belief that negative reinforcement (or no validation for the self) will continue in the future

APPLICATION OF THE NURSING PROCESS

ASSESSMENT

Major depressive disorder often goes unrecognized and underdiagnosed, yet early treatment can result in improved outcomes. Nurses at both the generalist and advanced practice levels are frequently in the position to screen and assess for signs of depression, thereby facilitating early and appropriate treatment.

General Assessment

Assessment Tools

Numerous standardized depression-screening tools that help assess the type and severity of depression are available. Common screening tools are the Beck Depression Inventory, the Hamilton Depression Scale, and the Geriatric Depression Scale. The Patient Health Questionnaire-9 (PHQ-9) is a short inventory that highlights predominant symptoms seen in depression. It is presented here because of its ease of use (Fig. 14.4) in primary care and community settings. Administering these tools at baseline and then again periodically allows clinicians to follow changes in the patient's symptoms and depression severity over time.

Assessment of Suicidality

The most dangerous aspect of major depressive disorder is a preoccupation with death. A patient may fantasize about her funeral or experience recurring dreams about death. Beyond these passive fantasies are thoughts of wanting to die. As a whole, all these negativistic thoughts are referred to as suicidal ideation. These thoughts may be relatively mild and fleeting or persistent and involve a plan. Suicidal ideation, especially those in which the patient has a plan and the means to carry the plan out, represents an emergency requiring immediate intervention (refer to Chapter 25). Suicidal thoughts are a major reason for hospitalization for patients with major depression.

Patients with major depressive disorder should always be evaluated for suicidal ideation. Risk for suicide is increased when depression is accompanied by hopelessness, substance use problems, a recent loss or separation, a history of past suicide attempts, and acute suicidal ideation. The following statements and questions help set the stage for assessing suicide potential:

- "You said you are depressed. Tell me what that is like for you."
- "When you feel depressed, what sort of thoughts do you have?"
- "Have you had thoughts about ending your life?"
- "Do you have a plan?"
- "Do you have the means to carry out your plan?"
- "Is there anything that would prevent you from carrying out your plan?"

Refer to Chapter 25 for a detailed discussion of suicide, critical risk factors, warning signs, and strategies for suicide prevention. Also see the Case Study and Nursing Care Plan.

CASE STUDY AND NURSING CARE PLAN

Depression

Ms. Glessner is a 35-year-old licensed practical nurse who is brought into the emergency department by her neighbor. Ms. Glessner reports that she has been depressed for as long as she can remember, yet she has become hopeless since her boyfriend left her. She has superficial cuts on her wrists. Her affect is blunted, she has poor eye contact, and is slumped in her chair.

Ms. Glessner is 5'5" and weighs 160 pounds. Her neighbor states that Ms. Glessner often stays awake late into the night, drinking alone and watching television. She sleeps through most of the day on the weekends.

After receiving treatment in the emergency department, Ms. Glessner is seen by a psychiatrist. The initial diagnosis is persistent depressive disorder with suicidal ideation and an order is written to admit her to the stress management unit.

Carrie, a registered nurse, admits Ms. Glessner to the unit from the emergency department.

Nurse: Hello, Ms. Glessner, I'm Carrie Wolfe. I'll be your primary nurse.
Ms. Glessner: Yeah…I don't need a nurse, a doctor, or anyone else. I just want to get away from this pain.
Nurse: You want to get away from your pain?

Ms. Glessner: Look at me. I'm fat…ugly… and I'm not good enough. No one wants me.
Nurse: No one wants you?
Ms. Glessner: My husband didn't want me… last week Jerry left me to go back to his wife.
Nurse: You think because Jerry went back to his wife that no one else could care for you?
Ms. Glessner: Well…he doesn't anyway.
Nurse: Who is in your life that supports you?
Ms. Glessner: No one…except my sons…I do love my sons, even though I don't often show it.
Nurse: Tell me more about your sons.

Carrie continues to speak with Ms. Glessner. Ms. Glessner talks about her sons with some affect and apparent affection. However, she continues to state that she does not think of herself as worthwhile.

Self-Assessment

Carrie is aware that when patients have depression, they can be negative, think life is hopeless, and be hostile toward those who want to help. When Carrie was

Continued

CASE STUDY AND NURSING CARE PLAN—cont'd

new to the unit, she was uncomfortable working with patients with depression. After working with this population for 2 years, she now looks forward to the improvement that can be made in people's lives.

Assessment
Subjective Data
- A recent break-up with her boyfriend
- Stays awake late at night, drinking by herself
- Poor self-image for 3 years since divorce
- Cares about her two sons
- "I just want to get away from this pain."
- "I'm fat and ugly."
- "Not good enough."

Objective Data
- Cuts on wrist
- 5'5" and 160 pounds
- Blunted affect

- Poor eye contact
- Slumped in the chair

Priority Diagnosis
Risk for suicide due to depression, loss of a relationship, and pain as evidenced by cuts on wrists, negative self-image, and drinking alone at night.

Outcome
Patient refrains from attempting suicide.

Planning
The most important element of care is in keeping the patient physically safe. Additional measures to address the emotional and situational factors that contributed to suicidal feelings should also be addressed, along with increasing coping strategies. As always, discharge is considered and outside support is identified.

Implementation
Ms. Glessner's plan of care is personalized as follows:

Short-Term Goal	Intervention	Rationale	Evaluation
1. Patient will remain safe while in the hospital.	1a. Observe patient every 15 min while she is suicidal. 1b. Remove all dangerous objects from patient.	1a. Patient safety is ensured. 1b. Impulsive self-harmful behavior is minimized.	**GOAL MET** Ms. Glessner experienced no suicide gestures or acts during the hospitalization.
2. Patient expresses at least one reason to live, and this is apparent by the second day of hospitalization.	2a. Spend regularly scheduled periods of time with patient throughout the day.	2a. This interaction reinforces that patient is worthwhile and builds up experience to begin to relate better to nurse on one-to-one basis.	**GOAL MET** By the end of the second day, she states that her sons are a reason to live and that she would never want to hurt them.
	2b. Assist patient in evaluating both positive and negative aspects of her life.	2b. A depressed person is often unable to acknowledge any positive aspects of life unless others point them out.	
	2c. Encourage appropriate expression of angry feelings.	2c. Providing for expression of pent-up hostility in a safe environment can reinforce more adaptive methods of releasing tension and may minimize need to act out self-directed anger.	
	2d. Accept patient's negativism.	2d. Acceptance enhances feelings of self-worth.	
3. Patient will identify two outside supports she can call upon if she feels suicidal in the future.	3a. Assist patient in identifying members of her support system.	3a. Strengths and weaknesses in support available can be evaluated.	**GOAL MET** By discharge, Ms. Glessner states that she will contact her oldest son or best friend if she becomes hopeless again. She also discussed joining a women's support group that meets once a week in a neighboring town.
	3b. Suggest community-based support groups she might wish to attend.	3b. Patient needs to be aware of community supports to use them.	

Evaluation
During the course of her work with Carrie, Ms. Glessner decides to go to some meetings of Parents Without Partners. She states that she is looking forward to getting back to work and feels more hopeful about life. She has also lost 3 pounds while attending Weight Watchers. She states, "I need to get back into the world."

PATIENT HEALTH QUESTIONNAIRE-9 (PHQ-9)

Over the last 2 weeks, how often have you been bothered by any of the following problems?	Not at all	Several days	More than half the days	Nearly every day
1. Little interest or pleasure in doing things	0	1	2	3
2. Feeling down, depressed, or hopeless	0	1	2	3
3. Trouble falling or staying asleep, or sleeping too much	0	1	2	3
4. Feeling tired or having little energy	0	1	2	3
5. Poor appetite or overeating	0	1	2	3
6. Feeling bad about yourself — or that you are a failure or have let yourself or your family down	0	1	2	3
7. Trouble concentrating on things, such as reading the newspaper or watching television	0	1	2	3
8. Moving or speaking so slowly that other people could have noticed? Or the opposite — being so fidgety or restless that you have been moving around a lot more than usual	0	1	2	3
9. Thoughts that you would be better off dead or of hurting yourself in some way	0	1	2	3

_0_ + _____ + _____ + _____

=Total score: _____

If you checked off any problems, how difficult have these problems made it for you to do your work, take care of things at home, or get along with other people?

Not difficult at all ☐	Somewhat difficult ☐	Very difficult ☐	Extremely difficult ☐

I confirm this information is accurate.	Patient's/Subject's initials:	Date:

A

PHQ-9 SCORING CARD FOR SEVERITY DETERMINATION

for health care professional use only

Scoring—add up all checked boxes on PHQ-9

Total Score	Depression Severity
0-4	None
5-9	Mild
10-14	Moderate
15-19	Moderately severe
20-27	Severe

B

Fig. 14.4 (A) Patient Health Questionnaire-9 (PHQ-9). (B) Scoring the PHQ-9. (Copyright 2005 by Pfizer, Inc. Developed by Drs. Robert L. Spitzer, Janet B. Williams, Kurt Kroenke, and colleagues.)

Key Assessment Findings

A depressed mood and anhedonia (i.e., inability to feel pleasure) are the key symptoms in depression. Anxiety, a common symptom of depression, has been found to be as high as 72% of patients with major depressive disorder in primary care (Zhou et al., 2017).

They also dwell on and exaggerate their perceived faults and failures and are unable to recognize their strengths and successes. If delusions are present, they are generally congruent with negative mood, such as being punished for past crimes or being a terrible person. Feelings of worthlessness, hopelessness, guilt, anger, and helplessness are common.

Depression and chronic pain are commonly seen together in primary care. Neurotransmitters for both problems are shared, as are nerve pathways, which can interact in a vicious cycle. Then there is the two-way interaction between pain and depression. Being in constant pain creates negative thinking overall and dampens brain chemistry, resulting in depression. On the other hand, depression magnifies pain and may also create a vulnerability to other physical problems.

Areas to Assess
Appearance

Grooming, dressing, and personal hygiene may be markedly neglected. People who usually take pride in their appearance and dress may allow themselves to look shabby and unkempt. They may neglect to bathe, change clothes, or engage in other basic self-care activities. The patient may make intermittent or even no eye contact. Posture tends to be slumped or hunched with head low and shoulders forward.

Behavior

Anergia, an abnormal lack of energy, may result in psychomotor retardation, in which movements are extremely slow, facial expressions are decreased, and gaze is fixed. The continuum of psychomotor retardation may range from slowed and difficult movements to complete inactivity and incontinence. Conversely, some patients experience psychomotor agitation, manifested in pacing, nail biting, finger tapping, or engaging in some other tension-relieving activity.

Vegetative signs of depression refer to alterations in those activities necessary to support physical life and growth (e.g., eating, elimination, sleeping, and sex). Appetite changes vary in individuals experiencing depression. Appetite loss is common, and sometimes patients can lose up to 5% of their body weight in less than a month. Other patients find they eat more often and complain of weight gain.

Changes in bowel habits are common. Constipation is seen most frequently in patients with psychomotor retardation. Diarrhea occurs less frequently, often in conjunction with psychomotor agitation or anxiety.

Sleep pattern disturbance is a hallmark sign of depression. Often, people experience insomnia, wake frequently, and have a total reduction in sleep, especially deep-stage sleep. Waking at 3 or 4 a.m. and then staying awake is common, as is sleeping for short periods only. The light sleep of a person with depression tends to prolong the agony of depression over a 24-hour period.

For some, sleep is increased (hypersomnia) and provides an escape from painful feelings. In any event, sleep is rarely restful or refreshing.

Sexual interest declines (loss of libido) during depression. Some men experience impotence. A decreased or absent interest in sex occurs in both men and women, which can further complicate marital and social relationships.

Mood

Mood is a term that describes a general emotional condition or state. Asking such questions as "How do you feel?" along with observing facial cues, voice tone, and posture can help you determine this general emotional condition in your patient. Unlike feelings and emotion, which tend to change more frequently, moods can last for an extended period of time, from several hours to several days. In depressive conditions, a depressed mood is evident for weeks. General terms that we use to describe mood are simply good and bad, although those words are not particularly useful from a clinical standpoint. More specific terms used to describe mood include euthymic (normal), euphoric (overly happy), angry, irritable, anxious, and apathetic.

Feelings and Emotions

In contrast to mood, feelings and emotions are more specific and can come and go quickly. They tend to be related to, and flow from, the mood. Feelings include worthlessness, guilt, helplessness, hopelessness, and anger.

- Feelings of worthlessness range from feeling inadequate to having an unrealistically negative self-evaluation. These feelings reflect the low self-esteem that is a painful partner to depression. Statements such as "I am no good" or "I'll never amount to anything" are common.
- Guilt is a nearly universal accompaniment to depression. A person may ruminate over present or past failings: "I was never a good parent," or "It's my fault that project at work failed." These thoughts tend to occur over and over again and are difficult for the patient to stop. These negative ruminations fill in the hours of lost sleep.
- Helplessness is demonstrated by a person's inability to solve problems in response to common concerns. In severe situations, helplessness may be evidenced by the inability to carry out the simplest tasks (e.g., grooming, doing housework, working, caring for children) because they seem too difficult to accomplish.
- With feelings of helplessness come feelings of hopelessness, which are particularly correlated with suicidality. Even though most depressive episodes are time limited, people experiencing them believe things will never change. This feeling of utter hopelessness can lead people to view suicide as a way out of constant mental pain.
- In contrast to the more apathetic feelings, anger and irritability are often more active by-products of depression. Anger may be expressed verbally and physically with aggression or destruction of property. Anger may also be directed inward, resulting in suicidal or otherwise self-destructive behaviors such as substance use, overeating, and smoking. These behaviors often reinforce feelings of low self-esteem and worthlessness.

One symptom of depression is referred to as anhedonia. Anhedonia (*an* "without" + *hedone* "pleasure" = inability to feel happy) means the absence of happiness or the inability to feel pleasure in aspects of life that once made a person happy. Social anhedonia is characterized by disinterest in interaction with others resulting in isolation. Physical anhedonia is the inability to experience physical pleasure in such activities as eating, touching, or sex.

Affect

Affect is the outward representation of a person's internal state and is an objective finding based on the nurse's assessment. Feelings of hopelessness and despair are reflected in the person's affect. Affect can be described as congruent with mood, that is, sad face and depressed mood. It can also be described as incongruent with mood, such as when a person is smiling despite a depressed mood. Patients with major depressive disorder commonly exhibit the following types of affect:

- Constricted affect refers to a reduction in the range and intensity of normal of expression.
- Blunted (or shallow) affect is more severe than constricted and represents a significant decrease in emotional reactivity.
- Flat affect is no or nearly no emotional expression or reactivity.

Speech

When patients are experiencing an episode of major depressive disorder, they tend to speak slowly and softly. Other characteristics of speech include monotone and lack of spontaneity.

Thought Processes

The patient may describe their thinking as slow. Thinking can be so severely impacted that we sometimes refer to it as **poverty of thought**. Responses may be slow or absent. During a conversation, you may have to repeat questions or comments in order to prompt the patient for a response. In severe depression, a person may become mute.

Thought Content and Perceptions

In profound depression, psychotic features—delusions and/or hallucinations—may be present. They may be mood-congruent and focus on depressive themes, mood-incongruent without depressive themes, or a combination of both. An example of a depressive delusional thought is, "I am responsible for Elvis Presley's death. I worked in a factory that made pill molds. Elvis died from an overdose. I deserve to die." Hallucinations, usually auditory, might be something like hearing critical voices, "You're not good enough" or "Your family deserves better." Psychosis increases the risk for suicide, self-harm, and other-directed violence.

Insight and Judgment

During a depressive episode, a person's ability to solve problems and think clearly is negatively affected. Judgment, or the ability to make reasonable decisions, is poor. This poor judgment leads to indecisiveness, which makes it difficult to make simple decisions, such as what to wear or what to eat.

Cognitive Changes

Major depressive disorder usually results in a decreased ability to think or concentrate and indecisiveness. This set of symptoms may be the primary mediator of functional impairment (Lam et al., 2014). These changes include deficits in attention, short-term and working memory, verbal and nonverbal learning, problem solving, processing speed, and auditory and visual processing. Cognitive deficits may linger even after successful treatment for the disorder and result in continued functional impairment.

Age Considerations
Assessment in Children and Adolescents

As children grow and develop, they may display a wide range of moods and behavior, making it easy to overlook signs of depression. The core symptoms of depression in children and adolescents are the same as for adults, which are sadness and loss of pleasure. What differs is how these symptoms are displayed. For example, a very young child may cry, a school-age child might withdraw, and a teenager may become irritable in response to feeling sad or hopeless. Younger children may suddenly refuse to go to school while adolescents may engage in substance use or sexual promiscuity and be preoccupied with death or suicide.

Assessment of Older Adults

Because they are more likely to complain of physical illness than emotional concerns, depression might be overlooked. Older patients actually do have comorbid physical problems, and it is difficult to determine whether fatigue, pain, and weakness are the result of an illness or depression. The Geriatric Depression Scale is a 30-item tool that is both valid and reliable in screening for depression in the older adult (Sheikh & Yesavage, 1986). Its "yes" or "no" format makes this scale easier to administer with patients with cognitive deficits. It can be helpful in determining suicidality in this population.

Self-Assessment

Patients with depression often reject the advice, encouragement, and understanding of the nurse and others. They often seem unresponsive to nursing interventions and resistant to change. If your assignment is to have a therapeutic interaction and your patient will not talk, you may feel like a failure. When this occurs, the nurse may experience feelings of frustration, hopelessness, and annoyance. These problematic responses can be altered in the following ways:

- Recognizing unrealistic expectations for yourself or the patient
- Identifying feelings that originate with the patient
- Understanding the roles biology and genetics play in major depressive disorder

As a student, your personal feelings should be recognized, named, and examined. You can discuss feelings with peers, staff, and faculty to separate personal feelings from those originating with the patient. Ultimately, supervision or peer support can increase your therapeutic potential and self-esteem while caring for individuals with depression.

ASSESSMENT GUIDELINES

Depression

1. Always evaluate the patient's risk of harm to self or others. Overt hostility is highly correlated with suicide.
2. Major depressive disorder may be secondary to many other disorders and medications. A thorough medical and neurological examination helps determine if the depression is primary or secondary to another disorder. Evaluate whether:
   - The patient is psychotic
   - The patient has taken drugs or alcohol
   - Medical conditions are present
   - The patient has a history of a comorbid psychiatric syndrome, such as an eating disorder, borderline personality disorder, or anxiety disorder.
3. Assess the patient's history of depression, what past treatments worked and did not work, and stressors that may have contributed to this episode.
4. Assess support systems, family, significant others, and the need for information and referrals.

NURSING DIAGNOSIS

Major depressive disorder is a complex disorder, and patients have a variety of needs. A high priority for the nurse is determining the risk of suicide, and the nursing diagnosis of *risk for suicide* is always considered. Refer to Chapter 25 for assessment guidelines and interventions for individuals with suicidal thoughts or plans. Other useful diagnoses are *impaired coping, social isolation, hopelessness, powerlessness, spiritual distress, and chronic low self-esteem. Vegetative signs of depression interfere with activities of daily living making impaired ability to perform hygiene, impaired sleep, impaired low nutritional intake, constipation,* and *impaired sexual functioning* useful diagnoses.

OUTCOMES IDENTIFICATION

The recovery model emphasizes that healing is possible and attainable for individuals with psychiatric disorders, including depression. Recovery is attained through partnerships between patients and healthcare providers who focus on the patient's strengths. Treatment goals are mutually developed based on the patient's personal needs and values, and interventions are evidenced-based. The recovery model is consistent with the focus on patient-centered care and is a key component of safe quality healthcare.

Major depressive disorder can be a recurrent and chronic illness. Care should be directed not only at resolution of the acute phase but also at long-term management. The nurse and the patient identify realistic outcome criteria and formulate concrete, measurable, short-term and long-term goals.

Table 14.2 identifies signs and symptoms commonly experienced in depression, offers potential nursing diagnoses, and suggests outcomes.

TABLE 14.2   Signs and Symptoms, Nursing Diagnoses, and Outcomes for Depression

Signs and Symptoms	Nursing Diagnoses	Outcomes
Previous suicidal attempts, putting affairs in order, giving away prized possessions, suicidal ideation (has plan, ability to carry it out), overt or covert statements regarding killing self, feelings of worthlessness, hopelessness, helplessness	*Risk for suicide*	Decreased suicide risk: Expresses feelings, verbalizes suicidal ideas, refrains from suicide attempts, plans for the future
Difficulty with simple tasks, inability to function at previous level, poor problem solving, poor cognitive functioning, verbalizations of inability to cope	*Impaired coping*	Improved coping: Identifies ineffective and effective coping, uses support system, uses new coping strategies, engages in personal actions to manage stressors effectively
Dull/sad affect, no eye contact, preoccupation with own thoughts, seeks to be alone, uncommunicative, withdrawn, feels rejected and not good enough	*Social isolation*	Decreased social isolation: Attends group meetings, interacts spontaneously with others, talks with the nurse in 1:1, demonstrates interest in engaging with family and others
Feelings of helplessness, hopelessness, powerlessness	*Hopelessness* *Powerlessness*	Decreased hopelessness/powerlessness: Expresses hope for a positive future, believes that personal actions impact outcomes, demonstrates optimism and describes plans for the future
Questioning meaning of life and existence, anger toward greater power, feeling abandoned, perceived suffering	*Spiritual distress*	Decreased spiritual distress: Shares feelings of connectedness with self, others, and a higher power, identifies meaning and purpose in life
Exaggerates negative feedback about self, excessive seeking of reassurance, guilt, indecisive and nonassertive behavior, poor eye contact, shame	*Chronic low self-esteem*	Improved self-esteem: Identifies strengths, verbalizes self-acceptance, participates in groups, expresses a personal judgment of self-worth
Vegetative signs of depression: grooming and hygiene deficiencies, significantly reduced appetite, changes in sleeping, eating, elimination, sexual patterns	*Impaired ability to perform hygiene* *Impaired sleep* *Impaired low nutritional intake* *Constipation* *Impaired sexual functioning*	Improved: Increases baseline personal care each day, reports adequate sleep, eating and elimination normalize, returns to a normal level of physiologic activity

International Council of Nursing Practice. (2019). *ICNP browser.* Retrieved from https://www.icn.ch/what-we-do/projects/ehealth/icnp-browser. ICNP® is owned and copyrighted by the International Council of Nurses (ICN). Reproduced with permission of the copyright holder.

PLANNING

The planning of care for patients with depression is geared toward the patient's phase of depression, particular symptoms, and personal goals. At all times students, nurses, and members of the healthcare team assess and monitor for the potential for suicide. Assessment of risk for self-harm (or harm to others) is ongoing. A combination of therapy (cognitive, behavioral, or interpersonal) and psychopharmacology is an effective approach to the treatment of depression across all age groups. Safety is always the highest priority.

IMPLEMENTATION

There are three phases in treatment and recovery from major depression:

1. The acute phase (6 to 12 weeks) is directed at reduction of depressive symptoms and restoration of psychosocial and work function. Hospitalization may be required, and medication or other biological treatments may be initiated.
2. The continuation phase (4 to 9 months) is directed at prevention of relapse through pharmacotherapy, education, and depression-specific psychotherapy.
3. The maintenance phase (1 year or more) of treatment is directed at prevention of further episodes of depression.

Depending on the risk factors for relapse, medication may be phased out or continued.

It is important to keep in mind that both the continuation and maintenance phases are geared toward maintaining the patient as a functional and contributing member of the community after recovery from the acute phase.

Counseling and Communication Techniques

Nurses often have difficulty communicating with patients without talking. However, some patients with depression are so withdrawn that they are unwilling or unable to speak and just sitting with them in silence may seem like a waste of time or be noticeably uncomfortable. As your anxiety increases, you may start daydreaming, feel bored, and believe that you should be doing something. It is important to be aware that this time can be meaningful, especially if you have a genuine interest in learning about and supporting the patient with depression.

It is difficult to say when a withdrawn patient will be able to respond, but certain techniques are known to be useful in guiding effective nursing interventions. Some communication techniques to use with a severely withdrawn patient are listed in Table 14.3. Counseling guidelines for use with patients with depression are offered in Table 14.4.

TABLE 14.3 Guidelines for Communication With Severely Withdrawn Persons

Intervention	Rationale
When a patient is silent, use the technique of making observations: "There are many new pictures on the wall." "You are wearing your new shoes."	When a patient is not ready to talk, direct questions can raise the patient's anxiety level and frustrate the nurse. Pointing to commonalities in the environment draws the patient into and reinforces reality.
Use simple, concrete words.	Slowed thinking and difficulty concentrating impair comprehension.
Allow time for the patient to respond.	Slowed thinking necessitates time to formulate a response.
Listen for covert messages, and ask about suicide plans.	People often experience relief and decrease in feelings of isolation when they share thoughts of suicide.
Avoid platitudes such as "Things will look up" or "Everyone gets down once in a while."	Platitudes tend to minimize the patient's feelings and can increase feelings of guilt and worthlessness because the patient cannot "look up" or "snap out of it."

TABLE 14.4 Guidelines for Counseling People With Depression

Intervention	Rationale
Help the patient question underlying assumptions and beliefs and consider alternate explanations to problems.	Reconstructing a healthier and more hopeful attitude about the future can alter depressed mood.
Work with the patient to identify cognitive distortions that result in a negative self-perception. For example:	Cognitive distortions reinforce a negative inaccurate perception of self and world.
1. Overgeneralizations	1. Taking one fact or event and making a general rule out of it ("He always..."; "I never...").
2. Self-blame	2. Consistently blaming self.
3. Mind reading	3. Despite a lack of evidence, assumes that others don't like him or her.
4. Discounting of positive attributes	4. Focusing on the negative.
Help the patient identify current coping skills and explore alternate coping skills.	Many depressed people use ineffective coping skills. Exploring and adopting alternate effective coping skills will improve the patient's outlook.
Encourage exercise, such as running and/or weightlifting.	Exercise can improve self-concept and improve the brain's neurochemistry.
Encourage formation of supportive relationships, such as individual therapy, support groups, and peer support.	Such relationships reduce social isolation and enable the patient to work on personal goals and relationship needs.
Provide information referrals, when needed, for religious or spiritual support (e.g., pastoral visits, readings, programs, tapes, community resources).	Spiritual and existential issues may be heightened during depressive episodes; many people find strength, support, and comfort in spirituality or religion.

Depressive Symptoms and Medical Errors in Physicians

Medical errors are a serious public health problem. They are a preventable source of needless suffering and even death. In a recent meta-analysis, researchers reviewed 11 studies, resulting in a combined sample size of more than 21,500. They found that physicians who screen positively for depression are at greater risk of committing errors. In addition, they found that physicians who made errors were also more likely to have depressive symptoms three months after the event.

Compounding this problem is the reluctance for physicians to seek treatment for major depressive disorder. One barrier to help seeking is fear of disclosure due to perceived personal, societal, and organizational stigma. Until quite recently, many state medical boards required applicants to report any psychiatric treatment. This practice resulted in people hiding conditions and also avoiding mental healthcare.

The authors call for organizational interventions aimed at reducing physicians' depressive symptoms. They also highlighted the need for institutional policies to remove barriers to delivering evidence-based treatments to physicians with depression.

Adapted from Pereira-Lima, K., Mata, D. A., Loureiro, S. R., Crippa, J. A., Bolsoni, L. M., & Sen, S. (2019). Association between physician depressive symptoms and medical errors: A systematic review and meta-analysis. *JAMA Network Open, 2*(11), e1916097.

Health Teaching and Health Promotion

A basic premise of the recovery model of mental illness is that individuals exercise personal control of treatment based on individual goals. Within this model, health teaching is paramount because it allows patients to make informed choices. Health teaching points include:

- Depression is an illness beyond a person's voluntary control.
- Although it is beyond voluntary control, depression can be managed through medication and lifestyle.
- Chronic illness management depends in large part on understanding personal signs and symptoms of relapse.
- Illness management depends on understanding the role of medication and possible medication side effects.
- Long-term management works best if the patient receives psychotherapy along with medication.
- Identifying and coping with the stress of interpersonal relationships—whether they are familial, social, or occupational—are key to stable illness management.

Including the family in discharge planning is also important. It helps the patient by:

- Increasing the family's understanding and acceptance of the family member with depression during the aftercare period
- Increasing the patient's use of aftercare facilities in the community
- Contributing to higher overall adjustment in the patient after discharge

Promotion of Self-Care Activities

Nursing measures for improving physical well-being and promoting adequate self-care are essential. Some effective interventions targeting physical needs in depression are listed in Table 14.5. Nurses in the community can work with family members to encourage a family member with depression to perform and maintain self-care activities.

Teamwork and Safety

Safe quality inpatient care requires the skills of a well-coordinated team. Treating a patient with depression requires the skills of nurses and prescribers. Other members of the team include mental health technicians, pharmacists, dietitians, social workers, and the patient's significant others.

Safety becomes the most important issue facing a team that cares for people with depression who may be at high risk for suicide. Suicide precautions are usually instituted and include the removal of all harmful objects such as "sharps" (e.g., razors, scissors, and nail files), strangulation risks (e.g., belts), and medication that can be used to overdose. Some patients with severe depression may need to have someone check on them frequently, perhaps every 15 minutes, or even have 1:1 observation. A full discussion of inpatient safety measures is provided in Chapter 4.

EVALUATION

Because each patient presents differently, outcome evaluation will be tailored to each patient's unique presentation. Based on your evaluation, modification of nursing diagnoses, goals, and interventions is made.

When suicidal ideation is present, the following questions should be addressed: Are these thoughts still present? How frequently do they occur? Does the patient have a plan? Is the patient able to stop suicidal thoughts and formulate alternatives to suicidal thoughts? If the depression is severe and the patient has demonstrated psychotic features, the nurse will ask about auditory hallucinations and evaluate for signs of delusions.

Basic self-care issues should be addressed. Is the patient taking in a sufficient number of calories and liquids? In an inpatient setting, the nurse will also evaluate the patient's sleep pattern. Is the patient able to fall asleep? Stay asleep? Has the number of hours of sleep increased since admission? What about personal hygiene and grooming?

Thought processes, self-esteem, and social interactions are evaluated because these areas are often problematic in people with depression. The nurse should assess self-esteem. How do you feel about yourself now as compared with when you were admitted? The nurse will evaluate negativity and if the patient is able to identify positive aspects of individual functioning.

TREATMENT MODALITIES

Biological Treatments

Pharmacotherapy

At the cellular level, mood disorders are caused by problems with neurotransmitters. It follows that medications that alter brain chemistry are an important component in their treatment. Antidepressant therapy is an effective strategy for most cases of major depressive disorder, particularly in severe cases. A combination of psychotherapies and antidepressant therapy is superior to either psychotherapy or psychopharmacological treatment alone (Institute for Clinical Systems Improvement, 2016).

▶ Neurobiology of Depression and the Effects of Antidepressants

Imbalance of neurotransmitters (serotonin and norepinephrine) contribute to depression in certain parts of the brain.

Prefrontal cortex regulates role in executive functions and emotional control and memory.

Limbic system regulates activities such as emotions, physical and sexual drives, and the stress response, as well as processing, learning, and memory (amygdala, hypothalamus, hippocampus).

Anterior cingulate cortex regulates heart rate and blood pressure. Other functions include decision making, emotional regulation, error detection, preparation for tasks, and executive functions.

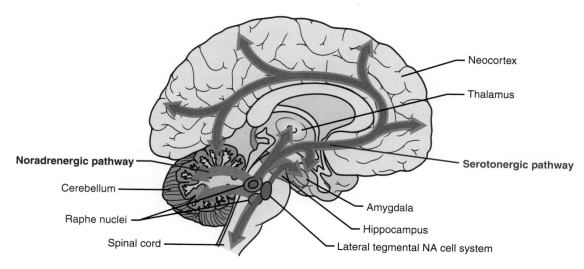

Noradrenergic pathway
The axons of these neurons project upward through the forebrain to the cerebral cortex, the limbic system, the thalamus, and the hippocampus.

Norepinephrine (NE) and the Noradrenergic System
Play a major role in mood and emotional behavior as well as energy, drive, anxiety, focus, and metabolism.

Serotonergic pathway
The axons of serotonergic neurons originate in the raphe nuclei of the brainstem and project to the cerebral cortex, the limbic system, cerebellum, and spinal cord.

Serotonin (5-HT) and the Serotonergic System
are involved in the regulation of pain, depression, pleasure, anxiety, panic arousal, sleep cycle, carbohydrate craving, and premenstrual syndrome.

Pharmacotherapy for Depression
Medications for depression include the selective serotonin reuptake inhibitors (**SSRIs**), serotonin norepinephrine reuptake inhibitors (**SNRIs**), serotonin antagonists and reuptake inhibitors (**SARIs**), norepinephrine dopamine reuptake inhibitor (**NDRI**), noradrenergic and specific serotonergic antidepressants (**NaSSAs**), tricyclic antidepressants (**TCAs**), and monoamine oxidase inhibitors (**MAOIs**).

All medications have similar efficacy. They are chosen by their safety profile and side effects. All have a delayed response, a discontinuation syndrome, and a Black Box Warning for suicidal thoughts and behaviors.

Patient's Problem	Example of Drug	Side-Effect Profile
Fatigue	Fluoxetine (SSRI)	Stimulates the CNS
Insomnia	Mirtazapine (NaSSA)	Substantial sedation
Sexual dysfunction	Bupropion (NDRI)	Enhances libido
Chronic pain	TCAs or duloxetine (SNRI)	Relieves pain

Antidepressants. Antidepressants can positively impact poor self-concept, social withdrawal, vegetative signs of depression, and activity level. Target symptoms include the following:
- Sleep disturbance (decreased or increased)
- Appetite disturbance (decreased or increased)
- Fatigue

- Decreased sex drive
- Psychomotor retardation or agitation
- Diurnal (i.e., daily cycle) variations in mood (often worse in the morning)
- Impaired concentration or forgetfulness
- Anhedonism

TABLE 14.5   Interventions Targeting the Vegetative Signs of Depression

Intervention	Rationale
Nutrition (Anorexia)	
Offer small, high-calorie, and high-protein snacks frequently throughout the day and evening.	Low weight and poor nutrition render the patient susceptible to illness. Small, frequent snacks are more easily tolerated than large plates of food when the patient is anorexic.
Offer high-protein and high-calorie fluids frequently throughout the day and evening.	These fluids prevent dehydration and can minimize constipation.
When possible, encourage family or friends to join the patient during meals.	Eating is a social event. This strategy reinforces the idea that someone cares, can raise the patient's self-esteem, and can serve as an incentive to eat.
Include the patient in choosing foods and drinks. Involve a dietitian if necessary.	The patient is more likely to eat the foods provided.
Weigh the patient weekly and observe the patient's eating patterns.	Monitoring the patient's status gives the information needed for revision of the intervention.
Sleep (Insomnia)	
Provide periods of rest after activities.	Fatigue can intensify feelings of depression.
Encourage the patient to get up and dress and to stay out of bed during the day.	Minimizing sleep during the day increases the likelihood of sleep at night and the establishment of healthy routines.
Encourage the use of relaxation measures in the evening (e.g., a warm bath, warm milk, soothing music or sounds).	These measures induce relaxation and sleep.
Provide decaffeinated coffee and soda.	Decreasing caffeine increases the possibility of sleep.
Self-Care Deficits	
Encourage the use of toothbrush, washcloth, soap, makeup, and shaving supplies.	Being clean and well groomed can improve self-esteem.
When appropriate, give step-by-step reminders, such as, "Wash the right side of your face, now the left."	Slowed thinking and difficulty concentrating make organizing simple tasks difficult.
Elimination (Constipation)	
Monitor intake and output, especially bowel movements.	Many depressed patients are constipated. If the condition is not addressed, fecal impaction can occur.
Offer foods high in fiber and provide periods of exercise.	Roughage and exercise stimulate peristalsis.
Encourage the intake of fluids.	Fluids help prevent constipation.
Evaluate the need for laxatives and enemas.	These measures prevent constipation.

A drawback of antidepressant drugs is that improvement in mood may take 1 to 3 weeks or longer. If a patient is acutely suicidal, electroconvulsive therapy (ECT) (discussed in detail later in this chapter) may be a reliable and effective alternative.

The goal of antidepressant therapy is the complete remission of symptoms. Often, the first antidepressant prescribed is not the one that will ultimately bring about remission. Aggressive treatment helps in finding the proper treatment. An adequate trial for the treatment of depression is 3 months. Individuals experiencing their first depressive episode are maintained on antidepressants for 6 to 9 months after symptoms of depression remit. Some people may have multiple episodes of depression or may have a chronic form and benefit from indefinite antidepressant therapy. Genetic testing holds some promise in individualizing antidepressant therapy (Box 14.2).

Antidepressants may precipitate a psychotic episode in a person with schizophrenia or a manic episode in a patient with bipolar disorder. Patients with bipolar disorder often receive a mood-stabilizing drug along with an antidepressant.

Antidepressants have demonstrated similar efficacy in pharmaceutical trials. Each of the antidepressants has different adverse effects, costs, safety issues, and maintenance

considerations. Selection of the appropriate antidepressant is based on the following considerations:

- Symptom profile of the patient
- Side-effect profile (e.g., sexual dysfunction, weight gain)
- Ease of administration
- History of past response
- Safety and medical considerations
- Genotyping (when available)

Table 14.6 provides an overview of antidepressants used in the United States.

Selective serotonin reuptake inhibitors. The SSRIs selectively block the neuronal uptake of serotonin (e.g., 5-HT, 5-HT_1 receptors). This blockage increases the availability of serotonin in the synaptic cleft. Refer to Chapter 3 for a more detailed discussion of how the SSRIs work.

SSRI antidepressant drugs have a relatively low side-effect profile compared with the older antidepressants (tricyclics—discussed later in this chapter). They do not create anticholinergic effects, dry mouth, blurred vision, or urinary retention, making it easier for patients to take these medications as prescribed. The SSRIs are effective in depression with anxiety features and depression with psychomotor agitation.

BOX 14.2 Genetic Testing for More Precise Antidepressant Selection?

Anyone who has ever been given or prescribed medication for depression can tell you that choosing the best drug is somewhat hit or miss. Some medications work, some do not. Some medications cause intolerable side effects. Why?

Of all the clinical factors that can alter a person's response to drugs—age, sex, weight, general health, and liver function—genetic factors account for about 42% of the variation (Perlis, 2014). One aspect of genetics is the way we metabolize medications. The way you metabolize is largely based on a genetic variation in the cytochrome P450 (CYP450) enzymes.

Genotyping tests can help to identify medications that are more likely to be processed. They identify four types of metabolizers:

- Poor—A missing enzyme causes slow metabolism that may result in a buildup of medication and significant side effects, such as serotonin syndrome. People in this category should avoid antidepressants.
- Intermediate—Reduced enzyme function in processing drugs causes a slower metabolism of drugs. Antidepressants will likely cause side effects and toxicity is a risk. Some depressive symptom relief can be expected, but not substantially.
- Extensive—People in this category have an expected range for metabolism. Medications will be effective and there will be few side effects.
- Ultrarapid—Medication is processed too quickly, before it has a chance to work. Antidepressants will either not work or will have to be used at higher doses.

The specific CYP450 enzyme with the most variation is CYP2D6. This enzyme processes common antidepressants, including fluoxetine (Prozac), paroxetine (Paxil, Pexeva), and venlafaxine (Effexor). The CYP2C19 enzyme is involved with metabolizing citalopram (Celexa) and escitalopram (Lexapro).

Despite the fact that several companies market this service, the jury is still out on whether clinicians should routinely use this testing in selecting medications. Large-scale studies are needed to clarify the usefulness of such tests.

From Perlis, R. H. (2014). Pharmacogenomic testing and personalized treatment of depression. *Clinical Chemistry, 60*(1), 53–59.

Indications. SSRIs are frequently the first-line treatment in depression. In addition to their use in treating depressive disorders, the SSRIs have been prescribed with success to treat some of the anxiety disorders—in particular, obsessive-compulsive disorder and panic disorder. Fluoxetine has been found to be effective in treating some women who suffer from premenstrual dysphoric disorder and bulimia nervosa. Paroxetine (Brisdelle) has FDA approval for treating vasomotor symptoms (hot flashes) of menopause.

Common adverse reactions. Agents that selectively enhance synaptic serotonin within the CNS may induce agitation, anxiety, sleep disturbance, tremor, sexual dysfunction (primarily anorgasmia), or tension headache. Autonomic reactions (e.g., dry mouth, sweating, weight change, mild nausea, and loose bowel movements) may also be experienced with the SSRIs.

Potential toxic effects. One rare and life-threatening event associated with SSRIs is serotonin syndrome. This syndrome is thought to be related to overactivation of the central serotonin receptors caused by either too high a dose or interaction with other drugs. The symptoms are many: abdominal pain, diarrhea, sweating, fever, tachycardia, elevated blood pressure, altered mental state (delirium), myoclonus (muscle spasms), increased motor activity, irritability, hostility, and mood change. Severe manifestations can induce hyperpyrexia (excessively high fever), cardiovascular shock, or death.

The risk of this syndrome seems to be greatest when an SSRI is administered in combination with a second serotonin-enhancing agent, such as a monoamine oxidase inhibitor (MAOI). A patient should discontinue all SSRIs for 2 to 5 weeks before starting an MAOI. Box 14.3 lists the signs of serotonin syndrome and gives emergency treatment guidelines. Box 14.4 is a useful tool for patient and family teaching about the SSRIs.

Serotonin norepinephrine reuptake inhibitors. The serotonin norepinephrine reuptake inhibitors (SNRIs) inhibit the reuptake of both serotonin and norepinephrine. Pharmacological side effects are similar to the SSRIs, although the SSRIs may be tolerated better. A few of the SNRIs—venlafaxine (Effexor), desvenlafaxine (Khedezla, Pristiq), and levomilnacipran (Fetzima)—may increase blood pressure.

Other newer antidepressants. Several other classifications of antidepressants have been introduced and have provided people with depression and prescribers with more options. The name of the classification describes the action of the antidepressants. They are the serotonin antagonists and reuptake inhibitors (SARIs), a norepinephrine dopamine reuptake inhibitor (NDRI), and a noradrenergic and specific serotonergic antidepressant (NaSSA). Chapter 3 provides more detail about these drug classifications.

Two other drugs have recently been approved for major depressive disorder that are not like any of the others previously discussed. They are esketamine and brexanolone.

Esketamine, an *N*-methyl-D-aspartate (NMDA) receptor antagonist, has FDA approval for treatment-resistant depression. It is also used off-label for acute suicidality (Witt et al., 2019). Unlike other antidepressants that affect serotonin, norepinephrine, or dopamine, esketamine affects glutamate by blocking it from binding to NMDA receptors. Esketamine is available as a nasal spray, Spravato, and is used along with an oral antidepressant.

Esketamine, formerly known as ketamine, is a Schedule III drug with some potential for abuse. It is a derivative of phencyclidine (PCP), which was developed as an anesthetic agent in the 1960s. Still used in some human surgical procedures, it is the most widely used anesthetic in veterinary medicine. Ketamine gained popularity as a club drug ("K" or "special K") in the 1980s and has been used as a date-rape drug. Due to risk of abuse or misuse, Spravato dispensing is limited to certified healthcare programs.

Patients should not eat 2 hours and should not drink 30 minutes prior to treatment due to the potential for nausea and vomiting. Elevated blood pressure is a side effect of treatment and blood pressure should be assessed prior to administration. Dissociation, that is, feeling disconnected from thoughts and surroundings, is another common side effect. Other side effects include dizziness, sedation, vertigo, numbness, anxiety, and feeling drunk. Some patients will have urological effects, such as, urgency or dysuria.

Monitoring for at least 2 hours after administration protects patients who are experiencing side effects, particularly increased blood pressure. They should not engage in potentially

TABLE 14.6   FDA-Approved Drugs for Major Depressive Disorder

Generic (Trade)	Action	Notes	Side Effects	Warnings
Selective Serotonin Reuptake Inhibitors (SSRIs)				
Citalopram (Celexa) Escitalopram (Lexapro) Fluoxetine (Prozac, Prozac Weekly) Paroxetine (Paxil, Paxil CR, Pexeva) Sertraline (Zoloft)	Block the synaptic reuptake of serotonin	First line of treatment for major depression Some SSRIs activate and others sedate; choice depends on patient symptoms Risk of lethal overdose minimized with SSRIs	Agitation, insomnia, headache, nausea and vomiting, sexual dysfunction, and hyponatremia	Discontinuation syndrome with dizziness, insomnia, nervousness, irritability, nausea, and agitation may occur with abrupt withdrawal (depending on half-life); taper slowly
Serotonin Norepinephrine Reuptake Inhibitors (SNRIs)				
Desvenlafaxine (Pristiq, Khedezla)	Blocks the synaptic reuptake of serotonin and norepinephrine	A metabolite of venlafaxine	Nausea, headache, dizziness, insomnia, diarrhea, dry mouth, sweating, constipation	Neonates with in utero exposure have required respiratory support and tube feeding
Duloxetine (Cymbalta)	Blocks the synaptic reuptake of serotonin and norepinephrine	FDA approved for use in generalized anxiety disorder	Nausea, dry mouth, insomnia, somnolence, constipation, reduced appetite, fatigue, sweating, blurred vision	May reduce pain associated with depression FDA approved for fibromyalgia, diabetic peripheral neuropathic pain, and chronic musculoskeletal pain
Levomilnacipran (Fetzima)	Blocks the synaptic reuptake of serotonin and norepinephrine	Unlike other SNRIs, inhibits reuptake of norepinephrine more than serotonin	Nausea, orthostatic hypotension, constipation, sweating, increased heart rate, palpitations, difficulty urinating, decreased appetite, sexual dysfunction	May increase the effects of anticoagulants
Venlafaxine (Effexor, Effexor XR)	Blocks the synaptic reuptake of serotonin and norepinephrine	Effexor is a popular next-step strategy after trying SSRIs	Hypertension, nausea, insomnia, dry mouth, sedation, sweating, agitation, headache, sexual dysfunction	Monitor blood pressure, especially at higher doses and with a history of hypertension Discontinuation syndrome with dizziness, insomnia, nervousness, irritability, nausea, and agitation may occur with abrupt withdrawal (depending on half-life); taper slowly
Serotonin Antagonists and Reuptake Inhibitors (SARIs)				
Nefazodone (generic only)	Blocks reuptake of serotonin	Lower risk of long-term weight gain than SSRIs or TCAs Lower risk of sexual side effects than SSRIs	Sedation, hepatotoxicity, dizziness, hypotension, paresthesias	Life-threatening liver failure is possible but rare; priapism of penis and clitoris is a rare but serious side effect
Trazodone (generic only) Trazodone ER	Moderate blockade of 5-HT synaptic reuptake	Significant sedative effect. Help with antidepressant-induced insomnia	Severe sedation, hypotension, nausea	Priapism has been reported
Vilazodone (Viibryd)	Blocks reuptake of serotonin and serotonergic ($5\text{-}HT_{1A}$) receptor partial agonist activity	Take this medication with food to reduce GI disturbances	Diarrhea, nausea, vomiting, dry mouth, dizziness, insomnia	Palpitations, ventricular premature beats, serotonin syndrome
Vortioxetine (Trintellix)	Blocks reuptake of serotonin	May improve memory and cognition	Constipation, nausea, vomiting	Hyponatremia, rare induction of manic states, serotonin syndrome
Norepinephrine Dopamine Reuptake Inhibitor (NDRI)				
Bupropion (Wellbutrin, Aplenzin, Forfivo XL, Zyban for smoking cessation)	Blocks the synaptic reuptake of norepinephrine and dopamine	Stimulant action may reduce appetite May increase sexual desire Used as an aid to quit smoking	Agitation, insomnia, headache, nausea and vomiting, seizures (0.4%)	High doses increase seizure risk, especially in people who are predisposed to them

TABLE 14.6 FDA-Approved Drugs for Major Depressive Disorder—cont'd

Generic (Trade)	Action	Notes	Side Effects	Warnings
Noradrenergic and Specific Serotonergic Antidepressant (NaSSA)				
Mirtazapine (Remeron)	Enhances the release of norepinephrine and serotonin by blocking α2-adrenergic receptors that normally inhibit norepinephrine and serotonin	Antidepressant effects equal SSRIs and may occur faster	Weight gain/appetite stimulation, sedation, dizziness, headache; sexual dysfunction is rare	Drug-induced somnolence exaggerated by alcohol, benzodiazepines, and other CNS depressants
Tricyclic Antidepressants (TCAs)				
Amitriptyline (generic only) Amoxapine (generic only) Desipramine (Norpramin) Doxepin (Sinequan) Imipramine (Tofranil) Maprotiline (generic only) Nortriptyline (Aventyl, Pamelor) Protriptyline (Vivactil) Trimipramine (Surmontil)	Inhibit the synaptic reuptake of serotonin and norepinephrine. Antagonize adrenergic, histaminergic, muscarinic receptors Amoxapine antagonizes dopamine receptors	Therapeutic effects similar to SSRIs, but side effects are more prominent May work better in melancholic depression and in people with comorbid medical conditions Some therapeutic serum levels may be monitored	Dry mouth, constipation, urinary retention, blurred vision, hypotension, cardiac toxicity, sedation	Lethal in overdose; use cautiously in older adults with cardiac disorders, elevated intraocular pressure, urinary retention, hyperthyroidism, seizure disorders, and liver or kidney dysfunction
Monoamine Oxidase Inhibitors (MAOIs)				
Isocarboxazid (Marplan) Phenelzine (Nardil) Selegiline (Emsam Transdermal System Patch) Tranylcypromine (Parnate)	Inhibits the enzyme monoamine oxidase, which normally breaks down neurotransmitters, including serotonin and norepinephrine	Efficacy similar to other antidepressants, but strict dietary (tyramine) restrictions and potential drug interactions make this drug class less desirable	Insomnia, nausea, agitation, and confusion; hypertensive crisis	Contraindicated in people taking SSRIs, used cautiously in people taking TCAs; tyramine-rich food could bring about a hypertensive crisis Many other strong drug and dietary interactions

US Food and Drug Administration. (2016). FDA online label repository. Retrieved from http://labels.fda.gov/; Burchum, J. R., & Rosenthal, L. D. (2016). *Lehne's pharmacology for nursing care* (9th ed.). St. Louis, MO: Elsevier.

BOX 14.3 Serotonin Syndrome: Signs and Interventions

Symptoms
- Hyperactivity or restlessness
- Tachycardia → cardiovascular shock
- Fever → hyperpyrexia
- Elevated blood pressure
- Altered mental states (delirium)
- Irrationality, mood swings, hostility
- Seizures → status epilepticus
- Myoclonus, incoordination, tonic rigidity
- Abdominal pain, diarrhea, bloating
- Apnea → death

Interventions
- Remove offending agent(s)
- Initiate symptomatic treatment
- Serotonin-receptor blockade with cyproheptadine, methysergide, propranolol
- Cooling blankets, chlorpromazine for hyperthermia
- Dantrolene, diazepam for muscle rigidity or rigors
- Anticonvulsants
- Artificial ventilation
- Induction of paralysis

hazardous activities such as driving until the next day after a full night of sleep.

Esketamine is initially dosed twice weekly for 4 weeks and tapered to once a week for 4 weeks. Week 9 and after dosing should be once every week or two. The least frequent dosing to maintain remission should be used.

Brexanolone (Zulresso) is the first and only FDA-approved medication specifically for postpartum depression. It is a neuroactive steroid and is thought to produce its effects by influencing GABA-A receptors. Brexanolone is a Schedule IV controlled substance with some abuse potential. It is only available to patients through a restricted distribution program.

Brexanolone is administered over a 60-hour (2.5 days) IV infusion. This one-time infusion offers the potential for rapid resolution of depressive symptoms of postpartum depression.

Hypoxia may occur and patients should be monitored through continuous pulse oximetry during treatment. Because of the potential for excessive sedation and sudden loss of consciousness, patients should be continuously monitored, especially during interactions with their child(ren). Other side effects include dry mouth, flushing, and hot flashes.

Tricyclic antidepressants. The tricyclic antidepressants (TCAs) inhibit the reuptake of norepinephrine and serotonin

BOX 14.4 Patient and Family Teaching: Selective Serotonin Reuptake Inhibitors

- May cause sexual dysfunction or lack of sex drive. Inform nurse or primary care provider if this occurs.
- May cause insomnia, anxiety, and nervousness. Inform nurse or primary care provider if this occurs.
- May interact with other medications. Tell primary care provider about other medications patient is taking (e.g., digoxin, warfarin). Selective serotonin reuptake inhibitors (SSRIs) should not be taken within 14 days of the last dose of a monoamine oxidase inhibitor.
- No over-the-counter drug should be taken without first notifying primary care provider.
- Common side effects include fatigue, nausea, diarrhea, dry mouth, dizziness, tremor, and sexual dysfunction or lack of sex drive.
- Because of the potential for drowsiness and dizziness, patient should not drive or operate machinery until these side effects are ruled out.
- Alcohol should be avoided.
- Liver and renal function tests should be performed and blood counts checked periodically.
- Medication should not be discontinued abruptly. If side effects become bothersome, patient should ask primary care provider about changing to a different drug. Abrupt cessation can lead to serotonin withdrawal.

Any of the following symptoms should be reported to the primary care provider immediately:
- Increase in depression or suicidal thoughts
- Rash or hives
- Rapid heartbeat
- Sore throat
- Difficulty urinating
- Fever, malaise
- Anorexia and weight loss
- Unusual bleeding
- Initiation of hyperactive behavior
- Severe headache

by the presynaptic neurons in the CNS. TCAs are viewed as second-line treatments for depression due to their adverse effects.

Common adverse reactions. Many of the side effects of TCAs are due to their secondary pharmacological actions. See Chapter 3 for more discussion of these actions. The sedative effects of the TCAs are attributed to the blockade of histamine receptors. Anticholinergic side effects include dry mouth, blurred vision, tachycardia, constipation, urinary retention, and esophageal reflux. They usually are not serious and are often transitory, but urinary retention and severe constipation require medical attention. Weight gain is also a common complaint among people taking TCAs.

Administering the total daily dose of TCA at night is beneficial for two reasons. First, most TCAs have sedative effects and thereby aid sleep. Second, the minor side effects occur while the individual is sleeping, which increases compliance with drug therapy.

Toxicity/overdose. TCA overdose carries a risk of death from cardiac conduction abnormalities: dysrhythmias, tachycardia, myocardial infarction, and heart block. Initial symptoms are CNS stimulation, including hyperpyrexia, delirium, hypertension, hallucinations, seizure, hyperreflexia,

and parkinsonian symptoms. This phase is followed by CNS depression. Immediate medical care is essential with TCA overdose. The TCAs should be used cautiously in suicidal patients since they are lethal in overdoses.

Contraindications. People who have recently had a myocardial infarction (or other cardiovascular problems), those with narrow-angle glaucoma or a history of seizures, and women who are pregnant should not be treated with TCAs except with extreme caution and careful monitoring.

Monoamine oxidase inhibitors. The enzyme monoamine oxidase is responsible for inactivating, or breaking down, monoamine neurotransmitters in the brain such as norepinephrine, serotonin, dopamine, and tyramine. When a person takes an MAOI, fewer amines get inactivated, resulting in an increase in the mood-elevating neurotransmitters.

Indications. MAOIs are considered third-line antidepressants due to their significant drug interactions and dietary restrictions. MAOIs with FDA approval are phenelzine (Nardil), tranylcypromine (Parnate), and isocarboxazid (Marplan). A transdermal patch, selegiline (Emsam), does not require strict dietary restrictions when used at its lowest dose.

Common adverse reactions. Some common and troublesome long-term side effects of the MAOIs are orthostatic hypotension, weight gain, edema, change in cardiac rate and rhythm, constipation, urinary hesitancy, sexual dysfunction, vertigo, overactivity, muscle twitching, hypomanic and manic behavior, insomnia, weakness, and fatigue.

Potential toxic effects. Inhibiting MAOI results in the inability to break down tyramine sufficiently. People who take MAOIs and eat tyramine-rich foods are at risk for a hypertensive crisis. This crisis results in severe hypertension that can lead to such events as a cerebrovascular accident, intracranial hemorrhage, and death. Blood pressure should be monitored during treatment with these drugs. Also, a reduction or elimination of foods and drugs that contain high amounts of tyramine needs to happen (Table 14.7 and Box 14.5).

The hypertensive crisis usually occurs within 15 to 90 minutes of ingestion of the offending substance. Early symptoms include irritability, anxiety, flushing, sweating, and a severe headache. The patient then becomes anxious, restless, and develops a fever. Eventually the fever becomes severe, seizures ensue, and coma or death is possible.

When a hypertensive crisis is suspected, immediate medical attention is crucial. If ingestion is recent, gastric lavage and charcoal may be helpful. Pyrexia is treated with hypothermic blankets or ice packs. Fluid therapy is essential, particularly with hyperthermia. A short-acting antihypertensive agent such as nitroprusside, nitroglycerine, or phentolamine may be used. Intravenous benzodiazepines are useful for agitation and seizure control.

Table 14.8 identifies common side effects and toxic effects of the MAOIs, and Box 14.6 can be used as an MAOI teaching guide for patients and their families.

Contraindications. The use of MAOIs may be contraindicated with each of the following:
- Cerebrovascular disease
- Hypertension and congestive heart failure

TABLE 14.7 Foods That Can Interact With Monoamine Oxidase Inhibitors

FOODS THAT CONTAIN TYRAMINE

Category	Unsafe Foods (High Tyramine Content)	Safe Foods (Little or No Tyramine)
Vegetables	Avocados, especially if overripe; fermented bean curd; fermented soybean; soybean paste	Most vegetables
Fruits	Figs, especially if overripe; bananas, in large amounts	Most fruits
Meats	Meats that are fermented, smoked, or otherwise aged; spoiled meats; liver, unless very fresh	Meats that are known to be fresh (exercise caution in restaurants; meats may not be fresh)
Sausages	Fermented varieties; bologna, pepperoni, salami, others	Nonfermented varieties
Fish	Dried or cured fish; fish that is fermented, smoked, or otherwise aged; spoiled fish	Fish that is known to be fresh; vacuum-packed fish, if eaten promptly or refrigerated only briefly after opening
Milk, milk products	Practically all cheeses	Milk, yogurt, cottage cheese, cream cheese
Foods with yeast	Yeast extract (e.g., Marmite, Bovril)	Baked goods that contain yeast
Beer, wine	Some imported beers, Chianti wines	Major domestic brands of beer; most wines
Other foods	Protein dietary supplements; soups (may contain protein extract); shrimp paste; soy sauce	

FOODS THAT CONTAIN OTHER NONTYRAMINE VASOPRESSORS

Food	Comments
Chocolate	Contains phenylethylamine, a pressor agent; large amounts can cause a reaction.
Fava beans	Contain dopamine, a pressor agent; reactions are most likely with overripe beans.
Ginseng	Headache, tremulousness, and mania-like reactions have occurred.
Caffeinated beverages	Caffeine is a weak pressor agent; large amounts may cause a reaction.

From Burchum, J. R., & Rosenthal, L. D. (2016). *Lehne's pharmacology for nursing care* (9th ed.). St. Louis, MO: Elsevier.

BOX 14.5 Drugs That Can Interact With Monoamine Oxidase Inhibitors

- Over-the-counter medications for colds, allergies, or congestion (any product containing ephedrine, phenylephrine hydrochloride, or phenylpropanolamine)
- Tricyclic antidepressants (imipramine, amitriptyline)
- Narcotics
- Antihypertensives (methyldopa, guanethidine, reserpine)
- Amine precursors (levodopa, L-tryptophan)
- Sedatives (alcohol, barbiturates, benzodiazepines)
- General anesthetics
- Stimulants (amphetamines, cocaine)

- Liver disease
- Consumption of foods containing tyramine, L-tryptophan, and dopamine (see Table 14.7)
- Use of certain medications (see Box 14.5)
- Recurrent or severe headaches
- Surgery in the previous 10 to 14 days
- Age younger than 16 years

Special populations

Antidepressant use by pregnant women. We know that antidepressants cross the placenta. Treatment of severe depression, particularly with suicidal ideation, must weigh out the risks versus the benefits. If antidepressant therapy is used during pregnancy, it should be a single medication (monotherapy) at the lowest effective dose, especially during the first trimester. SSRIs are considered an option with the exception of paroxetine (Paxil), which has a small association with fetal heart defects.

Antidepressant use by children and adolescents. In 2004, the FDA issued a black-box warning for all antidepressants. It alerted the public to an increased risk of suicidal thinking or attempts in children or adolescents taking antidepressants. Following the black-box warning, the number of prescriptions written for SSRIs for children, adolescents, and adults decreased (Friedman, 2014).

Unfortunately, suicide attempts increased after the black-box warning was instituted. The risk for suicide is greater in children and adolescents with depression who do not take antidepressants. To minimize the risk of suicide in persons taking antidepressants, close monitoring by healthcare professionals and patient/caregiver education are essential. Chapter 25 has a more detailed discussion of suicide risk factors and warning signs.

Antidepressants use by older adults. Polypharmacy and the normal metabolic processes of aging contribute to concerns about prescribing antidepressants for older adults. SSRIs are a first-line treatment for older adults, but this population has the potential for aggravated side effects. Starting doses are recommended to be half the lowest adult dose, with dose adjustments occurring no more frequently than every 7 days ("start low and go slow").

TABLE 14.8   Adverse Reactions to and Toxic Effects of Monoamine Oxidase Inhibitors

Adverse Reactions	Comments
Hypotension Sedation, weakness, fatigue Insomnia Changes in cardiac rhythm Muscle cramps Anorgasmia or sexual impotence Urinary hesitancy or constipation Weight gain	Hypotension is an expected side effect of monoamine oxidase inhibitors. Orthostatic blood pressures should be taken—first lying down, then sitting or standing after 1–2 min. This may be a dangerous side effect, especially in older adults who may fall and sustain injuries as a result of dizziness from the blood pressure drop.

Toxic Effects	Comments
Hypertensive crisis Severe headache Tachycardia, palpitations Hypertension Nausea and vomiting	Patient should go to local emergency department immediately—blood pressure should be checked. One of the following may be given to lower blood pressure: 5 mg intravenous phentolamine (Regitine) or sublingual nifedipine to promote vasodilation. Patients may be prescribed a 10-mg nifedipine capsule to carry in case of emergency.

BOX 14.6   Patient and Family Teaching: Monoamine Oxidase Inhibitors

- Tell the patient and family to avoid certain foods (especially those that are aged, cured, or ripened) and all medications (especially cold remedies) unless prescribed by and discussed with the patient's primary care provider.
- Give the patient a wallet card describing the monoamine oxidase inhibitor (MAOI) regimen.
- Instruct the patient to avoid Asian restaurants (sherry, brewer's yeast, and other contraindicated products may be used).
- Tell the patient to go to the emergency department immediately if he or she has a severe headache.
- Ideally, blood pressure should be monitored during the first 6 weeks of treatment (for both hypotensive and hypertensive effects).
- After the MAOI is stopped, instruct the patient that dietary and drug restrictions should be maintained for 14 days.

Integrative medicine. St. John's wort *(Hypericum perforatum)* is a flower that can be processed into tea or tablets. This herb may increase the amount of serotonin, norepinephrine, and dopamine in the brain, resulting in antidepressant effects. Studies of St. John's wort used in the treatment of depression provide mixed evaluations. It has generally been found to be as effective as antidepressants in the treatment of mild to moderate depression, but usefulness in severe depression has not been established (Carpenter, 2011).

Because St. John's wort is not regulated by the FDA, concentrations of the active ingredients may vary from preparation to preparation, which may account for some variation in research results. St. John's wort has the potential for adverse reactions when taken with other medications, particularly other antidepressants. Neither safety nor standardization of dose has been established. Therefore, it should be used with caution during pregnancy or in children.

Brain Stimulation Therapies

Electroconvulsive therapy. Despite being a highly effective somatic (physical) treatment for psychiatric disorders, ECT has a bad reputation. This may be due, in part, to past practices of restraining a conscious individual while having a full-blown seizure induced. In fact, before paralytic drugs, more than 30% of ECT patients experienced compression fractures of the spine (Welch, 2016). Given the current sophistication of anesthetic and paralytic agents, ECT is actually not dramatic at all.

Indications. ECT has FDA approval for depressive symptoms associated with major depressive disorder or bipolar disorder in patients aged 13 years and older. Using ECT for depressive symptoms accounts for about 65% of the procedures. However, the FDA does not regulate the practice of medicine. Practitioners may use ECT for other conditions, such as schizophrenia, schizoaffective disorder, and mania.

Risk factors. Using ECT requires clinicians to weigh the risk of using this method versus the risk of suicide and diminished quality of life. Several conditions pose risks and require careful workup and management. Because the heart can be stressed at the onset of the seizure and for up to 10 minutes after, careful assessment and management in hypertension, congestive heart failure, cardiac arrhythmias, and other cardiac conditions is warranted (Welch, 2016). ECT also stresses the brain as a result of increased cerebral oxygen, blood flow, and intracranial pressure. Conditions such as brain tumors and subdural hematomas may increase the risk of using ECT.

Procedure. The procedure is explained to the patient, and informed consent is obtained if the patient is being treated voluntarily. For a patient treated involuntarily, permission may be obtained from the next of kin although in some states treatment must be court-ordered. The patient is usually given a general anesthetic to induce sleep and a muscle-paralyzing agent to prevent muscle distress and fractures. These medications have revolutionized the comfort and safety of ECT.

Patients should have a pre-ECT workup, including a chest x-ray, electrocardiogram (ECG), urinalysis, complete blood count, blood urea nitrogen, and an electrolyte panel. Benzodiazepines should be discontinued since they will interfere with the seizure process.

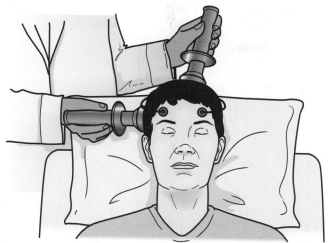

Fig. 14.5 Electroconvulsive therapy. (Photo from National Institute of Mental Health.)

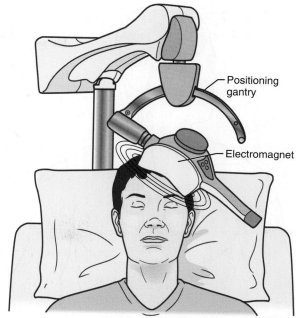

Fig. 14.6 Repetitive transcranial magnetic stimulation. (Photo from National Institute of Mental Health.)

An electroencephalogram (EEG) monitors brain waves, and an ECG monitors cardiac responses. Brief seizures (30 to 60+ seconds) are deliberately induced by an electrical current (as brief as 1 second) transmitted through electrodes attached to one or both sides of the head (Fig. 14.5).

The usual course of ECT for a patient with depression is two or three treatments per week to a total of 6 to 12 treatments. Continuation of ECT along with medication may help to decrease relapse rates.

Potential adverse reactions. Patients wake about 15 minutes after the procedure. The patient is often confused and disoriented for several hours. The nurse and family may need to orient the patient frequently during the course of treatment. Most people experience what is called retrograde amnesia, which is a loss of memory of events leading up to and including the treatment itself.

Repetitive transcranial magnetic stimulation. Repetitive transcranial magnetic stimulation (rTMS) is a noninvasive treatment modality. rTMS uses MRI-strength magnetic pulses to stimulate focal areas of the cerebral cortex.

Indications. In 2008, the FDA approved the use of rTMS to alleviate symptoms of mildly treatment-resistant depression. Treatment-resistant depression refers to people who have been unresponsive to at least one medication trial.

Risk factors. The only absolute contraindication to this procedure is the presence of metal in the area of stimulation. Cochlear implants, brain stimulators, or medication pumps are examples of metals that could interfere with the procedures. Patients with a history of seizure disorders should not be treated with high-frequency rTMS, but low-frequency procedures used to *treat* seizures do not appear to cause them (Keller et al., 2019).

Procedure. Outpatient treatment with rTMS takes about 30 minutes and is typically ordered for 5 days a week for 4 to 6 weeks. Patients are awake and alert during the procedure. An electromagnet is placed on the patient's scalp, and short, magnetic pulses pass into the prefrontal cortex of the brain

(Fig. 14.6). These pulses are similar to those used by MRI scanners but are more focused. The pulses cause electrical charges to flow and induce neurons to fire or become active. During rTMS, patients feel a slight tapping or knocking in the head, contraction of the scalp, and tightening of the jaws.

Potential adverse reactions. After the procedure, patients may feel pain on the scalp at the site of the stimulation due to muscle contraction. Headache, fatigue, and lightheadedness may occur. No neurological deficits or memory problems have been noted. Seizures are a rare complication of rTMS. Most of the common side effects of rTMS are mild and include scalp tingling and discomfort at the administration site.

Vagus nerve stimulation. The use of vagus nerve stimulation (VNS) originated as a treatment for epilepsy. Clinicians noted that in addition to decreasing seizures, VNS also seemed to improve mood in a population that normally experiences higher rates of depression. The theory behind VNS relates to the action of the vagus nerve, the longest cranial nerve, which extends from the brainstem to organs in the neck, chest, and abdomen. Electrical stimulation of the vagus nerve results in boosting the level of neurotransmitters, thereby improving mood and also enhancing the action of antidepressants.

Indications. Nearly a decade after VNS was approved for use in Europe, the FDA granted approval for VNS use in the United States for treatment-resistant depression. The efficacy of VNS in treating depression is still being established. Other potential applications of VNS include anxiety, obesity, and pain.

Procedure. The surgery to implant VNS is typically an outpatient procedure. A pacemaker-like device is implanted surgically into the left chest wall. The device is connected to a thin flexible wire that is threaded up and wrapped around the vagus nerve on the left side of the neck (Fig. 14.7). After

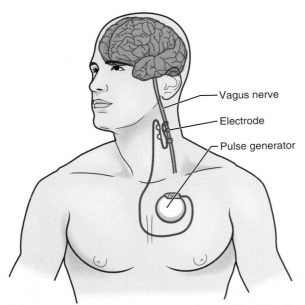

Fig. 14.7 Vagus nerve stimulation. (Photo from National Institute of Mental Health.)

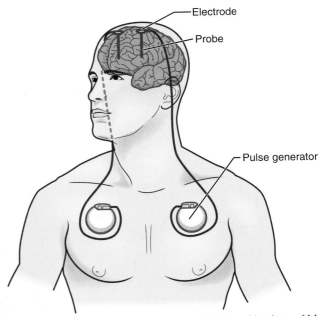

Fig. 14.8 Deep brain stimulation. (Photo from National Institute of Mental Health.)

surgery, an infrared magnetic wand is held against the chest while a personal computer or personal digital assistant is used to program the frequency of pulses. Pulses are usually delivered for 30 seconds, every 5 minutes, for 24 hours a day. Antidepressant action usually occurs in several weeks.

Potential adverse reactions. The implantation of VNS (see Fig. 14.7) is a surgical procedure, carrying with it the risks inherent in any surgical procedure (e.g., pain, infection, sensitivity to anesthesia). Side effects of active VNS therapy are due to the proximity of the lead on the vagus nerve, which is close to the laryngeal and pharyngeal branches of the left vagus nerve. Voice alteration and hoarseness are common side effects. Other side effects include neck pain, cough, paresthesia, and dyspnea, which tend to decrease with time. The device can be temporarily turned off at any time by placing a special magnet over the implant. This may be especially helpful when engaging in public speaking or heavy exercise.

Deep brain stimulation. **Deep brain stimulation (DBS)** is a treatment whereby electrodes are surgically implanted into specific areas of the brain to stimulate those regions identified to be underactive in depression. This treatment is considered to be invasive, but reversible.

Indications. DBS has FDA approval for Parkinson disease, and it has been approved for humanitarian use in treatment-resistant obsessive-compulsive disorder. It is used off-label in major depressive disorder.

Risk factors. DBS has a small risk factor of infection through the hardware in the system (Keller et al., 2019). Other potential problems include intracranial hemorrhage, seizures, stroke, confusion, and headache. It can also cause hypomania in patients with and without a history of bipolar disorder.

Procedure. As in VNS, a device is implanted in the chest wall designed to provide pulses of electrical stimulation. It differs from VNS in that electrodes are implanted directly into the brain to modify brain activity. DBS is being evaluated primarily in regard to treatment-resistant major depression. Fig. 14.8 illustrates DBS.

Other Therapeutic Modalities for Depression
Light Therapy

Light therapy has been researched for nearly 20 years and is accepted as a first-line treatment for SAD. In the *DSM-5* (2013), SAD is considered a subtype of major depressive disorder and listed as "with seasonal pattern." People with SAD often live in regions in which there are marked seasonal differences in the amount of daylight.

Light therapy's effectiveness is thought to be the influence of light on melatonin. Melatonin is secreted by the pineal gland and is necessary for maintaining and shifting biological rhythms. Exposure to light suppresses the nocturnal secretion of melatonin, which seems to have a therapeutic effect on people with SAD.

Ideal treatment consists of 30 to 45 minutes of exposure daily to a 10,000-lux light source. Morning exposure is best. However, success has been reported when exposure occurs at other times of the day or in divided doses. Anecdotal reports suggest that increasing the available light by adding additional light sources may also help to elevate mood. For those affected by SAD, light therapy has been found to be as effective in reducing depressive symptoms as medications. Negative side effects include headache and jitteriness.

Exercise

Exercise has biological, social, and psychological effects on symptoms of depression. Research shows that exercise increases the availability of serotonin in the brain. It has also been demonstrated to dampen the activity of the hypothalamic-pituitary-adrenocorticoid (HPA) axis, which is believed to be overly active in depression. People with depression who exercise regularly report feeling an elevated mood and greater happiness, and they become more socially involved. Additional benefits of exercise are that it is more easily accessed, less expensive, and results in fewer side effects than taking antidepressants.

Psychological Therapies

Like other advanced practice psychiatric professionals, psychiatric-mental health advanced practice registered nurses are usually qualified to diagnose, prescribe, and treat people with depressive disorders. One of the treatments that these nurses can provide is therapy, including individual and group therapy.

Individual Therapy

CBT, interpersonal therapy (IPT), time-limited focused psychotherapy, and behavioral therapy all are especially effective in the treatment of depression. However, only CBT and IPT demonstrate superiority in the maintenance phase. CBT helps people reconstruct their negative thought patterns and behaviors, leading to lasting mood improvements, whereas IPT focuses on working through personal relationships that may contribute to depression.

Group Therapy

Group therapy is a widespread modality for the treatment of depression. It increases the number of people who can receive treatment at a decreased cost per individual. Another advantage is that groups offer patients an opportunity to socialize and share common feelings and concerns, which decreases feelings of isolation, hopelessness, helplessness, and alienation. Therapy groups also provide a controlled environment in which patients can explore their patterns of interaction and response to others, which may contribute to or exacerbate their depression.

KEY POINTS TO REMEMBER

- Children and adolescents with disruptive mood dysregulation disorder had previously been diagnosed with bipolar disorder. Usually, children with this disorder grow up and are diagnosed with major depressive disorder or an anxiety disorder.
- Persistent depressive disorder is a low-level depression that tends to be chronic. Treatment for this disorder is similar to major depressive disorder.
- Premenstrual dysphoric disorder is diagnosed for women with physical discomfort and emotional symptoms similar to major depression. These symptoms disappear at the onset of menstruation.
- The symptoms of major depressive disorder are usually severe enough to interfere with a person's social or occupational functioning. A person with depression may or may not have psychotic symptoms. The most severe consequence of major depressive disorder is suicide.
- Many theories exist about the cause of depression. Biochemical abnormalities are strongly supported in the scientific community. The diathesis-stress theory suggests a dynamic interaction between psychosocial stressors and interpersonal events with neurochemical changes in the brain.
- Nursing assessment includes the evaluation of affect, thought processes (especially suicidal thoughts), mood, feelings, and physical behavior. The nurse also must be aware of the symptoms that may mask depression.
- Nursing diagnoses are numerous. Risk for suicide is always the priority diagnosis when suicidal ideation is present. Other common nursing diagnoses are *chronic low self-esteem, imbalanced nutrition, constipation, disturbed sleep pattern, ineffective coping,* and *disabled family coping.*
- Interventions include using specific principles of communication, planning activities of daily living, administering or participating in psychopharmacological therapy, maintaining a therapeutic environment, and teaching patients about the biochemical aspects of depression.
- Depression is often overlooked in children, adolescents, and older adults.
- Planning and interventions for patients with depression are based on the recovery model, which involves a therapeutic alliance with healthcare professionals to achieve outcomes based on individual patients' needs and values.
- Evaluation is ongoing throughout the nursing process, and patients' outcomes are compared with the stated outcome criteria and short-term and intermediate indicators. The care plan is revised when indicators are not being met.

CRITICAL THINKING

1. You are spending time with Mr. Plotsky, who is undergoing a workup for depression. He hardly makes eye contact, slouches in his seat, and wears a blank but sad expression. Mr. Plotsky has had numerous bouts of major depression in the past and says to you, "This will be my last depression. I will never go through this again."
   - Because safety is the first concern, what are the appropriate questions to ask Mr. Plotsky at this time?
   - In terms of behaviors, thought processes, activities of daily living, and ability to function at work and home, give examples of the kinds of signs and symptoms you might find when assessing a patient with depression.
   - Mr. Plotsky tells you that he has been on every medication there is, but none has worked. He asks you about the herb St. John's wort. What should you tell him about its effectiveness for severe depression, interactions with other antidepressants, and regulatory status?
   - What might be some somatic options for a person resistant to antidepressant medications?
   - Mr. Plotsky asks what causes depression. In simple terms, how might you respond to his query?
   - Mr. Plotsky tells you that he has never tried therapy because he thinks it is for weaklings. What information could you give him about various therapeutic modalities that have proven effective for other patients with depression?

2. You are working with Ms. Folk, a 28-year-old with major depression on long-term antidepressant therapy. She asks you about the possibility of pregnancy while taking her SSRIs.
   - What are some of the things Ms. Folk might want to consider about taking antidepressants if she plans to get pregnant?
   - If she decides to stop taking her antidepressants, what are some things she might do to help manage her depression?

CHAPTER REVIEW

1. Which response by a 15-year-old demonstrates a common symptom observed in patients diagnosed with major depressive disorder?
   a. "I'm so restless. I can't seem to sit still."
   b. "I spend most of my time studying. I have to get into a good college."
   c. "I'm obsessed with counting telephone poles as I drive by them."
   d. "I go to sleep around 11 p.m. but I'm always up by 3 a.m. and can't go back to sleep."

2. Which assessment question asked by the nurse demonstrates an understanding of comorbid mental health conditions associated with major depressive disorder? *Select all that apply.*
   a. "Do rules apply to you?"
   b. "What do you do to manage anxiety?"
   c. "Do you have a history of disordered eating?"
   d. "Do you think that you drink too much?"
   e. "Have you ever been arrested for committing a crime?"

3. Which nursing intervention focuses on managing a common characteristic of major depressive disorder associated with the older population?
   a. Conducting routine suicide screenings at a senior center.
   b. Identifying depression as a natural, but treatable result of aging.
   c. Identifying males as being at a greater risk for developing depression.
   d. Stressing that most individuals experience just a single episode of major depressive disorder in a lifetime.

4. Which characteristic identified during an assessment serves to support a diagnosis of disruptive mood dysregulation disorder? *Select all that apply.*
   a. Female
   b. 7 years old
   c. Comorbid autism diagnosis
   d. Outbursts occur at least once a week
   e. Temper tantrums occur at home and in school

5. Which chronic medical condition is a common trigger for major depressive disorder?
   a. Pain
   b. Hypertension
   c. Hypothyroidism
   d. Crohn disease

6. Tammy, a 28-year-old with major depressive disorder and bulimia nervosa, is ready for discharge from the county hospital after 2 weeks of inpatient therapy. Tammy is taking citalopram (Celexa) and reports that it has made her feel more hopeful. With a secondary diagnosis of bulimia nervosa, what is an alternative antidepressant to consider?
   a. Fluoxetine (Prozac)
   b. Isocarboxazid (Marplan)
   c. Amitriptyline
   d. Duloxetine (Cymbalta)

7. Cabot has multiple symptoms of depression, including mood reactivity, social phobia, anxiety, and overeating. With a history of mild hypertension, which classification of antidepressants dispensed as a transdermal patch would be a safe medication?
   a. Tricyclic antidepressants
   b. Selective serotonin reuptake inhibitors
   c. Serotonin and norepinephrine reuptake inhibitors
   d. Monoamine oxidase inhibitor

8. When a nurse uses therapeutic communication with a withdrawn patient who has major depressive disorder, an effective method of managing the silence is to:
   a. Meditate in the quiet environment
   b. Ask simple questions even if the patient will not answer
   c. Use the technique of making observations
   d. Simply sit quietly and leave when the patient falls asleep

9. The biological approach to treating depression with electrodes surgically implanted into specific areas of the brain to stimulate the regions identified to be underactive in depression is:
   a. Transcranial magnetic stimulation
   b. Deep brain stimulation
   c. Vagus nerve stimulation
   d. Electroconvulsive therapy

10. Two months ago, Natasha's husband died suddenly and she has been overwhelmed with grief. When Natasha is subsequently diagnosed with major depressive disorder, her daughter, Nadia, makes which true statement?
    a. "Depression often begins after a major loss. Losing dad was a major loss."
    b. "Bereavement and depression are the same problem."
    c. "Mourning is pathological and not normal behavior."
    d. "Antidepressant medications will not help this type of depression."

1. **d**; 2. **b, c, d**; 3. **a**; 4. **b, c, e**; 5. **a**; 6. **a**; 7. **d**; 8. **c**; 9. **b**; 10. **a**

NGN CASE STUDY AND QUESTIONS

Siddharth, 38 years old, is married and the father to three sons. He is admitted to the behavioral health unit for the treatment of major depressive disorder. He begins taking a selective serotonin reuptake inhibitor (SSRI). He is eventually discharged and treated on an outpatient basis.

Over the next year, he makes some progress, but medication seems to have little impact. Siddharth is motivated for treatment but is discouraged that nothing seems to help. The psychiatrist recommends repetitive transcranial magnetic stimulation (rTMS) on an outpatient basis as he tapers off medications.

1. In preparation for outpatient rTMS, the registered nurse gathers educational material for Siddharth and prepares for teaching. Identify essential educational information regarding this procedure. Select all that apply.
   a. rTMS is noninvasive.
   b. This procedure is thought to work through vagus nerve stimulation.

c. rTMS has US Food and Drug Administration (FDA) approval for depression.

d. The procedure is conducted with general anesthesia.

e. Seizures are a rare complication.

f. The only absolute contraindication for rTMS is metal in the skull, such as a cochlear implant.

Siddharth completed 6 weeks of rTMS therapy. He is taking sertraline (Zoloft), which he is tolerating well, along with psychotherapy. He found another job, with a good referral from his previous landscaping employer.

He still has bouts of both depression and anxiety. When he is tempted to drink, as he did before treatment, he resists this impulse by watching TV while overeating junk food. Siddharth reports no further suicide ideation, "…especially because of my new job, my awesome boys, and our whole, big ridiculous family."

Given these improvements, indicate which follow-up findings indicate successful achievement of outcomes. *Select all that apply.*

Follow-up Findings	Effective Outcomes
a. Resists impulse to drink alcohol	
b. Positive feelings for job, family, and community activities	
c. Feels anxious and depressed sometimes	
d. Overeats as a coping mechanism	
e. Continues psychotherapy and sertraline (Zoloft) regimen	
f. Gratitude and hope for future	
g. No further suicidal ideation	

NGN case study answers are on Evolve.

Visit the Evolve website for a posttest on the content in this chapter: http://evolve.elsevier.com/Varcarolis

REFERENCES

American Psychiatric Association. (2013). *Diagnostic and statistical manual of mental disorders* (5th ed.). Washington, DC: Author.

Beck, A. T., & Rush, A. J. (1995). Cognitive therapy. In H. I. Kaplan, & B. J. Sadock (Eds.), *Comprehensive textbook of psychiatry/VI (vol. 2)* (pp. 1847–1856). Baltimore, MD: Williams & Wilkins.

Carpenter, D. (2011). St. John's wort and S-adenosyl methionine as "natural" alternatives to conventional antidepressants in the era of the suicidality boxed warning: What is the evidence for clinically relevant benefit? *Alternative Medicine Health Review, 16*(1), 17–39.

Copeland, W. E., Angold, A., Costello, E. J., & Egger, H. (2013). Prevalence, comorbidity, and correlates of *DSM-5* proposed disruptive mood dysregulation disorder. *American Journal of Psychiatry, 170*(2), 173–179.

Flaster, M., Sharma, A., & Rao, M. (2013). Poststroke depression. *Topics in Stroke Rehabilitation, 20*(2), 139–150.

Friedman, R. A. (2014). Antidepressants' black-box warning 10 years later. *New England Journal of Medicine, 371,* 1666–1668.

Gillespie, C.F., & Nemeroff, C.B. (2005). Hypercortisolemia and depression. *Psychosomatic Medicine, 67,* S26–S28.

Institute for Clinical Systems Improvement. (2016). *Depression in primary care.* Retrieved from https://www.icsi.org/_asset/xm2nqq/DeprPC0216.pdf.

Keller, C., Bhati, M. T., Downar, J., & Etkin, A. (2019). Brain stimulation therapies. In L. W. Roberts (Ed.), *The American Psychiatric Association Publishing textbook of psychiatry* (pp. 861–898). Washington, DC: American Psychiatric Association.

Köhler–Forsberg, O., Lydholm, C. N., Hjorthoj, C., Nordentoft, M., Mors, O., & Benros, M. E. (2019). Efficacy of anti-inflammatory treatment on major depressive disorder or depressive symptoms. *Acta Psychiatrica Scandinavica, 139*(5), 404–419.

Krishnadas, R., & Cavanagh, J. (2012). Depression: An inflammatory illness? *Journal of Neurology, Neurosurgery, and Psychiatry, 83*(5), 495–502.

Lam, R. W., Kennedy, S. H., McIntyre, R. S., & Khullar, A. (2014). Cognitive dysfunction in major depressive disorder: Effects on psychosocial functioning and implications for treatment. *Canadian Journal of Psychiatry, 59*(12), 649–654.

Miller, G. E., & Cole, S. W. (2012). Clustering of depression and inflammation in adolescents previously exposed to childhood adversity. *Biological Psychiatry, 72*(1), 34–40.

Möller, H. J., Bandelow, B., Volz, H. P., Barnikol, U. B., Seifritz, E., & Kasper, S. (2016). The relevance of "mixed anxiety and depression" as a diagnostic category in clinical practice. *European Archives of Psychiatry and Clinical Neuroscience, 266*(8), 725–736.

National Institute of Mental Health. (2012). *Older adults: Depression and suicide facts* (fact sheet). Retrieved from http://www.nimh.nih.gov/health/publications/older-adults-and-depression/older-adults-and-depression_141998.pdf.

Parikh, S. V., Riba, M. B., & Greden, J. F. (2019). Depressive disorders. In L. W. Roberts (Ed.), *The American Psychiatric Association Publishing textbook of psychiatry* (pp. 307–340). Washington, DC: American Psychiatric Association.

Perlis, R.H. (2014). Pharmacogenomic testing and personalized treatment of depression. *Clinical Chemistry, 60*(1), 53–59.

Ryan, J., & Ancelin, M. (2012). Polymorphisms of estrogen receptors and risk of depression. *Drugs, 72*(13), 1725–1738.

Sheikh, J., & Yesavage, J. (1986). Geriatric depression scale (GDS): Recent evidence and development of a shorter version. *Clinical Gerontologist, 5*(1–2), 165–173.

Substance Abuse and Mental Health Services Administration. (2018). *Results from the 2017 National Survey on Drug Use and Health: Detailed tables.* Retrieved from https://www.samhsa.gov/data/sites/default/files/cbhsq-reports/NSDUHDetailedTabs2017/NSDUHDetailedTabs2017.htm#tab8-56A.

Vandeleur, C. L., Fassassi, S., Castelao, E., Glaus, J., Strippoli, M. F., Lasserre, A. M., et al. (2017). Prevalence and correlates of DSM05 major depressive and related disorders in the community. *Psychiatry Research, 250,* 50–58.

Welch, C. A. (2016). Electroconvulsive therapy. In T. A. Stern, M. Fava, T. E. Wilens, & J. F. Rosenbaum (Eds.), *Comprehensive clinical psychiatry* (2nd ed.). St. Louis, MO: Elsevier.

Witt, K., Potts, J., Hubers, A., Grunebaum, M. F., Murrough, J. W., Loo, C., et al. (2019). Ketamine for suicidal ideation in adults with psychiatric disorders: A systematic review and meta-analysis of treatment trials. *Australian and New Zealand Journal of Psychiatry, 54*(1), 29–45.

World Health Organization. (2019). *Depression.* Retrieved from https://www.who.int/news-room/fact-sheets/detail/depression.

Zhou, Y., Cao, Z., Yang, M., Xizoyan, X., Guo, Y., Fang, M., et al. (2017). Comorbid generalized anxiety disorder and its association with quality of life in patients with major depressive disorder. *Scientific Reports, 7,* 40511.

Anxiety and Obsessive-Compulsive Disorders

Margaret Jordan Halter

Visit the Evolve website for a pretest on the content in this chapter: http://evolve.elsevier.com/Varcarolis

OBJECTIVES

1. Compare and contrast the four levels of anxiety in relation to perceptual field, ability to solve problems, and other defining characteristics.
2. Identify defense mechanisms and consider one adaptive and one maladaptive (if any) use of each.
3. Describe the clinical manifestations of separation anxiety disorder, specific phobia, social anxiety disorder, panic disorder, agoraphobia, and generalized anxiety disorder.
4. Identify risk factors that may contribute to anxiety disorders.
5. Formulate four priority nursing diagnoses that can be used in caring for patients with an anxiety disorder.
6. Propose realistic outcome criteria for patients with an anxiety disorder.
7. Describe five basic nursing interventions used for patients with anxiety disorders.
8. Discuss the classes of medications used to treat anxiety disorders.
9. Describe psychological therapies for anxiety disorders.
10. Describe clinical manifestations of obsessive-compulsive disorder, body dysmorphic disorder, hoarding disorder, trichotillomania, and excoriation disorder.
11. Identify risk factors that may contribute to obsessive-compulsive disorders.
12. Formulate four priority nursing diagnoses that can be used in treating patients with obsessive-compulsive disorders.
13. Propose realistic outcome criteria for patients with obsessive-compulsive disorders.
14. Describe three basic nursing interventions used for patients with obsessive-compulsive disorders.
15. Discuss the classes of medications used to treat obsessive-compulsive disorders.
16. Describe psychological therapies for obsessive-compulsive disorders.

KEY TERMS AND CONCEPTS

agoraphobia
anxiety
compulsions

defense mechanisms
mild anxiety
moderate anxiety

obsessions
panic
severe anxiety

For most people, anxiety is a part of everyday life. "I felt really nervous when I couldn't find a parking space right before my final exam. I know I would have done better if that hadn't happened." For some people, however, anxiety-related symptoms become severely debilitating and interfere with normal functioning. "Today I got so worried I wouldn't find a parking space before the final exam, I stayed home." In this chapter, we will examine the concept of anxiety, defenses against anxiety, and an overview of anxiety disorders and their treatment.

ANXIETY

Anxiety is a universal human experience and is among the most basic of emotions. Anxiety is a feeling of apprehension, uneasiness, uncertainty, or dread resulting from a real or perceived threat. Fear is a reaction to a specific danger, whereas anxiety is a vague sense of dread related to an unspecified or unknown danger. However, the body reacts physiologically in similar ways to both anxiety and fear. Another important distinction between anxiety and fear is that anxiety affects us at a deeper level. It invades the central core of the personality and erodes feelings of self-esteem and personal worth.

Normal anxiety is a healthy reaction that is necessary for survival. Without anxiety, our ancestors would have had little motivation to run from the saber tooth tiger or hunt the mastodon. Anxiety provides the energy needed to carry out the tasks involved in living and striving toward goals. Anxiety motivates people to make and survive change. It prompts constructive behaviors, such as studying for an examination, being on time for a job interview, preparing for a presentation, and working toward a promotion.

An understanding of the levels and defensive patterns used in response to anxiety is basic to psychiatric–mental health nursing care. This understanding is essential for assessing and planning interventions to reduce a patient's level of anxiety (as well as one's own) effectively. With practice, you will become skilled at identifying levels of anxiety, understanding the defenses used to alleviate anxiety, and evaluating the possible stressors that contribute to increased levels of anxiety.

LEVELS OF ANXIETY

As discussed in Chapter 2, Hildegard Peplau played a profound role in shaping the specialty of psychiatric–mental health nursing: she identified anxiety as a key element in her theory of interpersonal relationships. Peplau (1968) developed a useful anxiety model consisting of four levels: mild, moderate, severe, and panic. The boundaries between these levels are not distinct, and the behaviors and characteristics of individuals experiencing anxiety can and often do overlap. Identification of a general level of anxiety is helpful in selecting interventions based on the *degree* of the patient's anxiety.

Mild Anxiety

Mild anxiety occurs in the normal experience of everyday living and allows an individual to perceive reality in sharp focus. A person experiencing a mild level of anxiety sees, hears, and grasps more information, and problem solving becomes more effective. Physical symptoms may include slight discomfort, restlessness, irritability, or mild tension-relieving behaviors (e.g., nail biting, foot or finger tapping, fidgeting).

Moderate Anxiety

As anxiety increases, the perceptual field narrows, and some details are excluded from observation. The person experiencing moderate anxiety sees, hears, and grasps less information and may demonstrate selective inattention, where only certain things in the environment are seen or heard unless they are pointed out. The ability to think clearly is hampered, but learning and problem solving can still take place, though not at an optimal level.

Sympathetic nervous system symptoms begin to kick in at this level. The individual may experience tension, a pounding heart, increased pulse and respiratory rates, perspiration, and mild somatic symptoms (e.g., gastric discomfort, headache, urinary urgency). Voice tremors and shaking may be noticed. Mild or moderate anxiety levels can be constructive because anxiety may be a signal that something in the person's life needs attention or is dangerous.

Severe Anxiety

The perceptual field of a person experiencing severe anxiety is greatly reduced. A person with severe anxiety may focus on one particular detail or on many scattered details and have difficulty noticing what is going on in the environment, even when another person points it out. Learning and problem solving are not possible at this level, and the person may be dazed and confused. Behavior is automatic and aimed at reducing or relieving anxiety. Somatic symptoms (e.g., headache, nausea, dizziness,

insomnia) often increase. Trembling and a pounding heart are common, and the person may experience hyperventilation and a sense of impending doom or dread.

Panic

Panic is the most extreme level of anxiety and results in markedly dysregulated behavior. Someone in a state of panic is unable to process what is going on in the environment and may lose touch with reality. The behavior that results may be manifested as pacing, running, shouting, screaming, or withdrawal. Hallucinations, which are false sensory perceptions, such as seeing something that is not really there or hearing voices, may be experienced. Physical behavior may become erratic, uncoordinated, and impulsive. Automatic behaviors are used to reduce and relieve anxiety, although such efforts may be ineffective. Acute panic may lead to exhaustion. See the Case Study and Nursing Care Plan for panic level anxiety on the Evolve website.

Review Table 15.1, which distinguishes among the levels of anxiety in regard to their (1) effects on perceptual field, (2) effects on problem solving, and (3) physical and other defining characteristics.

DEFENSES AGAINST ANXIETY

Sigmund Freud and his daughter, Anna Freud, outlined most of the defense mechanisms we recognize today. Defense mechanisms are automatic coping styles that protect people from anxiety and enable them to maintain their self-image by blocking feelings, conflicts, and memories. Although they operate all the time, defense mechanisms are not always apparent to the individual using them.

Adaptive use of defense mechanisms helps people to lower their levels of anxiety and to achieve their goals in acceptable ways. Maladaptive use of defense mechanisms occurs when one or several are used to excess, particularly immature defenses. Fig. 15.1 defines anxiety operationally and shows how defenses come into play.

Most defense mechanisms can be used in both healthy and unhealthy ways. People generally use a variety of defense mechanisms but not always to the same degree. Keep in mind that evaluating whether the use of defense mechanisms is adaptive or maladaptive is determined for the most part by their frequency, intensity, and duration of use. Table 15.2 describes defense mechanisms and provides examples of their adaptive and maladaptive uses.

ANXIETY DISORDERS

Individuals with anxiety disorders use rigid, repetitive, and ineffective behaviors to try to control their anxiety. The common element of such disorders is that those affected experience a degree of anxiety that interferes with personal, occupational, or social functioning.

Anxiety disorders are the most common mental health problems. About 19% of adults in the United States have an anxiety disorder. Table 15.3 summarizes the lifetime prevalence rates of anxiety disorders overall and by gender.

TABLE 15.1   Levels of Anxiety

Mild	Moderate	Severe	Panic
Perceptual Field			
Heightened perceptual field	Narrowed perceptual field Grasps less of what is going on	Greatly reduced and distorted perceptual field	Unable to attend to the environment
Focus is flexible and is aware of the anxiety	Focuses on the source of the anxiety Less able to pay attention	Focuses on details or one specific detail Attention is scattered	Focus is lost; may feel unreal (depersonalization) or that the world is unreal (derealization)
Ability to Solve Problems			
Able to work effectively toward a goal and examine alternatives	Able to solve problems but not at optimal level	Problem solving feels impossible Unable to see connections between events or details	Completely unable to process what is happening Disorganized or irrational reasoning
Mild and moderate levels of anxiety can alert the person that something is wrong and can stimulate appropriate action.		Severe and panic levels of anxiety prevent problem solving. Unproductive relief behaviors perpetuate a vicious cycle.	
Physical or Other Characteristics			
Slight discomfort Attention-seeking behavior Restlessness Easily startled Irritability or impatience Mild tension-relieving behavior (foot or finger tapping, lip chewing, fidgeting)	Voice tremors Change in voice pitch Poor concentration Shakiness Somatic complaints (urinary frequency, headache, backache, insomnia) Increased respiration, pulse, and muscle tension More tension-relieving behavior (pacing, banging hands on table)	Feelings of dread Confusion Purposeless activity Sense of impending doom More intense somatic complaints (chest discomfort, dizziness, nausea, sleeplessness) Diaphoresis (sweating) Withdrawal Loud and rapid speech Threats and demands	Experience of terror Immobility, severe hyperactivity, or flight Unintelligible communication or inability to speak Amplified or muffled sounds Somatic complaints increase (numbness or tingling, shortness of breath, dizziness, chest pain, nausea, trembling, chills, overheating, palpitations) Severe withdrawal Hallucinations or delusions Likely out of touch with reality

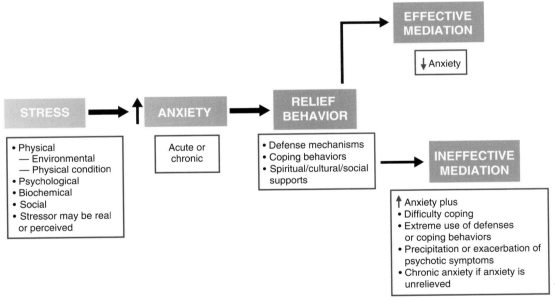

Fig. 15.1 Anxiety operationally defined.

Clinical Picture

According to the American Psychiatric Association (2013), anxiety disorders refers to a number of conditions, including the following:

- Separation anxiety disorder
- Specific phobia
- Social anxiety disorder (social phobia)
- Panic disorder
- Agoraphobia
- Generalized anxiety disorder

Separation Anxiety Disorder

Separation anxiety is a normal part of infant development that begins around 8 months of age, peaks at about 18 months, and begins to decline after that. People with **separation anxiety**

TABLE 15.2 Adaptive and Maladaptive Uses of Defense Mechanisms

Defense Mechanism	Adaptive Use	Maladaptive Use
Altruism is a largely unconscious motivation to feel caring and concern for others and act for the well-being of others.	A woman anonymously donates to her colleague's GoFundMe campaign.	A neighbor compulsively rescues cats and kittens to the detriment of the animals' and his own health and safety.
Compensation is used to counterbalance perceived deficiencies by emphasizing strengths.	A shorter-than-average man becomes assertively verbal and excels in business.	A woman drinks alcohol when her self-esteem is low to temporarily ease her discomfort.
Conversion is the unconscious transformation of anxiety into a physical symptom with no organic cause.	No example. Almost always a pathological defense.	A man becomes blind after seeing his wife enter a hotel room with another man.
Denial involves escaping unpleasant, anxiety-causing thoughts, feelings, wishes, or needs by ignoring their existence.	A man reacts to the death of a loved one by saying, "No, I don't believe you," to initially protect himself from the overwhelming news.	A woman whose husband died 3 years earlier still keeps his clothes in the closet and talks about him in the present tense.
Displacement is the transference of emotions associated with a particular person, object, or situation to another nonthreatening person, object, or situation.	A child yells at his teddy bear after being picked on by the school bully.	A child who is unable to acknowledge fear of his father becomes fearful of animals.
Dissociation is a disruption in consciousness, memory, identity, or perception of the environment that results in compartmentalizing uncomfortable or unpleasant aspects of oneself.	An art student is able to mentally separate herself from a noisy environment as she becomes absorbed in her work.	As the result of an abusive childhood and the need to separate from its realities, a woman finds herself perpetually disconnected from reality.
Identification is attributing to oneself the characteristics of another person or group. This may be done consciously or unconsciously.	An 8-year-old girl dresses up like her teacher and puts together a pretend classroom for her friends.	A boy dresses and talks like a neighborhood drug dealer and starts his own "gang."
Intellectualization is a process in which events are analyzed based on remote, cold facts and without passion, rather than incorporating feeling and emotion into the processing.	Despite having lost his farm to a tornado, a man analyzes his options and leads his child to safety.	A man responds to the death of his wife by focusing on the details of day care and operating the household rather than processing the grief with his children.
Projection refers to the unconscious rejection of emotionally unacceptable features and attributing them to others.	No example. This is considered an immature defense mechanism.	A woman who has repressed an attraction toward other women refuses to socialize. She fears that another woman will come on to her.
Rationalization consists of justifying illogical or unreasonable ideas, actions, or feelings by developing acceptable explanations that satisfy the teller and the listener.	An employee says, "I didn't get the raise because the boss doesn't like me."	A man who believes that his son was fathered by another man excuses his harsh treatment of the boy by saying, "He is lazy and doesn't listen to me," when that is not true.
Reaction formation is when unacceptable feelings or behaviors are controlled and kept out of awareness by developing the opposite emotion or behavior.	A recovering alcoholic constantly talks about the evils of drinking.	A woman who has an unconscious hostility toward her daughter is overprotective and hovers over her to protect her from harm, interfering with her normal growth and development.
Regression is reverting to an earlier, more primitive and childlike pattern of behavior that may or may not have been exhibited previously.	A 4-year-old boy with a new baby brother temporarily starts sucking his thumb and asking for a baby bottle.	A man who loses a promotion starts complaining to others, hands in sloppy work, misses appointments, and comes in late for meetings.
Repression is an unconscious exclusion of unpleasant or unwanted experiences, emotions, or ideas from conscious awareness.	After a marital fight, a man forgets his spouse's birthday.	A woman is unable to enjoy sex after having pushed out of awareness a traumatic sexual incident from childhood.
Splitting is the inability to integrate the positive and negative qualities of oneself or others into a cohesive image.	No example. Almost always a pathological defense.	A 26-year-old woman initially values her acquaintances yet invariably becomes disillusioned when they turn out to have flaws.
Sublimation is an unconscious process of transforming negative impulses into less damaging and even productive impulses.	A woman who is angry with her boss channels her feelings into housework until her house is sparkling clean.	No example. The use of sublimation is always constructive.
Suppression is the conscious decision to delay addressing a disturbing situation or feeling. For example, Jessica has studied for the state board examination for a week. She says, "I won't worry about paying my rent until after my exam tomorrow."	A businessman who is preparing to make an important speech is told by his wife that morning that she wants a divorce. Although visibly upset, he puts the incident aside until after his speech, when he can give the matter his total attention.	A woman who feels a lump in her breast shortly before leaving for a 3-week vacation puts the information in the back of her mind until after she returns from her vacation.
Undoing is when a person makes up for a regrettable act or communication.	After flirting with her male secretary, a woman brings her husband tickets to a concert he wants to see.	A man with rigid, moralistic beliefs and repressed sexuality is driven to wash his hands to gain composure when he is around attractive women.

TABLE 15.3   Lifetime Prevalence of Anxiety Disorders

	Percent	Female (%)	Male (%)
Specific phobia	12.5	15.8	8.9
Social anxiety disorder	12.1	13.0	11.1
Separation anxiety disorder	9.2	10.8	7.4
Generalized anxiety disorder	5.7	7.1	4.2
Panic disorder	4.7	6.2	3.1
Agoraphobia	1.3	1.6	1.1

TABLE 15.4   Clinical Names for Common Phobias

Clinical Name	Feared Object or Situation
Acrophobia	Heights
Agoraphobia	Open spaces
Astraphobia	Electrical storms
Claustrophobia	Closed spaces
Glossophobia	Talking
Hematophobia	Blood
Hydrophobia	Water
Monophobia	Being alone
Mysophobia	Germs or dirt
Nyctophobia	Darkness
Pyrophobia	Fire
Xenophobia	Strangers
Zoophobia	Animals

disorder exhibit developmentally inappropriate levels of concern over being away from a significant other. There may also be fear that something horrible will happen to the other person and that it will result in permanent separation. The anxiety is so intense that it distracts sufferers from their normal activities and causes sleep disruptions and nightmares. The separation anxiety is often manifested in physical symptoms, such as gastrointestinal disturbances and headaches.

Recently, clinicians have begun to recognize an adult form of separation anxiety disorder that may begin either in childhood or in adulthood. A person who is the subject of the attachment—a parent, a spouse, a child, or a friend—may become alienated due to the constant neediness and clinginess of the other. In fact, adults with this disorder often have extreme difficulties in romantic relationships and are more likely to be unmarried. Characteristics of adult separation anxiety disorder include harm avoidance, worry, shyness, uncertainty, fatigability, and a lack of self-direction. Fear of separation is accompanied by a significant level of discomfort and disability that impairs social and occupational functioning.

This problem is typically diagnosed before the age of 18, after about a month of symptoms. The 12-month prevalence rates of separation anxiety disorder in children, adolescents, and adults is 4%, 1.9%, and 0.9% to 1.9%, respectively. It is the most common anxiety disorder in children. Females are more likely to be affected.

Environmental stresses—such as a significant loss through death of a relative or pet, separation from significant others, or a change in environment by moving or immigration—can bring about symptoms of this disorder. A physical or sexual assault may also precede symptoms. Inherited traits such as neuroticism may play a role in separation anxiety disorder.

In children, this severe form of separation anxiety is often seen with generalized anxiety disorder and specific phobias. In adults, a range of disorders commonly coexist. They are depressive disorders, bipolar disorders, anxiety disorders, posttraumatic stress disorder, obsessive-compulsive disorder (OCD), and personality disorders.

Specific Phobias

A **specific phobia** is a persistent irrational fear of a specific object, activity, or situation that leads to a desire for avoidance or actual avoidance of the object, activity, or situation. Specific phobias are characterized by the experience of high levels of anxiety or fear in response to certain objects or situations—for example, dogs, spiders, heights, storms, water, blood, closed spaces, tunnels, and bridges.

Phobias compromise a person's daily functioning, and phobic people go to great lengths to avoid the feared object or situation. A phobic person may not be able to think about or visualize the object or situation without becoming severely anxious. The lives of people with phobias become more restricted as the phobic person gives up activities in order to avoid the phobic object. All too frequently, complications arise when sufferers try to decrease anxiety through self-medication with alcohol or drugs.

Consider the case of Daniel, who developed a profound fear of elevators after being trapped in one for 3 hours during a power outage. As his fear and anxiety intensified, it became necessary for him to use only stairs or escalators. He obsesses about the possibility that he will be forced to use an elevator in some social situation and avoids attending events where this may occur. It has reached a point where he cannot bear even to go inside a closet or small storage room. This fear of enclosed spaces is called *claustrophobia*. Other common phobias are listed in Table 15.4.

Twelve-month prevalence rates for specific phobias in children, adolescents, and adults are 5%, 16%, and 8%, respectively. Females are affected twice as often as males.

Animals, the environment, and situation-specific phobias are more common in females. Blood injury and injection (BII) phobia is experienced equally by males and females. This unique phobia is associated with a diphasic cardiovascular response that begins with tachycardia and then goes on to bradycardia, hypotension, diaphoresis, and fainting. BII phobia is a real concern as it prevents people from seeking healthcare.

Negative and traumatic experiences with the feared objects or situations lead to the fear. Phobic reactions tend to run in families. Having a first-degree relative with a specific phobia puts one at greater risk for having the same specific phobia.

Few people are seen in healthcare settings for the treatment of phobias. In general, such individuals seek help for comorbid conditions, including major depressive disorder, anxiety, substance use, somatic symptom disorders, and dependent personality disorder.

Social Anxiety Disorder

Social anxiety disorder, also called social phobia, is characterized by severe anxiety or fear provoked by exposure to a social or a performance situation that could be evaluated negatively by others. Situations that trigger this distress include fear of saying something that sounds foolish in public, not being able to answer questions in a classroom, looking awkward while eating or drinking in public, and performing badly on stage. Whenever possible, people with social anxiety disorder avoid such situations. If they are unable to avoid them, they endure the situation with intense anxiety and emotional distress.

Small children with this disorder may be mute and nervous and may hide behind their parents. Older children and adolescents may be paralyzed by fear of speaking in class or interacting with peers. Worry over saying the wrong thing or being criticized immobilizes them. Conversely, younger people may act out to compensate for this fear, making an accurate diagnosis more difficult. This anxiety often results in physical complaints that can help the person to avoid social situations, particularly school.

Fear of public speaking is the most common manifestation of social anxiety disorder. Interestingly, this disorder has afflicted famous singers and actors, including Barbra Streisand and Sir Laurence Olivier, both of whom were terrified that they might forget the words of songs or scripts.

The 12-month prevalence of social anxiety disorder is the same for children, adolescents, and adults—about 7%. As with many of the anxiety disorders, females are more likely to be affected.

Risk factors for social anxiety disorder include childhood mistreatment and adverse childhood experiences. The trait of shyness is also strongly heritable. Having parents who are shy carries a double risk of genetic transmission and parental modeling.

Chronic social isolation may increase the risk for major depressive disorder. Substance use disorders are common and may be related to the social isolation and inhibition caused by this illness. Bipolar disorder and body dysmorphic disorder are also comorbid. In children, comorbidities include high-functioning autism and selective mutism.

Panic Disorder

Panic attacks are the key feature of **panic disorder**. A **panic attack** is the sudden onset of extreme apprehension or fear, usually associated with feelings of impending doom. The feelings of terror present during a panic attack are so severe that normal functioning is suspended, the perceptual field is severely limited, and misinterpretation of reality may occur. People experiencing panic attacks may believe that they are losing their minds or having a heart attack. Typically, panic attacks come "out of the blue" (i.e., suddenly and not necessarily in response

to stress) and are extremely intense; they last a matter of minutes and then subside.

Unpredictability is a key aspect of panic disorder in children and adolescents. The attacks of panic seem to come out of nowhere, last about 10 minutes, and then subside. During the attack, the young person is less able to articulate its psychological aspects, such as fear. Such individuals may become avoidant of situations where help is not available, may develop feelings of hopelessness in controlling these attacks, and may become depressed. Alcohol or substance use is common among adolescents with this disorder.

People who experience these attacks begin to "fear the fear." They become so preoccupied with the possibility of future episodes that they avoid what could be pleasurable and adaptive activities, experiences, and obligations.

Major depressive disorder may occur before the onset of panic disorder or may arise at the same time. Substance use disorder frequently accompanies panic disorder, probably in an attempt to self-medicate. Nonpsychiatric disorders are also comorbid. They include hyperthyroidism, dizziness, cardiac arrhythmias, asthma, chronic obstructive pulmonary disease (COPD), and irritable bowel syndrome.

Table 15.5 outlines a generic nursing care plan for panic disorder. The *DSM-5* box contains diagnostic criteria for panic disorder.

DSM-5 CRITERIA FOR PANIC DISORDER

A. Recurrent unexpected panic attacks. A panic attack is an abrupt surge of intense fear or discomfort that reaches a peak within minutes; during the attack, four (or more) of the following symptoms occur:

Note: The abrupt surge can occur from a calm state or an anxious state.

1. Palpitations, pounding heart, or accelerated heart rate
2. Sweating
3. Trembling or shaking
4. Sensations of shortness of breath or smothering
5. Feelings of choking
6. Chest pain or discomfort
7. Nausea or abdominal distress
8. Feeling dizzy, unsteady, lightheaded, or faint
9. Chills or heat sensations
10. Paresthesias (numbness or tingling sensations)
11. Derealization (feelings of unreality) or depersonalization (being detached from oneself)
12. Fear of losing control or "going crazy"
13. Fear of dying

Note: Culture-specific symptoms (e.g., tinnitus, neck soreness, headache, uncontrollable screaming or crying) may be seen. Such symptoms should not count as one of the four required symptoms.

B. At least one of the attacks has been followed by 1 month (or more) of one or both of the following:

1. Persistent concern or worry about additional panic attacks or their consequences (e.g., losing control, having a heart attack, "going crazy").
2. A significant maladaptive change in behavior related to the attacks (e.g., behaviors designed to avoid having panic attacks, such as avoidance of exercise or unfamiliar situations).

C. The disturbance is not attributable to the physiological effects of a substance (e.g., a drug of abuse, a medication) or another medical condition (e.g., hyperthyroidism, cardiopulmonary disorders).

Continued

TABLE 15.5 Generic Care Plan for Panic Disorder

Priority diagnosis: Severe anxiety as evidenced by sudden onset of fear of impending doom or dying, increased pulse and respirations, shortness of breath, possible chest pain, dizziness, and abdominal distress.

Outcome criteria: Panic attacks will become less intense and time between episodes will lengthen.

Short-Term Goal	Intervention	Rationale
1. Patient's anxiety will decrease to moderate by (date).	1a. If hyperventilation occurs, instruct the patient to take slow, deep breaths. Breathing with the patient may be helpful. 1b. Keep expectations minimal and simple.	1a. Focus is shifted away from distressing symptoms. 1b. Anxiety limits one's ability to attend to complex tasks.
2. Patient will gain mastery over panic episodes by (date).	2a. Help the patient connect feelings before the attack with onset of attack: "What were you thinking about just before the attack?" "Can you identify what you were feeling just before the attack?" 2b. Help the patient to recognize symptoms as resulting from anxiety, not from a catastrophic physical problem. Examples: Explain physical symptoms of anxiety. Discuss the fact that anxiety causes sensations similar to those of physical events, such as a heart attack. 2c. Identify effective therapies for panic episodes. 2d. Teach the patient abdominal breathing, to be used immediately when anxiety is detected. 2e. Teach the patient to use positive self-talk, such as "I can control my anxiety." 2f. Teach the patient and family about any medication ordered to control the patient's panic attacks.	2a. Physiological symptoms of anxiety as the result of a stressor usually appear first. They are immediately followed by automatic thoughts, such as "I'm dying" or "I'm going crazy," which are distorted assessments. 2b. Factual information and alternative interpretations can help the patient recognize distortions in thought. 2c. Cognitive-behavioral treatment is highly effective. Antianxiety medication is appropriate. 2d. Breathing exercises break the cycle of escalating symptoms of anxiety. 2e. Cognitive restructuring is an effective way to replace negative self-talk. 2f. Patient and family need to know what the medication can do, what the side effects and toxic effects are, and whom to call if untoward reactions occur.

DSM-5 CRITERIA FOR PANIC DISORDER —contd

D. The disturbance is not better explained by another mental disorder (e.g., the panic attacks do not occur only in response to feared social situations, as in social anxiety disorder; in response to circumscribed phobic objects or situations, as in specific phobia; in response to obsessions, as in obsessive-compulsive disorder; in response to reminders of traumatic events, as in posttraumatic stress disorder; or in response to separation from attachment figures, as in separation anxiety disorder).

Reprinted with permission from American Psychiatric Association. (2013). *Diagnostic and statistical manual* (5th ed.). Washington, DC: Author.

Agoraphobia

The term **agoraphobia** is derived from the Greek *agora* ("open space") and phobia ("fear"). It refers to intense excessive anxiety or fear about being in places or situations from which escape might be difficult or embarrassing or where help might not be available. The feared places are avoided in an effort to control anxiety. Situations that are commonly avoided are being alone outside; being alone at home; traveling in a car, bus, or airplane; being on a bridge; and riding in an elevator. These situations may be seen as more tolerable with another person's company.

Avoidance behaviors can be debilitating and life constricting. Consider the effect on a father whose agoraphobia renders him unable to leave home and prevents him from seeing his child's high school graduation.

Nearly 2% of adolescents and adults experience agoraphobia in a given year. Some children may develop the disorder, but it typically begins in late adolescence or early adulthood. The ratio of females to males with agoraphobia is 2:1.

Adverse childhood experiences and stressful life events are associated with the development of agoraphobia. Families of origin are often described as emotionally cool and overprotective. Genetics are also implicated in this disorder. Agoraphobia has a strong heritability factor of 61%.

Before the onset of this fear-based disorder, many individuals will experience other anxiety disorders, such as phobias, panic, and social anxiety. After the onset of agoraphobia, individuals often experience depressive disorders and alcohol use disorder.

EVIDENCE-BASED PRACTICE

Talk Therapy for Social Anxiety May Preserve Cellular Health

Problem

Telomeres are compound structures found at the end of chromosomes. Attrition of telomeres is a hallmark of cellular aging. Shorter telomeres have been found in individuals with anxiety disorders such as social anxiety disorder.

Purpose of Study

To determine if cognitive-behavioral therapy (CBT) could counteract telomere shortening and improve social anxiety symptoms.

Methods

Participants were screened for social anxiety disorder prior to 9 weeks of online CBT and again thereafter. Researchers measured two telomere-protective blood elements—telomerase and the antioxidant enzyme glutathione peroxidase (GPx)—along with median telomere length.

Key Findings

- Social anxiety scores dropped significantly after the CBT modules were completed.
- Telomere length and telomerase activity did not increase after treatment.

- Increased telomerase activity was associated with decreased social anxiety.
- Lower pretreatment telomerase predicted subsequent symptom improvement.
- GPx activity increased following treatment, along with significant symptom improvement.

Implications for Nursing Practice

Exposing ourselves to new and fairly complex chemical research puts nurses in a position to appreciate the biological complexity of psychiatric disorders. Knowing that traditional talk therapy actually results in the preservation of telomeres and improved anxiety symptoms allows nurses to educate patients on its importance.

Mansson, K. N. T., Lindqvist, D., Yang, L. L., Svanborg, C., Isung, J., Nilsonne, G. ... Furmark, T. (2019). Improvement in indices of cellular protection after psychological treatment for social anxiety disorder. *Translational Psychiatry, 9*, 340.

Generalized Anxiety Disorder

The key pathological feature of **generalized anxiety disorder** is excessive worry. Children, teens, and adults may experience this worry, which is out of proportion to the true impact of events or situations.

Common worries in generalized anxiety disorder are inadequacy in interpersonal relationships, job responsibilities, finances, and health of family members. Because of this worry, huge amounts of time are spent in preparing for activities. Putting things off and avoidance are key symptoms and may result in lateness or absence from school or employment and overall social isolation. Family members and friends are overtaxed as the person with this disorder seeks continual reassurance and perseverates about meaningless details.

Sleep disturbance is common because the individual worries about the day's events and real or imagined mistakes, reviews past problems, and anticipates future difficulties. Fatigue is a noticeable side effect of this sleep deprivation.

The 12-month prevalence rate of generalized anxiety disorder is nearly 1% in adolescents and nearly 3% in adults. Over a lifetime, the risk of this disorder is 9%. The ratio of affected females to males is 2:1.

Parental overprotection and adverse experiences are associated with anxiety disorders. Genetics accounts for one-third of the risk of developing generalized anxiety disorder.

This anxiety problem is often comorbid with major depressive disorder. Other anxiety disorders frequently accompany generalized anxiety disorder.

Refer to Table 15.6 for a generic care plan for generalized anxiety disorder. The *DSM-5* box contains diagnostic criteria for generalized anxiety disorder.

TABLE 15.6 Generic Care Plan for Generalized Anxiety Disorder

Priority diagnosis: Impaired coping related to persistent anxiety, fatigue, difficulty concentrating.

Outcome criteria: Patient will maintain role performance.

Short-Term Goal	Intervention	Rationale
1. Patient will state that immediate distress is relieved by end of session.	1a. Stay with patient. 1b. Speak slowly and calmly. 1c. Use short simple sentences. 1d. Assure patient that you are in control and can assist him or her. 1e. Give brief directions. 1f. Decrease excessive stimuli; provide quiet environment. 1g. After assessing level of anxiety, administer appropriate dose of antianxiety drug as needed.	1a. Conveys acceptance and ability to give help. 1b. Conveys calm and promotes security. 1c. Promotes comprehension. 1d. Counters feeling of loss of control that accompanies severe anxiety. 1e. Reduces indecision. Conveys belief that patient can respond in a healthy manner. 1f. Reduces need to focus on diverse stimuli. Promotes ability to concentrate. 1g. Reduces anxiety and allows patient to use coping skills.
2. Patient will be able to identify precipitants of anxiety by (date).	2a. Encourage patient to discuss preceding events. 2b. Link, as the result of a stressor, patient's behavior to feelings. 2c. Teach a cognitive therapy principle: Anxiety is the result of automatic thinking with a dysfunctional appraisal of a situation. 2d. Ask questions that clarify and dispute illogical thinking: "What evidence do you have?" "Are you basing that conclusion on fact or feeling?" "What's the worst thing that could happen?" 2e. Encourage patient to provide an alternative interpretation.	2a. Promotes future change through identification of stressors. 2b. Promotes self-awareness. 2c. Provides a basis for behavioral change. 2d. Helps promote accurate cognition. 2e. Broadens perspective. Helps patient think in a new way about problem or symptom.
3. Patient will identify strengths and coping skills by (date).	3a. Identify what has provided relief in the past. 3b. Have patient write assessment of strengths. 3c. Reframe situation in ways that are positive.	3a. Provides awareness of self as individual with some ability to cope. 3b. Increases self-acceptance. 3c. Provides a new perspective and converts distorted thinking.

DSM-5 CRITERIA FOR GENERALIZED ANXIETY DISORDER

A. Excessive anxiety and worry (apprehensive expectation) occurring more days than not for at least 6 months about a number of events or activities (such as work or school performance).
B. The individual finds it difficult to control the worry.
C. The anxiety and worry are associated with three (or more) of the following six symptoms (with at least some symptoms having been present for more days than not for the previous 6 months):
   Note: Only one item is required for children.
   1. Restlessness or feeling keyed up or on edge
   2. Being easily fatigued
   3. Difficulty concentrating or mind going blank
   4. Irritability
   5. Muscle tension
   6. Sleep disturbance (difficulty falling or staying asleep, or restless, unsatisfying sleep)
D. The anxiety, worry, or physical symptoms cause clinically significant distress or impairment in social, occupational, or other important areas of functioning.
E. The disturbance is not attributable to the physiological effects of a substance (e.g., a drug of abuse, a medication) or another medical condition (e.g., hyperthyroidism).
F. The disturbance is not better explained by another mental disorder (e.g., anxiety or worry about having panic attacks in panic disorder, negative evaluation in social anxiety disorder, contamination or other obsessions in obsessive-compulsive disorder, separation from attachment figures in separation anxiety disorder, reminders of traumatic events in posttraumatic stress disorder, gaining weight in anorexia nervosa, physical complaints in somatic symptom disorder, perceived appearance flaws in body dysmorphic disorder, having a serious illness in illness anxiety disorder, or the content of delusional beliefs in schizophrenia or delusional disorder).

Reprinted with permission from American Psychiatric Association. (2013). *Diagnostic and statistical manual* (5th ed.). Washington, DC: Author.

TABLE 15.7 Common Medical Causes of Anxiety

System	Disorders
Respiratory	Chronic obstructive pulmonary disease Pulmonary embolism Asthma Hypoxia Pulmonary edema
Cardiovascular	Angina pectoris Arrhythmias Congestive heart failure Hypertension Hypotension Mitral valve prolapse
Endocrine	Hyperthyroidism Hypoglycemia Pheochromocytoma Carcinoid syndrome Hypercortisolism
Neurological	Delirium Essential tremor Complex partial seizures Parkinson's disease Akathisia Otoneurological disorders Postconcussion syndrome
Metabolic	Hypercalcemia Hyperkalemia Hyponatremia Porphyria

Other Anxiety Disorders

Selective mutism is a condition where children do not speak owing to fears of negative responses or evaluations. They tend to speak at home around immediate family members. When they are engaged in activities that do not require speech, these children seem comfortable.

Substance-induced anxiety disorder is characterized by symptoms of anxiety, panic attacks, obsessions, and compulsions that develop with the use of a substance (e.g., alcohol, cocaine, heroin, hallucinogens).

In **anxiety due to a medical condition**, the individual's symptoms of anxiety are a direct physiological result of a medical condition, such as hyperthyroidism, pulmonary embolism, or cardiac dysrhythmias. To determine whether the anxiety symptoms are due to a medical condition, a careful and comprehensive assessment of multiple factors is necessary. Refer to Table 15.7 for a list of medical disorders that may contribute to anxiety symptoms.

Cultural Considerations

Sociocultural variation in symptoms of anxiety disorders has been noted. In some cultures, individuals express anxiety through somatic symptoms, whereas in others, cognitive symptoms predominate. Panic attacks in Latin Americans and northern Europeans often involve sensations of choking, smothering, numbness, or tingling as well as fear of dying. In other cultural groups, panic attacks involve fear of magic or witchcraft. Social anxiety in Japanese and Korean cultures may relate to beliefs that the individual's blushing, eye contact, or body odor is offensive to others. Refer to Chapter 5 for more discussion of cultural issues.

CONSIDERING CULTURE

Attack of the Nerves in Hispanic People

Technology and the commonplace of travel have resulted in a "smaller" world. Psychiatric–mental health nurses in the United States will be exposed to culture-bound syndromes with which they may be unfamiliar.

One example of a culture-bound syndrome is *ataque de nervios*, or "attack of the nerves." This is a disorder found primarily among Hispanic populations in response to stressful events such as a death, acute family discord, or witnessing an accident. Symptoms are dramatic: sudden trembling, faintness, palpitations, out-of-control shouting, heat that moves from the chest to the head, and seizure-like activity. After the episode, the affected individual often has little memory of it. This disorder is more common among socially disadvantaged females with less than a high school education.

CONSIDERING CULTURE—cont'd

What do these symptoms sound like to you? Some clinicians and researchers believe that they are closely related to an anxiety disorder and could even be a form of panic attack. Unlike people who have panic attacks, individuals with this disorder are responding to a precipitating event, and they do not typically experience fear or apprehension before the attack.

Adapted from Chen, J. A., Durham, M. P., Madu, A., Trinh, N. H., Fricchione, G. L., & Henderson, D. C. (2018). Culture and psychiatry. In T. A. Stern, O. Freudenreich, F. A. Smith, G. L. Fricchione, & J. F. Rosenbaum (Eds.), *Massachusetts General Hospital comprehensive clinical psychiatry* (7th ed.). St. Louis, MO: Elsevier.

APPLICATION OF THE NURSING PROCESS

ASSESSMENT

General Assessment

People with anxiety disorders rarely need hospitalization unless they are suicidal. Most of these individuals are encountered incidentally in a variety of community settings. A common example is someone taken in for emergency care to rule out a heart attack when in fact the individual is experiencing a panic attack. It is essential to determine whether anxiety is the primary problem, as in an anxiety disorder, or secondary to another cause, such as medical condition or substance use.

Your assessment should be patient centered to be helpful or meaningful. First and foremost is the recognition that patients are the experts when it comes to their own illnesses. Elicit information about what has helped in the past. Identify expectations for the patient's personal participation in care and for the family's or significant other's participation in care. Assess for specific cultural, ethnic, and social backgrounds that may affect the care that you and the patient plan.

Objectively, a variety of scales are available to measure anxiety and anxiety-related symptoms. Phobias are measured on the Fear Questionnaire and panic symptoms are measured on the Panic Disorder Severity Scale. The Severity Measure for Generalized Anxiety Disorder in Adults is a popular tool for measuring anxiety (Fig. 15.2). High scores may indicate generalized anxiety disorder or panic disorder, although it is important to note that high anxiety scores may also point to major depressive disorder. Another measure, with identical assessment items, is available for people 11 to 17 years of age.

Self-Assessment

As a nurse working with an individual with an anxiety disorder, you may have feelings of frustration, especially if it seems that the symptoms are a matter of choice or under the patient's control. Consider your response to a person with phobias. The patient often acknowledges that the fear is exaggerated and unrealistic yet continues to engage in avoidant behavior.

Behavioral change is often accomplished slowly. The recovery process is different from what is seen in physical disorders, such as an infection. After being treated with antibiotics, an infection may improve in as little as 24 hours. Planning outcomes in small attainable steps can help to prevent you from

ASSESSMENT GUIDELINES

Anxiety

1. Ensure that a physical and neurological examination is conducted to help determine whether the anxiety is primary or secondary to another psychiatric disorder, medical condition, or substance use.
2. Determine the patient's current level of anxiety (mild, moderate, severe, or panic).
3. Assess for the potential for self-harm and suicidal ideation. People suffering from high levels of intractable anxiety may become desperate and attempt suicide.
4. Perform a psychosocial assessment. Always ask the person, "What is going on in your life that may be contributing to your anxiety?" The patient may identify a problem (stressful marriage, recent loss, stressful job, or school situation) that could be addressed by counseling.

feeling overwhelmed by a patient's slow progress and help the patient gain a sense of control.

NURSING DIAGNOSIS

The *International Council of Nursing Practice* ([ICNP] International Council of Nurses, 2019) provides nursing diagnoses that are useful for patients with anxiety disorders. Obviously, a nursing diagnosis of *anxiety*—with a specification of mild, moderate, severe, or panic—provides the basis for care. Other diagnoses useful in this population are *impaired socialization, fear, avoiding, impaired coping, separation anxiety,* and *chronic low self-esteem.*

OUTCOMES IDENTIFICATION

During the outcomes identification step in the nursing process, outcomes and goals—individualized to the patient and the patient's situation—are identified. Specific, measurable, and realistic statements are developed that will guide the evaluation phase of the nursing process. Priority setting is established in this step, ranking the order of importance and urgency.

Outcomes should directly address the problem state in the nursing diagnosis. For example, an outcome for a nursing diagnosis of *anxiety* (moderate) would logically be *reduced anxiety.* Likewise, the nursing diagnosis of *impaired socialization* would be paired with *improved socialization* as an outcome. Outcomes are linked with signs and symptoms and nursing diagnoses in Table 15.8.

PLANNING

If possible, the patient should be encouraged to participate actively in planning. By sharing decision making with the patient, you can increase the likelihood that the treatment regimen will be successful. Owning responsibility for health outcomes improves adherence. Shared planning is especially appropriate for someone with mild or moderate anxiety. When experiencing severe levels of anxiety, patients may be unable to participate in planning and the nurse may be required to take a more directive role.

IMPLEMENTATION

When you are working with patients with anxiety disorders, first determine what level of anxiety they are experiencing. A

Severity Measure for Generalized Anxiety Disorder—Adult

Name: _____ Age: _____ Sex: Male ☐ Female ☐ Date: _____

Instructions: The following questions ask about thoughts, feelings, and behaviors, often tied to concerns about family, health, finances, school, and work. **Please respond to each item by marking (✓ or x) one box per row.**

During the PAST 7 DAYS, I have...	Never	Occasionally	Half of the time	Most of the time	All of the time	Clinician use — Item Score
1 felt moments of sudden terror, fear, or fright	☐ 0	☐ 1	☐ 2	☐ 3	☐ 4	
2 felt anxious, worried, or nervous	☐ 0	☐ 1	☐ 2	☐ 3	☐ 4	
3 had thoughts of bad things happening, such as family tragedy, ill health, loss of a job, or accidents	☐ 0	☐ 1	☐ 2	☐ 3	☐ 4	
4 felt a racing heart, sweaty, trouble breathing, faint, or shaky	☐ 0	☐ 1	☐ 2	☐ 3	☐ 4	
5 felt tense muscles, felt on edge or restless, or had trouble relaxing or trouble sleeping	☐ 0	☐ 1	☐ 2	☐ 3	☐ 4	
6 avoided, or did not approach or enter, situations about which I worry	☐ 0	☐ 1	☐ 2	☐ 3	☐ 4	
7 left situations early or participated only minimally due to worries	☐ 0	☐ 1	☐ 2	☐ 3	☐ 4	
8 spent lots of time making decisions, putting off making decisions, or preparing for situations, due to worries	☐ 0	☐ 1	☐ 2	☐ 3	☐ 4	
9 sought reassurance from others due to worries	☐ 0	☐ 1	☐ 2	☐ 3	☐ 4	
10 needed help to cope with anxiety (e.g., alcohol or medication, superstitious objects, or other people)	☐ 0	☐ 1	☐ 2	☐ 3	☐ 4	
Total/partial raw score:						
Prorated total raw score: (if 1–2 items left unanswered)						
Average total score:						

Fig. 15.2 Methods of measuring the severity of generalized anxiety disorder in adults.

general framework for anxiety interventions can then be built on a solid foundation.

Mild to Moderate Levels of Anxiety

A person experiencing a mild to moderate level of anxiety is still able to solve problems. However, the ability to concentrate decreases as anxiety increases. A patient can be helped to focus and solve problems when you use specific nursing communication techniques such as asking open-ended questions, giving broad openings, and exploring and seeking clarification. Closing off topics of communication and bringing up irrelevant topics can increase a person's anxiety, making the nurse, not the patient, feel better.

Reducing the patient's anxiety level and preventing escalation to more distressing levels can be aided by providing a calm presence, recognizing the anxious person's distress, and being willing to listen. Evaluation of effective past coping mechanisms is also useful. Often, you can help the patient consider alternatives to problem situations and offer activities that may temporarily relieve feelings of inner tension. Table 15.9 identifies interventions that can be useful in helping people who are experiencing mild to moderate levels of anxiety.

TABLE 15.8   Signs and Symptoms, Nursing Diagnoses, and Outcomes of Anxiety-Related Disorders

Signs and Symptoms	Nursing Diagnoses	Outcomes
Separation from significant others, concern that a panic attack will occur, exposure to phobic object or situation, fear of panic attacks	*Anxiety (moderate, severe, panic)*	Reduced anxiety: Monitors intensity of anxiety, uses relaxation techniques, decreases environmental stimuli as needed, controls anxiety response, maintains role performance
Unable to attend social functions or become employed, anxiety interferes with the ability to work, avoidance behaviors (phobia, agoraphobia)	*Impaired coping*	Improved coping: Identifies ineffective coping patterns, asks for assistance, seeks information about illness and treatment, identifies multiple coping strategies, modifies lifestyle as needed

International Council of Nursing Practice. (2019). ICNP browser. Retrieved from https://www.icn.ch/what-we-do/projects/ehealth/icnp-browser. ICNP is owned and copyrighted by the International Council of Nurses (ICN). Reproduced with permission of the copyright holder.

Severe to Panic Levels of Anxiety

A person experiencing a severe to panic level of anxiety is unable to solve problems and may have a poor grasp of what is happening in the environment. Unproductive relief behaviors may take over, and the person may not be in control.

Priority nursing interventions are aimed at providing for the safety of the patient and others and to meet physical needs, such as the requirement for fluids and for rest to prevent exhaustion. Anxiety-reducing measures may take the form of guiding the person to a quiet environment. The use of medications and restraints/seclusion may have to be considered. As always, medications and restraints should be used only after other less restrictive interventions have failed to decrease a patent's anxiety to a safe level.

Because individuals experiencing severe to panic anxiety are unable to solve problems, the techniques suggested for communicating with people with mild to moderate levels of anxiety are not as effective at more severe levels. Patients experiencing severe to panic anxiety are out of control, so they need to know that they are safe from their own impulses. Firm, short, and simple statements are useful. Reinforcing commonalities in the environment and pointing out reality when there are distortions can also be useful interventions. Table 15.10 suggests some basic nursing interventions for patients with severe to panic anxiety.

Anxiety management and reduction are primary concerns for nurses working with patients who have anxiety disorders, but such patients may also have a variety of other needs. In developing a plan of care, the psychiatric–mental health registered nurse can utilize the *Psychiatric-Mental Health Nursing: Scope and Standards of Practice* (American Nurses Association [ANA] et al., 2014).

Guidelines for basic nursing interventions are as follows:

1. Use counseling, milieu therapy, promotion of self-care activities, pharmacotherapy, biological, and health teaching interventions.
2. Guide patients through slowing exercises along with progressive muscle relaxation.
3. Identify community resources that can offer the patient specialized treatment proven to be highly effective for people with a variety of anxiety disorders.
4. Identify community support groups for people with specific anxiety disorders and their families.

Counseling

Basic-level psychiatric–mental health registered nurses use counseling to reduce anxiety, enhance coping and communication skills, and intervene in crises. When patients request or prefer to use integrative therapies, the nurse can discuss pros and cons and provide teaching as appropriate.

Health Teaching and Health Promotion

Health teaching is a significant nursing intervention for patients with anxiety disorders. Patients may conceal symptoms for years before seeking treatment and often come to the attention of healthcare providers during a co-occurring problem. People with panic disorder and generalized anxiety disorder seem to be more motivated to get treatment than those with other anxiety disorders, and most seek help during the first year of symptoms (Wang et al., 2005).

Teaching about the specific disorder and available effective treatments is a major step toward improving the quality of life of those with anxiety disorders. Whether in a community or hospital setting, nurses can teach patients about the signs and symptoms of anxiety disorders, presumed causes or risk factors (especially substance use), medications, the use of relaxation techniques, and the benefits of psychotherapy.

Relaxation exercises for breathing or muscle groups are extremely useful in initiating a relaxation response. The relaxation response is the opposite of the stress response and results in a reduced heart rate and breathing and relaxed muscles. Refer to Chapter 10 for a description of different approaches to relaxation.

Teamwork and Safety

As mentioned earlier, most patients with anxiety disorders can be treated successfully as outpatients. Hospital admission is necessary only if severe anxiety or compulsive symptoms interfere with the individual's health or if the individual is suicidal. When hospitalization is necessary, the healthcare team can be especially effective by doing the following:

- Collaborating to develop a multidisciplinary treatment plan to address goals, interventions, and outcomes that includes the patient's input
- Evaluating and refining the plan of care at regular intervals
- Documenting the plan and other essential communication electronically through an interactive and secure system

TABLE 15.9 Interventions for Mild to Moderate Levels of Anxiety

Priority diagnosis: Anxiety (moderate) related to situational event or psychological stress, as evidenced by increase in vital signs, moderate discomfort, narrowing of perceptual field, and selective inattention.

Intervention	Rationale
Help the patient identify anxiety. "Are you comfortable right now?"	It is important to validate observations with the patient, name the anxiety, and start to work with the patient to lower anxiety.
Anticipate anxiety-provoking situations.	Escalation of anxiety to a more disorganizing level is prevented.
Use nonverbal language to demonstrate interest (e.g., lean forward, maintain eye contact, nod your head).	Verbal and nonverbal messages should be consistent. The presence of an interested person provides a stabilizing focus.
Encourage the patient to talk about feelings and concerns.	When concerns are stated aloud, problems can be discussed and feelings of isolation decreased.
Avoid closing off avenues of communication that are important to the patient. Focus on the patient's concerns.	When staff anxiety increases, changing the topic or offering advice is common but leaves the person isolated.
Ask questions to clarify what is being said. "I'm not sure what you mean. Give me an example."	Increased anxiety results in the scattering of thoughts. Clarification helps patients to identify their thoughts and feelings.
Help the patient to identify thoughts or feelings before the onset of anxiety. "What were you thinking right before you started to feel anxious?"	The patient is helped to identify thoughts and feelings, and problem solving is facilitated.
Encourage problem solving with the patient.[a]	Encouraging patients to explore alternatives increases their sense of control and decreases anxiety.
Help the patient to develop alternative solutions to a problem through role-play or modeling behaviors.	The patient is encouraged to try out alternative behaviors and solutions.
Explore behaviors that have worked to relieve the patient's anxiety in the past.	The patient is encouraged to mobilize successful coping mechanisms and strengths.
Provide outlets for working off excess energy (e.g., walking, playing ping-pong, dancing, exercising).	Physical activity can provide relief of built-up tension, increase muscle tone, and increase endorphin levels.

[a]Patients experiencing mild to moderate anxiety levels can solve problems.

TABLE 15.10 Interventions for Severe to Panic Levels of Anxiety

Priority diagnosis: Anxiety (severe, panic) related to perception of a severe threat as evidenced by verbal or physical acting out, extreme immobility, sense of impending doom, and inability to solve problems.

Intervention	Rationale
Maintain a calm manner.	Anxiety is communicated interpersonally. The quiet calm of the nurse can serve to calm the patient. The presence of anxiety can escalate anxiety in the patient.
Always remain with the person experiencing an acute, severe, or panic level of anxiety.	Alone with immense anxiety, a person feels abandoned. A caring face may be the patient's only contact with reality when confusion becomes overwhelming.
Minimize environmental stimuli. Move to a quieter setting, and stay with the patient.	Helps to minimize further escalation of the patient's anxiety.
Use clear and simple statements and repetition.	A person experiencing a severe to panic level of anxiety has difficulty concentrating and processing information.
Use a low-pitched voice; speak slowly.	A high-pitched voice can convey anxiety. Low pitch can decrease anxiety.
Reinforce reality if distortions occur (e.g., seeing objects that are not there or hearing voices when no one is present).	Anxiety can be reduced by focusing on and validating what is going on in the environment.
Listen for themes in communication.	In severe to panic levels of anxiety, verbal communication themes may be the only indication of the patient's thoughts or feelings.
Attend to physical and safety needs when necessary (e.g., need for warmth, fluids, elimination, pain relief, family contact).	High levels of anxiety may obscure the patient's awareness of physical needs.
Because safety is an overall goal, physical limits may have to be set. Speak in a firm, authoritative voice: "You may not hit anyone here. If you can't control yourself, we will help you."	A person who is out of control is often terrorized. Staff must offer the patient and others protection from destructive and self-destructive impulses.
Provide opportunities for exercise (e.g., walk with nurse, punching bag, ping-pong game).	Physical activity helps channel and dissipate tension and may temporarily lower anxiety.
When a person is constantly moving or pacing, offer high-calorie fluids.	Dehydration and exhaustion must be prevented.
Assess need for medication or seclusion after other interventions have been tried and have been unsuccessful.	Exhaustion and physical harm to self and others must be prevented.

- Identifying specific members of the treatment team to be responsible for carrying out specific actions of the plan
- Maximizing safety through the provision of calm and consistent care
- Stressing the value of unconditional positive regard
- Maintaining a safe environment with an atmosphere of low-level stimulation
- Providing ongoing education and training for the team to recognize escalating or problematic behaviors

Promotion of Self-Care Activities

Respecting patients' preferences for how involved they are in self-care while recognizing that they may require more or less guidance depending on their level of ability is a fine balance. Including the patient in care decisions is essential whenever possible. Patients with anxiety disorders are usually able to meet their own basic physical needs. Self-care activities that are most likely to be affected are discussed in the following sections.

Nutrition and Fluid Intake

Patients with high levels of anxiety are not focused on eating and drinking. Some phobic patients may be so afraid of germs that they cannot eat. In home settings, individuals who hoard may have created an environment that is so dysfunctional that normal intake may be impossible. Likewise, people who engage in ritualistic behaviors may be too involved with their rituals to take time to eat and drink. In general, a nutritious diet with snacks should be provided. Adequate intake should be firmly encouraged, but power struggles are to be avoided. Weighing patients frequently (e.g., three times a week) is useful in assessing nutrition.

Personal Hygiene and Grooming

Some patients with anxiety disorders are indecisive about bathing or about what clothing they should wear. For the latter, limiting the choice to two outfits may be helpful. In the event of severe indecisiveness, you may just have to present the patient with the clothing to be worn. You may also have to remain with the patient to give simple directions: "Put on your shirt. Now put on your slacks." Matter-of-fact support can help patients to perform as much of a task independently as possible. Encourage patients to express their thoughts and feelings about self-care. Such communication can provide a basis for future health teaching or for ongoing dialogue about the patient's abilities.

Sleep

Patients experiencing anxiety disorders frequently have difficulty sleeping, particularly in falling asleep. Patients with generalized anxiety disorder often experience sleep disturbance from nightmares. Those with separation anxiety disorder may have such profound fears that sleep seems impossible. They may perform rituals to the exclusion of resting and sleeping, thus becoming physically exhausted. Teaching about ways of promoting sleep (e.g., a warm bath, warm milk, and

relaxing music) and monitoring sleep through a sleep record can be useful. Chapter 19 offers an in-depth discussion of sleep disturbances.

EVALUATION

Identified outcomes serve as the basis for evaluation. In general, evaluation of outcomes for patients with anxiety disorders deals with questions such as the following:

- Is the patient experiencing a reduced level of anxiety?
- Does the patient recognize symptoms as anxiety related?
- Does the patient continue to display signs and symptoms such as obsessions, compulsions, phobias, worrying, or other symptoms of anxiety disorders? If these are still present, are they more or less frequent? More or less intense?
- Is the patient able to use new behaviors to manage anxiety?
- Does the patient perform self-care activities adequately?
- Can the patient maintain satisfying interpersonal relations?
- Is the patient able to assume usual roles?

TREATMENT MODALITIES
Biological Treatments
Pharmacotherapy

Several classes of medications have been found to be effective in the treatment of anxiety disorders. Table 15.11 identifies medications approved by the US Food and Drug Administration (FDA) for the treatment of anxiety disorders. Refer to Chapter 3 for a more detailed explanation of the actions of psychotropic medications.

Antidepressants. Selective serotonin reuptake inhibitors (SSRIs) are considered a first line of defense in most anxiety-related disorders. They include paroxetine (Paxil), fluoxetine (Prozac), escitalopram (Lexapro), and sertraline (Zoloft). Some exert more of an activating effect than others and may actually increase anxiety initially. Fluoxetine and sertraline tend to be the most activating. Paroxetine tends to have a more calming effect than the other SSRIs. Antidepressants have the secondary benefit of treating comorbid depressive disorders.

Venlafaxine (Effexor), a serotonin norepinephrine reuptake inhibitor (SNRI), is another first line of defense used in the treatment of several anxiety disorders. Another SNRI, duloxetine (Cymbalta), is effective in the treatment of generalized anxiety disorder. See Chapter 14 for a full discussion of antidepressants.

Antianxiety drugs. Antianxiety drugs are often used to treat the somatic and psychological symptoms of anxiety disorders. When moderate or severe anxiety is reduced, patients are better able to participate in the treatment of their underlying problems. Benzodiazepines are most commonly used because they have a quick onset of action. However, owing to the potential for dependence, these medications should be used only for short periods of time, or until other medications or treatments reduce symptoms.

An important nursing intervention is to monitor for side effects of the benzodiazepines, including sedation, ataxia, and decreased cognitive function. Paradoxical reactions—reactions that are the exact opposite of the intended responses—sometimes occur. Symptoms such as anxiety, agitation, talkativeness, and loss of impulse control may occur when medications of this class are used. Benzodiazepines are not recommended for patients with a substance use disorder. They are also not recommended for older adults owing to risk of delirium, falls, and fractures.

The decision to use benzodiazepines during pregnancy should be made by weighing the risk of fetal exposure versus the risk of an untreated anxiety disorder (US Department of Health and Human Services, 2012). Benzodiazepine use shortly before delivery can result in a dystonia and muscle weakness in the newborn known as floppy infant syndrome. Withdrawal symptoms in the neonate have been known to occur. Prenatal benzodiazepine exposure increases the risk of oral cleft lip and palate, although the absolute risk increases by only 0.01%. The FDA warns against breastfeeding while taking these drugs, since they pass into breast milk.

Box 15.1 summarizes important information for patient teaching.

Buspirone (BuSpar) is an alternative antianxiety medication that does not cause dependence, but it takes 2 to 4 weeks for it to reach its full effect. The drug may be used for long-term treatment and should be taken regularly. Side effects include dizziness, nausea, headache, nervousness, lightheadedness, and excitement.

Buspirone is not recommended for individuals with impaired hepatic or renal function, as increased plasma levels may result and the drug's half-life may be lengthened. There is no direct evidence that this medication poses a danger to the developing infant. However, the FDA recommends using the drug during pregnancy and breastfeeding only if clearly necessary.

Other classes of medications. Other classes of medications used to treat anxiety disorders include beta blockers, antihistamines, anticonvulsants, and antipsychotics. These agents are often added if the first course of treatment is ineffective. Beta-blockers block the receptors that, when stimulated, cause the heart to beat faster. They reduce the physical manifestations of anxiety by slowing the heart rate and reducing blushing; they have been used to treat social anxiety disorder.

BOX 15.1   Patient and Family Teaching: Antianxiety Drugs

1. Caution the patient about the following:
   Not to change the dose or frequency of medication without consulting the prescriber.
   These medications may make it unsafe to handle mechanical equipment (e.g., cars, saws, and machinery).
   Avoid using both alcoholic beverages and antianxiety medications, as this may lead to unsafe depressant effects.
   Avoid drinking beverages containing caffeine because they will decrease the desired effects of the drug.
   Review prescription medications and doses that may cause or increase anxiety (e.g., thyroid hormones, steroids, decongestants).
2. Discuss with the prescriber the risks to the fetus and the risk of untreated anxiety disorders should pregnancy occur or be considered.
3. Discuss breastfeeding with the prescriber because these drugs are excreted in breast milk and could have adverse effects on the infant.
4. Teach the patient that:
   Quitting a benzodiazepine after the first month of daily use may cause withdrawal symptoms such as insomnia, irritability, nervousness, dry mouth, tremors, convulsions, and confusion.
   Medications should be taken with or shortly after meals or snacks to reduce gastrointestinal discomfort.
   Drug interactions can occur: For example, antacids may delay absorption; cimetidine interferes with metabolism of benzodiazepines, causing increased sedation; central nervous system depressants, such as alcohol and barbiturates, cause increased sedation.

TABLE 15.11   Drugs for Anxiety Disorders Approved by the US Food and Drug Administration

Anxiety Disorder	Selective Serotonin Reuptake Inhibitors	Serotonin Norepinephrine Reuptake Inhibitors	Benzodiazepines	Other
Generalized anxiety disorder	Escitalopram (Lexapro) Paroxetine (Paxil)	Venlafaxine (Effexor) Duloxetine (Cymbalta)	Alprazolam (Xanax) Chlordiazepoxide (Librium) Clorazepate (Tranxene) Diazepam (Valium) Lorazepam (Ativan) Oxazepam (Serax)	Buspirone (BuSpar)
Panic disorder	Fluoxetine (Prozac) Paroxetine (Paxil) Sertraline (Zoloft)	Venlafaxine (Effexor)	Alprazolam (Xanax) Clonazepam (Klonopin)	
Social anxiety disorder	Paroxetine (Paxil) Sertraline (Zoloft)	Venlafaxine (Effexor)		

US Food and Drug Administration. (2020). *FDA label repository*. Retrieved from labels.fda.gov.

Anticonvulsants have shown some benefit in the management of generalized anxiety disorder and social anxiety disorder. Gabapentin (Neurontin) and pregabalin (Lyrica), for example, are commonly prescribed.

Antihistamines, such as hydroxyzine (Vistaril), are safe nonaddictive alternatives to benzodiazepines. They are an especially good choice for treating patients with substance use problems. Antipsychotic medications are also used in treating more severe symptoms of anxiety disorders.

There are no FDA-approved drugs for the treatment of separation anxiety disorder and specific phobia. Despite the lack of approval, these conditions are often treated with antidepressants, antianxiety agents, and the other classes of medications previously described.

Pharmacotherapy in children and adolescents. A few drugs are approved specifically for anxiety disorders in children and adolescents. The SNRI duloxetine (Cymbalta) has FDA approval for children aged 7 to 17 years for generalized anxiety disorder. Medications approved for other age groups are still prescribed off label. For example, SSRIs are used to treat generalized anxiety disorder, panic disorder, and social anxiety disorder, all with good results.

Integrative medicine. Chapter 35 identifies a number of complementary practices or integrative therapies that people use to cope with stress in their lives. Herbal therapy and dietary supplements are commonly used, yet they are not subject to the same rigorous testing as prescription medications. Also, herbs and dietary supplements may not be uniformly prepared or dosed, and there is no guarantee of bioequivalence of the active compound among preparations. Problems that can arise with the use of psychotropic herbs include toxic side effects and herb-drug interactions. Nurses and other healthcare providers should stay current regarding these popular products in order to help their patients make informed decisions.

One example is kava, which is derived from the roots of *Piper methysticum,* a South American plant. Kava is used as a sedative with antianxiety effects. As an alternative to seeking professional care, people with anxiety disorders may try kava in the belief that herbs are safer than medications, but this herb has a dark side. In 2010, the FDA issued a warning regarding the risk of liver damage from kava, which is known to dramatically inhibit the P450 liver enzyme necessary for the metabolism of many medications. This inhibition can lead to liver failure, especially when kava is taken along with alcohol or other medications such as central nervous system depressants (antianxiety agents fall into this category).

Psychological Therapies

Psychiatric–mental health advanced practice registered nurses, like other advanced practice psychiatric professionals, are qualified to conduct individual and group psychotherapy. Two important forms of therapy for anxiety disorders are behavioral therapy and cognitive-behavioral therapy.

Behavioral Therapy

There are currently several forms of **behavioral therapy**, all of which involve teaching and physical practice of activities to decrease anxious or avoidant behavior in the following ways:

- **Modeling:** The therapist or significant other acts as a role model to demonstrate appropriate behavior in a feared situation, and then the patient imitates it. For example, the role model rides in an elevator with a patient who has claustrophobia.
- **Systematic desensitization:** The patient is gradually introduced to a feared object or experience through a series of steps, from the least frightening to the most frightening (graduated exposure). The patient is taught to use a relaxation technique at each step when the anxiety becomes overwhelming. For example, a patient with agoraphobia would start with opening the door to the house to go out on the steps and would then advance to attending a movie in a theater. The therapist may start with imagined situations in the office before moving on to in vivo (live) exposures.
- **Flooding:** Unlike systematic desensitization, this method exposes the patient to a large amount of an undesirable stimulus in an effort to extinguish the anxiety response. The patient learns through prolonged exposure that survival is possible and that anxiety diminishes spontaneously.
- **Thought stopping:** Through this technique a negative thought or obsession is interrupted. The patient may be instructed to say "Stop!" out loud when the idea comes to mind or to snap a rubber band worn on the wrist. This distraction briefly blocks the automatic undesirable thought and cues the patient to select an alternative, more positive idea. After learning the exercise, the patient gives the command silently.

Cognitive-Behavioral Therapy

Cognitive-behavioral therapy combines cognitive therapy with specific behavioral therapies to reduce the anxiety response. Cognitive-behavioral therapy includes cognitive restructuring, psychoeducation, breath restraining and muscle relaxation, teaching of self-monitoring for panic and other symptoms, and in vivo (real-life) exposure to feared objects or situations.

The cognitive model of anxiety disorder is based on the premise that people with these disorders overestimate the danger of situations and underestimate their own ability to handle them (Stein & Sareen, 2019). Therefore, triggering situations lead to catastrophic automatic thoughts. Patients are taught to monitor the thoughts that occur prior to anxiety responses, learn to challenge these thoughts, and replace them with a more realistic appraisal.

OBSESSIVE-COMPULSIVE DISORDERS

OCDs are a group of related disorders that all have obsessive-compulsive characteristics. Obsessions are thoughts, impulses, or images that persist and recur so that they cannot be dismissed from the mind even though the individual attempts to do so. Obsessions often seem senseless to the individual who experiences them (they are said to be ego dystonic), and their presence causes severe anxiety.

Compulsions are ritualistic behaviors individuals feel driven to perform in an attempt to reduce anxiety or prevent an imagined calamity. Performing the compulsive act temporarily reduces anxiety, but because the relief is only temporary, the compulsive act must be repeated again and again.

Until 2013, the American Psychiatric Association considered OCD an anxiety disorder, and it was a part of the anxiety disorders chapter in the *Diagnostic and Statistical Manual of Mental Disorders*, 4th edition. In the latest edition, *DSM-5*, OCD is grouped along with conditions that all have prominent obsessions and compulsions. These associated disorders were in a variety of other chapters in the previous edition of the *DSM*. The obsessive-compulsive and related disorders include the following:

- Obsessive-compulsive disorder
- Body dysmorphic disorder
- Hoarding disorder
- Trichotillomania (hair pulling) disorder
- Excoriation (skin picking) disorder

Obsessive-Compulsive Disorder

Obsessive-compulsive behavior exists along a continuum. Most sufferers may experience mildly obsessive-compulsive symptoms, such as nagging doubts as to whether a door is locked or the stove is turned off. These doubts require the person to go back to check the door or stove. Mild compulsions about timeliness, orderliness, and reliability are valued traits in US society.

At the pathological end of the continuum is **obsessive-compulsive disorder (OCD)**, with symptoms that occur on a daily basis and may involve issues of sexuality, violence, contamination, illness, or death. Pathological obsessions or compulsions cause marked distress to individuals who often feel humiliation and shame regarding these behaviors.

The rituals are time-consuming and interfere with normal routines, social activities, and relationships with others. Severe OCD occupies so much of the individual's mental process that the performance of cognitive tasks is impaired. English soccer player David Beckham has shared his struggle with OCD. He has a compulsion to count his clothes and line his magazines up in a straight line. Examples of common obsessions and compulsions are given in Table 15.12.

The 12-month prevalence of OCD is 1.2%. Females are slightly more affected, but males have an earlier age of onset (about 25% before age 10). Onset after age 35 is rare.

Sexual and physical abuse or trauma in childhood increase the risk of this disorder. Some children develop OCD along with a postinfectious autoimmune syndrome. Genetics are strongly associated with this disorder. First-degree relatives have twice the risk. Early-onset OCD results in a 10 times greater risk of the disorder appearing in first-degree relatives.

OCD tends to occur along with anxiety disorders 76% of the time. Other comorbid conditions for OCD include major depressive disorder, bipolar disorder, and eating disorders. About 30% of individuals with this problem also have a tic disorder.

See the *DSM-5* box for diagnostic criteria.

DSM-5 CRITERIA FOR OBSESSIVE-COMPULSIVE DISORDER

A. Presence of obsessions, compulsions, or both.
   Obsessions are defined by (1) and (2):
   1. Recurrent and persistent thoughts, urges, or images that are experienced, at some time during the disturbance, as intrusive and unwanted, and that in most individuals cause marked anxiety or distress.
   2. The individual attempts to ignore or suppress such thoughts, urges, or images or to neutralize them with some other thought or action (i.e., by performing a compulsion).
   3. Compulsions are defined by (1) and (2):
   4. Repetitive behaviors (e.g., handwashing, ordering, checking) or mental acts (e.g., praying, counting, repeating words silently) that the individual feels driven to perform in response to an obsession or according to rules that must be applied rigidly.
   5. The behaviors or mental acts are aimed at preventing or reducing anxiety or distress or preventing some dreaded event or situation; however, these behaviors or mental acts are not connected in a realistic way with what they are designed to neutralize or prevent or are clearly excessive.
   Note: Young children may not be able to articulate the aims of these behaviors or mental acts.
B. The obsessions or compulsions are time-consuming (e.g., take more than 1 hour per day) or cause clinically significant distress or impairment in social, occupational, or other important areas of functioning.
C. The obsessive-compulsive symptoms are not attributable to the physiological effects of a substance (e.g., a drug of abuse, a medication) or another medical condition.
D. The disturbance is not better explained by the symptoms of another mental disorder (e.g., excessive worries, as in generalized anxiety disorder; preoccupation with appearance, as in body dysmorphic disorder; difficulty discarding or parting with possessions, as in hoarding disorder; hair pulling, as in trichotillomania; skin picking, as in excoriation disorder; stereotypes, as in stereotypic movement disorder; ritualized eating behavior, as in eating disorders; preoccupation with substances or gambling, as in substance-related and addictive disorder; preoccupation with having an illness, as in illness anxiety disorder; sexual urges or fantasies, as in paraphilic disorders; impulses, as in disruptive, impulse-control, and conduct disorders; guilty ruminations, as in major depressive disorder; thought insertion or delusional preoccupations, as in schizophrenia spectrum and other psychotic disorders; or repetitive patterns of behavior, as in autism spectrum disorder.

Reprinted with permission from American Psychiatric Association. (2013). *Diagnostic and statistical manual* (5th ed.). Washington, DC: Author.

Body Dysmorphic Disorder

Body dysmorphic disorder was first described over a century ago and, just as then, it continues to be a challenge to treat. Patients with body dysmorphic disorder are commonly seen in community, psychiatric, cosmetic surgery, and dermatological settings. Although such patients tend to have a normal appearance, their preoccupation with an imagined defective body part results in obsessional thinking and compulsive behavior such as mirror checking and camouflaging. Their levels of insight vary. People may be well aware that their thoughts are distorted, or they may be completely sure about the existence of the defect.

False assumptions about the importance of appearance, fear of rejection by others, perfectionism, and the conviction of being disfigured lead to overwhelming emotions of

TABLE 15.12 Common Obsessions and Compulsions

Type of Obsession	Example	Accompanying Compulsion
Losing control and religious concerns	A middle-age man worries, "If I go to church, what will stop me from blurting out obscenities?"	Despite his desire to attend services, has not gone to church in 2 years.
Harm	"If I don't turn the light switch off, the room will catch on fire, and my mom will die while I am at school," worries a 9-year-old girl.	Returns to her room four times before school, checks that the light is turned off, and taps the four sides of the light switch.
Unwanted sexual thoughts	A young man has a recurrent thought: "What if I get a sexually transmitted disease from a prostitute during sleepwalking?"	Ritualistically locks the doors of the house with a key each night and hides his wallet.
Perfectionism	"My work is never second best," proclaims an administrative assistant.	Gets to work early, leaves work late, never has a messy desk, always completes tasks.
Violence	A man repeatedly has the thought "I should kill her" when he sees a blonde woman.	Abruptly turns head away from women and squints eyes to try to avoid seeing blondes.
Contamination	A woman ruminates, "Everything is covered in germs."	Avoids touching all objects; scrubs hands if forced to touch any object.
Superstitions	"All lists need to end in an even number," thinks a college professor.	Adds or deletes items from tests, agendas, and other numbered items.

disgust, shame, and depression. Patients are frequently concerned with their skin, hair, nose, stomach, teeth, weight, and breasts/chest. Men tend to be concerned with body build and the appearance of their genitals. Women focus on the appearance of their skin, stomach, weight, breasts, buttocks, thighs, legs, hips, and toes.

Often, the patient keeps the disorder secret for many years. The disorder is chronic and response to treatment is limited. Suicide risk is high in this population.

The prevalence of body dysmorphic disorder is slightly higher in females (2.5%) than males (2.2%). The incidence of this problem is higher among patients seeking cosmetic surgery, dermatology treatment, adult orthodontia, and oral/maxillofacial surgery.

Individuals with this disorder often come from homes where they were subjected to abuse and neglect. Body dysmorphic disorder seems to be related to OCD, because first-degree relatives often share those conditions.

The most common comorbid disorder is major depressive disorder, which usually comes on after body dysmorphic disorder. Social anxiety disorder, OCD, and substance use disorders are also seen with this disorder.

Hoarding Disorder

Have you ever reached the point where there is just too much clutter in your closet and you proceed to sort through it and make stacks labeled "keep," "give away," and "donate"? You probably have, and for most of us this is neither a pleasant nor a painful experience. For individuals with **hoarding disorder**, it would be extremely distressing. In fact, the accumulation of belongings that may have little or no value prevents some people from leading normal lives. In their homes, belongings cover every available surface and fill every drawer, cupboard, and closet. Usually, family and other guests can (or will) no longer visit. The problem may progress to the point where the home is nearly uninhabitable owing to unsafe and/or unsanitary conditions. Individuals who hoard may or may not be aware of the

problem and how the quest to collect has consumed their lives and alienated others.

It is difficult to determine the age of onset of this disorder, as children do not have the means to add to their collections, as adults do. Symptoms usually emerge in adolescence, begin to interfere with functioning in the 20s, and significantly impair functioning in the 30s. The condition worsens with each decade of life. Although more women are treated for hoarding disorder, it is likely that men are affected at much the same rate but do not seek treatment. Estimates of prevalence in the United Kingdom is about 1.5% (Nordsletten et al., 2013).

Indecisiveness is associated with hoarding. Stressful life events seem to precede the onset of symptoms. The disorder is strongly heritable, with a twin concordance rate (percentage of time one twin will be affected when the other one is) of 50%.

Nearly all hoarders (75%) also experience major depressive and/or anxiety disorders. Not surprisingly, about 20% of these individuals also have OCD. It is the presence of these other disorders that may cause them to seek treatment because they resist seeing hoarding as a problem.

Trichotillomania and Excoriation Disorder

Two OCDs are collectively known as body-focused repetitive behaviors. **Trichotillomania (hair-pulling disorder)** and **excoriation disorder (skin-picking disorder)** are two distressing problems that may result in varying degrees of disability, social stigma, and altered appearance. Either of these activities is irresistible to the individual, who typically tries to hide it. These disorders have been linked to symptoms of OCD. They occur more often in children than in adults and may begin as early as 1 year of age.

Trichotillomania (tricho·til·lo·ma·nia) may be one of the oldest recorded psychiatric problems. The phrase "I was so annoyed that I wanted to pull my hair out" attests to the anxiety-related component of the disorder. Typically it is the hair of the head, but it may be hair anywhere on the body, including eyebrows, eyelashes, pubic areas, axillae, and limbs. The amount of hair removed ranges from small patches to completely naked skin. For some, the pain brought on by hair pulling reduces their anxiety, as is the case of those who engage in cutting. Most individuals may be unaware of their behavior until they notice a wad of hair close by.

Trichophagia, or secretly swallowing the pulled hair, is common in this disorder. This may lead to hair masses, or trichobezoars, in the gastrointestinal system. The masses can be fatal if they progress to abdominal obstruction or perforation. You may be interested to know that this last condition is also referred to as the Rapunzel syndrome.

The disorder may begin in childhood, adolescence, or even adulthood and may last for weeks to decades. The 12-month prevalence in adolescents and adults is about 2%. Females are affected more frequently than males, with a ratio around 10:1. There is no gender difference among children.

The disorder seems to run in families. Individuals with relatives who have OCD tend to have higher rates of trichotillomania. People who pull their hair obsessively also often have major depressive disorder. Trichotillomania is often accompanied by excoriation disorder.

The skin-picking of **excoriation** (ex·co·ri·ay·shun) **disorder** is typically confined to the face, although other areas of the body may be targeted. As with hair pulling, the individual may engage in skin picking as a way to deal with stress and relieve anxiety, whereas others may engage in this activity without thinking about it. Most people occasionally pick at their skin, nails, and scabs. However, people with skin-picking disorder damage their skin. Fingers and fingernails are the usual implements, but nail cutters, tweezers, and the person's teeth may also be used. The most common areas of focus are the face, head, cuticles, back, arms and legs, and hands and feet. Complications include pain, sores, scars, and infections.

The lifetime prevalence of this problem is 1.4%, and 75% of those affected are females. The onset is in adolescence and frequently begins with conditions such as acne.

A risk factor for this disorder is having relatives with OCD. Excoriation disorder is often accompanied by OCDs and trichotillomania.

Other Compulsive Disorders

Substance-induced obsessive-compulsive and related disorders are characterized by obsessions and compulsions that develop with the use of a substance or within a month of stopping use of the substance. This diagnosis is based on a thorough history, physical examination, and laboratory findings. Drugs used to treat the movement disorders in Parkinson's disease have been reported to cause obsessions with gambling, irresistible urges for sex, and out-of-control spending. Substances that may cause obsessive-compulsive symptoms include the following:
- Amphetamines
- Cocaine
- Levodopa (L-dopa)
- Other stimulants/dopamine agonists
- Heavy metals
- Second-generation antipsychotics

In **obsessive-compulsive or related disorders due to a medical condition**, the individual's symptoms of obsessions and compulsions are a direct physiological result of a medical condition. To determine whether the symptoms are due to a medical condition, a careful and comprehensive assessment of multiple factors is necessary. Evidence must be present in the history, physical examination, or laboratory findings for this diagnosis. Medical conditions that may cause obsessive-compulsive symptoms include (Dougherty et al., 2019) the following:
- Cerebrovascular accident
- Central nervous system (CNS) neoplasm/tumor
- Head injury
- CNS infection (usually but not always streptococcal)

APPLICATION OF THE NURSING PROCESS
ASSESSMENT

People with OCDs rarely need hospitalization unless they are suicidal or have compulsions that cause injury (e.g., cutting self, causing infected sores from picking).

Objectively, a variety of scales are available to measure OCDs, and most can be found online. The American Psychiatric Association's comprehensive online list of assessment measures includes tools that one can access. An example of a tool for measuring severity of obsessive-compulsive behaviors is found in Fig. 15.3.

Self-Assessment

As a nurse working with an individual with an OCD, you may have feelings of frustration. This is especially true if it seems that the symptoms are a matter of choice or under the patient's control. The rituals of the patient with OCD may seriously slow your ability to complete certain nursing tasks within the usual time.

You may be mystified by body dysmorphic disorder: "How could anyone be that focused on her face and undergo so many plastic surgeries?" People who compulsively hoard may cause you to feel disgust: "They found dead animals in his house." The body-focused repetitive disorders may be severe and result in a badly altered appearance: "Why doesn't she just stop that?" It helps to remember that all of these OCDs are biologically based and similar to a faulty video loop that keeps playing back over and over.

NURSING DIAGNOSIS

The International Council of Nursing Practice (ICNP, 2019) provides nursing diagnoses that are useful for patients with OCDs. All of these disorders result in dysfunctional anxiety. Therefore, the nursing diagnosis *anxiety* can be applied to any patient with obsessions and compulsions. Likewise, *obsession* and *compulsive behavior* also apply to this group of disorders.

In the case of OCD with frequent handwashing, trichotillomania with hair pulling, and excoriation disorder with skin

The OCI-R is a self-rating scale that is designed to assess the severity and type of symptoms of those potentially dealing with OCD. The following statements refer to experiences that many people have in their everyday lives. Select the answer that best describes **how much** that experience has **distressed** or **bothered** you during the **past month.**

	Not at All	A Little	Moderately	A Lot	Extremely
1. I have saved up so many things that they get in the way.					
2. I check things more often than necessary.					
3. I get upset if objects are not arranged properly.					
4. I feel compelled to count while I am doing things.					
5. I find it difficult to touch an object when I know it has been touched by strangers or certain people.					
6. I find it difficult to control my own thoughts.					
7. I collect things that I don't need.					
8. I repeatedly check doors, windows, drawers, etc.					
9. I get upset if others change the way I have arranged things.					
10. I feel I have to repeat certain numbers.					
11. I sometimes have to wash or clean myself simply because I feel contaminated.					
12. I am upset by unpleasant thoughts that come into my mind against my will.					
13. I avoid throwing things away because I am afraid I might need them later.					
14. I repeatedly check gas and water taps and light switches after turning them off.					
15. I need things to be arranged in a particular way.					
16. I feel that there are good and bad numbers.					
17. I wash my hands more often and longer than necessary.					
18. I frequently get nasty thoughts and have difficulty in getting rid of them.					

Fig. 15.3 Obsessive-Compulsive Inventory–Revised (OCI-R). (Adaped from Foa, E. B., Huppert, J. D., Leiberg, S., Langner, R., Kichic, R., Hajcak, G., & Salkovskis, P. M. [2002]. The obsessive-compulsive inventory: Development and validation of a short version. *Psychological Assessment, 14*[4], 485–496.)

picking, *impaired skin integrity* and *risk for self-destructive behavior* may be priority diagnoses. *Disturbed body image* is an ideal diagnosis for body dysmorphic disorder. As with the anxiety disorders, other diagnoses useful in this population are *impaired socialization, fear, impaired coping,* and *chronic low self-esteem.*

OUTCOMES IDENTIFICATION

As we address the problem identified in the nursing diagnosis, specific outcomes become logical. Addressing the diagnoses in the previous paragraphs would result in the following:

- Reduced anxiety
- Improved skin integrity
- Reduced self-destructive behavior
- Improved body image
- Improved socialization
- Reduced fear
- Improved coping
- Improved self-esteem

PLANNING

Developing a patient-centered plan includes the patient as partner. Patients with OCDs tend to be resistant addressing dysfunctional behaviors. They will, however, discuss how the illness has affected their lives. As medication begins to alleviate the most severe obsessions and resultant compulsions, patients tend to become less resistive.

IMPLEMENTATION

Some patients, especially those with OCD, may be excessively neat and engage in time-consuming rituals associated with bathing and dressing. Hygiene, dressing, and grooming may take several hours.

As previously stated, maintenance of skin integrity may become a problem when the rituals involve excessive washing and the patient's skin becomes fissured and infected. Skin integrity is also a concern for individuals who pull their hair or pick at their skin.

Patients with severe OCD may be so involved with the performance of rituals that they may suppress the urge to void and defecate. Urinary tract infections and constipation may result. Interventions may include creating a regular schedule for taking the patient to the bathroom.

EVALUATION

OCDs disrupt an individual's ability focus on important and normal aspects of life. When you are evaluating a patient who has been obsessing and behaving compulsively, the acid test as to whether improvement is occurring is by assessing functioning and distress. Often, these improvements are quite small, but they should be recognized and affirmed. Families may be quite disrupted by the symptoms of these disorders, and evaluation of the families is an essential part of care.

TREATMENT MODALITIES

Biological Treatments

Pharmacotherapy

Several medications have FDA approval for the treatment of OCD. Most of these drugs are SSRIs, including fluoxetine (Prozac), fluvoxamine (Luvox), paroxetine (Paxil), and sertraline (Zoloft). Another approved drug, clomipramine (Anafranil), is part of one of the older classes called tricyclic antidepressants. While every medication used for OCD may not have FDA approval, they are still commonly prescribed. This includes other SSRIs and the SNRI venlafaxine (Effexor). Antipsychotic medications are sometimes used in conjunction with antidepressants to reduce severe symptoms.

There are no FDA-approved medications for body dysmorphic disorder, hoarding disorder, trichotillomania, or excoriation disorder. However, the same medications used for OCD—the SSRIs—are used to address the obsessive-compulsive features of these other disorders.

Pharmacotherapy for children and adolescents. Several drugs are approved specifically for OCD in children and adolescents. The FDA has approved four medications with age stipulations for their use. They are fluoxetine (Prozac) for ages 7 to 17, fluvoxamine (Luvox) for ages 8 to 17, sertraline (Zoloft) for ages 6 to 17, and clomipramine (Anafranil) for ages 10 to 17. Other non–FDA approved SSRIs are also used off label.

Brain-Based Therapies

Besides medication, there are few biological treatments available to disrupt the course of an OCD. Surgery has been used for those most severely affected. Gamma knife surgery is used to purposely cause irreversible damage, or a lesion, in a specific area of the brain, thus disconnecting overactive circuits or regions.

A reversible surgical treatment used for OCD is deep brain stimulation (DBS). The FDA approved DBS as an adjunct to medications in treatment-resistant OCD in adults who have failed at least three SSRI trials. In DBS, electrodes are surgically placed bilaterally in the subthalamic nucleus of the brain. Then, an implanted pulse generator in the chest activates a low-dose current for a specified period of time (several months in some cases). In a recent meta-analysis of studies about DBS for OCD, it was reported to result in a 39% reduction of obsessive-compulsive symptoms (Vicheva et al., 2020). Adverse events were reported as generally mild. However, there have been incidents of intracerebral hemorrhage and infection.

Psychological Therapies

Certain nonpharmacological therapies seem to be particularly useful for OCDs. These therapies are done by advanced practice professionals such as nurse practitioners, psychologists, and social workers.

- **Exposure and response prevention:** This first-line cognitive-behavioral intervention is used for obsessive-compulsive behaviors. First, the patient is exposed to stimuli that trigger the specific OCD symptoms. For patients with contamination fears, this might involve having them touch a doorknob or faucet handle. Patients then prevent themselves from performing the compulsive ritual of handwashing. The patient learns that anxiety does subside even when the ritual is not completed. After trying this in the office, the patient learns to set time limits at home to gradually lengthen the time between rituals until the urge fades away.
- **Flooding:** This method exposes the patient to a large amount of an undesirable stimulus in an effort to extinguish the response. The patient learns through prolonged exposure that survival is possible and that anxiety diminishes spontaneously. For example, an obsessive patient who usually touches objects with a paper towel may be forced to touch objects with a bare hand for 1 hour. By the end of that period, the anxiety level is expected to be lower.

▶ Neurobiology of Anxiety Disorders and the Effects of Antianxiety Medications

An imbalance of certain neurotransmitters are thought to disrupt specific brain regions that contribute to various anxiety disorders.

Frontal cortex: Cognitive interpretations (e.g., potential threat)

Hypothalamus: Activation of the stress response (fight-or-flight response)

Hippocampus: Associated with memory related to fear responses

Amygdala: Fear, especially related to phobic and panic disorders

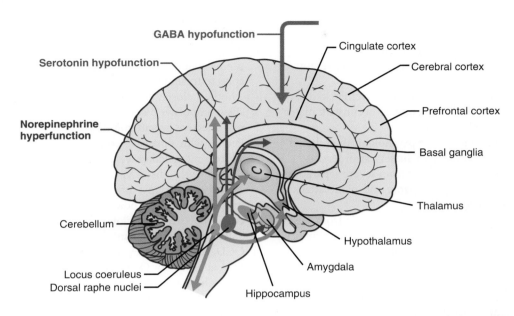

Serotonin is found in the midbrain, ventral tegmental area (VTA), cerebral cortex, and hypothalamus. Helps regulate mood, sleep, sexual desire, appetite, and inhibits pain. In anxiety disorders it is believed that there are reduced levels of serotonin transmission. Low levels of serotonin are believed to play a role in anxiety disorders as well as depression.

Gamma-aminobutyric acid (GABA) is widely distributed in the brain. GABA slows neuron activity which plays a role in lowering anxiety and also effects memory. There appears to be strong support that problems with the GABA neurotransmitter system in the brain is related to anxiety disorders.

Norepinephrine is found in the midbrain, VTA, cerebral cortex, and hypothalamus. Plays a role in sensitization, fear conditioning, stress response (increases blood pressure and heart rate). Excessive and unregulated norepinephrine thought to be related to anxiety disorders

Antianxiety Agent	How It Works	Examples of Use
Selective serotonin reuptake inhibitors (SSRIs)–first-line treatment	Blocks reuptake of serotonin-increasing levels in the brain	Paroxetine (Paxil)—helpful in generalized anxiety disorder (GAD)
Serotonin norepinephrine reuptake inhibitors (SNRIs)–first-line treatment	Blocks reuptake of both serotonin and norepinephrine in the brain	Venlafaxine (Effexor)—mixed anxiety/depression, anxiety, and nerve pain
Noradrenergic drugs	Propranolol—blocks adrenergic receptor activity Clonidine—reduces adrenergic activity	Propranolol—short-term relief of social anxiety and performance anxiety Clonidine—anxiety disorders, panic attacks
Benzodiazepines	Binds to benzodiazepine receptors, facilitates action of GABA, slowing neural transmission thus lowering anxiety	Alprazolam (Xanax)—may be used short term to treat panic disorder and agoraphobia
Buspirone (BuSpar)	Functions as a serotonin 5-HT$_{1A}$ receptor partial agonist resulting in antianxiety and antidepressant effects	Buspirone's reduces symptoms of GAD in 1-2 weeks with limited misuse potential

KEY POINTS TO REMEMBER

- Anxiety has an unknown or unrecognized source, whereas fear is a reaction to a specific threat.
- Peplau operationally defined four levels of anxiety (mild, moderate, severe, and panic). The patient's perceptual field, ability to learn, and other characteristics are different at each level.
- Defenses mechanisms can be adaptive or maladaptive. Generally, overuse of any one defense mechnism, particularly the immature defense mechanisms, results in maladaptive responses.
- Anxiety disorders are the most common psychiatric disorders in the United States and frequently co-occur with major depressive disorder or substance use.
- Research has identified biological, psychological, and environmental factors in the etiology of anxiety disorders.
- Patients with anxiety disorders suffer from severe separation anxiety, social anxiety, feelings of panic and panic attacks, and debilitating generalized anxiety.
- Embarrassment and shame often prevent people from seeking psychiatric help. Instead, they may present to primary care providers with multiple somatic complaints.
- Understanding the levels of anxiety will help in planning basic care, including how much direction your patient will need, what precautions should be taken to prevent harm, and how able your patient is to learn.
- Basic-level nursing interventions for anxiety include counseling, health teaching and health promotion, providing a safe milieu, and promotion of self-care activities.
- Selective serotonin reuptake inhibitors are considered the first line of treatment with anxiety-related disorders. Other antidepressants, antianxiety agents, beta blockers, antihistamines, anticonvulsants, and antipsychotics are also used to treat anxiety disorders.
- Advanced practice providers such as as nurse practitioners use behavioral and cognitive-behavioral psychological therapies to treat anxiety disorders.
- Another closely related set of disorders are the obsessive-compulsive disorders, in which anxiety results in abnormal selective overattention.
- People with obsessive-compulsive disorders tend to resist addressing maladaptive thoughts and behaviors.
- People with obsessive-compulsive disorders suffer from excessive worrying, uncontrollable rituals, distorted body images, unhealthy hoarding, and dysfunctional body-focused repetitive behaviors.
- SSRIs and a tricyclic antidepressant have FDA approval for OCD. Brain therapies such deep brain stimulation also have FDA approval for OCD. The other obsessive-compulsive disorders have no FDA-approved treatments.
- Advanced practice psychological interventions are behaviorally based.

CRITICAL THINKING

1. Tiffany, a teenager with obsessive-compulsive disorder, washes her hands until they are cracked and bleeding. Your nursing goal is to promote healing of her hands. What interventions will you plan?
2. Corey is a senior in college and is taking his final examinations for an engineering course. The professor catches him copying from the examination of his willing partner, Katie, and takes his exam away. Corey's heart immediately begins to pound, his pulse and respiration rates increase, and he has to wipe perspiration from his hands and face several times. He feels like vomiting and has a throbbing in his head.

   After the examination, he approaches the professor but has difficulty focusing. When he starts to speak, his voice trembles. Corey says that Katie suggested that cheating is no big deal, that he needed to do it to be competitive, and that it was done all the time. Corey goes on to say that this "silly exam" doesn't mean anything anyway and that he already passed the important courses. He tells the professor, "I thought you were the greatest, and now I see that you're a fool."

   The professor remains calm and explains that regardless of Corey's thoughts on this matter, he was, in fact, caught cheating, and he will have to take responsibility for his actions. The professor will refer Corey to the disciplinary board. When Corey realizes how serious this incident is, he flips out and yells at the professor and calls him offensive names. Another professor walking past the classroom witnesses this encounter.

   a. Identify the level of anxiety Corey was experiencing once he was caught cheating, and describe the signs and symptoms that helped you determine this level.

   b. Identify and define five defense mechanisms Corey used to lessen his anxiety.

   c. Given the circumstances once Corey was caught, how could he have reacted more responsibly, using healthier coping defenses?

3. This is Logan's third emergency department visit in a week. He is experiencing severe anxiety accompanied by many physical symptoms. He clings to you, desperately crying, "Help me! Help me! Don't let me die!" Diagnostic tests have ruled out a physical disorder. The patient outcome has been identified as "Patient's anxiety level will be reduced to moderate/mild within 1 hour."

   a. What interventions should you use? Be comprehensive in your approach.

   b. Logan is given an appointment at the anxiety disorders clinic. How will you explain the importance of keeping the clinic appointment? Are there any factors you would have to consider while providing patient education?

4. Liz is a patient with generalized anxiety disorder. She has a history of substance use and is now recovering from alcohol use disorder. During a clinic visit, she tells you that she plans to ask the psychiatrist to prescribe diazepam (Valium) to use when she feels anxious. She asks whether you think this is a good idea. How would you respond? What action could you take?

CHAPTER REVIEW

1. The nurse is providing care for a patient demonstrating behaviors associated with moderate levels of anxiety. What question should the nurse ask initially in attempting to help the patient de-escalate the anxiety?
   a. "Do you know what will help you manage your anxiety?"
   b. "Do you need help to manage your anxiety?"
   c. "Can you identify what was happening when your anxiety began to increase?"
   d. "Are you feeling anxious right now?"

2. Which patient is at increased risk for the development of anxiety and will require frequent assessment by the nurse? *Select all that apply.*
   a. Exacerbation of asthma signs and symptoms
   b. History of peanut and strawberry allergies
   c. History of chronic obstructive pulmonary disease
   d. Current treatment for unstable angina pectoris
   e. History of a traumatic brain injury

3. Which medication should the nurse be prepared to educate patients on when they are prescribed a selective serotonin reuptake inhibitor (SSRI) for panic attacks?
   a. Alprazolam (Xanax)
   b. Fluoxetine (Prozac)
   c. Clonazepam (Klonopin)
   d. Venlafaxine (Effexor)

4. Which statement or statements made by the nurse demonstrates an understanding of the effective use of relaxation therapy for anxiety management? *Select all that apply.*
   a. "Relaxation therapy's main goal is to prevent exhaustion by removing muscle tension."
   b. "Muscle relaxation promotes the relaxation response."
   c. "Show me how you learned to deep breathe in yesterday's therapy session."
   d. "You've said that going to group makes you nervous, so let's start relaxing now."
   e. "I've given you written descriptions of the various relaxation exercises for you to review."

5. To maximize the therapeutic effect, which lifestyle practice should the nurse discourage for a patient who has recently been prescribed an antianxiety medication?
   a. Eating high-protein foods.
   b. Using acetaminophen without first discussing it with a healthcare provider
   c. Taking medications after eating dinner or while having a bedtime snack
   d. Buying a large coffee with sugar and extra cream each morning on the way to work

6. In a parent-teacher conference, the school nurse meets with the parents of a profoundly shy 8-year-old girl. The parents hold hands, speak softly, respond briefly, and have poor eye contact. The nurse recognizes that the child is most likely exposed to parental modeling and
   a. The inherited shyness trait
   b. A lack of affection in the home
   c. Severe punishment by the parents
   d. Is afraid to say something foolish

7. Isabel is a straight-A student, yet she suffers from severe test anxiety and seeks medical attention. The nurse interviews Isabel and develops a plan of care. The nurse recognizes effective teaching about mild anxiety when Isabel states the following:
   a. "I would like to try a benzodiazepine for my anxiety."
   b. "If I study harder, my anxiety level will go down."
   c. "Mild anxiety is okay because it helps me to focus."
   d. "I have fear that I will fail at college."

8. The activity of gamma-aminobutyric acid (GABA) contributes to a slowing of neural activity. Which of the following drugs facilitate the action of GABA?
   a. Benzodiazepines
   b. Antihistamines
   c. Anticonvulsants
   d. Noradrenergics

9. Samantha is a new patient at the mental health clinic and is seeking assistance for what she describes as "severe anxiety." In addition to daily self-medicating with alcohol, Samantha describes long-term use of herbal kava. The nurse practitioner knows that kava is associated with inhibiting P450 and orders which of the following tests?
   a. Electrocardiogram
   b. Liver enzymes
   c. Glomerular filtration rate
   d. Complete blood count

10. A homebound patient diagnosed with agoraphobia has been receiving therapy at home. The nurse recognizes effective teaching when the patient states the following:
    a. "I may never leave the house again."
    b. "Having groceries delivered is very convenient."
    c. "My risk for agoraphobia is increased by my family history."
    d. "I will go out again someday, just not today."

1. c; 2. a, c, d, e; 3. b; 4. b, c, d, e; 5. d; 6. a; 7. c; 8. a; 9. b; 10. c

NGN CASE STUDY AND QUESTIONS

Jasmine is a 19-year-old student who visits the university health center. She shares that, before an exam this semester, she experienced sweating, shortness of breath, abdominal pain, and the sensation of her heart being "in her throat." She found out later she got a grade of "D" on the exam, which alarmed her. She says, "I've always gotten Bs, and this is a subject I'm good at."

The symptoms scared her so much that over the next month, she began avoiding class for fear of feeling like that again. When she did attend class one day, she reports feeling tightness in her chest and her heart started pounding. As she began to breathe faster, she just said a silent prayer to not freak out, waiting for class to be over so she could get out of there. "Now I don't go to class. I just read and watch movies in my dorm—it's terrible. When I even think about classes and exams, I get stomach aches and nausea." She begins to cry and says, "Even when I don't *think* I'm anxious, I'm afraid of *getting* anxious. I want to go to school and get my degree. I just don't know what to do."

1. Identify the assessment findings that will require follow-up by the nurse. *Select all that apply.*
   a. Lives in the dorm
   b. Pounding heart
   c. Praying to calm herself
   d. Abdominal pain
   e. Feeling of doom
   f. Crying
   g. Shortness of breath
   h. Chest discomfort
   i. Intellectual deficit for field of study
   j. Grade of D on an important exam
2. Choose the *most likely* options to complete the following statement.
   Jasmine is diagnosed with a moderate panic disorder. Based on her strong desire to continue attending school, the

priority outcome is to ____1____. The nurse will assist the student to accomplish this goal by focusing on ____2____, as well as ___3___.

Options for 1	Options for 2	Options for 3
a. Develop multiple coping strategies to offset or reduce panic episodes	a. Explaining that anxiety causes sensations similar to those of a heart attack.	a. Developing a plan to help the student avoid situations that can cause anxiety
b. Identify feelings that lead to impaired socialization	b. Assisting student in achieving a grasp of what is happening in the environment	b. Monitoring and controlling anxiety responses
c. Become increasingly able to focus on what is happening in her environment so that she can function in it	c. Helping the student overcome maladaptive avoidant behaviors	c. Teaching that symptoms result from anxiety, not from a catastrophic physical problem

NGN case study answers are on Evolve.

Visit the Evolve website for a posttest on the content in this chapter: http://evolve.elsevier.com/Varcarolis

REFERENCES

American Nurses Association, American Psychiatric Nurses Association, & International Society of Psychiatric-Mental Health Nurses. (2014). *Psychiatric-mental health nursing: Scope and standards of practice* (2nd ed.). Silver Spring, MD: NurseBooks.org.

American Psychiatric Association. (2013). *Diagnostic and statistical manual of mental disorders* (5th ed.). Washington: D.C. Author.

Dougherty, D. D., Wilhelm, S., & Jenike, M. A. (2019). Obsessive-compulsive and related disorders. In L. W. Roberts (Ed.), *The American Psychiatric Association Publishing textbook of psychiatry* (7th ed.) (pp. 371–392).

International Council of Nurses. (2019). ICNP browser. Retrieved from https://www.icn.ch/what-we-do/projects/ehealth/icnp-rowser.

Nordsletten, A. E., Reichenberg, A., Hatch, S. L., Fernandez de la Cruz, L., Pertusa, A., Hotopf, M., et al. (2013). Epidemiology of hoarding disorder. *British Journal of Psychiatry* [online]. Retrieved from http://bjp.rcpsych.org/content/early/2013/10/17/bjp.bp.113.130195.short.

Peplau, H. E. (1968). A working definition of anxiety. In S. F. Burd, & M. A. Marshall (Eds.), *Some clinical approaches to psychiatric nursing* (pp. 323–327). New York, NY: Macmillan.

Stein, M. B., & Sareen, J. (2019). Anxiety disorders. In L. W. Roberts (Ed.), *Textbook of psychiatry* (7th ed.) (pp. 341–370). Washington, DC: American Psychiatric.

US Department of Health and Human Services. (2012). *Use of psychiatric medications in pregnancy and lactation.* Retrieved from https://www.guideline.gov/summaries/summary/12490.

Vicheva, P., Butler, M., & Shotbolt, P. (2020). Deep brain stimulation for obsessive-compulsive disorder: A systematic review of randomized controlled trials. *Neuroscience & Biobehavioral Reviews, 109*, 129–138.

Wang, P. S., Berglund, P., Olfson, M., Pincus, H. A., Wells, K. B., & Kessler, R. C. (2005). Failure and delay in initial treatment contact after first onset of mental disorders in the national co-morbidity survey replication. *Archives of General Psychiatry, 62*, 603–613.

16

Trauma, Stressor-Related, and Dissociative Disorders

Audrey M. Beauvais and Kathleen Wheeler

Visit the Evolve website for a pretest on the content in this chapter: http://evolve.elsevier.com/Varcarolis

OBJECTIVES

1. Describe reactive attachment disorder and disinhibited social engagement disorder and general care for both attachment disorders.
2. Describe the symptoms, epidemiology, comorbidity, and etiology of posttraumatic stress disorder in children and adolescents.
3. Discuss at least five of the neurobiological changes that occur with trauma.
4. Apply the nursing process to the care of children and adolescents who are experiencing posttraumatic stress disorder.
5. Identify pharmacological and psychological treatment modalities for posttraumatic stress disorder in children and adolescents.
6. Describe the symptoms, epidemiology, comorbidity, and etiology of posttraumatic stress disorder in adults.
7. Apply the nursing process to the care of adults who are experiencing posttraumatic stress disorder.
8. Identify pharmacological and psychological treatment modalities for posttraumatic stress disorder in adults.
9. Describe symptoms, general nursing care, and treatment modalities for acute stress disorder.
10. Identify the clinical picture, epidemiology, and risk factors for adjustment disorder.
11. Describe dissociative amnesia and depersonalization/derealization disorder.
12. Describe dissociative identity disorder in terms of symptoms, prevalence, comorbidity, and risk factors.
13. Apply the nursing process to the care of individuals who are experiencing dissociative identity disorder.

KEY TERMS AND CONCEPTS

alternate personality (alter)
depersonalization
derealization
dissociation

eye movement desensitization and
  reprocessing
flashbacks
neuroplasticity

resilience
trauma-informed care
window of tolerance

Traumatic life events are associated with a wide range of psychiatric and other medical disorders. Traumatic events are not always as extraordinary as war and may be as common as interpersonal trauma, sexual abuse, physical abuse, severe neglect, emotional abuse, repeated abandonment, or sudden and traumatic loss in childhood, adolescence, or adulthood (Wheeler, 2014).

Our understanding of the long-term physiological and psychological effects of trauma has expanded, and effective treatments are available. However, people who need these treatments do not always get the care that they need. Trauma-informed care is a treatment framework that involves recognizing and responding to the effects of all types of trauma. Integrating trauma-informed care into all healthcare settings can reduce the pervasive and damaging effects of trauma.

Trauma-informed competencies for undergraduate nursing education support compassionate care for patients. The competencies include enhancing resilience in nurses as well as for patients. While the competencies were developed for undergraduate nursing education, they are foundational for graduate and specialty nursing practice. Table 16.1 contains the primary competencies for each domain.

This chapter begins with a discussion of two child-specific trauma-related disorders—reactive attachment disorder and disinhibited social engagement disorder (American Psychiatric Association, 2013). The other trauma disorders that will be addressed are:

- Posttraumatic stress disorder (PTSD)
- Acute stress disorder
- Adjustment disorder

TABLE 16.1 Trauma and Resilience Competencies for Undergraduate Nursing

Domain and Competency	Content
Self-Resilience: Demonstrate participation in and maintenance of self-care, managing stress, and supportive relationships with others.	Self-care, work/life balance, bullying, workplace incivility, lateral violence, vicarious trauma
Resilience: Incorporate a strength-based approach in working with patients, families, and communities affected by trauma.	Components of resilience, somatic mindfulness, resilience narratives ABCs (active coping, building strength, cognitive awareness and social support)
Knowledge: Explain the effects of adverse childhood experiences on risk-related morbidity and mortality.	Neurobiological changes that occur as a result of trauma, HPA dysregulation
Assessment: Ask patients if they have experienced neglect, substance use by a caregiver, physical or sexual abuse, and how that has affected their health.	Stigma, self-stigma, patient narrative
Diagnosis: Identify nursing diagnoses for those who have experienced trauma.	Powerlessness Hopelessness Impaired coping
Interventions: Apply best practices in providing holistic care to individuals and families with a history of trauma.	Individual and community resources, barriers to access resources, trauma-informed care
Evaluation: Involve the patient with a history of trauma in evaluating progress toward measurable individualized goals.	Specific, measurable, achievable, realistic, and timely (SMART) objectives
Ethics/Culture/Policy: Advocate for the patient/family/community with a history of trauma.	#MeToo movement, organizational culture, institutional betrayal, sociocultural trauma, gun violence, gender, differences in the experience of trauma, LBGTQ community trauma

Wheeler, K., & Phillips, K. (2019). The development of trauma and resilience competencies for nursing education. *Journal of the American Psychiatric Nurses Association*. Retrieved from https://www.acesconnection.com/blog/trauma-and-resilience-competencies-for-nursing-education

Dissociative disorders are also related to trauma—specifically, early interpersonal trauma. The second part of this chapter addresses dissociative disorders, which are (APA, 2013):

- Dissociative amnesia
- Depersonalization/derealization disorder
- Dissociative identity disorder

TRAUMA-RELATED DISORDERS

ATTACHMENT DISORDERS

Attachment disorders are psychiatric conditions in children who have problems with emotional attachments to others. They are caused by a grossly inadequate nurturing environment deficient in bonding experiences with a primary caregiver by the age of 8 months. Children with **reactive attachment disorder** have a consistent pattern of inhibited and emotionally withdrawn behavior. The child rarely seeks comfort or responds to comfort with adult caregivers when distressed.

Another seemingly opposite, but closely related response to inadequate parenting is manifested in **disinhibited social engagement disorder**. Children with this disorder demonstrate no normal fear of strangers. They seem to be unfazed in response to separation from a primary caregiver. Younger children may allow unfamiliar people to pick them up, feed them, or play with them. These children tend to be overly friendly and are usually willing, or even eager, to go with someone they do not know.

Reactive attachment disorder and disinhibited social engagement disorder are rare. The rates of these problems have been estimated at 1% of all children under the age of 5. Even in high-risk situations such as foster care or institutional settings, these conditions are fairly rare. Reactive attachment disorder only occurs in around 10% of these children, and disinhibited social engagement disorder occurs in about 20% of this population.

Risk factors for attachment disorders are a combination of neurobiology and environment. Attachment at its most basic level ensures survival of the species. Lack of attachment is counter to such a basic drive. In an infant, the brain's right hemisphere develops far earlier than the left. It is essential in regulating body functions and coping with stress. The right hemisphere is also responsible for the very human qualities of processing social and emotional information and promoting attachment. Early relationships are particularly important for healthy neural development and lifelong social connection and attachment. Disruption of this process occurs when there is a severe absence of reliable and nurturing caregivers.

Tizard (1977) conducted a classic study related to attachment. Twenty-six children living in an institutional setting were provided with play areas, books, and basic needs. They were not provided with an adequate ratio of caregivers to children. To make matters worse, caregivers were actually instructed not to form attachments with the children. Yet after 4 years, 8 of the 26 children managed to form some attachment with caregivers. However, 8 of the children became emotionally unresponsive, and 10 of the children became indiscriminately social and attention-seeking. These responses are reflective of reactive attachment disorder and disinhibited social engagement disorder.

Risk factors for attachment disorder include institutional living situations, as previously discussed. Frequently changing foster homes or experiencing shifts in primary caregivers also puts a child at risk. Impaired parenting due to severe psychiatric problems, criminal behavior, or substance use disorders also disrupts essential bonding experiences. Prolonged separation from caregivers or parents due to such events as extended hospitalization also puts children at risk for attachment disorders. Without treatment, attachment disorders may have lifelong consequences, including lack of trust or not feeling secure in friendships and partnerships. However, children tend to be naturally resilient and, with support, can learn to develop healthy relationships. Children with attachment disorders benefit from a comprehensive psychiatric assessment. A physical assessment is essential to rule out physical causes of withdrawn or overly outgoing behavior.

Treatment always involves both the child and the caregivers in individual and family therapy. A primary goal of care is to strengthen the relationship between the child and caregiver. A safe and stable living environment is also essential to improving attachment behaviors.

POSTTRAUMATIC STRESS DISORDER IN CHILDREN AND ADOLESCENTS

Clinical Picture

Posttraumatic stress disorder (PTSD) in preschool children may manifest as a reduction in play—play that includes aspects of the traumatic event, social withdrawal, and negative emotions such as fear, guilt, anger, horror, sadness, shame, or confusion. Children may blame themselves for the traumatic event. In addition, there may be a feeling of detachment or estrangement from others and diminished interest or participation in significant activities. Often, there is irritability, aggressive or self-destructive behavior, sleep disturbances, problems concentrating, and hypervigilance.

Epidemiology

Prevalence rates for PTSD in children have not been reported. However, research on adolescents indicates a lifetime prevalence of 5% (National Institute of Mental Health, 2017). According to the US Department of Veterans Affairs (2018a), approximately 15% to 43% of children and teens experience trauma. Of those, more girls than boys go on to develop PTSD—3% to 15% and 1% to 6%, respectively. Nearly 100% of children who witness their parent's murder or sexual assault will develop PTSD. Other alarming statistical relationships with PTSD are for children who are sexually abused (90%), exposed to a shooting at school (77%), and see community violence in urban settings (35%).

Comorbidity

Children and adolescents who have suffered toxic stress and trauma often meet the criteria for more than one diagnostic category. Even if a child does not have sufficient symptoms for a diagnosis of PTSD, he can still suffer from overwhelming nightmares or difficulties with trust, phobias, somatic problems, impulse control, and identity issues. Learning and attention problems, behavioral problems, sleep disorders, depression, suicide attempts, dissociation, and substance-abuse problems are all significant comorbidities (Scheidell et al., 2018). These comorbidities expose children to an endless cycle of medications, punishments, and inadequate responses that revictimize and stigmatize them.

Risk Factors
Biological Factors
Genetic. Genetic variability is thought to play a role in stress reactivity, with epigenetic factors modulating the expression of

genotype. A twin study examined the genetic and environmental risk factors associated with PTSD symptoms (Wolf et al., 2018). Genetic factors provide evidence for a single spectrum of traumatic stress, showing resilience at one end and high symptom severity at the other. This finding has implications for the quest to find trauma-related genetic markers. Another study that looked at earthquake survivors also supports that PTSD is associated with genetic factors (Xiao et al., 2019).

Neurobiological. Neural connections between the limbic system and prefrontal cortex are established between 10 and 18 months of age, and these neural pathways play a crucial role in modulating arousal and emotional regulation. Normally, information from the environment is taken in through our senses, matched against previous experiences, and processed. Experiences are integrated into adaptive memory neural networks in a way that allows for connection with other memory networks.

Normal stress responses. In a normal stress response, the hyperarousal in the sympathetic system is balanced by the parasympathetic system. When a person senses danger through the eyes or ears (or both), this information is sent to the amygdala. The amygdala interprets the sensory input. Neuronal circuits connect the amygdala to the prefrontal lobe in the cortex. The prefrontal lobe serves as the translator of the emotion so that amygdala activation can be modulated. The prefrontal association area keeps track of where information has been stored in long-term memory. This area is then responsible for retrieving and integrating memories with sensory input for decision making.

Trauma stress responses. Repeated stress and trauma can cause changes in the brain as well as hormonal imbalances in the body (Iacona & Johnson, 2018). When experiencing trauma, the hypothalamus emits corticotropin-releasing hormone (CRH). CRH subsequently attaches to the CRH receptor on the pituitary gland, causing the pituitary to release adrenocorticotropic hormone (ACTH). ACTH subsequently triggers the adrenal cortex to release cortisol, a stress hormone. The cortisol then attaches to glucocorticoid receptors until a particular blood level is achieved (Nugent et al., 2016). Glucocorticoid receptors play a role in the feedback loop for the hypothalamic-pituitary-adrenal (HPA) axis.

Recurrent experiences with trauma or stress will result in frequent activation of the HPA axis, which leads to elevated levels of stress hormones (Iacona & Johnson, 2018). Elevated stress hormones influence the immune and inflammatory systems (Nugent et al., 2016). Frequent activation of the HPA axis when the brain is developing can result in gene expression that may ultimately influence adult emotional and cognitive behavior and functioning (Hornor, 2017).

Following exposure to violence and trauma, the parasympathetic response triggers a hypoaroused state with dysregulation of the hypothalamic-pituitary-adrenal axis that may result in dissociation. **Dissociation** is a disconnection of thoughts, emotions, sensations, and behaviors connected with a memory. Some dissociation is considered a normal experience for most people, such as when we zone out during a movie or when driving. However, severe dissociation, or mindflight, occurs for those who have suffered significant trauma (Pearce et al., 2017).

The episodic failure of dissociation causes intrusive symptoms such as flashbacks, thus dysregulating cortisol, resulting in either too much or too little of the hormone.

Polyvagal theory suggests that the autonomic nervous system is not limited to a fight-or-flight response to threat. Instead, there are actually three different responses (Porges, 2011). The sympathetic and parasympathetic systems are governed by the tenth cranial nerve, or vagus nerve, which sends and receives information between the body and the brain. This information is carried by two major vagus nerves (ventral and dorsal) with two branches (myelinated and unmyelinated). The responses are as follows:

1. Myelinated ventral vagal responses are activated during social or intellectual engagement when the individual is "on," in a state of pleasant, not overwhelming arousal. This state serves as a gentle break by inhibiting sympathetic responses of the autonomic system.
2. Unmyelinated ventral vagus responses are activated when we perceive a threat. The attending sympathetic arousal symptoms of rapid heart rate and rapid respiration prepare the person for fight-or-flight responses. After many hours, days, or months, the body cannot sustain this state.
3. The third response is the dorsal vagal response that occurs to dampen down the sympathetic nervous system. This is a parasympathetic response, with the heart rate and respiration slowing down and a decrease in blood pressure. Animals in the wild illustrate the ultimate dorsal vagal shutdown by playing dead when extremely threatened.
4. Subjectively, a person may just want to sleep or escape through mind-numbing activities and stay in this hypoaroused or depressed state alternating with a hyperaroused or anxious state. This theory provides an explanation of why many people with PTSD also suffer from depression.

Environmental Factors

To a greater degree than adults, children are dependent on others. It is this dependency in tandem with the neuroplasticity (malleability) of the developing brain that increases vulnerability to adverse life experiences. External factors in the environment can either support or put stress on children and adolescents and shape development. Young persons are vulnerable in an environment in which systems (e.g., schools, court systems) and adults (e.g., parents, counselors) have power and control. Parents model behavior and provide the child with a view of the world. If parents are abusive, rejecting, or overly controlling, the child may suffer detrimental effects during the period of development when the trauma occurs. Fortunately, most children who suffer a traumatic and stressful event develop normally.

Poverty, parental substance use, and exposure to violence are receiving increased attention and place minority children at greater risk for trauma and stress. A study by Soylu and colleagues (2018) found ethnic and racial disparities in health insurance, services, and quality of care among children. Differences in cultural expectations, presence of stresses, and lack of support by the dominant culture may have profound effects and increase the risk of mental, emotional, and academic problems. Family stability may provide cushioning effects in the face of poverty and adversity.

EVIDENCE-BASED PRACTICE

Resilience Intervention for Traumatic Experiences

Problem

Traumatic experiences can cause recurrent intrusive visual memories that are disruptive and distressing. Post trauma preventative interventions are lacking.

Purpose of Study

The purpose of this study was to determine if an intervention involving a computer game would reduce intrusive memories of real-world trauma, in patients visiting an acute care emergency department following a traumatic motor vehicle accident compared with an attention-placebo control.

Methods

The sample included 71 patients who used emergency department services after experiencing a motor vehicle accident and met the criteria for PTSD. The patients were randomly assigned to an intervention group or a control group. The intervention group was asked to remember the accident and describe the worst moments. After sharing their memories, participants played a computer game for at least 10 min.

Members of the control group were given activity logs, in which they wrote about activities they participated in during their time in the emergency department. For example, they could document that they read, talked, received treatment, texted, and completed crossword puzzles. They also documented the amount of time spent on each activity, which had to be at least 10 min.

Outcome assessments—number of intrusive memories, posttraumatic distress—were completed at 1 week and 1 month following the accident by patients in both groups.

Key Findings

Participants in the intervention group who played the computer game experienced reduced intrusive memories overall and a more rapid decline of intrusive memories.

Implications for Nursing Practice

This brief "therapist-free" computer game intervention is feasible and acceptable in conjunction with therapy. Evaluating this intervention with a larger sample that includes children and adolescents is important.

Iyadurai, L., Blackwell, S. E., Meiser-Stedman, R. M., Watson, P. C., Bonsali, M. B., Geddes, J. R., et al. (2018). Preventing intrusive memories after trauma via a brief intervention involving Tetris computer game play in the emergency department: A proof-of-concept randomized controlled trial. *Molecular Psychiatry, 23,* 674–682.

Children brought up in a chaotic or non-nurturing environment suffer neurological consequences that are long-lasting and difficult to remediate (Shonkoff & Garner, 2012). Toxic stress and adverse childhood experiences (ACEs) have been found to result in lifelong consequences for both psychological and physical health (Dowd, 2017). Trauma in early childhood also plays a role in the intergenerational transmission of disparities in health outcomes.

Despite negative environmental factors, some children thrive and grow into successful and healthy adults. The term resilience refers to positive adaptation, or the ability to maintain or regain mental health despite adversity. Studies have shown that factors that enhance resilience are the presence of social support as well as protective factors that include collectivism (Ariapooran et al., 2018).

APPLICATION OF THE NURSING PROCESS

ASSESSMENT

A traumatized child or adolescent may experience delayed development if care is not available. It is important for nurses working in schools, community settings, and juvenile detention centers to assess for PTSD and environmental safety for young people who have been traumatized or experienced abuse and a history of violence.

The type of data collected depends on the setting, the severity of the presenting problem, and the availability of resources. However, assessment is an ongoing process throughout treatment. Methods of collecting data include interviewing, screening, testing (neurological, psychological, intelligence), observing, and interacting with the child or adolescent. Histories are taken from multiple sources, including parents, other caregivers, the child or adolescent, and other adults, such as teachers, when possible. A genogram can document family composition, history, and relationships (refer to Chapter 35).

The assessment of the mental status of children and adolescents provides information about the child's state at the time of the examination and identifies problems with thinking, feeling, and behaving. Broad categories to assess include safety, general appearance, socialization, activity level, speech, coordination and motor function, affect, manner of relating, intellectual function, thought processes and content, and characteristics of play.

The observation-interaction part of a mental health assessment begins with a semistructured interview in which the nurse asks the young person about the home environment, parents, and siblings, and about the school environment, teachers, and peers. In this format, children are free to describe problems and give information about their developmental history. Play activities, such as games, drawings, and puppets, are used for younger children who cannot respond to a direct approach. The initial interview is key to observing interactions among the child, caregiver, and siblings (if available) and to building trust and rapport.

Essential assessment data include posttraumatic symptoms such as:

- Nightmares and night terrors
- Intrusive traumatic thoughts and memories
- Re-experiencing or flashbacks
- Numbing
- Avoidance of stimuli associated with the traumatic event

Another area of assessment includes the presence of self-injurious behaviors due to anxiety and negative emotional states. Children and adolescents may experience somatic symptoms such as headaches, stomachaches, or pain; memory problems include amnesia, forgetfulness, difficulty concentrating, or trance states. The child may disturbingly re-enact the trauma in play.

Specific assessment tools may include instruments such as the Child Dissociative Checklist (Putnam et al., 1993), Trauma Symptoms Checklist for Children (Briere, 1996), and the Child Sexual Behavior Inventory (Friedrich et al., 2001). Advanced practice professionals such as a nurse practitioner or a psychologist usually administer these assessment tools. However, parents and teachers may complete structured questionnaires and behavior checklists to track progress.

Developmental Assessment

Developmental testing should also be conducted for young children since significant developmental delays may occur. The developmental assessment provides information about the child or adolescent's maturational level. Is the child behaving and functioning at his chronological age, or are there areas where the child lags behind the norms and peers?

The Denver II Developmental Screening Test for infants and children up to 6 years of age is a popular assessment tool (Frankenburg et al., 1992). For adolescents, tools may be tailored to specific areas of assessment, such as neuropsychological, physical, hormonal, and biochemical. Some computer-based screening tools for children and adolescents are used in primary care settings to gather sensitive information.

Abnormal findings in the developmental and mental status assessments may be temporary. The nurse working with parents may handle stress-related behaviors or minor regressions. However, as young people use maladaptive behaviors over time, they become more vulnerable to developing other psychiatric disorders. Early intervention is essential to reduce further disability.

NURSING DIAGNOSIS

After a comprehensive trauma assessment, priority nursing diagnoses are identified (International Council of Nurses [ICN], 2019). The first is *post trauma response,* which directly addresses the medical problem of PTSD. The second priority diagnosis is *impaired caregiver-child attachment.* This diagnosis identifies a disruption of the attachment process between caregiver and child. The third is *impaired adolescent development.* This diagnosis refers a 25% or more in the areas of social behavior, self-regulatory behavior, cognition, language, and motor skills.

OUTCOME IDENTIFICATION

To the best of our ability and the patient's ability, patients should be involved in the development of outcomes and goals. Outcomes should be aimed at reducing the problem identified in the nursing diagnoses. They should be patient-focused, stated in positive terms, and include a timeline. Based on the diagnoses in the previous paragraph, overall outcomes would be:

1. Improved response to trauma
2. Improved caregiver-child attachment
3. Improved adolescent development

Smaller goals are also included to break down the steps to reach the outcomes.

IMPLEMENTATION

Stages for Implementation

Nurses and other licensed healthcare providers are mandated by law to report all instances of suspected abuse of a minor to the local child protective services. The overall treatment plan for trauma includes psychobiological, psychological, and family goals within a staged treatment protocol.

The staged model of treatment for trauma includes the following:

Stage 1: Providing safety and stabilization through creating a safe, predictable environment; stopping self-destructive behaviors; providing education about trauma and its effects.

Stage 2: Reducing arousal and regulating emotion through symptom reduction and memory work; finding comfort from others; tolerating affect; integrating disavowed emotions and accepting ambivalence; overcoming avoidance; improving attention and decreasing dissociation; working with memories; and transforming memories.

Stage 3: Developmental skills catch-up by enhancing problem-solving skills; nurturing self-awareness; social skills training; and developing a value system. Interventions in this phase should focus on teaching coping skills to deal with trauma, supporting efforts to achieve socially appropriate goals, and facilitating the development of and integration into healthy social support systems.

Treatment strategies for the traumatized child are designed to modulate arousal so that the child is helped to stay within a window of tolerance. The **window of tolerance** is a term that means a balance between sympathetic and parasympathetic arousal (Porges, 2011). Traumatized children have difficulty shifting their emotional and physiological state to accommodate different environments and social contexts. They alternate between hyperarousal (anxiety, fear, hyperactivity, aggression) and hypoarousal (withdrawal, isolation, numbness). Increasing the child's ability to self-regulate through specific strategies designed to mediate these arousal states while providing a nurturing safe environment supports a sense of well-being and competency.

Interventions

Since the child with trauma has suffered significant disconnection and fragmentation of relationships with self and others, the most important healing ingredient is that of relationship and connection to others. Connection, caring, and management of the patient's anxiety are essential to provide the foundation so that integration is possible. Box 16.1 identifies interventions appropriate for a child who has suffered a specific trauma.

Interventions for a traumatized young person are used in a variety of settings: inpatient, residential, outpatient, day treatment, outreach programs in schools, and home visits. Many of the modalities can encompass activities of daily living, learning activities, multiple forms of play and recreational activities, and interactions with adults and peers.

Often, traumatized children feel responsible for what happened to them and are frightened by flashbacks and amnesia. Some children may use an imaginary friend as a coping

---

BOX 16.1 Trauma Interventions for a Child With Posttraumatic Stress Disorder

Definition: Use of an interactive helping process to resolve a trauma experienced by a child.

Establish trust and safety in the therapeutic relationship.
Use developmentally appropriate language to explore feelings.
Teach relaxation techniques before trauma exploration to restore a sense of control over thoughts and feelings.
Help the child to identify and cope with feelings through the use of art and play to promote expression.
Involve the parents or appropriate caretakers in one-on-ones, unless they are the cause of the trauma.
Educate the child and parents about the grief process and response to the trauma.
Assist parents in resolving their own emotional distress about the trauma.
Coordinate with social workers for protections as indicated.

---

mechanism. While this imaginary friend was adaptive during the trauma, the child should understand that this friend is really a part of the self and not a separate person. In such a case, explain to the child that sometimes when really bad things happen, our brain helps us by forgetting and creating special parts of ourselves.

In addition to teaching about the recovery process and normalizing the experiences, traumatized children need to learn strategies to regulate emotion and arousal levels. Teaching deep breathing techniques and mindfulness techniques helps decrease arousal levels and restore natural rhythms. Soothing strategies that redirect behavior might also include warm baths, singing, distraction, listening to music, guided imagery, and using a low, calming voice. These strategies help the child to manage feelings. Talking about feelings and helping the child to identify emotions is essential. Teaching the family how to set limits without being harsh helps the child to feel in control.

EVALUATION

Treatment is effective when:
1. The child's safety has been maintained.
2. Anxiety has been reduced, and stress is handled adaptively.
3. Emotions and behavior are appropriate for the situation.
4. The child achieves normal developmental milestones for his or her chronological age.
5. The child is able to seek out adults for nurturance and help when needed.

TREATMENT MODALITIES

Biological Treatments

Pharmacotherapy

Medicating children works best when combined with another treatment, such as EMDR therapy or cognitive behavioral therapy (CBT). Medications that target specific symptoms or comorbidities such as attention-deficit/hyperactivity disorder (ADHD) or major depressive disorder can enhance the child or adolescent's potential for growth and may make a real difference in a family's ability to cope and quality of life.

Psychological Therapies

Advanced practice mental health clinicians and advanced practice psychiatric-mental health registered nurses are qualified to conduct individual and group psychotherapy. International guidelines recommend the use of CBT and eye movement desensitization and reprocessing (EMDR) therapy as first-line treatments for the treatment of traumatized children (WHO, 2013). CBT uses a range of strategies—such as psychoeducation, behavior modification, cognitive therapy, exposure therapy, and stress management—to help the child manage behavior and change maladaptive beliefs and thoughts.

EMDR therapy is an evidence-based therapy used to treat children and adults (Wheeler, 2014). EMDR therapy helps people process traumatic memories. People are encouraged to think about the traumatic event while also focusing on other stimulation, such as eye movements, audio tones, or tapping. EMDR may work through neurological and physiological changes that help to process and integrate traumatic memories. Specific protocols have been developed for the treatment of children, and even if the child does not remember what happened, EMDR therapy can be helpful. As a licensed mental health provider, advanced practice psychiatric nurses can become certified to use EMDR through additional training.

POSTTRAUMATIC STRESS DISORDER IN ADULTS

Clinical Picture

As in children, PTSD in adults is characterized by persistent re-experiencing of a highly traumatic event. This event involves actual or threatened death or serious injury to self or others. Responses of intense fear, helplessness, or horror are felt. PTSD may occur after any traumatic event that is outside the range of usual experience. Examples of PTSD-inducing events include:

- Military combat, prisoner-of-war experience, or being taken hostage
- Crime-related events, such as bombing, assault, mugging, or rape
- Natural disasters, such as floods, tornadoes, and earthquakes
- Human disasters, such as automobile, airline, and train accidents

An often-overlooked cause of PTSD is being diagnosed with a life-threatening illness or being treated for a serious illness, particularly in the intensive care unit. PTSD symptoms can begin a month after exposure, but a symptom delay of months or years is not uncommon.

As in children, the major features of PTSD include the following:

1. Re-experiencing the trauma through recurrent intrusive recollections of the event or dreams about the event. Flashbacks are dissociative experiences during which the event is relived along with vivid sensory input.
2. **Avoidance** of stimuli associated with the trauma, causing the individual to avoid talking about the event or avoid activities, people, or places that arouse memories of the trauma. This avoidance is accompanied by feelings of detachment, emptiness, and numbing.
3. Persistent symptoms of increased arousal, as evidenced by irritability, difficulty sleeping, difficulty concentrating, **hypervigilance**, or exaggerated startle response.
4. **Alterations in mood**, such as chronic depression, negative appraisals, and lack of interest in previously pleasurable activities (APA, 2013).

The flashbacks and hypervigilance of PTSD can be terrifying. When the person recalls a traumatic memory, physiological reactions—a sensation of terror in the stomach, heart palpitations, and muscles tensing—occur. The person often does not know where these sensations are coming from and attributes them to present circumstances, and thus the past becomes the present. Because of the changes in the brain, the individual can fluctuate radically from moments of overstimulation and anxiety to moments of complete shutdown and depression. Just when the person feels at rest, as while asleep, intrusive flashbacks occur. People who suffer from PTSD begin to feel permanently damaged and often hate themselves for feeling so needy and helpless. Difficulty with interpersonal, social, or occupational relationships nearly always accompanies PTSD, and trust is a common issue.

Epidemiology

Epidemiological studies indicate that about 60% of men and 50% of women have at least one trauma in their lifetime (US Department of Veterans Affairs, 2018b). Men are more likely to have experienced physical assaults, accidents, disasters, combat, and witnessing injury or death. Women are more likely to experience child sexual abuse and/or sexual assault. Approximately 8% of the population have PTSD at some time in their lives.

Not everyone who experiences trauma will develop PTSD. An individual's response to a disturbing event is highly individual. It depends on such factors as the person's age, developmental stage, coping skills, support system, cognitive deficits, and preexisting neural physiology.

Comorbidity

The more ACEs, the more medical and mental illness occurs in adulthood. Also, while short-term dissociation may actually be adaptive during a distressing event, the tendency toward persistent dissociation may be another significant risk factor (Bryant et al., 2011). Consequences of ACE include obesity, sexually transmitted diseases, alcoholism, severe and persistent mental illness, psychosis, substance use, eating disorders, sleep disorders, dissociative disorders, and anxiety and depressive disorders (Dowd, 2017).

Comorbidities for adults with PTSD include major depressive disorder, anxiety disorders, sleep disorders, and dissociative disorders. Often, substances are used to try to manage the feelings and symptoms.

Risk Factors

See the earlier discussion on biological factors in trauma-related disorders for children.

APPLICATION OF THE NURSING PROCESS

ASSESSMENT

Screening tools for PTSD in adults include the Primary Care PTSD Screen for DSM-5 (PC-PTSD-5) (Prins et al., 2015) and the PTSD Checklist (PCL-5) (Weathers et al., 2013). A more comprehensive assessment is indicated for those who initially screen positive.

Additional history about the time of onset, frequency, course, severity, level of distress, and degree of functional impairment is important. Further assessment for suicidal or violent ideation, family and social supports, insomnia, social withdrawal, functional impairment, current life stressors, medication, past medical and psychiatric history, and a mental status exam are indicated (refer to Chapter 7). The diagnosis of PTSD involves a comprehensive clinical interview that assesses all symptoms collectively.

NURSING DIAGNOSIS

Priority nursing diagnoses are identified after a comprehensive assessment. As with children, the priority diagnosis is post trauma response, which directly addresses the medical problem of PTSD (ICN, 2019). Other nursing diagnoses are useful with this disorder. They include:

- Anxiety (moderate, severe, panic)
- Impaired coping
- Social isolation
- Insomnia
- Sleep deprivation
- Hopelessness
- Chronic low self-esteem
- Self-care deficit

OUTCOMES IDENTIFICATION

A general outcome for post trauma response is simply an improved response to trauma.

Goals for trauma-related disorders for adults include the following:

1. The patient is able to manage anxiety as demonstrated by the use of relaxation techniques, adequate sleep, and the ability to maintain a role or work requirements.
2. The patient experiences enhanced self-esteem, as demonstrated by maintenance of grooming/hygiene, maintenance of eye contact, positive statements about self, and acceptance of self-limitations.
3. The patient exhibits an enhanced ability to cope as demonstrated by a decrease in physical symptoms, an ability to ask for help, and seeking information about treatment.

IMPLEMENTATION

A stage model of treatment as previously described for children is the standard for trauma treatment for adults. It begins with providing safety and stabilization through a safe and predictable environment. Reducing arousal and regulating emotion can be taught through strategies such as deep breathing, imagery, and mindfulness exercises. Improving socialization by connecting the person to support groups, family, and friends reduces feelings of isolation and poor self-esteem.

Nurses can be helpful by encouraging the patient to develop a narrative of the event and the meaning of the event to the person. The person often feels guilty and responsible for the event, and the nurse, as a witness through listening and reflecting back to the person their concerns, can gently suggest that the person was not responsible for what happened. By sharing their experiences, patients can begin to heal and integrate what happened into their lives.

Health Teaching and Health Promotion

Educating the person and family about PTSD is important to normalize the situation. Often, people think they are going crazy and do not understand that theirs is a normal reaction to an abnormal event. You can provide reassurance that reactions to trauma do not indicate personal failure or weakness.

The patient and family should be informed that trauma symptoms can present in a variety of ways. Symptoms such as interpersonal problems with family and friends, occupational problems, and substance use are often present. In addition, strategies to improve coping, enhance self-care, and facilitate recognition of symptoms are essential teaching topics. Providing patients with instructions in simple relaxation techniques such as slow and deep breathing helps patients self-regulate. Patients who are being discharged should be made aware of community supports and be provided with a referral for follow-up care.

EVALUATION

Treatment is effective when:

1. The patient recognizes symptoms as related to the trauma
2. The patient is able to use newly learned strategies to manage anxiety
3. The patient experiences no flashbacks or intrusive thoughts about the traumatic event
4. The patient is able to sleep adequately without nightmares
5. The patient can assume usual roles and maintains satisfying interpersonal relationships

(See Case Study and Nursing Care Plan 16.1.)

TREATMENT MODALITIES

Biological Treatments

Pharmacotherapy

While the primary treatment for PTSD is trauma-focused psychotherapy, there are some medications used for this condition. Antidepressants can help with symptoms of depression and anxiety. They also help with sleep problems and concentration. The selective serotonin reuptake inhibitors (SSRIs) sertraline (Zoloft) and paroxetine (Paxil) are FDA approved for the treatment of PTSD.

Other antidepressants that are prescribed off label include fluoxetine (Prozac) and venlafaxine (Effexor). Nefazodone (Serzone), imipramine (Tofranil), and phenelzine (Nardil) are suggested if other medications are ineffective (US Department of Veterans Affairs and Department of Defense, 2017). Due to a lack of evidence for efficacy and known adverse effects and associated risks, atypical antipsychotics as well as citalopram (Celexa), amitriptyline (Elavil), topiramate (Topamax), and lamotrigine (Lamictal) are not recommended for the treatment of PTSD.

Psychological Therapies

Evidence-based treatments for PTSD include trauma-focused psychotherapy that may include components of exposure and/or cognitive restructuring and EMDR therapy. EMDR is discussed under the child and adolescent with PTSD section. These modalities are often combined with anxiety management/stress reduction that focuses on the alleviation of symptoms. Other helpful strategies include brief psychodynamic psychotherapy, imagery, relaxation techniques, hypnosis, and group therapy. Refer to Chapter 2 for more information about these therapies.

CASE STUDY AND NURSING PLAN

A distraught wife brings Mr. Blake, 46, to the emergency department after she finds him writing a suicide note and planning to shoot himself with a handgun. Mr. Blake is subdued, shows minimal effect, and his breath has the distinct odor of alcohol. When asked about suicidal thoughts, he states that he is worthless and that his wife and family would be better off if he were dead. The decision is made to hospitalize him to protect him from danger to himself.

Mr. Blake's wife provides further history. Her husband is a construction contractor who served in the US National Guard during the Iraq War. He lost half his squad from a roadside bombing, narrowly escaping with his life. He walks with a permanent limp due to the attack. Upon returning home, he showed no signs of anxiety and refused offers of crisis treatment, stating, "I was in a war. I can handle stress." But 6 months later, Mrs. Blake noticed that her husband had trouble sleeping, his mood was irritable or withdrawn, he avoided news reports on television, and he started to drink daily. He complained of nightmares but would not talk to her about his fears. He only agreed to go to his primary care nurse practitioner to request sleeping medication.

Mr. Blake was admitted to the psychiatric unit, and his care was assigned to Ms. Dawson, a registered nurse. She observes that Mr. Blake is quiet and passive as he is oriented to the unit but that he looks around vigilantly and is easily startled by sounds on the unit.

Self-Assessment

Ms. Dawson is a registered nurse with an associate's degree and 3 years of experience on this unit. Initially, she feels sympathy for Mr. Blake, and he reminds her of her Uncle James, who served in Vietnam. She is concerned because his suicide plan was lethal and he is guarded in his speech, not revealing his thoughts or feelings. Ms. Dawson implements suicide precautions. She knows that she will demonstrate an attitude of hope and acceptance to him to develop trust.

Assessment

Screening tools include the Primary Care PTSD Screen for *DSM-5* (PC-PTSD-5; Prins et al., 2015), Impact of Events Scale (IES; Horowitz et al., 1979; Box 16.2), Impact of Events Scale-Revised (IES-R; Weiss & Marmar, 1996), and the PTSD Checklist (PCL; Lang & Stein, 2005). A more comprehensive assessment is indicated for those who initially screen positive.

Additional history about the time of onset, frequency, course, severity, level of distress, and degree of functional impairment is important. Further assessment for suicidal or violent ideation, family and social supports, insomnia, social withdrawal, functional impairment, current life stressors, medication, past medical and psychiatric history, and a Mental Status Exam are indicated (refer to Chapter 7). The diagnosis of PTSD involves a comprehensive clinical interview that assesses all symptoms collectively.

Objective Data	Subjective Data
Hypervigilance	Sleep difficulty, nightmares
Alcohol on breath	Alcohol use
Irritable	Feels estranged from wife and children
Withdrawn mood	Avoids news coverage with potential for emergency reports
Constricted range of affect	Suicide plan
	"I don't deserve to live; I should have died with the others."
	"You can't stop me."

Diagnosis

The initial plan is to maintain safety for Mr. Blake while encouraging him to express feelings and recognize that his situation is not hopeless. His nursing diagnosis is: *Risk for suicide as evidenced by suicidal plan and verbalization of intent.*

Outcomes Identification

Patient will have a decreased suicide risk.

Planning

The initial plan is to maintain safety for Mr. Blake while encouraging him to express feelings and recognize that his situation is not hopeless.

Implementation

Mr. Blake's plan of care is personalized as follows:

Short-Term

Goal	Intervention	Rationale	Evaluation
1. Patient will speak to staff whenever experiencing self-destructive thoughts.	1a. Administer medications with mouth checks. 1b. Provide ongoing surveillance of patient and environment. 1c. Use direct, nonjudgmental approach in discussing suicide. 1d. Provide illness teaching regarding PTSD.	1a. Addresses risk of hiding medications. 1b. Provides one-to-one monitoring for safety. 1c. Encourages increased self-control. 1d. Shows acceptance of patient's situation with respect. 1e. Offers reality of treatment.	**GOAL MET** After 8 h, patient contracts for safety every shift and starts to discuss feelings of self-harm.

Continued

Short-Term Goal	Intervention	Rationale	Evaluation	Short-Term Goal	Intervention	Rationale	Evaluation
2. Patient will express feelings by the third day of hospitalization.	2a. Interact with patient at regular intervals to convey caring and openness and to provide an opportunity to talk. 2b. Use silence and listening to encourage expression of feelings. 2c. Be open to expressions of loneliness and powerlessness. 2d. Share observations or thoughts about patient's behavior or response.	2a. Encourages development of trust. 2b. Shows positive expectation that patient will respond. 2c. Allows patient to voice these uncomfortable feelings. 2d. Directs attention to here-and-now treatment situation.	GOAL MET By second day, patient occasionally answers questions about feelings and admits to anger and grief.	3. Patient will express will to live by discharge from unit.	3a. Listen to expressions of grief. 3b. Encourage patient to identify own strengths and abilities. 3c. Explore with patient previous methods of dealing with life problems. 3d. Assist in identifying available support systems. 3e. Refer to spiritual advisor of individual's choice.	3a. Supports patient, communicating that such feelings are natural. 3b. Affirms patient's worth and potential to survive. 3c. Reinforces patient's past coping skills and ability to problem solve now. 3d. Addresses fact that anxiety has narrowed patient's perspective, distorting reality about loved ones. 3e. Allows opportunity to explore spiritual values and self-worth.	GOAL MET By third day, patient becomes tearful and states that he does not want to hurt his wife and daughter.

Evaluation

See individual outcomes and evaluation within the care plan.

ACUTE STRESS DISORDER

Acute stress disorder (ASD) may develop after exposure to a highly traumatic event, such as those listed in the prior section on PTSD. ASD is diagnosed 3 days to 1 month after the traumatic event. To be diagnosed with ASD, the individual must display 8 out of the following 14 symptoms either during or after the traumatic event:

- A subjective sense of numbing
- Derealization (a sense of unreality related to the environment)
- Inability to remember at least one important aspect of the event
- Intrusive distressing memories of the event
- Recurrent distressing dreams
- Feeling as if the event is recurring
- Intense prolonged distress or physiological reactivity
- Avoidance of thoughts or feelings about the event
- Sleep disturbances
- Hypervigilance
- Irritable, angry, or aggressive behavior
- Exaggerated startle response
- Agitation or restlessness

VIGNETTE: Olivia, a 22-year-old college student, is sexually assaulted by a family acquaintance. After being brought into the emergency department by a friend, she describes feeling detached from her body and being unaware of her surroundings during the assault, "as though it took place in a vacuum." She displays virtually no affect (i.e., she does not cry or appear anxious, angry, or sad). Olivia finds it difficult to concentrate on the examiner's questions. After a week, Olivia still feels as though her mind is detached from her body; she reports having difficulty sleeping, not being able to concentrate, and startling whenever anyone touches her.

APPLICATION OF THE NURSING PROCESS

ASSESSMENT

A nursing assessment for acute stress disorder is similar to that of PTSD. One key difference is that individuals who have recently experienced trauma may have more difficulty sharing their symptoms. Furthermore, this population is more likely to experience derealization, which makes a person less secure in the environment. These problems result in a need for for a non-rushed and reassuring approach to assessment.

BOX 16.2   Impact of Events Scale

On (date) _____, you experienced a motor vehicle accident. Below is a list of comments made by people after stressful life events. Please check each item, indicating how frequently these comments were true for you DURING THE PAST 7 DAYS. If they did not occur during that time, please mark the "not at all" column.

I thought about it when I didn't mean to.
   Not at all
   Rarely
   Sometimes
   Often

I avoided letting myself get upset when I thought about it or was reminded of it.
   Not at all
   Rarely
   Sometimes
   Often

I tried to remove it from memory
   Not at all
   Rarely
   Sometimes
   Often

I had trouble falling asleep or staying asleep, because pictures or thoughts about it came into my mind.
   Not at all
   Rarely
   Sometimes
   Often

I had waves of strong feelings about it.
   Not at all
   Rarely
   Sometimes
   Often

I had dreams about it.
   Not at all
   Rarely
   Sometimes
   Often

I stayed away from reminders of it.
   Not at all
   Rarely
   Sometimes
   Often

I felt as if it hadn't happened or it wasn't real.
   Not at all
   Rarely
   Sometimes
   Often

I tried not to talk about it.
   Not at all
   Rarely
   Sometimes
   Often

Pictures about it popped into my mind.
   Not at all
   Rarely
   Sometimes
   Often

Other things kept making me think about it.
   Not at all
   Rarely
   Sometimes
   Often

I was aware that I still had a lot of feelings about it, but I didn't deal with them.
   Not at all
   Rarely
   Sometimes
   Often

I tried not to think about it.
   Not at all
   Rarely
   Sometimes
   Often

Any reminder brought back feelings about it.
   Not at all
   Rarely
   Sometimes
   Often

My feelings about it were kind of numb.
   Not at all
   Rarely
   Sometimes
   Often

Horowitz, M., Wilner, N., & Alvarez, W. (1979). Impact of events scale: A measure of subjective stress. *Psychosomatic Medicine, 41*, 209–218.

Screening tools used for PTSD such as the PC-PTSD-5 are also used to gauge the severity of symptoms in acute stress disorder. A specific self-reporting Acute Stress Disorder Scale (Bryant, 2016) is useful in indexing acute stress disorder. It is also predictive for the subsequent development of PTSD.

NURSING DIAGNOSIS

As with PTSD, the priority nursing diagnosis is *post trauma response*. Other appropriate nursing diagnoses for a patient with ASD (ICN, 2019) are *impaired adaptation* and *anxiety (specify level)*.

OUTCOMES IDENTIFICATION

Addressing the prioritized nursing diagnoses results in outcomes such as:
1. Reduced response to trauma
2. Improved adaptation
3. Decreased anxiety

IMPLEMENTATION

The nurse's role in caring for a patient with ASD involves primarily establishing a therapeutic relationship with the person, helping the person to problem solve, connecting the person to supports such as family and friends, educating about ASD, coordination of care through collaboration with others, ensuring and maintaining safety, and monitoring response and/or adherence to treatment.

EVALUATION

See the Evaluation section for PTSD provided previously.

TREATMENT MODALITIES

Psychological Therapies

CBT has been found to be effective in reducing the subsequent development of PTSD for people with ASD (Hsih & MacKinnon, 2017). Other promising therapies for ASD include specialized protocols for EMDR therapy, the EMDR Protocol for Recent Critical Incidents (EMDR-PRECI) (Jarero, Artigas, & Luber, 2011), the Recent Event Protocol (Luber, 2009), and the Recent Traumatic Episode Protocol (R-TEP) (Shapiro & Laub, 2008).

ADJUSTMENT DISORDER

A milder, less specific version of ASD and PTSD is **adjustment disorder**. Like ASD and PTSD, it is precipitated by a stressful event. However, the event—including retirement, chronic illness, or a breakup—may not be as severe and may not be considered a traumatic event. Adjustment disorder may be diagnosed immediately or within 3 months of exposure.

Symptoms of adjustment disorder run the gamut of all forms of distress, including guilt, depression, anxiety, and anger. These feelings may be combined with other manifestations of distress, including physical complaints, social withdrawal, impaired occupational function, and academic decline.

Losing a loved one due to death may result in a specific type of adjustment disorder. Complicated grieving occurs during the 12-month period of time after the loss of a loved one. This type of adjustment disorder is manifested by intense yearning and longing for the deceased. It is accompanied by deep sorrow and emotional pain or preoccupation with the deceased or the circumstances of the death. In addition, the person may feel anger, a diminished sense of self, emptiness, difficulty in relationships, and in planning future activities.

The prevalence of adjustment disorder varies widely, depending on the setting. For example, in a general acute care unit, adjustment disorders occurred in 12% of the patients. On a post cardiac surgery floor, up to 50% of the population were diagnosable with adjustment disorders (Strain, 2018). Within community samples, about 2% to 8% of children, adolescents, and older adults have adjustment disorders.

The standard intervention for adjustment disorders is psychotherapy, which may include reality orientation, crisis intervention, family therapy, or group treatment. The goal of any of these interventions is to encourage verbalization of emotions related to the stressors. Depressive symptoms associated with adjustment disorders are generally treated with antidepressants, and anxiety symptoms are treated with benzodiazepines.

DISSOCIATIVE DISORDERS

Dissociative disorders occur after significant adverse experiences and traumas. The predominant response is a severe interruption of consciousness. Dissociation is an unconscious defense mechanism that protects the individual against overwhelming anxiety through an emotional separation. However, this separation results in disturbances in memory, consciousness, self-identity, and perception.

Mild, fleeting dissociative experiences are relatively common for all of us. For example, we say we are on "auto-pilot" when we drove home from work and cannot recall the last 15 minutes before reaching the house.

These common experiences are distinctly different from the processes of pathological dissociation. Dissociation is involuntary and results in failure of the normal control over a person's mental processes and normal integration of conscious awareness (Spiegel et al., 2011). Dimensions of a memory that should be linked are not and are fragmented. For example, a person may be aware of a sound or smell, but these sensations would not be linked to the actual event itself, leaving the person fearful and/or confused. In addition, the person may re-enact, as well as re-experience, trauma without consciously knowing why.

Symptoms of dissociation may be either positive or negative. Positive symptoms refer to unwanted additions to mental activity, such as flashbacks. Negative symptoms refer to deficits, such as memory problems or the inability to sense or control different parts of the body. Dissociation may be protective in that it decreases the immediate distress of the trauma and also continues to protect the individual from full awareness of the disturbing event.

This protective aspect of dissociation can be seen in children who continue to be attached to caretakers who are abusive or neglectful. Dissociation allows them to fragment the good from the bad. Memories of abuse and neglect may become compartmentalized, and often do not intrude into awareness until later in life during stressful situations.

Epidemiology

The prevalence of dissociative disorders occurring at some time during a person's life in the United States is fairly high, with a range from 2% to 10% (International Society for the Study of Trauma and Dissociation [ISSTD], 2012). Patients with these disorders usually seek treatment for another problem, such as anxiety or depression.

Risk Factors

Childhood physical, sexual, or emotional abuse and other traumatic life events are associated with adults experiencing dissociative symptoms. Dissociative symptoms, or "mindflight," actually reduce disturbing feelings and protect the person from full awareness of the trauma.

Biological Factors

Genetic. Although genetic variability is thought to play a role in stress reactivity, dissociation is thought to be largely due to extreme stress or environmental factors.

Neurobiological. Research suggests that the limbic system is involved in the development of dissociative disorders. Animal studies show that early, prolonged detachment from the caretaker negatively affects the development of the limbic system. Traumatic memories are processed in the limbic system, and the hippocampus stores this information. Individuals with dissociative disorders have increased activation of the orbital frontal cortex that inhibits activation of the amygdala and insular cortex as well as the hippocampal areas (Spiegel et al., 2011).

Cognitive Factors

One of the most primitive ego defense mechanisms is dissociation. The theory of structural dissociation of the personality proposes that patients with complex trauma have different parts of their personality, the apparently normal part and the emotional part, that are not fully integrated with each other (Steele et al., 2005). Each part has its own responses, feelings, thoughts, perceptions, physical sensations, and behaviors. These different parts may not be aware of each other, with only one dominant personality operating depending on the situation and circumstance of the moment.

Environmental Factors

Dissociative disorders are responses to acute overwhelming trauma and as such are due to environmental factors. These may include any experience that is overwhelming to the person, such as a motor vehicle accident, combat, emotional/verbal abuse, incest, neglectful or abusive caregivers, imprisonment, and many other types of traumatic events.

Cultural Considerations

Certain culture-bound disorders exist in which there is a high level of activity, a trancelike state, and running or fleeing, followed by exhaustion, sleep, and amnesia regarding the episode. These syndromes include *piblokto*, seen in native people of the Arctic; *frenzy* witchcraft among the Navajo; and *amok* among Western Pacific natives. These syndromes, if observed in individuals native to the corresponding geographical areas, should be differentiated from dissociative disorders.

🌐 CONSIDERING CULTURE

Are Dissociative Disorders Equally Distributed Across Cultures?

Culture-bound syndromes of psychiatric disorders are common. These syndromes are a combination of psychiatric and somatic symptoms that are recognizable diseases only within a specific culture. Researchers who have studied dissociative disorders extensively have concluded that pathological dissociation and dissociative disorders occur at comparable rates in different cultures. They conclude that pathological dissociation in response to traumatic events is a universal phenomenon.

Adapted from Kruger, C. (2019). Culture, trauma, and dissociation: A broadening perspective for our field. *Journal of Trauma & Dissociation, 21*(1), 1–13.

DISSOCIATIVE AMNESIA

Dissociative amnesia is marked by the inability to recall important personal information, often of a traumatic or stressful nature; this lack of memory is too pervasive to be explained by ordinary forgetfulness. In dissociative amnesia, autobiographical memory is available but is not accessible. In contrast, a patient with generalized amnesia is unable to recall information about his or her entire lifetime. The amnesia may also be localized (the patient is unable to remember all events in a certain period) or selective (the patient is able to recall some but not all events in a certain period).

A subtype of dissociative amnesia is **dissociative fugue**, which is characterized by sudden, unexpected travel away from the customary locale and inability to recall one's identity and information about some or all of the past. In rare cases, an individual with dissociative fugue assumes a whole new identity. During a fugue state, individuals tend to lead rather simple lives, rarely calling attention to themselves. After a few weeks to a few months, they may remember their former identities and then become amnesic for the time spent in the fugue state. Usually, a dissociative fugue is precipitated by a traumatic event. In fugue states, individuals often function adequately in their new identities by choosing simple, undemanding occupations and having few intimate social interactions. Patients with amnesia, in contrast to those with fugue, may be more dysfunctional.

ACEs are risk factors for the development of dissociative amnesia. An increasing number, severity, frequency of these experiences, and level of violence make this disorder more likely.

Dissociative amnesia is also fairly common, with a prevalence of about 2% to 7%. Dissociative amnesia may occur in any age group, from children to adults. The amnesia is often related to trauma, and memory returns spontaneously after the individual is removed from the stressful situation (ISSTD, 2012).

Dissociative amnesia may be comorbid with a conversion disorder or a personality disorder. Dissociative fugue may co-occur with PTSD.

There are no specific treatments for dissociative amnesia (Maldonado & Spiegel, 2019). Anxiety-reducing medications such as benzodiazepines may be used short term. Usually, dissociative amnesia reverts spontaneously, particularly when the stressful situation has been resolved or when the person is exposed to cues from the past. Since patients with these symptoms tend to be highly hypnotizable, hypnosis is used to regress the patient back to the time before the amnesia commenced.

> **VIGNETTE:** A young woman found wandering in a Florida park is partly dressed and poorly nourished. She has no knowledge of who she is. Her parents identify her 2 weeks later when she appears in an interview on a national television show. She had just broken up with her boyfriend of 3 years.

DEPERSONALIZATION/DEREALIZATION DISORDER

Depersonalization/derealization disorder results in persistent or recurrent episodes of depersonalization, derealization, or both. **Depersonalization** is an extremely uncomfortable feeling of being an observer of one's own body or mental processes. Feelings of unreality, detachment, or unfamiliarity with parts of self or the whole self are features of this disorder. A patient may feel detached from his entire self, aspects of himself, including feelings, thoughts, body parts, or sensations.

In **derealization**, the focus is on the outside world. It is the recurring feeling that one's surroundings are unreal or distant. The person may feel like she is walking around in a fog, bubble, or dream. It may feel like there is an invisible veil between her and the rest of the world. Visual distortions are manifested in blurriness, changes in the visual field (widened or narrowed), and altered size of objects. Auditory distortions include the muting or heightening of sound.

Some people suffer episodes of these problems that come and go, while others have episodes that begin with stressors and eventually become constant. Patients describe these experiences as very distressing.

Most people experience transient symptoms of this disorder. The lifetime prevalence of depersonalization/derealization disorder is about 2%. The gender ratio is about 1:1. Most people who develop this disorder do so before the age of 20.

ACEs such as emotional abuse and neglect are associated with depersonalization/derealization disorder. Severe stress and illegal drug use are usually the precipitants of an episode.

Depersonalization/derealization disorder occurs comorbidly with major depressive disorder and anxiety disorders. Three personality disorders—avoidant, borderline, and obsessive-compulsive—commonly have symptoms of depersonalization/derealization.

Depersonalization and derealization are often short-lived and go away on their own without treatment. However, some treatment modalities have been used with success, including self-hypnosis and CBT (Maldonado & Spiegel, 2019). Pharmacotherapy is used to treat comorbid disorders and symptoms, such as antianxiety agents and antidepressants. Repetitive transcranial magnetic stimulation (rTMS) has been used successfully in the treatment of this disorder as well.

> **VIGNETTE:** Elizabeth, a 42-year-old executive, gasps as she looks in the mirror. She can't believe the changes in her appearance. She thinks that her body looks wavy and out of focus. She says that it feels as though she is floating in a fog and her feet are not actually touching the ground. "I wonder if I am really awake or if my life is a dream." As she is admitted to the stress-management unit, Elizabeth confides to the nurse that her son has recently been charged with insider trading in the stock market and that he may be facing a lengthy jail sentence.

DISSOCIATIVE IDENTITY DISORDER

The essential feature of **dissociative identity disorder** is the presence of two or more distinct personality states that recurrently take control of behavior. Each **alternate personality (alter)** has its own pattern of perceiving, relating to, and thinking about the self and the environment. It is believed that severe sexual, physical, or psychological trauma in childhood predisposes an individual to the development of dissociative identity disorder.

Dissociative identity disorder is characterized by at least two identity states: one is a state or personality that functions on a daily basis and blocks access and responses to traumatic memories. A second or more state, referred to as an *alter state*, is fixated on traumatic memories. These separate states are due to the activation of increased endogenous opioids that prevent high arousal states at times of severe threat (Lanius, Paulson, & Corrigan, 2014). This response is mediated by the dorsal vagal parasympathetic response, such as occurs in mammals who freeze when threatened and play dead.

Each alter is a complex unit with its own memories, behavioral patterns, and social relationships that dictate how the person acts when that personality is dominant. Often, the original or primary personality is moralistic, while the alters are pleasure-seeking and nonconforming. The alter personalities may behave as individuals of a different sex, race, or religion. The dominant hand and the voice may also be different. Intelligence and even electroencephalographic (EEG) findings may also be altered.

Typical cognitive distortions include the insistence that alternate personalities inhabit separate bodies and are unaffected by the actions of one another. The primary personality or host is usually not aware of the alters and is perplexed by lost time and unexplained events. Experiences such as finding unfamiliar clothing in the closet, being called a different name by a stranger, or not having childhood memories are characteristic of dissociative identity disorder. Alters may be aware of the existence of each other to some degree. The transition from one personality to another (switching) occurs during times of stress and may range from a dramatic to a barely noticeable event. Some patients experience the transition when awakening. Shifts may last from minutes to months, although shorter periods are more common.

Several movies and TV shows with individuals diagnosed with dissociative identity disorder have been produced. They include the classic *Sybil* (1976), *Fight Club* (1999), *Me, Myself and Irene* (2000), *Hereditary* (2018), and the television series *The United States of Tara* (2009–2011).

The exact prevalence of dissociative identity disorder is difficult to determine. Since switching from one personality to another happens infrequently, clinicians do not have the opportunity to observe this switching. Therefore, given the unusual symptoms, many people are misdiagnosed as having a psychotic disorder, such as schizophrenia.

The 12-month prevalence of dissociative identity disorder is 1.5%. Dissociative identity disorder may occur at any age but is diagnosed slightly more frequently in adult females than in adult males.

Individuals with dissociative identity disorder usually have comorbid conditions. Most patients will also exhibit PTSD. Other disorders that are highly comorbid include depressive disorders, avoidant and borderline personality disorders, conversion disorder, somatic symptom disorder, eating disorders, substance use disorders, obsessive-compulsive disorder, and sleep disorder.

Risk factors for dissociative identity disorder include physical and sexual abuse. About 90% of people with the disorder experienced childhood abuse and neglect (APA, 2013). Other traumatizing experiences, such as severe medical illness and other mental disorders, are considered risk factors.

Suicide risk is extremely high—up to 70% of outpatients with this disorder have attempted suicide (APA, 2013). Assessment of previous suicide behavior may be extremely difficult due to the presence of more than one personality state.

APPLICATION OF THE NURSING PROCESS

ASSESSMENT

For a diagnosis of dissociative identity disorder to be made, medical and neurological illnesses, substance use, and other psychiatric disorders are ruled out. The assessment should include objective data from physical examination, EEG, imaging studies, and specific questions to identify dissociative symptoms.

Scales are useful to assess dissociation. They include the Dissociative Experience Scale (DES; Bernstein & Putnam, 1986), the Somatoform Questionnaire (SDQ; Nijenhuis, Spinhoven, Van Dyck, Van der Hart, & Vanderlinden, 1996), and the Dissociative Disorders Interview Schedule (DDIS; Ross et al., 1989). The latter two are available online.

These assessment tools are important because a psychiatric interview will often miss the presence of dissociation. By definition, dissociative periods involve lapses of memory that a person may be aware of, and patients with dissociative disorders do not know what they do not know. Specific information about identity, memory, consciousness, life events, mood, suicide risk, and the impact of the disorder on the patient and the family are important dimensions to assess.

Assessing patients' ability to identify themselves requires more than asking them to state their names. Changes in patient behavior, voice, and dress might signal the presence of an alternate personality. Referring to the self by another name or in the third person and using the word *we* instead of *I* are indications that the patient may have assumed a new identity. The nurse should consider the following when assessing memory:

1. Can the patient remember recent and past events?
2. Is the patient's memory clear and complete or partial and fuzzy?
3. Is the patient aware of gaps in memory, for example, a lack of memory for events such as a graduation or a wedding?
4. Do the patient's memories place the self with a family, in school, or in an occupation?
5. Does the patient ever lose time or have blackouts?
6. Does the patient ever find herself or himself in places with no idea how she or he got there?

History

The nurse gathers information about events in the person's life. Has the patient sustained a recent injury, such as a concussion? Does the patient have a history of epilepsy, especially temporal lobe epilepsy? Does the patient have a history of early trauma, such as physical, mental, or sexual abuse? If dissociative identity disorder is suspected, pertinent questions include the following:

1. Have you ever found yourself wearing clothes you cannot remember buying?
2. Have you ever had people you didn't know approach you as though they were old friends?
3. Does your ability to engage in activities such as sports, creative tasks, or mechanical work seem to change?
4. Do you have memories about your childhood?

Mood

Many patients with dissociative identity disorder seek help when the primary personality is depressed. The nurse also observes for mood shifts. When alternate identities of dissociative identity disorder take control, their predominant moods may be different from that of the principal personality. If the alternate identities shift frequently, marked mood swings may be noted.

Impact on Patient and Family

Losing time results in confusion for the patient. This confusion along with disorganization make employment extremely difficult. Families find it difficult to accept the seemingly erratic behaviors of the patient. The patient's memory loss interferes with normal relationships. Families often direct considerable attention toward the patient but may exhibit concern over having to assume roles that were once assigned to the patient.

Suicide Risk

Whenever lives have been substantially disrupted, patients may have thoughts of suicide. The nurse gathering data should be alert for expressions of hopelessness, helplessness, or worthlessness and for verbalization or other behavior of an alternate identity that indicates the intent to engage in self-destructive or self-mutilating behaviors.

Self-Assessment

It is natural to experience feelings of skepticism while caring for patients who are diagnosed with dissociative identity disorder. You may find it difficult to believe in the authenticity of the symptoms the patient is displaying. A sense of inadequacy may accompany the need to be ready to interact in a therapeutic way with whichever personality is in control at the moment. However, some nurses experience feelings of fascination and are caught up in the intrigue of caring for a patient with multiple identities.

Feelings of inadequacy can also arise when the establishment of a trusting relationship occurs slowly. It is important to remember that the patient with a dissociative disorder has often experienced relationships in which trust was betrayed. When alters struggle for control and attempt to embarrass or harm each other, crises are common. Preparing for the unexpected, including the possibility of a suicide attempt, means constant hypervigilance by staff, and such observational demands can eventually lead to fatigue. Caring for a patient with a dissociative disorder can generate anxiety in any of the following situations:

1. When a patient who has regained memory develops panic-level anxiety
2. When a patient becomes assaultive because of extreme confusion or panic-level anxiety

3. When a patient attempts self-harm by acting out against the primary personality or other personalities

If the patient manifesting symptoms of a dissociative disorder has been involved in the commission of a crime, the medical record is likely to be a court exhibit. You may experience concern over that fact or be angry if you believe the patient is faking illness to avoid being found guilty of the crime. Supervision should always be available for nursing staff and clinicians caring for a patient with a dissociative disorder. By discussing feelings and the plan of care with the treatment team or peers, the nurse can better ensure objective and appropriate care for the patient.

ASSESSMENT GUIDELINES

Dissociative Identity Disorder

1. Assess for a history of self-harm.
2. Evaluate the level of anxiety and signs of dissociation.
3. Identify support systems through a psychosocial assessment.

NURSING DIAGNOSIS

The overall medical goal for dissociative identity disorder is the integration of personalities into a single personality. ICN (2019) nursing diagnoses include *disturbed personal identity*, *impaired role performance*, and *anxiety* (*specify level*).

OUTCOMES IDENTIFICATION

Overall outcomes will be based on the nursing diagnosis. Therefore, based on the diagnoses named above, the outcomes will be:
1. Improved personal identity
2. Improved role performance
3. Reduced anxiety

PLANNING

The setting and presenting problem influence the planning of nursing care for the patient with a dissociative disorder. However, a phase-oriented treatment model is recommended and includes the following (ISSTD, 2012):

Phase 1: Establishing safety, stabilization, and symptom reduction

Phase 2: Confronting, working through, and integrating traumatic memories

Phase 3: Identity integration and rehabilitation

The nurse will most often encounter the patient in times of crisis (i.e., when the patient is admitted to the hospital for suicidal or homicidal behavior). The care plan will focus on Phase 1 strategies to ensure safety and crisis intervention. The patient may also come for the treatment of a comorbid depression or anxiety disorder in the community setting. Planning will address the presenting complaint with appropriate referrals for treatment of the dissociative disorder.

IMPLEMENTATION

Healing trauma can be thought of as a process of integration and linking neural networks that have become disconnected during an overwhelming event. Basic-level interventions are aimed at offering emotional presence during the recall of painful experiences, providing a sense of safety, and encouraging an optimal level of functioning. *NIC* topics that offer relevant interventions include *anxiety reduction*, *coping enhancement*, *self-awareness enhancement*, *self-esteem enhancement*, and *emotional support*. Refer to Table 16.2 for examples of basic-level interventions.

TABLE 16.2 Basic-Level Nursing Interventions for Dissociative Disorders

Intervention	Rationale
Provide an undemanding, simple routine.	Reduces anxiety
Ensure patient safety by providing safe, protected environment and frequent observation.	Sense of bewilderment may lead to inattention to safety needs; some alters may be thrill-seeking, violent, or careless
Confirm the identity of patient and orientation to time and place.	Supports reality and promotes ego integrity
Encourage patient to do things for self and make decisions about routine tasks.	Enhances self-esteem by reducing sense of powerlessness and reduces secondary gain associated with dependence
Assist with major decision making until memory returns.	Lowers stress and prevents patient from having to live with the consequences of unwise decisions
Support patient during the exploration of feelings surrounding the stressful event.	Helps lower the defense of dissociation used by patient to block awareness of the stressful event
Do not flood patient with data regarding past events.	Memory loss serves the purpose of preventing severe to panic levels of anxiety from overtaking and disorganizing the individual
Allow patient to progress at own pace as memory is recovered.	Prevents undue anxiety and resistance
Provide support through empathetic listening during disclosure of painful experiences.	Can be healing, while minimizing feelings of isolation
Teach patient grounding techniques, such as taking a shower, deep breathing, touching fabric on chair, exercising, or stomping feet.	Helps to keep the person in the present and decrease dissociation
Accept patient's expression of negative feelings.	Conveys permission to have negative or unacceptable feelings
Teach stress-reduction methods.	Provides alternatives for anxiety relief
If patient does not remember significant others, work with involved parties to reestablish relationships.	Helps patient experience satisfaction and relieves sense of isolation

Health Teaching and Promotion

Patients with dissociative disorders need to be educated about their illness and given ongoing instruction about coping skills and stress management. Normalizing experiences by explaining to the patient that his or her symptoms are adaptive responses to past overwhelming events is important. Often, the victim of childhood trauma feels as if he or she is a bad person and grows up with the false negative belief that the abuse was deserved punishment.

Teaching **grounding techniques** that bring the person's awareness back to noticing real things in the present helps counter dissociative episodes. Examples of grounding techniques can include the following: stomping one's feet on the ground, taking a shower, holding an ice cube, exercising, deep breathing, counting beads, or touching fabric or upholstery on a chair. Patients should also be taught to keep a daily journal to increase their awareness of feelings and to identify triggers to dissociation. If a patient has never written a journal, the nurse should suggest beginning with a 5- to 10-minute daily writing exercise.

EVALUATION

Overall, treatment effectiveness for dissociative identity disorder is "integration," coordinated functioning among alternate identities to promote optimal functioning (ISSTD, 2012). This occurs primarily through long-term psychotherapy.

In general, treatment for trauma-related disorders is considered successful when outcomes are met. The evaluation of treatment is positive when:

1. Patient safety has been maintained.
2. Anxiety has been reduced, and the patient has returned to a functional state.
3. Integration of the fragmented memories has occurred.
4. New coping strategies have permitted the patient to function at a better level.
5. Stress is handled adaptively, without the use of dissociation.

TREATMENT MODALITIES

Biological Treatments

Pharmacotherapy

There are no specific medications for patients with dissociative disorders, but appropriate medications are often prescribed for the hyperarousal and intrusive symptoms that accompany PTSD and dissociation (ISSTD, 2012). These might include antidepressant medication, anxiolytics, and antipsychotics. Substance use disorders and suicidal risk, which are common, must be assessed carefully in selecting safe and appropriate pharmacotherapy. In the acute setting, the nurse may witness dramatic memory retrieval in patients with dissociative amnesia or fugue after treatment with intravenous benzodiazepines.

Psychological Therapies

Advanced practice nurses and other skilled licensed mental health professionals use CBT, psychodynamic psychotherapy, exposure therapy, modified EMDR therapy, hypnotherapy, neurofeedback, ego state therapies, somatic therapies, and medication to treat patients with dissociative disorders. Advanced training is needed to treat these patients effectively as such, and ongoing supervision is suggested.

Somatic Therapy

Dissociation causes people to experience a distressing fragmentation of consciousness and a sense of separation from themselves. Disturbances of perception, sensation, autonomic regulation, and movement are common for those who have suffered significant trauma, since trauma is often stored physically in the body. Verbal and bodily psychotherapies are seen as complementary by the discipline of dance movement therapists in working with traumatized dissociative patients in emotional recovery (Colace, 2017; Koch & Harvey, 2012).

A specific type of somatic psychotherapy, sensorimotor psychotherapy, combines talking therapy with body-centered interventions and movement to address the dissociative symptoms inherent in trauma (Buckley, Punkanen, & Ogden, 2018). This type of therapy is integrated into phase-oriented trauma treatment to facilitate symptom reduction and stability, to integrate the traumatic memory, and to restore the person's ability to stay in the present moment. This therapy is based on the premise that the body, mind, emotions, and spirit are interrelated, and a change at one level results in changes in the others. Awareness, focusing on the present, and recognizing touch as a means of communicating are some of the principles of this therapy. During psychotherapy sessions, the patient is asked to describe the physical sensations he or she is experiencing. The goal is to safely disarm the pathological defense mechanism of dissociation and replace it with other resources, especially body awareness and mindfulness.

▮ KEY POINTS TO REMEMBER

- Childhood trauma changes the brain and can cause medical and psychological problems in adulthood.
- A phase model of treatment is most effective, with safety and stabilization first.
- Evidenced-based treatments for trauma are EMDR therapy and CBT.
- Understanding patients as traumatized changes the conversation from "What is wrong with this person?" to "What happened to this person?"
- Trauma fractures and fragments memory; healing involves connection and integration.

- Trauma is stored in the body and often manifests as physical symptoms.
- Dissociative disorders involve a disruption in consciousness with significant impairments in memory, identity, and perception of self.
- Assessment is especially important in clarifying the history and course of past symptoms as well as obtaining a complete picture of the current physical, mental, and safety status.
- Patients with dissociative disorders are often misdiagnosed with depression, schizophrenia, or borderline personality disorder.

- Psychotherapy is the treatment of choice for trauma, with medication prescribed only to ameliorate symptoms.
- Patients with trauma-related disorders are often treated on an outpatient basis, except during a period of crisis such as suicidal risk.
- Crisis intervention is important for stabilization; referral for psychotherapy to attain sustained improvement in level of functioning is typically necessary.

CRITICAL THINKING

1. Jeanne is a 48-year-old woman with dissociative identity disorder who was admitted to the crisis unit for a short-term stay after a suicide threat. On the unit, she has repeated the statement that she will kill herself to get rid of "all the others"—meaning her alters.
   a. How do you think the staff reacts to working with patients such as Jeanne?
   b. What do you believe needs to be done to protect Jeanne?
2. Cyrus is an 8-year-old child who was in a devastating earthquake and came to the outpatient clinic with his parents because he was having nightmares and trouble sleeping. How would you explain what is happening to Cyrus?
3. Erich, a 24-year-old man, returned from the Afghan War last month and has become increasingly irritable, isolated, and depressed. His wife says he does not want to go anywhere and won't leave his home for days at a time. In the interview with the nurse at the clinic, Erich indicates that he feels helpless, anxious, and jumpy. The mental healthcare provider assigns a diagnosis of posttraumatic stress disorder. Identify priorities in providing care for this patient and develop a nursing care plan.

CHAPTER REVIEW

1. Nick, a construction worker, is on duty when a nearly completed wall suddenly falls, crushing a number of his co-workers. Although badly shaken initially, he seemed to be coping well. About 2 weeks after the tragedy, he begins to experience tremors, nightmares, and periods during which he feels numb or detached from his environment. He finds himself frequently thinking about the tragedy and feeling guilty that he was spared while many others died. Which statement about this situation is most accurate?
   a. Nick has acute stress disorder and will benefit from antianxiety medications.
   b. Nick is experiencing posttraumatic stress disorder (PTSD) and should be referred for outpatient treatment.
   c. Nick is experiencing anxiety and grief and should be monitored for PTSD symptoms.
   d. Nick is experiencing mild anxiety and a normal grief reaction; no intervention is needed.
2. You are caring for Susannah, a 29-year-old who has been diagnosed with dissociative identity disorder. She was recently hospitalized after coming to the emergency department with deep cuts on her arms with no memory of how this occurred. The priority nursing intervention for Susannah is:
   a. Assist in recovering memories of abuse.
   b. Maintain 1:1 observation.
   c. Teach coping skills and stress-management strategies.
   d. Refer for integrative therapy.
3. You are caring for Connor, an 8-year-old boy who has been diagnosed with reactive attachment disorder. Which of the following nursing outcomes would be the most appropriate to achieve?
   a. Increases ability to self-control and decreases impulsive behaviors.
   b. Avoids situations that trigger conflicts.
   c. Expresses complex thoughts.
   d. Writes or draws feelings in a journal.

4. Ashley is a 21-year-old college student who was sexually assaulted at a party. She was seen in the local emergency department and referred for counseling after being diagnosed by the provider on call as having acute stress disorder. Which of the following treatment modalities would you expect to see used in therapy with Ashley?
   a. Aversion therapy
   b. Stress-reduction therapy
   c. Cognitive behavioral therapy
   d. Short-term classical analysis therapy
5. Jamie, age 24, has been diagnosed with a dissociative disorder following a traumatic event. Jamie's mother asks you, "Does this mean my daughter is now crazy?" Your best response would be:
   a. "People with dissociative disorders are out of touch with reality, so in that way, your daughter is now mentally ill. Don't worry. Treatment is available."
   b. "Jamie will most likely need long-term intensive inpatient treatment to deal with her traumatic memories as well as to work through her delusions."
   c. "Most mental health providers are skeptical about dissociative disorders and aren't sure they truly exist. Jamie may be making up her symptoms as a cry for help."
   d. "Jamie is dealing with the anxiety associated with the trauma by separating herself from it. With treatment, she can get back to her previous level of functioning."
6. A young child is found wandering alone at a mall. A male store employee approaches and asks where her parents are. She responds, "I don't know. Maybe you will take me home with you?" This sort of response in children may be due to:
   a. A lack of bonding as an infant
   b. A healthy confidence in the child
   c. Adequate parental bonding
   d. Normal parenting

7. During a routine health screening, a grieving widow whose husband died 15 months ago reports emptiness, a loss of self, difficulty thinking of the future, and anger at her dead husband. The nurse suggests bereavement counseling. The widow is most likely suffering from:
   a. Major depression
   b. Normal grieving
   c. Adjustment disorder
   d. Posttraumatic stress disorder
8. Maggie, a child in protective custody, is found to have an imaginary friend, Holly. The foster family shares this information with the nurse. The nurse teaches the family members about children who have suffered trauma and knows her teaching was effective when the foster mother states:
   a. "I understand that imaginary friends are abnormal."
   b. "I understand that imaginary friends are a maladaptive behavior."
   c. "I understand that imaginary friends are a coping mechanism."
   d. "I understand that we should tell the child that imaginary friends are unacceptable."
9. The school nurse has been alerted to the fact that an 8-year-old boy routinely play acts as a police officer, "locking up" other children on the playground to the point where the children get scared. The nurse recognizes that this behavior is most likely an indication of:
   a. The need to dominate others
   b. Inventing traumatic events
   c. A need to develop close relationships
   d. A potential symptom of traumatization
10. A pregnant woman is in a relationship with a male who routinely abuses her. Her unborn child may engage in high-risk behavior as a teen as a result of:
    a. Maternal stress
    b. Parental nurturing
    c. Appropriate stress responses in the brain
    d. Memories of the abuse

1. a; 2. b; 3. d; 4. c; 5. d; 6. a; 7. c; 8. c; 9. d; 10. a

NGN CASE STUDY AND QUESTIONS

Three months after experiencing a motor vehicle accident that took the life of his wife and young son, Kevin, aged 35, is seen in the emergency department. He reports intrusive memories of the crash that cause heart palpitations and a sensation of terror he feels in the pit of his stomach. He reports feeling irritable, especially at work. He is unable to concentrate because he keeps "seeing the accident in my head." He asks for sleeping pills, saying, "Some nights the nightmares are so bad that I give up and go watch TV until it's time to go to work." He reports having no appetite, does not want to do anything, and feels detached from everyone he knows. At 6'2" he has lost 5 pounds from an original weight of 225 pounds.

When asked about a support system, including family and friends, he says, "I killed them, didn't I?" The nurse notes that his respirations increase, his voice shakes, and he is on the edge of tears, when he says, "I just can't talk about this anymore."

He is a moderate smoker and reports a slight increase in cigarettes smoked per day, "...but not that much." He has a history of physical abuse from a stepfather who was removed from the home when the patient was a child and one episode of major depressive disorder after a job layoff 7 years ago. He denies a return of the depressive symptoms once he got a new job—until now.

1. Indicate which actions listed in the left column would be included in the plan of care.

Actions	Plan of Care
a. Help determine the true cause of the crash to attain clarity.	
b. Explain the pathophysiology of posttraumatic stress disorder (PTSD).	
c. Teach deep breathing, imagery, and mindfulness exercises.	
d. Recommend a refresher course in safe driving to build confidence.	
e. Discourage the expression of negative thoughts that may contribute to depressive feelings.	
f. Prepare for eye movement desensitization and reprocessing (EMDR) therapy.	
g. Prepare for electroconvulsive therapy (ECT).	

2. The patient is expected to begin trauma-focused psychotherapy tomorrow as the primary means of treatment for PTSD. In the meantime, the provider has prescribed medication. Tonight, the nurse prepares to give the patient's first medication after admission to the behavioral health unit.

   Identify the medications that will be (1) administered (appropriate or necessary), (2) held until needed, and (3) contraindicated (contact the healthcare provider). Only one selection can be made for each drug.

Medication	1. Administer	2. Hold Until Needed	3. Contraindicated
Sertraline (Zoloft) once daily			
Acetaminophen (Tylenol) prn headache			
Aripiprazole (Abilify) once daily			
Risperidone (Risperdal) at bedtime			

NGN case study answers are on Evolve.

Visit the Evolve website for a posttest on the content in this chapter: http://evolve.elsevier.com/Varcarolis

REFERENCES

Ainsworth, M. D. (1967). *Infancy in Uganda*. Baltimore, MD: Johns Hopkins.

American Psychiatric Association. (2013). *DSM-5 table of contents*. Retrieved from http://www.psychiatry.org/dsm5.

Ariapooran, S., Heidari, S., Asgari, M., Ashtarian, H., & Khezeli, M. (2018). Individualism-collectivism, social support, resilience and suicidal ideation among women with the experience of the death of a young person. *International Journal of Community Based Nursing & Midwifery*, 6(3), 250–259.

Bernstein, E. M., & Putnam, F. W. (1986). Development, reliability, and validity of a dissociation scale. *Journal of Nervous and Mental Disease*, 174(12), 727–735.

Bowlby, J. (1988). *A secure base: Clinical applications of attachment theory*. London, UK: Routledge.

Briere, J. (1996). *The trauma symptom checklist for children*. Retrieved from http://www4.parinc.com/Products/Product.aspx?ProductID5TSCC.

Bryant, R., Friedman, M., Spiegel, D., Ursano, R., & Strain, J. (2011). A review of acute stress disorder in DSM-V. *Depression and Anxiety*, 28, 802–817.

Bryant, R.A. (2016). *Acute stress disorder: What it is and how to treat it*. New York, NY: Guilford Press.

Buckley, T., Punkanen, M., & Ogden, P. (2018). The role of the body in fostering resilience: A sensorimotor psychotherapy perspective. *Body, Movement and Dance in Psychotherapy*, 13(4), 225–233.

Colace, E. (2017). Dance movement therapy and developmental trauma: Dissociation and enactment in a clinical case study. *Body, Movement and Dance in Psychotherapy*, 12(1), 36–49.

Dowd, M. D. (2017). Early adversity, toxic stress, and resilience: Pediatrics for today. *Pediatric Annals*, 46(7), e246–e249.

Frankenburg, W. K., Dodds, J., Archer, P., Shapiro, H., & Bresnick, B. (1992). The Denver II: A major revision and restandardization of the Denver Developmental Screening Test. *Pediatrics*, 89(1), 91–97.

Friedrich, W., Gerber, P., Koplin, B., Davis, M., Giese, J., Mykelebust, C., et al. (2001). Multimodal assessment of dissociation in adolescents: Inpatients and juvenile sex offenders. Sexual Abuse. *Journal of Research and Treatment*, 13, 167–177.

Hornor, G. (2017). Resilience. *Journal of Pediatric Health Care*, 31(3), 384–390.

Horowitz, M., Wilner, N., & Alvarez, W. (1979). Impact of Events Scale: A measure of subjective stress. *Psychosomatic Medicine*, 41, 209–218.

Hsih, K. W., & MacKinnon, D. (2017). *John Hopkins psychiatry guide: Acute stress disorder*. Retrieved from https://www.hopkinsguides.com/hopkins/view/Johns_Hopkins_Psychiatry_Guide/787067/all/Acute_Stress_Disorder.

Iacona, J., & Johnson, S. (2018). Neurobiology of trauma and mindfulness for children. *Journal of Trauma Nursing*, 25(3), 187–191.

International Council of Nurses. (2019). *International Classification for Nursing Practice*. Retrieved from https://www.icn.ch/sites/default/files/inline-files/ICNP2019-DC.pdf.

International Society for the Study of Trauma and Dissociation. (2012). Guidelines for treating dissociative identity disorder in adults (3rd rev.). *Journal of Trauma and Dissociation*, 12(2), 115–187.

Jarero, I., Artigas, L., & Luber, M. (2011). The EMDR protocol for recent critical incidents: Application in a disaster mental health continuum of care context. *Journal of EMDR Practice and Research*, 5(3), 82–94.

Koch, S. C., & Harvey, S. (2012). Dance/movement therapy with traumatized dissociative patients. In S. C. Koch, T. Fuchs, M. Summa,

& C. Muller (Eds.), *Body memory, metaphor and movement* (pp. 369–386). Philadelphia, PA: John Benjamins.

Lang, A., & Stein, M. B. (2005). An abbreviated PTSD checklist for use as a screening instrument in primary care. *Behaviour Research and Therapy*, 43, 585–594.

Lanius, U.F., Paulson, S.L., & Corrigan, F.M. (2014). Dissociation: Cortical deafferentation and the loss of self. In U.F. Lanius, S.L., Paulsen, & F.M. Corrigan (Eds.), *Neurobiology and treatment of traumatic dissociation: Toward an embodied self* (pp. 5-28). New York, NY: Springer.

Luber, M. (2009). *Eye movement desensitization and reprocessing scripted protocols: Basics and special situations*. New York, NY: Springer.

Maldonado, J. R., & Spiegel, D. (2019). Dissociative disorders. In L. W. Roberts (Ed.), *The American Psychiatric Association Publishing textbook of psychiatry* (7th ed.) (pp. 437–474). Washington, DC: American Psychiatric Association.

National Child Traumatic Stress Network. (2014). *Pediatric medical traumatic stress toolkit for health care providers*. Retrieved at https://www.nctsn.org/sites/default/files/resources//pediatric_toolkit_for_health_care_providers.pdf.

National Institute of Mental Health (NIMH). (2017). Post-traumatic stress disorder. Retrieved from https://www.nimh.nih.gov/health/statistics/post-traumatic-stress-disorder-ptsd.shtml.

Nijenhuis, E. R. S., Spinhoven, P., Van Dyck, R., Van der Hart, O., & Vanderlinden, J. (1996). The development and the psychometric characteristics of the Somatoform Dissociation Questionnaire (SDQ-20). *Journal of Mental and Nervous Disease*, 184, 688–694.

Nugent, N. R., Goldberg, A., & Uddin, M. (2016, January). Topical review: The emerging field of epigenetics: Informing models of pediatric trauma and physical health. *Journal of Pediatric Psychology*, 41(1), 55–64.

Pearce, J., Simpson, J., Berry, K., Bucci, S., Moskowitz, A., & Varese, F. (2017). Attachment and dissociation as mediators of the link between childhood trauma and psychotic experiences. *Clinical Psychology & Psychotherapy*, 24(6), 1304–1312.

Porges, S. W. (2011). *The polyvagal theory*. New York, NY: W.W. Norton.

Prins, A., Bovin, M. J., Kimerling,R., Kaloupek, D. G, Marx, B. P., Pless Kaiser, A., & Schnurr, P. P. (2015). *Primary Care PTSD Screen for DSM-5 (PC-PTSD-5)*. Retrieved from https://www.ptsd.va.gov/professional/assessment/screens/pc-ptsd.asp.

Putnam, F. W., Helmers, K., & Trickett, P. K. (1993). Development, reliability, and validity of a child dissociation scale. *Child Abuse & Neglect*, 17, 731–742.

Ross, C. A., Heber, S., Norton, G. R., Anderson, D., Anderson, G., & Barchet, P. (1989). The dissociative disorders interview schedule: A structured interview. *Dissociation*, 2, 169–189.

Scheidell, J., Quinn, K., McGorray, S., Frueh, B., Beharier, N., Cottler, L., et al. (2018). Childhood traumatic experiences and the association with marijuana and cocaine use in adolescence through adulthood. *Addiction*, 113(1), 44–56.

Shapiro, E., & Laub, B. (2008). Early EMDR Intervention (EEI): A summary, a theoretical model, and the Recent Traumatic Episode Protocol (R-TEP). *Journal of EMDR Practice and Research*, 2(2), 79–96.

Shonkoff, J. P., & Garner, A. S. (2012). The lifelong effects of early childhood adversity and toxic stress. *Pediatrics*, 129(1), 232–246.

Soylu, T. G., Elashkar, E., Aloudah, F., Ahmed, M., & Kitsantas, P. (2018). Racial/ethnic differences in health insurance adequacy and consistency among children. *Journal of Public Health Research*, 7(1), 1280.

Spiegel, D., Loewenstein, R., Lewis-Fernandez, R., Sar, V., Simeon, D., Vermetten, E., et al. (2011). Dissociative disorders in DSM-5. *Depression and Anxiety, 28*, 824–852.

Steele, K., van der Hart, O., & Nijenjuis, E. (2005). Phase-oriented treatment of structural dissociation in complex traumatization: Overcoming trauma-related phobias. *Journal of Trauma and Dissociation, 6*(3), 11–53.

Strain, J. J. (2018). Adjustment disorders. *Psychiatric Times, 35*(2), 25–27.

Tizard, B. (1977). *Adoption: A second chance.* London, UK: Open Books.

US Department of Veterans Affairs. (2018a). *PTSD: How common is PTSD in children and teens?* Retrieved from https://www.ptsd.va.gov/understand/common/common_children_teens.asp.

US Department of Veterans Affairs. (2018b). *PTSD: How common is PTSD in adults?* Retrieved from https://www.ptsd.va.gov/understand/common/common_adults.asp.

US Department of Veterans Affairs and Department of Defense. (2017). *VA/DOD Clinical Practice Guideline for the management of posttraumatic stress disorder and acute stress disorder.* Retrieved from https://www.healthquality.va.gov/guidelines/MH/ptsd/VA-DoDPTSDCPGFinal012418.pdf.

Weathers, F. W., Litz, B. T., Keane, T. M., Palmieri, P. A., Marx, B. P., & Schnurr, P. P. (2013). *The PTSD Checklist for DSM-5 (PCL-5).* Retrieved from www.ptsd.va.gov.

Weiss, D.S., & Marmar, C.R. (1996). The Impact of Event Scale—Revised. In J. Wilson & T.M. Keane (Eds.), *Assessing psychological trauma and PTSD* (pp. 399-411). New York, NY: Guilford.

Wheeler, K. (2014). *Psychotherapy for the advanced practice psychiatric nurse: A how-to guide for evidence-based practice* (2nd ed.). New York, NY: Springer.

World Health Organization. (2013). *Guidelines for the management of conditions specifically related to stress.* Geneva, Switzerland: Author.

Wolf, E. J., Miller, M. W., Sullivan, D. R., Amstadler, A. B., Mitchell, K. S., Goldberg, J., et al. (2018). A classical twin study of PTSD symptoms and resilience: Evidence for a single spectrum of vulnerability to traumatic stress. *Depression and Anxiety, 35*(2), 132–139.

Xiao, Y., Liu, D., Liu, K., Wu, C., Zhang, H., Niu, Y., et al. (2019). Association of DRD2, 5-HTTLPR, and 5-HTTVNTR gene polymorphisms with posttraumatic stress disorder in Tibetan adolescents: A case control study. *Biological Research for Nursing, 21*(3), 286–295.

17

Somatic Symptom Disorders

Lois Angelo

🌐 Visit the Evolve website for a pretest on the content in this chapter: http://evolve.elsevier.com/Varcarolis

OBJECTIVES

1. Describe the clinical manifestations of each of the somatic symptom disorders, including somatic symptom disorder, illness anxiety disorder, conversion disorder, and psychological factors affecting medical condition.
2. Discuss risk factors for the development of somatic symptom disorders.
3. Analyze the impact of childhood trauma on adult somatic preoccupation.
4. Describe how anxiety, anger, depression, and loneliness trauma can result in physical distress.
5. Identify specific treatment modalities for each of the somatic symptom disorders.
6. Apply the nursing process to individuals with somatic symptom disorders.
7. Discuss the concept of resilient coping and how it affects somatic symptoms.
8. Describe five psychosocial interventions for the care of the patient who has a somatic symptom disorder.
9. Identify psychological therapies that an advanced practice psychiatric–mental health registered nurse may use to manage somatic symptom disorders.
10. Differentiate factitious disorder and malingering from the other somatic symptom disorders.

KEY TERMS AND CONCEPTS

loneliness
malingering

resilient coping
self-compassion

somatization

Soma is the Greek word for "body." Somatization is the psychological and emotional expression of stress through physical symptoms. More specifically, instead of feeling anxiety, depression, or irritability, some individuals experience head, back and chest pain, paralysis, unexplained skin rashes, and other symptoms. Many factors, including biological, cognitive, psychological, and social factors, play a role in the development of somatic symptoms.

While it is important for psychiatric nurses to understand somatic disorders, patients do not usually seek psychiatric care for their symptoms. Typically, primary care and other medical settings encounter individuals with these disorders. Therefore, it is important for nurses who work outside of psychiatric settings to be aware of the influence of the environment, stress, individual lifestyle, a support network, and coping skills of each patient.

This chapter will address four primary somatic symptom and related disorders (American Psychiatric Association [APA], 2013). These disorders are:

- Somatic symptom disorder
- Illness anxiety disorder
- Conversion disorder
- Psychological factors affecting medical condition

Each disorder will be discussed in terms of the clinical picture, epidemiology, comorbidity, risk factors, guidelines for nursing care, and treatment. The nursing process will be applied and a case study will be provided.

Two other conditions, factitious disorder and malingering, will be addressed separately. Unlike the other conditions, these conditions are under conscious control. Nursing care and responses will reflect this difference.

SOMATIC SYMPTOM DISORDER

Somatic symptom disorder is characterized by a focus on somatic (physical) symptoms, such as pain or fatigue, to the point of excessive concern, preoccupation, and fear. Patients' suffering is authentic, and they typically experience a high level of functional impairment. In the previous edition of the *DSM*, individuals with these symptoms were usually diagnosed with hypochondriasis. Now, about 75% of patients who formerly matched the criteria for hypochondriasis are subsumed under the somatic symptom disorder label (APA, 2013). The other 25% have high illness anxiety in the absence of somatic symptoms. These individuals are now diagnosed with illness anxiety disorder, which will be discussed later. Criteria for somatic symptom disorder are listed in the *DSM-5* box.

DSM-5 CRITERIA FOR SOMATIC SYMPTOM DISORDER

A. One or more somatic symptoms that are distressing or result in significant disruption of daily life.

B. Excessive thoughts, feelings, or behaviors related to the somatic symptoms or associated health concerns as manifested by at least one of the following:
1. Disproportionate and persistent thoughts about the seriousness of one's symptoms
2. Persistently high level of anxiety about health or symptoms
3. Excessive time and energy devoted to these symptoms or health concerns

C. Although any one somatic symptom may not be continuously present, the state of being symptomatic is persistent (typically more than 6 months).

Specify if:

With predominant pain (previously pain disorder): This specifier is for individuals whose somatic symptoms predominantly involve pain.

Specify if:

Persistent: A persistent course is characterized by severe symptoms, marked impairment, and long duration (more than 6 months).

Specify current severity:

Mild: Only one of the symptoms specified in Criterion B is fulfilled.

Moderate: Two or more of the symptoms specified in Criterion B are fulfilled.

Severe: Two or more of the symptoms specified in Criterion B are fulfilled plus there are multiple somatic complaints (or one very severe somatic symptom).

From the American Psychiatric Association. (2013). *Diagnostic and statistical manual of mental disorders* (5th ed.). Washington, DC: Author.

In somatic symptom disorder, there tends to be a high level of help seeking. Unfortunately, this contact with healthcare professionals rarely eases the patient's concerns. Common symptoms for primary care visits are chest pain, fatigue, dizziness, headache, swelling, back pain, shortness of breath, insomnia, abdominal pain, and numbness. Health-related quality of life is frequently severely impaired, and patients see their bodily symptoms as unduly threatening, harmful, or troublesome, often fearing the worst about their health.

While multiple symptoms are common, sometimes one severe symptom is present. Usually that symptom is pain. Pain response is individual and difficult to measure objectively. Low back pain is one of the most common musculoskeletal conditions worldwide and may be somatic in origin. In a study of US college students, factors such as feeling sad, exhausted, and overwhelmed were associated with the presence of low back pain (Ahmed, 2017).

Children tend to experience one prominent symptom, most commonly recurrent abdominal pain, headache, fatigue, and nausea. While children may have somatic complaints, they do not worry about the seriousness of the condition.

When the care provider is unable to find an explanation for the symptoms, patients feel discounted and misunderstood. There is, in fact, some basis for these feelings. Providers tend to use less patient-centered communication in this population as compared with patients with more straightforward symptoms, even though their visits are longer. A "difficult" patient may receive a somatic diagnosis more readily than a "pleasant" patient, which could contribute to an inadequate workup. The strongest predictor of misdiagnosing somatic disorders is the primary care provider's dissatisfaction with the clinical encounter (Huang & McCarron, 2011).

BOX 17.1 Self-Compassion Scale Short Form

Please read each statement carefully before answering.

Indicate how often you behave in the stated manner, using the following scale:

Almost never 1 2 3 4 5 Almost always

How I typically act towards myself in difficult times:

____1. When I fail at something important to me, I become consumed by feelings of inadequacy.

____2. I try to be understanding and patient toward those aspects of my personality I don't like.

____3. When something painful happens, I try to take a balanced view of the situation.

____4. When I'm feeling down, I tend to feel like most other people are probably happier than I am.

____5. I try to see my failings as part of the human condition.

____6. When I'm going through a very hard time, I give myself the caring and tenderness I need.

____7. When something upsets me, I try to keep my emotions in balance.

____8. When I fail at something that's important to me, I tend to feel alone in my failure.

____9. When I am feeling down, I tend to obsess and fixate on everything that's wrong.

____10. When I feel inadequate in some way, I try to remind myself that feelings of inadequacy are shared by most people.

____11. I'm disapproving and judgmental about my own flaws and inadequacies.

____12. I'm intolerant and impatient toward those aspects of my personality I don't like.

Coding Key: Self-kindness: 2, 6; Self-judgment: 11, 12; Common humanity: 5, 10; Isolation: 4, 8; Mindfulness: 3, 7; Over-identification: 1, 9.

Subscale scores are computed by calculating the mean of subscale item responses.

To compute a total self-compassion score, reverse score the negative subscale items—self-judgment, isolation, and over-identification (i.e., 1 = 5, 2 = 4, 3 = 3, 4 = 2, 5 = 1)—then compute a total mean.

Raes, F.E., Pommier, K.D., Neff, D., & Van Gucht, D. (2011). Construction and factorial validation of a short form of the Self-Compassion Scale. *Clinical Psychology and Psychotherapy, 18*(3), 250–255.

Individuals who somaticize tend to be hard on themselves and have limited self-compassion. Self-compassion is a protective factor that fosters emotional resilience and is particularly relevant to the study of human adaptation to life adversity and stress (Muris & Petrocchi, 2016). Self-compassion is the tendency to be caring, warm, and understanding toward ourselves when faced with personal shortcomings, inadequacies, or failures. Low self-compassion is associated with physical and psychological symptoms and reduced health-related quality of life. The Self-Compassion Scale is provided in Box 17.1.

Epidemiology

Determining how common somatic symptom disorder is requires an educated guess since patients do not seek treatment for it. Among adults, the prevalence may be about 5% to 7% (APA, 2013). The prevalence is probably higher in females since they report more somatic symptoms than males.

Comorbidity

Anxiety disorders and major depressive disorders are commonly comorbid with somatic symptom disorder. Medical illnesses may also be comorbid and result in higher degrees of impairment than would be expected from the illness alone.

Risk Factors

Biological Factors

Genetic. Personality traits are inherited and associated with somatic symptom disorder. The trait of negative affectivity (neuroticism) is a risk factor in the development of this disorder.

Environmental Factors

Stressful events are often the precipitant for the development of somatic symptoms and anxiety. Lack of education and a low socioeconomic status put people at greater risk for the development of this disorder.

Guidelines for Nursing Care

- Develop a strong therapeutic relationship.
- Provide education regarding the manifestations of somatic symptom disorder.
- Provide consistent reassurance.
- Support the family when possible and include them in education regarding the disorder.
- Encourage a healthy lifestyle, such as sleep hygiene, regular exercise, positive thinking, assertive techniques, massage/acupuncture, and hobbies.
- Resist the temptation to concentrate on psychosocial issues too early in the planning process and initially concentrate on current bodily symptoms.
- Focus on the development of self-compassion and internal locus of control.

TREATMENT MODALITIES

A strong and supportive approach is helpful for reducing fears. Care providers should be careful to avoid repetitive and unnecessary laboratory tests and diagnostic procedures (Scher & Shwarts, 2019).

Besides hypnotherapy, which has been shown to be strongly efficacious, there is no single treatment approach (Henningsen, 2018). However, as with most psychiatric conditions, cognitive-behavioral therapy in conjunction with medication may be beneficial. Tricyclic antidepressants such as amitriptyline and selective serotonin reuptake inhibitors (SSRIs) such as fluoxetine (Prozac) have been used with success (Scher & Shwarts, 2019).

ILLNESS ANXIETY DISORDER

Illness anxiety disorder is characterized by extreme worry and fear about the possibility of having a disease. This worry leads to frequent self-scanning for signs of illness. Actual symptoms and complaints of symptoms are either mild or absent. As mentioned in the somatic symptom disorder discussion, about 25% of people formerly diagnosed with hypochondriasis are now

diagnosed with illness anxiety disorder based on high health anxiety.

Thoughts about illness may be intrusive and hard to dismiss even when patients realize their fears are unrealistic. Constantly talking about health and possible illness is common. Some individuals with this disorder are reassurance seekers and some are care avoiders. Reassurance seekers make frequent medical appointments to be sure that their symptoms are nothing. For example, a man who obsesses about skin cancer will make multiple trips to a variety of providers to have his skin assessed. The avoiders do everything they can to prevent interaction with healthcare providers to eliminate confirmation of illness.

DSM-5 CRITERIA FOR ILLNESS ANXIETY DISORDER

A. Preoccupation with having or acquiring a serious illness.

B. Somatic symptoms are not present or, if present, are only mild in intensity. If another medical condition is present or there is a high risk for developing a medical condition (e.g., strong family history is present), the preoccupation is clearly excessive or disproportionate.

C. There is a high level of anxiety about health, and the individual is easily alarmed about personal health status.

D. The individual performs excessive health-related behaviors (e.g., repeatedly checks his or her body for signs of illness) or exhibits maladaptive avoidance (e.g., avoids doctor appointments and hospitals).

E. Illness preoccupation has been present for at least 6 months, but the specific illness that is feared may change over that period of time.

F. The illness-related preoccupation is not better explained by another mental disorder, such as somatic symptom disorder, panic disorder, generalized anxiety disorder, body dysmorphic disorder, obsessive-compulsive disorder, or delusional disorder, somatic type.

Specify whether:

Care-seeking type: Medical care, including physician visits or undergoing tests and procedures, is frequently used.

Care-avoidant type: Medical care is rarely used.

From the American Psychiatric Association. (2013). *Diagnostic and statistical manual of mental disorders* (5th ed.). Washington, DC: Author.

The course of illness anxiety disorder is chronic and relapsing, with symptoms becoming amplified during times of increased stress. Depression may play a role in increasing concerns. Care providers may suggest a consultation with a mental health professional, but the patient typically refuses it.

Overall, the illness anxiety patient uses about 41% to 78% more healthcare services per year than patients with well-defined medical conditions (Fink, 2010). It is important that clinicians possess basic skills in identifying and treating this disorder. If patient health concerns are addressed at an early stage, repeated consultations, multiple trials of medications, and medical examinations can be prevented.

Exposure to media that urge us to use certain health screens or suggest we talk to our doctor about specific medications may also contribute to fears about health. Social media in particular seems to increase fears. For example, following a large-scale trauma or disaster, the use of Twitter and YouTube is

BOX 17.2   The UCLA Loneliness Scale

1=Never 2=Rarely 3=Sometimes 4=Always

1. How often do you feel unhappy doing so many things alone?
2. How often do you feel you have no one to talk to?
3. How often do you feel you cannot tolerate being so alone?
4. How often do you feel as if no one understands you?
5. How often do you find yourself waiting for people to call or write?
6. How often do you feel completely alone?
7. How often do you feel unable to reach out and communicate with those around you?
8. How often do you feel starved for company?
9. How often do you feel it is difficult for you to make friends?
10. How often do you feel shut out and excluded by others?

Scoring

A total score is computed by adding up the response to each question. The average loneliness score on the measure is 20. A score of 25 or higher reflects a high level of loneliness. A score of 30 or higher reflects a very high level of loneliness.

From Ausin, B., Munoz, M., Martin, T., Perez-Santos, E., & Castellanos, M. A. (2018). Confirmatory factor analysis of the Revised UCLA Loneliness Scale (UCLA LS-R) in individuals over 65. *Aging and Mental Health, 23*(3), 345–351.

significantly associated with higher stress responses (Goodwin, Palgi, Lavenda, Hamama-Raz, & Ben-Ezra, 2015).

Loneliness stems from a perceived social isolation and results in an unpleasant emotional response. It triggers a maladaptive threat response in older adults creating greater self-focus, often leading to symptoms of illness anxiety (Barnett, Moore, & Archuleta, 2019). Box 17.2 has a scale that is commonly used in the quantification of loneliness.

Epidemiology

One- to two-year prevalence of illness anxiety disorder has been estimated at about 1.3% to 10%. Males and females are equally affected by this disorder.

Comorbidity

Most people with illness anxiety disorder will have a comorbid psychiatric disorder. Anxiety disorders—including generalized anxiety disorder, panic disorder, obsessive-compulsive disorder, and depressive disorders—are frequently comorbid. Personality disorders and somatic symptom disorder are also more common in this population.

Risk Factors

Cognitive Factors

Anger, aggression, or hostility that had its source in past losses or a disappointment may be expressed as a need for help and concern from others. Illness anxiety may also be a defense against guilt or low self-esteem. In the patient's view, the somatic symptoms may often serve as a deserved punishment.

Environmental Factors

Illness anxiety disorder often follows a major life stress or a health threat that turns out well. A history of adverse childhood experience, such as abuse or illness, may predispose adults to this disorder.

Guidelines for Nursing Care

- Develop a therapeutic relationship with the patient.
- During counseling, allow time to discuss illness concerns, but limit the amount of time in favor of other topics, such as education.
- Emphasize and reassure the patient that psychiatric care will supplement medical care and not replace it.
- Encourage socialization in unit or program activities since loneliness is associated with illness anxiety.

TREATMENT MODALITIES

Medication may be used to provide symptomatic measures, such as nonsteroidal pain relief, laxatives, and complementary medicine. Since illness anxiety disorder's major symptom is anxiety, SSRIs may provide relief.

Electroconvulsive therapy (ECT), particularly with older adults with concurrent depression, has been successful (Wong et al., 2017). Cognitive-behavioral therapy (CBT), particularly internet-delivered cognitive-behavioral therapy (iCBT), provides an effective and also accessible treatment option for people with illness anxiety (Newby et al., 2018).

CONVERSION DISORDER

Conversion disorder, also known as functional neurological disorder, manifests itself as neurological symptoms in the absence of a neurological diagnosis. Conversion disorder is marked by the presence of deficits in voluntary motor or sensory functions, including paralysis, blindness, movement disorder, gait disorder, numbness, paresthesia (tingling or burning sensations), loss of vision or hearing, or episodes resembling epilepsy.

In conversion disorder, emotional conflicts or stressors are transferred to physical symptoms. This transfer may have a physical basis. Some MRI studies suggest that patients with conversion disorder have an abnormal pattern of cerebral activation (Feinstein, 2011).

One of the most striking aspects of conversion disorder is that many patients show a lack of emotional concern about often dramatic symptoms. This response is called la belle indifference (lah bel an-dif-er-ahns), or "the grand" indifference. Imagine someone casually discussing sudden blindness. Despite the calm response of the afflicted, care providers should assume there is an organic cause to the symptoms until physical pathology has been ruled out.

Epidemiology

Lifetime prevalence of conversion disorder ranges from 2 to 5 per 100,000 people (APA, 2013). In neurology clinics, the rate climbs to 5%. This disorder is up to three times more common in females.

Comorbidity

Psychiatric comorbidity is present in about 74% of patients with conversion disorder (Akyuz, Gokalp, Erdiman, Oflaz, & Karsidag, 2017). The most common conditions are major depressive disorder at 50% and dissociative disorder at about 48%.

Risk Factors

Biological Factors

Physiological. Individuals who actually have a neurological disease with symptoms similar to those originating from the conversion symptom are at higher risk. For example, a patient with epileptic seizures may be at greater risk for nonepileptic seizures.

Neurobiological. Conversion disorder may have a biological basis. Hypometabolism in the dominant hemisphere and hypermetabolism in the nondominant hemisphere may lead to impaired hemispheric communication (Sadock, Sadock, & Ruiz, 2015). Excess cortisol may set off negative feedback loops between the cerebral cortex and the brainstem. This cortical output may inhibit the patient's awareness of bodily sensations, thereby resulting in sensory deficits.

Cognitive Factors

Psychoanalytic theory once dominated medical thinking about somatization, which Sigmund Freud considered a "mysterious leap from mind to body" (Stone, Vuilleumier, & Friedman, 2010). Psychoanalytic theorists viewed the psychogenic complaints of pain, illness, or loss of physical function as a cover-up for conflicted feelings and/or unwelcome experiences. Transforming anxiety into a physical symptom is symbolically related to the conflict.

For example, in conversion disorder, conversion symptoms allow a forbidden wish or urge to be partly expressed but sufficiently disguised so that the individual does not have to face the unacceptable wish. The symptoms also permit the individual to communicate a need for special treatment or consideration from others. Psychogenic blindness or hearing loss may represent the symbolic statement "I can't face this knowledge." For example, after a woman overheard friends discussing her husband's sexual infidelity, she developed total deafness.

Environmental Factors

Current studies attribute conversion symptoms to purely biological factors and to psychological and traumatic factors such as childhood abuse (in particular, child sexual abuse) and family dysfunction, all of which are likely shaped by a combination of genetic programming and environmental factors involving childhood development.

Guidelines for Nursing Care

- Develop a therapeutic relationship.
- Avoid direct confrontation of the conversion symptom.
- Provide reassurance and support for the patient's feelings and beliefs.
- Encourage socialization.
- Explore alternate and adaptive coping mechanisms.

TREATMENT MODALITIES

If symptoms are severely distressing and result in disability, an aggressive approach to treatment may be required. Narcoanalysis using medication such as amobarbital in an interview setting may result in immediate cessation of symptoms (Scher and Shwarts, 2019). Hypnosis may also result in rapid resolution.

Body-oriented psychological therapy (BOPT) utilizes nonverbal expressive behavior, body awareness, and movement to facilitate a change process linking the expression of emotions, such as repressed anger and conflicts (Papadopoulos & Rohricht, 2018). The playfulness in BOPT fosters creative capabilities and symbolic enactments of trauma to explore alternative coping strategies.

Other treatments include dialectical behavior therapy (DBT). DBT encourages skills to target emotional dysregulation, distress tolerance, and interpersonal conflicts (Bullock, Mirza, Forte, & Trockel, 2015). Psychodrama is a less common group therapy in which role-playing is used to acknowledge, re-experience, and explore issues with a goal of improving insight and correcting problematic responses. This psychotherapy has been used along with pharmacotherapy in the treatment of conversion disorder (Ozlem et al., 2018).

Physical therapy may be used for motor symptoms. Physical therapy not only helps with increased function but can also provide additional psychological support via an ongoing, positive,

EVIDENCE-BASED PRACTICE

Do People Who Somaticize Have an External Locus of Control?

Problem

People with somatization seek validation of symptoms by healthcare providers, resulting in distress for patients, frustration for clinicians, and wasted healthcare resources. A need for validation may be related to locus of control. Individuals with an internal locus of control believe that they control their health, and can take steps to become healthy again. Conversely, individuals with an external locus of control believe that external forces such as doctors have control and authority over their health.

Purpose of Study

To determine the role of health locus of control in patients with somatic disorders.

Method

Data were collected from 100 patients at a private clinic. The Patient Health Questionnaire and the Multidimensional Health Locus of Control (MHLC) scale was used. The MHLC scale measures four types of beliefs about health locus of control:

1. I am directly responsible for my condition getting better or worse.
2. Most things that affect my condition happen to me by chance.
3. Following doctor's orders to the letter is the best way to keep my condition from getting any worse.
4. The type of help I receive from other people determines how soon my condition improves.

Key Findings

- The higher the internal locus of control, the lower the severity of somatization.
- Lower internal locus of control is associated with increased utilization of the healthcare system.

Implications for Nursing Practice

One of the key interventions for registered nurses is in promoting self-care and self-advocacy. Helping patients recognize their own ability to manage symptoms through education and anxiety-reducing techniques will support them in developing stronger coping techniques.

Bhargava, T., & Pandey, R. (2016). Effect of health locus of control on patient with somatization. *International Journal of Indian Psychology, 4*(1).

caring relationship with a physical therapist (Mesaroli et al., 2019).

PSYCHOLOGICAL FACTORS AFFECTING MEDICAL CONDITION

Both medical and mental health professionals recognize the interrelationships between medical and psychiatric comorbidities. Psychological factors may increase the risk of medical disease or they may magnify and adversely affect a medical condition. For example, there is a growing body of evidence that links psychiatric disorders with cardiovascular disease. Major depressive disorder is a risk factor in the occurrence of coronary heart disease (Marwijk et a;., 2015). An association between depression and cancer incidence has been suggested since the time of the ancient Greeks. Depression is such a powerful condition that it is associated with increased risk of death from nearly all major medical causes (Zivin et al., 2015).

Table 17.1 identifies common medical conditions that are negatively affected by stress.

Epidemiology

It is unclear how widespread the effects of psychological factors on medical conditions are. Virtually all diseases and conditions are affected by psychological and behavioral factors. We do know from a medical billing standpoint that diagnoses

TABLE 17.1   Common Medical Conditions Negatively Affected by Stress

Medical Condition	Incidence	Genetic and Biological Correlates	Common Precipitating Factors	Holistic Therapies in Addition to Medical Management
Cardiovascular disease (e.g., coronary heart disease)	Rates higher in males until age 60 years Rates higher in white population than in African American population	Family history of cardiac disease a risk factor Other risk factors include hypertension, increased serum lipid levels, obesity, sedentary lifestyle, and cigarette smoking Psychosocial risk factors (stress, depression, loneliness) High anxiety risk in patient with prior cardiac events	Often, myocardial infarction occurs after sudden stress preceded by a period of losses, frustration, and disappointments	Relaxation training, stress management, group social support, and psychosocial intervention Support groups for type A personalities and type A modification helpful Anxiolytics (benzodiazepines) and antidepressants when indicated
Peptic ulcer (caused by *Helicobacter pylori* infection)	Occurs in 12% of men, 6% of women (more prevalent in industrialized societies)	Infection with *H. pylori* is associated with 95%–99% of peptic ulcers Both peptic and duodenal ulcers cluster in families, but separately from each other	Periods of social tension and increased life stress After losses; often after menopause	Biofeedback can alter gastric acidity; cognitive-behavioral approaches are used to reduce stress (stress management)
Cancer	Men: most common in lung, prostate, colon, and rectum Women: most common in breast, uterus, colon, and rectum Death rate higher in men (especially African American men) than in women	Genetic evidence suggests dysfunction of cellular proliferation Familial patterns for breast cancer, colorectal cancer, stomach cancer, melanoma	Prolonged and intensive stress Stressful life events (e.g., separation from or loss of significant other 2 years before diagnosis) Feelings of hopelessness, helplessness, and despair (depression) may precede the diagnosis of cancer	Relaxation (e.g., meditation, autogenic training, self-hypnosis) Visualization Psychological counseling Support groups Massage therapy Stress management
Tension headache	Occurs in 80% of population when under stress Begins at end of workday or early evening		Associated with anxiety and depression	Psychotherapy usually prescribed for chronic tension headaches Learning to cope or avoiding tension-creating situations or people Relaxation techniques, stress management techniques, cognitive restructuring techniques
Essential hypertension	Rates higher in males until age 60 years	Family history of cardiac disease and hypertension a risk factor	Life changes and traumatic life events Stressful job (e.g., air traffic controller) Hypothesized to be found more in areas of social stress and conflict	Behavioral feedback, stress reduction techniques, meditation, yoga, hypnosis Note: Pharmacological treatment considered primary for treatment of hypertension

of psychological factors affecting medical conditions are more common than diagnoses of somatic symptom disorders.

Risk Factors
Environmental Factors
Loneliness and weak interpersonal connections are associated with negative health outcomes. They result in a lifespan similar to that caused by smoking 15 cigarettes a day and even greater than that associated with obesity. High levels of loneliness are associated with exaggerated blood pressure and inflammatory reactivity to acute stress. This, in turn, damages blood vessels and other tissues, increasing the risk of heart disease, diabetes, joint disease, and premature death (Murthy, 2020). There are indications that loneliness may also be related to blunted cardiac, cortisol, and immune responses (Brown, Gallagher, & Creaven, 2017).

Adverse childhood experiences (ACEs) have been shown to contribute to more negative health outcomes in adulthood. Childhood trauma associated with physical or sexual violence is consistently linked with physical disorders later in life (Greenberg, 2017). Prolonged trauma, especially in childhood, can cause neurobiological changes such as alterations in the volume and activity levels of major brain structures (Meichenbaum, 2017). Resilient coping is the ability to "bounce back" from adversity. Highly resilient subjects show less distress and physical symptoms despite reported childhood adversities in comparison to those with low resilient coping abilities (Beutel et al., 2015).

Guidelines for Nursing Care
- Develop a therapeutic relationship.
- Teach the importance of positive affective responses to individuals who use negative behaviors in their interactions since negativity is associated with worse outcomes.
- Consistently assess ACEs in both children and adult patients.
- Include the concept of resilience on a regular basis in health teaching with both children and adults.
- Focus on the patient's connections to family, friends, and community to avoid prolonged periods of loneliness.

TREATMENT MODALITIES

Provide treatment for anxiety, depression, and loneliness, as they are identified as risk factors for multiple illnesses, particularly those related to cardiovascular disease.

APPLICATION OF THE NURSING PROCESS

ASSESSMENT

The assessment of patients with somatization disorders is a complex process that requires careful and complete documentation. This section outlines several areas that are important in the assessment of a patient with a suspected somatic symptom disorder.

ASSESSMENT GUIDELINES
Somatic Symptom Disorders
1. Assess for nature, location, onset, characteristics, and duration of the symptom(s).
2. Explore past history of ACEs.
3. Identify symptoms of anxiety, depression, and past trauma that may be contributing to somatic symptoms and the ability to meet basic physical and safety/security needs.
4. Determine current quality of life, social support, and coping skills, including spirituality.
5. Identify any secondary gain that the patient is experiencing from symptom(s).
6. Explore the patient's cognitive style and ability to communicate feelings and needs.
7. Assess current psychosocial and biological needs.
8. Screen for misuse of prescribed medication and substance use.

Assessment should begin with collection of data about the nature, location, onset, character, and duration of the symptom or symptoms. A thorough medical and psychosocial history is also essential. Assessment of nutrition, fluid balance, and elimination needs should be a high priority, as patients with somatic symptom disorders often complain of gastrointestinal distress, diarrhea, constipation, and anorexia.

Fig. 17.1 provides a useful tool to quantify somatic symptoms. This measure was adapted from the Patient Health Questionnaire Physical Symptoms.

In addition, nurses should gather information about patients' ability to meet their own basic needs. Rest, comfort, activity, and hygiene needs may be altered as a result of patient problems such as fatigue, weakness, insomnia, muscle tension, pain, and avoidance of diversional activity. Safety and security needs may be threatened by patient experiences of blindness, deafness, loss of balance and falling, and anesthesia of various parts of the body.

During assessment, it is important to determine whether symptoms are under the patient's voluntary control. Somatization symptoms are not under the individual's voluntary control. Although the relationship between symptoms and interpersonal conflicts may be obvious to others, the patient cannot see it.

Symptom reporting will vary, depending upon the disorder. Patients with conversion disorder may matter-of-factly report having a sudden loss in function of a body part: "I woke up this morning and couldn't move my arm." In contrast, patients with somatic symptom disorder and illness anxiety disorder usually discuss their symptoms in dramatic terms. They may use colorful metaphors and exaggerations: "The pain was searing, like a hot sword slicing across my forehead." "My symptoms are so rare that I've stumped hundreds of doctors."

Table 17.2 provides an outline for a psychosocial assessment of a patient with a medical condition. You perform a psychosocial assessment in tandem with a thorough physical workup and mental-status examination.

Level 2—Somatic Symptom—Adult Patient
Adapted from the Patient Health Questionnaire Physical Symptoms (PHQ-15)

Instructions: On the DSM-5 Level 1 cross-cutting questionnaire that you just completed, you indicated that *during the past 2 weeks* you (the individual receiving care) have been bothered by "unexplained aches and pains," and/or "feeling that your illnesses are not being taken seriously enough" at a mild or greater level of severity. The questions below ask about these feelings in more detail and especially how often you (the individual receiving care) have been bothered by a list of symptoms <u>during the past 7 days.</u> Please respond to each item by marking (✓ or x) one box per row.

During the <u>past 7 days</u>, how much have you been bothered by any of the following problems?	Not bothered at all (0)	Bothered a little (1)	Bothered a lot (2)
1 Stomach pain	☐	☐	☐
2 Back pain	☐	☐	☐
3 Pain in your arms, legs, or joints (knees, hips, etc.)	☐	☐	☐
4 Menstrual cramps or other problems with your periods *WOMEN ONLY*	☐	☐	☐
5 Headaches	☐	☐	☐
6 Chest pain	☐	☐	☐
7 Dizziness	☐	☐	☐
8 Fainting spells	☐	☐	☐
9 Feeling your heart pound or race	☐	☐	☐
10 Shortness of breath	☐	☐	☐
11 Pain or problems during sexual intercourse	☐	☐	☐
12 Constipation, loose bowels, or diarrhea	☐	☐	☐
13 Nausea, gas, or indigestion	☐	☐	☐
14 Feeling tired or having low energy	☐	☐	☐
15 Trouble sleeping	☐	☐	☐

Fig. 17.1 Somatic symptom—adult patient.

Coping Skills

Assessing how a patient has dealt with adversity in the past provides information about coping skills available for use now and in the future. Healthcare workers can also support the patient in gaining additional coping skills that may help an individual better manage a healthier lifestyle.

Spirituality and Religion

Spirituality or religion may play an important role in many patients' lives. Support from a priest, pastor, rabbi, or other religious leader may be indicated, especially in a case of spiritual distress. Beliefs and practices are forces that promote resilience; the practice of healthy coping depends upon the capacity to create meaning from life experiences.

Cultural Considerations

The type and frequency of somatic symptoms vary across cultures. For example, West Indians (Caribbean) attribute somatic symptoms to chronic overwork and the irregularity of daily

TABLE 17.2   Psychosocial Assessment of Patients With Medical Conditions

Areas to Assess	Specific Questions to Ask
Social Supports and Cultural Issues	
Family	What were the effects of the patient's illness, treatments, and recovery on the family in the past?
Friends	Who can the patient share painful feelings with?
	Does the patient have friends to joke and laugh with?
	Are there people the patient believes would stand by him or her?
Religious or spiritual beliefs	Does the patient find comfort and support in spiritual practices?
	Is the patient a member of a spiritual or religious group in the community (church, temple, other place of worship)?
	Does the patient find inner peace and strength in religious or spiritual practices?
	Does the patient believe that life has value, meaning, and direction?
	Does the patient feel a connection with the universe?
	I [often/sometimes/seldom] believe in a power greater than myself.
Cultural beliefs	Does the patient use specific culture-oriented treatments or remedies?
	Do the patient's cultural beliefs allow for adequate treatment by Western medical standards?
Work	Are there colleagues at work the patient can count on for support?
Concurrent Physical Conditions Affecting Psychosocial Well-Being	
Physical pain	Is the patient in pain?
	How does the patient cope with the pain?
	Is the pain disabling?
	Are there pain-reducing techniques that might help?
Major illness	Does the patient have a co-occurring major illness that will negatively affect the current condition?
	Is the patient undergoing treatments that are affecting daily life more than expected?
	Are there interventions that would help the patient better cope with the sequelae of the illness and treatments?
	Has the patient been hospitalized in the past? How many times? For what? How did the patient cope?
Addictions and mental health	Does the patient have a co-occurring mental health problem (depression, anxiety, compulsions)?
	Has the patient suffered a mental disease in the past?
	Does the patient participate in any compulsive behavior (e.g., smoking, overworking, excessive spending, gambling, cybersex)?
	Does the patient abuse substances (alcohol, drugs [illicit, over-the-counter, prescription])?

living. These somatic symptoms include dizziness, fatigue, joint pain, and muscle tension. Patients from Korea may explain some distress as *hwa-byung*, a syndrome of both somatic and depressive symptoms, commonly attributed to suppressed anger or rage (Edwards et al., 2010).

In some cultures, certain physical symptoms are believed to be the result of spells being cast. Spellbound individuals often seek the help of traditional healers in addition to modern medical staff. The medical provider may diagnose a non-life-threatening somatic symptom disorder, whereas the traditional healer may offer an entirely different explanation and prognosis. The individual may not show improvement until the traditional healer removes the spell.

In the US immigrant population, primary care visits are often due to responses to traumatic events. Immigrants frequently experience multiple traumatic events, both intentional and unintentional, in premigration and postmigration life. It is important for primary care providers evaluating immigrants to be aware of the possible link between somatization symptoms reported by the patient and undisclosed traumatic experiences.

🌐 CONSIDERING CULTURE

Somatic Symptoms in Immigrants and Refugees

Immigrants and refugees, as well as patients from ethnic and racial minorities, frequently seek care for a spectrum of physical and psychological symptoms. These symptoms are best understood within the context of their cultural background and experiences.

Carlos is a 27-year-old from El Salvador. He fled his native country after finding out that his name was on a death squad list for execution. Nine months after his arrival in the United States, he learned his wife was killed during an attempt to extract information about Carlos's whereabouts.

Carlos visited a primary care provider at a community clinic. He described multiple symptoms, including weakness, which caused him to be terminated from his temporary job. He also complained of abdominal pain, chest pain, insomnia, and weight loss. After extensive diagnostic studies, Carlos's primary care provider could find no physical cause for his symptoms.

He was then referred to a psychiatric nurse practitioner (NP). The NP diagnosed somatic symptom disorder and prescribed a low-dose antidepressant along with individual therapy.

Carlos grew more aware of the emotional factors that exacerbated his symptoms and developed new coping strategies. He joined a group of local Central American refugees, where he was encouraged to write and to recite poetry as a therapeutic tool. During the following months, his somatic symptoms gradually decreased.

Communication

Patients with somatization symptoms generally have difficulty communicating their emotional needs. Although they are able to describe their physical symptoms, they frequently do not verbalize feelings, especially those related to anger, guilt, and dependence. The somatic symptom may be the patient's chief means of communicating emotional needs.

Self-Assessment

Working with patients with somatization illnesses can be frustrating and unsatisfying. When a physiological basis for the patient's symptoms is absent, you may wonder why this patient is taking up valuable time that might better be spent on a "sick" patient. You may feel resentment or anger toward such a patient. Negative feelings occur whether the patient is being cared for in a medical setting or in a psychiatric setting.

It is helpful to remember that the symptom the patient is experiencing feels real, even though the objective data may not support a physiological basis. It is important for you to recognize your thoughts and feelings while monitoring your words or body language. Ultimately, your increased self-awareness and increased skill will help you provide strong and consistent care for this population.

NURSING DIAGNOSIS

The *International Classification for Nursing Practice* (ICNP) (2019) provides nursing diagnoses that are useful for patients with somatic symptom disorders. *Difficulty coping* is a priority in this population. Other potential nursing diagnoses include *anxiety, risk for loneliness, powerlessness, hopelessness, chronic low self-esteem, impaired socialization, pain, impaired family process,* and *risk for suicide*.

OUTCOMES IDENTIFICATION

Because shared decision making promotes goal attainment, the patient should participate in identifying desired outcomes. Outcome criteria must be realistic and attainable. Structuring outcomes in small steps helps the patient see concrete evidence of progress. Table 17.3 describes signs and symptoms, potential nursing diagnoses, and outcomes for somatic symptom disorders.

IMPLEMENTATION

Psychosocial Interventions

Because patients are seldom admitted to psychiatric care settings specifically for treatment of somatic disorders, long-term interventions usually take place on an outpatient basis. The nurse may initiate short-term planning if the patient is admitted to a medical-surgical unit. Such a stay is usually brief, and discharge will occur after the results of diagnostic tests are negative.

Patients who somaticize often do not mention psychological symptoms and attribute their symptoms to physical problems when consulting healthcare providers. Somatization is common in primary care, but providers are not confident in managing it and often prescribe unnecessary treatments. Because comorbidities between somatic disorders and major depressive disorder and anxiety disorders are common in primary care, it is essential that an integrated model of care exist between psychiatric care providers and medical clinicians.

Initially, nursing interventions should focus on establishing a helping relationship with the patient. The therapeutic relationship is vital to the success of the care plan given (1) the patient's resistance to the concept that no physical cause for the symptom exists and (2) the patient's tendency to go from caregiver to caregiver. To be successful, therapeutic interventions address ways to help the patient have needs met without resorting to somatization.

Since multiple providers may be involved in the management of this disorder, good communication among treating clinicians is required to maintain a consistent approach. In an ideal situation, a multidisciplinary team of caretakers, including an advanced practice psychiatric–mental health registered nurse who provides consultation to nurses outside of psychiatry, would be involved in the treatment of patients with somatization illnesses. Using the data from the holistic assessment, nurse clinicians, along with a physician, are in a position to provide useful and effective interventions.

People who have distressing symptoms are vulnerable to a variety of psychosocial stresses. How they cope with these stresses may make the difference between living with an acceptable quality of life and giving in to despair, withdrawal, helplessness, or hopelessness. Nurses are in a position to assess and understand patients' psychosocial stressors, identify needed coping skills, and teach stress-management techniques. Nurses can play an important role not only in managing patients' immediate care but also in helping patients improve their ability to cope and increase their quality of life during the course of somatic disorders.

TABLE 17.3 Signs and Symptoms, Nursing Diagnoses, and Outcomes for Somatic Symptom Disorders

Signs and Symptoms	Nursing Diagnoses	Outcomes
Ineffective coping strategies, insufficient access of social support, insufficient problem-solving skills, inability to meet role expectations	Difficulty coping	Improved coping: Identifies ineffective coping patterns, identifies alternate coping strategies, uses support system
Presence of secondary gains by adoption of sick role	Pain, acute or chronic	Reduced pain: Recognizes associated symptoms of pain, reports pain control
Absence of support system, disabling condition, preoccupation with own thoughts, friends and family alienated by physical obsessions	Impaired socialization	Improved socialization: identifies support system, willing to call on others for assistance, identifies a support group
Nonassertive behavior, exaggerates negative feedback about self, excessive seeking of reassurance, repeatedly unsuccessful in life events	Chronic low self-esteem	Improved self-esteem: Verbalizes positive regard for self, describes self as successful, strong beliefs that decisions and actions control health outcomes

Patients can learn various effective **coping skills** such as assertiveness training, cognitive reframing, problem-solving skills, and social supports. Nurses are in key positions to assess, educate, or provide referrals to a patient to enable healthier ways of looking at and dealing with illness. Teaching relaxation techniques, such as progressive muscle relaxation, meditation, guided imagery, and breathing exercises, promotes self-care and provides a distraction from obsessive somatic thoughts.

⚡ HEALTH POLICY

Primary Care and Mental Health Services: A Call for Integration

For many patients seen in primary healthcare, there is no evidence of physical disease. Due to the interrelated nature of mental and physical treatment, integration of behavioral and physical care makes sense. In addition, integrating mental health services into primary healthcare results in less stigmatization. Because primary healthcare services are not associated with any specific health conditions, individuals reduce the stigma when seeking mental healthcare from a primary healthcare provider.

In the Netherlands, several models have been developed to integrate behavioral health and primary care. They launched the Depression Initiative Primary Mental Health Collaborative Care Model. This model consists of a primary care provider prescribing an antidepressant, a psychiatrist available for consult, and a nurse case manager who monitors patient progress and provides behavioral healthcare. The Netherlands expects that 80% of mental disorders will be treated in the primary care setting.

Psychiatric–mental health nurses can bring a strong perspective in assessing and managing both physical and mental health needs in such integrated care settings. Advocating for models such as the one used in the Netherlands is an important aspect of leadership in nursing.

Pincus, H.A., Jun, M., Franx, G., van der Feltz-Cornelis, C., Ito, H., & Mossialos, E. (2015). How can we link general medical and behavioral healthcare? *Psychiatric Services, 66*(8), 775-777.

The following interventions have all been shown to positively affect a patient's recovery:

- Educating the patient regarding specific treatments
- Referring the patient to community support groups or systems
- Teaching patients more effective coping skills that take into consideration patients' values, preferences, and lifestyle
- Focusing on a patient's strengths and reinforcing coping skills that work (e.g., prayerfulness, participation in hobbies, relaxation techniques)
- General recommendations for healthcare providers in working with patients with somatic symptoms include six key elements for effective relationships and treatment:
  1. Provide continuity of care.
  2. Avoid unnecessary tests and procedures.
  3. Provide frequent, brief, and regular office visits.
  4. Always conduct a physical examination.
  5. Avoid making disparaging comments such as "Your symptoms are all in your head."
  6. Set reasonable therapeutic goals such as maintaining function despite ongoing pain.

Promotion of Self-Care Activities

When somatization is present, the patient's ability to perform self-care activities may be impaired, and nursing intervention is necessary. In general, interventions involve the use of a matter-of-fact approach to support the highest level of self-care of which the patient is capable.

For patients manifesting paralysis, blindness, or severe fatigue, an effective nursing approach is to support patients while expecting them to support themselves. For example, the patient who demonstrates paralysis of an arm can be expected to eat using the other arm. To encourage the patient experiencing blindness to feed himself, he can be told where food is located in reference to numbers on an imaginary clock on his plate. These strategies are effective for reducing secondary gain.

Assertiveness training is often identified as appropriate teaching for patients with somatic symptom disorders. The use of assertiveness techniques gives patients a direct means of getting needs met, thereby decreasing the need for somatic symptoms. Teaching an exercise regimen, such as doing range-of-motion exercises for 15 to 20 minutes daily and taking regular walks, if possible, can help the patient feel in control, increase endorphin levels, and help decrease anxiety.

Table 17.4 provides basic-level interventions for somatic symptom disorders.

Case Management

"Doctor shopping" is common among patients with somatization illnesses. Patients may go from provider to provider, clinic to clinic, or hospital to hospital, hoping to establish a physical basis for their distress. Repeated computed tomographic scans, magnetic resonance images, and other diagnostic tests are often documented in the medical record.

Case management can help limit healthcare costs associated with such visits. The case manager can recommend to the primary care provider that the patient be scheduled for brief appointments every 4 to 6 weeks at set times, rather than on demand, and that laboratory tests be avoided unless they are absolutely necessary. The patient who establishes a relationship with the case manager often feels less anxiety because the patient has someone to contact and knows that a healthcare expert is a partner.

EVALUATION

Evaluation of patients with somatization illnesses is a straightforward process when you have written measurable behavioral outcomes clearly and realistically. For these patients, you might often find that goals and outcomes are only partially met. Patients are likely to report the continuing presence of somatic symptoms, but they often say they are less concerned about the symptoms. Families frequently report relatively high satisfaction with outcomes, even without total eradication of the patient's symptoms.

TREATMENT MODALITIES

Psychological Therapies

Advanced practice registered nurses use CBT, the most evidence-based approach for the treatment of somatic disorders. CBT helps patients find ways to reframe their thoughts, gain control of their situation, and break what can become a self-fulfilling cycle of pain, despair, and health-seeking behaviors. Refer to Chapter 2 for a more complete explanation of CBT. Table 17.5 provides a summary of advanced practice interventions.

TABLE 17.4 Basic-Level Interventions for Somatic Symptom Disorders

Intervention	Rationale
Offer explanations and support during diagnostic testing.	Reduces anxiety while ruling out organic illness
After physical complaints have been investigated, avoid further reinforcement (e.g., do not take vital signs each time patient complains of palpitations).	Directs focus away from physical symptoms
Spend time with patient at times other than when patient summons nurse to voice physical complaint.	Rewards non-illness-related behaviors and encourages repetition of desired behavior
Observe and record frequency and intensity of somatic symptoms. (Patient or family can give information.)	Establishes a baseline and later enables evaluation of effectiveness of interventions
Do not imply that symptoms are not real.	Acknowledges that symptoms are real to the patient
Shift focus from somatic complaints to feelings or to neutral topics.	Conveys interest in patient as a person rather than in patient's symptoms; reduces need to gain attention via symptoms
Assess secondary gains "physical illness" provides for patient (e.g., attention, increased dependency, and distraction from another problem).	Allows these needs to be met in healthier ways and thus minimizes secondary gains
Use matter-of-fact approach to patient exhibiting resistance or covert anger.	Avoids power struggles; demonstrates acceptance of anger and permits discussion of angry feelings
Have patient direct all requests to case manager.	Reduces manipulation
Help patient look at effect of illness behavior on others.	Encourages insight; can help improve intrafamily relationships
Show concern for patient while avoiding fostering dependency needs.	Shows respect for patient's feelings while minimizing secondary gains from "illness"
Reinforce patient's strengths and problem-solving abilities.	Contributes to positive self-esteem; helps patient realize that needs can be met without resorting to somatic symptoms
Teach assertive communication.	Provides patient with a positive means of getting needs met; reduces feelings of helplessness and need for manipulation
Teach patient stress-reduction techniques, such as meditation, relaxation, and mild physical exercise.	Provides alternate coping strategies; reduces need for medication

CASE STUDY AND NURSING CARE PLAN

Somatic Symptom Disorder

Cara, age 49, a recently divorced mother of twin teenage daughters, works as a copy editor for a local newspaper. She has been trying to sell her house to downsize after her daughters graduate from high school next year. Cara feels "nervous most of the time" and states that she only leaves the house for work or to do grocery shopping. She reports no social life and states, "I don't have any friends."

She reports being been referred to a variety of specialists who found no evidence of organic origins of her pathophysiology. Today, she went to the emergency department with tachycardia in normal sinus rhythm, shortness of breath, and fatigue. All diagnostic tests were normal.

Cara agreed to attend an intensive outpatient program (IOP) three mornings each week. After 2 days in the IOP, she has not engaged in treatment. She is worried about losing her job if she does not return to work soon. She is frustrated that her fatigue and physical symptoms are continuing. "My mood is fine, but my body is a major problem."

Self-Assessment

Heather is a registered nurse with 3 years of experience in the IOP. She recognizes her own feelings of frustration toward Cara for refusing to identify emotional concerns and wanting to leave the program and return to work.

Heather realizes she has to monitor her emotional reactions to Cara and adopt a matter-of-fact approach to encourage the patient to be more assertive, self-aware, and independent. Heather plans to actively support Cara in creating her discharge plan.

Assessment

Subjective Data

- No history of diagnosed physical illness or psychiatric disorders.
- Onset of symptoms coincides with a divorce and impending graduation of her daughters.
- Complains of shortness of breath and a rapid heart rate.

- "I don't have any friends."
- States she's "nervous most of the time" and only leaves the house for work or to do grocery shopping.
- "My mood is fine, but my body is the major problem."

Objective Data

- Vital signs are within normal limits.
- Diagnostic tests are negative.

Nursing Diagnoses

1. *Dysfunctional grief* due to the loss of significant other and anticipatory losses of children and home, as evidenced by multiple somatic symptoms, anxiety, and depressed mood.
2. *Impaired socialization* due to fatigue/pain as evidenced by decreased contact and interaction with family and friends.

Outcomes Identification

1. Improved grieving
   a. Patient will identify and express emotions without physical symptoms.
   b. Patient will describe the process of grief.
2. Improved socialization
   a. Patient will seek out a trusted staff member to discuss concerns.
   b. Patient will initiate a social contact with two patients.

Planning

The initial plan is to encourage Cara to explore feelings related to recent and impending losses and to develop a support system.

Implementation

The plan of care for Cara is personalized as follows:

Continued

CASE STUDY AND NURSING CARE PLAN—cont'd

Short-Term Goal	Intervention	Rationale	Evaluation
1. Patient will identify levels of anxiety in at least three situations and encounters with IOP patients and staff.	1. Teach the patient techniques to identify and manage anxiety.	1. Identifying anxiety and anxiety reduction techniques helps manage distress and provides patient with self-care behaviors, thereby enhancing self-esteem.	**GOAL MET**
2. Patient will develop a contract in conjunction with staff to plan for behavior change.	2. Develop a relationship with the patient that includes a mutually agreed upon contract that details expected changes in behaviors.	2. A concrete means to keep track of patient actions will enhance self-direction and independent actions.	**GOAL MET**
3. Patient will seek support from staff and patients when feelings of anxiety become difficult to handle or physical symptoms increase.	3. Educate the patient about sharing feelings of loss with staff, friends, and family members.	3. Communication and expression of feelings with family and friends helps alleviate stress and often provides a more supportive environment.	**GOAL MET**
4. Patient will make a list with contacts and phone numbers of community resources of interest to her.	4. Assist in the identification of available support systems.	4. Patients are more successful with stressful life events if there is adequate support.	**GOAL MET**
5. Patient will utilize the therapeutic milieu to increase her ability to express feelings.	5. Support expression of feelings via the arts, such as writing, music, and role-playing.	5. Various forms of artistic expression encourage the promotion of feelings.	**GOAL MET**
6. Patient will be active in unit activities.	6. Assist the patient in identification of appropriate diversional activities.	6. Diversional activities assist the patient to be less attentive to inner turmoil. The patient is more likely to use activities that are of specific interest.	**GOAL MET**
7. Patient will challenge negative and self-defeating thoughts and replace them with positive thoughts.	7. Encourage the patient to use positive self-talk, such as, "I can do this one step at a time," "Right now I need to stretch and breathe," and "I don't need to be perfect."	7. Cognitive techniques focus on changing behaviors and feelings by changing thoughts. Replacing negative thoughts with positive ones helps to decrease anxiety.	**GOAL MET**

Evaluation
After spending 3 weeks in the IOP, Cara developed a trusting relationship with one staff person and two patients. Heather arranged a family meeting with Cara and her daughters where Cara was able to express her feelings. Her daughters expressed their concerns and emotions about leaving home as well. Cara also became more active in expressing her grief, particularly in the assertiveness and anger-management classes. Cara felt the music group amazingly improved her mood. Following discharge from the IOP, Cara decided to take piano lessons and also enrolled in some of her town's adult education classes. She is meeting more people in the community.

Many of Cara's symptoms have decreased. In particular, there have been no further episodes of tachycardia. Cara will continue to see her nurse therapist weekly, work on assertiveness skills, identification and expression of feelings, and a healthier lifestyle.

FACTITIOUS DISORDER

Whereas other somatic disorders are not under conscious control, people with a **factitious disorder** consciously pretend to be ill to have their emotional needs met and achieve the status of patient. The term *factitious* comes from the Latin word meaning artificial or contrived. Patients with this disorder artificially, deliberately, and dramatically fabricate symptoms or self-inflict injury with the goal of assuming the sick role. Similar to substance use disorders, this problem is compulsive, and individuals consciously conceal the true nature of their alleged illness through deception. Factitious disorder results in disability and immeasurable costs to the healthcare system.

The contrived illness may be physical or psychiatric. Examples of manufactured illnesses include bleeding, fever, hypoglycemia, seizures, hallucinations, and even cancer. Individuals with factitious disorder may report depression and suicidality after the death of a spouse despite the fact that the death never occurred or they were never even married (APA, 2013).

An older term for factitious disorder is **Munchausen syndrome**, which was named for Baron von Münchausen

(1720–97). He was an 18th-century German officer with a reputation for fabricating outrageous tales, such as traveling to the moon, riding a cannonball, or fighting a 40-foot crocodile.

Factitious Disorder Imposed on Self

Admission to the hospital often begins in the emergency department with a dramatic description of an illness using unusually proper medical terminology. The patient is often reluctant for professionals to speak with family members, friends, or previous healthcare providers. Once admitted, the patient is frequently demanding and requests specific treatments and interventions. Negative test results are often followed by new symptoms. If the healthcare team sets limits and does not follow through with requests, the patient may become angry and accuse the staff of incompetence and maltreatment.

Patients go from one primary care provider or hospital to another. Serious complications and sepsis may result from self-injections of toxins such as *E. coli*. Patients may have "crisscrossed" or "railroad-track" abdomens due to scars from numerous exploratory surgeries to investigate unexplained symptoms. In the extreme, amputations may even result from this disorder.

TABLE 17.5 Advanced Practice Interventions for Somatic Symptom Disorders

Disorder	Course	Interventions
Somatic symptom disorder	Chronic and relapsing	Consistent primary care provider with regular patient visits, limited tests Group therapy Cognitive-behavioral therapy
Illness anxiety disorder	Chronic and relapsing, but 50% of patients improve	Cognitive-behavioral therapy Insight-oriented therapy Group therapy Psychopharmacological management for comorbid conditions Stress management
Conversion disorder	Usually acute onset; resolves quickly	Suggest that the conversion symptom will gradually improve Behavioral therapy Insight-oriented therapy Hypnosis Antianxiety drugs
Psychological factors affecting medical condition	Acute and chronic; variable resolution	Treat psychiatric symptoms Tailor treatment to address both the psychological symptom and the medical condition
Factitious disorder	Highly treatment resistant	Confrontation is counterproductive Emphasis on management over cure Legal interventions may be necessary in the case of factitious disorder imposed on another

BOX 17.3 Dee Dee Blanchard: Factitious Disorder Imposed on Another

A famous example of this disorder is Dee Dee Blanchard, who subjected her daughter, Gypsy Rose (born in 1991), to a childhood of horrendous abuse. Among other problems, Dee Dee claimed that her daughter had muscular dystrophy, apnea, and seizures. As a result, Gypsy Rose was confined to a wheelchair in public, was fed with a feeding tube, slept with a breathing machine, and was given anticonvulsants for nonexistent seizures. Among the unnecessary surgeries performed on the child were the removal of her salivary glands and procedures on her eyes. She lost teeth due to the salivary gland removal. By the time that Gypsy Rose was a young adult, she wanted out of this dismal situation. In 2015, Gypsy Rose and a man she had met on the internet plotted the death of Dee Dee by stabbing. She was subsequently sentenced to 10 years in prison, a place where Gypsy Rose considers to have more freedom than she did in her early life.

Factitious Disorder Imposed on Another

The most insidious form of factitious disorder is **factitious disorder imposed on another** (also known as Munchausen syndrome by proxy), in which a caregiver deliberately falsifies illness in a vulnerable dependent. The diagnosis is imposed on the perpetrator and not the victim. People with this disorder may receive awards such as insurance money or other compensation. Even in the absence of awards, they do it for the purpose of attention and excitement and to perpetuate the relationship with the healthcare providers of that dependent. The parent or guardian is frequently a healthcare worker or someone with knowledge of the healthcare system.

The disorder results in unnecessary medical visits and sometimes-harmful medical procedures. Examples of this falsified problem include inducing premature delivery by rupturing the amniotic sac with a fingernail, infant apnea and sudden infant death, and introducing microorganisms into a child's wound. Falsification of illnesses results in extreme pain, surgical procedures, and even the death of dependents (Box 17.3).

Epidemiology

Epidemiological studies estimate an incidence rate for factitious disorders of 0.8% to 1.3%. Explanation for the low incidence rate includes the belief that a large number of cases are missed due to frequent denial of factitious disorder behaviors, the challenge to differentiate between real and feigned illness, and the fact that many patients often flee the healthcare setting. Factitious disorder, however, is more prevalent than previously recognized, with suggestions that up to 6% of healthcare provider contacts may involve factitious disorder. Nurses should consider this diagnosis in complicated patients, especially those with a history of emotional or physical distress, excessive dependence, and resistance to discharge.

Comorbidity

People with factitious disorders tend to complain of physical problems, although some patients may also try to convince clinicians that they have a psychiatric disorder. Patients may describe symptoms of depression, dissociation, conversion, and psychoses and seek treatment for these problems. According to some reports, substance use, borderline personality disorders, and sexual disorders are frequently present along with a normal to high intelligence quotient (IQ) and an intimate knowledge of the healthcare system.

Risk Factors
Biological Factors

Research points to brain dysfunction as a possible source of the symptoms of factitious disorders (Sadock, Sadock, & Ruiz, 2015). Specifically, impaired information processing is a potential cause. There does not seem to be a genetic pattern, and there are no abnormalities in electroencephalographic studies among people with factitious disorder.

Cognitive Factors

It is difficult to determine or understand the psychological basis of these disorders because of the patients' intention to skew the facts. There is some evidence that persons with these disorders suffered abuse and neglect as children and may have been hospitalized more frequently than is typical (Sadock, Sadock, & Ruiz, 2015). These hospitalizations may have been perceived as a refuge from a chaotic home life. Patients with factitious disorders may have a masochistic side and feel a need to be punished through painful procedures.

Nursing Care Associated With Factitious Disorders

Nurses who work with patients with factitious disorders—patients who intentionally and consciously fake illnesses—are often angry and resentful. After all, there are patients who really need care and have no control over how sick they are, and then there are patients with factitious disorders who are probably causing their own problems.

In cases of self-directed factitious disorder and particularly other-directed factitious disorder, the nurse must consider safety. Nurses must carefully monitor patients who may purposefully inflict damage to themselves and report suspicious activities to the healthcare team for discussion. It is essential that the nurse share any information that may prevent a person or a vulnerable and unsuspecting child from undergoing unnecessary surgery or treatments.

New coping strategies should permit the patient to function at a higher level, and the patient should handle stress adaptively without the desire or need for the pretense of a physiological disorder.

TREATMENT MODALITIES

CBT focusing on childhood trauma may be useful. People with factitious disorder do not benefit from various medical interventions such as antidepressants and/or antipsychotics.

MALINGERING

While not a specific mental disorder, malingering is mentioned here as a condition related to factitious disorders. **Malingering** is a consciously motivated act of fabricating an illness or exaggerating symptoms. This is done for secondary gain to become eligible for such things as disability compensation, committing fraud against insurance companies, obtaining prescription medications, evading military service, or receiving a reduced prison sentence. Reported pains are vague and hard for clinicians to prove or disprove, such as back pain, stomach ailments, headache, or toothache.

Malingering is likely more common in men than in women. It is nearly impossible to determine the prevalence of malingering due to the concealment of its origins. Childhood neglect and abuse are possible causes. A childhood history of frequent illnesses, especially those that result in hospitalization, may also be present in people who develop this disorder. Malingering is associated with antisocial, narcissistic, and borderline personality disorders.

KEY POINTS TO REMEMBER

- There is irrefutable evidence that emotional conditions may precipitate and often increase the severity of physical symptoms. Likewise, physical illnesses are often accompanied by a spectrum of emotional responses.
- Somatic symptom disorders are characterized by the presence of multiple real physical symptoms with or without an identifiable medical illness.
- Somatic symptom disorders are responses to psychosocial stress, although the patient often shows no insight into the potential stressors.
- The course of somatic symptom disorders may be brief, with acute onset and spontaneous remission, or chronic, with a gradual onset and prolonged impairment.
- The nursing assessment is especially important to identify symptoms of ACEs, depression, anxiety, posttraumatic
stress disorder, and substance use that are contributing to the somatic symptom disorder.
- Interventions target both the psychological and medical problems to increase adherence to the care regimen, maximize quality of life, promote healing, and minimize healthcare costs.
- The advanced practice psychiatric–mental health registered nurse is in a key position to assist other healthcare personnel to view patients in an integrated approach in both inpatient and outpatient settings.
- Factitious disorders, in contrast to other somatic disorders, are under conscious control. Nurses are challenged to provide care for persons who are pretending to have disorders when there are others with real illnesses who need their time.

CRITICAL THINKING

A patient with suspected somatic symptom disorder has been admitted to the medical-surgical unit after an episode of chest pain with possible electrocardiographic changes. While on the unit, she frequently complains of palpitations, asks the nurse to check her vital signs, and begs staff to stay with her. Some nurses take her pulse and blood pressure when she asks.

Others evade her requests. Most of the staff try to avoid spending time with her.

1. Consider why staff members wish to avoid her. How would you feel as a nurse in this situation?
2. Design interventions to cope with the patient's behaviors. Give rationales for your interventions.

CHAPTER REVIEW

1. The care plan of a patient diagnosed with a somatic disorder includes the nursing diagnosis *impaired coping*. Which patient behavior demonstrates a successful outcome for that nursing diagnosis?
   a. Showers and dresses in clean clothes daily
   b. Calls a friend to talk when feeling lonely
   c. Spends more time talking about pain in her abdomen
   d. Maintains focus and concentration

2. Which patient is at greatest risk for developing a stress-induced myocardial infarction?
   a. A patient who lost a child in an accidental shooting 24 hours ago
   b. A woman who has begun experiencing early signs of menopause
   c. A patient who has spent years trying to sustain a successful business
   d. A patient who was diagnosed with chronic major depressive disorder 10 years ago

3. What precipitating emotional factor has been associated with an increased incidence of cancers? *Select all that apply.*
   a. Anxiety
   b. Job-related stress
   c. Acute grief
   d. Feelings of hopelessness and despair from depression
   e. Prolonged, intense stress

4. You are caring for Aaron, a 38-year-old patient diagnosed with somatic symptom disorder. When interacting with you, Aaron continues to focus on his severe headaches. In planning care for Aaron, which of the following interventions would be appropriate?
   a. Call for a family meeting with Aaron in attendance to confront Aaron regarding his diagnosis.
   b. Educate Aaron on alternative therapies to deal with pain.
   c. Improve reality testing by telling Aaron that you do not believe that the headaches are real.
   d. After a limited discussion of physical concerns, shift focus to feelings and effective coping skills.

5. Living comfortable and materialistic lives in Western societies seems to have altered the original hierarchy proposed by Maslow in that:
   a. Once lower-level needs are satisfied, no further growth feels necessary.
   b. Self-actualization is easier to achieve with financial stability.
   c. Esteem is more highly valued than safety.
   d. Focusing on materialism reduces interests in love, belonging, and family.

6. Diane, a 63-year-old mother of three, was brought to the community psychiatric clinic. Diane and her son had a bitter fight over finances. Ever since, Diane has been complaining of "a severe pain in my neck." She has seen several doctors who cannot find a physical basis for the pain. The nurse knows that:
   a. Showing concern for Diane's pain will increase her obsessional thinking.
   b. Diane's symptoms are manipulative and under conscious control.
   c. Diane believes there is a physical cause for the pain and will resist a psychological explanation.
   d. Diane is trying to make her son feel bad about the argument.

7. Conversion disorder is described as an absence of a neurological diagnosis that manifests in neurological symptoms. Channeling of emotions, conflicts, and stressors into physical symptoms is thought to be the cause of conversion disorder. Which statement is true?
   a. People with conversion disorder are extremely upset about often dramatic symptoms.
   b. Abnormal patterns of cerebral activation have been found in individuals with conversion disorder.
   c. An organic cause is usually found in most cases of conversion disorder.
   d. Symptoms can be turned off and on depending on the patient's choice.

8. Melanie is a 38-year-old female admitted to the hospital to rule out a neurological disorder. The testing was negative, yet she is reluctant to be discharged. Today she has added lower back pain and a stabbing sensation in her abdomen. The nurse suspects a factitious disorder in which Melanie may:
   a. Consciously be trying to maintain her role of a sick patient.
   b. Not recognize her unmet needs to be cared for.
   c. Protect her child from illness.
   d. Recognize physical symptoms as a coping mechanism.

9. You are caring for Yolanda, a 67-year-old patient who has been receiving hemodialysis for 3 months. Yolanda reports that she feels angry whenever it is time for her dialysis treatment. You attribute this to:
   a. Organic changes in Yolanda's brain.
   b. A flaw in Yolanda's personality.
   c. A normal response to grief and loss.
   d. Denial of the reality of a poor prognosis.

10. Lucas is a nurse on a medical floor caring for Kelly, a 48-year-old patient with newly diagnosed type 2 diabetes. He realizes that depression is a complicating factor in the patient's adjustment to her new diagnosis. What problem has the most potential to arise?
    a. Development of agoraphobia
    b. Treatment nonadherence
    c. Frequent hypoglycemic reactions
    d. Sleeping rather than checking blood sugar

1. **b**; 2. **d**; 3. **d, e**; 4. **d**; 5. **d**; 6. **c**; 7. **b**; 8. **a**; 9. **c**; 10. **b**

NGN CASE STUDY AND QUESTIONS

Cynthia is a 64 year old who is admitted to the emergency department (ED) after a near-lethal dose of acetaminophen (Tylenol). Despite the severity of the overdose, she avoids questions about it. Instead, she focuses on physical symptoms, especially mild abdominal pain and concern over bowel movements. She states she has not seen her primary care provider, a nurse practitioner, in several years. "I'm afraid of what I'll find out." Her electronic medical record shows that Cynthia had surgery to remove a benign breast tumor 10 months ago.

She shares a detailed chart tracking vegan intake and bowel movements that she developed after her mother died from colon cancer 2 years ago. When asked how she has been dealing with her grief since then, she says, "Not very well. I'm sad and feel lonely. I think it's worse because I've been so worried about my own symptoms." Regarding a support system, she says, "I am an only child. Taking care of mother, I was too busy to go out. And now, of course, since I am ill, I can't deal with other people. Can you recheck my blood pressure? I think it's really high."

Vital signs—including blood pressure—are normal. All ED tests and imaging demonstrate no evidence of gastrointestinal pathology. The ED provider suspects that Cynthia has illness anxiety disorder.

1. Identify the assessment findings that require the nurse to follow up. *Select all that apply.*
   a. Reports occasional abnormal bowel movements
   b. Had recent benign tumor diagnosis
   c. Reports mild abdominal discomfort
   d. Excessive health-related behaviors
   e. Preference for veganism
   f. Maladaptive avoidance
   g. Family history of colon cancer
   h. Symptoms present for at least 9 months

2. Based on the patient's condition, the patient's *priority* problems include which of the following? *Select all that apply:*
   a. Accidentally overdosed on acetaminophen for symptom relief
   b. Expresses difficulty coping with loss of mother and expresses loneliness
   c. Reports having no other family or friends
   d. Displays nutritional deficits
   e. Keeps a detailed food and bowel movement diary
   f. Excessive concern about elevated blood pressure in the absence of symptoms or values
   g. Says that socializing would just make her more nervous

NGN case study answers are on Evolve.

🌐 Visit the Evolve website for a posttest on the content in this chapter: http://evolve.elsevier.com/Varcarolis

REFERENCES

Ahmed, H. (2017). *Psychosocial symptoms as predictors for persistent pain in temporomandibular disorder* (Master's thesis). University of Washington, US. Retrieved from https://pdfs.semanticscholar.org/b220/14ef3843c1181025590e57c6170e5743ee94.pdf.

Akyuz, F., Gokalp, P. G., Erdiman, S., Oflaz, S., & Karsidag, C. (2017). Conversion disorder comorbidity and childhood trauma. *Archives of Neuropsychiatry, 54*(1), 15–20.

American Psychiatric Association. (2013). *Diagnostic and statistical manual of mental disorders* (5th ed.). Washington, DC: Author.

Barnett, M., Moore, J. W., & Archuleta, W. P. (2019). A loneliness model of hypochrondriasis among older adults: The mediating role of intolerance of uncertainty and anxious symptoms. *Archives of Gerontology and Geriatrics, 83*, 86–90.

Beutel, M., Tibubos, A. N., Klein, E. M., Schmutzer, G., Reiner, I., Kocalevent, R. D., & Brähler, E. (2015). Childhood adversities and distress—The role of resilience in a representative sample. *PLOS ONE, 12*(3), e0173826.

Bhargava, T., & Pandey, R. (2016). Effect of health locus of control on patient with somatization. *International Journal of Indian Psychology, 4*(1).

Brown, E. G., Gallagher, S., & Creaven, A. M. (2017). Loneliness and acute stress reactivity: A systematic review of psychophysiological studies. *Psychophysiology, 55*(5), e13031.

Bullock, K. D., Mirza, N., Forte, C., & Trockel, M. (2015). Group dialectical-behavior therapy skills training for conversion disorder with seizures. *Journal of Neuropsychiatry and Clinical Neurosciences, 27*(3), 240–243.

Edwards, T., Stern, A., Clarke, D. D., Ivbijaro, G., & Kasney, L. M. (2010). The treatment of the patient with medically unexplained symptoms in primary care: A review of the literature. *Mental Health in Family Medicine, 7*(4), 209–221.

Feinstein, A. (2011). Conversion disorder: advances in our understanding. *CMAJ, 183*(8), 915–920.

Fink, P. (2010). The outcome of health anxiety in primary care: A two-year follow up study on healthcare costs and self-rated health. *PloS ONE, 5*(3), e9873.

Goodwin, R., Palgi, Y., Lavenda, O., Hamama-Raz, Y., & Ben-Ezra, M. (2015). Association between media use, acute stress disorder, and psychological distress. *Psychotherapy and Psychosomatics, 84*, 253–254.

Greenberg, D. B. (2017). *Somatization: Epidemiology pathogenesis, clinical features, medical evaluation, and diagnosis. Official report from Uptodate.* Wolters Kluwer.

Henningsen, Peter (2018). Somatic symptom disorder and illness anxiety. In J. L. Levenson (Ed.), *Textbook of psychosomatic medicine* (pp. 35–37). Washington, DC: American Psychiatric Association.

Huang, H., & McCarron, R. M. (2011). Medically unexplained symptoms: Evidence-based interventions. *Current Psychiatry, 10*(7), 17–31.

Marwijk, H. W. J., Kooy, K. G., Stehouwer, C. D., Beekman, A. T., & van Hout, H. P. (2015). Depression increases the onset of cardiovascular disease over and above other determinants in older primary care patients, a cohort study. *BMC Cardiovascular Disorders, 15*, 40.

Meichenbaum, D. (2017). *Evolution of cognitive behavioral therapy.* New York, NY: Routledge.

Mesaroli, G., Munns, C., & DeSouza, C. (2019). Evidence-based practice: Physiotherapy for children and adolescents with motor symptoms of conversion disorder. *Physiotherapy: Canada, 71*(4), 400–402.

Muris, P., & Petrocchi, N. (2016). Protection or vulnerability? A meta-analysis of the relations between the positive and negative components of self-compassion and psychopathology. *Clinical Psychology and Psychotherapy*. Retrieved from http://self-compassion.org/wp-content/uploads/2016/04/Muris.Petrocchi2015.pdf.

Murthy, V.H. (2020). *Together: The healing power of human connection in a sometimes lonely world*. Harper Wave.

Newby, J. M., Smith, J., Uppal, S., Mason, E., Mahoney, A. E. J., & Andrews, G. (2018). Internet-based cognitive behavioral therapy versus psychoeducation control for illness anxiety disorder and somatic symptom disorder. *Journal of Consulting and Clinical Psychology*, 86(1), 89–98.

Özlem, K. K., Akgul, S., & İzci, F. (2018). An approach to conversion disorder with comorbid major depression using pharmacotherapy and psychodrama techniques. *Journal of Psychiatry and Neurological Sciences*, 4(31), 413–420.

Papadopoulos, N. L. R., & Rohricht, F. (2018). A single case report of body oriented psychological therapy for a patient with chronic conversion disorder. *The Arts in Psychotherapy*, 61, 38–43.

Sadock, B. J., Sadock, V. A., & Ruiz, P. (2015). *Synopsis of psychiatry* (11th ed.). Philadelphia, PA: Wolters Kluwer.

Scher, L. M., & Shwarts, E. (2019). Somatic symptom and related disorders. In L. W. Roberts (Ed.), *The American Psychiatric Association Publishing textbook of psychiatry* (7th ed.) (pp. 475–496). Washington, DC: American Psychiatric Association.

Stone, J., Vuilleumier, P., & Friedman, J. H. (2010). Conversion disorder: Separating "how" from "why." *Neurology*, 74(3), 190–191.

Wong, M. M. C., Pang, P. F., & Yiu, M. G. C. (2017). Hypochondriacal delusion in an elderly man with good response to ECT but complicated by febrile reaction. *Archives of Depression and Anxiety*, 3(2), 038–041.

Zivin, K., Yosef, M., Miller, E. M., Valenstein, M., Duffy, S., Kales, H. C., & Kim, H. M. (2015). Association between depression and cause specific death: A retrospective cohort study in the Veterans Health Administration. *Journal of Psychosomatic Research*, 78(4), 324–331.

18

Eating and Feeding Disorders

Rachel M. Childs and Carissa R. Enright

Visit the Evolve website for a pretest on the content in this chapter: http://evolve.elsevier.com/Varcarolis

OBJECTIVES

1. Compare and contrast the signs and symptoms of anorexia nervosa, bulimia nervosa, and binge-eating disorder.
2. Describe the biological, cognitive, and environmental factors associated with eating disorders.
3. Apply the nursing process to patients with anorexia nervosa, bulimia nervosa, and binge-eating disorders.
4. Identify three life-threatening conditions, stated in terms of nursing diagnoses, in a patient with an eating disorder.
5. Identify two realistic outcome criteria for a patient with anorexia nervosa, bulimia nervosa, and binge-eating disorder.
6. Describe biological treatments and psychological therapies for eating disorders.
7. Describe three feeding disorders: pica, rumination disorder, and avoidant/restrictive food intake disorder.

KEY TERMS AND CONCEPTS

body mass index (BMI)	lanugo	refeeding syndrome
ideal body weight	pica	rumination

Of all the psychiatric disorders, eating disorders may be the most perplexing and potentially the most lethal. Eating and sharing food is usually a pleasurable and culturally important aspect of human life. Consequently, it may be difficult for us to understand why someone would engage in potentially lethal behaviors in order to avoid this experience or to lose weight. Although there are many theories to date, research is ongoing in the effort to understand the biopsychosocial components that cause and maintain eating disorders.

Eating disorders represent a multidimensional set of symptoms and behaviors occurring along a spectrum, similar to our current understanding of autism (Goldschmidt et al., 2018). Following onset, eating disorder symptoms can wax and wane over the life span, much like depression, schizophrenia, or substance use disorders. Patients with eating disorders move along a spectrum both in intensity of symptoms and in the type of eating disorder behavior. Although a patient's eating disorder may start with restriction, it may progress to binging and then binging and purging.

In this chapter, we focus on the three main eating disorders: anorexia nervosa, bulimia nervosa, and binge-eating disorder (American Psychiatric Association, 2013). A summary of characteristics of these disorders is included in Box 18.1. After discussing the eating disorders, we also briefly review feeding disorders.

ANOREXIA NERVOSA

Clinical Picture

Individuals with **anorexia nervosa** have an intense fear of gaining weight. Often, there is a misperception that individuals with anorexia refuse to eat despite being hungry. However, evidence suggests that people with anorexia experience significant differences in sensation of taste, appetite, and satiety, which help to perpetuate the disorder (Kerr et al., 2016). Whereas healthy controls experience great satisfaction or comfort following the consumption of foods and in the presence of fullness, an individual coping with anorexia may experience fear, anxiety, panic, or depression.

To prevent these negative emotions, people with anorexia may engage in restriction along with other compensatory behaviors. Such behaviors are acts an individual utilizes to make up for the effects of eating or to mitigate previous intake (National Eating Disorder Association, 2018). Purging is a type of compensatory behavior. Although most of us think of self-induced vomiting when we hear the word *purging*, it also refers to excessive exercise, the use of laxatives or stimulants, or of thyroid medications aimed at decreasing weight (Mehler & Andersen, 2017).

Anorexia nervosa is difficult to treat. Even when remission is achieved, the 1-year relapse rate is approximately 50%. Even after 4 years, up to 40% of patients continue to meet some criteria for anorexia (Harrington et al., 2015). Recovery is

BOX 18.1 Characteristics of Eating Problems

Anorexia Nervosa	Bulimia Nervosa	Binge Eating
Intense fear of weight gain	Recurrent episodes of uncontrollable binging	Recurrent episodes of uncontrollable binging without compensatory behaviors
Distorted body image	Inappropriate compensatory behaviors: vomiting, laxatives, diuretics, or exercise	Binging episodes induce guilt, depression, embarrassment, or disgust
Restricted calories with significantly low BMI	Self-image largely influenced by body image	
Subtypes:		
Restricting (no consistent bulimic features)		
Binge/eating/purging type (primarily restriction, some bulimic behaviors)		

BMI, Body mass index.

evaluated as a stage in the process rather than a fixed event. Factors that influence the stage of recovery include the percentage of weight restoration, extent to which self-worth is defined by shape and weight, and functional impairment in the patient's personal life.

The *DSM-5* box contains the criteria for anorexia nervosa.

DSM-5 CRITERIA FOR ANOREXIA NERVOSA

A. Restrictions of energy intake relative to requirements, leading to a significantly low body weight in the context of age, sex, developmental trajectory, and physical health. Significantly low weight is defined as a weight less than minimally normal or, for children and adolescents, less than that minimally expected.

B. Intense fear of gaining weight or becoming fat or persistent behavior that interferes with weight gain, even though already at a significantly low weight.

C. Disturbance in the way in which one's body weight or shape is experienced, undue influence of body weight or shape on self-evaluation, or persistent lack of recognition of the seriousness of the current low body weight.

Specify whether:

(F50.01) Restricting type: During the last 3 months, the individual has not engaged in recurrent episodes of binge-eating or purging behavior (i.e., self-induced vomiting or the misuse of laxatives, diuretics, or enemas). This subtype describes presentations in which weight loss is accomplished primarily through dieting, fasting, and/or excessive exercise.

(F50.02) Binge-eating/purging type: During the last 3 months, the individual has engaged in recurrent episodes of binge-eating or purging behavior (i.e., self-induced vomiting or the misuse of laxatives, diuretics, or enemas).

From American Psychiatric Association. (2013). *Diagnostic and statistical manual of disorders* (5th ed.). Washington, DC: Author.

Epidemiology

The estimated lifetime prevalence of anorexia nervosa is 0.5%, with a median age of onset of 18 years (Hudson et al., 2012). Actual prevalence must be higher, as individuals may conceal symptoms. In fact, research indicates that less than half of individuals with anorexia seek help for the disorder (Rosenvinge &

Petterson, 2015). Anorexia nervosa commonly begins during adolescence or in young adults. It is uncommon for it to occur before puberty or after age 40.

Anorexia is more prevalent among females than males. Depending on environment, however, this ratio can narrow or expand. For example, in a hospital setting, the ratio of females to males is 10:1. In community samples, the ratio decreases to 3:1 (Mehler & Andersen, 2017).

Regardless of gender, disordered eating is more common among athletes who participate in sports that emphasize aesthetics or leanness for advantage in competition (Joy et al., 2016). These sports include running, gymnastics, wrestling, rowing, and figure skating.

The prevalence of eating disorders may also be higher among individuals who identify themselves as lesbian, gay, bisexual, transgender, and/or queer (or questioning) (LGBTQ). In a recent survey of youth who identify as LGBTQ, about 54% had been diagnosed with an eating disorder (Trevor Project, 2018). For straight transgender respondents, anorexia was the most common type of eating disorder.

Comorbidity

Comorbidities commonly associated with anorexia nervosa include the following:

- Bipolar disorder
- Anxiety disorders
- Depressive disorders
- Obsessive compulsive disorder
- Posttraumatic stress disorder (PTSD) and other trauma-related disorders
- Alcohol or substance use disorder

Risk Factors

Biological Factors

Genetic. The heritability of anorexia nervosa is estimated to be 50% to 60% (Yilmaz, Hardaway, & Bulik, 2015). Researchers have explored the correlation between anorexia nervosa and other genetic variations among nearly 17,000 people with anorexia and about 55,000 healthy controls (Watson et al., 2019). They found genetic correlations between anorexia, major depressive disorder, anxiety disorders, obsessive-compulsive disorder, and schizophrenia. They also found a correlation between anorexia and variations in glucose and lipid metabolism, which may indicate differences in metabolism following food restriction. These variations may be predisposing factors for anorexia's onset and maintenance.

Neurobiological

Neurotransmitters. Tryptophan, an amino acid essential to serotonin synthesis, is available only through diet. A normal diet boosts serotonin in the brain and regulates mood. Temporary declines in dietary tryptophan may actually relieve symptoms of anxiety and dysphoria and provide a reward for caloric restriction. However, continued malnutrition will result in a physiological dysphoria. This cycle of temporary relief, followed by more dysphoria, sets up a positive feedback loop that reinforces disordered eating behavior. The dietary need for tryptophan may also explain why antidepressants that boost serotonin do not improve mood symptoms until after a patient has been restored to 90% of optimal weight.

The body responds to prolonged nutritional deprivation by activating the hypothalamus. This results in the release of cortisol and dopamine and the modulation of dopamine receptors. It is a survival response meant to elicit a drive for food. Individuals with anorexia nervosa interpret these physiological responses as threats to their control. Consequently, they may experience panic, anxiety, or fear and be increasingly motivated to avoid these internal states by intensifying efforts at restriction (Frank et al., 2019).

Neuroanatomy. Functional magnetic resonance imaging (fMRI) studies demonstrate variations in neuroanatomy that may be present before and after the onset of anorexia nervosa. Individuals with anorexia nervosa have less in gray and white matter in the central nervous system (Zipfel et al., 2015). They exhibit decreases in the size and/or function of portions of the hypothalamus, basal ganglia, and somatosensory cortex. Regions of the insula, amygdala, and dorsolateral prefrontal cortex appear larger or experience greater activation in comparison to observations in healthy controls (Brownell & Walsh, 2017). The insula is a portion of the brain associated with interoceptive awareness or the ability to receive, interpret, and appraise internal sensations like satiety or fullness.

Cognitive Factors

Anorexia nervosa is an ego-syntonic disorder. That is, the affected individuals value their disorder. Although they know that their actions are potentially harmful, they believe that the benefits outweigh the harm (Mehler & Andersen, 2017). Anxious and perfectionistic temperaments are aligned with a need for control and progress toward an unrealistic ideal of thinness.

Compared with healthy controls, patients with anorexia struggle significantly with emotional identification, regulation, and processing (Brownell & Walsh, 2017). Therefore, they tend to exhibit low distress tolerance and deficits in behavioral control in response to distress.

Environmental Factors

Culture exerts an influence on the development of self-concept and satisfaction with body size. Anorexia nervosa is associated with cultures that value thinness. Increasingly, social media are exerting influence on the dominant culture. YouTube anorexia-related videos were studied by Sidani and colleagues (2016). Unfortunately, approximately one-third of these videos were judged to favor or encourage fasting behaviors. Even worse, these "pro anorexia" or "pro ana" videos were more likely to receive high ratings than videos that describe the health risks associated with this illness.

APPLICATION OF THE NURSING PROCESS

ASSESSMENT

Patients with anorexia nervosa often do not see a problem with their behavior. Typically, they are seen in healthcare settings under duress from concerned family or friends, who insist that they get treatment. They may also seek care for significant physical declines and other alarming symptoms.

Box 18.2 lists thoughts and behaviors associated with anorexia nervosa, and Table 18.1 identifies clinical signs and symptoms of anorexia nervosa along with their causes.

General Assessment

Patients with anorexia are underweight and may have a growth of fine, downy hair called **lanugo** on the face and back. They will also have mottled, cool skin on the extremities and low blood pressure, pulse, and temperature readings consistent with a malnourished, dehydrated state. Usually, electrolytes will not deviate far from the normal ranges. However, if patients are engaged in purging, they may experience severe electrolyte imbalances.

Body mass index (BMI) is the gauge used to determine the severity of this disorder. According to the American Psychiatric

---

BOX 18.2 Thoughts and Behaviors Associated With Anorexia Nervosa

- Terror of gaining weight
- Preoccupation with thoughts of food
- View of self as fat even when emaciated
- Peculiar handling of food: cutting food into small bits
- Pushing pieces of food around plate
- Possible development of rigorous exercise regimen
- Possible self-induced vomiting, use of laxatives and diuretics
- Cognition so disturbed that individual judges self-worth by weight

---

TABLE 18.1 Possible Signs and Symptoms of Anorexia Nervosa

Clinical Presentation	Cause
Low weight	Caloric restriction, excessive exercising
Amenorrhea	Low weight
Yellow skin	Hypercarotenemia
Lanugo	Starvation
Cold extremities	Starvation
Peripheral edema	Hypoalbuminemia and refeeding
Muscle weakening	Starvation, electrolyte imbalance
Constipation	Starvation
Abnormal laboratory values (low triiodothyronine, thyroxine levels)	Starvation
Abnormal computed tomographic scans, electroencephalographic changes	Starvation
Cardiovascular abnormalities (hypotension, bradycardia, heart failure)	Starvation, dehydration
	Electrolyte imbalance
Impaired renal function	Dehydration
Hypokalemia (<3.5 mEq/L)	Starvation
Anemic pancytopenia	Starvation
Decreased bone density	Estrogen deficiency, low calcium intake

Association (2013), the disorder is considered mild with a BMI of 17 or more, moderate with a BMI of 16 to 17, severe with a BMI of 15 to 16, and extreme when the BMI is less than 15.

Self-Assessment

When you are caring for a patient with anorexia, you may underestimate the severity of the obsessive-compulsive nature of the illness. You may believe that the behaviors are mostly self-imposed. However, the patient views these behaviors as essential to her security and safety as well as a means to avoid negative feelings. Think about aspects of your own life that make you feel safe, comfortable, and in control. Can you imagine being asked to give them up abruptly? It helps to remember how afraid such patients are of losing control. It also helps to remember that anorexia nervosa is a complex disorder associated with biological processes that support its continuation.

📄 ASSESSMENT GUIDELINES

Anorexia Nervosa

1. Determine the patient's perception of the problem, or chief complaint.
2. Perform a complete nursing assessment, including orthostatic vital signs, review of systems, and general appearance.
3. Gather a psychosocial history, including screening for suicide or self-harm behaviors.
4. Assess nutritional pattern and fluid intake.
5. Assess daily activities, including exercise.
6. Review laboratory testing, including the following:
   - Electrolyte levels
   - Glucose level
   - Thyroid function tests
   - Complete blood count
   - Electrocardiogram (ECG)
   - Dual energy x-ray absorptiometry (DEXA) to measure bone density
   - Erythrocyte sedimentation rate (ESR)
   - Creatine phosphokinase (CPK)
7. Determine the patient's goals of treatment.

NURSING DIAGNOSIS

Nursing diagnoses may include *impaired low nutritional intake*, *impaired cardiac output*, *electrolyte imbalance*, and *fluid imbalance*, all of which should be addressed in order of severity. Other nursing diagnoses include *impaired body image*, *impaired coping*, *chronic low self-esteem*, and *risk for powerlessness*.

OUTCOMES IDENTIFICATION

Outcomes are patient centered and ideally developed along with the patient or with someone who can represent the patient. The most important outcome is the attainment of a safe weight. Table 18.2 identifies signs and symptoms commonly experienced with anorexia nervosa, offers potential nursing diagnoses, and suggests outcome criteria for evaluation.

PLANNING

Planning depends on the acuity of the patient's situation. In general, two criteria for hospitalization include extreme electrolyte imbalance or weights below 75% of **ideal body weight**. The plan is then to provide immediate medical stabilization, most likely on an inpatient unit. Other criteria for hospitalization include less than 10% body fat, a daytime heart rate of less than 50 beats per minute, a systolic blood pressure of less than 90, a temperature of less than 96°F, and arrhythmias. If a specialized eating disorder unit is not available, hospitalization on a cardiac or medical unit is usually brief. These hospitalizations provide only limited weight restoration and address such acute complications as electrolyte imbalance and dysrhythmias and acute psychiatric symptoms such as severe depression and suicidality.

Severely malnourished patients may need treatment on a medical unit for therapeutic nutrition. During prolonged starvation, the body adapts to preserve function and prevent muscle breakdown, switching from glucose-based energy to fat- and protein-based energy. When nutrients are restored, insulin stimulates glycogen, fat, and protein synthesis, a process that requires minerals such as phosphate and magnesium. In severely malnourished patients, a potentially lethal **refeeding syndrome** may occur. This complication may result in abnormalities of fluid balance and glucose metabolism as well as hypophosphatemia, hypomagnesemia, and hypokalemia. Thiamine deficiency can also occur. Nutrients are reintroduced slowly in order to avoid this syndrome.

Once a patient is medically stable, the plan addresses the issues underlying the eating disorder. The plan of care will include individual, group, and family therapy as well as pharmacotherapy and nutritional therapy in varying degrees depending on the phase of illness.

Discharge planning is a critical component of treatment and should include the patient's family or chosen social support group. While they are completing discharge planning, nurses may take steps to facilitate patients' connections with community resources. Such resources may be related to living arrangements, school, work, financial aid applications to state and/or federal programs, and outpatient treatment.

IMPLEMENTATION

Treatment for anorexia may occur in inpatient, day treatment programs, and outpatient environments. Regardless of setting, treatment will consist of psychosocial interventions, pharmacotherapy, psychotherapy, nutrition, and medical intervention.

If patients are in a state of crisis, they may be admitted to an inpatient psychiatric facility or a specialized eating disorder treatment facility. No matter the setting, the initial focus depends on the results of a comprehensive assessment. Acute psychiatric symptoms, such as suicidal ideation, are immediately addressed.

After resolving acute symptoms, the patient with anorexia begins a weight restoration program that allows for incremental weight gain. Based on the patient's height, a treatment goal is set at 90% of ideal body weight. Specially trained dieticians will assist in developing a daily meal plan and caloric intake. While increasing daily intake, the patient is confronting what were

TABLE 18.2   Signs and Symptoms, Nursing Diagnoses, and Outcomes for Anorexia Nervosa

Signs and Symptoms	Nursing Diagnoses	Outcomes
Emaciation, dehydration, arrhythmias, inadequate intake, dry skin, decreased blood pressure, decreased urine output, increased urine concentration, weakness	Impaired low nutritional intake Impaired cardiac output Electrolyte imbalance Fluid imbalance	Improved nutritional intake, cardiac output, electrolyte balance, and fluid balance: Nutrients are ingested and absorbed to meet metabolic needs; cardiac pump supports systemic perfusion pressure; electrolytes are in balance; fluids are in balance
Excessive self-monitoring, describes self as fat despite emaciation	Impaired body image	Positive body image: Congruence between body reality, body ideal, and body presentation; satisfaction with body appearance
Destructive behavior toward self, poor concentration, inability to meet role expectations, inadequate problem solving	Impaired coping	Effective coping: Reports decrease in anxiety, uses personal support system, uses effective coping strategies, reports increase in psychological comfort
Indecisive behavior, lack of eye contact, passive, reports feelings of shame, rejects positive feedback about self	Chronic low self-esteem	Positive self-esteem: Verbalizes a positive level of confidence, makes informed life decisions, expresses independence with decision-making processes

International Council of Nursing Practice (ICN). (2019). *ICNP browser.* Retrieved from https://www.icn.ch/what-we-do/projects/ehealth/icnp-browser. ICNP® is owned and copyrighted by the ICN. Reproduced with permission of the copyright holder.

once considered terrifying realities and exposure to specific changes to weight or body size can trigger decompensation. Patients are generally weighed two to three times a week in this environment to gauge progress. Often, the patient stands on the scale backward to decrease anxiety over weight gain.

The milieu of an eating-disorder unit is purposefully organized to assist the patient in establishing more adaptive behavior patterns and normalization of eating. The highly structured environment provides precise meal times and adherence to the selected menu. Close observation before and after meals as well as monitoring weight, movement, and bathroom trips are critical.

Patients may also need monitoring on bathroom trips after seeing visitors and after any hospital pass to ensure they have not had access to and ingested any laxatives or diuretics. Close monitoring and development of specific parameters for movement or exercise are also warranted. These plans are individualized and based on the patient's ability to safely withstand activity while on the unit.

During inpatient care, patients will be part of and participate in the unit's milieu. In this setting, the patient should feel accepted and safe from judgmental evaluations. The focus should be on the eating behaviors and underlying feelings of anxiety, dysphoria, low self-esteem, and lack of control.

Outpatient partial hospitalization is an option for patients who have been stabilized. In this setting patients are in a clinical setting during the day and then go home to practice skills in the afternoon. Outpatient treatment continues if the patient maintains a contracted weight, normal range of vitals, and increased abstinence from eating disordered behaviors. A patient deviating from the treatment agreement may need to return to a higher level of care in an inpatient or residential environment.

Families frequently report feeling powerless during decompensation and in early recovery. They are often unaware of the biological origins of eating disorders. As such, strategies they used to address the disorder in the past, such as forcing the patient to eat, negotiating or begging the patient to eat, and removing free choice or privacy to encourage eating have failed. They commonly have feelings of frustration, hopelessness, or

despair. A significant part of the recovery process will include rebuilding relationships with family. The nurse plays an integral role in this process by providing family members with education about the illness and treatment.

⊕ CONSIDERING CULTURE

Does Religion or Faith Affect Disordered Eating?

In a survey including 687 Sydney University students, individuals completed a web-based survey designed to let researchers examine the association between religiosity/spirituality and the presence of disordered eating or related psychopathology.

All the participants were women, on average of 21 years of age. About 70% identified as having some degree of religiosity, and about 85% identified as having some degree of spiritual or personal existential belief. Existential beliefs were conceptualized as a personal belief of hope, optimism, meaning, and peace. Results were as follows:

- Lower levels of religiosity were associated with higher levels of body dissatisfaction.
- Desire for thinness was negatively correlated with the presence of both religious and existential beliefs.
- Existential or personal and to a lesser extent spiritual beliefs were associated with lower levels of disordered eating psychopathology.

Culturally sensitive nursing care requires that nurses seek to understand a patient's cultural, religious, and personal beliefs and background. Through this lens, the nurse can begin to understand what influences may be contributing to patients' disordered eating pathology and what strengths can be emphasized to support the patient in treatment. In this way, the nurse will be able to understand and treat patients as they would like to be treated.

Adapted from Akrawi, D., Bartrop, R., Surgenor, L., Shanmugam, S., Potter, U., & Touyz, S. (2017). The relationship between spiritual, religious, and personal beliefs and disordered eating psychopathology. *Translational Developmental Psychiatry, 5*(1).

Health Teaching and Health Promotion

People with anorexia may need support in basic skills. Some of these skills include learning how to create meal plans, shop at the grocery store, and navigate various social or familial situations. In order to accomplish these tasks, patients need help to develop healthy coping, communication, problem-solving, and decision-making skills. As patients approach their goal weight, plans should be made and tested for how to navigate home, social, educational, and occupational environments.

Teamwork and Safety

Patients admitted to an inpatient unit designed to treat eating disorders participate in a combination of therapeutic modalities provided by an interprofessional team. These modalities normalize eating patterns and begin to address the medical, family, and social issues raised by the illness.

EVALUATION

Evaluation is a fluid and continuous process. Further, it is composed of short-term indicators along the way. These indicators provide a daily guide for gauging success and are continually reevaluated for their appropriateness. The Case Study and Nursing Care Plan later in this chapter presents a patient with anorexia nervosa.

TREATMENT MODALITIES
Biological Treatments
Pharmacotherapy

There are no drugs approved by the US Food and Drug Administration (FDA) for the treatment of anorexia nervosa. Research does not support the use of pharmacological agents to treat the core symptoms (Harrington et al., 2015). Consequently, psychotropic medication is utilized to treat associated symptoms or other co-occurring disorders. Some of these medications may include selective serotonin reuptake inhibitors (SSRIs), antianxiety agents, second-generation antipsychotics, and mood stabilizers.

Integrative Therapy

Patients may benefit from integrative approaches that can be used in conjunction with traditional eating disorder treatment (Fogarty, Smith, & Hay, 2016). These approaches include yoga, massage, acupuncture, or bright light therapy. The nurse can play a vital role in providing education regarding how these therapies can be incorporated and in setting realistic expectations for their efficacy.

Psychological Therapies

Psychiatric–mental health advanced practice registered nurses are prepared to assess, diagnose, and treat patients with anorexia nervosa. Some psychiatric advanced practice nurses even specialize in eating disorders. They can provide educational and supportive individual, group, or family therapy and can also facilitate the more complex group therapy.

There is no empirical evidence to support any specific psychotherapy model in adults with anorexia nervosa. However, in adolescent patients with anorexia, there is evidence to support its use. Insight-oriented individual therapy, where patients are encouraged to learn more about themselves, has been demonstrated to be effective (Lock, 2015). Family approaches, especially family-based treatment (F-BT), has been demonstrated to be more effective than individual therapy. F-BT is an outpatient 6- to 12-week treatment that helps parents disrupt their child's starvation and excessive exercise and encourage the child to develop a more constructive approach to weight.

Advanced practice nurses may provide adolescents with anorexia nervosa with adolescent-focused therapy (AFT). This model focuses on self-monitoring of eating and weight gain that is supported by the therapeutic relationship with the nurse or other advanced practice therapist. Cognitive behavioral therapy (CBT), which helps to identify automatic negative thoughts and to challenge them, has also been used with success in this population.

CASE STUDY AND NURSING CARE PLAN
Anorexia Nervosa

Brad is a 21-year-old and a division one collegiate track star with plans to attend medical school after graduation. He is brought to the inpatient eating disorders unit of a psychiatric research hospital by his two older brothers, who physically support him on both sides. He is profoundly weak, holding his head up with his hands.

During the intake interview, Brad denies being underweight and says, "I need treatment because I keep fainting during training." He is particularly concerned about definition in his legs. "I check my legs every night. I'm so afraid of getting fat or slowing down." A self-described perfectionist, Brad comments, "I don't like to let my times slip, I know I can go faster, and I don't want anyone to see me as weak."

Self-Assessment

Mindy Jacobs, a registered nurse, is assigned to care for Brad. Three years earlier, when she began working on the unit, she had difficulty with overidentifying with patients. During college, Mindy was a swimmer and also struggled with restriction. However, after undergoing treatment, she did well. She seeks guidance from her nursing supervisor and the multidisciplinary team. This support allows her to maintain appropriate boundaries while creating therapeutic relationships with patients.

Assessment
Subjective Data
- Denies being underweight: "I need treatment because I keep fainting during training."
- "I check my legs every night. I'm so afraid of getting fat or slowing down."

- "I don't like to let my times slip, I know I can go faster and I don't want anyone to see me as weak."

Objective Data
- Height: 62 inches (5 feet, 2 inches)
- Weight: 58 pounds—50% of ideal body weight
- Blood pressure: 74/50 mm Hg
- Pulse: 54 beats per minute
- Hemoglobin: 9 g/dL
- Cachexia; pale, fine lanugo
- Sad facial expression

Priority Nursing Diagnosis
Impaired low nutritional intake related to restriction of caloric intake secondary to extreme fear of weight gain.

Outcomes Identification
Patient will reach 75% of ideal weight (92 pounds) by discharge.

Planning
The initial plan is to address Brad's unstable physiological state.

Implementation
Brad's care plan is personalized as follows:

Continued

Short-Term Goal	Intervention	Rationale	Evaluation
1. Patient will gain a minimum of 2 pounds and a maximum of 3 pounds weekly through inpatient stay.	1a. Acknowledge the emotional and physical difficulty patient is experiencing. Use patient's extreme fatigue to engage cooperation in the treatment plan. 1b. Weigh daily for the first week, then three times a week. Weigh in underwear only. No oral intake, including water, before the morning weigh-in. 1c. Do not negotiate weight with patient or reweigh. Patient may not want to look at the scale. 1d. Measure orthostatic vital signs TID until stable, then daily. Repeat ECG and laboratory tests until stable. 1e. Provide a pleasant, calm atmosphere at mealtimes. Patient should be told the specific times and duration (usually a half hour) of meals. 1f. Administer liquid supplement as ordered. 1g. Observe patient during meals to prevent hiding or throwing away of food and for at least 1 hour after eating to prevent purging. 1h. Be empathetic with patient's struggle to give up control of eating and weight as he is expected to make minimum weight gain on a regular basis. Permit patient to verbalize feelings at these times. 1i. Monitor patient's weight gain. A weight gain of 2–3 pounds/week is medically acceptable. 1j. Provide teaching regarding healthy eating as the basis of a healthy lifestyle. 1k. Use a cognitive-behavioral approach to address patient's fears regarding weight gain. Identify and examine distorted thoughts. 1l. As patient approaches his target weight, he should be encouraged to make his own menu choices. 1m. Emphasize the social nature of eating. Encourage conversation during mealtimes that does not involve the topics of food or exercise. 1n. Focus on the patient's strengths, including his work in normalizing his weight and eating habits. 1o. Challenge the patient by incorporating different types of planned exercise when patient reaches target weight. 1p. Encourage patient to apply all the knowledge, skills, and gains made from the various individual, family, and group therapy sessions.	1a. The first priority is to establish a therapeutic relationship. 1b. These measures ensure that the weight being taken is accurate. 1c. The patient may try to control and sabotage treatment by exercising in his room before bed. 1d. As the patient begins to gain weight, his cardiovascular status improves to within normal range and monitoring becomes less frequent. 1e. Mealtimes become episodes of high anxiety; knowledge of the regulations decreases tension, particularly when the patient has given up so much control by entering treatment. 1f. The patient may be unable to eat solid food at first. 1g. The primary goal is to promote good nutrition and a healthy weight; external control is required initially. Cognitive and behavioral changes will occur gradually. 1h. Patient is expected to gain at least 0.5 pound on a specific schedule, usually three times a week (Monday, Wednesday, Friday). 1i. Weight gain of more than 5 pounds in 1 week may result in pulmonary edema. 1j. Healthy aspects of eating (e.g., increased energy rather than gaining weight) are reinforced. 1k. Confronting irrational thoughts and beliefs is crucial to changing eating behaviors. 1l. Patient can assume more control of his meals, which is empowering for the patient with anorexia. 1m. Eating as a social activity, shared with others and with participation in conversation, serves as both a distraction from obsessive preoccupations and a pleasurable event. 1n. The patient who is beginning to normalize his weight and eating behaviors has met a major milestone. Activities other than eating are explored as sources of gratification. 1o. The patient experiences a strong drive to exercise; this measure accommodates this drive by planning a reasonable amount. 1p. The patient has been receiving intensive therapy and education, which have provided the tools and techniques needed to maintain healthy behaviors.	**WEEK 1:** The patient increases his caloric intake with liquid supplement only. The patient is unable to eat solid food. The patient does not gain weight. The patient remains hypotensive, bradycardic, and anemic (hemoglobin [HGB] = 9 g/dL). **WEEK 2:** The patient gains 2 pounds drinking liquid supplements and taking only minimal solid food. The patient remains hypotensive and bradycardic (HGB = 10 g/dL). **WEEK 3:** The patient gains 1 pound drinking liquid supplements. He selects a meal plan but is unable to eat most of solid food. The patient's blood pressure (BP) = 84/60 mm Hg; pulse = 68 beats per minute, regular; HGB = 11 g/dL. **WEEKS 4–6:** The patient gains an average of 2.5 pounds/week. Patient samples more of the solid food from meal plan. Patient's BP = 90/60 mm Hg; pulse = 68 beats per minute, regular; HGB = 11.5 g/dL. **WEEK 7:** The patient weighs 71 pounds (almost 60% of his ideal body weight); calories come mostly from the liquid supplements. Patient selects balanced meals, eating more varied solid food: turkey, carrots, lettuce, fruit. The patient's HGB = 12.5 g/dL; normal range of BP and pulse are maintained. The patient continues to increase participation in the social aspects of eating. **WEEKS 8–12:** The patient gains an average of 2.5 pounds/week and weighs 82 pounds (approx. 68% of his ideal body weight). The patient is eating more varied solid food, but most of his caloric intake still comes from liquid supplements. The patient maintains normal vital signs and HGB levels. Patient maintains social interaction during mealtimes and snacks. **WEEKS 13–16:** The patient has reached a medically stable weight at the end of 16th week—92 pounds (75% of his ideal body weight). The patient continues to eat more solid food with relatively less liquid supplement. The patient is not able to participate in a planned exercise program until he reaches 85% of his ideal body weight.

Evaluation

By the end of the 16th week, Brad has achieved a stable weight of 92 pounds. His BMI is 16.8, which is underweight, but is approaching an acceptable level for Brad's frame and age. His vital signs and hemoglobin levels are consistently within normal levels. He is participating in therapy and consistently communicating satisfaction with his body appearance.

BMI, Body mass index, *ECG*, electrocardiogram.

BULIMIA NERVOSA

Clinical Picture

Individuals with **bulimia nervosa** engage in repeated episodes of binge eating. Binge eating is eating between 1500 and 5000 calories within any 2-hour period. The binge eating is followed by compensatory behaviors such as self-induced vomiting; misuse of laxatives, diuretics, or other medications; fasting; or excessive exercise. This disorder is characterized by a significant disturbance in the individual's perception of body shape and weight. The *DSM-5* box contains specific criteria for the diagnosis of bulimia nervosa.

DSM-5 CRITERIA FOR BULIMIA NERVOSA

A. Recurrent episodes of binge eating. An episode of binge eating is characterized by both of the following:
  1. Eating, in a discrete period of time (e.g., within any 2-hour period), an amount of food that is definitely larger than what most individuals would eat in a similar period of time under similar circumstances.
  2. A sense of lack of control over eating during the episode (e.g., feeling that one cannot stop eating or control what or how much one is eating).
B. Recurrent inappropriate compensatory behavior to prevent weight gain, such as self-induced vomiting; misuse of laxatives, diuretics, or other medications; fasting; or excessive exercise.
C. The binge eating and inappropriate compensatory behaviors both occur, on average, at least once a week for 3 months.
D. Self-evaluation is unduly influenced by body shape and weight.
E. The disturbance does not occur exclusively during episodes of anorexia nervosa.

From American Psychiatric Association. (2013). *Diagnostic and statistical manual of disorders* (5th ed.). Washington, DC: Author.

EVIDENCE-BASED PRACTICE

Can Yoga Reduce Premeal Anxiety?

Problem
For individuals with eating disorders, the pre- and postmeal periods are associated with negative affect, high anxiety, panic, and an increased likelihood of engagement in compensatory behaviors that can impede recovery.

Purpose of Study
The purpose of this study was to explore the impact of yoga on negative affect in residents in an eating disorder program.

Methods
Thirty-eight individuals in a residential eating disorder treatment program were randomized to an intervention or control group. The treatment group participated in 50 minutes of yoga before dinner for 5 days. The control group participated in other scheduled activities. Negative affect was assessed before and after meals.

Key Findings
- Yoga significantly reduced premeal negative affect compared with treatment as usual.
- Yoga also reduced postmeal negative affect in the intervention group, but not significantly.
- Anxiety in the intervention group decreased significantly as compared with the control group over the study's 5 days.

Implications for Nursing Practice
Being aware that negative emotions can increase disordered eating around mealtimes will help nurses to develop interventions to counter them. Yoga is one intervention that can be recommended to patients with eating disorders. Other relaxation-inducing interventions—such as meditation, guided imagery, and mindfulness—can reduce mealtime anxiety.

Pacanowski, C. R., Diers, L., Crosby, R. D., & Neumark-Sztainer, D. (2017). Yoga in the treatment of eating disorders within a residential program: A randomized controlled trial. *Eating Disorders, 25*(1), 37–51.

Epidemiology

The 12-month prevalence of bulimia nervosa among young women is 1% to 1.5%. The lifetime incidence of bulimia nervosa for women is 2.3%, and the lifetime incidence for men is 0.5% (Rosenvinge & Petterson, 2015). Bulimia commonly begins in later adolescence; the prevalence then peaks into young adulthood. Onset of bulimia nervosa is rare in children younger than 12 years of age and in adults above age 40.

Comorbidity

Comorbidities commonly associated with bulimia nervosa include the following:
- Depressive disorders
- Anxiety disorders
- Bipolar disorder
- Alcohol and substance use disorders
- PTSD and other trauma-based disorders
- Borderline personality disorder

Risk Factors
Biological Factors
Genetic. The heritability of bulimia nervosa is estimated at 60% (Bulik et al., 2019). Further, gene variations responsible for serotonin transport and monoamine oxidase (MAO) enzyme activity have been implicated in patients who experience both bulimia and borderline personality disorder (McDonald, 2019). Similarities between these two disorders have also been found in epigenetic studies, which showed methylation of genes associated with stress response, regulation of nutritional intake, and impulsivity or craving behaviors.

Neurobiological
Neurotransmitters. Cycles of binging and purging may have an association with neurotransmitters, specifically serotonin and dopamine. As already mentioned, there is evidence pointing to impaired transport of serotonin, which contributes to an altered sensation of satiety or fullness. In addition, researchers have found that in some parts of the brain, serotonin modulates dopamine. Dopamine is a neurotransmitter associated with motivation for action and perception of reward. As a result of decreased or impaired serotonin transport, these patients may experience increased dopamine in parts of the brain, which can cause an increased sensitivity and motivation, despite risks, to seek rewards

(Pearson et al., 2015). Outside of serotonin and dopamine, purging by self-induced vomiting may increase plasma endorphin levels. The feeling of well-being or relief that some patients feel after vomiting may be due to these endorphins, which may further reinforce the behavior.

Neuroanatomy. Corticostriatal circuits in individuals with bulimia nervosa, as compared with those in healthy controls, do not function normally. These circuits include the orbitofrontal, prefrontal, and insular cortices (Donnelly et al., 2018). Altered functioning in corticostriatal circuits can interfere with the way in which individuals with bulimia respond to negative stimuli. For example, when confronted with negative stimuli, they have less input from the prefrontal cortex and altered function in the orbitofrontal cortex. This causes them to be less able to develop or choose responses with consideration to long-term consequences (Pearson et al., 2015).

Because of these differences, when faced with negative stimuli or input from the amygdala, an individual may choose a strategy that seeks to immediately reduce a negative effect without considering long-term consequences. Alternatively, these neuroanatomical differences lead to impaired reward processing in the brain, leading individuals to prefer immediate reward over delayed gratification.

Cognitive Factors

The psychological roots of bulimia nervosa have been explained by some theorists as poor early attachment with parents and later problems with attachment in friendships and intimate relationships (Cooper, 2003). Parents of affected offspring were described as negative and unsupportive of independence in their offspring.

Given the much higher prevalence of bulimia among females, it makes sense that theories focusing on gender would be developed. One theory posits that women with bulimia reject their traditional maternal roles. Yet another theory suggests that bulimia is associated with high scores on such femininity measures as passivity, dependence, and need for approval. Going in a third direction is the explanation that women with bulimia aspire to take on a masculine role.

From a cognitive perspective, people with bulimia tend to evaluate themselves based on shape and weight. They view being overweight negatively and are rigid in their beliefs. Types of distorted thinking for people with bulimia include black-and-white thinking, excessive generalization, and errors of attribution.

Environmental Factors

Internalization of a thin body ideal increases the risk for weight worries, which in turn increase the risk for bulimia nervosa. Weight-based teasing or bullying can also increase the likelihood of bulimia. As referenced earlier, the experience of trauma can increase the likelihood of developing an eating disorder, and this is particularly true in the case of emotional abuse and development of bulimia nervosa (Bakalar et al., 2015).

APPLICATION OF THE NURSING PROCESS

ASSESSMENT

General Assessment

Initially, patients with bulimia nervosa do not appear to be physically ill. They are often at or close to ideal body weight. However, as the assessment continues, the physical problems become apparent. If the patient has been inducing vomiting, she may have developed enlarged parotid glands, dental erosion, and dental caries. Calluses on the knuckles or back of the hand due to repeated self-induced vomiting is known as the Russell sign. Esophageal involvement in the form of esophageal tears or a history of esophagitis may be the result of repeated exposure to stomach acids through vomiting.

The psychosocial history may reveal great difficulties with personal, interpersonal, and familial relationships. Personality traits associated with this eating disorder include low self-esteem, depressive symptoms, social anxiety, and being overly anxious as a child.

Box 18.3 lists several thoughts and behaviors associated with bulimia nervosa, and Table 18.3 identifies possible signs and symptoms and their causes.

> **VIGNETTE:** During the initial assessment, the nurse wonders if Brittany is actually in need of hospitalization on the eating disorders unit. The nurse is struck by how well the patient appears; she seems healthy and is both well dressed and articulate.
>
> Brittany tells of restricting her intake of food until early evening, when she shops for food and begins to binge. Once home, she immediately induces vomiting. For the remainder of the evening and into the early morning hours, she "zones out" while watching television and binge eating. Periodically, she goes to the bathroom to vomit. She does this about 15 times during the night.
>
> The nurse admitting Brittany reminds her of the goals of the hospitalization, including interrupting the binge-purge cycle and normalizing eating. The nurse further explains to Brittany that she has the support of the eating disorder treatment team and the milieu of the unit to help her recover.

Self-Assessment

Patients are sensitive to the perceptions of others regarding this illness. They may feel significant shame and feel out of control. As you build a therapeutic relationship, try to empathize with the patient's feelings of low self-esteem and dysphoria. If you believe

> ### BOX 18.3 Thoughts and Behaviors Associated With Bulimia Nervosa
>
> - Binge-eating behaviors
> - Often self-induced vomiting (or laxative or diuretic use) after bingeing
> - History of anorexia nervosa in one-fourth to one-third of individuals
> - Depressive signs and symptoms
> - Problems with interpersonal relationships
> - Self-concept
> - Impulsive behaviors
> - Increased levels of anxiety and compulsivity
> - Possible substance use disorders
> - Possible impulsive stealing

TABLE 18.3 Signs and Symptoms of Bulimia Nervosa

Clinical Presentation	Cause
Normal to slightly low weight	Excessive caloric intake with purging, excessive exercising
Dental caries, tooth erosion	Vomiting (HCl reflux over enamel)
Parotid swelling	Increased serum amylase levels
Gastric dilation, rupture	Binge eating
Calluses, scars on hand (Russell sign)	Self-induced vomiting
Peripheral edema	Rebound fluid, especially if diuretic used
Muscle weakening	Electrolyte imbalance
Abnormal laboratory values (electrolyte imbalance, hypokalemia, hyponatremia)	Purging: vomiting, laxative and/or diuretic use
Cardiovascular abnormalities (cardiomyopathy, electrocardiographic changes)	Electrolyte imbalance—**can lead to death**
Cardiac failure (cardiomyopathy)	Ipecac intoxication
Seizure	Purging via self-induced vomiting: lowers seizure threshold

the patient is not being honest about active binge eating or purging, you may become frustrated. After all, you are there to help, and it may seem as though you are doing all the work. It is important to discuss your concerns with the patient and work together with her or him to develop a solution. The patient may benefit from using a journal to record feelings and behaviors or self-administering a screening tool and sharing the results on a daily basis. An accepting, nonjudgmental approach will help to build trust.

ASSESSMENT GUIDELINES

Bulimia Nervosa

1. Determine the patient's perception of the problem or chief complaint.
2. Perform a complete nursing assessment, including vital signs, review of systems, and general appearance.
3. Gather a psychosocial history.
4. Assess the patient's nutritional pattern and fluid intake.
5. Assess the patient's binging and purging patterns with direct questions.
6. Assess the patient's daily activities, including exercise.
7. Review the patient's laboratory tests, including the following:
   - Electrolyte levels
   - Glucose level
   - Thyroid function tests
   - Complete blood count
   - Electrocardiogram (ECG)
8. Determine the patient's goals for treatment.

NURSING DIAGNOSIS

Nursing diagnoses that relate to disordered eating and weight-control behaviors should be chosen. Problems resulting from purging are a first priority because electrolyte and fluid balance and cardiac function are affected. Common nursing diagnoses include *impaired cardiac output, impaired body image, impaired coping, risk for powerlessness, chronic low self-esteem,* and *risk for social isolation.*

OUTCOMES IDENTIFICATION

Outcomes criteria are linked to the diagnoses listed previously. Table 18.4 provides an overview of signs and symptoms, nursing diagnoses, and associated outcomes for individuals with bulimia nervosa.

PLANNING

As in the case of the patient with anorexia nervosa, the nurse prioritizes care that addresses life-threatening complications. Criteria for inpatient hospitalization include syncope, serum potassium of less than 3.2 mEq/L, serum chloride of less than 88 mEq/L, esophageal tears, arrhythmias, intractable vomiting, and hematemesis (vomiting blood). Suicide risk in this population also requires hospitalization.

> **VIGNETTE:** Iris weighs 85% of her ideal body weight. She has a history of diuretic use and becomes edematous when she stops using them. The nurse tells Iris that the edema is related to the use of diuretics and that it will go away after she discontinues them. Iris cannot tolerate the weight gain and the accompanying edema that occurs when she stops taking diuretics. She restarts the diuretics, perpetuating the cycle of fluid retention and the risk of kidney damage. The nurse empathizes with Iris's inability to tolerate the feelings of anxiety and dread she experiences because of her markedly swollen extremities.

IMPLEMENTATION

Inpatient units designed to treat eating disorders are especially structured to interrupt the cycle of binge eating and purging and to normalize eating habits. The patient also begins therapy to examine the underlying conflicts and body dissatisfaction that help to sustain the illness. Evaluation for treatment of comorbid disorders, including major depressive disorder and substance use, is also undertaken. In most cases of substance use disorder, the treatment of the eating disorder follows the treatment for substance use.

Counseling

Compared with patients who have anorexia, patients with bulimia nervosa establish a therapeutic alliance with the nurse more readily. This is because they want help. Patients with bulimia experience their bulimic behaviors as problematic and incongruent with how they see themselves otherwise.

Health Teaching and Health Promotion

Health teaching focuses not only on the eating disorder but also on meal planning, maintenance of a healthy diet, and daily movement. Additionally, the nurse provides psychoeducation about the impact of cognitive distortions and development of positive coping skills to address disordered thoughts. This preparation lays the foundation for the second phase of treatment, in which the nurse carefully plans challenges to the patient's newly developed skills.

Once patients reach their therapeutic goals, it is recommended that they seek long-term care to solidify them. Continued therapy can help them address the attitudes and perceptions that may perpetuate the disordered eating symptoms.

TABLE 18.4 Signs and Symptoms, Nursing Diagnoses, and Outcomes for Bulimia Nervosa

Signs and Symptoms	Nursing Diagnoses	Outcomes
Electrolyte imbalances, esophageal tears, cardiac problems, excessive vomiting, self-destructive behaviors	*Impaired cardiac output* *Electrolyte imbalance*	Improved cardiac output: Cardiac pump supports systemic perfusion pressure; electrolytes are in balance
Obsession with body, denial of problems, dissatisfied with appearance	*Impaired body image*	Improved body image: Congruence between body reality, body ideal, and body presentation; satisfaction with body appearance
Obsessed with food, substance use, impulsive responses to problems; inappropriate use of laxatives, diuretics, enemas, fasting, inadequate problem solving	*Impaired coping*	Improved coping: Demonstrates effective coping, reports decrease in stress, uses personal support system, uses effective coping strategies, reports increase in psychological comfort
Loss of control with the binge-purge cycle, feelings of shame and guilt, views self as unable to deal with events, excessive seeking of reassurance	*Chronic low self-esteem*	Positive self-esteem: Verbalizes a positive level of confidence, makes informed life decisions, expresses independence with decision-making processes
Absence of supportive significant others, hides eating behaviors from others, reports feeling alone	*Risk for social isolation*	Decreased social isolation: Willing to call on others for assistance, develops a confidant relationship, feels a sense of belonging

International Council of Nursing Practice (ICN). (2019). *ICNP browser*. Retrieved from https://www.icn.ch/what-we-do/projects/ehealth/icnp-browser. ICNP® is owned and copyrighted by the ICN. Reproduced with permission of the copyright holder.

Teamwork and Safety

The structured milieu of an inpatient unit can help to interrupt the binge-purge cycle and other disordered or self-injurious behaviors. To do this, treatment plans and observation prior to and after meals to prevent purging are used. During this time, patients are learning to experience life without the behaviors that previously helped them to cope. Consequently, patients may experience irritability, activation, or depression as they may now be fully confronting disturbing thoughts or emotions for the first time.

EVALUATION

Evaluation of treatment effectiveness is ongoing. Outcomes are revised with the patient as necessary to reach the desired outcomes. The Case Study and Nursing Care Plan later in this chapter presents a patient with bulimia nervosa.

TREATMENT MODALITIES

Biological Treatments

Pharmacotherapy

Fluoxetine (Prozac), an SSRI antidepressant, is the only FDA-approved medication for the treatment of bulimia nervosa in adult patients. This drug can be helpful for people with bulimia even in the absence of depressive symptoms. Fluoxetine doses tend to be higher when used for this eating disorder in comparison to major depressive disorder. When used off label (not specifically approved for bulimia nervosa), most antidepressant medications are more effective than a placebo in reducing binge and purge behaviors (McElroy et al., 2019).

Other antidepressants have shown efficacy in the treatment of bulimia nervosa at the same dose as used for depression. They include the following:

- SSRIs sertraline (Zoloft), paroxetine (Paxil), and citalopram (Celexa)
- The tricyclic antidepressants imipramine (Tofranil), nortriptyline (Pamelor), and desipramine (Norpramin)

- The monoamine oxidase inhibitor tranylcypromine (Parnate)

Bupropion (Wellbutrin) is contraindicated in patients diagnosed with bulimia owing to the increased risk of seizure. Serotonin norepinephrine reuptake inhibitors (SNRIs) have not been evaluated through randomized controlled trials in patients with bulimia. Research is exploring the potential for second-generation antipsychotics, antiepileptics, and/or opioid antagonists for decreasing symptoms associated with bulimia.

Psychological Therapies

Psychiatric–mental health advanced practice registered nurses are qualified to use the evidence-based CBT, which is considered a first-line treatment for bulimia. When patients eliminate bulimic behaviors, issues of self-worth and interpersonal functioning become more prominent. Restructuring faulty perceptions and helping individuals develop accepting attitudes toward themselves and their bodies are the primary focus of therapy. If early improvement is not seen with CBT, an antidepressant should be added.

Advanced practice nurses may use a mixed method approach for treatment refractory patients. Additional modalities which have been explored and found to be helpful include dialectical behavioral therapy (DBT), interpersonal therapy (IPT), and acceptance and commitment therapy (ACT) (Mehler & Andersen, 2017).

BINGE-EATING DISORDER

Clinical Picture

Individuals with **binge-eating disorder** engage in episodes of increased intake that occur beyond the point of satiety and cause distress afterward. These individuals do not regularly use the compensatory behaviors that are seen in patients with bulimia nervosa. Although individuals who start binge eating may be of normal weight, repeated binge eating inevitably causes obesity in this cohort. The *DSM-5* box contains criteria for binge-eating disorder.

Bulimia Nervosa

Kaitlyn, a 40-year-old college graduate, has been working as a teacher for 15 years. Her childhood was marked by emotional neglect and sexual abuse (via a family friend) that began when she was 13 years old; her eating disorder was related to that history. In her admission interview, she expresses concern that her behaviors were interfering with her performance at school, but she says, "I can't stand to be fat." Despite this, Kaitlyn is motivated to change. "I'm ashamed that I can't control my binging and purging—I know it's not good. I hate myself." She is being admitted to a partial hospitalization program that specializes in treating eating disorders. Kaitlyn is diagnosed with bulimia nervosa.

Self-Assessment

Matthew, an experienced nurse in the area of eating disorders, is assigned as case manager for Kaitlyn. Matthew enjoys working with patients with bulimia because he believes that he can help them to manage their condition. Taking a trauma-informed approach, Matthew asks a female nursing technician to accompany him while he meets with Kaitlyn for the first time to discuss the program and parameters for treatment. Wanting to make sure that Kaitlin would feel safe and supported as she begins treatment, he asks her whether she would feel comfortable working with a male care provider.

Assessment

Subjective Data

- "I can't stand to be fat."
- "I'm ashamed that I can't control my binging and purging—I hate myself."

Objective Data

- Height: 65 inches (5 feet 5 inches)
- Weight: 127 pounds—95% of ideal body weight
- Blood pressure: 120/80 mm Hg sitting; 90/60 mm Hg standing
- Pulse: 70 beats per minute sitting; 96 beats per minute standing
- Potassium level 2.7 mmol/L (normal range, 3.3–5.5 mmol/L)
- ECG: abnormal—consistent with hypokalemia
- Erosion of teeth enamel, enlarged parotid glands

Priority Diagnosis

Risk for injury related to binge eating and purging as evidenced by low potassium and other physical changes.

Outcomes Identification

Kaitlyn will demonstrate an ability to regulate her eating patterns, resulting in a consistently normal electrolyte balance.

Planning

Kaitlyn is admitted to a partial hospitalization program designed for patients with eating disorders. She attends the program 3 or 4 days a week and participates in individual and group therapy.

Implementation

Kaitlyn's care plan is personalized as follows:

Short-Term Goal	Intervention	Rationale	Evaluation
1. Patient will identify signs and symptoms of low potassium (K⁺) level, and K⁺ level will remain within normal limits throughout hospitalization.	1a. Educate patient regarding the ill effects of self-induced vomiting on K^+ level.	1a. Health teaching is crucial to promoting self-care.	**WEEK 1:** Patient begins to select balanced meals. Patient demonstrates knowledge of untoward effects of vomiting and K⁺ deficiency. Patient begins to demonstrate understanding of repetitive nature of binge-purge cycle.
	1b. Educate patient about binge-purge cycle and its self-perpetuating nature. 1c. Teach patient that fasting sets one up to binge eat.	1b, 1c. The compulsive nature of the binge-purge cycle is maintained by the sequence of intake restriction, hunger, bingeing, purging accompanied by feelings of guilt, and then repetition of the cycle over and over.	
	1d. Explore thoughts that trigger binge behavior.	1d. If the patient understands that the thoughts that trigger binge behavior are irrational, such thoughts can be challenged.	**WEEK 2:** Patient begins to challenge irrational thoughts and beliefs. Patient continues to plan nutritionally balanced meals including dinner at home. Patient begins to sample "forbidden foods" and discuss thoughts and attitudes about same.
	1e. Challenge irrational thoughts and beliefs about "forbidden" foods.	1e. Challenge forces the patient to examine her thinking and beliefs.	**WEEK 3:** Patient discusses triggers to binge and resultant behavior. Patient continues to challenge irrational thoughts and beliefs in individual and group sessions. Patient plans meals including "forbidden foods."
	1f. Teach patient to plan and eat regularly scheduled balanced meals.	1f. This teaching helps to ensure success in maintaining abstinence from binge-purge activity.	**WEEK 4:** Patient reports no binge-purge behaviors at day program or outside. Patient demonstrates understanding of repetitive nature of binge-purge cycle. Patient continues to challenge irrational thoughts and beliefs.

Evaluation

At the end of 4 weeks, Kaitlyn reports no binge-purge cycles and her potassium level remains consistently within normal limits. She is beginning to plan meals and to challenge irrational thoughts and beliefs.

DSM-5 CRITERIA FOR BINGE-EATING DISORDER

A. Recurrent episodes of binge eating. An episode of binge eating is characterized by both of the following:
   1. Eating, in a discrete period of time (e.g., within any 2-hour period), an amount of food that is definitely larger than what most people would eat in a similar period of time under similar circumstances.
   2. A sense of lack of control over eating during the episode (e.g., a feeling that one cannot stop eating or control what or how much one is eating).
B. The binge-eating episodes are associated with three (or more) of the following:
   1. Eating much more rapidly than normal
   2. Eating until feeling uncomfortably full
   3. Eating large amounts of food when not feeling physically hungry
   4. Eating alone because of feeling embarrassed by how much one is eating
   5. Feeling disgusted with oneself, depressed, or very guilty afterward
C. Marked distress regarding binge eating is present.
D. The binge eating occurs, on average, at least once a week for 3 months.
E. The binge eating is not associated with the recurrent use of inappropriate compensatory behavior, as in bulimia nervosa, and does not occur exclusively during the course of bulimia nervosa or anorexia nervosa.

From American Psychiatric Association. (2013). *Diagnostic and statistical manual of disorders* (5th ed.). Washington, DC: Author.

Epidemiology

Binge-eating disorder is the most common eating disorder. The 12-month prevalence of binge-eating disorder for US adults is 1.6% in females and 0.8% in males. For women, the lifetime incidence of binge-eating disorder is 3.6% and the lifetime incidence for men is 2.1% (Rosenvinge & Petterson, 2015). The prevalence of binge-eating disorder is higher in overweight populations (3%) than in the general population (2%). All racial and ethnic groups seem to be represented fairly equally.

Comorbidity

The rate of psychiatric comorbidity is high in binge-eating disorder. Approximately 79% of people with this disorder have another psychiatric disorder (Kessler et al., 2013). A lifetime history of two or more comorbid disorders occurs in 49% of people. The most prevalent comorbid conditions are as follows:
1. Specific phobia (37%)
2. Social phobia (32%)
3. Posttraumatic stress disorder (26%)
4. Alcohol abuse or dependence (21%)

Risk Factors
Biological Factors
Genetic. Heritability for binge eating is estimated at 41% to 57%, depending on the criteria used (Himmerich et al., 2019). There have been limited genetic studies in regard to this disorder. However, one study noted genetic alterations associated with both binge eating and alcoholism (Bulik et al., 2019).

Neurobiological. As in the case of patients diagnosed with bulimia nervosa, patients with binge eating have also exhibited altered processing in the orbitofrontal cortex (Donnelly et al., 2018). This area affects impulse control and inhibition of behaviors. Individuals with binge-eating disorder also show decreased activation in the prefrontal cortex and insula, which can lead to altered perceptions of satiety and reward sensitivity (Brownell & Walsh, 2017).

Cognitive Factors

Individuals with high impulsivity and reward sensitivity may experience an addictive response to certain foods, as in the case of substance use disorders (Schulte et al., 2016). The foods that seem to be particularly addictive are high-sugar and high-fat foods. Body dissatisfaction, low self-esteem, and difficulty coping with feelings can also contribute to binge-eating disorder.

Environmental Factors

Social pressures to be thin, which are typically influenced through media, can trigger emotional eating. Social weight stigma, which is stereotyping or discrimination based on a person's body, is common in the United States and perpetuates the cycle of binging.

A history of trauma, particularly emotional neglect, increases the risk of binge eating. In patients pursuing bariatric surgery, over 35% reported lifetime prevalence of binge eating (Quilliot et al., 2019). In comparison with controls, this group of patients was significantly more likely to have experienced psychological trauma. Adverse experiences were predominantly related to emotional neglect or abuse for both males and females in this study.

A history of food insecurity, which is the result of not having reliable access to a sufficient quantity of nutritious and affordable food, is associated with binge-eating disorder. Food insecurity can lead to both poor nutritional intake as well as increased risk of overeating and obesity (Rasmusson et al., 2018).

APPLICATION OF THE NURSING PROCESS
ASSESSMENT

Although obesity puts patients at risk for diabetes, hypertension, and heart disease, hospitalization to treat the binge eating itself is not usually indicated. Because the stomach must accommodate larger than normal volumes during a binge, there are also associated gastrointestinal problems. In addition to helping patients reduce their binge eating, the nurse will have to help them manage the gastric symptoms associated with the disorder.

General Assessment

To some extent, all people with obesity have periods when their eating feels out of control; to the nurse, the amount of food such patients consume during meals may look larger than normal. This presents a major challenge to distinguishing between people who are obese due to metabolic or lifestyle causes and those who engage in binge eating.

Self-Assessment

It is common for people to believe that obesity is a personal flaw of failing to control eating and exercise habits. It is helpful to remember that binge-eating disorder has a more complex origin that includes biological pathology.

 ASSESSMENT GUIDELINES

Binge-Eating Disorder

1. Determine the patient's perception of the problem or chief complaint.
2. Perform a complete nursing assessment, including vital signs, review of systems, and general appearance.
3. Gather a psychosocial history.
4. Assess the nutritional pattern.
5. Assess the history of weight cycling (i.e., gains and losses).
6. Collect a careful history of binge-eating triggers, foods, and frequency.

NURSING DIAGNOSIS

Impaired high nutritional intake is usually the most appropriate initial nursing diagnosis for individuals with binge-eating disorder. Other nursing diagnoses may include *impaired body image, impaired coping, anxiety, chronic low self-esteem, risk for powerlessness,* and *risk for social isolation.*

OUTCOMES IDENTIFICATION

To evaluate the effectiveness of treatment, establish outcome criteria to measure treatment results. You should include patients when developing outcomes to empower them to be active participants in their care. Table 18.5 provides a summary of signs and symptoms, nursing diagnoses, and general outcomes for binge-eating disorder.

PLANNING

Care planning may include a focus on rebuilding daily intake, balancing frequency and volume. In addition, plans will focus

on inclusion of healthy movement and physical activity at a slow pace. Nurses may also encourage patient's further examination of the emotional components associated with a binge episode. With greater insight, patients can begin developing positive coping mechanisms which address underlying emotional issues or maladaptive behaviors.

Physically, episodes of abnormal eating cause gastrointestinal problems associated with the periodic dilation of the stomach. These patients have significant difficulties with heartburn, dysphagia, bloating, and abdominal pain as well as with diarrhea, urgency, constipation, and a feeling of anal blockage. The nurse will have to help patients manage dysregulation of the entire gastrointestinal tract.

IMPLEMENTATION

Although obesity puts patients in this population at risk for diabetes, hypertension, and heart disease, hospitalization to treat the binge eating itself is not indicated. Treatment is usually provided in an outpatient setting. Unless you are working in an outpatient setting, it is not likely that you will have a patient being treated specifically for binge-eating disorder. In inpatient settings, you may work with patients being treated with a comorbid condition such as major depressive disorder along with binge-eating disorder.

When they are caring for an individual with binge–eating disorder, nurses are careful to avoid judgmental terms that can decrease the patient's likelihood of engagement in treatment or recovery. In terms of preference for terminology, individuals who struggle with binge eating find the terms *unhealthy weight* or *unhealthy BMI* preferable to or less stigmatizing than weight problem or heavy (Lydecker et al., 2016).

It is important to know that binge eating is not about the food, it is about coping with emotion. Counseling a person should proceed empathetically, allowing sufficient time for the expression of feelings. Encourage the patient to track what was happening and feelings prior to binge eating. Once the patient is consciously aware of

TABLE 18.5	Signs and Symptoms, Nursing Diagnoses, and Outcomes for Binge-Eating Disorder		
Signs and Symptoms	**Nursing Diagnoses**	**Outcomes**	
Dysfunctional eating pattern, eating in response to internal cues, sedentary lifestyle, weight significantly over ideal for height and frame, intake exceeds metabolic need	*Impaired high nutritional intake*	Nutrient intake meets metabolic needs	
Embarrassment due to weight gain, fear of negative reactions by others, attempts to hide weight gain, body dissatisfaction	*Impaired body image*	Congruence between body reality, body ideal, and body presentation; satisfaction with body appearance	
Eats as a coping method, absence of other more effective coping methods, eats even when full	*Impaired coping*	Demonstrates effective coping, reports decrease in stress, uses personal support system, uses effective coping strategies, reports increase in psychological comfort	
Feelings of discomfort or dread, feelings of inadequacy, focused on self, increased wariness, irritability, heart pounding, increased blood pressure and pulse	*Anxiety*	Verbalizes a positive level of confidence; makes informed life decisions, expresses independence with decision-making processes	
Loss of control of eating, feelings of shame and guilt, views self as unable to deal with events	*Chronic low self-esteem* *Risk for powerlessness*	Verbalizes a positive level of confidence; makes informed life decisions, expresses independence with decision-making processes	
Absence of supportive significant others, eats normally in the presence of others, hides eating behaviors, reports feeling alone	*Risk for social isolation*	Willing to call on others for assistance, develops a confidant relationship, feels a sense of belonging	

International Council of Nursing Practice (ICN). (2019). *ICNP browser.* Retrieved from https://www.icn.ch/what-we-do/projects/ehealth/icnp-browser. ICNP® is owned and copyrighted by the ICN. Reproduced with permission of the copyright holder.

particular events and emotions that are triggers for out-of-control eating, other responses and coping mechanisms can be practiced.

For this population, socializing has often become uncomfortable and avoidance often becomes the dominant mode of responding to invitations. Additionally, staying away from other people allows the individual the privacy to engage in binge eating. Social isolation can be addressed by exploring community activities, groups that can be joined, and the reestablishment of neglected relationships. Developing small goals provides an incremental approach to changing unhealthy avoidance. For example, a patient-centered and patient-driven goal may be to try one new activity, such as a lunch with a friend or participation in a yoga class once a week.

Health Teaching and Health Promotion

Patients struggling with binge-eating disorder have been using food to regulate their mood and will have to learn new coping strategies for the challenges in their lives. Education centered on healthy eating and exercise will have to be reinforced within a caring nurse-patient relationship. At first, the focus of change will be the binge eating itself. Once abstinence has been established, the focus may change to slow and steady weight loss to improve the person's overall health.

Box 18.4 presents relevant interventions for the management of eating disorders.

EVALUATION

Evaluation of treatment effectiveness is ongoing, and outcomes are revised with the patient's input as necessary. The Case Study and Nursing Care plan presents a patient with bulimia nervosa and illustrates the evaluation component of care.

TREATMENT MODALITIES

Biological Treatments

Pharmacotherapy

Because of their efficacy with bulimia nervosa, researchers have studied the use of SSRIs at or near the high end of the dosage range to treat binge-eating disorder. Although these medications seem to help in the short term, patients regained significant weight after stopping them. Some evidence has been found to support SNRIs, including duloxetine (Cymbalta) or venlafaxine (Effexor XR) in the treatment of patients with comorbid binge-eating disorder and major depressive disorder (Brownell & Walsh, 2017). Other medications that are under investigation include the tricyclic antidepressants and antiepileptic agents.

Lisdexamfetamine dimesylate (Vyvanse) is a stimulant used to treat attention-deficit/hyperactivity disorder. It also has FDA approval for the treatment of moderate to severe binge-eating disorder in adults. Lisdexamfetamine is correlated with a significantly lower risk of relapse in binge episodes compared with placebo at 6-month follow-up (Brownell & Walsh, 2017). In adults with binge-eating disorder, the most common side effects are dry mouth, insomnia, decreased appetite, increased heart rate, constipation, feeling jittery, and anxiety. The FDA includes a black box warning on lisdexamfetamine's label due to concern for "abuse and dependence."

BOX 18.4 Interventions for the Management of Eating Disorders

Teamwork
- Collaborate with other members of healthcare team to develop treatment plan.
- Involve patient and/or significant others in the treatment plan.
- Work with team to set a target weight.
- Consult with a dietitian to determine caloric intake necessary to attain and/or maintain target weight.
- Encourage patient to discuss food preferences with dietitian.
- Meet with the healthcare team on a regular basis to evaluate the patient's progress.

Monitoring
- Monitor objective measures such as vital signs and electrolyte levels as needed.
- Weigh on a routine basis at the same time of day and after urinating.
- Monitor daily caloric intake and intake and output of fluids.
- Encourage self-monitoring of daily caloric intake.
- Observe patient during and after meals and snacks.
- Accompany patient to bathroom during designated observation times following meals and snacks.
- Limit time spent in bathroom.
- Monitor physical activity to reduce excessive exercise.

Support
- Use motivational interviewing and contracting with the patient to increase ownership of healthcare goals.
- Provide reinforcement for weight gain and behaviors that promote weight gain.
- Provide education regarding relaxation techniques.
- Use counseling to discuss feelings as the patient integrates new eating behaviors, changing body image, and lifestyle changes.
- Encourage patient use of daily logs to record feelings and circumstances surrounding eating disordered behavior.
- Assist the patient and significant others, as appropriate, to examine and resolve personal issues that may contribute to the eating disorder.
- Assist patient to develop a self-esteem that is compatible with a healthy body weight.

Promote Increasing Independence
- Allow opportunity to make limited choices about meal planning and movement as weight gain progresses in desirable manner.
- Initiate maintenance phase of treatment when patient has achieved target weight and has consistently shown desired eating behaviors for designated period of time.
- Place responsibility for choices about eating and physical activity with patient, as appropriate.
- Institute a treatment program and follow-up care (medical, counseling) for home management.

Surgical Interventions

Bariatric surgery is a controversial option for the treatment of obesity due to binge-eating disorder. Potential complications from this surgery require individuals to consider it carefully (Mitchell et al., 2015). Such complications include impaired fasting glucose levels, high triglycerides, and urinary incontinence.

Bariatric surgery is generally unsuccessful for patients with comorbid binge-eating disorder. Although most patients experience a short-term postsurgical reduction in symptoms of depression and anxiety, these symptoms tend to return to previous levels (Spirou et al., 2020). As the stomach expands after surgery, binge eating behaviors may resume. If a patient with binge-eating disorder does opt for bariatric surgery, the surgery should be accompanied by and followed with counseling and/or psychotherapy to improve the patient's emotional responses to food.

Psychological Therapies

Psychiatric–mental health advanced practice registered nurses can be instrumental in providing care to this population. CBT, dialectical behavior therapy, and IPT have all been associated with reductions in binge frequency (Mehler & Andersen, 2017).

CASE STUDY AND NURSING CARE PLAN

Binge-Eating Disorder

John is a 29-year-old lawyer who been overeating since he was 10 years old. He seeks treatment at a community mental health center because he has recently felt more depressed, stating, "1 I eat anything in sight." He also says, "1 wish I wouldn't wake up in the morning."

Self-Assessment
Bernice is the nurse assigned to John. She is new to the community mental health center; her experience as a psychiatric nurse is primarily with people with serious mental illness. During Bernice's initial contact with John, she recognizes some negative feelings toward John because of his weight. Bernice does some research and learns that binge-eating disorder is an illness, just as schizophrenia is.

Assessment
Subjective Data
- Uncontrollable eating pattern
- Recently felt more depressed
- History of overeating since age of 10
- "I'll eat anything in sight."

- "I wish I wouldn't wake up in the morning."

Objective Data
- Height: 61 inches (5 feet 1 inch)
- Weight: 200 pounds—180% of ideal weight
- Sad facial expression

Priority Diagnosis
Impaired high nutritional intake related to compulsive overeating, including episodes of binging.

Outcomes Identification
Patient will normalize eating pattern and achieve a specific target weight according to a predetermined plan.

Implementation
John's care plan is personalized as follows:

Short-Term Goal	Intervention	Rationale	Evaluation
1. Patient will demonstrate at least two coping strategies that result in adhering to a structured meal schedule.	1a. The advanced practice nurse uses cognitive-behavioral therapy to address weight issues and disordered eating. Asks the patient to begin keeping a journal.	1a. Cognitive-behavioral techniques can be useful in addressing automatic behaviors. Recording what, when, and where one eats begins to identify patterns that can be modified.	**WEEK 1:** Patient selects a meal plan with structured times and places; begins journal and maintains it consistently. Begins to share feelings about eating.
	1b. Teach the patient to structure and plan ahead for times and places where he will have his meals and snacks for the day.	1b. Organization and structure can allow for a different choice.	**WEEK 2:** Patient is able to adhere to structured meal schedule approximately 25% of the time. Patient expresses feelings of tension regarding this schedule; some modifications are made to allow the patient to be more successful. Patient shares contents of journal, which she consistently maintains. Weight is unchanged; patient was unable to change pattern of exercise.
	1c. Teach patient to eat small amounts more frequently to avoid rebound binge eating. 1d. Review the nutritional content of dietary intake to ensure consumption of a balanced diet.	1c, 1d. Extended periods of abstinence, restrictive dietary intake, or a very low-calorie diet can result in rebound overeating.	**WEEK 3:** Patient is adhering to schedule 50% of the time. Patient shares journal entries and relates thoughts and feelings concerning eating. Patient achieves 1 pound of weight loss. Patient is beginning to walk for a half hour as part of his daily routine.
	1e. Review journal with patient to identify areas for improvement in adhering to the treatment plan. 1f. Explore thoughts and feelings he is experiencing about this new regimen. 1g. Identify thoughts, beliefs, and underlying assumptions that reinforce disordered eating patterns. 1h. Establish a once-a-week schedule of weighing.	1e. The journal is an important tool in modifying eating behaviors. 1f, 1g. Nurse must be empathetic and supportive of the patient's experience, which is one of struggle accompanied by feelings of tension. 1h. From day to day, there may be minimal or no weight reduction, which can lead to discouragement.	**WEEK 4:** Patient continues to adhere to his structured schedule approximately 75% of the time. Patient walks regularly, experiencing a greater sense of well-being. Patient thinks he is up to the challenge of continuing the plan to normalize his eating pattern and increase his energy expenditure. Patient's weight is 196 pounds (−4 pounds); he acknowledges that progress has been and will continue to be slow.

Evaluation
At the end of 4 weeks, John's weight is 196 pounds. He adheres to a structured meal plan 75% of the time and has increased his exercise by incorporating daily walks into his routine.

FEEDING DISORDERS

We have all witnessed children with picky eating habits. However, children with feeding disorders take this problem to an extreme. The three feeding disorders are **pica, rumination disorder,** and **avoidant/restrictive food intake disorder**. It is important to note that although these conditions generally begin early in life, all three can begin at any age. Box 18.5 identifies the diagnostic criteria for these disorders.

Pica

Pica is defined as the ingestion of substances that have no nutritional value, such as dirt or paint. Among institutionalized children, the prevalence of this disorder may be as high as 26%. Pica usually begins in early childhood and lasts for a few months. Eating nonfood items may interfere with eating nutritional items. Eating nonfood items can also be dangerous. Paint may contain lead, which can cause brain damage. Objects that cannot be digested, such as stones, can cause intestinal blockage. Sharp objects such as paper clips or nails can cause intestinal damage or laceration. Bacteria from dirt or other soiled objects can lead to serious infection and dental problems. Enamel on teeth may be eroded from taking in and chewing on abrasive and erosive substances.

The prevalence of pica is unknown. Among people with intellectual disabilities, pica is more common, and it increases with the severity of the condition. Onset is generally in childhood, but the condition can also appear in adolescence or adulthood. Males and females are affected equally.

Monitoring of the individual's eating behavior is obviously an essential aspect of treating this problem. Behavioral interventions such as rewarding appropriate eating can be helpful.

Rumination Disorder

Rumination is characterized by undigested food being returned to the mouth. It is then rechewed, reswallowed, or spit out. **Rumination disorder** may be diagnosed after 1 month of symptoms. The symptoms frequently remit spontaneously but may become habitual and result in severe malnutrition and even death.

Prevalence statistics are not available. As with pica, ruminating behaviors occur more frequently among people with intellectual disabilities. Rumination can begin at any age. In infants, the onset is usually between 3 and 12 months. Childhood neglect is a predisposing factor to the development of this disorder.

Interventions include repositioning infants and small children during feeding. Improving the interaction between caregiver and

BOX 18.5   Characteristics of Feeding Problems

Pica	Rumination	Avoidant/Restrictive
Eating nonfood items after maturing past toddlerhood	Regurgitation with rechewing, reswallowing, or spitting	Avoiding or restricting foods starting in childhood
Not culturally sanctioned	No GI or medical reason	Significantly low BMI
Not part of any other mental illness	Not part of other mental illness or eating disorder	Dependent on enteral feeding or experiencing nutritional deficiencies
		No distortion of body image
		Not medically explained or part of any other mental illness

BMI, Body mass index; *GI,* gastrointestinal.

child and making mealtimes a pleasant experience often reduce rumination. Distracting the child when the behavior starts can also be helpful. Family therapy may be required.

Avoidant/Restrictive Food Intake Disorder

Up to 40% of all toddlers will experience mealtime difficulties that resolve spontaneously with or without caregiver support and education. In **avoidant/restrictive food intake disorder,** the consequences are serious and can result in significant weight loss, nutritional deficiency, dependence on supplements or enteral feeding, and marked interference with functioning. Children and adolescents who have not completed their growth may not grow along their developmental trajectory.

In some people, food avoidance may be related to strong dislikes related to sensory qualities of food. Appearance, color, smell, texture, temperature, and taste are implicated in food refusal.

About 5% to 20% of children without other disorders may have feeding disorders. Prematurity, failure to thrive, autism, and genetic syndromes result in ranges of 40% to 80% with feeding disorders (Romano et al., 2015). There are no unifying etiologies for food refusal, but personal anxiety and family anxiety seem to be risk factors.

Males and females are equally affected by this eating disorder of infancy and early childhood. When food avoidance is comorbid with autism, males are more likely to be affected.

The primary treatment modality is some form of behavioral modification to increase regular food consumption. Families caring for a child with a feeding disorder often need support and education in specific behavioral techniques, but family therapy is not usually necessary. The treatment of anxiety and depressive symptoms may be helpful in some cases.

KEY POINTS TO REMEMBER

- Risk for and maintenance of eating disorders is influenced by an interplay between neurobiological, psychological, environmental, and social factors.
- Neurobiological theories focus on neurotransmitters and neuroanatomy in the brain that regulate mood, hunger, reward, decision making, and interoception.
- Given the degree of heritability, genetic vulnerabilities may predispose people toward eating disorders.

- Anorexia nervosa is a potentially life-threatening eating disorder that includes severe underweight; low blood pressure, pulse, and temperature; dehydration; and dysrhythmias.
- Anorexia can be treated with milieu therapy, psychotherapy, pharmacotherapy, nutritional intervention, and health promotion across a variety of treatment environments.

- Although patients with bulimia nervosa are typically within the normal weight range or slightly above, they are still at high risk for physical decompensation and serious injury.
- Assessment of the patient with bulimia nervosa may show enlargement of the parotid glands, dental erosion, and caries if the patient has induced vomiting.
- Acute care may be necessary when life-threatening complications such as gastric rupture, electrolyte imbalance, and cardiac dysrhythmias are present.
- The goal of interventions is to interrupt the binge-purge cycle; these interventions may include psychotherapy, skills training, or pharmacotherapy.
- Therapy is part of long-term treatment to address coexisting major depressive disorder, substance use, and/or personality disorders.

- Effective treatment for obese patients with binge-eating disorder includes binge abstinence, improvement of depressive symptoms, and achievement of an appropriate weight for the individual.
- Patients with binge-eating disorder often have upper and lower GI problems that bring them to medical professionals for management.
- Feeding disorders have multiple etiologies and are often associated with developmental delays of childhood.
- Feeding disorders may result in significant nutritional deficiencies and can be fatal. Behavioral interventions to increase appropriate food consumption are the primary treatments.

CRITICAL THINKING

1. Logan, a 19-year-old wrestler, experienced a rapid decrease in weight after his coach told him that he would have to lose weight or miss a match. Logan is 6 feet 2 inches tall; over a period of 4 months he went from his usual 176 pounds down to 132 pounds. He is brought to the emergency department with a pulse of 40 beats per minute and severe arrhythmias. His laboratory workup reveals severe hypokalemia. He has become extremely depressed, saying, "I'm too fat ... I don't want anything to eat. If I gain weight, my life will be ruined. There is nothing to live for if I can't wrestle." Logan's parents are startled and confused, and his best friend is worried but feels powerless to help Logan. "I tell Logan he needs to eat or he will die ... I tell him that he is a skeleton, but he refuses to listen to me. I don't know what to do."
   a. Which physical and psychiatric criteria suggest that Logan should be hospitalized immediately?
   b. What are some of the questions you would eventually ask Logan as you evaluate his biopsychosocial functioning?
   c. What are your feelings toward someone with anorexia? Can you make a distinction between your thoughts and feelings toward women with anorexia and those toward men with anorexia?
   d. What are some things you could do for Logan's parents and friend in terms of offering them information, support, and referrals? Identify specific referrals.

   e. Identify at least five criteria that, if met, would indicate that Logan was improving.
2. You and Heather have been close friends since nursing school and are now working on the same surgical unit. Heather tells you that she has made several suicide attempts in the past. Today, you come upon her bingeing off the unit; when she sees you she looks embarrassed and uncomfortable. Several times you notice that she spends time in the bathroom, and you hear sounds of retching. In response to your concern, she admits that she has been binge-purging for several years but that now she is getting out of control and feels profoundly depressed.
   a. Although Heather does not show any physical signs of bulimia nervosa, what would you look for when you are assessing an individual with bulimia?
   b. What kinds of emergencies could result from binging and purging?
   c. What would be the most useful type of psychotherapy provided by an advanced practice caregiver for Heather initially, and what issues would have to be addressed?
   d. What new skills does a person with bulimia have to learn to lessen the compulsion to binge and purge?
   e. What would be some signs that Heather is recovering?

CHAPTER REVIEW

1. Which patient statement acknowledges the characteristic behavior associated with a diagnosis of pica?
   a. "Nothing could make me drink milk."
   b. "I'm ashamed of it, but I eat my hair."
   c. "I haven't eaten a green vegetable since I was 3 years old."
   d. "I regurgitate and rechew my food after almost every meal."
2. In evaluating an eating disorder, what physical criterion for hospital admission would you consider?
   a. A daytime heart rate of less than 50 beats per minute
   b. An oral temperature of 100°F or more
   c. 90% of ideal body weight
   d. Systolic blood pressure greater than 130 mm Hg

3. In considering the need for monitoring, which intervention should the nurse implement for a patient with anorexia nervosa? *Select all that apply.*
   a. Provide scheduled portion-controlled meals and snacks.
   b. Congratulate patients for weight gain and behaviors that promote weight gain.
   c. Limit time spent in the bathroom during periods when the patient is not under direct supervision.
   d. Promote exercise as a method to increase appetite.
   e. Observe patient during and after meals/snacks to ensure that adequate intake is achieved and maintained.

4. Which intervention will promote independence in a patient being treated for bulimia nervosa?
   a. Have the patient monitor daily caloric intake and intake and output of fluids.
   b. Encourage the patient to use behavior modification techniques to promote weight gain behaviors.
   c. Ask the patient to use a daily log to record feelings and circumstances related to urges to purge.
   d. Allow the patient to make limited choices about eating and exercise as weight gain progresses.
5. Which patient statement supports the diagnosis of anorexia nervosa?
   a. "I'm terrified of gaining weight."
   b. "I wish I had a good friend to talk to."
   c. "I've been told that I drink way too much alcohol."
   d. "I don't get much pleasure out of life anymore."
6. Obesity can be the end result of a binge-eating disorder. The nurse understands that the best treatment option in persons with a binge-eating disorder is
   a. Bariatric surgery
   b. Coping strategies
   c. Avoidance of public eating
   d. Appetite suppression medications
7. Taylor, a psychiatric registered nurse, orients Regina, a patient with anorexia nervosa, to the room where she will be assigned during her stay. After getting Regina settled, the nurse informs Regina of the following:
   a. "I need to go through the belongings you have brought with you."
   b. "You can use the scale in the back room when you need to."
   c. "You will be eating five times a day here."
   d. "The daily structure is based around your desire to eat."
8. Safety measures are of concern in treating eating disorders. Patients with anorexia nervosa are supervised closely to monitor the following: *Select all that apply.*
   a. Foods that are eaten
   b. Attempts at self-induced vomiting
   c. Relationships with other patients
   d. Weight
9. Malika has been overweight all her life. Now an adult, she has health problems related to excessive weight. Seeking weight-loss assistance at a primary care facility, Malika is surprised when the nurse practitioner suggests the following:
   a. A trial of SSRI antidepressant therapy
   b. Mild exercise to start, increasing in intensity over time

   c. Removing snack foods from the home
   d. Medication treatment for hypertension
10. Malika agrees to try losing weight according to the nurse practitioner's outlined plan. Additional teaching is warranted when Malika states that
   a. "I am willing to admit that I am depressed."
   b. "Psychotherapy will be a part of my treatment."
   c. "I prefer to have a gastric bypass rather than use this plan."
   d. "My comorbid conditions may improve with weight loss."

1. **b**; 2. **a**; 3. **a, c, e**; 4. **d**; 5. **a**; 6. **b**; 7. **a**; 8. **a, b, d**; 9. **a**; 10. **c**

NGN CASE STUDY AND QUESTIONS

Sophia, a severely underweight 13-year-old, is admitted to the psychiatric unit of a children's hospital after losing consciousness after a 2-day fast. She averts her eyes during the intake interview. Sophia's mother reports that she is obsessed with the fear of falling behind in school. She regularly skips breakfast. After gymnastics practice 3 days a week, she immediately goes to bed and falls asleep without supper. When she does join the family for dinner, Sophia rearranges the food on her plate to appear half-eaten. The patient reports muscle weakness and cramping, fatigue, and constipation.

When asked how fatigue affects her schoolwork, the patient expresses dissatisfaction with earning low As. Sophia's mother reports the patient's internet browser history consists of websites encouraging anorexic behaviors. The mother expresses despair and reports that this behavior resembles her own eating problems in adolescence. The patient responds, "I never do anything right...really, no matter what I do, I can't win."

Vital signs and lab values are:
- Blood pressure 90/50
- Heart rate 40 bpm
- Body mass index (BMI) 17.5
- High urine specific gravity
- Potassium 3.2 mEq/L
- Sodium 130 mEq/L

After seeing the patient, the healthcare provider assigns a diagnosis of anorexia nervosa.

The patient responds, "But that's not possible. I'm too fat."

1. Identify the nursing actions as 1—indicated (appropriate or necessary), 2—contraindicated (could be harmful), or 3—nonessential (not necessary) for the patient's care at this time. *Only one selection can be made for each nursing action.*

Nursing Action	1.Indicated	2. Contraindicated	3. Nonessential
a. Establish a therapeutic nurse/patient relationship that respects personal boundaries			
b. Begin refeeding in a structured environment, including precise time and duration of meals			
c. Minimize the social nature of eating; focus conversation on the texture and tastes of the food			
d. As the patient approaches the goal weight, encourage her to prepare a meal for a loved one			
e. Weigh patient three times daily after each meal, in underwear only, for the first week			
f. Set a goal for the patient to achieve a 5-pound weight gain in 1 week			
g. Regard evaluation as taking place over time rather than as a fixed event			

2. Once Sophia is medically stable, which action will the nurse plan to implement? *Select all that apply.*

Actions	Implement
a. Initiate recovery with FDA-approved medications for anorexia nervosa.	
b. Educate the patient regarding integrative approaches that may be used, along with the need to contact healthcare providers before using herbal therapy.	
c. Use the patient's fatigue to engage cooperation in the treatment plan.	
d. Ensure that the patient consumes vegetables and other high-fiber foods within the first 3 days to relieve constipation.	
e. Prioritize family-based treatment (F-BT) over individual therapies.	
f. Seek to understand the patient's culture and personal belief system.	

NGN case study answers are on Evolve.

Visit the Evolve website for a posttest on the content in this chapter: http://evolve.elsevier.com/Varcarolis

REFERENCES

American Psychiatric Association (APA). (2013). *Diagnostic and statistical manual of mental disorders* (5th ed.). Washington, DC: Author.

Bakalar, J. L., Shank, L. M., Vannucci, A., Radin, R. M., & Tanofsky-Kraff, M. (2015). Recent advances in developmental and risk factor research on eating disorders. *Current Psychiatry Reports, 17*(6), 42.

Brownell, K. D., & Walsh, B. T. (2017). *Eating disorders and obesity: A comprehensive handbook.* New York, NY: Guilford.

Bulik, C. M., Blake, L., & Austin, J. (2019). Genetics of eating disorders: What the clinician needs to know. *Psychiatric Clinics, 42*(1), 59–73.

Cooper, M. (2003). *The psychology of bulimia nervosa: A cognitive perspective.* Oxford, UK: Oxford.

Donnelly, B., Touyz, S., Hay, P., Burton, A., Russell, J., & Caterson, I. (2018). Neuroimaging in bulimia nervosa and binge eating disorder: A systematic review. *Journal of Eating Disorders, 20,* 6.3.

Fogarty, S., Smith, C., & Hay, P. (2016). The role of complementary and alternative medicine in the treatment of eating disorders: A systematic review. *Eating Disorders, 21,* 179–188.

Frank, G., DeGuzman, M., & Shott, M. (2019). Motivation to eat and not to eat: The psycho-biological conflict in anorexia nervosa. *Physiology & Behavior, 206,* 185–190.

Goldschmidt, A. B., Crosby, R. D., Cao, L., Moessner, M., Forbush, K. T., et al. (2018). Network analysis of pediatric eating disorder symptoms in a treatment-seeking, transdiagnostic sample. *Journal of Abnormal Psychology, 127*(2), 251.

Harrington, B. C., Jimerson, M., Haxton, C., & Jimerson, D. C. (2015). Initial evaluation, diagnosis, and treatment of anorexia nervosa and bulimia nervosa. *American Family Physician, 91*(1), 46–52.

Himmerich, H., Bentley, J., Kan, C., & Treasure, J. (2019). Genetic risk factors for eating disorders: An update and insights into pathophysiology. *Therapeutic Advances in Psychopharmacology, 12*(9).

Hudson, J. I., Hiripi, E., Pope, H. G., & Kessler, R. C. (2012). The prevalence and correlates of eating disorders in the national comorbidity survey replication. *Erratum in Biological Psychiatry, 72*(2), 164.

Joy, E., Kussman, A., & Nattiv, A. (2016). 2016 Update on eating disorders in athletes: A comprehensive narrative review with a focus on clinical assessment and management. *British Journal of Sports Medicine, 50*(3), 154–162.

Kerr, K. L., Moseman, S. E., Avery, J. A., Bodurka, J., Zucker, N. L., & Simmons, W. K. (2016). Altered insula activity during visceral interoception in weight-restored patients with anorexia nervosa. *Neuropsychopharmacology, 41*(2), 521–528.

Kessler, R. C., Berglund, P. A., Chiu, W. T., Deitz, A. C., Hudson, J. I., Shahly, V., et al. (2013). The prevalence and correlates of binge eating disorder in the World Health Organization World Mental Health Surveys. *Biological Psychiatry, 73*(9), 904–914.

Lock, J. (2015). An update on evidenced-based psychosocial treatments for eating disorders in children and adolescents. *Journal of Clinical Child and Adolescent Psychology*, 44(5), 707–721.

Lydecker, J. A., Galbraith, K., Ivezaj, V., White, M. A., Barnes, R. D., Roberto, C. A., et al. (2016). Words will never hurt me? Preferred terms for describing obesity and binge eating. *International Journal of Clinical Practice*, 70(8), 682–690.

McDonald, S. (2019). Understanding the genetics and epigenetics of bulimia nervosa/bulimia spectrum disorder and comorbid borderline personality disorder (BN/BSD-BPD): A systematic review. *Eating and Weight Disorders*, 24(5), 799–814.

McElroy, S. L., Guerdjikova, A. I., Mori, N., & Romo-Nava, F. (2019). Progress in developing pharmacologic agents to treat bulimia nervosa. *CNS Drugs*, 33(1), 31–46.

Mehler, P. S., & Andersen, A. E. (2017). *Eating disorders: A guide to medical care and complications*. Baltimore, MD: Johns Hopkins.

Mitchell, J. E., King, W. C., Pories, W., Wolfe, B., Flum, D. R., et al. (2015). Binge eating disorder and medical comorbidities in bariatric surgery candidates. *International Journal of Eating Disorders*, 48(5), 471–476.

National Eating Disorder Association. (2018). *Glossary*. Retrieved from https://www.nationaleatingdisorders.org/learn/glossary.

Pearson, C. M., Wonderlich, S. A., & Smith, G. T. (2015). A risk and maintenance model for bulimia nervosa: From impulsive action to compulsive behavior. *Psychological Review*, 122(3), 516–535.

Quilliot, D., Brunaud, L., Mathieu, J., Quenot, C., Sirveaux, M. A., Kahn, J. P., et al. (2019). Links between traumatic experiences in childhood or early adulthood and lifetime binge eating disorder. *Psychiatry Research*, 276, 134–141.

Rasmusson, G., Lydecker, J. A., Coffino, J. A., White, M. A., & Grilo, C. M. (2018). Household food insecurity is associated with binge–eating disorder and obesity. *International Journal of Eating Disorders*, 52(1), 28–35.

Romano, C., Hartman, C., Privitera, C., Cardile, S., & Shamir, R. (2015). Current topics in the diagnosis and management of the pediatric non organic feeding disorders (NOFEDs). *Clinical Nutrition*, 34(2), 195–200.

Rosenvinge, J., & Petterson, G. (2015). Epidemiology of eating disorders part II: An update with a special reference to the DSM-5. *Advances in Eating Disorders*, 3(2), 198–220.

Schulte, E. M., Grilo, C. M., & Gearhardt, A. N. (2016). Shared and unique mechanisms underlying binge eating disorder and addictive disorders. *Clinical Psychology*, 44, 125–139.

Sidani, J. E., Shensa, A., Hoffman, B., Hanmer, J., & Primack, B. A. (2016). The association between social media use and eating concerns among US young adults. *Journal of the Academy of Nutrition and Dietetics*, 116(9), 1465–1472.

Spirou, D., Raman, J., & Smith, E. (2020). Psychological outcomes following surgical and endoscopic bariatric procedures: A systematic review. *Obesity Reviews*, 21(6), e12998.

The Trevor Project. (2018). *Eating disorders among LGBTQ youth: A 2018 national assessment*. Retrieved from https://www.nationaleatingdisorders.org/sites/default/files/nedaw18/NEDA%20-Trevor%20Project%202018%20Survey%20-%20Full%20Results.pdf.

Watson, H. J., Yilmaz, Z., Thornton, L. M., Hübel, C., Coleman, J. R., Gaspar, H. A., et al. (2019). Genome-wide association study identifies eight risk loci and implicates metabo-psychiatric origins for anorexia nervosa. *Nature Genetics*, 51(8), 1207–1214.

Yilmaz, Z., Hardaway, J. A., & Bulik, C. M. (2015). Genetics and epigenetics of eating disorders. *Advances in Genomics and Genetics*, 5, 131–150.

Zipfel, S., Giel, K. E., Bulik, C. M., Hay, P., & Schmidt, U. (2015). Anorexia nervosa: Aetiology, assessment, and treatment. *Lancet Psychiatry*, 2(12), 1099–1111.

19

Sleep-Wake Disorders

Margaret Jordan Halter

 Visit the Evolve website for a pretest on the content in this chapter: http://evolve.elsevier.com/Varcarolis

OBJECTIVES

1. Discuss the impact of inadequate sleep on overall physical and mental health.
2. Describe the social and economic impact of sleep disturbance and chronic sleep deprivation.
3. Recognize the risks to personal and community safety imposed by sleep disturbance and chronic sleep deprivation.
4. Describe normal sleep physiology and explain the variations in normal sleep.
5. Identify the major categories and medical diagnoses for sleep disorders.
6. Identify the predisposing, precipitating, and perpetuating factors for patients with insomnia.
7. Apply the nursing process in caring for individuals with sleep disorders.
8. Describe the use of two assessment tools in the evaluation of patients experiencing sleep disturbance.
9. Formulate three nursing diagnoses for patients experiencing a sleep disturbance.
10. Develop a teaching plan for a patient with insomnia disorder incorporating principles of sleep restriction, stimulus control, and cognitive behavioral therapy.
11. Develop a care plan for the patient experiencing sleep disturbance, incorporating basic sleep hygiene principles.
12. Identify biological and psychological treatment modalities used for sleep disorders.

KEY TERMS AND CONCEPTS

basal sleep requirement
cataplexy
circadian drive
excessive sleepiness
hypersomnolence
narcolepsy

sleep architecture
sleep continuity
sleep deprivation
sleep drive
sleep efficiency
sleep fragmentation

sleep hygiene
sleep latency
sleep restriction
stimulus control

Sleep and sleep disorders are receiving increased attention in the medical, nursing, research, and social science literature. Achieving sufficient quality sleep is now recognized as a key determinant of health and well-being. The national health promotion and disease prevention initiative, *Healthy People 2020,* included sleep health in the list of current health topics, making sleep a national health priority. *Healthy People 2030* continued the practice.

⚓ HEALTH POLICY

Healthy People 2030 *and Sleep*

Healthy People 2030 continues to make sleep health a priority for the national health agenda. This priority was underscored with a goal to "improve health, productivity, well-being, quality of life, and safety by helping people get enough sleep." Core objectives for sleep are identified as:
1. Reduce the rate of vehicular crashes that are due to drowsy driving.

2. Increase the proportion of adults with sleep apnea symptoms who get evaluated by a healthcare provider.
3. Increase the proportion of adults who get enough sleep
4. Increase the proportion of high school students who get sufficient sleep.
5. Increase the proportion of children who get sufficient sleep.
6. Increase the proportion of infants who are put to sleep on their back.
7. Increase the proportion of infants who are put to sleep in a safe sleep environment.
8. Increase the proportion of secondary schools with a start time of 8:30 or later.

Nurses can be instrumental in advancing the sleep goals of *Healthy People 2030.* As 24/7 care providers, nurses can assess for sleep problems, educate patients about sleep requirements, and promote a restful environment in patient care areas. As healthcare advocates, nurses can bring forth or support policy change that brings the problems of inadequate sleep and its consequences into sharp focus.

US Department of Health and Human Services. (2020). *Healthy People 2030.* Retrieved from https://health.gov/healthypeople/objectives-and-data/browse-objectives/sleep.

The National Center on Sleep Disorder Research (NCSDR) was established in 1996 to facilitate research, training, health information dissemination, and other activities with respect to the basic understanding of sleep and sleep disorders. Under the guidance of the NCSDR and other organizations such as the National Sleep Foundation (NSF) and the American Academy of Sleep Medicine (AASM), there has been exponential growth in the scientific understanding of sleep over the past two decades.

Formal training in sleep or sleep disorders within medical and nursing education is limited, and the number of trained clinicians and researchers continues to be insufficient (Institute of Medicine, 2006). Awareness among healthcare providers regarding the prevalence and burden of sleep disruption and the problem of inadequate sleep is underappreciated, and providers do not routinely screen for sleep disturbance or inquire about overall sleep quality. Consequently, sleep disturbances may not be recognized, diagnosed, managed, and treated.

SLEEP

For many people, sleep becomes an expendable commodity. In a fast-paced society, sleep is often forfeited, and people subject themselves to schedules that disrupt normal sleep physiology. The amount of time spent working, engaging in academic activities, and traveling to and from work and school are the strongest determinants of total sleep time. The more time devoted to other activities, the less time spent sleeping. Table 19.1 provides recommendations for sleep based on age.

TABLE 19.1 Sleep Duration Recommendations

Age	Recommended	May Be Appropriate	Not Recommended
Newborn <3 months	14–17 h	11–13 h 18–19 h	<11 h >19 h
Infants 4–11 months	12–15 h	10–11 h 16–18 h	<10 h >18 h
Toddlers 1–2 years	11–14 h	9–10 h 15–16 h	<9 h >16 h
Preschoolers 3–5 years	10–13 h	8–9 h 14 h	<8 h >14 h
School-aged 6–13 years	9–11 h	7–8 h 12 h	<7 h >12 h
Teenagers 14–17 years	8–10 h	7 h 11 h	<7 h >11 h
Young Adults 18–25 years	7–9 h	6 h 10–11 h	<6 h >11 h
Adults 26–64 years	7–9 h	6 h 10 h	<6 h >10 h
Older Adults ≥65 years	7–8 h	5–6 h 9 h	<5 h >9 h

National Sleep Foundation. (2016). *Recommended hours of sleep by age.* Retrieved from https://www.sleepfoundation.org/press-release/national-sleep-foundation-recommends-new-sleep-times.

The NSF's annual *Sleep in America* poll measures specific topics related to sleep each year. In 2019, they administered the poll alongside a sleep health index, which measured sleep health status based on measures of sleep duration, sleep quality, and disordered sleep. US adults scored an average of 77 on a 0 to 100 scale. Scores were 6 to 11 points higher for individuals with the most regular sleep times and wake times than for those with the most varied sleep and wake times. Fig. 19.1 demonstrates the association between feeling well rested on weekdays based by sleep health status.

Not only are hours asleep important, but consistency of sleep, too, is important. Going to bed at roughly the same time and waking at roughly the same time is correlated with feeling well rested in the morning (NSF, 2020). When people with the strictest sleep schedules are compared with those who have the most variable sleep schedules, the strict sleepers are 1.5 times more likely to feel well rested. These same individuals can also afford to shift 1 hour of their sleep schedules without ill effects the next day.

Consequences of Sleep Loss

The major consequence of acute or chronic sleep reduction is **excessive sleepiness**. Excessive sleepiness is a subjective self-report of difficulty staying awake. Individuals with this problem believe that it is serious enough to impact social and work functioning and increase the risk for accident or injury. Sleep restriction may be caused by a disruption of the normal sleep cycle as seen in shift work, underlying sleep disorders, medications, alcohol and substance use, and medical and psychiatric disorders.

We need only to look to our own experiences with acute or total sleep loss to recognize its consequences. After a poor night's sleep, we feel tired, lethargic, and out of synch. The effects of chronic sleep loss may be less obvious but may have a greater overall impact on health and well-being. A discrepancy between hours of sleep obtained and hours of sleep required for optimal functioning is referred to as **sleep deprivation**. Sleep deprivation has widespread implications for quality of life, health, and safety. Because there can be considerable individual variability

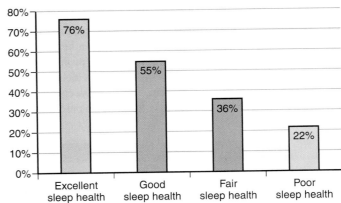

Fig. 19.1 Feeling well rested by sleep on weekdays by sleep health status. (National Sleep Foundation. [2019]. *NSF's 2019 Sleep in America poll shows disciplined sleepers reap reward.* Retrieved from https://www.sleepfoundation.org/press-release/nsfs-2019-sleep-america-poll-shows-disciplined-sleepers-reap-reward.)

in total sleep need, the term *sleep deprivation* applies when sleep loss is accompanied by impaired functioning.

Neurocognitive symptoms of chronic sleep deprivation can mimic psychiatric symptoms, highlighting the importance of a comprehensive sleep evaluation for patients with mental health disorders. For example, a person with a psychotic disorder may experience increased symptoms, such as hearing voices or experiencing disorganized thought. A clinician may respond by increasing antipsychotic medications. However, a careful evaluation of sleep habits may reveal a lack of stable housing and unsafe sleeping conditions.

Short-term consequences of sleep disruption include increased stress responsivity, somatic pain, reduced quality of life, emotional distress and mood disorders, and cognitive, memory, and performance deficits. Long-term consequences of sleep disruption in otherwise healthy individuals include cardiovascular disease, weight-related issues, metabolic syndrome, type 2 diabetes mellitus, and colorectal cancer. All-cause mortality is also increased with sleep disturbances.

Children and adolescents are most vulnerable to the negative effects of sleep deprivation. Behavioral problems and impaired cognition are associated with sleep disruption in children. For adolescents, emotional and social health, school performance, and risk-taking behaviors are impacted by sleep disruption.

Sleep loss may play a role in the increased prevalence of diabetes and obesity. Explanations for this increase have to do with alterations in glucose metabolism and decreased energy expenditure. Sleep deprivation also results in an increased appetite. This may be due, in part, to a dysregulation of leptin, a hormone that regulates satiety or feelings of fullness, and ghrelin, a hormone that regulates hunger.

Safety

Sleep loss diminishes safety and results in the loss of lives and property. Sleep deprivation can produce psychomotor impairments equivalent to those induced by alcohol consumption at or above the legal limit. Daytime wakefulness in excess of 17 to 19 hours can produce psychomotor deficits equivalent to blood alcohol concentrations (BACs) between 0.05% and 0.1% while the legal limit in most states is 0.08% (Insurance Institute for Highway Safety, 2012).

Acute or chronic sleep deprivation can result in episodes of microsleep lasting from 1 second up to 10 seconds when a tired person is trying to stay awake. Many of us have experienced this when sitting in a class or in a meeting. Such lapses can lead to lower capabilities and efficiency of task performance and increased risk for errors.

Some of the most devastating environmental and human tragedies of our time can be linked to human error due to sleep loss and fatigue. The grounding of the Exxon Valdez, the nuclear meltdown at Three Mile Island, and the explosion of the Union Carbide chemical plant in India are prime examples.

Sleepiness with driving has become a national epidemic. The 2011 NSF *Sleep in America Poll* (NSF, 2011) indicates that an alarming 52% of respondents admitted to driving while sleepy.

Another incredible statistic is that one-third of Americans report falling asleep while driving once or twice a month (Centers for Disease Control, 2010). In order to address this dangerous practice, researchers have been exploring eye tracking technology to assess vigilance in drivers to provide early warning of fatigue and drowsiness (Zandi et al., 2019).

Financial Burden

Although researchers have tried to quantify the financial burden associated with sleep disruption, there are relatively few comprehensive data available on the economic burden of sleep-wake disorders. However, considering the prevalence, impact on overall health and quality of life, and the indirect costs associated with property loss and damage, the economic burden is considerable.

Among the conditions that have been studied in terms of economic burden include sleep apnea and insomnia. Sleep loss due to undiagnosed obstructive sleep apnea among US adults carries an economic price tag of about $150 billion (AASM, 2016). This amount includes $87 billion in lost productivity, $26 billion in motor vehicle accidents, and $6.5 billion in workplace accidents. People who sleep less than 6 hours a night due to insomnia are significantly less productive than those sleeping 7 to 9 hours (Hafner et al., 2016). These same individuals also lose around 6 working days to absenteeism per year more than a worker who sleeps between 7 and 9 hours.

Irregular Sleep

Not only are humans designed to require a certain number of hours of sleep; we seem to be programmed for consistency in sleep. Sticking to a regular bedtime and wake-up schedule keeps us healthier. Irregularity and high day-to-day variability in sleep duration and timing has metabolic consequences such as lower high-density lipoprotein (HDL) cholesterol; higher waist circumference; and increased blood pressure, total triglycerides, and fasting glucose (Huang & Redline, 2019).

Too Much Sleep

In regard to sleep, too much of a good thing is not necessarily better. Similar to lack of sleep, excessive sleep—more than 9 hours in adults—can lead to a variety of health consequences, including stroke risk. In a study of almost 32,000 adults for 6 years, researchers found that compared with 7 to 8 hours a night, sleeping 9 or more hours increased the risk for stroke by 23% (Zhou et al., 2019). They also found that midday napping for 90 minutes or more was associated with a 25% increased stroke risk compared to napping 30 minutes or less. The biggest risk was when respondents slept more than 9 hours and napped more than 90 minutes. They were 85% more likely to have a stroke.

Childhood obesity is associated with sleeping too much. Long sleep duration may impair whole-body metabolism and increase the risk of obesity (Nascimento-Ferreira et al., 2020). As with sleep deprivation, adults who sleep 10 or more hours have a much higher risk for metabolic syndrome, which includes excess abdominal fat, hypertension, low levels of HDL cholesterol, high fasting blood glucose, and high triglycerides.

Besides metabolic issues, excessive sleep has been linked to depression, headaches, and a greater risk of dying from a medical condition. A question that arises when considering the topic of too much sleep is: What is cause and what is effect? That is, does sleeping too much cause problems or is sleeping too much a sign of other problems? Typically, there are reasons for sleeping too much. They include sleep apnea, restless legs syndrome, bruxism (teeth grinding), pain, narcolepsy, and hypersomnolence.

In this chapter, we review the components of normal sleep, sleep regulation, and functions of sleep. Following this review, we discuss the most common sleep disturbances encountered in the clinical environment, with a focus on their relationship to psychiatric illness. The nurse's role in the assessment and management of patients with sleep disturbances is explored.

Normal Sleep Cycle

Sleep is a dynamic neurological process that involves complex interaction between the central nervous system and the environment. Behaviorally, sleep is associated with low or absent motor activity, a reduced response to environmental stimuli, and closed eyes. Neurophysiologically, sleep is categorized according to specific brain wave patterns, eye movements, and general muscle tone. Sleep is measured through an electroencephalogram (EEG) and consists of two distinct physiological states: non–rapid eye movement (NREM) sleep and rapid eye movement (REM) sleep.

Non–Rapid Eye Movement Sleep

NREM sleep is divided into three stages (N1, N2, N3) and is characterized by progressive or deeper sleep. Stage 1 (N1) is a brief transition between wakefulness and sleep. It comprises between 2% to 5% of total sleep time. The time it takes to fall asleep is referred to as *sleep latency*. During stage 1 sleep, body temperature declines and muscles relax. Slow rolling eye movements are common. People lose awareness of their environment but are generally easily aroused. Stage 2 (N2) sleep occupies 45% to 55% of total sleep time. During this period, heart rate and respiratory rate decline. Arousal from stage 2 sleep requires more stimuli than stage 1.

Stage 3 (N3) is known as slow wave sleep or delta sleep. Slow wave sleep is relatively short and constitutes only about 13% to 23% of total sleep time. It is characterized by further reduction in heart rate, respiratory rate, blood pressure, and response to external stimuli. The three stages of NREM sleep make up 75% to 80% of total sleep time. Stage 3 sleep is considered to be "restorative sleep," as it is a time of reduced sympathetic activity.

Rapid Eye Movement Sleep

REM sleep comprises 20% to 25% of total sleep time. REM sleep is characterized by reduction and absence of skeletal muscle tone (muscle atonia), bursts of REM, myoclonic twitches of the facial and limb muscles, reports of dreaming, and autonomic nervous system variability. The atonia in REM sleep is thought to be a protective mechanism to prevent the acting out of nightmares and dreams. Fig. 19.2 shows the EEG patterns characteristic of these sleep stages.

Non–Rapid Eye Movement and Rapid Eye Movement Patterns

In the adult, sleep normally begins with NREM sleep. Continuous EEG recordings of sleep demonstrate an alternating cycle between NREM and REM sleep. There are typically four to six cycles of NREM and REM sleep occurring over 90- to 120-minute intervals across the sleep period.

There is also a distinct organization to sleep, with NREM predominating the first half of the sleep period and REM sleep predominating during the second half. The shortest REM period occurs 60 to 90 minutes after sleep onset and lasts only for several minutes. The longest REM period occurs at the end of the sleep period and can last up to an hour. This is the reason why many people remember dreaming upon awakening.

The structural organization of NREM and REM sleep is known as sleep architecture and is often displayed graphically as a *hypnogram*. Fig. 19.3 is a hypnogram depicting the normal progression of the stages of sleep in an adult. The visual depiction of sleep is helpful in identifying sleep continuity (i.e., the distribution of sleep and wakefulness across the sleep period), as well as changes in sleep that may occur as a result of aging, illness, or certain medications.

Disruption of sleep stages as indicated by excessive amounts of stage 1 sleep, multiple brief arousals, and frequent shifts in sleep staging is known as sleep fragmentation. Fig. 19.4 is a hypnogram of a patient with a complaint of insomnia, indicating multiple brief arousals.

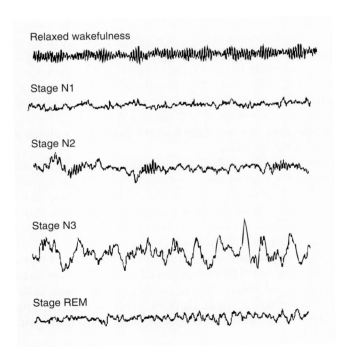

Fig. 19.2 Stages of sleep. *REM*, Rapid eye movement. (Reprinted with permission of Sleep Health Centers, Boston, MA.)

The function of alternations between NREM and REM sleep is not yet understood. We do know that irregular cycling, absent sleep stages, and sleep fragmentation are associated with many psychiatric disorders, sleep disorders, and medication effects. For example, in patients with depression, the latency period to REM sleep is frequently reduced, as is the percentage of slow wave sleep. Patients with narcolepsy frequently enter sleep through REM sleep rather than NREM sleep. Benzodiazepines tend to suppress slow wave sleep, whereas serotonergic drugs such as antidepressants suppress REM sleep.

Life Cycle Sleep Patterns

Sleep architecture changes over the lifespan. The percentage in each stage of sleep, as well as the overall sleep efficiency or ratio of sleep duration to time spent in bed, varies according to age. For example, infants sleep 16 to 18 hours a day, enter sleep through REM (not NREM) sleep, and spend up to 50% of sleep time in REM sleep. The percentage of REM sleep decreases to 20% to 25% by age 3 and stays relatively constant throughout the lifespan. The amount of slow wave sleep is maximal in young children and declines with age to almost none, particularly in men. This results in a tendency for middle-of-the-night awakenings and reduced sleep efficiency with age (Bliwise, 2011).

Regulation of Sleep

The regulation of sleep and wakefulness is believed to be a complex interaction between two processes, one that promotes

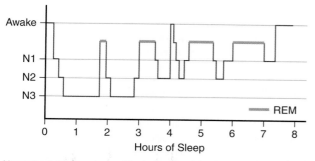

Normal adult hypnogram with slow wave sleep (N3) most prominent early in the sleep cycle and REM increasing throughout the sleep cycle.

Fig. 19.3 Hypnogram depicting the progression of the sleep stages of an adult. *REM*, Rapid eye movement.

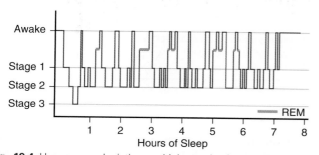

Fig. 19.4 Hypnogram depicting multiple awakenings and sleep fragmentation.

sleep—known as the homeostatic process or sleep drive—and one that promotes wakefulness, known as the circadian process or circadian drive. The homeostatic process is dependent on the number of hours a person is awake. The longer the period of wakefulness, the stronger the sleep drive. During sleep, the sleep drive gradually dissipates.

Circadian drives are near–24-hour cycles of behavior and physiology generated and influenced by endogenous and exogenous factors and are wake-promoting. The exogenous factors are various clues from the environment known as *zeitgebers* (time-givers) that help set our internal clock to a 24-hour cycle. The strongest external cue for wakefulness is light, whereas darkness is the cue for sleep. Other environmental cues include the timing of social events such as meals, work, or exercise.

A *master biological clock* is located in the suprachiasmatic nucleus (SCN) of the hypothalamus. This clock regulates not only sleep but also a host of other biological and physiological functions within the body. Information about the lighting conditions of the external environment is relayed to the SCN from the retina. The SCN also receives information from the thalamus and the midbrain. These two pathways transmit photic and nonphotic information to the circadian clock through an expansive network. In addition to regulating sleep-wake cycles, they also exert control over endocrine regulation, body temperature, metabolism, autonomic regulation, psychomotor and cognitive performance, attention, memory, and emotion (Czeisler et al., 2011).

In addition to the circadian and homeostatic processes, several neurotransmitter systems are responsible for sleep and wakefulness. The wakefulness neurotransmitters are dopamine, norepinephrine, serotonin, acetylcholine, histamine, glutamate, and hypocretin/orexin. Sleep-promoting neurotransmitters include adenosine, gamma-aminobutyric acid (GABA), and galanin (Carney et al., 2011). Any medication that crosses the blood-brain barrier may have effects on sleep and wakefulness through modulation of these neurotransmitters.

It is important to appreciate the neurotransmitters involved in sleep and wakefulness. Many of the medications used in psychiatry manipulate these neurotransmitter systems. For example, amphetamines—which promote wakefulness—increase the release of dopamine and norepinephrine. Caffeine (methylxanthine)—which promotes alertness—functions by blocking the sleep-promoting neurotransmitter adenosine. Patients report both difficulty sleeping and drowsiness when beginning treatment with antidepressants classified as selective serotonin reuptake inhibitors (SSRIs).

Functions of Sleep

Despite remarkable advances in the understanding of sleep disorders and the biological and physiological process of sleep, very little is known about the true function of sleep. Most of the information regarding the function of sleep comes to us from animal models of sleep deprivation and human models of partial sleep deprivation. Based on these models, several theories are proposed and include brain tissue restoration, body restoration (NREM sleep), energy conservation, memory reinforcement and consolidation (REM sleep), regulation of immune function, metabolism and regulation of certain hormones, and thermoregulation (Arun et al., 2014).

Sleep Requirements

Sleep architecture and efficiency may change over time, but there is little change in the amount of sleep required once we reach adulthood. Sleep requirements vary from individual to individual and to some degree are probably genetically mediated. While most adults require 7 to 8 hours of sleep for optimal functioning, there is a small percentage of individuals defined as *long sleepers* (requiring 10 or more hours per night) and *short sleepers* (requiring less than 5 hours per night). The amount of sleep necessary to feel fully awake and able to sustain normal levels of performance is known as the basal sleep requirement.

Unfortunately, many people allow circumstances to dictate the amount of sleep obtained. However, there is a simple way to determine your basal sleep requirement. The first step is to establish a routine bedtime. Then, allow yourself to sleep undisturbed without an alarm for several days. This is usually best accomplished during an extended period of leisure time, such as during a vacation. The average of several nights' undisturbed sleep is a good estimate of the basal sleep requirement. Activity trackers can help you fine-tune your understanding of that mysterious world of sleep. They provide such information as length of time to fall asleep, number of times restless, number of times awake, and the number of steps you take during hours of sleep.

DIAGNOSING SLEEP DISORDERS

Sleep testing is often indicated for patients complaining of sleep disturbance or excessive sleepiness that impairs social and vocational functioning. There are four common diagnostic procedures used in the evaluation of sleep disorders:

1. **Polysomnography** is the most common sleep test and is used to diagnose and evaluate patients with sleep-related breathing disorders and nocturnal seizure disorders. It usually involves one or two nights of sleep in a lab with electrodes and monitors placed on the head, chest, and legs. Technicians record brain wave activity, eye movement, muscle tone, heart rhythm, and breathing.

2. The **multiple sleep latency test (MSLT)** is a daytime nap test used to objectively measure sleepiness in a sleep-conducive setting. Polysomnography and MSLT performed on the day after polysomnography evaluation are routinely indicated in patients suspected of having narcolepsy.

3. The **maintenance of wakefulness test (MWT)** evaluates a patient's ability to remain awake in a situation conducive to sleep. It is used to document adequate alertness in individuals with careers such as airline pilots, for which sleepiness would pose a risk to public safety.

4. **Actigraphy** involves using a wristwatch-type tracker that records body movement over a period of time and is helpful in evaluating sleep patterns and sleep duration. It is used in patients with circadian rhythm disorders and insomnia.

CLINICAL PICTURE

In this chapter, you will review the major categories of sleep disorders. The American Psychiatric Association (2013) identifies the following disorders:

- Insomnia disorder
- Hypersomnolence disorder
- Narcolepsy
- Breathing-related sleep disorders
- Circadian rhythm disorders
- NREM sleep arousal disorders
- Nightmare disorder
- REM sleep behavior disorder
- Restless legs syndrome
- Substance-induced sleep disorders

Insomnia Disorder

Insomnia is characterized by dissatisfaction with quantity or quality of sleep. It is the most common sleep disorder and may affect up to 45% of adults (Sadock et al., 2015). Females are more frequently affected, as are older adults. *DSM-5* criteria for insomnia disorders are listed in the *DSM-5* box.

DSM-5 CRITERIA FOR INSOMNIA DISORDER

A. A predominant complaint of dissatisfaction with sleep quantity or quality associated with one (or more) of the following symptoms:
  1. Difficulty initiating sleep. (In children, this may manifest as difficulty initiating sleep without caregiver intervention.)
  2. Difficulty maintaining sleep, characterized by frequent awakenings or problems returning to sleep after awakenings. (In children, this may manifest as difficulty returning to sleep without caregiver intervention.)
  3. Early-morning awakening with inability to return to sleep.
B. The sleep disturbance causes clinically significant distress or impairment in social, occupational, educational, academic, behavioral, or other important areas of functioning.
C. The sleep difficulty occurs at least three nights per week.
D. The sleep difficulty is present for at least 3 months.
E. The sleep difficulty occurs despite adequate opportunity for sleep.
F. The insomnia is not better explained by and does not occur exclusively during the course of another sleep-wake disorder (e.g., narcolepsy, a breathing-related sleep disorder, a circadian rhythm sleep-wake disorder, a parasomnia).
G. The insomnia is not attributable to the physiological effects of a substance (e.g., a drug of abuse, a medication).
H. Coexisting mental disorders and medical conditions do not adequately explain the predominant complaint of insomnia.
Specify if:
With nonsleep disorder mental comorbidity, including substance use disorders
With other medical comorbidity
With other sleep disorder

From the American Psychiatric Association. (2013). *Diagnostic and statistical manual of mental disorders* (5th ed.). Washington, DC: Author.

In addition to a thorough medical, psychiatric, and substance use history, it is helpful to use Spielman's **3P model of insomnia** to comprehensively assess the causes of insomnia, suggest appropriate interventions, and provide rationales for treatment (Spielman & Glovinsky, 2004). This model suggests that there are three factors that contribute to the insomnia complaint: **predisposing**, **precipitating**, and **perpetuating** factors (Fig. 19.5).

Predisposing factors are individual factors that create a vulnerability to insomnia. These may include a prior history of poor-quality sleep, history of depression and anxiety, or a state of hyperarousal. Patients at risk to develop insomnia may describe themselves as light sleepers and night owls. **Precipitating** factors are external events that trigger insomnia. Personal and vocational difficulties, medical and psychiatric disorders, grief, and changes in role or identity (as seen with retirement) are examples. **Perpetuating** factors are sleep practices and attributes that maintain the sleep complaint, such as excessive caffeine or alcohol use, spending excessive amounts of time in bed or napping, and worrying about the consequences of insomnia.

Nursing care for patients experiencing insomnia will be addressed later in the chapter. Medication for its treatment will also be discussed.

Hypersomnolence Disorder

Hypersomnolence disorder is associated with excessive daytime sleepiness and has a prevalence of about 5% to 10% of individuals who seek help in sleep disorder clinics. Hypersomnolence disorder is chronic (3 months or more) and begins in young adulthood. It affects males and females equally.

The patient with hypersomnolence reports recurrent periods of sleep or unintended lapses into sleep, frequent napping, a prolonged main sleep period of greater than 9 hours, nonrefreshing nonrestorative sleep regardless of amount of time slept, and difficulty with full alertness during the wake period. Excessive sleepiness significantly impairs social and vocational functioning by impacting the person's ability to participate in and enjoy relationships and function in the workplace. Cognitive impairment is common, as is an increased risk for accident or injury associated with the sleepiness.

Treatment for hypersomnolence disorders focuses on maintaining a regular sleep-wake schedule with an ample sleep opportunity. Some individuals will improve if they allow for an extended sleep opportunity of 10 or more hours. Pharmacotherapy with long-acting amphetamine-based stimulants such as methylphenidate and

nonamphetamine-based stimulants such as modafinil (Provigil) are helpful.

Narcolepsy

People with *narcolepsy* have an uncontrollable urge to sleep. This relatively rare phenomenon affects less than 0.05% of the general population. Narcolepsy seems to occur slightly more frequently in men. It usually begins before young adulthood and persists throughout the lifespan.

Symptoms of narcolepsy include disturbed nighttime sleep with multiple middle-of-the-night awakenings and automatic behaviors characterized by memory lapses. Patients with narcolepsy generally feel refreshed upon awakening, but within 2 or 3 hours begin to feel sleepy again. Individuals with other hypersomnia disorders generally do not feel rested or refreshed regardless of the amount of sleep obtained. Measuring levels of hypocretin, a neuropeptide that regulates arousal and wakefulness, in cerebrospinal fluid can provide an objective marker for this diagnosis.

Narcolepsy may be accompanied by cataplexy. Cataplexy refers to brief episodes of bilateral loss of muscle tone while maintaining consciousness. These episodes are usually triggered by strong emotions such as anger, fear, frustration, and joy, or even the act of laughing. This terrifying symptom may last for up to several minutes, and recovery is generally immediate and complete. Cataplexy is probably due to the occurrence of REM sleep paralysis during wakefulness. Cataplexy occurs in about half of all people with narcolepsy. Some people have one or two episodes in their whole lives, while other people may have up to 20 episodes a day. It can have a major impact on people's social lives, functioning, and even safety.

Two other classic symptoms of narcolepsy are:
- Hypnagogic hallucinations—false auditory, visual, and tactile sensations. They occur at the transition from wakefulness to sleep.
- Sleep paralysis—an inability to move or speak during the transition from sleep to wakefulness.

Treatment for narcolepsy includes naps, exercise, and a balanced diet. Medications with US Food and Drug Administration (FDA) approval for excessive daytime sleepiness include the stimulants modafinil (Provigil), armodafinil (Nuvigil), methylphenidate, and amphetamine.

Pitolisant (Wakix) and solriamfetol (Sunosi) are two nonstimulant medications used to treat excessive daytime sleepiness associated with narcolepsy. Pitolisant is a histamine-3 receptor antagonist/inverse agonist. Common side effects include insomnia, nausea, and anxiety. Solriamfetol is a dopamine and norepinephrine reuptake inhibitor. Both dopamine and norepinephrine are wakefulness neurotransmitters. It is contraindicated with use of monoamine oxidase inhibitors. Monitor blood pressure and heart rate in patients receiving solriamfetol.

Depending on its severity, cataplexy can be treated with medications and achieve excellent responses. Sodium oxybate (Xyrem) is a central nervous system depressant with FDA approval for both excessive daytime sleepiness and cataplexy in patients 7 years of age and older. It helps to restore normal sleep architecture at night, which, in turn, may improve daytime

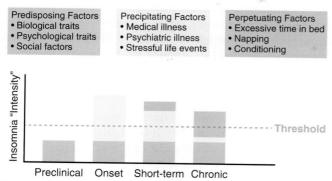

Fig. 19.5 Spielman's 3P Model of Insomnia. (From Spielman, A., & Glovinsky, P. [2004]. A conceptual framework of insomnia for primary care providers: Predisposing, precipitating, and perpetuating factors. *Sleep Medicine Alert, 9*[1], 1–6.)

alertness. Some SSRIs and tricyclic antidepressants are used off-label for this condition with good results. They may work by suppressing REM sleep associated with the paralysis.

Breathing-Related Sleep Disorders

The most common disorder of breathing and sleeping is obstructive sleep apnea hypopnea syndrome. It affects about 2% of children and 2% to 20% of adults—rates increase with age. More men than women are affected. This type of apnea is strongly associated with obesity.

This problem is characterized by repeated episodes of upper airway collapse and obstruction that result in sleep fragmentation. Essentially, patients with obstructive sleep apnea are not able to sleep and breathe at the same time. Typical symptoms include loud disruptive snoring, apnea episodes witnessed by others, and excessive daytime sleepiness. Diagnosis is determined by clinical evaluation and polysomnography. Treatment is with continuous positive airway pressure (CPAP) therapy.

Additional breathing-related sleep disorders include central sleep apnea and sleep-related hypoventilation. Central sleep apnea is the cessation of respiration during sleep. This problem is due to instability of the respiratory control system, and there is no compensatory response. Central sleep apnea is seen in older individuals, those with advanced cardiac or pulmonary disease, or those with neurological disorders. Sleep-related hypoventilation is associated with sustained oxygen desaturation during sleep in the absence of apnea or respiratory events. This problem is seen in individuals with morbid obesity, lung parenchymal disease, or pulmonary vascular pathology.

Circadian Rhythm Sleep Disorders

Circadian rhythm sleep disorders occur when there is a misalignment between the timing of the individual's normal circadian rhythm and external factors that affect the timing or duration of sleep. Diagnosis is determined by clinical evaluation, sleep diaries, and actigraphy. Treatment is with aggressive lifestyle management strategies aimed at adapting to or modifying the required sleep schedule. Examples include:

- Delayed sleep phase type—A delay of more than 2 hours between desired time of sleep and actual sleep. Results in delays in waking. Rare in the general population, more common in adolescents (about 7%).
- Advanced sleep phase type—Sleep begins several hours earlier and ends several hours earlier than desired. This problem is thought to affect about 1% of middle-age adults and becomes more common with age.
- Irregular sleep-wake type—Sleep is sporadic and fragmented. The longest sleep period lasts about 4 hours and tends to occur between 2:00 a.m. and 6:00 a.m. It is associated with brain disorders such as Alzheimer disease and disruptive environments such as hospitals.
- Non–24-hour sleep-wake type—Characterized by a mismatch of the 24-hour environment and the person's internal clock. Sleep tends to occur later and later, eventually resulting in daytime sleeping. This problem is rare in sighted people but is a significant problem for up to 70% of blind individuals. Medication is specifically approved for this problem—tasimelteon (Hetlioz)—which works by increasing melatonin.
- Shift work type—Working outside of the normal work hours (late evening and night) results in excessive sleepiness at work and impaired sleep at home. It is estimated to occur in up to 10% of night shift workers.

> **VIGNETTE:** Sarah had been living with treatment-resistant schizophrenia for many years. Despite multiple medication trials, she was frequently hospitalized. Last year, she was started on clozapine (Clozaril) and within a few months experienced a dramatic reduction in psychotic symptoms.
>
> Despite careful monitoring of her dietary intake and weight by her group home staff, Sarah began to experience weight gain while taking the clozapine. Staff also began to notice a change in her sleeping patterns. She complained of frequently waking in the night and having a morning headache and sore throat. When she returned home from work in the afternoon, it was not unusual for her to have a nap for 60 minutes or longer.
>
> While home on a family visit, her mother noted loud snoring and discussed this with the psychiatrist. Polysomnography was performed, which demonstrated a severe degree of obstructive sleep apnea, most likely related to her recent weight gain. CPAP therapy was initiated, and she was able to return to her baseline level of functioning.

Non–Rapid Eye Movement Sleep Arousal Disorders

Non–rapid eye movement (NREM) sleep arousal disorders include sleepwalking and sleep terrors. Because individuals in the NREM phase of sleep are not experiencing the loss of muscle tone that characterizes REM sleep, unsafe activities may occur.

Sleepwalking, or somnambulism, consists of a sequence of complex behaviors that begin in the first third of the night during NREM sleep. Individuals leave the bed and walk about without full consciousness or later memory. The individual may dress, go to the bathroom, leave the house, and, in some extreme cases, drive a car.

This problem tends to run in families and is rare in adults (Sadock et al., 2015). It is very common in children between the ages of 4 and 8. Typically, it disappears in adolescence.

Because of the possibility of accident or injury, a sleep specialist should always evaluate somnambulism. Polysomnography is sometimes indicated to rule out the possibility of an underlying disorder of sleep fragmentation. Treatment consists of instructing the patient and family regarding safety measures such as alarms or locks on windows and doors and gating stairways. Attention to sleep hygiene, limiting alcohol before bed, obtaining adequate amounts of sleep, and stress reduction are helpful. Benzodiazepines are frequently prescribed when the risk for accident or injury is likely.

Sleep terrors refer to sudden terrified near-awakenings. Sleep terrors tend to run in families. It is a fairly rare disorder and typically presents between the ages of 4 to 12. Sleep terrors may occur in response to fever or central nervous system depressant withdrawal (Sadock et al., 2015).

Typically, the episodes begin with sitting up in bed followed by a panicked scream. The person is unresponsive to stimuli, is overcome with anxiety, and may vocalize incoherently. There is a tremendous degree of autonomic arousal and intense fear. Sleepwalking may accompany this problem. Sleep terrors generally occur during the first third of the sleep episode arising out of slow wave sleep. Afterward, there is no recollection of dream content.

Sleep terrors are addressed by exploring areas of stress that can be managed. Regular sleep habits (e.g., going to bed at the same time each night) may help reduce their occurrence. Medication is rarely used, but benzodiazepines may be helpful in the short term.

Nightmare Disorder

Nightmare disorder is characterized by long frightening dreams from which people awaken scared. Nightmare disorder begins in preschool. It tends to increase until males reach the age of 13; for females, it tends to increase until the age of 29. About 6% of adults have monthly nightmares.

The nightmares almost always occur during REM sleep and usually after a long REM period late in the night. A nightmare disorder may be diagnosed with repeated occurrences of extremely unsettling dreams that are remembered well upon awakening. Risk factors for nightmares include frequent past adverse events, sleep problems, and a familial disposition for sleep disturbances.

Polysomnography is sometimes necessary to rule out the possibility of an underlying disorder of sleep fragmentation, such as obstructive sleep apnea. Treatment for nightmare disorder and night terrors is dependent on the frequency and severity of the symptoms, as well as the underlying cause. Treatment with hypnotic therapy is sometimes indicated. Many patients do well with lifestyle modification measures, attention to sleep hygiene, and stress reduction.

Rapid Eye Movement Sleep Behavior Disorder

REM sleep behavior disorder is characterized by elaborate motor activity associated with dreaming. These patients are actually acting out their dreams. Comedian Mike Birbiglia (2010) shares his experience of dreaming: he was standing on a podium accepting an Olympic medal when he was actually falling off of a tall bookcase in his living room. Another incident occurred while he was on tour and staying in a hotel room. In order to avoid a guided missile headed toward his room, he jumped from a second story window and ended up with 33 stitches.

The prevalence of REM behavior disorder is about 0.5% in the general population. It is most frequently seen in elderly men. It may also be the heralding symptom of neurological pathology such as Parkinson's disease. Serotonergic medications such as SSRIs or selective norepinephrine reuptake inhibitors (SNRIs) can induce or exacerbate episodes.

Diagnosis is determined by clinical evaluation and polysomnography with video recording. Treatment focuses on patient and sleep partner safety. Placing the mattress on the floor is sometimes necessary to prevent injury as a result of falling out of bed. The use of an intermediate-acting benzodiazepine can be helpful, especially in cases of severe disruption to the sleep partner and concerns about safety.

VIGNETTE: A primary care provider refers an 80-year-old man with Parkinson's disease to a sleep clinic. The patient's wife became concerned when on several occasions she awoke to find him shouting and thrashing in the bed. It appeared that he was acting out his dreams. The patient reported no memory of these events and had no particular sleep complaint. During one of these episodes, he knocked over the bedside lamp and struck her. When he was awoken, he reported that he was dreaming there was an intruder in the house and he was attempting to save her. A polysomnography examination demonstrated an absence of the muscle atonia normally seen in REM sleep, confirming a diagnosis of REM sleep behavior disorder. He was treated with a low dose of a benzodiazepine and given instructions regarding personal and sleep partner safety.

Restless Legs Syndrome

Restless legs syndrome is a sensory and movement disorder characterized by an uncomfortable sensation in the legs (occasionally, the arms and trunk are affected) accompanied by an urge to move. The prevalence rate is about 2% to 7%. Females tend to be affected by this problem more than men. Most of this gender difference is due to the increased risk of restless legs syndrome in pregnancy. Twelve percent of pregnant women are affected, and about half of those affected continue to experience restless legs syndrome postpartum (Hubner et al., 2013). Most people with this disorder had symptoms before adulthood.

Symptoms begin or worsen during periods of inactivity and are relieved or reduced by physical activity, such as walking, stretching, or flexing. Symptoms are worse in the evening and at bedtime and can have a significant impact on the individual's ability to fall asleep and stay asleep. SSRIs or SNRIs may precipitate restless legs syndrome. First-generation antihistamines (e.g., diphenhydramine) and dopamine blockers (e.g., antipsychotics) can also worsen symptoms.

The cause of restless legs syndrome is unknown. Evidence suggests that it may be related to dysfunction of the brain's basal ganglia circuits that use the neurotransmitter dopamine. Also, some patients with this condition have low levels of serum ferritin (iron), which plays a role in dopamine synthesis. This disorder tends to run in families and has a high concordance rate in monozygotic twins (Jiménez-Jiménez, Alonso-Navarro, Garcia-Martin, & Agundez, 2018). Although the causative gene(s) have not been identified, variants of several genes have been associated with restless legs syndrome risk.

Diagnosis is determined by clinical evaluation. Many patients with restless legs syndrome also have periodic limb movements of sleep that are observed during polysomnography.

Many dopamine receptor agonists are FDA approved for the treatment of restless legs syndrome. Examples are ropinirole (Requip), pramipexole (Mirapex), and rotigotine (Neupro). Unfortunately, long-term use of these drugs can lead to augmentation, or worsening, of symptoms. Another FDA-approved drug is gabapentin enacarbil (Horizant), an anticonvulsant. Iron deficiencies are treated with iron supplements. Levodopa is used off-label for intermittent restless legs syndrome.

A nonpharmacological treatment for restless legs syndrome is Relaxis. It is a pad that works by providing counterstimulation of the legs in the form of vibration that slowly tapers off through the night. Individuals who have had a deep vein thrombosis within the past 6 months should not use this treatment.

VIGNETTE: Kathy is a 32-year-old woman referred by her primary care provider for a psychiatric evaluation for complaints of anxiety and restlessness. She reported feeling fine during the day, but in the evening, she felt nervous and anxious. The symptoms always started at the same time. As soon as she would settle down for the evening to watch television, she would begin to have a restless sensation in her legs that would make her jump up and pace up and down. She described the sensation as having "soda pop fizzing through my veins." Sometimes she would go out for a walk at night even if it was very late to "calm down." These episodes began to occur almost nightly, and as a result, she was having difficulty getting a good night's sleep. She began to dread the approach of darkness. A full clinical evaluation suggested the diagnosis of restless legs syndrome. A course of the dopamine agonist pramipexole (Mirapex) was initiated in the evening with dramatic improvement in symptoms and total resolution of her sleep complaint.

Substance-Induced Sleep Disorder

A substance-induced sleep disorder can result from the use or recent discontinuance of a substance or medication. While it is quite obvious that many prescriptions and over-the-counter medications may affect sleep, there is less appreciation for the effects of commonly used substances on sleep. Alcohol, nicotine, and caffeine all have an impact on sleep quantity and quality.

- **Alcohol**—despite its great soporific (sleep-inducing) effects—decreases deep sleep (stage 3) and REM sleep and is responsible for middle-of-the-night awakenings with difficulty returning to sleep.
- **Nicotine** is a central nervous system stimulant, increasing heart rate, blood pressure, and respiratory rate. As nicotine levels decline through the night, patients wake in response to mild withdrawal symptoms. Patients should be reminded to remove nicotine delivery patches at bedtime.
- **Caffeine** blocks the neurotransmitter adenosine, promoting wakefulness. It increases sleep latency, reduces slow wave sleep, and acts as a diuretic, causing middle-of-the-night awakening for urination.

⊕ CONSIDERING CULTURE

Sleep Cafes in Japan

Japanese companies were looking for a way to increase quality and productivity. One common-sense solution was to support midday catnaps. Nestlé Japan opened the Suimin Café in a fifth floor Tokyo building. Beds and chairs are separated by cloth partitions. For under 10 US dollars, customers are provided with a cup of coffee and a 30-min nap. The caffeine kicks in about the time the nap ends. Probably not coincidentally, the coffee provides a marketing outlet for the chocolate giant, Nestlé. For longer naps, from 1 to 3 h, customers are provided with a decaffeinated cup of coffee before sleeping and a fully caffeinated one after.

The cafés have proven to be popular, and there is often a line to get in.

Adapted from Matsumoto, C. (2019). Japan's sleep cafes: Trying lying down on the job. *Financial Times.* Retrieved from https://www.ft.com/content/75c523c2-c35d-11e9-a8e9-296ca66511c9.

COMORBIDITY

Multiple studies suggest that sleeping less than 6 hours per night may have a significant impact on cardiovascular, endocrine, immune, and neurological function. Short sleep duration has been associated with obesity, cardiovascular disease and hypertension, impaired glucose tolerance and diabetes, and mood disturbance (Cappuccio et al., 2010).

Many sleep disorders increase the risk for the development of certain medical conditions. For example, obstructive sleep apnea has been associated with hypertension, diabetes, cardiovascular disease, and stroke (Tracova et al., 2008). Individuals with neurological disease, such as Alzheimer's and Parkinson's diseases, frequently experience sleep disturbance that worsens with the progression of the illness. Sleep disturbance is a major factor contributing to nursing home placement in patients with dementia.

Virtually all psychiatric disorders are associated with sleep disturbance. Nearly all individuals with major depressive disorder or bipolar disorder will report some type of a sleep disturbance over the course of the illness. In addition, there is evidence to demonstrate that sleep disruption itself may be a precipitating factor in triggering mood and other psychiatric disorders and increases the risk to relapse, making the identification and management of sleep disturbance in patients with affective disorders critical. Of special concern is that depressed patients with sleep disturbances demonstrate greater degrees of suicidal ideation.

Sleep disturbance is common in patients with alcoholism, and insomnia occurs in most patients in early recovery and persists for months or even years. Sleep disturbance increases the risk for relapse to alcohol abuse. Targeting sleep disturbance during recovery may support continued abstinence.

EVIDENCE-BASED PRACTICE

Does Gender Impact Nursing Students' Sleep?

Problem

Sleeping problems, such as insomnia, excessive daytime sleepiness, and poor-quality sleep, are common among nursing students and are closely linked with academic performance.

Purpose

This cross-sectional study explored the relationship between sleeping problems and academic performance and to determine if there were any gender-specific effects.

Methods

A total of 492 undergraduate nursing students, 103 male and 389 female, in Indonesia were the sample. Participants completed the following tools: the Pittsburgh Sleep Quality Index (PSQI), Insomnia Severity Index, Epworth Sleepiness Scale, Morningness-Eveningness Questionnaire, and the Beck Depression Inventory. Grade point average was used as a measure of academic performance.

Key Findings

- In male nursing students, the prevalence of poor sleep quality, insomnia, and daytime sleepiness was 66.0%, 45.6%, and 24.3%, respectively.
- In female nursing students, the prevalence of poor sleep quality, insomnia, and daytime sleepiness was 71.5%, 52.4%, and 28.8%, respectively.
- Insomnia in females was the only variable that was significantly associated with poor academic performance.

Implications for Nursing Practice
Sleep disturbances are too common for both male and female nursing students. This study highlights the importance of adequate sleep for everyone, but it seems to be especially true for females. Insomnia is a treatable condition and is seemingly crucial in supporting a strong academic performance. Also, if nurses are to provide quality and non–sleep-impaired care to their patients, they first need to care for themselves.

Dwi Marta, O. F., Kuo, S., Bloomfield, J., Lee, H., Ruhyanudin, F., Poynor, M. Y., et al. (2020). Gender differences in the relationships between sleep disturbances and academic performance among nursing students. *Nurse Education Today*, 85, 104270.

APPLICATION OF THE NURSING PROCESS

Regardless of the clinical environment or the presenting complaint, all patients can benefit from an evaluation of their sleep. Assessment of the patient's sleep allows the nurse to identify short- and long-term health risks associated with sleep disorders and sleep deprivation, provide health teaching and counseling regarding sleep needs, and improve clinical outcomes in patients experiencing a sleep disturbance.

The major focus of this section of the chapter is insomnia. However, you will find helpful information for anyone experiencing a sleep-wake disorder.

ASSESSMENT

General Assessment

Sleep Patterns

Patients frequently do not report sleep difficulties or discuss their sleep-related concerns with care providers. People tend to minimize or adapt to the consequences of sleep disturbance. Furthermore, there is a lack of appreciation about the impact sleep disturbance and sleep deprivation have on overall functioning and health. Many patients do not complain of sleep disturbance directly but rather complain of associated symptoms such as fatigue, decreased concentration, mood disturbance, or physical ailments.

When assessing an individual who has a sleep complaint, it is important to recognize the 24-hour nature of the sleep disturbance. Sleep disturbance is not confined to the 7 or 8 hours devoted to sleep. Sleep diaries (Fig. 19.6) are helpful in identifying sleep patterns and behaviors that may be contributing to the sleep complaint. Assigning the patient the homework of

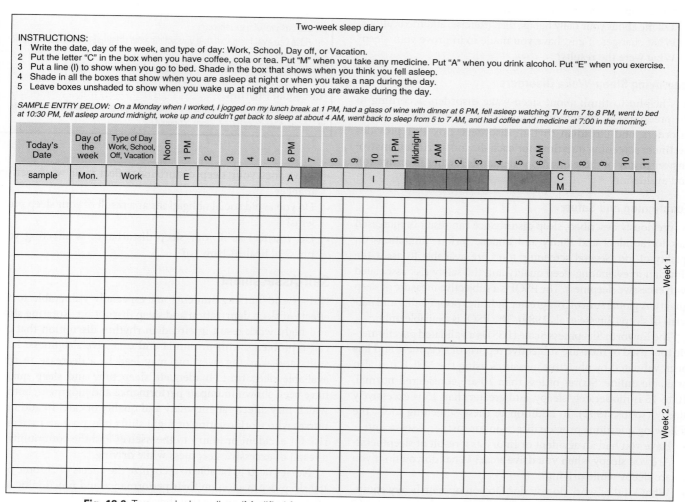

Fig. 19.6 Two-week sleep diary. (Modified from the American Academy of Sleep Medicine. Retrieved from http://www.sleepeducation.com/pdf/sleepdiary.pdf.)

completing a sleep diary for 2 weeks will help guide the assessment and direct the plan of care.

The following questions and comments provide direction for the assessment:

- When did you begin having trouble with sleep? Have you had trouble with sleep in the past?
- Describe your prebedtime routine. What are the activities you customarily engage in before sleep?
- Describe your sleeping environment. Are there things in your sleep environment that are hampering your sleep (such as noise, light, temperature, or overall comfort)?
- Do you use your bedroom for things other than sleep or sexual activity (such as working, eating, or watching television)?
- What time do you go to bed? How long does it take to fall asleep?
- Once asleep, does middle-of-the-night awakening disturb you? If so, what wakes you up? Are you able to return to sleep?
- If you are unable to sleep, what do you do?
- What time do you wake up? What time do you get out of bed?
- How much time do you actually think you sleep?
- Do you sleep longer on weekends or days off?
- Do you nap? If so, for how long? Do you feel refreshed after napping?
- Can you identify any stress or problem that may have initially contributed to your sleep difficulties?
- Tell me about your daily habits, diet, exercise, and medications.
- What changes, if any, have you made to improve your sleep? What were the results?

Identifying Sleep-Wake Disorders

It is helpful to think about sleep-wake disorders according to the predominant symptoms of insomnia, hypersomnia, arousal disorders, and circadian rhythm disorders. Box 19.1 provides pertinent screening questions for each diagnosis. An affirmative answer to any of these questions demands further investigation and evaluation.

Functioning and Safety

As previously described, sleep disturbance can result in increased risk for accident and injury and impose serious limitations on quality of life. Several screening tools are available to assist the clinician in evaluating sleep quality and the safety risk associated with excessive sleepiness. The PSQI is a subjective measure of sleep quality. A global sum of 5 or greater indicates poor quality and patterns of sleep (Buysse et al., 1989). The PSQI is available online.

The Epworth Sleepiness Scale (ESS) is a validated psychometric tool used to measure subjective reports of sleepiness and has been validated by objective measures using the MSLT. It is also available online. Scores of less than 10 are considered normal, 10 to 15 is moderately sleepy, and greater than 15 is excessively sleepy (Johns, 1991). In addition to these screening tools, the following questions provide direction for further assessment:

- Have you had an accident or injury as a result of sleepiness?
- Are you sleepy when you drive a car? What do you do if you are sleepy while driving?
- What kind of work do you do? Do you operate heavy equipment or machinery? How many hours a week do you work? How long is your commute?

BOX 19.1   Sleep Disorders Screening Questions

Insomnia
- Do you have difficulty with falling asleep, staying asleep, or early-morning awakenings?
- Do you feel refreshed and restored in the morning?
- Have you noticed any problems with your energy, mood, concentration, or work quality as a result of your sleep problem?

Hypersomnia
- Obstructive sleep apnea hypopnea syndrome: Have you ever been told that you snore or that it looks as if you stop breathing in your sleep?
- Restless legs syndrome: Do you have an unpleasant or uncomfortable sensation in your legs (or arms) that prevents you from sleeping or wakes you up from sleep and makes you want to move?
- Narcolepsy: Do you have episodes of sleepiness you cannot control? Have you experienced episodes where you were unable to move as you were about to fall asleep or wake up (sleep paralysis)? Unexplained muscle weakness after a strong emotion (cataplexy)? Have you ever seen or heard something that you knew was not real as you were falling asleep or waking up from sleep (hypnogogic hallucination)?
- Primary hypersomnia: Do you ever feel unrested even after an extended sleep period?

Arousal
- Have you ever been told that you have done anything unusual in your sleep, such as walking or talking?
- Have you ever been told that you act out your dreams? (REM sleep behavior disorder)
- Have you been troubled by nightmares or disturbing dreams?

Circadian Rhythm
- Is your desired sleep schedule in conflict with your social and vocational goals?
- What is your preferred sleep schedule?

- How does your sleep disturbance affect your work performance?
- Do you avoid social obligations as a result of your sleep problems?
- Do you feel as if your sleep disturbance is affecting your physical health? How so?

Self-Assessment

Nurses and nursing students are especially vulnerable to the effects of sleep deprivation and sleep disruption. Rotating shifts and night work result in circadian rhythm disruption that can cause problems with insomnia and excessive sleepiness. Long shifts and working overtime may lead to a decrease in total available sleep time. Inadequate sleep time and sleep quality have been shown to impair performance and judgment, both of which may affect patient safety and quality of care. In addition, nurses who work rotating or night shifts may pose an increased risk for accident or injury to themselves and the community as a result of excessive sleepiness while driving.

Nurses need to be able to recognize the effects of chronic partial sleep deprivation on their performance and functioning and take measures to ensure that they are well rested and able to provide safe and competent care. Self-evaluation for a possible sleep disorder and ability to cope with the rigors of shift work is warranted. Consultation with a sleep professional is indicated if there is significant disruption to sleep, physical and mental health, job performance, job satisfaction, and social functioning. Attention to issues of sleep hygiene, limiting overtime, limiting shift work to 8 hours, and obtaining 7 to 8 hours of sleep within a 24-hour period are essential for personal, patient, and community safety.

NURSING DIAGNOSIS

There are several specific International Classification for Nursing Practice (ICNP) (International Council of Nurses, 2019) nursing diagnoses for sleep disturbances. They are *insomnia, hypersomnia, sleep deprivation, risk for impaired sleep, impaired sleep, nightmares, sleep walking, risk for apnea,* and *apnea.*

OUTCOMES IDENTIFICATION

Outcomes are aimed at improving or reducing the risk for the problem or the problem itself. Table 19.2 provides signs and symptoms, nursing diagnoses, and short-term and long-term indicators for these categories.

PLANNING

The majority of patients with sleep disorders are treated in the community. The exceptions are cases in which the patient has a primary psychiatric disorder or a medical condition that requires hospitalization. Because long-standing sleep problems are associated with significant occupational, social, interpersonal, psychiatric, and medical conditions, the treatment is multifaceted and frequently requires a team approach under the leadership of a sleep disorder specialist. The role of the nurse is generally to conduct a full assessment, provide support to the patient and family while the appropriate interventions are determined, and teach the patient and family strategies that may improve sleep.

IMPLEMENTATION

Counseling

The nurse's counseling role begins with the assessment of the sleep disorder. The nurse's questions and responses provide support to the patient and family, as well as assurance that the sleep problems are amenable to treatment. The distress caused by chronic sleep difficulties results in hopelessness for many patients. Through the nurse's counseling approach, this hopelessness is identified and countered with encouragement, positive suggestions, and the belief that the patient will be able to manage sleep difficulties.

Health Teaching and Health Promotion

The nurse's role in health teaching cannot be overemphasized. Many people minimize the importance of their sleep and even boast about how little sleep they need to get by. This means that they also do not recognize the importance of a sleep routine or consider factors that influence good sleep. In addition, there are many myths regarding what constitutes "good sleep" and what factors contribute to sleep quality (Box 19.2). The nurse may also be involved in teaching relaxation techniques such as meditation, guided imagery, progressive muscle relaxation, or controlled breathing exercises. Use of these techniques has been linked to sustained benefits for patients with primary insomnia.

Modifying poor sleep habits and establishing a regular sleep-wake schedule can be accomplished using sleep diaries (see Fig. 19.6). As previously mentioned, a period of 2 weeks is helpful in establishing overall sleep patterns and determining overall sleep efficiency ([time in bed divided by total sleep time] × 100). After reviewing sleep diaries, patients are sometimes surprised to discover that their sleep problems are not as bad as previously believed.

Sleep restriction, or limiting the total sleep time, creates a temporary mild state of sleep deprivation and strengthens

BOX 19.2 Sleep Hygiene

- Maintain a regular sleep-wake schedule.
- Develop a presleep routine that signals the end of the day.
- Reserve the bedroom for sleep and a place for intimacy.
- Create an environment that is conducive to sleep (taking into consideration light, temperature, and clothing).
- Avoid clock watching.
- Limit caffeinated beverages to one or two a day and none in the evening.
- Avoid heavy meals before bedtime.
- Use alcohol cautiously and avoid use for several hours before bed.
- Avoid daytime napping.
- Exercise daily, but not right before bed.

TABLE 19.2 Signs and Symptoms, Diagnoses, and Outcomes for Sleep Disorders

Signs and Symptoms	Nursing Diagnoses	Outcomes
Absenteeism, changes in affect and energy; reports changes in mood, quality of life, concentration, and sleep; reports lack of energy, sleep disturbances, early wakening	Insomnia	Improved sleep: Successful sleep induction, appropriate hours of sleep, consistent sleep pattern, minimal awakening
Acute confusion, agitation, anxiety, apathy, fatigue, poor concentration, irritability, lethargy, malaise, perceptual disorders, slowed reaction	Sleep deprivation	Adequate quantity of sleep: Balance between work and sleep, minimal awakening, feeling restored after sleep, sleeping between 7 and 9 h on average
Changes in normal sleep pattern, decreased ability to function, dissatisfaction with sleep, awakening, no difficulty falling asleep, not feeling well rested	Impaired sleep	Adequate quantity and quality of sleep: Minimal awakening, feeling restored after sleep

International Council of Nursing Practice. (2019). *ICNP browser*. Retrieved from https://www.icn.ch/what-we-do/projects/ehealth/icnp-browser.
ICNP® is owned and copyrighted by the International Council of Nurses (ICN). Reproduced with permission of the copyright holder.

the sleep homeostatic drive. This helps decrease sleep latency and improves sleep continuity and quality. If, for example, a sleep diary indicates that your patient is in bed for 8 hours but sleeping only 6 hours, sleep is restricted to 6 hours, and the bedtime and wake time are adjusted accordingly. The sleep time should not be reduced below 5 hours, regardless of sleep efficiency, and patients should be cautioned about the dangers of sleepiness with driving while undergoing a trial of sleep restriction. Once sleep efficiency is improved, total sleep time is gradually increased by 10- to 20-minute increments.

EVALUATION

Evaluation is based on whether or not the patient experiences improved sleep quality as evidenced by decreased sleep latency, fewer nighttime awakenings, a shorter time to get back to sleep after awakening, and improvement in daytime symptoms of sleepiness. This evaluation is accomplished through patient report and patient maintenance of a sleep diary. Just as important as objective changes in the patient's sleep pattern is the patient's perception that there has been an improvement. Objectively, the improvement may be quite modest, but the patient may no longer feel *controlled by* sleep, but instead has *control over* sleep through lifestyle changes and a better sleep routine.

TREATMENT MODALITIES

Successful treatment of insomnia involves an integration of the basic principles of sleep hygiene (conditions and practices that promote continuous and effective sleep), behavioral therapies, and, in some instances, the use of hypnotic medication.

Biological Treatments

Pharmacotherapy

Generally, long-term sleeping pill use is discouraged because nonpharmacological treatments have shown superior efficacy in reducing insomnia. Other classifications of drugs used for insomnia are antidepressants, anticonvulsants, and antihistamines, which are used off-label without specific approval from the FDA. Second-generation antipsychotics improve sleep in people using them as indicated for other problems, such as schizophrenia. Table 19.3 provides an overview of pharmacological treatment of insomnia.

Hypnotic medication is always used with caution, and over-the-counter sleeping aids have limited effectiveness. Melatonin, a naturally occurring hormone, is a popular over-the-counter

TABLE 19.3 FDA-Approved Drugs for Insomnia

Generic (Trade) Name	Onset of Action (Min.)	Duration of Action	USE IN INSOMNIA		
			DFA	DMS	Habit Forming
Benzodiazepines					
Estazolam (ProSom)	15–60	Intermediate	✓	✓	Yes; all drugs in this class are schedule IV
Flurazepam (Dalmane)[a]	30–60	Long	✓	✓	
Quazepam (Doral)[a]	20–45	Long	✓	✓	
Temazepam (Restoril)	45–60	Intermediate	–	✓	
Triazolam (Halcion)	15–30	Short	✓	–	
Nonbenzodiazepine Receptor Agonists					
Eszopiclone (Lunesta)	60	Intermediate	✓	✓	Yes; all drugs in this class are schedule IV
Zaleplon (Sonata)	15–30	Ultra Short	✓	–	
Zolpidem					
Immediate release (Ambien)	30	Short	✓	–	
Immediate release (Intermezzo)[b]	30	Short	–	✓	
Extended release (Ambien CR)	30	Intermediate	✓	✓	
Melatonin Receptor Agonists					
Ramelteon (Rozerem)	30	Short	✓	–	No
Orexin Receptor Antagonists					
Lemborexant (Dayvigo)	15–20	Intermediate	✓	✓	Yes; schedule IV
Suvorexant (Belsomra)	30	Intermediate	✓	✓	Yes; schedule IV
Tricyclic Antidepressant					
Doxepin (Silenor)	>60	Intermediate	–	✓	No

DFA, Difficulty falling asleep; *DMS*, difficulty maintaining sleep.

[a]Because of its long duration of action, this drug is generally not recommended.

[b]A sublingual taken in the middle of the night when there are at least 4 hours left to sleep.

US Food and Drug Administration. (2020). Drugs@FDA: FDA-approved drugs. Retrieved from https://www.accessdata.fda.gov/scripts/cder/daf/.

product. To date, there are few data to support its use in the management of insomnia disorder, but new research into prolonged-release forms of melatonin are demonstrating some promise.

Somatic Interventions

Functional magnetic resonance imaging studies indicate that the prefrontal cortex is overly active with insomnia. Racing thoughts interfere with the individual's ability to sleep. The Cerêve Sleep System has FDA approval and significantly reduced sleep latency from stage 1 to stage 2 in clinical trials. It is a software-controlled bedside device that is placed on the forehead. A fluid-filled pad cools the forehead and reduces activity in the cerebral cortex.

Psychological Therapies

Advanced practice psychiatric–mental health nurses are qualified to conduct psychotherapy. A specific type of cognitive behavioral therapy (CBT) for insomnia (CBT-I) has been developed. Educational, behavioral, and cognitive components target factors that perpetuate insomnia over time (Morin, 2004). The first objectives are to provide education regarding sleep and sleep needs and to help the patient to set realistic expectations regarding sleep. Patients should be asked what they believe constitutes healthy sleep and have any misconceptions clarified. Determining the total number of hours spent sleeping typically has little value. Many patients are stuck on a set number of sleep hours rather than on the quality of sleep obtained. Focusing on the number of hours slept rather than the quality of sleep and daytime functioning increases the insomnia experience.

Stimulus control is a behavioral intervention that involves some interventions previously discussed with sleep hygiene. Adherence to five basic principles that decrease the negative associations between the bed and bedroom and strengthen the stimulus for sleep is essential. Patients should be instructed to:
1. Go to bed only when sleepy.
2. Use the bed or bedroom only for sleep and intimacy (no television, reading, or other activities in the bedroom).
3. Get out of bed if unable to sleep and engage in a quiet-time activity, such as reading or crossword puzzles (no television, work, or computer).
4. Maintain a regular sleep-wake schedule, with getting up at the same time each day being the most important factor.
5. Avoid daytime napping. If napping is necessary to avoid accident or injury, it should be limited to 20 to 30 minutes maximum, and a timer should be set.

Other objectives of CBT-I are aimed at identifying and correcting maladaptive attitudes and beliefs about sleep that perpetuate insomnia. For example, patients frequently amplify the consequences of their insomnia and attribute most daytime experiences to their sleep complaint. They may rationalize maladaptive coping behaviors such as excessive time in bed to "catch up" on lost sleep and may exhibit unrealistic expectations about sleep. The nurse offers alternative interpretations regarding the sleep complaint to assist the patient to think about insomnia in a different way, empowering the patient to be in control of sleep. Because CBT-I approaches are not immediately effective and may take several weeks of practice before improvement is seen, success is dependent on both a high degree of motivation in patients and a commitment on the part of the practitioner.

KEY POINTS TO REMEMBER

- Sleep disturbance has major implications for overall health, quality of life, and personal and community safety.
- Research into the physiology of normal sleep, as well as sleep disorders, is expanding.
- Virtually all patients with a mood disorder will report sleep disturbance; recognition and treatment of sleep disturbance in patients with psychiatric disorders improves clinical outcomes.

- Regardless of the clinical environment or the presenting complaint, all patients can benefit from an evaluation of their sleep needs.
- Primary insomnia can be effectively treated with nonpharmacological interventions such as CBT-I, sleep restriction, stimulus control, and attention to issues of sleep hygiene. Long-term pharmacological management is generally not indicated.

CRITICAL THINKING

1. Anthony is a 46-year-old who complains of waking frequently at night. Consequently, he is tired all day and knows that he has not been functioning as well as he should. Whenever he can manage it, he goes out to his car at lunchtime to take a 60-minute nap, because he has fallen asleep at his desk and been given a disciplinary warning. He is drinking 2 to 3 cups of coffee in the afternoon so that he does not feel sleepy while driving home.
   a. What questions would you ask to determine if Anthony might have a sleep disorder?
   b. What recommendations will you make to improve his sleep hygiene?

   c. What instructions and education should you give this patient regarding personal and community safety?
2. Your patient, Vivian, has been using temazepam (Restoril) for several years to treat insomnia. She has been reading that long-term use of hypnotics is not healthy or productive and wants to quit taking them. However, she is focused on needing 9 hours of sleep each night and is extremely worried about what will happen when she discontinues the temazepam.
   a. What instructions would you provide to Vivian regarding stimulus control, sleep restriction, and cognitive restructuring of her sleep complaint?

b. Identify alternative pharmacological therapies.

3. Mrs. Levine is a 72-year-old woman with a history of major depressive disorder. She takes fluoxetine (Prozac) and has experienced significant relief from depression. While reviewing her medications, she tells you she is using a variety of over-the-counter (OTC) sleep aids because she has been having some difficulty sleeping recently. These OTC products include diphenhydramine, melatonin, valerian, and something that her neighbor gave her to try.

a. In light of the patient's age and history of depression, what are your concerns?

b. What further assessment is required?

c. What specific question would you need to ask concerning her use of Prozac?

d. What instructions and education will you provide?

CHAPTER REVIEW

1. Which patient statement supports a diagnosis of narcolepsy?
   a. "My wife tells me I snore at night."
   b. "I sleepwalk several nights a week."
   c. "I have no control over when I fall asleep."
   d. "My legs feel funny, and that keeps me awake."

2. Madelyn, a 29-year-old patient recently diagnosed with major depressive disorder, comes to the mental health clinic complaining of continued difficulty sleeping. One week ago, she was started on a selective serotonin reuptake inhibitor (SSRI), fluoxetine (Prozac), for her depressive symptoms. When educating Madelyn, your response is guided by the knowledge that:
   a. SSRIs such as fluoxetine more commonly cause hypersomnolence as opposed to difficulty sleeping.
   b. The sleep problem is caused by the depression and is unrelated to the medication.
   c. The neurotransmitters involved in sleep and wakefulness are the same neurotransmitters targeted by many psychiatric medications and may be affecting her sleep.
   d. The medication should be discontinued since sleep is the most important element to her recovery.

3. Which behaviors will the nurse encourage a patient diagnosed with insomnia disorder to adopt? *Select all that apply.*
   a. Avoiding exercising at bedtime
   b. Avoiding napping during the day
   c. Eating a hearty snack at bedtime
   d. Getting up at the same time each day
   e. Moving the clock so it is not visible from the bed

4. Which treatment is typically prescribed for primary insomnia? *Select all that apply.*
   a. Cognitive behavioral therapy–insomnia (CBT-I)
   b. Intravenous medication for sedation
   c. Stimulus control
   d. Sleep restriction
   e. Sleep hygiene measures

5. Light projected into the retina is believed to trigger changes in sleep patterns and quality of sleep. Therefore, the nurse should suggest:
   a. Not reading within an hour of bedtime.
   b. Exercising before bedtime in a darkened environment.
   c. Limiting use of electronic devices in the hour before bedtime.
   d. Dimming the screen on cellphones and computers in the evening.

6. Sleep disturbances are often overlooked or undiagnosed due to:
   a. A lack of formal nurse and physician training in sleep disturbances.
   b. Patients not often accurately describing sleep disturbance patterns.
   c. The belief that sleep disturbance is a necessary part of hospitalization.
   d. Patients hiding the fact that they have issues with sleep.

7. Many people allow life circumstances to dictate their amount of sleep instead of recognizing sleep as a priority. Which statement will the nurse recognize as progress in the patient's sleep hygiene program?
   a. "I go to bed even if I am not sleepy, hoping I will fall asleep."
   b. "I have one glass of red wine at bedtime each night."
   c. "I take a nap each day to 'catch up' on my sleep deficit."
   d. "I have removed the television from my bedroom."

8. Larry is a 50-year-old man who works about 60 hours per week. He arrives at the clinic seeking assistance with a weight gain of 50 pounds over the past year. Larry admits to sleeping 4 to 5 hours a night. The nurse recognizes that the weight gain may be related to:
   a. A new onset of diabetes.
   b. Suspected cardiovascular disease.
   c. Dysregulation of hormones that influence appetite.
   d. Comorbidity of depression with obesity.

9. Sleep deprivation is considered a safety issue that results in loss of life and property. Psychomotor impairments of sleep deprivation are similar to symptoms caused by:
   a. Sleeping in excess of 10 hours.
   a. Misuse of caffeine products.
   c. Alcohol consumption.
   d. Working more than 40 hours per week.

10. The stage of sleep known as rapid eye movement or REM sleep is characterized by atonia and myoclonic twitches in addition to the actual rapid movement of the eyes. Atonia is thought to be a protective mechanism as it:
    a. Limits physical movements.
    b. Prevents nightmares.
    c. Enhances the dream state.
    d. Regulates the autonomic nervous system.

1. **c**; 2. **c**; 3. **a, b, d, e**; 4. **a, c, d, e**; 5. **c**; 6. **a**; 7. **d**; 8. **c**; 9. **c**; 10. **a**

NGN CASE STUDY AND QUESTIONS

Joshua is a 45-year-old man who has no trouble going to sleep but wakes between 1:00 and 3:00 a.m. and has difficulty going back to sleep. He admits being anxious about current events and to spending "too much time" arguing with friends and family members on social media in the evening. He then wakes up during the night worrying and watches TV until he can fall back asleep. Because he has a history of intermittent depression, his partner has urged him to stop watching the news and to limit his social media participation. Assessment data show normal vital signs and a body mass index of 27.

The patient's partner reports that Joshua's snoring is most alarming because it is followed by intervals of not breathing. The patient reports that he gets sleepy at his desk during the day, so he uses his lunch hour to take a nap. He admits to loss of concentration when trying to work. "I read the same stuff over and over again and can't take it in." When asked how long he thinks he sleeps at night, he says, "probably 4 hours a night on average."

1. Choose the *most likely* options to complete the following statement.

    Because of this patient's partner's observations, this patient is most likely to benefit from ____1____ which involves ____2____ in order to ___3___.

Options for 1	Options for 2	Options for 3
a. Polysomnography	**a.** A wristwatch-type tracker to record body movement over a period of time	**a.** Measure daytime sleepiness in a sleep-conducive setting
b. Multiple sleep latency test (MSLT)	**b.** A monitored daytime nap	**b.** Document daytime alertness

Options for 1	Options for 2	Options for 3
c. Actigraphy	**c.** Overnight use of electrodes and monitors	**c.** Evaluate sleep patterns and circadian rhythm
d. Maintenance of wakefulness test (MWT)	**d.** A low-light video camera to monitor patient's ability to remain awake midday	**d.** Record brain wave activity, eye movement, muscle tone, heart rhythm, and breathing

Testing shows that Joshua has borderline mild sleep apnea. He is instructed in good sleep hygiene, but no further action will be taken at this time. The patient will be assessed again in nine months for possible continuous positive airway pressure (CPAP) interventions. In the meantime, Joshua and the treatment team will focus on developing better sleep hygiene to counteract insomnia.

2. Which recommendation will the nurse be *most likely* to discuss with the healthcare provider to incorporate into this patient's plan of care right now? *Select all that apply.*
   a. Iron supplementation
   b. Long-term benzodiazepine therapy
   c. Engagement in cognitive-behavioral therapy for insomnia (CBT-I)
   d. Sleep restriction
   e. Stimulus control
   f. Administration of methylphenidate or modafinil (Provigil)

NGN case study answers are on Evolve.

Visit the Evolve website for a posttest on the content in this chapter: http://evolve.elsevier.com/Varcarolis

REFERENCES

American Academy of Sleep Medicine. (2016). *Economic impact of obstructive sleep apnea.* Retrieved from https://j2vjt3dnbra3ps7ll1clb4q2-wpengine.netdna-ssl.com/wp-content/uploads/2017/10/sleep-apnea-economic-crisis.pdf.

American Psychiatric Association. (2013). *Diagnostic and statistical manual of mental disorders* (5th ed.). Washington, DC: Author.

Arun, S., Sathiamma, S., & Bindu, K. (2014). Current understanding on the neurobiology of sleep and wakefulness. *International Journal of Clinical and Experimental Psychology, 1*(1), 3–9.

Birbiglia, M. (2010). *Sleepwalk with me.* New York, NY: Simon and Schuster.

Bliwise, D. (2011). Normal aging. In M. Kryger, T. Roth, & W. Dement (Eds.), *Principles and practice of sleep medicine* (5th ed.). Philadelphia, PA: Saunders.

Buysse, D. J., Reynolds, C. F., III, Monk, T. H., Berman, S. R., & Kupfer, D. J. (1989). The Pittsburgh Sleep Quality Index: A new instrument for psychiatric practice and research. *Psychiatry Research, 28*(2), 193–213.

Cappuccio, E., Miller, M., & Lockley, S. (2010). *Sleep, health, and society: From aetiology to public health.* Oxford, UK; New York, NY: Oxford University Press.

Carney, R., Berry, R., & Geyer, J. (2011). *Clinical sleep disorders* (2nd ed.). Philadelphia, PA: Lippincott Williams & Wilkins.

Centers for Disease Control. (2010). Youth risk behavior surveillance—United States, 2009. *Morbidity and Mortality Weekly Report, 59*(SS-5), 1–142.

Czeisler, C., Buxton, O., & Khalsa, S. (2011). The human circadian system and sleep-wake regulation. In M. Kryger, T. Roth, & W. Dement (Eds.), *Principles and practice of sleep medicine* (5th ed.). Philadelphia, PA: Saunders.

Hafner, M., Stepanek, M., Taylor, J., Troxel, W. M., & van Stolk, C. (2016). *Why sleep matters: The economic costs of insufficient sleep.* Retrieved from rand_rr1791.pdf.

Huang, T., & Redline, S. (2019). Cross-sectional and prospective associations of actigraphy-assessed sleep regularity with metabolic abnormalities: The multi-ethnic study of atherosclerosis. *Epidemiology/Health Services Research, 42*(8), 1422–1429.

Hubner, A., Krafft, A., Gadient, S., Werth, E., Zimmermann, R., & Bassetti, C. L. (2013). Characteristics and determinants of restless legs syndrome in pregnancy. *Neurology, 80*(8), 738–742.

Institute of Medicine. (2006). *Sleep disorders and sleep deprivation: An unmet public health problem.* Washington, DC: The National Academies Press.

Insurance Institute for Highway Safety. (2012). *DUI/DWI laws.* Retrieved from http://www.iihs.org/laws/dui.aspx.

International Council of Nurses. (2019). *International Classification for Nursing Practice catalog.* Retrieved from https://www.icn.ch/sites/default/files/inline-files/ICNP2019-DC.pdf.

Jiménez-Jiménez, F. J., Alonso-Navarro, H., Garcia-Martin, E., & Agundez, J. A. G. (2018). Genetics of restless legs syndrome: An update. *Sleep Medicine Reviews, 39,* 108–121.

Johns, M. W. (1991). A new method for measuring daytime sleepiness: The Epworth Sleepiness Scale. *Sleep, 14,* 540–545.

Morin, C. (2004). Cognitive-behavioral approaches to the treatment of insomnia. *Journal of Clinical Psychiatry, 65*(Suppl. 16), 33–40.

Nascimento-Ferreira, M. V., Cesar, A., DeMoraes, F. L., Torres-Leal, & Carvalho, H. B. (2020). Modulation and consequences of sleep duration in child obesity. In R. R. Watson, & V. R. Preedy (Eds.), *Neurological modulation of sleep* (pp. 95–101). London, UK: Academic Press.

National Sleep Foundation. (2011). *2011 NSF Sleep in America Poll.* Retrieved from https://sleepfoundation.org/sites/default/files/sleepinamericapoll/SIAP_2011_Summary_of_Findings.pdf.

National Sleep Foundation. (2020). *Can you change your circadian rhythm.* Retrieved from https://www.sleepfoundation.org/circadian-rhythm/can-you-change-your-circadian-rhythm.

Sadock, B. J., Sadock, V. A., & Ruiz, P. (2015). *Kaplan and Sadock's synopsis of psychiatry.* Philadelphia, PA: Wolters Kluwer.

Spielman, A., & Glovinsky, P. (2004). A conceptual framework of insomnia for primary care providers: Predisposing, precipitating, and perpetuating factors. *Sleep Medicine Alert, 9*(1), 1–6.

Tracova, R., Dorkova, Z., Molcanyiova, A., Radikova, Z., Klimes, I., & Tkac, I. (2008). Cardiovascular risk and insulin resistance in patients with obstructive sleep apnea. *Medical Science Monitor, 14*(9), CR438–CR444.

Zandi, A. S., Quddus, A., Prest, L., & Comeau, F. J. E. (2019). Non-intrusive detection of drowsy driving based on eye tracking data. *Transportation Journal, 2673*(6), 247–257.

Zhou, L., Yu, K., Yang, L., Wang, H., Xiao, Y., Qiu, G., & Zhang, X. (2019). Sleep duration, midday napping, and sleep quality and incident stroke. *Neurology, 94*(4), e345–e356.

20

Sexual Dysfunction, Gender Dysphoria, and Paraphilic Disorders

Margaret Jordan Halter

 Visit the Evolve website for a pretest on the content in this chapter: http://evolve.elsevier.com/Varcarolis

OBJECTIVES

1. Describe the four phases of the sexual response cycle.
2. Describe clinical manifestations of each major sexual dysfunction.
3. Consider the impact of medical problems and medications on normal sexual functioning.
4. Describe biological and cognitive factors related to sexual dysfunction.
5. Apply the nursing process to caring for individuals with sexual dysfunction.
6. Discuss the importance of nurses being knowledgeable about and comfortable discussing topics pertaining to sexuality.
7. Describe pharmacological treaments and psychological therapies available for sexual dysfunction.
8. Identify the clinical picture of gender dysphoria in children and adults.
9. Describe general nursing care and support for people with gender dysphoria.
10. Discuss biological treatment (e.g., pharmacotherapy, surgical intervention) and psychological therapy for gender dysphoria.
11. Identify sexual preoccupations considered to be paraphilic disorders.
12. Discuss personal values and biases regarding sexuality and sexual behaviors.
13. Develop a plan of care for individuals diagnosed with sexual disorders.
14. Discuss treatment modalities for individuals with paraphilic disorders.

KEY TERMS AND CONCEPTS

asexuality
gender identity

sex reassignment surgery
sexual dysfunction

sexual response cycle

The practice of professional nursing requires us to engage in matter-of-fact discussions with patients regarding topics generally considered to be extremely private and personal. We perform head-to-toe assessments during which we inquire about everything from headaches and sore throats to difficulties urinating and problems with constipation. The realities of providing physical care necessitate becoming comfortable with a number of skills that concern privacy and modesty, such as performing breast examinations, initiating urinary catheters, and inserting rectal medications.

Despite a sort of learned fearlessness when it comes to addressing other intimate issues, the topic of sexuality is often a source of discomfort not only for nurses but also other healthcare providers. Although most of us recognize that addressing sexuality is part of holistic care, many do not routinely include the topic when they are doing assessments. Nursing curricula typically have a deficiency in training nurses in the fundamentals of sexuality and nursing care. Patients want to know how, for example, medications or treatments will affect their relationships and ability to have satisfying sex lives. Nurses can normalize such issues and foster opportunities to address feelings and fears.

Views regarding sexuality are based on our individual beliefs about ourselves as women and men, mothers and fathers, and generative individuals who create and give to society. Multiple factors—including societal attitudes and traditions, parental views, cultural practices, spiritual and religious teaching, socioeconomic status, and education—affect our sexual beliefs and behaviors and also our attitudes toward the sexual behaviors of others, including our patients.

Health promotion and disease prevention are key responsibilities for nurses. Nurses should be educated to assess a patient's sexuality and be prepared to educate, dispel myths, assist with values clarification, refer to appropriate care providers when indicated, and share resources. These actions can alleviate or decrease patient illness and suffering and reduce healthcare costs through prevention. As a nursing student, you are introduced to complex aspects of sexual behavior that should help facilitate thoughtful discussion of the topic, make you aware of your personal beliefs, and help you consider the broader perspective of sexual issues as they exist in contemporary society.

This chapter addresses two general categories related to sexuality. In the first half of the chapter, we examine the normal sexual response cycle, clinical disorders related to the disruption or malfunction of this cycle, and guidelines for nursing care. In the second half of the chapter, we focus on problems related to sexual preoccupation. These problems may be sources of discomfort and distress to the person experiencing them (e.g., gender dysphoria) and may be a source of pain and trauma for others whose rights are violated (e.g., pedophilia).

SEXUALITY

Phases of the Sexual Response Cycle

Before looking more closely at sexual dysfunctions, we will first review the **sexual response cycle**. According to the early experts in sexuality and sexual functioning, Masters and Johnson (1966), there are four distinct phases:

- Phase 1: Desire
- Phase 2: Excitement
- Phase 3: Orgasm
- Phase 4: Resolution

Desire

Many factors may affect interest in sexual activity, including age, physical and emotional health, availability of a sexual partner, and the context of an individual's life. In fact, for a number of individuals, the lack of sexual desire is not a source of distress either to the person or the partner. In such a situation, decreased or absent sexual desire is not viewed as an illness. Furthermore, desire is not a necessary component of sexual functioning.

 CONSIDERING CULTURE

Female Genital Mutilation and Sexual Functioning

Female genital mutilation (FGM) is the surgical altering of female sexual organs for nonmedical reasons. The World Health Organization (2016) condemns this practice, as does the United Nations. An estimated 100 to 140 million females are currently living with the consequences of this surgery, which occurs between birth and 15 years of age. It is performed to decrease libido (ensuring chastity and fidelity to spouses), prevent premarital sex, uphold a cultural tradition, or make the girl more feminine and beautiful by removing parts that are considered "male."

The actual practice of FGM varies depending on what structures are removed or altered.

Type 1: *Clitoridectomy.* Partial or total removal of the clitoris.

Type 2: *Excision.* Partial or total removal of the clitoris and the labia minora with or without excision of the labia majora.

Type 3: *Infibulation.* The most extreme form of FGM involves the removal of all external genitalia and stitching the labia together. A small opening allows for urination and menstruation.

Type 4: All other harmful nonmedical procedures to genitalia include pricking, piercing, incising, scraping, and cauterizing.

The surgery is often done ritualistically and in unsanitary conditions with a razor blade that may be reused. The immediate effects are severe pain and infection. Afterward, girls and women suffer recurrent urinary tract infections, cysts, infertility, and childbirth complications. Clitoridectomy results in altered sexual responsiveness. Sexual activity is often associated with dyspareunia (painful intercourse).

The procedure occurs mainly in Africa, the Middle East, and Asia. It is increasingly protested and restricted by law, leading in some families to take their daughters abroad for "vacation cutting." Some US doctors suggest that parents should be allowed to have their daughters' genitals ritually nicked to prevent more extreme versions of FGM (Arora & Jacobs, 2016).

Clinicians in the United States also encounter females who have already undergone these procedures. Few healthcare providers are prepared to deal with these mutilation and sexual problems. Developing a trusting relationship with patients who have been subjected to this custom includes understanding the type of mutilation as well as the culture in which it occurs.

Adapted from Arora, K. S., & Jacobs, A. J. (2016). Female genital alteration: A compromise solution. *Journal of Medical Ethics, 42(3),* 148–154. World Health Organization. (2016). *Female genital mutilation.* Retrieved from http://www.who.int/(3)mediacentre/factsheets/fs241/en/.

According to Levine (2010), there are three components to desire: drive, motive, and values. He refers to *drive* as the biologically motivated interest based in the cerebral cortex and the limbic and endocrine systems that prompts a focus on the sexually appealing aspects of another, physiological response, and plotting for connection. *Motive* is less physiological and more psychological and is based on choices, aspirations, and motives for interpersonal connection. This is the area that clinicians often target for intervention. *Values* impact sexuality by imparting certain familial, religious, and cultural beliefs and guidelines for responses and behaviors. It is a significant part of an individual's programming beginning in adolescence. For adults, these values are fairly enduring, but they may shift depending on other motivations.

Invariably there is a difference in sex drive within a relationship, and negotiations almost always occur. Low sexual desire may be a source of frustration, both for the one experiencing it and also for the partner. It is sometimes associated with psychiatric or medical conditions. Conversely, excessive sexual desire becomes a problem when it creates difficulties for the partner or when such excessive desire drives the person to demand sexual compliance from a partner or to force it on an unwilling one.

Testosterone, normally present in the circulation of both males and females but at a much higher level in males, appears to be essential to sexual desire in both men and women. Estrogen does not seem to have a direct effect on sexual desire in women. A secondary effect, however, may be present in the requirement of estrogen for the maintenance of normal vaginal elasticity and lubrication.

Excitement

The excitement phase of the normal human sexual response cycle is that period of time during which sexual tension continues to increase from the preceding level of sexual desire. Traditionally, penile erection and vaginal lubrication have been used as indicators of the presence of sexual excitement. If erection or lubrication does not occur in what, for that individual, is a sexually stimulating and appropriate situation, then there has been an inhibition of sexual excitement regardless of the causative factors.

Orgasm

The orgasm phase of the human sexual response cycle is attained only at high levels of sexual tension in both women and men. Sexual tension (also described as sexual arousal) is produced by a combination of mental activity—including thoughts, fantasies, and dreams—and erotic stimulation of erogenous areas, which may be more or less specific for each individual. Most men require some penile stimulation and most women some clitoral stimulation, either directly or indirectly, to produce the high levels of sexual tension necessary for orgasm to occur.

Some women who have experienced one orgasm may have repeated orgasms during the continuation of the same sexual activity. The occurrence of multiple orgasms depends on the maintenance of high levels of sexual tension through continued stimulation. On the other hand, once men ejaculate as a part of orgasm, they go through a refractory period. This is the time required to produce another ejaculate, which varies primarily with age. In a young man, this refractory period is measured in minutes, whereas in an older man it may last several hours.

Resolution

During the resolution phase, sexual tension developed in prior phases subsides to baseline levels provided that sexual stimulation has ceased. The physiological changes that occurred during the earlier phases of the response cycle now tend to dissipate. This is a period of psychological vulnerability and can either be experienced as a period of pleasurable afterglow or described as being uncomfortably emotionally exposed. With the restoration of normal pulse, respiratory rate, and blood pressure, individuals frequently experience increased perspiration.

SEXUAL DYSFUNCTION

Sexual dysfunction is an extremely common problem that involves the disturbance in the desire, excitement, or orgasm phases of the sexual response cycle or pain during sexual intercourse. It may prevent or reduce a person's ability to enjoy sex and can be classified according to the phase of the sexual response cycle in which it occurs. In evaluating a patient with a sexual dysfunction, a physical assessment—including laboratory studies—is performed before exploring psychological factors such as emotional issues, life situation, and experiences. Sexual dysfunctions can be the result of physiological problems, interpersonal conflicts, or a combination of both. Stress of any kind can adversely affect sexual function.

Clinical Picture

Seven major classes of sexual dysfunction include the following:
- Female sexual interest/arousal disorder
- Male hypoactive sexual desire disorder
- Erectile disorder
- Female orgasmic disorder
- Delayed ejaculation
- Premature ejaculation
- Genitopelvic pain/penetration disorder

Sexual dysfunction may be a lifelong problem or acquired. Some individuals have problems from sexual maturity onward. Conversely, some individuals have normal sexual functioning and then experience a disturbance in functioning. Also, sexual dysfunction can be generalized or situational. Some people have a generalized sexual dysfunction no matter the type of stimulation, situation, or partner. For others, the dysfunction is situational and depends on the type of stimulation, situation, or partner.

In addition to these disorders and conditions, there is substance/medication-induced dysfunction and sexual dysfunction that is not classified (American Psychiatric Association [APA], 2013).

It is important to note that individuals may not have a desire for sexual relations. This is called asexuality, which may be a distinct form of sexual orientation. Asexuality is different from celibacy, which is a conscious choice to abstain from sex even though the desire is there. Asexuality is experiencing no sexual attraction, although there may be romantic interest. If being straight, or heterosexual, is attraction to the opposite sex and being gay or lesbian is the attraction to the same sex, then asexuality describes the preference for no sexual attraction. People who are asexual may have an interest in cuddling and physical contact but no interest in sex, and asexual individuals may be in relationships and negotiate for sex or simply do without.

Sexual Desire Disorders

Female sexual interest/arousal disorder. The female version of low sexual desire includes the descriptors *interest* and *arousal*. This combination places the disorder across both the "desire" and "excitement" categories (see the following section). **Female sexual interest/arousal disorder** is characterized by emotional distress caused by absent or reduced interest in sexual fantasies, sexual activity, pleasure, and arousal. Some women experience these symptoms their whole lives, whereas others may gradually become less interested in sexual activity. The symptoms must be present for at least 6 months for a woman to be diagnosed with this disorder.

Reasons for the disorder may be clear, such as having an abusive mate. In other cases, it is a baffling problem to both the woman and her partner. The cause may be a combination of neurobiological, hormonal, and psychosocial factors. Dopamine, progesterone, estrogen, and testosterone play an excitatory role, whereas serotonin, prolactin, and opioids inhibit sexual desire.

Sexual desire may decrease with age, in women particularly after menopause. The incidence of female sexual disinterest/arousal is thought to be fairly widespread, although exact prevalence rates are not available. However, a disorder is diagnosed only with this criterion: "the symptoms … cause clinically significant distress in the individual." When distress is factored in, prevalence estimates are markedly lower (APA, 2013, p. 435).

Comorbid conditions associated with decreased sexual desire in women are depression, thyroid problems, anxiety, and urinary incontinence. Pain from medical problems such as arthritis and inflammatory bowel conditions is also associated with reduced interest and arousal.

Male hypoactive sexual desire disorder. The male version of low interest in sex is called **male hypoactive sexual desire disorder**. It is characterized by a deficiency or absence of sexual fantasies or desire for sexual activity. For a man to be diagnosed with this disorder, the symptoms must have been present for at least 6 months.

The source of this disorder may be physiological, psychological, or a combination of both. Hormonal imbalance, particularly testosterone deficiency, may be an issue. Depression is often implicated in a lack of desire for sexual intimacy in men.

Lack of sexual desire occurs more frequently in older males. About 6% of men between 18 and 24 years of age compared with 41% of those between 66 and 74 have this problem. Male hypoactive sexual disorder is associated with major depressive disorder and endocrinological factors such as hyperprolactinemia.

Sexual Excitement Disorders

Erectile disorder. **Erectile disorder** (also called *erectile dysfunction* and *impotence*) refers to failure to obtain and maintain an erection sufficient for sexual activity. Although most men occasionally experience this problem, it is a disorder only if it happens on 75% of sexual occasions and has been present for at least 6 months.

This problem may be a rare lifelong condition in which a man has never been able to obtain an erection sufficient for intercourse. It may also be an acquired condition in which a man has previously been able to have sexual intercourse but has lost the ability.

Aging is associated with erectile disorder. The prevalence in men younger than 40 years of age is about 2%. Men above age 60 experience significant erectile problems at a rate of about 40%.

Other conditions associated with erectile disorder include premature ejaculation and male hypoactive sexual desire disorder. Diseases that affect the vascular, neurological, and/or endocrine systems are implicated in this disorder. They include dyslipidemia, cardiovascular disease, hypogonadism, multiple sclerosis, and diabetes mellitus.

Orgasmic Disorders

Female orgasmic disorder. Study of the female orgasm is more complicated than that of the male orgasm, which results in a noticeable ejaculation. Additionally, reproduction is not associated with the female orgasm. Comparing female and male responses to orgasm, men are more focused on performance, whereas women tend to be focused on the subjective quality of having sex. Some women are uncertain whether orgasm has even occurred.

Female orgasmic disorder is sometimes referred to as *inhibited female orgasm* or *anorgasmia* and is defined as the recurrent or persistent inhibition of female orgasm. It is manifested by the recurrent delay in or absence of orgasm after a normal sexual excitement phase achieved by masturbation or coitus. For it to be considered a clinically significant problem, it must have occurred for at least 6 months during most sexual encounters. Orgasmic difficulties cause clinically significant distress in the woman.

It may be a lifelong disorder (never having achieved orgasm) or may be acquired (having had at least one orgasm and then having had difficulties). Most cases are lifelong rather than acquired, and once a woman learns how to achieve orgasm it is unusual to lose this capacity. Acquired anorgasmia in women tends to be associated with painful intercourse during or after menopause.

Psychological factors—including fears of pregnancy, rejection, or loss of control—are associated with anorgasmia. Other factors may include hostility toward or from men and cultural/societal restrictions.

The prevalence of orgasmic problems in women is estimated to be between 10% and 42%. Only a portion of women experience distress due to diminished orgasms or lack of orgasm and therefore would not be diagnosed with female orgasmic disorder. Medical conditions such as multiple sclerosis, pelvic nerve damage, and spinal cord injuries can result in problems with orgasm. Psychiatric conditions, such as major depressive disorder, are associated with anorgasmia. Some medications, such as selective serotonin reuptake inhibitors (SSRIs), are known to delay or prevent orgasm. Vulvovaginal atrophy and dryness associated with menopause can result in pain, thus preventing sexual pleasure.

Delayed ejaculation. In **delayed ejaculation**, formerly referred to as *male orgasmic disorder*, *inhibited orgasm*, or *retarded ejaculation*, a man achieves ejaculation during partnered sexual activity only with great difficulty. To be diagnosed with this condition, symptoms must have persisted for a minimum duration of 6 months.

A man with a *lifelong delayed ejaculation* has never been able to ejaculate during sexual activity. This uncommon condition may result from a rigid background in which sex is believed to be a sin. Physically, it is associated with age-related loss of fast-conducting peripheral sensory nerves and decreased sex steroid secretion.

Acquired delayed ejaculation develops after previously normal functioning and is fairly common. Interpersonal problems may be the cause. Physical conditions, substance use, and prescribed medication may also cause this problem and should be assessed.

Delayed ejaculation is the least common male sexual complaint. Most men experience periods of sexual activity without ejaculation. However, less than 1% of men complain of problems lasting at least 6 months. Major depressive disorder, diabetes, and late-onset hypogonadism are comorbidites for delayed ejaculation (Abdel-Hamid & Ali, 2018). Age-related disease treatments (e.g. surgical, medical, radiation) can also impact ejaculatory function.

Premature ejaculation. In **premature ejaculation**, a man persistently or recurrently achieves orgasm and ejaculation before he wishes to. Diagnosis is made when a man regularly ejaculates before or immediately after the penis enters the vagina. Symptoms must be present for at least 6 months for a man to be diagnosed with this problem. There is no disorder in women that corresponds to premature ejaculation.

The *Diagnostic and Statistical Manual of Mental Disorders,* fifth edition (*DSM-5*) (APA, 2013), specifically states that premature ejaculation occurs during vaginal penetration, which obviously refers to a man and a woman. However, sexual activity can be generalized to include other activities, such as oral or anal sex between a man and a woman or between a man and a man.

Physical factors may be involved. Some men may be more tactilely sensitive and respond more intensely to stimulation. Psychological factors include fear about performance and stressful relationships where the man feels hurried. Considerations as to age, newness of the relationship, and how often the man has intercourse should be assessed.

Although this problem is fairly uncommon in the general population (1%–3%), about 35% to 40% of men who are treated for sexual disorders complain of premature ejaculation. Individuals with lifelong problems often have some anxiety disorders. Acquired premature ejaculation is associated with prostatitis, thyroid disease, or drug withdrawal, as from opioids.

Genitopelvic Pain/Penetration Disorder

The group of disorders previously diagnosed in the psychiatric community included a problem called *dyspareunia,* which referred to pelvic and/or vaginal pain during or after intercourse. It also included vaginismus, or involuntary constriction of the muscles of the vagina. Researchers believed that the distinction between the two disorders is too blurry and therefore combined them into a single disorder.

Genitopelvic pain/penetration disorder interferes with penile insertion or penetration during intercourse. It may even be elicited during a normal gynecological examination with a speculum. Women experiencing these problems become fearful that pain and spasms will occur during the next sexual encounter. This fear compounds the problem by increasing anxiety and muscle tension.

About 15% of North American women report pain during sexual intercourse/penetration. This is associated with relationship distress due to avoidance of sexual activities. Pain during penetration is associated with physical problems such as urinary/vaginal infection, endometriosis, irritable bowel syndrome, and constipation.

> **VIGNETTE:** Jessica, a computer programmer, had recently had a baby and was looking forward to renewing her love life with her husband. She said, "My husband would barely begin penetration, and the pain would be awful. The whole area just clenched up." She continued, "I had never had any problems before, and I didn't think I would because I'd had a cesarean, so I didn't think that anything would change. 'Good grief, that hurts,' I thought. 'What is wrong with me?' We were both terribly upset."

Other Sexual Dysfunctions and Problems

Sexual dysfunction due to a general medical condition includes sexual desire disorders, orgasm disorders, and sexual pain

---

> **BOX 20.1 Sexual Dysfunction in Women: The Viagra Effect**
>
> Experts in psychiatric disorders are expressing concern that women may be overdiagnosed with disorders in sexual function based on criteria in the *Diagnostic and Statistical Manual of Mental Disorders* (APA, 2013). Normal variations in sexual interest, along with variability within the life cycle, should be taken into consideration when these diagnoses are made.
>
> A safeguard in the criteria for female sexual interest/arousal disorder stipulates that emotional distress must be experienced. However, the advent of pharmacological innovations such as sildenafil (Viagra), which improve sexual performance in men, should be factored into this emotional distress. Expectations on the part of men as treated partners, researchers, and pharmaceutical leaders set the social stage for the overdiagnosis of female sexual dysfunction in women. Only a generation ago, both partners in a couple were aging and experiencing a reduction in sexual interest and appetite. Now, pharmacotherapy may have created a mismatch between treated men and untreated women.

disorders. The cause of each is related to a medical condition, such as cardiovascular, neurological, or endocrine disease.

The diagnosis *substance-induced sexual dysfunction* is used when evidence of substance intoxication or withdrawal is apparent from the history, physical examination, or laboratory findings. Specified substances include alcohol, amphetamines or related substances, cocaine, opioids, sedatives, hypnotics, antianxiety agents, and other known and unknown substances. Abused recreational substances can have a variety of effects on sexual functioning. In small doses, many substances enhance sexual performance. With continued use, sexual difficulties become the norm.

Sexual dysfunction not elsewhere classified is a category that covers sexual dysfunctions that cannot be classified under one of the other categories. Typically, this is because their presentation is not quite strong enough to meet the criteria for a disorder or because there is not enough information to make a diagnosis.

Box 20.1 provides a discussion regarding the influence of pharmacological treatment for men and psychiatric diagnoses for sexual dysfunction in women.

Risk Factors
Biological Factors

Aging appears to be a factor in the prevalence of all sexual dysfunction among both men and women. In addition, a variety of physical conditions are related to sexual dysfunction; these are summarized in Table 20.1.

Cognitive Factors

Pioneers in the study of human sexuality include Helen Singer Kaplan (1929–95). According to Kaplan (1974), sexual dysfunctions are the result of a combination of factors, including the following:

- Misinformation or ignorance regarding sexual and social interaction
- Unconscious guilt and anxiety regarding sex

TABLE 20.1   Medical Conditions and Surgical Procedures That Cause Sexual Dysfunction

System/State	Organic Disorders	Sexual Impairment
Endocrine	Hypothyroidism, adrenal dysfunction, hypogonadism, diabetes mellitus	Low libido, erectile dysfunction, decreased vaginal lubrication
Vascular	Hypertension, atherosclerosis, stroke, venous insufficiency, sickle cell disease	Erectile disorder with intact ejaculation and libido
Neurological	Spinal cord damage, diabetic neuropathy, herniated lumbar disc, alcoholic neuropathy, multiple sclerosis, temporal lobe epilepsy	Sexual disorder—early signs: low or high libido, erectile dysfunction, impaired orgasm
Genital	*Male*—Priapism, Peyronie disease, urethritis, prostatitis, hydrocele	Low libido, erectile dysfunction
	Female—Imperforate hymen, vaginitis, pelvic inflammatory disease, endometriosis	Genitopelvic pain, low libido, decreased arousal
Systemic	Renal, pulmonary, hepatic, advanced malignancies, infections	Low libido, erectile dysfunction, decreased arousal
Psychiatric	Major depressive disorder	Low libido, erectile dysfunction
	Bipolar disorder (manic phase)	Increased libido
	Generalized anxiety disorder, panic disorder, posttraumatic stress disorder (PTSD)	Low libido, erectile dysfunction, lack of vaginal lubrication, anorgasmia
	Obsessive-compulsive disorder (OCD)	Low libido, erectile dysfunction, lack of vaginal lubrication, anorgasmia, "anti-fantasies" focusing on the negative aspects of a partner
	Schizophrenia	Low desire, bizarre sexual fantasies
	Personality disorders (borderline, obsessive-compulsive, histrionic)	Low libido, erectile dysfunction, premature ejaculation, anorgasmia
Surgical-postoperative	*Male*—Prostatectomy, abdominal-perineal bowel resection	Impotence, no loss of libido, ejaculatory impairment
	Female—Episiotomy, vaginal prolapse repair, oophorectomy	Genitopelvic pain, decreased lubrication
	Male and female—Leg amputation, colostomy, ileostomy	Mechanical difficulties in sex, low self-image, fear of odor

Adapted from Shafer, L. C. (2018). Sexual disorders or sexual dysfunction. In T. A. Stern, O. Freudenreich, F. A. Smith, G. L. Fricchione, & J. F. Rosenbaum (Eds.), *Handbook of general hospital psychiatry* (7th ed., pp. 279–290). Philadelphia, PA: Elsevier.

- Anxiety related to performance, especially with erectile and orgasmic dysfunction
- Poor communication between partners about feelings and what they desire sexually

Additional factors have been identified to explain sexual dysfunction. Unacknowledged or unidentified sexual orientation may lead to poor performance with the opposite sex, or the presence of one sexual problem may lead to another. For example, difficulty maintaining an erection may lead to hypoactive sexual desire. Education seems to have a buffering effect, and people who have more education have fewer sexual problems and are less anxious about issues pertaining to sex.

APPLICATION OF THE NURSING PROCESS

ASSESSMENT

General Assessment

Sexual assessment includes both subjective and objective data. Many psychiatric hospitals use a nursing history tool that is biologically oriented and has few questions on sexual functioning. Health history questions pertaining to the reproductive system may be limited to menstrual history, parity, history of sexually transmitted diseases, method of contraception, and questions regarding safe sex practices. There may be a few vague questions about sexual functioning or sexual concerns.

Patients may cue the nurse into the presence of sexual concerns without explicitly verbalizing them. Box 20.2 presents a discussion of these cues.

The nurse may ask the patient if there is concern in the area of sexual functioning. Generally, it is more comfortable for the patient if the nurse first asks questions in a general manner and then proceeds to the patient's experience. For example, the nurse might say, "Some people who are prescribed this medication find that it makes it difficult to achieve an erection. Have you had this problem?" This general approach allows the patient to feel that he is not alone in what he is experiencing. Table 20.2 provides facilitative statements for the interviewer conducting a sexual assessment.

The sexual history includes the patient's perception of physiological functioning and behavioral, emotional, and spiritual aspects of sexuality. It also includes cultural and religious beliefs with regard to sexual behavior and sexual knowledge base. During the assessment, both the nurse and the patient are free to ask questions and clarify information. It is reasonable to defer lengthy sexual health assessment when acute psychiatric symptoms prevent a calm, thoughtful discussion. As symptoms subside and rapport is developed, the assessment may be resumed. With experience, the nurse will be able to identify those patients who are at greater risk for difficulties in sexual functioning. This includes patients with a history of certain medical problems or surgical procedures (see Table 20.1) and patients taking some drugs (Table 20.3).

BOX 20.2 Patient Cues That May Indicate Concerns About Sexuality

Nonverbal Behaviors
- Showing discomfort by blushing, looking away, making tight fists, fidgeting, crying
- Openly engaging in overt sexual behaviors (e.g., touching one's own body parts, masturbating, exposing one's genitals, making sexually suggestive sounds)

Verbal Behaviors
- Telling sexually explicit jokes
- Making sexual comments about the nurse
- Asking inappropriate questions about the nurse's sexual activity
- Discussing sexual exploits
- Expressing concern about relationship with partner:
  - "I don't feel the same about my partner."
  - "My partner doesn't feel the same about me."
  - "We're not as close."
  - "Our relationship has changed."
  - "My personal life has changed."
- Expressing concern that sexuality has been diminished (e.g., feeling less of a man, less of a woman):
  - "I've lost my manhood."
  - "I'm not as desirable as I once was."
- Expressing concern over lack of sexual desire:
  - "I'm not interested in sex anymore."
  - "My desire has changed."
  - "I'm not the man/woman I used to be."
  - "We don't click anymore."
- Expressing concern over sexual performance:
  - "I've lost my power."
  - "What will happen to my ability to perform?"
  - "I can't perform like I used to."
- Expressing concern about one's love life:
  - "My love life has changed."
  - "The spark is gone."
- Expressing concern over the sexual impact of drugs, surgery, or some other medical treatment:
  - "Will this drug interfere with my sex life?"
  - "Will I still be able to perform sexually after surgery?"

Self-Assessment

The nurse's discomfort in assessing sexual history may be due to poor training, inexperience, inadequate time, or the belief that sexual history is not important. Indeed, you may experience discomfort exploring sexual issues with patients, fearing that this discussion will be personally embarrassing and embarrassing to the patient. You may fear that you will not know what questions to ask or wonder why the questions should be asked.

Concerns related to age and gender differences are understandable. Maybe your patient is approximately your age and of the opposite sex. In this case, you might wonder whether talking about sexuality is inappropriate or whether the patient might decide that you are a little too interested. Discussing issues related to sexuality with people who are your parents' or grandparents' age may also create a level of discomfort, especially if you grew up in a home where such topics were avoided.

Remembering your position as a professional and addressing the topics in a tone and manner appropriate for a professional will increase your comfort as well as the patient's. Also, letting the patient know *why* you are asking such personal questions will increase openness and cooperation. For example, "People who are depressed sometimes find that their mood affects their sexual desire. Because you have been depressed, have you noticed a change in your interest in sex?" Sometimes, a subtler approach that shifts the focus away from the patient can be helpful. "Because you have been depressed, has your husband felt as if you were less interested in him?"

Perhaps the most helpful consideration is recognizing that assessing sexuality is part of holistic nursing care. Your role and responsibility lie in helping patients to deal with their responses to illness and/or the treatment of their illness. Understanding your patient's concerns, acknowledging the patient's discomfort, and providing useful feedback will enhance your professional abilities to care for your patient and perhaps even improve your self-understanding.

ASSESSMENT GUIDELINES

Sexual Dysfunction

1. A sexual assessment should be conducted in a setting that provides privacy and eliminates distractions.
2. Although note taking may be necessary for the beginner, it can be distracting to the patient and interrupts the flow of the interview. When note taking is necessary, it should be unobtrusive and kept to a minimum.
3. The interviewer should be aware of personal biases and attitudes that could block an open discussion of sexual issues.
4. Good eye contact, a relaxed posture, and friendly facial expressions facilitate the patient's comfort and communicate openness and receptivity on the part of the nurse.

NURSING DIAGNOSIS

A comprehensive assessment may reveal areas of sexual concern and dysfunction in the patient. These data are analyzed to determine the appropriate nursing diagnoses. A priority nursing diagnosis (International Council of Nurses, 2019)

A priority nursing diagnosis is *impaired sexual functioning* (International Council of Nurses, 2019). This diagnosis refers to the state in which an individual experiences a change in sexual function during the sexual response phases of desire, excitation, and/or orgasm. The change is viewed as unsatisfying, unrewarding, or inadequate and may be due to a variety of factors, including the following:
- Major depressive disorder
- Intimate partner abuse
- Altered body function from medication
- The process of aging

Other nursing diagnoses that may accompany sexual dysfunctions include *relationship problem*, *situational* or *chronic low self-esteem*, and *negative self-image*. Lack of information about normal sexual functioning can be addressed by *lack of knowledge of sexual functioning*. Because the dysfunction may be brought on by physiological problems, other diagnoses such as *substance use* or *urinary tract infection* may target the underlying problem.

TABLE 20.2 Facilitative Statements for the Interviewer Conducting a Sexual Assessment

Purpose	Facilitative Statement
To provide a rationale for a question	"As a nurse, I'm concerned about all aspects of your health. Many individuals have concern about sexual matters, especially when they are sick or having other health problems."
To give statements of generality or normality	"Most people are hesitant to discuss…" "Many people worry about feeling…" "Many people have concerns about…"
To identify sexual dysfunction	"Most people have difficulties at some time with their sexual relationships. What have yours been?"
To obtain information	"Are you sexually active? What has been your pattern of sexual activity?"
To identify sexual myths	"While growing up, most of us have heard some sexual myths or half-truths that continue to puzzle us. Are there any that come to mind?"
To determine whether being gay is a source of conflict	"What is your/your family's attitude toward being gay?"
To identify an older person's concerns about sexual function	"What is your understanding about sexuality during the later years? How has the passage of time affected your sexuality (sex life)?"
To obtain and give information (miscellaneous areas)	"Frequently, people have questions about…" "What questions do you have about…" "What would you like to know about…"
To close the history	"Is there anything further in the area of sexuality that you would like to discuss now?"

TABLE 20.3 Drugs That Can Cause Sexual Dysfunction

Category	Drug	Sexual Side Effects
Cardiovascular drugs	Methyldopa	Amenorrhea, breast enlargement, gynecomastia, lactation, impotence, decreased libido
	Thiazides	Impotence
	Clonidine	Erectile dysfunction, decreased libido
	Propranolol	Impotence, Peyronie disease
	Digoxin	Gynecomastia
	Clofibrate	Decreased libido, impotence
Gastrointestinal drugs	Cimetidine	Decreased libido, impotence, gynecomastia, reduced sperm count
	Methantheline bromide	Impotence
Sedatives	Alcohol	Decreased libido, delayed ejaculation, gynecomastia, testicular atrophy
Antianxiety drugs	Alprazolam Diazepam	Decreased libido, decreased orgasm, impotence, delayed ejaculation
Antipsychotics	First-generation antipsychotics	Amenorrhea, galactorrhea, retarded or retrograde ejaculation, impotence, gynecomastia
	Second-generation antipsychotics	Amenorrhea, galactorrhea, abnormal ejaculation, impotence, galactorrhea, gynecomastia
Antidepressants	SSRIs	Decreased libido, delayed or absent orgasm, delayed ejaculation, erectile dysfunction
	SNRIs	Decreased libido, delayed or absent orgasm, erectile dysfunction, abnormal ejaculation
	SARIs (trazodone)	Priapism (sustained erection in the absence of sexual stimuli)
	Tricyclics	Breast enlargement, decreased orgasm, erectile dysfunction
	MAOIs	Vaginal dryness, inhibited orgasm, erectile dysfunction, inhibited orgasm
Antimanic drugs	Lithium	Erectile dysfunction

MAOI, Monoamine oxidase inhibitor; *SSRI*, selective serotonin reuptake inhibitor; *SNRI*, serotonin norepinephrine reuptake inhibitor; *SARI*, serotonin antagonist and reuptake inhibitor.
US Food and Drug Administration. (2016). *Drugs*. Retrieved from http://www.fda.gov/Drugs/default.htm.

OUTCOMES IDENTIFICATION

A specific overall outcome for *impaired sexual functioning* is *improved sexual functioning* or even *effective sexual functioning*. *Relationship problem* is paired with *improved relationship*. Nursing outcomes for the self-esteem diagnoses related to self-image would be aimed at improvement as well. The *knowledge* diagnosis is paired with *improved knowledge about sexual functioning*. Regarding the physiological diagnoses, outcomes for *substance use* or *urinary tract infection* would be *no substance use* and *no urinary tract infection*.

Table 20.4 lists signs and symptoms, nursing diagnoses, and outcomes for sexual dysfunction.

TABLE 20.4 Signs and Symptoms, Diagnoses, and Outcomes of Sexual Dysfunction		
Signs and Symptoms	**Nursing Diagnoses**	**Outcomes**
Alteration in achieving perceived sex role, alteration in relationship with significant other, changes in sexual activities and/or behaviors	*Impaired sexual functioning*	Effective sexual functioning: Attains sexual arousal, sustains arousal through orgasm, adapts sexual techniques as needed, expresses ability to be intimate, communicates comfortably with partner
Feeling like a failure in terms of sexuality, embarrassment due to inability to be intimate	*Negative self-image*	Improved self-image: Addresses the underlying problems for altered functioning, accepts sexual limitations, develops other methods to fulfill intimacy needs

International Council of Nursing Practice. (2019). ICNP browser. Retrieved from https://www.icn.ch/what-we-do/projects/ehealth/icnp-browser. ICNP® is owned and copyrighted by the International Council of Nurses (ICN). Reproduced with permission of the copyright holder.

PLANNING

The planning of nursing care for a patient with a sexual dysfunction may occur as part of care for a coexisting disorder. Nurses prepared at the basic level may encounter such patients when they are being treated for a variety of conditions in any setting.

IMPLEMENTATION

It is essential for nurses who work in psychiatry—and almost any specialty area in nursing, including oncology, cardiology, and neurology—to understanding sexual function and dysfunction. All nurses must be able to facilitate a discussion with the patient about sexuality. To be a facilitator, the nurse must be nonjudgmental, have a basic knowledge of sexual functioning, and have the ability to conduct a basic sexual assessment. Once the assessment has been completed, the nurse must know when and to whom to refer the patient with a sexual complaint. Depending on the nature of the problem, the patient may need a referral to a professional such as a marital counselor, psychiatrist, gynecologist, urologist, clinical nurse specialist, or pastoral counselor.

Box 20.3 provides a list of sample interventions for sexual counseling.

Health Teaching and Health Promotion

An area of teaching in which nurses can be most helpful involves medication. Nurses should help patients weigh the pros and cons of any type of pharmacotherapy and its impact on sexual functioning. Many drugs cause sexual side effects, and psychotropic medications used for psychiatric disorders are common offenders. Nurses tend to ignore or minimize the sexual side effects associated with these medications, perhaps in an attempt to promote adherence. Helping patients to evaluate for themselves the benefits versus risks of pharmacotherapy empowers them to choose the best course of action. Such a patient-centered approach increases patients' ability to be informed consumers of mental health services.

EVALUATION

Evaluation of expected outcomes relates to the level of control and personal satisfaction achieved. Acceptance of sexual dysfunction (e.g., impotence) as being part—but not necessarily the defining characteristic—of sexual behavior can result in greater satisfaction. The degree to which negative attitudes about sex are no longer problematic is also important.

EVIDENCE-BASED PRACTICE

Sexual Dysfunction in Young Women

Problem

Sexual dysfunction can be a lifelong problem that has its roots in adolescence or young adulthood. Owing to social taboos and privacy concerns, clinicians may not address this problem.

Purpose of Study

The purpose of this study was to determine the extent of sexual dysfunction among female university students.

Methods

This descriptive cross-sectional study analyzed data from a population of 18- to 29-year-olds. The Female Sexual Functioning Index (FSFI) was used to assess sexual functioning in 310 participants. One variable that was examined was whether each participant had or had not engaged in recent sexual activity. Other predictors of female sexual dysfunction were also explored.

Key Findings

- The FSFI was about 35% in non–sexually active females.
- The FSFI was about 42% in sexually active females.
- Increased risk for female sexual dysfunction was associated with younger age (18–21 years), prior psychiatric diagnosis, and self-reported problems with arousal.

Implications for Nursing Practice

Moving from home to the university setting can be an unsettling experience and a landmark of young adulthood. During this time, students have far greater freedom and begin to develop their views of themselves sexually. Nurses in clinics and other settings can be seen as safe resources and may be influential by providing education and support, thus helping young women to understand their bodies.

Chapa, H. O., Fish, J. T., Hagar, C., & Wilson, T. (2018). Prevalence of female sexual dysfunction among women attending college presenting for gynecological care at a university student health center. *Journal of American College Health, 68*(1), 52–60.

TREATMENT MODALITIES

Biological Treatments

Pharmacotherapy

Treatments for sexual dysfunction are increasingly being advanced by the pharmaceutical industry. Despite the fact that women with sexual dysfunction greatly outnumber men, most of the available pharmacological treatments for sexual dysfunction are intended for men.

Two medications are approved by the US Food and Drug Administration (FDA) for the treatment of premenopausal women with acquired generalized hypoactive sexual desire disorder. Flibanserin (Addyi) boosts dopamine and norepinephrine (both responsible for sexual excitement) while decreasing levels of serotonin. Flibanserin is dosed at bedtime because it poses risks of hypotension, syncope, and sedation. In 2019, the FDA approved a melanocortin receptor agonist, bremelanotide (Vyleesi), which is a subcutaneous injection given at least 45 minutes prior to sexual activity for up to eight times in a month. Testosterone pills, patches, and gels are also prescribed off label for treating sexual dysfunction in women. Table 20.5 summarizes treatments for sexual dysfunction.

Pharmacotherapy may *cause* sexual dysfunction; therefore, medications may have to be evaluated for change or dose reduction. Several strategies for combating antidepressant-induced sexual dysfunction include the following:

- Waiting to see whether sexual side effects decrease over the course of several weeks
- Reducing the dose of the antidepressant
- Planning for sexual activity before taking the antidepressant if the dosing is once a day
- For men, using a phosphodiesterase inhibitor such as sildenafil citrate (Viagra)
- Switching to an antidepressant with a more favorable side-effect profile, such as mirtazapine (Remeron), bupropion (Wellbutrin), or vilazodone (Viibryd).

BOX 20.3   Interventions for Counseling About Sexual Functioning

- Establish a therapeutic relationship based on trust and respect.
- Provide privacy and safeguard confidentiality.
- Discuss the effect of health on sexuality.
- Discuss the effect of medications (if any) on sexuality.
- Replace myths with facts regarding sexuality.
- Provide reassurance that sexual practices with consent are healthy.
- Include the partner in counseling as much as possible.
- If necessary, refer the patient to an advanced practice professional or a sex therapist.

TABLE 20.5   Pharmacotherapy, Cognitive Approaches, and Other Treatments for Sexual Dysfunction

Sexual Disorder	Pharmacotherapy	Cognitive Approaches	Other Treatments
Male hypoactive sexual desire disorder	Transdermal testosterone for hypogonadism or low testosterone levels Antidepressants (if depressed)	Individual therapy Couples therapy Education	
Female sexual interest/arousal disorder	Flibanserin (Addyi)[a] Bremelanotide (Vyleesi)[a] Alprostadil cream Testosterone	CBT Sex therapy Sensate focus exercises	EROS-CTD clitoral suction device* Water soluble lubrication (e.g., K-Y Jelly)
Male erectile disorder	Sildenafil (Viagra)[a], tadalafil (Cialis)[a], vardenafil (Levitra)[a], avanafil (Stendra)[a] are PDE-5 inhibitors Alprostadil (MUSE),[a] papaverine, vasoactive intestinal polypeptide/-phentolamine are penile injection and intraurethral suppository Testosterone (for hypogonadism)	Individual therapy Couples therapy Sensate focus exercises Group therapy Hypnotherapy Systematic desensitization	Vacuum pump Surgical implantation of penile prostheses
Female orgasmic disorder	Sildenafil (Viagra) or other PDE-5 inhibitor Bupropion (Wellbutrin)	CBT Masturbation training Couples CBT Kegel vaginal exercises	
Male orgasmic disorder	Sildenafil (Viagra)	Masturbatory training Systematic desensitization	
Premature ejaculation	SSRIs, especially paroxetine (Paxil) to delay or retard ejaculation	Start-stop technique Squeeze technique Increased sexual frequency	Topical anesthetics Condoms
Genitopelvic pain/penetration disorder	Ospemifene (Osphena)[a] for postmenopausal vaginal dryness Antianxiety medication	CBT Physical therapy Education Systematic desensitization Pelvic floor exercises Vaginal dilation exercises Surgical excision of hypersensitive tissue	Water soluble lubrication (e.g., K-Y Jelly) Topic anesthetics (e.g., lidocaine) Botulinum toxin

[a]FDA approved.

Psychological Therapies

Advanced practice psychiatric–mental health registered nurses can be qualified to treat sexual dysfunction through advanced training and certification. General therapies include psychoanalytic therapy, couples therapy, group therapy, and hypnotherapy. Some specific therapies available for sexual dysfunction include the following.

- **Sensate focus:** A therapeutic treatment in which patients progress from general touching and cuddling without intercourse to more intimate forms of expression
- **Behavioral therapy:** Useful for men with premature ejaculation when psychogenic or relationship factors are present—often best combined with medication in an integrated treatment program
- **Systematic desensitization:** Relaxation exercises combined with sexual anxiety–producing stimuli.
- **Masturbation training:** Especially helpful for women who have never had an orgasm. This approach helps women learn about their bodies and their sexual responsiveness.

> **VIGNETTE:** Maria, 67 years old, was widowed many years ago. She was recently approached by a 75-year-old widower who proposed marriage. Maria is concerned about the sexual implications of a marriage so late in life. She confides to her nurse practitioner, "I really haven't even thought about sex for so many years. I know Joe is just an old goat. He's always after me to take my clothes off." After discussing the possibility of a physiological cause for her lack of interest in sex, Maria's nurse practitioner gives her small doses of testosterone. Within a remarkably short time, Maria stops referring to Joe as "an old goat" and begins talking about how great life can be with the right partner.

GENDER DYSPHORIA

Clinical Picture

When we inquire about the birth of an infant, we want to know if it is a boy or a girl. We are asking about the child's gender (i.e., whether its chromosomes are XX or XY). However, **gender identity**, the sense of maleness or femaleness, is not usually established until a child is about 3 years of age.

People tend to be comfortable with the fact that they are male or female. Unfortunately, biological assignment does not necessarily determine whether individuals think of themselves as male or female. When biological sex differs from gender identity, such individuals may suffer from **gender dysphoria**, or feelings of unease about their incongruent maleness or femaleness. A man might describe himself as "a woman trapped in a man's body."

Symptoms in children include expressions of desire to be the opposite sex. Some children insist that they *are* the opposite sex and ask their families to call them by another name. Only a small percentage of children who display gender dysphoria characteristics will continue to show these characteristics into adolescence or adulthood. More intense childhood symptoms are associated with persistence of the dysphoria into adulthood (Steensma et al., 2013).

Teenagers and adults may also verbalize a desire to be the other sex and to be treated as such. Dressing up and passing for the opposite sex is common. Adolescents may dread the appearance of secondary sexual characteristics and (along with adults) may seek hormones or surgery to alter their masculinity or femininity. These individuals do not usually consider themselves to be homosexual. The biological female who falls in love with a woman believes that she is actually a man who loves a woman.

Epidemiology

While once considered a fairly rare condition, there is evidence to suggest that gender dysphoria has increased in the last couple of decades (Zucker, 2017). In childhood, the prevalence of birth-assigned males with gender dysphoria is more common. In adolescents, there has been a recent change in the sex ratio to one favoring birth-assigned females. In a 2014 study (Dhejne et al., 2014), sexual reassignment by gender was tracked over a period of 50 years. During that time, 429 male-to-females and 252 female-to males underwent this procedure.

Comorbidity

Children with gender dysphoria may also have anxiety, impulse-control problems, be disruptive, and have depressive disorders. Autism spectrum disorder has also been associated with gender dysphoria. In adolescents and adults, anxiety disorders are most common, followed by mood disorders. Substance use and self-destructive behavior are also common parallels found in people suffering from gender dysphoria.

Risk Factors
Biological Factors

Although biological factors are not thought to *cause* this problem, they are believed to influence its development. Hormones may play a role, as decreased levels of testosterone in males and increased levels in women are associated with gender dysphoria.

There is some evidence to suggest a genetic linkage. Heylens et al., (2012) studied concordance rates in monozygotic (identical) and dizygotic (fraternal) twins. Monozygotic twins had a concordance rate for gender dysphoria at 39%. This means that 39% of the time, when one twin has the problem, the other does too. No concordance was found for fraternal twins. Foreman et al., (2019) also found a significant association between several genes involved in sex hormone signaling and gender dysphoria.

Cognitive Factors

Learning theorists suggest that the absence of same-sex role models may contribute to gender dysphoria. In this scenario, caregivers provide either covert or overt approval for cross-gender identification and behaviors.

Psychoanalytic theorists have posited that male children who are deprived of their mothers seek to internally meld or become one with their mothers. This melding prevents them from developing fully as separate entities.

Nursing Care for Gender Dysphoria

Individuals dealing with gender dysphoria may feel profound social and internal guilt and shame. "I am disgusted by how hairy my body is" and "I have never wanted to be macho; I have always been sensitive and caring." A nursing diagnosis that goes along with this problem includes *gender identity disturbance* due to incongruence between expressed (felt) and assigned (inborn) gender. A specific outcome for this diagnosis is improved gender identity. Goals include seeking social support, using healthy coping behaviors to resolve sexual identity issues, and acknowledging and accepting one's sexual identity.

TREATMENT MODALITIES

Biological Treatments

Pharmacotherapy

Pharmacological interventions in adolescents may be used to delay puberty. Supporters of this reversible approach suggest that this gives adolescents time to explore gender-related issues. See the following box titled "Health Policy" for a further discussion of this treatment method.

Adults with gender dysphoria may choose to take hormones to alter their chemistry toward their preferred gender. A female who would like to become a male takes testosterone. In the first 6 months, this results in skin oiliness and acne, fat redistribution, cessation of menses, clitoral enlargement, vaginal atrophy, and amenorrhea (Yarbrough, 2019). Within a year, testosterone users experience the growth of facial and body hair, loss of scalp hair, increasing muscle mass, and deepening of the voice. When a male takes estrogen, within the first 2 months his libido declines and spontaneous erections decrease. Within 3 to 6 months of taking transfeminine hormone, he will experience softening of the skin, decreased testicular volume, less muscle, more fat on the hips, and breast growth.

◤ HEALTH POLICY

Should Puberty Be Delayed in Children With Gender Dysphoria?

Injections or implantation of gonadotropin-releasing hormone (GnRH) agonists to reversibly block the onset of puberty in youth with gender dysphoria is a relatively new practice. Previously, these drugs were reserved for precocious (abnormally early) puberty or children with short stature to increase adult height.

Proponents of puberty blocking believe that GnRH gives young persons more time to explore their options and participate in mental health therapy before secondary sex characteristics develop. They contend that by so doing, better psychological functioning will result.

Opponents say that puberty blockers are harmful. Eight state legislatures have introduced bills to restrict transgender treatment for minors; these laws hold providers criminally liable for using this treatment for gender dysphoric disorder. A defeated South Dakota house bill aimed to prohibit the use of pubertal blocks for children aged 16 years or younger. The ability and competence of a child to make such a decision is also raised as an argument against such treatment.

Guideline Directed Care. (2020). Controversial pubertal blocker legislation may bring unintended consequences for children. *Endocrine Today*. Retrieved from https://www.healio.com/endocrinology/reproduction-androgen-disorders/news/online/%7B425a065b-91e4-42f6-bdae-df8c299ba0eb%7D/controversial-pubertal-blocker-legislation-may-bring-unintended-consequences-for-children.

Surgical Treatment

When gender dysphoria in adults and even adolescents is severe and intractable, sex reassignment surgery is an option. If the patient is considered appropriate for sex reassignment, psychotherapy is usually initiated to prepare him or her for the cross-gender role. Patients are then instructed to live in the cross-gender role before surgery—including going to work or attending school—to determine whether they can interact successfully with members of society in the cross-gender mode.

Legal and social arrangements are made, such as changing the patient's name on legal documents. The patient may seek new employment if it is necessary to leave a former job because of discrimination. Relationship issues—such as what to tell parents, children, and former spouses—must be addressed. Males are instructed to have electrolysis and to practice female behaviors. Females are instructed to cut their hair, bind or conceal their breasts, and similarly take on a male identity.

If these measures are successful and the patient still wishes reassignment, hormone treatment is begun. After a period of time on hormone therapy, the patient may be considered for surgical reassignment if it is still desired.

In men, surgery may include removal of the penis (penectomy) and testes (orchiectomy) and the addition of a vagina (vaginoplasty). In females, surgical procedures may include the removal of the breasts (mastectomy), optional removal of the uterus (hysterectomy) and ovaries (oophorectomy), and the construction of a penis (phalloplasty) in females. Efforts to create an artificial penis have met with mixed results.

Do people regret having sex reassignment surgery? In a study by Dhejne and colleagues (2014), regret for the surgery was found in only about 2% of people who had opted for it. Still, psychotherapy is indicated after surgery to help the patient adjust to the surgical changes and to discuss issues of sexual functioning and satisfaction. Box 20.4 describes a case of sex reassignment gone wrong.

Psychological Therapies

Children

There is no consensus as to the best approach in treating children. However, the goal is to optimize the child's psychological adjustment and well-being. One approach is to let the child identify with the opposite gender and provide support for the stresses of familial and peer responses (e.g., bullying). Another is to accept the parents' goal of having the child accept his natal gender and then working on making him comfortable it. In this approach, family dynamics are also examined for their role in perpetuating the cross-gender behavior. Another family-directed approach is to provide supportive therapy while waiting to see whether the dysphoria will continue.

Adolescents and Adults

Gender dysphoria in adolescents will likely continue into adulthood. Individual and family therapy can be helpful. Adolescents will need help with coping skills to deal with harassment. Long-term psychotherapy is recommended to address gender dysphoria and comorbid conditions (Shafer, 2018). A thorough psychological evaluation is commonly required before sex reassignment.

BOX 20.4 Nature or Nurture? A Case of Sex Reassignment Gone Wrong

Accidents in early infancy may result in sex reassignment. One such fascinating and tragic case is that of David Reimer, a Canadian-born identical twin whose penis was destroyed as the result of a botched circumcision. With the advice of healthcare professionals, the child underwent surgical reassignment and later received hormonal therapy in puberty to induce the development of breasts and secondary female sex characteristics.

The family psychologist proclaimed the reassignment from male to female a success and concluded that gender identity was primarily based on socialization. However, David never felt comfortable. He rejected his female designation of Brenda and began living his life as a male at age 14. Shortly after that he learned about his biological gender. Subsequently, he had the reassignment surgically reversed, married a woman, and became stepfather to her three children.

However, David always felt uncomfortable and ultimately committed suicide. His case bolstered support for the biological influence of prenatal and early-life exposure to male hormones on gender identity. David Reimer's life is chronicled in the book *As Nature Made Him*, which raises questions about gender reassignment and the modification of a nonconsenting minor's genitals.

From Colapinto, J. (2006). *As nature made him: The boy who was raised as a girl*. New York, NY: HarperCollins.

PARAPHILIC DISORDERS

People do not consciously decide what arouses them sexually. Rather, during the maturation process, they discover the nature of their own sexual orientation and interests. Individuals differ from one another in terms of the types of partners they find to be erotically appealing and the types of behaviors they find to be erotically stimulating. They also differ in the intensity of the sexual drive, in the degree of difficulty they experience in trying to resist sexual urges, and in their attitudes about whether or not such urges should be resisted.

Sexual disorders include many forms of **paraphilic disorders**. The word *paraphilia* is derived from the Greek *para*, meaning "beside," and *philos*, meaning "loving." The paraphilic disorders include acts or sexual stimuli that are outside of what society considers normal but are required by some individuals to experience desire, arousal, and orgasm. Criteria for being diagnosed with this category of disorders include symptom occurrence for at least 6 months. A disorder is characterized by the fact that it causes discomfort in the individual or persistent risk or danger to themselves or others.

A small segment of individual with paraphilic disorders actually commit sexual offenses. However, many people who meet the criteria for paraphilic disorders do not act on their sexual feelings (Sorrentino, 2016).

Exhibitionistic Disorder

Exhibitionistic disorder is the illegal and intentional display of one's genitals in a public place. Most cases of **exhibitionism** involve a man exposing himself to a woman or women. This may occur as a man walks around exposed in a busy shopping mall or exposes himself on a doorstep after ringing the doorbell.

Excitement results from anticipation of the act, and the individual masturbates while or after exposing himself. The exhibitionist becomes aroused by observers' responses of shock and even disgust, and some fantasize that the person will also be aroused by the experience and actually want to be with the exhibitionist sexually.

On the other hand, some people with exhibitionistic disorder may experience deep shame and judge themselves by the same standard that society does and consider themselves to be perverts. They may cover their actions and live in intense fear that they will be recognized and thus shame themselves and their families.

Although these behaviors are illegal, they are apparently engaged in more for shock value than as a precursor to sexual assault or rape. Actual contact is rarely sought. Because few people are arrested for this behavior after age 40, we speculate that it resolves with age.

As with the other paraphilic disorders, the prevalence rate is unknown. However, based on general populations, the highest prevalence rate is estimated at 2% to 4% in males and much lower in females.

Comorbidities are based on criminal convictions of individuals who have exposed themselves; therefore, they might not be generalizable to all exhibitionists. Such comorbidities include depression, bipolar, anxiety, and substance use disorders. Hypersexuality, other paraphilic disorders, attention-deficit/hyperactivity disorder, and antisocial personality disorder are also comorbid.

Fetishistic Disorder

The term *fetish* is derived from the Portuguese word *feitico*, which means "obsessive fascination." **Fetishistic disorder** is characterized by a sexual focus on objects—such as shoes, gloves, pantyhose, and stockings—that are intimately associated with the human body. Preferred items are shoes, leather or latex items, and underclothing. Basically, fetishism means becoming aroused by something that would not normally arouse other people.

This disorder is far more common in men and is almost unheard of in women. Fetishes may replace sexual partners, or the fetish may be a component of sexual activity. Fetishes may become all-consuming and destructive. Many people have fetishes. However, to be diagnosed with a fetishistic disorder, the person must experience significant distress or overall impairment in functioning due to the fetish.

Frotteuristic Disorder

Rubbing or touching a nonconsenting person characterizes **frotteuristic disorder**. In fact, the word *frotteurism* originates from the French word *frotter*, which means to "rub or scrape." The disorder is usually seen in men. The behavior typically occurs in busy public places, particularly in subways and on buses, where the individual can escape after touching his victim. People with this disorder often have no close relationships, and this sort of aggressive contact is their only means of sexual gratification.

Up to 30% of adult males may engage in frotteuristic acts. About 10% to 14% of adult males in outpatient paraphilic treatment settings meet the criteria for frotteuristic disorder.

Comorbid conditions include other paraphilic disorders, especially exhibitionistic disorder. Conduct disorder, antisocial personality disorder, depression, bipolar, anxiety, and substance use disorders also co-occur.

Pedophilic Disorder

Pedophilic disorder is, unfortunately, the most common paraphilic disorder. It involves a predominant or exclusive sexual interest in prepubescent children (generally 13 years of age or younger). Sexual fantasies can lead some individuals to seek physical contact with these sexually immature children. A subtype of this disorder refers to pubescents between ages 11 and 14. Termed *hebephilia*, this attraction is unacceptable in most cultures and represents a profound violation of the boundaries of childhood. Those who criticize the pathologizing of attraction to pubescent young people—that is, by calling it a mental disorder—say that adults commonly have a sexual interest in this age group and that it is a legal issue, not a disorder.

For the definition of pedophilia to be met, the perpetrator must be at least 16 years of age and at least 5 years older than the victim. The nature of the child molestation can range from undressing and looking at the child, to genital fondling or oral sex, to penetration, and even to torture.

The population prevalence for pedophilic disorder is unknown owing to its illegality. The highest prevalence is estimated to be 3% to 5% of the male population. The prevalence among females is likely to be a fraction of the male prevalence.

There is a wide range of comorbid disorders. They include substance use disorders and depression as well as bipolar, anxiety, and antisocial personality disorder and other paraphilic disorders.

Sexual Sadism Disorder and Sexual Masochism Disorder

The term **sadism** is derived from the name of the Marquis de Sade (1740–1814), a well-known French writer who was obsessed with sexual violence. **Sexual sadism** disorder involves the achievement of sexual satisfaction from the physical or psychological suffering (including humiliation) of the victim. The sadist inflicts pain and suffering on (usually) nonconsenting people.

Consenting partners of sadists may be sexual masochists. **Sexual masochism** involves the achievement of sexual satisfaction by being humiliated, beaten, bound, or otherwise made to suffer. Sexual masochistic practices are more common among men than among women. In either case, participants tend to know that this is a "game," and actual humiliation or pain is avoided.

The prevalence of sexual sadism and masochism is unknown. Comorbidities of both disorders include other paraphilic disorders.

Transvestic Disorder

In **transvestic disorder**, sexual satisfaction is achieved by dressing in the clothing of the opposite gender. This behavior is related to **fetishism** but often goes beyond the use of one particular object. Generally, this behavior develops early in life and is associated with someone with whom the person is closely associated, whether in a loving relationship or through abuse. Unlike gender dysphoria, there are no sexual orientation issues, and people with transvestic disorder do not desire a sex change. Transvestites are usually heterosexual. Many cross dress only in specific sexual situations, and they often receive the cooperation and support of their partners. This paraphilic disorder is more common among men than among women. Over time, some men, as well as some women, with transvestic disorder desire to dress and live permanently as the opposite sex.

The prevalence of transvestic disorder is not known. Less than 3% of males report having been sexually aroused by dressing in women's attire.

Transvestism is frequently comorbid with other paraphilic disorders. The most common are fetishism and masochism. Autoerotic asphyxia by cutting off one's air supply during orgasm is associated with transvestism in a high proportion of fatal cases.

Voyeuristic Disorder

Voyeurism is another illegal activity that begins in adolescence or early adulthood. It is characterized by seeking sexual arousal through viewing, usually secretly, other people in intimate situations (e.g., naked, in the process of disrobing, or engaging in sexual activity). In the language of the layperson, this behavior is called being a *peeping Tom*. **Voyeuristic disorder** often begins in adolescence and may become a chronic condition and the only type of sexual activity for the person. Voyeurism may be driven by anger and a need to retaliate. Typically, people who engage in voyeurism also engage in other compulsive sexual behavior and are frequently addicted to pornography and going to strip clubs.

As in the case of exhibitionism, a person who engages in voyeurism may also be consumed by dissonance. The drive to engage in this activity does not make sense, considering the lengths to which the voyeur goes and the risks taken. "Why am I throwing away 2 or 3 hours staring through these binoculars on the off chance that I will see somebody naked when I can rent a movie, buy a magazine, or even find a real relationship? I must be such a loser." As with all obsessions and compulsions, the shame and anxiety are temporarily relieved by engaging in the very activity that brings it about.

Voyeuristic acts are the most common of the illegal sexual behaviors. Exact prevalence rates are difficult to determine owing to the hidden nature of the problem. An estimated lifetime prevalence of voyeurism is about 12% in males and 4% in females.

Comorbid conditions associated with voyeurism include other hypersexuality and other paraphilic disorders, especially exhibitionism. Other psychiatric conditions such as depression, anxiety, bipolar disorder, and substance use disorders are commonly seen along with this disorder. Attention-deficit/hyperactivity disorder, conduct disorder, and antisocial personality disorder are also frequently comorbid.

Paraphilic Disorder Not Otherwise Specified

Other paraphilic disorders include various problems that do not meet the criteria for the categories already described. The following are included in this grouping:

- **Telephone scatalogia disorder:** Obscene phone calling to an unsuspecting person or sending obscene messages or video images by e-mail.
- **Necrophilic disorder:** Obsession with having a sexual encounter with a cadaver.
- **Zoophilic disorder:** Incorporation of animals into sexual activity.
- **Coprophilic disorder:** Fixation on feces in sexual encounters.
- **Klismaphilic disorder:** Sexual activity that incorporates enemas.
- **Urophilic disorder:** Sexual activity that involves urinating on one's partner or being urinated on.
- **Hypoxyphilia:** Desire to achieve an altered state of consciousness secondary to hypoxia while experiencing orgasm; a drug such as nitrous oxide may be used to produce hypoxia.

Many of the people involved in nonstandard sexual practices feel no need for therapy because their sexual activities are carried out with a consenting adult partner and they are neither illegal nor physically or emotionally harmful to either partner. If, however, the person is experiencing relationship difficulties, wishes to change the sexual behaviors, becomes involved in illegal activity, or is physically or emotionally harming others or being harmed, therapy is indicated.

Epidemiology

Although the paraphilic disorders are uncommon, the repetitive and consuming nature of the disorders make their occurrence highly frequent. Most people with paraphilic disorders are Caucasian males; in about 50% of these individuals, the onset of the paraphilic arousal is before age 18 years. The average age of onset is between 8 and 12. The behaviors associated with the disorder tend to peak in the decade between 15 and 25 years of age and then become virtually nonexistent by age 50. Patients with paraphilic disorders often have more than one paraphilia, which can occur simultaneously or at different points in their lives.

Risk Factors
Biological Factors

A variety of theories attempt to identify what predisposes an individual to the development of paraphilic disorders, but these theories are far from conclusive, as they have focused primarily on violent offenders. Sexual problems can result from head trauma. Patients who have experienced head trauma with damage to the frontal lobe of the brain may display symptoms of promiscuity, poor judgment, inability to recognize triggers that

set off sexual desires, and poor impulse control. Inappropriate sexual arousal has also been linked to abnormal levels of androgens.

Cognitive Factors

Psychoanalytic theories suggest that castration anxiety results in the safer substitution of a symbolic object for the mother, which results in fetishism and transvestism. The need for a safe substitute may result in extreme behaviors, such as pedophilia, exhibitionism, and voyeurism.

Learning theorists explain paraphilic disorders in terms of timing and reinforcement. During vulnerable periods, especially puberty, sexual exploration is common. If it is pleasurable and there are no negative consequences, the activity becomes reinforced and is repeated. For example, if an adolescent boy experiments sexually with a 7-year-old boy, does not get caught, and continues to fantasize, he may develop arousal to young boys.

Cognitive theorists identify paraphilic disorders as being based on cognitive distortions. Errors in thought make it seem acceptable for deviant and destructive sexual behaviors to occur. For example, belief that there is agreement on the part of a child makes it okay in the individual's mind to have relations with her; or watching others engage in sexual relations may seem to be okay "as long as no one gets hurt." Perhaps the perpetrator of exhibitionistic behavior believes that young girls may get as excited as he does when he exposes himself.

▌APPLICATION OF THE NURSING PROCESS

ASSESSMENT

General Assessment

Patients with paraphilic disorders are rarely hospitalized as a direct result of their condition. However, people with paraphilic disorders may be overrepresented in psychiatric care settings due to the frequency of comorbid psychiatric conditions that are undoubtedly exacerbated by the sexual disorder. Inpatient treatment is necessary for individuals who are suicidal, potentially violent, or unable to take care of themselves. Suicide risk may be high if they feel exposed or confronted. If patients are charged with a crime or have been arrested, they may be incarcerated subsequent to hospitalization. Nurses who work in forensic settings such as prisons and jails may care for inmates who are imprisoned because of the consequences of paraphilic disorders. Major depressive disorder with substance use and suicidal ideation are common comorbid conditions and should be assessed using the principles outlined in Chapters 22 and 25.

During a thorough intake assessment, you may discover symptoms of one of the paraphilic disorders. For example, you may ask a patient about his family, and he may remark, "My wife and I aren't getting along so great lately." As you explore this area of concern further, he reveals, "My wife wants to do the same old boring things … you know … sexually, all the time." As the assessment continues, you may learn that he is focused on sadistic activities, is obsessed with pornography, and is no longer interested in relations with his wife.

Self-Assessment

It is reasonable for students to read descriptions of sexual disorders and feel repelled by paraphilic behaviors. It is also common to respond with frustration, anger, and hostility toward people with disorders that involve victims, such as sexual masochism and pedophilia. Providing care for someone who has abused others may be nearly impossible for certain individuals. We may have known someone who was the victim of a voyeur or a pedophile or we may personally have been victimized. Exploring paraphilic disorders, even in an academic context, may evoke significant distress. At this point, talking with a faculty member, a primary care provider, or a mental health professional can be helpful and important and may even result in better personal understanding and coping.

📄 ASSESSMENT GUIDELINES

Paraphilic Disorders

1. Assess the potential for self-harm, because patients with paraphilic disorders may become despondent and be more likely to consider suicide.
2. The main focus of the assessment should be on the presenting problem (e.g., major depressive disorder with suicidal ideation).
3. Elicit the patient's perception of the impact of the sexual disorder on the current illness.

NURSING DIAGNOSIS

Nursing diagnoses for individuals with paraphilic disorders include *risk for suicide, risk for violence, impaired impulse control*, and *problematic sexual behavior*. Other diagnoses should be considered depending on the comorbid psychiatric condition that has precipitated the admission.

OUTCOMES IDENTIFICATION

General outcomes are aimed at reversing or attenuating the nursing diagnoses. Thus, the outcome for *risk for suicide* would be *decreased suicide risk*. Table 20.6 lists the signs and symptoms, nursing diagnoses, and outcomes for paraphilic disorders.

PLANNING

The setting and presenting problem influence the planning of nursing care for the patient with a paraphilic disorder. The basic-level registered nurse may encounter such a patient during treatment for a comorbid condition, especially when the patient is admitted to the hospital for suicidal thoughts and behavior. Sometimes, psychiatric care and treatment are mandated, as when a voyeur or exhibitionist gets caught.

The care plan will focus on safety and crisis intervention. The patient may also be treated for comorbid depression or anxiety disorders in the community setting. Planning will address the major complaint along with the sexual disorder.

IMPLEMENTATION

Interventions are aimed at offering a nonjudgmental emotional presence while exploring identity issues, self-esteem, and anxiety and encouraging an optimal level of functioning. Patients with a potential for violating the boundaries of others may require closer observation and firm limit setting. Box 20.5 lists examples of basic-level interventions for paraphilic disorders.

Health Teaching and Health Promotion

Education is typically geared toward reducing symptoms from the presenting problem, typically depression and anxiety. Patients with paraphilic disorders can be taught to journal their feelings and to begin to identify triggers for pathological behavior.

TABLE 20.6 Signs and Symptoms, Diagnoses, and Outcomes for Paraphilic Disorders		
Signs and Symptoms	**Nursing Diagnoses**	**Outcomes**
Shame when dressing like a woman, fears loss of community respect, wife found a suicide note, increasingly unable to control sexual impulses	*Risk for suicide*	Decreased suicide risk: Expresses a determination to live and a sense of control; identifies strategies to manage his urges, refrains from self-destructive urges
Lacks interest in his spouse, feels an increasing attraction to prepubescent girls, history of arrests	*Risk for violence (sexual)*	No violence: Identifies triggers for maladaptive sexual fantasies and describes techniques to control these fantasies; practices self-restraint of sexual urges and behaviors
History of exposing self to others, deep remorse and shame over behavior, wants to control the fantasies, urges, and resultant behaviors	*Impaired impulse control*	Improved impulse control: Identifies feelings that lead to impulsive actions, consequences of actions, and alternatives; practices self-restraint of impulsive behaviors
Problematic sexual urges, preoccupation with unacceptable sexual urges, dysfunctional adult sexual relationships	*Problematic sexual behavior*	No problematic sexual behavior: Identifies triggers to unacceptable urges, works to decrease urges, refocuses on healthy sexual thoughts

International Council of Nursing Practice. (2019). *ICNP browser.* Retrieved from https://www.icn.ch/what-we-do/projects/ehealth/icnp-browser. ICNP® is owned and copyrighted by the International Council of Nurses (ICN). Reproduced with permission of the copyright holder.

BOX 20.5 Interventions for Paraphilic Disorders

Problematic Sexual Behavior

- Emphasize that although sexual urges may occur, they can be reduced, refocused, or even eliminated.
- Discuss the negative effect that such behavior has on others.
- Encourage the expression of feelings about past crises.
- Provide opportunities for other caregivers to process their feelings about working with patients with probematic sexual behaviors.

Improvement of Self-Esteem

- Encourage the patient to identify personal strengths.
- Assist in setting realistic goals to achieve higher self-esteem.
- Help the patient to accept dependence on others as appropriate.
- Explore previous achievements of success.
- Encourage the patient to identify and accept new challenges.

Improvement of Support Systems

- Assist in identifying problems resulting from lack of support systems.
- Encourage verbalization of feelings regarding seeking support systems.
- Identify specific supports that might be realistically attained.
- Identify steps needed to improve support systems and provide community resources.

Teamwork and Safety

When the patient who has a paraphilic disorder is in a crisis that requires hospitalization, providing a safe environment is fundamental. All patients on a psychiatric inpatient unit should be informed on admission about unit rules regarding personal contact between patients and between patients and staff. Limit setting is done consistently when it is needed, and staff work together as a team to this end.

Individuals with paraphilic disorders tend to isolate themselves. The unit environment may be a challenge. Sharing meals with others may cause discomfort, and patients may wonder how others may perceive them. A particular challenge may be interacting in formal group settings and the expectation of participation. But the group setting may actually provide patients with the greatest opportunity for growth. They have the opportunity to experience other group members as humans with feelings, and they may learn how much pain personal violations have caused them. The group setting provides other people who empathize with the patient's current distress and allows the patient to see that others face similar distress and challenges.

EVALUATION

Essential evaluative criteria for paraphilic disorders include maintaining the safety of others and self, reducing and/or eliminating urges and behaviors that result in discomfort and shame, and improving interpersonal relationships. Despite progress, people with sexual impulse disorders, especially those that involve victims, may be required to continue treatment, which has been demonstrated to reduce recidivism (relapse into the offending behavior).

TREATMENT MODALITIES

Biological Treatments

Pharmacotherapy

No medications have FDA approval for the treatment of paraphilic disorders. However, two classes of pharmacological agents, antiandrogens and serotonergic antidepressants, may be prescribed off label for paraphilic disorders. Medication is not used without other concomitant interventions. Drugs that reduce levels of testosterone may be used to treat sex offenders. The drugs that are frequently used are progestin derivatives, including medroxyprogesterone acetate (MPA; an analog of progesterone) and cyproterone acetate (CPA; an inhibitor of testosterone). Both of these drugs act to decrease libido and reduce compulsive deviant sexual behavior. They work best in patients with paraphilic disorders and a strong sexual drive, such as pedophiles and exhibitionists, and less well in those with a weak sexual drive or an antisocial personality (Balon, 2019).

SSRIs are also used off label without specific FDA approval in the treatment of paraphilias. Fluoxetine (Prozac) has been used successfully to treat patients with exhibitionism, voyeurism, and pedophilia and people who have committed rape. These drugs may work to improve mood, reduce impulsivity, decrease sexual obsessions, and cause sexual dysfunction. In addition to fluoxetine, other drugs, such as clomipramine (Anafranil) and fluvoxamine (Luvox), have been used in the treatment of sexual obsessions, addictions, and paraphilic disorders.

Psychological Therapies

The usual treatment plan for working with patients with paraphilic disorders is cognitive behavioral therapy. An attempt is made to help the person learn a new sexual response pattern that will eliminate the need for the activity that is causing the problem. Techniques range from positive reinforcement for appropriate object choices to aversion techniques, in which mild electrical shocks may be applied for inappropriate choices. Other treatment modalities include psychodynamic techniques designed to help the patient understand the origin of the paraphilia.

Advanced practice psychiatric–mental health registered nurses may seek specialized training to enable them to work effectively with patients with paraphilic disorders.

KEY POINTS TO REMEMBER

- Sexual dysfunction is an extremely common problem that involves a disturbance in the desire, excitement, or orgasm phases of the sexual response cycle or pain during sexual intercourse.
- Sexual problems have the potential to disrupt meaningful relationships.
- Healthcare workers are often uncomfortable asking questions related to sexuality. Providing professional and holistic care requires that nurses include this vital area of assessment.
- Certain medical and surgical conditions and some drugs result in a variety of sexual dysfunctions, including low libido, impotence, erectile dysfunction, anorgasmia, and priapism.

- There are distinctions between biological sex and gender identity. Gender dysphoria is a strong and persistent cross-gender identification accompanied by anxiety, discomfort, and unhappiness.
- The term *paraphilia* identifies repetitive or preferred sexual fantasies or behaviors that involve the preference for use of a nonhuman object, repetitive sexual activity with humans involving real or simulated suffering or humiliation, and repetitive sexual activity with nonconsenting partners.
- Paraphilic disorders include exhibitionistic disorder, fetishistic disorder, frotteuristic disorder, pedophilic disorder, sexual masochism disorder, sexual sadism disorder, transvestic disorder, voyeuristic disorder, and paraphilic disorders not otherwise specified.
- In addition to conducting sexual assessments, nurses are involved in milieu management, counseling, education, and medication management.
- Advanced-practice nurses and other mental healthcare professionals may specialize in the area of sexual counseling, treatment, and psychotherapy.

CRITICAL THINKING

1. As a nurse on an adolescent psychiatric–mental health nursing unit, you will often encounter teenagers who are misinformed about their growth and development as well as sexuality. What information would you include in a series of teaching sessions that would help these adolescents acquire a better understanding of the developmental changes they are going through?
2. To understand your own beliefs, answer these questions:
   a. Are you comfortable with your own sexuality? With that of others?
   b. Are you judgmental?
   c. Could you be helpful to someone who has a sexual disorder?
   d. What factors have influenced your beliefs and values regarding sexuality?
   e. What do you think is the impact of sexually explicit online content, television, music videos, and movies on your sexual attitudes, values, and beliefs?
3. During a one-to-one session, Mrs. Chase, a patient who was admitted to your inpatient unit with major depressive disorder and generalized anxiety disorder, confides her concern about her 17-year-old son, Alex. She becomes tearful and says, "I don't know what I've done wrong. Alex was arrested for exposing himself to a girl at school. I'm worried that he may begin doing even worse things."
   a. Provide Mrs. Chase with information regarding Alex's condition and his probable prognosis.
   b. What sort of feelings about Alex within yourself would you have to be aware of in order to give Mrs. Chase the best possible care?

CHAPTER REVIEW

1. Which patient statement suggests a concern over one's ability to perform sexually?
   a. "My partner and I aren't as close as we once were."
   b. "I'm not as desirable as I once was."
   c. "My personal life has changed a lot."
   d. "I'm not the partner I used to be."
2. The nurse should plan to educate male patients who are taking selective serotonin reuptake inhibitors (SSRIs) on the possible development of which common side effect?
   a. Impotence
   b. Gynecomastia
   c. Decreased libido
   d. Premature ejaculation
3. Which medications are currently approved for the treatment of male erectile disorder? *Select all that apply.*
   a. Sildenafil (Viagra)
   b. Flibanserin (Addyi)
   c. Tadalafil (Cialis)
   d. Vardenafil (Levitra)
   e. Avanafil (Stendra)
4. Which statement describes a common sexual side effect of diazepam (Valium)?
   a. "I'm just not interested in sex as much."
   b. "I'm experiencing vaginal dryness."
   c. "I am having prolonged erections."
   d. "My breasts have gotten larger."
5. Obtaining a sexual history can be embarrassing for the patient and practitioner. Experience with addressing the topic can help, as can which of the following?
   a. Using informal language familiar to the patient's age group
   b. Avoiding specifics and focusing the interview on general topics
   c. Avoiding eye contact
   d. Using a professional tone of voice and a relaxed posture
6. Which patient has the greatest risk for suicide?
   a. A patient who expresses the inability to stop searching the internet for child pornography.
   b. A patient who reports having lost interest in having a sexual relationship with his wife.
   c. A patient with a history of exposing himself to female strangers on the bus.
   d. A patient whose attraction to prepubescent girls has increased.
7. When Melissa was a small child, she insisted that she was a boy, refused to wear dresses, and wanted to be called Mitch. As Melissa reached puberty, she no longer displayed a desire to be male. This change in identity is considered
   a. Gender dysphoria
   b. Reaction formation
   c. Normal
   d. Early transgender syndrome

8. Phillip, a 63-year-old male, has exposed his genitals in public for all of his adult life, but the act has lost some of the former thrill. A rationale for this change in his experience may be
   a. An increasing sense of shame
   b. Disgust over his lack of control
   c. Desire waning with age
   d. Progression into actual assault
9. A male arrested for inappropriate sexual contact in a subway car denies the allegation. On interviewing the man, the nurse suspects frotteuristic disorder due to his
   a. Lack of relationships
   b. Overall aggressive nature
   c. Criminal history including robbery
   d. Intense hatred of women
10. Pedophilic disorder is the most common paraphilic disorder where adults who have a primary or exclusive sexual preference for prepubescent children. A subset of this disorder is termed hebephilia and is defined as attraction to
    a. Infants
    b. Pubescent individuals
    c. Teens between the ages of 15 and 19
    d. Males only

1. **d**; 2. **c**; 3. **a, c, d, e**; 4. **a**; 5. **d**; 6. **a**; 7. **c**; 8. **c**; 9. **a**; 10. **b**

NGN CASE STUDY AND QUESTIONS

Sophia is a 26-year-old being admitted to a psychiatric unit for treatment of severe major depressive disorder. During the intake assessment, Sophia reports experiencing sexual dysfunction. Although she experienced satisfying intimacy in the first 4 years of marriage, she states that her interest in sexual activity has diminished. Several months ago, Sophia began treatment with a combination therapy of bupropion (Wellbutrin) and citalopram (Celexa) for depression. With further questioning, the patient reports getting anxious before sex, stating, "I just want to get it over with as soon as possible. Please don't tell my husband—I don't want to hurt his feelings. Our relationship is wonderful other than this problem I am having."

Sophia's vital signs and laboratory tests are within normal limits. She has a peanut allergy and an allergy to penicillin.

Based on further evaluation, in addition to major depressive disorder, the admitting psychiatrist diagnoses female sexual interest/arousal disorder.

1. The registered nurse continues to assess Sophia. What physical conditions, if present, could be relevant to this patient's sexual dysfunction? *Select all that apply.*
   a. Major depressive disorder
   b. Peanut allergy
   c. Thyroid condition
   d. Urinary incontinence
   e. Penicillin sensitivity
   f. Endometriosis
   g. Arthritis
   h. Inflammatory bowel disease
   i. Parkinson's disease
   j. Scoliosis
2. Which finding will indicate effectiveness of this patient's treatment for female sexual interest/arousal disorder? *Select all that apply.*
   a. Achieves a satisfactory level of control of her sexual activity and response
   b. Recognizes that she will need lifelong estrogen replacement.
   c. Reports personal satisfaction with her sexuality
   d. Reports that sexual dysfunction is no longer present

NGN case study answers are on Evolve.

Visit the Evolve website for a posttest on the content in this chapter: http://evolve.elsevier.com/Varcarolis

REFERENCES

Abdel-Hamid, I. A., & Ali, O. I. (2018). Deleayed ejaculation: Pathophysiology, diagnosis, and treatment. *World Journal of Men's Health, 36*(1), 22–40.

American Psychiatric Association. (2013). *DSM-5 table of contents.* Retrieved from http://www.psychiatry.org/dsm5.

Balon, R. (2019). Paraphilic disorders. In L. W. Roberts (Ed.), *Textbook of psychiatry* (pp. 749–767). Washington, DC: American Psychiatric Association.

Dhejne, C., Oberg, K., Arver, S., & Landen, M. (2014). An analysis of all applications for sex reassignment surgery in Sweden, 1960–2010: Prevalence, incidence, and regrets. *Archives of Sexual Behavior, 43*(8), 1535–1545.

Foreman, M., Hare, L., York, K., Balakrishnan, K., Sanchez, F. J., & Harte, F., et al. (2019). Genetic link between gender dysphoria and sex hormone signaling. *Journal of Clinical Endocrinology & Metabolism, 104*(2), 390–396.

Heylens, G., DeCuypere, G., Zucker, K. J., Schelfaut, C., Elaut, E., & Vanden Bossche, H., et al. (2012). Gender identity disorder in twins: A review of the case report literature. *Journal of Sexual Medicine, 9*(3), 751–757.

International Council of Nurses. (2019). *International Classification for Nursing Practice Catalog.* Retrieved from https://www.icn.ch/sites/default/files/inline-files/ICNP2019-DC.pdf.

Kaplan, H. S. (1974). *The new sex therapy: Active treatment of sexual dysfunctions.* New York, NY: Brunner/Mazel.

Levine, H. B. (2010). What patients mean by love, intimacy, and sexual desire. In H. B. Levine, C. B. Risen, & S. E. Althof (Eds.), *Handbook of clinical sexuality for mental health professionals* (pp. 41–56). New York, NY: Taylor and Francis.

Masters, W. H., & Johnson, V. E. (1966). *Human sexual response.* Boston, MA: Little, Brown.

Shafer, L. C. (2018). Sexual disorders or sexual dysfunction. In T. A. Stern, O. Freudenreich, F. A. Smith, G. L. Fricchione, & J. F. Rosenbaum (Eds.), *Handbook of general hospital psychiatry.* (7th ed.) (pp. 279–290). Philadelphia, PA: Elsevier.

Sorrentino, R. (2016). DSM-5 and paraphilias: What psychiatrists need to know. *Psychiatric Times.* Retrieved from http:/www.psychiatrictimes.com/dsm-5-0/dsm-5-and-paraphilias-what-psychiatrists-need-know/page/0/1.

Steensma, T., McGuire, J. K., Kreukels, B. P. C., Beekman, A. J., & Cohen-Kettinis, P. T. (2013). Factors associated with desistence and persistence of childhood gender dysphoria. *Child and Adolescent Psychiatry*, *52*(6), 582–590.

Yarbrough, E. (2019). Gender dysphoria. In L. W. Roberts (Ed.), *Textbook of psychiatry* (9th ed.) (pp. 597–611). Washington, DC: American Psychiatric Association.

Zucker, K. J. (2017). Epidemiology of gender dysphoria and transgender identity. *Sexual Health*, *14*(5), 404–411.

21

Impulse Control Disorders

Sandra S. Yaklin and Margaret Jordan Halter

🌐 Visit the Evolve website for a pretest on the content in this chapter: http://evolve.elsevier.com/Varcarolis

OBJECTIVES

1. Describe the clinical manifestations of oppositional defiant disorder, conduct disorder, intermittent explosive disorder, pyromania, and kleptomania.
2. Describe the biological, cognitive, and environmental factors related to the development of impulse control disorders.
3. Compare your feelings with those of someone else in your class about working with a person who has an impulse control disorder.
4. Formulate three nursing diagnoses for impulse control disorders and identify patient outcomes for each.
5. Identify person-centered nursing interventions for each of the impulse control disorders.
6. Identify pharmacotherapy and psychological therapies used for oppositional defiant disorder, conduct disorder, and intermittent explosive disorder.

KEY TERMS AND CONCEPTS

adverse childhood experiences (ACEs)
callousness

cognitive behavioral therapy (CBT)
dialectical behavioral therapy (DBT)

expressed emotion

The development of a psychiatric illness can be devastating to the person affected and to significant others. Disorders such as autism and schizophrenia can alter the entire direction of a person's life, yet it is usually evident that there is a psychiatric basis to the disorders. Comparatively, people with impulse control disorders may seem like children whose parents cannot control them or adults who simply do not choose to control their behavior.

Disruptive, impulse control, and conduct disorders are characterized by aggressive behaviors and emotions. Problems relating to others in socially acceptable ways result in a lack of healthy relationships, leaving the individual isolated and the family devastated. The behaviors related to these disorders can have severe criminal consequences and long-lasting negative personal impacts.

Recognizing and treating aggressive and impulsive behaviors while a person is young can prevent further problems and avoid interactions with the criminal justice system. Unfortunately, stigma and misconceptions around mental illness may cause individuals and their families to conceal these conditions. Concealment can limit help-seeking and professional care, preventing timely intervention. Unfortunately, without professional care, many young people end up interfacing with the criminal justice system, where treatment may or may not take place.

According to the American Psychiatric Association (APA, 2013), major disorders considered under this umbrella include the following:

- Oppositional defiant disorder
- Conduct disorder
- Intermittent explosive disorder

Two other disorders included in the disruptive, impulse-control, and conduct disorders section of the *Diagnostic and Statistical Manual of Mental Disorders*, 5th edition *(DSM-5)* are pyromania and kleptomania. These conditions are briefly addressed following the other disorders.

OPPOSITIONAL DEFIANT DISORDER

Clinical Picture

A certain amount of oppositional behavior and contrariness is normal and developmentally appropriate for children and early adolescents. For instance, 2-year-old children and early adolescents often assert their growing autonomy by saying "No!" However, there are also children and adolescents whose behavior exceeds the boundaries of what is socially acceptable. **Oppositional defiant disorder** affects both emotions (e.g., anger and irritation) and behaviors (e.g., argumentativeness and defiance).

A child or adolescent with oppositional defiant disorder is not just difficult or defiant. This disorder impairs the child's life and makes school functioning, friendships, and family life extremely difficult. The behaviors may be confined to only one setting or, in more severe cases, present in multiple settings such as both at home and in school. Children and adults with oppositional defiant disorder show a preference for large rewards and pay little attention to increasing penalties.

Left untreated, most children outgrow this disorder, especially if the child receives treatment for comorbid conditions such as attention-deficit/hyperactivity disorder (ADHD) and parents receive parent training. However, some do not improve and continue to experience social difficulties, conflicts with authority figures, and academic problems that affect their whole lives.

Some children with oppositional defiant disorder may progress to conduct disorder, discussed later in this chapter. Both are related to conflict with adults and authority. The difference between the two is that conduct disorder is more severe and includes aggression toward people or animals, destruction of property, stealing, and deceit. Also, the emotional dysregulation (e.g., anger, irritability) in oppositional defiant disorder is not present in conduct disorder.

The APA (2013) differentiates between emotional (e.g., anger), behavioral (e.g., defiance), and spiteful/vindictive (e.g., revenge seeking) behaviors. This system is important, as emotional symptoms tend to be linked to current or future mood and anxiety disorders, whereas spiteful and vindictive behaviors are predictive of future conduct disorder and delinquency. Diagnostic criteria for oppositional defiant disorder are listed in the *DSM-5* box.

DSM-5 CRITERIA FOR OPPOSITIONAL DEFIANT DISORDER

A. A pattern of angry/irritable mood, argumentative/defiant behavior, or vindictiveness lasting at least 6 months as evidenced by at least four symptoms from any of the following categories and exhibited during interaction with at least one individual who is not a sibling.

Angry/Irritable Mood
1. Often loses temper
2. Is often touchy or easily annoyed
3. Is often angry and resentful

Argumentative/Defiant Behavior
4. Often argues with authority figures or, for children and adolescents, with adults
5. Often actively defies or refuses to comply with requests from authority figures or with rules
6. Often deliberately annoys others
7. Often blames others for his or her mistakes or misbehavior

Vindictiveness
8. Has been spiteful or vindictive at least twice within the previous 6 months.

Note: The persistence and frequency of these behaviors should be used to distinguish a behavior within normal limits from a behavior that is symptomatic. For children below 5 years of age, the behavior should occur on most days for a period of at least 6 months unless otherwise noted (criterion A8). For individuals 5 years of age or older, the behavior should occur at least once per week for at least 6 months unless otherwise noted (criterion A8). Although these frequency criteria provide guidance on a minimal level of frequency to define symptoms, other factors should also be considered, such as whether the frequency and intensity of the behaviors are outside a normative range for the individual's developmental level, gender, and culture.

B. The disturbance in behavior is associated with distress in the individual or others in his or her immediate social context (e.g., family, peer group, work colleagues) or it impacts negatively on social, educational, occupational, or other important areas of functioning.

C. The behaviors do not occur exclusively during the course of a psychotic, substance use, depressive, or bipolar disorder. Also, the criteria for disruptive mood dysregulation disorder are not met.

Specify *current severity:*

Mild: Symptoms are confined to only one setting (e.g., at home, at school, at work, with peers).

Moderate: Some symptoms are present in at least two settings.

Severe: Some symptoms are present in three or more settings.

From the American Psychiatric Association. (2013). *Diagnostic and statistical manual of mental disorders* (5th ed.). Washington, DC: Author.

Epidemiology

Oppositional defiant disorder is typically diagnosed around 8 years of age, but it may be seen as early as age 3 and usually not later than early adolescence. The prevalence of oppositional defiant disorder is globally consistent and similar across race and ethnicity. The lifetime prevalence is nearly 13%.

Males are diagnosed three times more often than females (Loeber et al., 2009). Various factors may account for this gender difference. For example, some traits of the disorder are seen more in boys than in girls, as boys are more likely to annoy and blame others and girls argue more. Additionally, clinicians may view and judge an individual's display of behavior differently depending on the person's gender. For example, it may be more socially appropriate in many cultures for a boy to express aggression than for a girl to do so.

Comorbidity

The most common condition associated with oppositional defiant disorder is ADHD, with rates reaching nearly 40%. Anxiety and depressive disorders are also commonly present in this population.

Oppositional defiant disorder shares criteria with disruptive mood dysregulation disorder, a depressive disorder. Its symptoms include a chronic negative mood and temper outbursts. Symptoms tend to be more severe in disruptive mood dysregulation disorder. If the individual meets the criteria for this disorder, a diagnosis of oppositional defiant disorder is not given. Mayes and colleagues (2016) do not support two separate diagnoses. They suggest that disruptive mood dysregulation disorder should be classified as a specifier for oppositional defiant disorder rather than a separate diagnosis.

Risk Factors
Biological Factors
Genetic. Oppositional defiant disorder tends to manifest at a young age, and more than 100 studies have supported that aggressive and antisocial behavior has a 40% to 60% genetic basis (Raine, 2014). Many individuals diagnosed with this disorder have a family history of another mental illness.

Neurobiological. A growing body of research supports the neurobiological basis of aggressive behavior. In individuals with oppositional defiant disorder, gray matter is less dense in the left prefrontal cortex, an area associated with impulse control and self-regulation (Fahim et al., 2012). Noordermeer and colleagues (2016) analyzed controlled studies that used both structural magnetic resonance imaging (sMRI) and functional MRI (fMRI) in individuals diagnosed with oppositional defiant disorder. These individuals had smaller brain structures and lower brain activity in the bilateral amygdala, bilateral insula, right striatum, left medial/superior frontal gyrus, and left precuneus. These deficits suggest impaired cognitive control over emotional behavior.

Oppositional defiant disorder has been associated with other brain abnormalities. Hyporeactivity of the amygdala to negative stimuli and altered serotonin and noradrenaline neurotransmission have also been found (Matthys et al., 2012). These abnormalities may reduce the ability of children, adolescents, and adults to make associations between inappropriate behaviors and future punishment. Altered dopamine function may also render them hyposensitive to rewards that most people commonly seek.

Physiological. During times of stress, people experience increased cortisol activity. Individuals with oppositional defiant disorder demonstrate reduced cortisol reactivity to stress (Matthys et al., 2012). Additionally, they experience sympathetic nervous system hyporeactivity to incentives and low basal heart rate during times of sensation seeking. These states may make such individuals prone to sensation-seeking behavior, such as defying authority, breaking rules, and abusing substances.

Oppositional defiant disorder is not always associated with a low resting heart rate. Schoorl and colleagues (2016) studied resting heart rates in boys 8 to 12 years of age with this disorder. A high resting heart rate and high skin conductance levels were associated with reactive aggression. A low resting heart rate and low skin conductance levels were associated with proactive aggression. These findings suggest that there are variants of this disorder.

Cognitive Factors

Learning theory suggests that negative symptoms are acquired. Children mirror the negative reinforcement methods used by parents and other people in positions of power. Individuals may also manifest oppositional defiance to get the attention and reactions they crave from parents, even if it is a negative sort of attention.

From the perspective of developmental theory, problems begin as early as toddlerhood and then continue. Children and teens with oppositional defiant disorder may be displaying developmental issues that last beyond the toddler years.

Environmental Factors

Adverse childhood experiences (ACEs) are associated with oppositional defiant disorder and other impulse control disorders that continue into adulthood (Horn et al., 2019). ACEs include family distress, inadequate parenting, and problems with attachment. Conflict in the marriage is more important than whether or not the parents separate. Children from larger and impoverished families are also at risk.

Although we know that coercive or inconsistent parental behavior and child abuse are correlated with the development of disruptive behaviors, the directionality of causation is not always one way. That is, child abuse may be both the cause of oppositional defiance and the result of oppositional defiance. Although parents may have provided consistent parenting to a child with a mild temperament, having a child with a difficult temperament or ADHD can result in harsh and inconsistent parenting. A further complication is that children with this disorder tend to have a low sensitivity to punishment, which makes them less able to associate behaviors with punishments.

Other factors—such as socioeconomic status, neighborhood violence, and lack of structure within the home—all contribute some risk toward the development of this disorder.

EVIDENCE-BASED PRACTICE

Oppositional Defiant Disorder...in Adults?

Problem

Although clinicians have speculated that oppositional defiant disorder persists into adulthood, more research is needed to understand how this disorder affects adults. It is likely that adults may be affected by negative functional outcomes.

Purpose of Study

This study was conducted to explore the prevalence and associated impairments of oppositional defiance disorder symptoms in young adults.

Methods

College students between the ages of 18 and 24 were the subjects in this study. Two large samples of 1792 and 1497 students completed self-report scales of oppositional defiant disorder symptoms, other psychiatric diagnoses, and functional impairments. Researchers explored the association between high levels of oppositional defiant symptoms, social and authority-related impairments, and online antagonistic behavior.

Findings

- In the two samples, the proportions of individuals reporting four or more symptoms of oppositional defiant disorder were about 3.4% and 4.1%, respectively.
- Gender did not affect the prevalence.
- Higher oppositional defiance severity was associated with social impairment, more conflict with authority figures, and antagonistic behaviors online.

Why Should Nurses Be Interested in This Study?

Knowing that oppositional defiant disorder does not always disappear after adolescence may help nurses to understand mystifying oppositional symptoms in young adults. Based on Erikson's theory of psychosocial development (see Chapter 2), the task of college students is the achievement of intimacy versus living in isolation. Limited social outlets along with time spent flaming online do not support the achievement of intimacy and may also affect college performance. Nurses are often in a position to recognize these problems and to support patients with oppositional symptoms.

Johnston, O. G., Derella, O. J., & Burke, J. D. (2018). Identification of oppositional defiant disorder in young adult college students. *Journal of Psychopathology and Behavioral Assessment, 40,* 563–572.

CONDUCT DISORDER

Clinical Picture

Conduct disorder is a persistent pattern of behavior in which the rights of others are violated and societal norms or rules are disregarded. The behavior is usually abnormally aggressive and can frequently lead to the destruction of property or physical injury. Individuals with this disorder initiate physical fights and engage in bullying. They may steal or use a weapon to intimidate or hurt others. Coercion into an activity against another's will, including sexual activity, is characteristic of this disorder. These behaviors are enduring patterns and continue over a period of 6 months and beyond.

People affected by this disorder may have normal intelligence but tend to skip class or disrupt school so much that they fall behind and may fail, be expelled, or drop out. Complications associated with conduct disorder include juvenile delinquency, drug and alcohol abuse and dependency, and juvenile court involvement. People with conduct disorder crave excitement and do not worry as much about consequences as others do.

Although the literature tends to focus on children and adolescents with conduct disorder, adults can also be diagnosed with this condition. In adults, conduct disorder has similar characteristics of aggression, destruction of property, stealing, deceitfulness, and criminal behavior.

There are two subtypes of conduct disorder—child onset versus adolescent onset—both of which can occur in mild, moderate, or severe forms.

Childhood-onset conduct disorder occurs before age 10 and occurs mostly in males. These boys are physically aggressive, have poor peer relationships, show little concern for others, and lack feelings of guilt or remorse. They tend to interpret others' intentions as hostile and believe that their own aggressive responses are justified.

Violent children also often display antisocial reasoning, such as "he deserved it," when they are rationalizing aggressive behaviors. Children with childhood-onset conduct disorder attempt to project a strong image, but they actually have low self-esteem. Limited frustration tolerance, irritability, and temper outbursts are hallmarks of this disorder. Individuals with childhood-onset conduct disorder are more likely to have problems that persist through adolescence. Without intensive treatment, they may later, as adults, develop antisocial personality disorder.

In adolescent-onset conduct disorder, no clinically significant symptoms are present before age 10. Affected adolescents tend to act out in the context of their peer group through sexual behavior, substance use, or risk-taking behaviors. Males are more likely to fight, steal, vandalize, and have school discipline problems. Girls tend to lie, be truant, run away, misuse substances, and be sexually promiscuous. The male-to-female ratio is not as high as for the childhood-onset type, indicating that more girls become aggressive during this period of development.

A subset of people with conduct disorder exhibit the especially dangerous qualities of being callous and unemotional. **Callousness** is characterized by a lack of empathy and being unconcerned about the feelings of others. Expression of guilt is absent except when the individual is facing punishment. School and family obligations are unimportant to affected individuals. Callousness may be a predictor of future antisocial personality disorder in adults (Burke et al., 2010). Unemotional traits include a shallow, unexpressive, and superficial affect.

Diagnostic criteria for conduct disorder are listed in the *DSM-5* box.

DSM-5 CRITERIA FOR CONDUCT DISORDER

A. A repetitive and persistent pattern of behavior in which the basic rights of others or major age-appropriate societal norms or rules are violated as manifested by the presence of at least three of the following 15 criteria in the past 12 months from any of the following categories with at least one criterion present in the past 6 months:

Aggression to People and Animals
1. Often bullies, threatens, or intimidates others
2. Often initiates physical fights
3. Has used a weapon that can cause serious physical harm to others (e.g., a bat, brick, broken bottle, knife, gun)
4. Has been physically cruel to people
5. Has been physically cruel to animals
6. Has stolen while confronting a victim (e.g., mugging, purse snatching, extortion, armed robbery)
7. Has forced someone into sexual activity

Destruction of Property
8. Has deliberately engaged in fire setting with the intention of causing serious damage
9. Has deliberately destroyed others' property (other than by fire setting)

Deceitfulness or Theft
10. Has broken into someone else's house, building, or car
11. Often lies to obtain goods or favors to avoid obligations (i.e., "cons" others)
12. Has stolen items of nontrivial value without confronting a victim (e.g., shoplifting but without breaking and entering; forgery)

Serious Violations of Rules
13. Often stays out at night despite parental prohibitions, beginning before age 13 years
14. Has run away from home overnight at least twice while living in the parental or parental surrogate home or once without returning for a lengthy period
15. Is often truant from school beginning before age 13 years

B. The disturbance in behavior causes clinically significant impairment in social, academic, or occupational functioning.

C. If the individual is age 18 years or older, criteria are not met for antisocial personality disorder.

Specify whether:
Childhood-onset type: Individuals show at least one symptom characteristic of conduct disorder before age 10 years.
Adolescent-onset type: Individuals show no symptom characteristic of conduct disorder before age 10 years.
Unspecified onset: Criteria for a diagnosis of conduct disorder are met, but there is not enough information available to determine whether the onset of the first symptom was before or after age 10 years.
Specify if: With limited prosocial emotions
Specify current severity: mild, moderate, or severe

From the American Psychiatric Association. (2013). *Diagnostic and statistical manual of mental disorders* (5th ed.). Washington, DC: Author.

Epidemiology

Conduct disorder carries a lifetime prevalence of nearly 7%. This may be higher in urban settings as compared with rural areas. Childhood onset is more common in males than in females, but in adolescent onset, the numbers are nearly equal. This disorder seems to be stable across races and ethnicities. The diagnosis of conduct disorder is four times more common among individuals who have previously been diagnosed with oppositional defiant disorder (Loeber et al., 2009).

Comorbidity

ADHD and oppositional defiant disorder are both common among people with conduct disorder. The combination of both predicts worse outcomes. Conduct disorders are often comorbid with one or more of the following disorders: specific learning disorder, anxiety disorders, depressive or bipolar disorders, and substance use disorders.

Risk Factors

Biological Factors

Genetic. Conduct disorder seems to be influenced by genetic factors. The risk is increased in children with a biological parent or a sibling with the disorder. However, it is difficult to tease out the contribution of genetics versus that of a traumatic environment. Do people inherit traits associated with antisocial behavior or do they learn to be antisocial by the intergenerational mirroring of characteristics? One study points to a mix of genetic inheritance and environmental factors. Salvatore and Dick (2018) found that a genetic predisposition may increase an individual's selection of higher-risk environments (e.g., rule-violating peers, dangerous activities, and unsafe areas). These environments may differentially methylate conduct disorder candidate genes, thereby modifying the function of the genes and affecting gene expression.

Neurobiological. Adolescents with conduct disorder have been found to have significantly reduced gray matter in the anterior insulate cortex and the left amygdala. The insulate cortex is believed to be involved in emotion and empathy, and the amygdala helps process emotional reactions and rewards (Byrd et al., 2014). Individuals with conduct disorder who display limited prosocial emotions, specifically those who are callous and unemotional, have more folds in the cortical insula (Fairchild et al., 2015).

Brain changes in people with conduct disorder are not simply structural, they are also functional. Investigators asked children with conduct disorder who displayed callousness to respond to images of others being harmed. Functional MRIs indicated that the children experienced diminished blood flow in the region of the brain associated with empathy and emotional response as compared with healthy controls (Michalska et al., 2015).

Environmental Factors

As in the case of oppositional defiant disorder, conduct disorder is highly associated with ACEs. ACEs commonly found with conduct disorder include parental rejection and neglect, inconsistent parenting with harsh discipline, early institutional living, chaotic home life, large family size, an absent father, antisocial family members, and alcohol and substance use at home. Social factors include peer rejection, violent neighborhoods, and association with delinquent peers.

INTERMITTENT EXPLOSIVE DISORDER

Clinical Picture

Intermittent explosive disorder is a pattern of behavioral outbursts characterized by an inability to control one's aggressive impulses. The aggression can be verbal or physical and is targeted toward other people, animals, property, or even oneself.

Anything can trigger the aggressive reaction to the situation. A man may be unable to locate his favorite video game and impulsively punches his fist through a pane of glass. He may tear his room apart, break furniture, or damage costly property. As the rage continues, he may attack anyone who intervenes and will often cause injury. The explosive anger may occur during a competitive sport, such as lashing out at opposing baseball fans when his team loses.

A pattern that commonly emerges is going from rage to remorse. The first stage is tension and arousal based on some environmental stimulus, such as someone driving too slowly in the passing lane on the expressway. This is followed by explosive behavior and aggression. A response to the slow driver may be hitting the gas and dangerously passing the person on the shoulder of the road. Immediately after, the person feels a sense of relief and release, taking satisfaction by looking at the offender in the rearview mirror and delivering a negative hand signal. Delayed consequences include feelings of remorse, regret, and embarrassment over the aggressive behavior. After the event, reality may set in. "Wow, I just risked my life to pass an 80-year-old man to get to a party that will go on for hours. I have to stop doing this."

This disorder can impair a person's functioning by leading to problems with interpersonal relationships as well as occupational difficulties. It can lead to legal problems as well. Significant problems with physical health, such as hypertension and diabetes, have been linked to this disorder (McCloskey et al., 2010). Being in a heightened state of stress and agitation for a prolonged period of time may be correlated with these outcomes.

Individuals with intermittent explosive disorder may feel a range of emotions—not just anger—stronger than that felt by other people. The problem is a general form of emotional dysregulation, and explosive anger is just one manifestation (Fettich et al., 2015).

Epidemiology

Lifetime prevalence of intermittent explosive disorder is about 7%. It is more common in males than in females (McCloskey et al., 2010). This disorder tends to begin in childhood and is more prevalent in people below 50 years of age.

Comorbidity

The most commonly associated comorbid conditions associated with intermittent explosive disorder are depressive disorders, anxiety disorders, and substance use disorders. Antisocial and borderline personality disorder, ADHD, and a history of the other disruptive disorders (e.g., conduct disorder, oppositional defiant disorder) are also associated with this disorder.

Risk Factors
Biological Factors
Physiological. Individuals with intermittent explosive disorder have been found to have higher than normal levels of the inflammatory markers C-reactive protein and interleukin-6 present in the blood during times of infection (Coccaro et al., 2014). These markers may facilitate aggression by modulating certain neurotransmitters. Research demonstrates a direct correlation between high levels of these markers and actual measures of aggression. Also, higher levels of the hormone testosterone have been associated with intermittent explosive disorder.

Neurobiological. Intermittent explosive disorder is associated with the loss of neurons in both the amygdala and hippocampus. These changes may play a role in the pathophysiology of impulsive aggression (Coccaro et al., 2015). Abnormalities in serotonin in the limbic area of the brain have been found in individuals with this diagnosis.

Environmental Factors
Intermittent explosive disorder is associated with trauma, particularly conflict and violence in the family of origin. Being exposed to violence at an early age makes it more likely that, as the child matures, the behavior will be repeated. It is common for these families to have a history of addiction and substance use disorder.

Impulsivity and aggression are distinctive characteristics of intermittent explosive disorder and are also risk factors for suicide (self-aggression). Childhood maltreatment is a factor strongly associated with impulsive aggression. Physical abuse is a specific risk factor for developing intermittent explosive disorder (Fanning et al., 2014). Sexual abuse is also associated with the development of this disorder.

⊕ CONSIDERING CULTURE

Are Veterans at Risk for Intermittent Explosive Disorder?

Military training and culture reinforce risk factors for violent behavior. Experiencing trauma and violence increases the risk for violent behavior and predisposes veterans to posttraumatic stress disorder (PTSD), which is associated with aggressive and suicidal behavior. Researchers have discovered that there is significant overlap between PTSD and intermittent explosive disorder. These findings have a tremendous impact on caring for these veterans, since this particular comorbidity results in a subgroup of individuals with very high levels of aggressive behavior and a high rate of suicide attempts, which was 41.4% in the sample studied. Screening for intermittent explosive disorder may aid in identifying individuals at risk for aggressive and suicidal behavior.

Adapted from Fanning, J. R., Lee, R., & Coccaro, E. F. (2016). Comorbid intermittent explosive disorder and posttraumatic stress disorder: Clinical correlates and relationship to suicidal behavior. *Comprehensive Psychiatry, 70,* 125–133.

PYROMANIA AND KLEPTOMANIA

Two problems related to impulse control disorders are pyromania and kleptomania. **Pyromania** is described as repeated deliberate fire setting. The person experiences tension or becomes excited before setting a fire and shows a fascination with or unusual interest in fire and its contexts, such as matches. The person also experiences pleasure or relief on setting a fire, witnessing a fire, or participating in the aftermath of a fire. The fire setting is done solely to bring this relief and/or pleasure and not for other reasons, such as to conceal a crime.

Pyromania occurs more often in males, particularly those who have poor social skills and learning difficulties (APA, 2013). Individuals with pyromania often have a history of alcohol or substance use. Juvenile fire setting is usually associated with conduct disorder or ADHD.

Kleptomania is a repeated failure to resist urges to steal objects not needed for personal use or monetary value. For example, a person may take books even though he cannot read or take baby outfits considered cute even though she has no children and has enough money to buy them. As in pyromania, the person experiences a buildup of tension before taking the object with feelings of relief or pleasure following the theft. Some research has explored whether this disorder is more closely linked to other addictive behaviors, such as substance use disorder, since the person is acting to satisfy a compulsion (Talih, 2011).

Kleptomania is associated with other impulse control disorders and impulse control–related problems, such as impulsive buying. It is also associated with mood disorders, such as major depressive disorder, anxiety disorders, eating disorders (particularly bulimia nervosa), and personality disorders.

Table 21.1 provides a summary of the characteristics of impulse control disorders.

▌APPLICATION OF THE NURSING PROCESS

ASSESSMENT

General Assessment
Some individuals with disruptive, impulse control, and conduct disorders may be in the healthcare system based on severe symptoms and a need to stabilize them. Patients with these disorders may also be in the healthcare system based on comorbid disorders such as ADHD, anxiety, major depressive disorder, or substance use disorder. Careful assessment is important to separate and understand the problems. With children, interviewing the parents along with the child and then separately will enrich the value of the assessment.

Suicide Risk
To determine the cause of the distress and the risk of violence, the nurse must listen carefully to any person expressing the wish to hurt self or others. The primary predictor of suicidal risk is a past suicide attempt. Impulsivity and aggression in this population make the possibility of suicide attempts more

TABLE 21.1 Characteristics of Impulse Control Disorders

Disorder	Age of Onset	Lifetime Prevalence	Gender	Clinical Features	Notes
Oppositional defiant disorder	Childhood/adolescence; usually diagnosed around age 8	12.6%	More males	Angry/irritable mood. Argumentative defiant behavior. Vindictiveness. Despite behavior, the person recognizes that others have rights and that there are rules.	May become conduct disorder in later years.
Conduct disorder	Childhood onset (<10 years) worse prognosis. Adolescent onset (no symptoms before age 10)	6.8%	Childhood onset: more males. Adolescent onset: equal	Unimpulsive violation of the rights of others, aggression to people and animals, destruction of property, deceitfulness, violates rules.	More criminal involvement. May be a precursor to antisocial personality disorder.
Intermittent explosive disorder	May be diagnosed at age 6; mean age of onset, 13–21 years	7.3%	More males	Impulsive and unwarranted emotional outbursts, violence, destruction of property.	Early treatment may prevent worsening pathology.

Merikangas, K. R., He, J., Burstein, M., Swanson, S. A., Avenevoli, S., Cui, L. ... Swendsen, J. (2010). Lifetime prevalence of mental disorders in U.S. adolescents: Results from the National Comorbidity Survey Replication—Adolescent supplement. *Journal of the American Academy of Adolescent Psychiatry, 49*(10), 980–989.

likely. Areas to explore in assessing suicidal risk include the following:

- Past suicidal thoughts, threats, or attempts
- Existence of a plan, lethality of the plan, and accessibility of the methods for carrying out the plan
- Feelings of hopelessness, changes in level of energy
- Circumstances, state of mind, and motivation
- Viewpoints about suicide and death (e.g., Has a family member or friend attempted or completed suicide?)
- Depression and other moods or feelings (e.g., anger, guilt, rejection)
- History of impulsivity, poor judgment, or decreased ability to make decisions
- Drug or alcohol use
- Prescribed medications and recent adherence issues
- Assessment of strengths, protective factors, and effective coping skills

For the younger person with oppositional defiant disorder or conduct disorder, a distorted concept of death and immature ego functions complicate an assessment of the lethality of a suicide plan. For instance, a child who is highly suicidal may believe that a few aspirin tablets will cause death. The incorrect judgment about the lethality does not diminish the seriousness of the intent. Some teens may make a pact to kill themselves or may become upset after a friend has committed suicide or died accidentally. Early intervention is essential, and parents must understand that suicidal thoughts or self-threatening behavior (e.g., cutting, reckless driving, binge drinking) must be taken seriously and evaluated by mental health professionals as an emergency.

Assessment Tools

There are a variety of tools that you can use to increase your understanding of the important facets of these disorders. Also, they can help you to share information with colleagues and families of patients.

Oppositional defiant and conduct disorder in young people can be examined more carefully with the questions in Fig. 21.1. They are subsets of an ADHD scale. For both scales individually, scores of 2 to 3 are considered to be indicative of a problem.

📋 ASSESSMENT GUIDELINES

Oppositional Defiant Disorder

1. Identify issues that result in power struggles and triggers for outbursts—when they begin and how they are handled.
2. Assess the child's or adolescent's view of his or her behavior and its impact on others (e.g., at home, at school, and with peers). Explore the child's or adolescent's feelings of empathy and remorse.
3. Explore the degree to which the child or adolescent can exercise control and take responsibility, solve problems, and plan to handle things more effectively in the future. Assess barriers, the motivation to change, and the use of potential rewards to engage the patient.

Conduct Disorder

1. Assess the seriousness, types, and initiation of disruptive behavior and how it has been managed.
2. Assess anxiety, aggression and anger levels, motivation, and the ability to control impulses.
3. Assess moral development, problem solving, belief system, and spirituality for the ability to understand the impact of hurtful behavior on others, to empathize with others, and to feel remorse.
4. Assess the ability to form a therapeutic relationship and engage in honest and committed therapeutic work leading to observable behavioral change (e.g., signing a behavioral contract, drug testing, and living according to "home rules").
5. Assess for substance use (past and present).

Intermittent Explosive Disorder

1. Assess the history, frequency, and triggers for violent outbursts.
2. Identify times in which the patient was able to maintain control despite being in a situation in which the patient might normally lose control of emotions.
3. Explore actual and potential sources of support at home and socially.
4. Assess for substance use (past and present).

Oppositional Defiant Disorder	Never	Occasionally	Often	Very Often
1. Argues with adults	0	1	2	3
2. Loses temper	0	1	2	3
3. Actively disobeys or refuses to follow an adult's request or rules	0	1	2	3
4. Bothers people on purpose	0	1	2	3
5. Blames others for his or her mistakes or misbehaviors	0	1	2	3
6. Is touchy or easily annoyed by others	0	1	2	3
7. Is angry or bitter	0	1	2	3
8. Is hateful and wants to get even	0	1	2	3

Conduct Disorder	Never	Occasionally	Often	Very Often
1. Bullies, threatens, or scares others	0	1	2	3
2. Starts physical fights	0	1	2	3
3. Lies to get out of trouble or to avoid jobs	0	1	2	3
4. Skips school without permission	0	1	2	3
5. Is physically unkind to people	0	1	2	3
6. Has stolen things that have value	0	1	2	3
7. Destroys others' property on purpose	0	1	2	3
8. Has used a weapon that can cause serious harm (bat, knife, brick, gun)	0	1	2	3
9. Is physically mean to animals	0	1	2	3
10. Has set fire on purpose to do damage	0	1	2	3
11. Has broken into someone else's home, business, or car	0	1	2	3
12. Has stayed out at night without permission	0	1	2	3
13. Has run away from home overnight	0	1	2	3
14. Has forced someone into sexual activity	0	1	2	3

Fig. 21.1 Screening for disruptive behaviors: Vanderbilt Attention-Deficit/Hyperactivity Disorder Diagnostic Teacher Rating Scale. (From Wolraich, M. L., Feurer, I. D., Hannah, J. N., Baumgaertel, A., & Pinnock, T. Y. [1998]. Obtaining systematic teacher reports of disruptive behavior disorders utilizing DSM-IV. *Journal of Abnormal Child Psychology, 26*[2], 141–152.)

Self-Assessment

People with impulse control disorders have behaviors that are objectionable to most others. Concerns for personal, emotional, and physical safety may be real or exaggerated depending on the nature of the patient's behavior. These concerns should be addressed, and steps should be taken to provide the safest environment for care.

Negative attitudes may be directed at the patient because the caretaker feels that behavior is controllable and that the patient is choosing not to get better. Our ethical and professional responsibility to provide equal care to all people extends to this population. An empathetic view of people with these disorders is necessary, particularly considering their environments of origin and history of constant negative responses from others.

NURSING DIAGNOSIS

Children, adolescents, and adults with oppositional defiant disorder, conduct disorder, and intermittent explosive disorder display disruptive behaviors that are impulsive, angry/aggressive, and often dangerous. Therefore, nursing diagnoses would include *impaired impulse control, risk for suicide, aggressive behavior*, and *risk for violence* (International Council of Nurses, 2019). These individuals are treatment nonadherent, do not follow age-appropriate social norms, and have inappropriate ways of meeting their needs. Corresponding to these problems, nursing diagnoses would include *nonadherence to safety regime*, *impaired child/adolescent development*, and *impaired coping*. Parenting problems such as inconsistent or harsh punishment can be addressed with the nursing diagnosis *impaired parenting*.

OUTCOMES IDENTIFICATION

Outcomes for impulse control disorders relate specifically to reversing the diagnosis that has been identified. Whenever possible, outcomes should be centered on the patient and agreed upon by both the nurse and patient or the patient's designee.

Signs and symptoms, nursing diagnoses, and associated outcomes for people with impulse control disorders are paired in Table 21.2.

IMPLEMENTATION

Interventions for severe oppositional defiant, conduct, and intermittent explosive disorders focus on correcting firmly entrenched patterns such as blaming others and denial of responsibility for personal actions. Children, adolescents, and adults with these disorders also must generate more mature and adaptive coping mechanisms and prosocial goals, a process that is gradual and cannot be accomplished during short-term treatment.

General interventions include the following:
1. Promote a climate of safety for the patient and for others.
2. Establish rapport with the patient.
3. Set limits and expectations.
4. Consistently follow through with consequences of rule breaking.
5. Provide structure and boundaries.
6. Provide activities and opportunities for achievement of goals to promote a sense of purpose.

When caring for individuals with impulse control disorders, it is important to remember the adverse environmental conditions associated with these counterproductive behaviors. Recognizing these harsh environments supports nurses in providing trauma-informed care. Trauma-informed care promotes an environment of healing and recovery rather than unintentionally retraumatizing the patient. An attitude of "what happened to you?" versus "what is wrong with you?" sets the stage for compassionate care.

Oppositional youth are generally treated on an outpatient basis, using individual, group, and family therapy, with much of the focus on parenting issues. In conduct disorder, inpatient hospitalization for crisis intervention, evaluation, and treatment planning as well as transfer to therapeutic foster care, group homes, or long-term residential treatment are often needed. Patients with intermittent explosive disorder may be treated on an inpatient basis, particularly if they are facing employment and relationship consequences of angry outbursts.

Teamwork and Safety

During inpatient stays, part of teamwork and the promotion of safety is the monitoring of dynamics between staff and patients. Safety is compromised when a power struggle exists between staff, patients, and family members. The term **expressed emotion** refers to the qualitative amount of emotion displayed, usually in the context of family interactions. In the context of the treatment environment, strongly expressed emotion is a major cause of aggressive responses from patients with impulse control disorders.

Violence increases when staff act in an authoritarian or confrontational way or engage in power struggles. Body language such as standing too close and tone of voice can indicate aggression on the part of staff. Arbitrary or poorly explained denial of privileges can trigger violent retaliation. Strongly expressed emotion includes criticisms, resentment, or annoyance about patient behavior.

Staff who use moderately expressed emotion calmly communicate in a way that reduces confrontation and decreases the need for seclusion and restraint and also decreases relapse in the

TABLE 21.2 Signs and Symptoms, Nursing Diagnoses, and Outcomes for Impulse Control Disorders

Signs and Symptoms	Nursing Diagnoses	Outcomes
History of suicide attempts, aggression and impulsivity, conflictual interpersonal relationships; states, "If I have to stay here, I'm going to kill myself."	*Risk for suicide*	Decreased suicide risk: Expresses feelings, verbalizes suicidal ideas, refrains from suicide attempts, plans for the future
Rigid body posture, clenches fists and jaw, paces, invades others' personal space, history of cruelty to animals and fire setting, adverse childhood experiences. States "I don't get mad, I get even."	*Risk for violence*	No violence: Identifies harmful impulsive behaviors, controls impulses, refrains from aggressive acts, identifies social support
Hostile laughter, projects responsibility for behavior onto others, grandiosity, difficulty establishing relationships. States, "That nurse pushed me over the edge."	*Impaired impulse control*	Improved impulse control: Identifies ineffective and effective coping, identifies and uses support system, uses new coping strategies
Rejection of child or hostility toward child, abuse, neglect, inconsistent discipline. Caregiver states, "We've given up on him."	*Impaired parenting*	Effective parenting: Parent/caregiver participates in the therapeutic program, learns effective parenting skills

patient. The best way to communicate with a potentially hostile patient includes the following techniques:

- Using nonthreatening body posture and a flat, neutral tone of voice (never an angry tone of voice) when correcting behavior
- Using matter-of-fact, easy-to-understand words
- Consistently setting limits
- Avoiding personal terms (such as "I" or "you") in setting limits

Seclusion and Restraint

Seclusion and restraint may be necessary as a last resort when one is working with patients who have impulse control disorders. The use of a time out or a quiet area may be helpful in reducing the stimuli of the environment. Refer to Chapter 6 for more information related to seclusion and restraint.

Box 21.1 provides a summary of techniques to manage disruptive behaviors.

Health Teaching and Health Promotion

When the patient is a child or adolescent, ideally families will be actively engaged and be given support in using parenting skills to provide nurturance and set consistent limits. They can be taught techniques for behavior modification, monitoring medication for therapeutic effects, collaborating with teachers to foster academic success, and setting up a home environment that is consistent, structured, and nurturing to promote the achievement of normal developmental milestones. If families are abusive, drug dependent, or highly disorganized, the child may require out-of-home placement.

The following nursing interventions are helpful in working with parents and caregivers:

- Explore the impact of the child's behaviors on family life and of the other members' behavior on the child.
- Help the immediate and extended family to access available and supportive individuals and systems.
- Discuss how to make the home a safe environment, especially with regard to weapons and drugs; attempt to talk to members individually if possible.
- Discuss realistic behavioral goals and how to set them; explore potential problems.
- Teach behavior modification techniques. Role-play them with the parents in different problem situations that might arise with their child.
- Give support and encouragement as parents learn to apply new techniques.
- Provide education about medications.
- Refer patients, parents, or other caregivers to local self-help groups.
- Advocate with the educational system if special education services are needed.

EVALUATION

Patients with impulse control disorders exhibit an inability to self-regulate. Care is aimed at providing external boundaries and a safe environment. Ideally, patients on inpatient units demonstrate increased levels of self-regulation and ability to interact appropriately with others. In outpatient and community settings, patients will progress incrementally from aggressive

---

BOX 21.1 Techniques for Managing Disruptive Behaviors

Behavioral contract: A patient-centered verbal or written agreement between the patient and nurse or other parties (e.g., family, treatment team, teacher) about behaviors, expectations, and needs. The contract is periodically evaluated and reviewed and typically coupled with rewards and other contingencies, positive and negative.

Counseling: Verbal interactions teach, coach, or maintain adaptive behavior and provide positive reinforcement. It is most effective for motivated patients and those with well-developed communication and self-reflective skills.

Modeling: A method of learning behaviors or skills by observation and imitation that can be used in a wide variety of situations. It is enhanced when the modeler is perceived to be similar (e.g., age, interests) and attending to the task is required.

Role playing: A counseling technique in which the nurse, the patient, or a group of patients act out a specified script or role to enhance their understanding of that role, learn and practice new behaviors or skills, and practice specific situations. It requires well-developed expressive and receptive language skills.

Planned ignoring: When the staff determines behaviors not to be safe and only attention seeking, they may be ignored. Additional interventions may be used in conjunction (e.g., positive reinforcement for on-task actions).

Physical distance and touch control: Whereas touching and closeness may have a positive effect on many patients, patients with oppositional defiant, intermittent explosive, and conduct disorders may need increased personal space and feel threatened by touch.

Redirection: A technique used after an undesirable or inappropriate behavior to engage or reengage an individual in an appropriate activity. It may involve the use of verbal directives (e.g., setting firm limits), gestures, or physical prompts.

Positive feedback: Emotional support and positive feedback are good for anyone, but they are particularly helpful for individuals who rarely receive such attention.

Clarification as intervention: Sometimes, misunderstandings are the source of frustration and potential loss of control. Helping the patient to understand the environment and what is happening can reduce feelings of vulnerability and the urge to strike out.

Restructuring: Changing an activity in a way that will decrease the stimulation or frustration (e.g., shorten the 1:1 session or change to a physical activity). This requires flexibility and planning to have an alternative in mind in case the activity is not going well.

Limit setting: Involves giving direction, stating an expectation, or telling the patient what is required. This should be done firmly, calmly, without judgment or anger, preferably in advance of problem behaviors occurring, and consistently when in a treatment setting among multiple staff.

Simple restitution: Refers to a procedure in which an individual is required or expected to correct the adverse environmental or relational effects of misbehavior by restoring the environment to its prior state, making a plan to correct actions with the nurse, and implementing the plan (e.g., apologizing to the people harmed, fixing the chairs that are upturned). Simple restitution is not punitive in nature, and typically additional interventions are involved (e.g., counseling).

Physical restraint: Seclusion and restraint may be necessary.

and impulsive behavior and move onto considering the rights of others and behaviors that are in control.

TREATMENT MODALITIES

Biological Treatments

Pharmacotherapy

The US Food and Drug Administration (FDA) has not approved any drugs for the treatment of oppositional defiant disorder, conduct disorder, or intermittent explosive disorder. Pharmacotherapy is often aimed at symptoms such as outbursts, anger, and aggression. Managing these symptoms may help individuals with impulse control disorders better respond to therapeutic interventions (Wu et al., 2015, p. 135).

Divalproex sodium (Depakote), a mood stabilizing and anticonvulsant medication, has been shown to reduce reactive aggression and irritability in oppositional defiant disorder. Five classes of medications are used for children and adolescents with conduct disorder; antidepressants, mood stabilizers/anticonvulsants, stimulants, antipsychotics, and adrenergic medications all show some efficacy (Taylor et al., 2019). Aripiprazole (Abilify) and risperidone (Risperdal) are two second-generation antipsychotics that have some proven efficacy in diminishing aggression associated with conduct disorder.

Several medications are used off-label (i.e., not for their intended use) for intermittent explosive disorder. Selective serotonin reuptake inhibitors (SSRIs) such as fluoxetine (Prozac) are used; escitalopram (Lexapro) has also been shown to improve social cognition, empathy, and understanding of others (Cremers et al., 2016). Mood stabilizers, such as lithium or some of the anticonvulsant agents, may be used along with an SSRI to increase its beneficial effects.

Second-generation antipsychotics such as aripiprazole (Abilify) may also exert a calming effect on the outbursts associated with intermittent explosive disorder. Beta-blocking medications may also help calm individuals with intermittent explosive disorder by slowing the heart rate and reducing blood pressure. However, benzodiazepine medications should be avoided because they may further reduce inhibitions and self-control in much the same way as alcohol does.

Psychological Therapies

Advanced practice psychiatric–mental health registered nurses and other professionals with advanced training—such as psychiatrists, psychologists, counselors, and social workers—use specialized psychosocial interventions. These interventions target pathology associated with impulse control disorders. The overall goals are to (1) help patients maintain control of their thoughts and behaviors and (2) help families to function more adaptively.

Cognitive Behavioral Therapy

Cognitive behavioral therapy (CBT) is an evidence-based treatment approach that can be used for children, adolescents, and adults on an individual or group basis. It is a talk therapy that focuses on a patient's feelings, thoughts, and behaviors and is based on the idea that by changing our thoughts to be more realistic and positive, we can change the way we experience life.

Trauma-focused cognitive behavioral therapy (TF-CBT) addresses the specific emotional needs of children, adolescents, adults, and families who are trying to overcome the effects of early trauma. TF-CBT is sensitive to the unique problems of patients with posttraumatic stress and mood disorders that result from violence, abuse, or loss. If the patient is a child, non-offending caregivers are often brought into treatment that also uses principles of family therapy.

Psychodynamic Psychotherapy

One of the older treatment approaches, psychodynamic psychotherapy, continues to have relevance. Its focus is on underlying feelings and motivations and explores conscious and unconscious thought processes. In working with impulse control problems, the therapist may help the patient to uncover underlying feelings and reasons behind rage or anger. This may help patients to develop better ways to think about and control their behavior.

Dialectical Behavioral Therapy

A specific kind of cognitive behavioral treatment that has a focus on impulse control is dialectical behavioral therapy (DBT). Skills taught include mindfulness, emotional regulation, distress tolerance, and personal effectiveness. Shelton and colleagues (2011) found a DBT-Corrections Modified version of this therapy to be effective in reducing physical aggression in incarcerated adolescents.

Parent-Child Interaction Therapy

Another evidence-based approach is parent-child interaction therapy (PCIT). Therapists such as advanced practice nurses sit behind one-way mirrors and coach parents through an earbud audio device while they interact with their children. The advanced practice nurse or other advanced practice provider (e.g., psychiatrist, psychologist, counselor, or therapist) can suggest strategies that reinforce positive behavior in the child or adolescent. The goal is to improve parenting strategies and thereby reduce problematic behavior.

Parent Management Training

Parent management training (PMT). Parents of children with oppositional defiant disorder and conduct disorder tend to engage in patterns of negative interactions, ineffective harsh punishments, emotionally charged commands and comments, and poor modeling of appropriate behaviors. Treating children and adolescents, parental intervention is an essential component of care. PMT is used to (1) help parents manage their offspring's behavior, (2) learn and use successful discipline techniques, and (3) promote positive behaviors in their children (Taylor et al., 2019). This evidence-based treatment is for children aged 2 to 14 with mild to severe behavioral problems. Home visits and programs such as Head Start can also reduce future oppositional behaviors and delinquency.

Social Skills Training

Children and adolescents benefit from therapy that will help them to be more flexible and learn how to interact more positively and effectively with peers. This type of training works best when it is conducted in a group setting that allows for interaction and feedback. Individuals with intermittent explosive disorder tend to attribute the actions of others as being hostile. Social skills training helps them to more accurately interpret the motivations of others.

Multisystemic Therapy

Of all the treatment approaches presented in this list, MST is the most extensive. This evidence-based approach is an intensive family- and community-based program that takes into consideration all of the environments of violent juvenile offenders. Therapists work with caregivers who are on call 24 hours a day, 7 days a week to go where the child is. Hanging out with friends is replaced with healthy activities such as sports or recreational activities. MST can improve family functioning, school performance, and peer relationships and can build meaningful social supports.

KEY POINTS TO REMEMBER

- Impulse control disorders include oppositional defiant disorder, conduct disorder, and intermittent explosive disorder. These are disorders of impulse that are seen in mental healthcare settings and in the criminal justice system.
- Chaotic and punitive environments are strongly correlated with the development of these disorders.
- Impulsivity and aggression in this population make the possibility of suicide attempts and other-directed violence more likely. Continual assessment of suicidal risk and other-directed violence is an essential component of care.
- Nurses are often attracted to healthcare to help people who want and need their assistance. Patients with impulse control disorders may create a level of discomfort, as they resist help and seem to be self-defeating and unkind. Remembering the tragic etiology of these disorders helps to increase empathy and therapeutic responses.

- Nursing diagnoses are focused on protection of self and others from impulsive and premeditated acts, improvement of coping skills, and development of an increased self-esteem.
- The three most important interventions with this population are to promote a climate of safety for the patient and for others, establish rapport with the patient, and set limits and expectations.
- An important concept in working with impulse control disorders is expressed emotion. To create a positive atmosphere of teamwork and safety, expressed emotion on the part of caregivers should be low to prevent emotional and behavioral reactivity.
- Seclusion and restraint may be necessary to protect the patient with an impulse control disorder and others during times of unsafe escalation.
- A variety of advanced practice interventions should be considered for this population. Most of them are evidence based and effective.

CRITICAL THINKING

1. Jacob is a 14-year-old adolescent who has been diagnosed with conduct disorder.
   a. Explain to one of your classmates his probable behaviors in terms of (1) aggression toward others, (2) destruction of property, (3) deceitfulness, and (4) violation of rules.
   b. What are the outcomes for this disorder?
   c. List at least seven ways in which you could support Jacob's parents. What are some community referrals you could give them in your own locale?
2. Mallory is a 17-year-old adolescent; she is being admitted to the adolescent psychiatric unit after several weeks of

impulsive behaviors, such as extensive cutting and running away from home.
   a. Put the following areas of assessment in order of priority and provide the rationale for your choices:
      1. Suicide risk
      2. Current coping skills
      3. Skin integrity/risk for infection
      4. Childhood development
      5. Current family relationships
   b. Identify at least three appropriate nursing diagnoses for Mallory based on the previously provided information.
   c. Name three nursing interventions to support the nursing diagnosis of ineffective coping.

CHAPTER REVIEW

1. Which statement made by a 9-year-old child after hitting a classmate is a typical comment associated with childhood conduct disorder?
   a. "I'm sorry, I won't hit him again."
   b. "He deserved it for being a sissy."
   c. "I didn't think I hit him very hard."
   d. "He hit me first. You just didn't see it."

2. What assessment data would support a diagnosis of conduct disorder? *Select all that apply.*
   a. Evidence of social isolation
   b. Arrested twice for disorderly conduct
   c. Expresses difficulty in keeping employment
   d. Demonstrates objective signs of phobia
   e. Exhibits signs of chronic self-mutilation

3. Which event experienced in the patient's childhood increases the risk of the development of behaviors associated with intermittent explosive disorder?
   a. Orphaned at age 4
   b. Physically abused from ages 3 to 10
   c. Born with a chronic congenital disorder
   d. Has one parent who has been diagnosed with obsessive-compulsive disorder

4. What is a common behavior observed in a patient diagnosed with intermittent explosive disorder? *Select all that apply.*
   a. Short attention span.
   b. Threatens suicide.
   c. Often purges after eating.
   d. Uses alcohol to excess.
   e. States, "Everyone is out to get me."

5. When the nurse is discussing oppositional defiant disorder with a group of parents, what information about the disorder should be included? *Select all that apply*
   a. Classic symptoms, including anger, irritation, and defiant behavior.
   b. The fact that children generally outgrow the behaviors without formal treatment.
   c. That severity is considered mild when symptoms are present in only one setting.
   d. That the disorder is diagnosed equally in both males and females.
   e. That the terms *argumentative* and *defiant* are often used to describe the patient.

6. Tommy, a 12-year-old boy admitted to the pediatric psychiatric unit, has recently been diagnosed with conduct disorder. In the activity room, the games he wanted to play were already in use. He responded by threatening to throw furniture and to hurt those who had the game he wanted. Nancy, a registered nurse, recognizes that Tommy's therapy must include which of the following?
   a. Consistency in implementing the consequences of breaking rules
   b. Empathetic reasoning when Tommy acts out in the activity room
   c. Teaching Tommy the benefits of socializing
   d. Solitary time so that Tommy can think about his actions

7. Santiago, an adolescent in a treatment facility, is loudly displaying anger with a visiting family member in the day room. It is obvious to the nurse that this pattern has played out before. Violence is often escalated when family members or authority figures
   a. Use a soft tone of voice to gain control of the situation
   b. Move away from the agitated person in fear
   c. Use simple words to communicate
   d. Engage in a power struggle

8. The impulse control spectrum can begin in childhood and continue on into adulthood, often morphing into criminal behaviors. Working with patients diagnosed with these disorders, the best examples of expressed emotion by the nursing staff are
   a. Low to prevent emotional reactions
   b. Matched to the patient's level of emotion

   c. Flat without evidence of any emotional output
   d. High in expression to improve therapeutic patient emotions

9. Claude is a new nurse on the psychiatric unit. He asks a senior nurse on staff for advice in working with patients with oppositional defiant disorder. Which statement reflects advice on solid therapeutic communication?
   a. "When you are correcting behavior, use a loud firm tone."
   b. "Use language beyond the patient's education level."
   c. "When you are setting limits, be specific and outline the consequences."
   d. "Aggressive body language will make the patients respect your position."

10. Childhood-onset conduct disorder is thought to be a precursor to which of the following psychiatric conditions?
    a. Antisocial personality disorder
    b. Bipolar disorder
    c. Schizophrenia
    d. Dissociative identity disorder

1. **b**; 2. **a, b, c**; 3. **b**; 4. **a, b, d**; 5. **a, b, c, e**; 6. **a**; 7. **d**; 8. **a**; 9. **c**; 10. **a**

NGN CASE STUDY AND QUESTIONS

Tyler is a 14-year-old male who is brought to the school nurse-counselor after a pattern of fighting, bullying, vandalizing school property, and skipping class. Last week, he was suspended from school after being found smoking marijuana in the restroom. Today, on his first day back in school, he provokes a fight in the cafeteria in the process of taking another student's lunch pass. He was then sent to the counselor, who was puzzled by his records. Until 1 year ago, upon entering seventh grade, he earned good grades and had no behavior problems at school.

Eventually, the school nurse suggests a psychiatric referral, which results in a recommendation for inpatient evaluation and care. Once admitted to the pediatric behavioral unit, the advanced practice provider diagnoses Tyler with conduct disorder and attention-deficit/hyperactivity disorder (ADHD).

1. For each assessment finding, indicate whether it is a characteristic of 1—conduct disorder, 2—ADHD, or 3—unrelated to either diagnosis. *Only one selection can be made for each assessment finding.*

Assessment Findings	1. Conduct Disorder	2. Attention-Deficit/ Hyperactivity Disorder	3. Unrelated to Either Diagnosis
a. Violates rights of others nonimpulsively			
b. Does not listen when spoken to directly			

Assessment Findings	1. Conduct Disorder	2. Attention-Deficit/ Hyperactivity Disorder	3. Unrelated to Either Diagnosis
c. Acts with vindictiveness			
d. Displays argumentative behavior			
e. Impulsively uses people's belongings without permission			
f. Acknowledges but rebels against rules and rights			
g. Shows aggression toward people and animals			
h. Destroys property			

Patient Finding	1. Achieved	2. Not Achieved	3. Unrelated
a. Stops himself from responding aggressively 40% of the time			
b. Shows aggression when others are using recreational equipment that he wants, particularly the basketball equipment			
c. Eats finger foods and refuses to eat whole meals if he does not like them			
d. Chooses social support from a favorite staff member; becomes agitated if that individual is busy			
e. Expresses hatred towards parents, then laughs and says nothing more			
f. Verbalizes suicidal thoughts for the first time and is willing to talk about them			

2. Tyler spends 7 days in the hospital and is nearing the end of inpatient treatment. The interprofessional treatment team meets to evaluate his progress.

Identify the patient findings that demonstrate that progress in meeting outcomes was 1—achieved, 2—not achieved, or 3—unrelated. *Only one selection can be made for each patient finding.*

NGN case study answers are on Evolve.

Visit the Evolve website for a posttest on the content in this chapter: http://evolve.elsevier.com/Varcarolis

REFERENCES

American Psychiatric Association. (2013). *DSM-5 table of contents.* Retrieved from http://www.psychiatry.org/dsm5.

Burke, J. D., Waldman, I., & Lahey, B. B. (2010). Predictive validity of childhood oppositional defiant disorder and conduct disorder: Implications for the DSM-V. *Journal of Abnormal Psychology, 119*(4), 739–751.

Byrd, A. L., Loeber, R., & Pardini, D. A. (2014). Antisocial behavior, psychopathic features and abnormalities in reward and punishment processing in youth. *Clinical Child and Family Psychology Review, 17*(2), 125–156.

Coccaro, E. F., Royce, L., & Coussons-Read, M. (2014). Elevated plasma inflammatory markers in individuals with intermittent explosive disorder and correlation with aggression in humans. *JAMA Psychiatry, 71*(2), 158–165.

Coccaro, E. F., Lee, R., McCloskey, M., Csernansky, J. G., & Wang, L. (2015). Morphometric analysis of amygdala and hippocampus shape in impulsively aggressive and healthy control subjects. *Journal of Psychiatric Research, 69*, 80–86.

Cremers, H., Lee, R., Keedy, S., Phan, K. L., & Coccaro, E. (2016). Effects of escitalopram administration on face processing in intermittent explosive disorder: An fMRI study. *Neuropsychopharmacology, 41*(2), 590–597.

Fahim, C., Fiori, M., Evans, A. C., & Perusse, D. (2012). The relationship between social defiance, vindictiveness, anger, and brain morphology in eight-year-old boys and girls. *Social Development, 21*(3), 592–609.

Fairchild, G., Toschi, N., Hagan, C. C., Goodyer, I. M., Calder, A. J., & Passamonti, L. (2015). Cortical thickness, surface area, and folding alterations in male youths with conduct disorder and varying levels of callous–unemotional traits. *NeuroImage: Clinical, 8*, 253–260.

Fanning, J. R., Meyerhoff, J. J., Lee, R., & Coccaro, E. F. (2014). History of childhood maltreatment in intermittent explosive disorder and suicidal behavior. *Journal of Psychiatric Research, 56*, 10–17.

Fettich, K. C., McCloskey, M. S., Look, A. E., & Coccaro, E. F. (2015). Emotion regulation deficits in intermittent explosive disorder. *Aggressive Behavior, 41*(1), 25–33.

Horn, S. R., Leve, L. D., Levitt, P., & Fisher, P. A. (2019). Childhood adversity, mental health, and oxidative stress: A pilot study. *PloS one, 14*(4), e0215085.

International Council of Nurses. (2019). *ICNP browser.* Retrieved from https://www.icn.ch/what-we-do/projects/ehealth/icnp-browser.

Loeber, R., Burke, J., & Pardini, D. A. (2009). Perspectives on oppositional defiant disorder, conduct disorder, and psychopathic features. *Journal of Child Psychology and Psychiatry, 50*(1-2), 133–142.

Matthys, W., Vanderschuren, L. J. M. J., Schutter, D. J. L. G., & Lochman, J. E. (2012). Impaired neurocognitive functions affect social learning processes in oppositional defiant disorder and conduct disorder: Implications for interventions. *Clinical Child and Family Psychology Review, 15*(3), 234–246.

Mayes, S. D., Waxmonsky, J. D., Calhoun, S. L., & Bixler, E. O. (2016). Disruptive mood dysregulation disorder symptoms and association with oppositional defiant and other disorders in a general population child sample. *Journal of Child and Adolescent Psychopharmacology, 26*(2), 101–106.

McCloskey, M. S., Noblett, K. L., Deffenbacher, J. L., Gollan, J. K., & Coccaro, E. F. (2008). Cognitive-behavioral therapy for intermittent explosive disorder: A pilot randomized clinical trial. *Journal of Consulting Clinical Psychology, 76*(5).

McCloskey, M. S., Kleabir, K., Berman, M. E., Chen, E. Y., & Coccaro, E. F. (2010). Unhealthy aggression: intermittent explosive disorder and adverse physical health outcomes. *Health Psychology, 29*(3), 324–332.

Michalska, K. J., Zeffiro, T. A., & Decety, J. (2015). Brain response to viewing others being harmed in children with conduct disorder symptoms. *Journal of Child Psychology and Psychiatry, 57*(4), 510–519.

Noordermeer, S. D., Luman, M., & Oosterlaan, J. (2016). A systematic review and meta-analysis of neuroimaging in oppositional defiant disorder (ODD) and conduct disorder (CD) taking attention-deficit hyperactivity disorder (attention-deficit/hyperactivity disorder) into account. *Neuropsychology Review, 26*(1), 44–72.

Raine, A. (2014). *The anatomy of violence: The biological roots of crime.* New York, NY: Vintage Books.

Salvatore, J. E., & Dick, D. M. (2018). Genetic influences on conduct disorder. *Neuroscience-Biobehavoral Reviews, 91*(91), 100.

Schoorl, J., Van Rijn, S., De Wied, M., Van Goozen, S. H. M., & Swaab, H. (2016). Variability in emotional/behavior problems in boys with oppositional defiant disorder or conduct disorder. *European Child and Adolescent Psychiatry, 25*, 821–830.

Shelton, D., Kesten, K., Zhang, W., & Trestman, R. (2011). Impact of a dialectic behavior therapy-corrections modified upon behaviorally challenged incarcerated male adolescents. *Journal of Child and Adolescent Psychiatric Nursing, 24*(2), 105–113.

Talih, F. R. (2011). Kleptomania and potential exacerbating factors: A review and case report. *Innovations in Clinical Neuroscience, 8*(10), 35–39.

Taylor, B. P., Schlussel, D., & Hllander, E. (2019). Disruptive, impulsive-control, and conduct disorders. In L. W. Roberts (Ed.), *Textbook of psychiatry* (7th ed.) (pp. 613–645). Washington, DC: American Psychiatric Association.

Wu, T., Howells, N., Burger, J., Lopez, P., Lundeen, R., & Sikkenga, A. V. (2015). Conduct disorder. In G. M. Kapalka (Ed.), *Treating disruptive disorders: A guide to psychological, pharmacological, and combined therapies.* Devon, UK: Routledge.

22

Substance-Related and Addictive Disorders

Margaret Jordan Halter and Jill Espeilin

 Visit the Evolve website for a pretest on the content in this chapter: http://evolve.elsevier.com/Varcarolis

OBJECTIVES

1. Define addiction, intoxication, tolerance, and withdrawal.
2. Define substance use disorder as a chronic disease.
3. Explain the system used by the Drug Enforcement Agency (DEA) to rank drugs on a schedule.
4. Describe the neurobiological process that occurs in the brain and neurotransmitters involved with substance use.
5. Identify potential co-occurring substance use disorders and other psychiatric disorders.
6. Describe the major groups of substance-related and addictive disorders in terms of use, intoxication, withdrawal, overdose, and treatment.
7. Identify types of problematic drinking.
8. Describe alcohol intoxication, withdrawal, and treatment.
9. Discuss the wide range of damaging effects from alcohol use and misuse.
10. Identify relevant nursing diagnoses for alcohol use disorder specifically and substance use disorders in general.
11. Identify pharmacotherapy and psychological therapies in treating alcohol use disorder.
12. Apply the nursing process to caring for an individual with alcohol use disorder.
13. Describe the continuum of care for substance use disorders from detoxification to relapse prevention.

KEY TERMS AND CONCEPTS

addiction
codependence
co-occurring disorders
intoxication

process addictions
Screening, Brief Intervention, and
    Referral to Treatment (SBIRT)
substance use disorder

tolerance
withdrawal

Substance use disorders are not illnesses of choice. They are complex diseases of the brain characterized by craving, seeking, and using regardless of consequences. Continuous substance use results in actual changes in brain structure and brain function. Substance use disorders are chronic and relapsing. They result in compromised executive function circuits that mediate self-control and decision making.

Historically, substance use disorders and psychiatric disorders were treated in separate systems of care. Individuals received care for mental health problems in the psychiatric system while treatment for substance disorders took place in specialized chemical dependency units or separate facilities. If both mental health and substance use disorders were present, the treatment might occur concurrently in different settings or as back-to-back treatment in one system followed by the other. Currently, the trend is to integrate treatment, and facilities increasingly provide services for co-occurring disorders.

Due to the magnitude of substance use disorders, agencies at the national level have been created to address them. The lead federal agency devoted to research regarding drug use is the National Institute on Drug Abuse (NIDA). Its mission is to advance science on the causes and consequences of drug use and addiction and to apply that knowledge to improve individual and public health (NIDA, 2015). Similar to NIDA, the Substance Abuse and Mental Health Administration's (SAMHSA, 2018) mission includes reducing the impact of substance misuse and also reducing the impact of mental illness on communities in the United States.

It is important for all nurses, regardless of their practice specialty area, to develop an understanding of the complex disease of substance use disorders. In this chapter, you are provided with an overall picture of substance use disorders, concepts central to this problem, and risk factors for its development. We will review the clinical picture for each of the substance addictions and one process addiction and discuss associated treatment. Finally, we focus specifically on alcohol use disorder and apply the nursing process to it.

SUBSTANCE USE DISORDERS

Substance use disorders were once described in terms of "substance abuse" and "substance dependence." The distinction between substance abuse and dependence was based on abuse being mild or an early phase and dependence as a more severe manifestation. Yet, in practice, abuse could be quite severe and the difference was deemed negligible. In the *Diagnostic and Statistical Manual of Mental Disorders*, fifth edition (*DSM-5*) (American Psychiatric Association [APA], 2013), the categories of substance abuse and substance dependence were merged into a single category: substance use disorder. The APA defines a substance use disorder as a pathological use of a substance that leads to a disorder of use. Symptoms fall into four major groups:

1. Impaired control
2. Social impairment
3. Risky use
4. Physical effects (i.e., intoxication, tolerance, and withdrawal)

Substance use disorders encompass a broad range of products that human beings take into their bodies through various means, such as swallowing, inhaling, and injecting. They range from fairly harmless and innocent-seeming substances such as caffeine to absolutely illegal mind-altering drugs such as LSD. No matter the substance, use disorders share many commonalities, intoxication characteristics, and withdrawal attributes.

The *DSM-5* (APA, 2013) provides diagnostic criteria for the following psychoactive substances:

- Alcohol
- Caffeine
- Cannabis
- Hallucinogen
- Inhalant
- Opioid
- Sedative, hypnotic, and antianxiety medication
- Stimulant
- Tobacco

In addition to substances, behaviors, too, are gradually being recognized as addictive. These behavioral addictions are also called process addictions. In process addictions, there are no substances but rather a behavior or the feeling brought about by the relevant action. While the physical signs of drug addiction do not accompany these types of addictions, compulsive actions activate the reward or pleasure pathways in the brain similarly to substances. The first process addiction, gambling, was officially announced as a disorder in 2013 (APA). Internet gaming, social media use, shopping, and sexual activity are also process addictions that may rise to the level of a disorder in future *DSM* editions.

Concepts Central to Substance Use Disorders
Addiction

A term that people commonly use to describe substance use disorders is addiction. Addiction is a chronic medical condition with roots in the environment, neurotransmission, genetics, and life experiences (**American Society of Addiction Medicine, 2019**). Like other chronic diseases, there are cycles of relapse and remission. Ultimately, without treatment, addiction is progressive and often results in disability or premature death.

Substance use and compulsive behaviors associated with substance use continue, even though they result in harmful consequences. Individuals with addictions are unable to consistently abstain from the substance or activity. They are also unwilling or unable to recognize the extent to which the addictions are creating serious problems in functioning, interpersonal relationships, and emotional responses.

Intoxication

When people are in the process of using a substance to excess, they are experiencing intoxication. Intoxication may manifest itself in a variety of ways depending on the physiological response of the body to the substance being used. Individuals who are using substances are considered to be under the influence, intoxicated, or high. Terminology may vary, depending on the substance and the population who is using it. For example, alcohol causes one to be drunk, while marijuana makes you stoned.

Tolerance

People with substance use disorders experience tolerance to the effects of the substances. Tolerance occurs when a person no longer responds to the drug in the way that the person initially responded. It takes a higher dose of the drug to achieve the same level of response achieved initially. Some substances, such as cocaine, cause rapid physiological tolerance. Other substances, such as prescription pain medications, may result in tolerance after weeks or months of use.

Withdrawal

Withdrawal is a set of physiological symptoms that occur when a person stops using a substance. Withdrawal is specific to the substance being used, and each substance will have its own characteristic syndrome. Substance-specific withdrawal can be mild or life threatening. The same substance, or one with a similar action, may be taken to avoid or relieve withdrawal symptoms. The more intense symptoms a person has, the more likely the person is to start using the substance again to avoid the symptoms. Behavioral addictions such as gambling result in psychological withdrawal symptoms, including cravings, sleep disruption, anxiety, and depression.

Scheduled Drugs

Drugs are classified into five categories, or schedules, based on the drug's acceptable medical use and the drug's misuse potential. The lower the schedule number, the higher the potential for misuse. The DEA (n.d.) classifies drugs in the following way:

- Schedule I drugs carry a high potential for abuse and have no acceptable medical use. Examples are heroin and lysergic acid diethylamide (LSD).
- Schedule II drugs have a high potential for abuse, are considered dangerous, and are available only by prescription. Examples include methadone, meperidine (Demerol), and methylphenidate (Ritalin).
- Schedule III drugs have a low to moderate potential for misuse and are available only by prescription. Examples are testosterone, acetaminophen/codeine (Tylenol with codeine), and buprenorphine (Suboxone).

- Schedule IV drugs are low-risk drugs and are available by prescription. Examples of schedule IV drugs are alprazolam (Xanax), lorazepam (Ativan), and propoxyphene/acetaminophen (Darvocet).
- Schedule V drugs contain limited quantities of certain narcotics for the treatment of diarrhea, coughing, and pain. Examples are atropine/diphenoxylate (Lomotil), guaifenesin and codeine (Robitussin AC), and pregabalin (Lyrica), available over-the-counter.

See Table 22.1 for information on commonly misused drugs.

Epidemiology

The National Survey on Drug Use and Health Survey (SAMHSA, 2019) is conducted annually in the United States. Participants

TABLE 22.1	Commonly Misused Drugs	
Substance	**Administration**	**Acute Effects/Health Risks**
Nicotine	Smoked, snorted, chewed	*Increased blood pressure and heart rate* Chronic lung disease, cardiovascular disease, stroke, cancers of the mouth, pharynx, larynx, esophagus, stomach, pancreas, cervix, kidney, bladder, and acute myeloid leukemia, adverse pregnancy outcomes, addiction
Alcohol	Swallowed	*Low doses: Euphoria, mild stimulation, relaxation, lowered inhibitions* *High doses: Drowsiness, slurred speech, nausea, emotional volatility, loss of coordination, visual distortions, impaired memory, loss of consciousness, respiratory arrest, seizures, coma, death* Increased risk of injuries, violence, fetal damage, depression, neurological deficits, hypertension, liver and heart disease, addiction, fatal overdose
Marijuana	Smoked, swallowed	*Euphoria, relaxation, slowed reaction time, distorted sensory perception, impaired balance and coordination, increased heart rate and appetite, impaired learning, memory, anxiety, panic attacks, psychosis/cough*
Hashish	Smoked, swallowed	Frequent respiratory infections, possible mental health decline, addiction
Heroin (Diacetylmorphine)	Injected, smoked, snorted	*Euphoria, drowsiness, impaired coordination, dizziness, confusion, nausea, sedation, feeling of heaviness in the body, slowed or arrested breathing*
Opium	Swallowed, smoked	Constipation, endocarditis, hepatitis, HIV, addiction, fatal overdose
Cocaine (Cocaine hydrochloride)	Snorted, smoked, injected	*Increased heart rate, blood pressure, body temperature, metabolism, feelings of exhilaration, increased energy, mental alertness, tremors, reduced appetite, irritability, anxiety, panic, paranoia, violent behavior, psychosis*
Amphetamine (Biphetamine, Dexedrine)	Swallowed, snorted, smoked, injected	Weight loss, insomnia, cardiac or cardiovascular complications, stroke, seizures, addiction
Methamphetamine (Desoxyn)	Swallowed, snorted, smoked, injected	Cocaine: Nasal damage from snorting Methamphetamine: Severe dental problems
Methylenedioxy-methamphetamine (MDMA)	Swallowed, snorted, injected	*Mild hallucinogenic effects, increased tactile sensitivity, empathic feelings, lowered inhibition, anxiety, chills, sweating, teeth clenching, muscle cramping* Sleep disturbances, depression, impaired memory, hyperthermia, addiction
Flunitrazepam (Rohypnol), similar to benzodiazepine chemically	Swallowed, snorted	*Sedation, muscle relaxation, confusion, memory loss, dizziness, impaired coordination* Addiction
Gamma-hydroxybutyrate (GHB)	Swallowed	*Drowsiness, nausea, headache, disorientation, loss of coordination, memory loss* Unconsciousness, seizures, coma
Ayahuasca, a brew that includes chacruna or chagropanga, dimethyltryptamine (DMT)–containing plants	Listed in the FDA's poisonous plant database Brewed as a tea	*Strong hallucinations, altered vision and auditory perceptions, increased blood pressure, vomiting, diarrhea*
Dimethyltryptamine (DMT) synthetic drug	White or yellow powder, smoked, swallowed	*30–60 min of intense hallucinations, depersonalization, high blood pressure, rapid eye movements, agitation, seizures*
Lysergic acid diethylamide (LSD)	Swallowed, absorbed through mouth tissues	*Altered states of perception and feeling, hallucinations, nausea, increased body temperature, heart rate, blood pressure, loss of appetite, sweating, sleeplessness, numbness, dizziness, weakness, tremors, impulsive behavior, rapid shifts in emotion* Flashbacks, hallucinogen persisting perception disorder
Mescaline	Swallowed, smoked	*Altered states of perception and feeling, hallucinations, nausea, increased body temperature, heart rate, blood pressure, loss of appetite, sweating, sleeplessness, numbness, dizziness, weakness, tremors, impulsive behavior, rapid shifts in emotion*

TABLE 22.1 Commonly Misused Drugs—cont'd

Substance	Administration	Acute Effects/Health Risks
Psilocybin	Swallowed	*Altered states of perception and feeling, hallucinations, nausea, nervousness, paranoia, panic*
Ketamine (Ketalar)	Injected, snorted, smoked	*Feelings of being separate from one's body and environment, impaired motor function, analgesia, impaired memory, delirium, respiratory depression and arrest, death* Anxiety, tremors, numbness, memory loss, nausea
Phencyclidine (PCP) and analogs	Swallowed, smoked, injected	*Feelings of being separate from one's body and environment, impaired motor function, analgesia, psychosis, aggression, violence, slurred speech, loss of coordination, hallucinations* Anxiety, tremors, numbness, memory loss, nausea
Salvia divinorum	Chewed, swallowed, smoked	*Feelings of being separate from one's body and environment, impaired motor function* Anxiety, tremors, numbness, memory loss, nausea
Dextromethorphan (DXM)	Swallowed	*Feelings of being separate from one's body and environment, impaired motor function, euphoria, slurred speech, confusion, dizziness, distorted visual perceptions* Anxiety, tremors, numbness, memory loss, nausea
Hallucinogens/other compounds		
Anabolic steroids	Injected, swallowed, applied to skin	*No intoxication effects* Hypertension, blood clotting and cholesterol changes, liver cysts, hostility and aggression, acne; in adolescents premature stoppage of growth; in males, prostate cancer, reduced sperm production, shrunken testicles, breast enlargement; in females, menstrual irregularities, development of beard and other masculine characteristics
Inhalants Solvents, propellants, thinners, and fuels	Inhaled through nose or mouth	*Varies by chemical—stimulation, loss of inhibition, headache, nausea or vomiting, slurred speech, loss of motor coordination, wheezing* *Cramps, muscle weakness, depression, memory impairment, damage to cardiovascular and nervous systems, unconsciousness, sudden death*
Prescription pain relievers	Capsules, liquid, injected, swallowed, smoked, snorted	Drowsiness, lethargy, euphoria, slow breathing, death
Prescription sedatives	Pill, capsule, liquid, injected, swallowed	Drowsiness, slurred speech, poor concentration, low blood pressure, decrease respiratory rate
Prescription Stimulants		
Amphetamine (Adderall, Benzedrine)	Tablet, chewable, liquid, swallowed, smoked, injected	*Increased alertness, increased blood pressure and heart rate, narrowed blood vessels, increased blood sugar*
Methylphenidate (Concerta, Ritalin)	Liquid, tablet, chewable tablet, capsule Swallowed, snorted, smoked, injected, chewed	Long-term high doses: heart problems, psychosis, anger

National Institute on Drug Abuse. (2016). *Commonly abused drug chart*. Retrieved from http://www.drugabuse.gov/drugs-abuse/commonly-abused-drugs/commonly-abused-drugs-chart.

who are 12 years or older are randomly selected for an in-person interview. Data from this survey are the primary source for national drug use statistics and trending. Based on these data, SAMSHA estimates that about 165 million people (about 60%) used substances (i.e., tobacco, alcohol, or illicit drugs) within the last month. Illicit drugs refer to both recreational drugs and the nonmedical or nonprescribed use of prescription drugs.

The number of people with actual substance use disorders was estimated at about 20.3 million. This number includes about 15 million people with an alcohol use disorder and about 8 million people with an illicit drug use disorder. The most common illicit drug was marijuana use disorder, with about 4.5 million people. Opioid use disorder was estimated at 2.0 million

people, which includes 1.7 million people using prescription pain relievers and 0.5 million using heroin (Fig. 22.1).

Comorbidity

Comorbidity refers to two or more disorders occurring in the same person at the same time with potential interactions and exacerbation (worsening) of symptoms. Co-occurring disorders may include any combination of two or more substance use disorders and psychiatric disorders identified in the *DSM-5*.

The National Survey on Drug Use and Health Survey (SAMHSA, 2019) classifies mental disorders as either "any mental illness" or "serious mental illness." Any mental illness ranges from no impairment to mild, moderate, or even severe

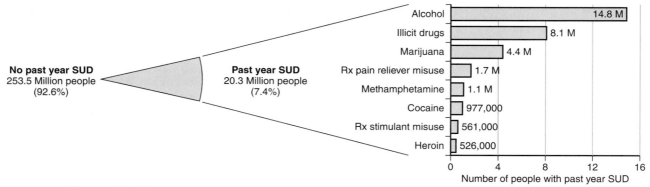

Fig. 22.1 People aged 12 or older with a past year substance use disorder (SUD): 2018. (Adapted from Substance Abuse and Mental Health Services Administration. [2019]. *Key substance use and mental health indicators in the United States.* Retrieved from https://www.samhsa.gov/data/sites/default/files/cbhsq-reports/NSDUHNationalFindingsReport2018/NSDUHNationalFindingsReport2018.htm#sud.)

impairment. Serious mental illness indicates serious functional impairment, which substantially interferes with major life activities. In 2018, about 9 million (3.7%) adults were estimated to have any mental illness and at least one substance use disorder. About 3 million (1.3%) of adults had co-occurring serious mental illness and a substance use disorder in the past year.

Risk Factors
Biological Factors
Genetic. There appears to be a genetic underlying vulnerability to addiction that expresses itself in a variety of substances. Substance use disorders such as cannabis, cocaine, and opiates definitely run in families. Twin studies support heritability in substance use disorders. Estimates range from 30% to 40% for hallucinogens and stimulants, and as high as 70% to 80% for cocaine and opiates (Ebert, Finn, & Smoller, 2016)

Neurobiological. Researchers have found neurotransmitters associated with substance use disorders. The opioids, for example, act on opioid receptors. People with too little natural opioid activity or too much opioid antagonism might be prone to self-medicating through the use of opioid drugs. Even people who originally had normal opioid function will develop altered function with repeated use of external opioids, to the point where taking the drug makes them feel normal again.

The major neurotransmitters involved in developing substance use disorders are the opioid, catecholamine (especially dopamine), and gamma-aminobutyric acid (GABA) systems (Sadock et al., 2015). The dopaminergic neurons in the ventral tegmental area (VTA) are especially important in the sensation of reward.

Environmental Factors
Many chronic stressors have their roots in socioeconomic factors. Poverty raises the risk of an unfavorable living environment, lack of parental supervision, poor educational resources, and impaired support systems. A cycle of negative environmental events often begins within disadvantaged neighborhoods, increasing stress and anxiety along with a lack of or negative social ties, which contributes to depression. Coping mechanisms may include drugs and acting out behaviors, leading to destructive consequences and interaction with the legal system.

Clinical Picture
Caffeine
Caffeine is the most widely used psychoactive substance in the world. According to the APA (2013), unlike the other substances discussed in this chapter, excessive caffeine use is not an official use disorder. However, caffeine can result in intoxication, overdose, and withdrawal. Excessive use is associated with many psychiatric problems, including bipolar disorders, eating disorders, and sleep disorders.

The stimulatory effects of caffeine may begin as early as 15 minutes after ingesting the drug and last as long as 6 hours. The average cup of coffee has about 95 mg of caffeine, although commercially prepared coffee such as Starbucks contains much more. Energy drinks may contain upward of 300 mg of caffeine, and energy shots can have more than 400 mg.

Caffeine intoxication. The prevalence of caffeine intoxication in the United States is about 7%. Caffeine intoxication occurs after the recent consumption of caffeine, usually at a high dose (or doses) of more than 250 mg.

Caffeine intoxication is characterized by behavioral symptoms such as restlessness, nervousness, excitement, agitation, rambling speech, and inexhaustibility. Physical symptoms of intoxication are flushed face, diuresis, gastrointestinal disturbance, muscle twitching, tachycardia, or cardiac arrhythmia. These symptoms are distressing to the individual and result in the impairment of normal areas of functioning. Individuals with tolerance are less sensitive to intoxication.

Caffeine overdose and treatment. Lethal overdoses of caffeine from coffee or tea are rare due to the amount of fluid that would be required to reach toxic levels (Murray & Traylor, 2019). However, energy drinks and over-the-counter products such as diet aids, decongestants, bronchodilators, or stay-awake preparations are increasingly implicated in overdose. Children and adolescents are especially vulnerable to caffeine overdose from attractive-looking energy drinks, which may also be gateway drugs to other substances. Breastfeeding babies are also at risk from mothers who ingest excessive caffeine.

Caffeine overdose is characterized by fever, tachycardia or bradycardia, and hypertension initially, followed by hypotension (Murray & Traylor, 2019). Extremely high doses of

▶ **Neurobiology of Heroin Use**

When a person injects, smokes, or snorts heroin the drug travels quickly to the brain through the bloodstream. In the brain, the heroin is converted to morphine by enzymes.

Morphine binds to opiate receptors in certain areas within the reward pathway including the ventral tegmental area (VTA), nucleus accumbens, and cortex. Morphine also binds to areas involved in the pain pathway including the thalamus, brainstem, and spinal cord.

The Reward Pathway

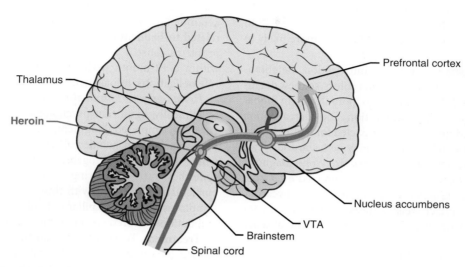

Brain Dysfunction

Addiction develops when the neurons adapt to exposure of the drug and only function normally in the presence of the drug. Many of the heroin or morphine withdrawal symptoms are generated when the opiate receptors in the thalamus and brainstem are deprived of morphine. Withdrawal can be very serious and the abuser will use the drug again to avoid the symptoms.

Tolerance to the analgesic (pain reducing) properties of heroin or morphine no longer respond to the drug in the initial way. Tolerance occurs in the pain passage pathway that includes the thalamus and the spinal cord. These areas are important in sending pain messages and are responsible for the analgesic effects of morphine. However, a person does not fully develop tolerance to the respiratory depressive effects of heroin/morphine.

When morphine binds to opiate receptors, it inhibits an enzyme, adenylate cyclase, that coordinates the firing of impulses. After repeated opiate receptor activation by morphine, the enzyme adapts so that the morphine can no longer cause changes in cell firing.

Overdose is particularly lethal due to respiratory depression. To reduce deaths from overdose, naloxone (Narcan) is used by both healthcare providers and the general public. This drug is a pure opioid antagonist with no pharmacological properties. After intranasal, intravenous, subcutaneous, and intramuscular injection, it temporarily (30–90 minutes) binds with them. Its binding ability is stronger than morphine's so it can push the morphine off the receptor and reverse the effects of morphine. Duration of action is short compared with many opioids, so repeated administration may be required.

caffeine may result in grand mal seizures, and respiratory failure may cause death. Pupillary mydriasis (dilation), muscular rigidity and hyperreflexia, nausea, and vomiting are common. Neurologically, patients may have disorganized thinking, agitation, delusions, hallucinations, and seizures due to ischemia from vasoconstriction.

Treatment for caffeine overdose is generally supportive. Hydration may be oral or intravenous. Gastric lavage can be used to remove excess caffeine, or activated charcoal can bind caffeine if the ingestion is recent. Beta-blockade is used for tachycardia. Vasopressors can help maintain blood pressure without worsening tachycardia.

Caffeine withdrawal. Caffeine withdrawal is not associated with serious medical problems or the need for intervention. Removal of caffeine from the daily routine results in headache, drowsiness, irritability, and poor concentration. Some people experience flu-like symptoms, such as nausea, vomiting, and muscle aches. Symptoms occur within 12 to 24 hours after the last dose, peak in 24 to 48 hours, and resolve within 1 week.

Cannabis Use Disorder

Cannabis, or marijuana, is a widely used drug. It is the third most commonly used psychoactive drug in the United States after alcohol and illicit drugs (SAMHSA, 2019). It comes from the dried leaves, flowers, stems, and seeds of the hemp plant, *Cannabis sativa.* A chemical, delta-9-tetrahydrocannabinol (THC), is responsible for its mind-altering effects. The concentrated form of cannabis is known as hashish.

Synthetic cannabinoids of THC, dronabinol (Marinol) and nabilone (Cesamet), are prescribed to treat nausea caused by chemotherapy for cancer and boost appetite in patients with AIDS. The US Food and Drug Administration (FDA, 2018) also approved Epidiolex (cannabidiol, CBD) for rare forms of epilepsy. Unlike THC, CBD does not cause intoxication. As of 2020, cannabis for medical use was legal in 33 states, and marijuana for recreational use was legal in 11 states (Burke & Gould, 2020). Despite its legal status, the DEA continues to consider cannabis to be a Schedule I substance, meaning it has no legitimate medical use. Advocates are seeking to change this designation.

The 12-month prevalence of cannabis use disorder in adolescents is about 3.5% and about 1.5% in adults (APA, 2013). Rates tend to decrease with age, with rates highest among 18 to 29 years of age and lowest after age 65. Males are more likely to be affected.

Cannabis intoxication. Cannabis intoxication heightens users' sensations. They experience brighter colors, see new details in common stimuli, and time seems to go more slowly. In higher doses, they experience depersonalization and derealization (Sadock et al., 2015). Motor skills are impacted for 8 to 12 hours, and driving and the use of machinery may be hazardous. Two of the following physical symptoms are required for a diagnosis of cannabis intoxication: conjunctival injection (red eyes from vessel dilation), increased appetite, dry mouth, and tachycardia. Hallucinations with intact reality testing may occur, or auditory, visual, or tactile illusions may occur in the absence of delirium.

Modern cannabis is quite different from previous generations of the substance. Before the 1990s, the THC content was less than 2% (Stuyt, 2018). In the 1990s, the content doubled to 4%, and between 1995 and 2015, there was a 212% increase in THC content in the marijuana flower. In 2017, popular strains found in dispensaries had a range of THC content from 17% to 28%. The increased potency can make cannabis preparations more dangerous and more likely to result in addiction. Ingested cannabis is also more difficult to gauge due to the delayed onset of action.

Cannabis withdrawal. Withdrawal from cannabis is comparatively late—within 1 week of cessation. Symptoms include irritability, anger, aggression, anxiety, restlessness, and depressed mood. Because people often use marijuana as a sleep aid, insomnia and disturbing dreams may develop without it. Decreased appetite may lead to weight loss. Physical symptoms of marijuana withdrawal include at least one of the following: abdominal pain, shakiness, sweating, fever, chills, or headache.

Treatment. Abstinence and support are the main principles of treatment for cannabis use disorder. Hospitalization or outpatient care may be required. Individual, family, and group therapies can provide support. Antianxiety medication may be useful for short-term relief of withdrawal symptoms. Patients with underlying anxiety and depression may respond to antidepressant therapy.

Hallucinogen Use Disorder

Hallucinogens are, by definition, intoxicants. They cause a profound disturbance in reality. Hallucinogens are associated with flashbacks, panic attacks, psychosis, delirium, and mood and anxiety disorders. They are both natural and synthetic substances. Hallucinogens are classified as Schedule I controlled substances, meaning that they have no medical use and carry a high abuse potential. The 12-month prevalence of hallucinogen use is estimated at 1.50% in individuals ages 12 to 17, 6.90% in individuals ages 18 to 25, and 1.30% in individuals ages 26 and older (SAMHSA, 2019).

Hallucinogens are found in some plants and mushrooms (or their extracts) or can be man-made. They are commonly divided into two broad categories: classic hallucinogens (e.g., LSD) and dissociative drugs (e.g., phencyclidine [PCP] and ketamine; see Table 22.1). The APA identifies two use disorders related to hallucinogens—PCP and other hallucinogens. Both problems cause a clinically significant impairment or distress within a 12-month period, including craving, difficulty with role obligations, impairment, and tolerance.

Hallucinogen intoxication. Intoxication is characterized by clinically significant psychological and behavioral changes. Paranoia, impaired judgment, intensification of perceptions, depersonalization, and derealization are commonly experienced while using hallucinogens. Illusions, hallucinations, and synesthesia (e.g., hearing colors or seeing sounds) are particularly prominent with this type of intoxication. Physical symptoms include pupillary dilation, tachycardia, sweating, palpitations, blurred vision, tremors, and incoordination.

Treatment. Treatment for hallucinogen intoxication includes talking the patient down. This refers to reassurance that the symptoms are caused by the drug and that the symptoms will subside. Patient and provider safety are essential goals. Physical restraint may be necessary. In severe cases, an antipsychotic such as haloperidol (Haldol) or a benzodiazepine such as diazepam (Valium) can be used in the short term.

Phencyclidine intoxication. PCP intoxication is a medical emergency that can result in dangerous and violent side effects. People under the influence of this drug can be belligerent, assaultive, impulsive, and unpredictable. Significant physical manifestations of this drug include nystagmus (involuntary eye movements), hypertension, tachycardia, diminished response to pain, ataxia (loss of voluntary muscle control), dysarthria (unclear speech), muscle rigidity, seizures, coma, and hyperacusis (sensitivity to sound). Hyperthermia and seizure activity may also occur. Management of individuals intoxicated by PCP is primarily supportive.

Treatment. Patients who have ingested PCP cannot be talked down and may require restraint. A calming medication such as a benzodiazepine may be administered intramuscularly or intravenously. Mechanical cooling may be necessary for severe hyperthermia.

Hallucinogen withdrawal. There is no official withdrawal diagnosis or pattern with prolonged hallucinogen use. However, hallucinogen persisting perception disorder may be experienced during periods of sobriety, particularly from LSD. The prevalence of this problem among hallucinogen users is about 4%. The hallmark of this problem is the reexperiencing of perceptual symptoms that were experienced while intoxicated. These symptoms are distressing and impair the individual from normal functioning for weeks, months, or even years.

Inhalant Use Disorder

Volatile hydrocarbons are toxic gases inhaled through the nose or mouth to enter the bloodstream. Common household products with chemicals that share similar pharmacological properties include:

- Solvents for glues and adhesives
- Propellants found in aerosol paint sprays, hair sprays, and shaving cream
- Thinners, such as paint products and correction fluids
- Fuels, such as gasoline and propane

Most people who use inhalants usually do so for a short period of time. Some users continue their use, despite knowing that this practice is causing serious problems. Characteristics of out-of-control inhalant use are using more and more, craving, and tolerance. Inhalants cause failure in major life roles and problems in interpersonal relationships. "Sudden sniffing death" from cardiac arrhythmias may occur with inhalants, particularly with butane and propane.

This disorder is primarily one that occurs in youth. About 662,000 adolescents, or 2.7%, aged 12 to 17 were past-year users of inhalants (SAMHSA, 2019). Among young adults aged 18 to 25, estimates include about 495,000 users, or 1.5%. Only about 0.4% of adults older than 26 are past-year users, a statistic that represents 846,000 adults.

Inhalant intoxication. Small doses of inhalants result in disinhibition and euphoria. High doses can cause fearfulness, illusions, auditory and visual hallucinations, and a distorted body image. Apathy, diminished social and occupational functioning, impaired judgment, and impulsive and aggressive behavior accompany intoxication.

Physical responses to inhalant intoxication include nausea, anorexia, nystagmus, depressed reflexes, and diplopia. High doses and long exposure can lead to stupor, unconsciousness, and amnesia. Delirium, dementia, and psychosis are also serious side effects from inhalant use. Although withdrawal is not considered a disorder in the *DSM-5* (APA, 2013), some users develop a withdrawal syndrome when ceasing inhalant use.

Treatment. Inhalant intoxication usually does not require any treatment. Serious and potentially fatal responses such as coma, cardiac arrhythmias, or bronchospasm do happen. A psychotic response can be induced by inhalant intoxication. This self-limiting (a few hours to a few weeks) problem may require careful use of haloperidol (Haldol) to manage severe agitation.

Opioid Use Disorder

Opioid misuse, particularly with heroin and prescription drugs, is a chronic relapsing disorder. In opioid use disorders, cravings result in larger amounts and longer periods of time being devoted to the drug and increasing tolerance to its effects. The use of this substance results in significant impairment in life roles, interpersonal conflict, and puts a person in physically hazardous situations.

In 2018, an estimated 2.0 million people aged 12 or older had an opioid use disorder, which corresponds to 0.7% of the population (SAMHSA, 2019). Opioid use usually begins in the late teens or early 20s and peaks from 18 to 25 years of age. Increasing age is associated with fewer affected individuals, probably due to early mortality and a cessation of use after

age 40. Being female and having a higher level of education are protective factors. Table 22.2 identifies the prevalence of opioid use by ages, gender, Hispanic origin and race, and education (SAMHSA, 2019).

Opioid intoxication. People intoxicated on opioids exhibit psychomotor retardation, drowsiness, slurred speech, altered mood (withdrawn to elated), and impaired memory and attention (Nisavic & Nejad, 2018). Physical symptoms of acute intoxication include miosis (pinpoint pupils) and decreased bowel sounds. Respiratory rates and blood pressure are reduced and heart rates are normal to low. Skin disruptions in the form of track marks or fresh injection sites may confirm IV drug use.

Opioid overdose. Death attributable to opioids usually stems from respiratory arrest due to the respiratory depressant effect of the drug. Symptoms of overdose include unresponsiveness, slow respiration, coma, hypothermia, hypotension, and bradycardia. Three symptoms—coma, pinpoint pupils, and respiratory depression—are strongly suggestive of overdose.

Opioid overdose treatment. Treatment for an overdose begins with promoting breathing by aspirating secretions, inserting an airway, and mechanical ventilation. Naloxone (Narcan), a specific opioid antagonist, has FDA approval for opioid overdose and can be given intranasally, intramuscularly, subcutaneously, or intravenously. Increased respirations and pupillary dilation should happen quickly. Too much naloxone may produce withdrawal symptoms. Duration of action for naloxone is short compared with many opioids, so repeated administration may be required.

Opioid withdrawal. Withdrawal symptoms for opioids occur after a reduction or cessation of heavy opioid use, or after an opioid antagonist has been administered (discussed as follows). Symptoms of withdrawal include mood dysphoria, nausea, vomiting, diarrhea, muscle aches, fever, and insomnia. Other classic symptoms of withdrawal are lacrimation (watery eyes), rhinorrhea (runny nose), pupillary dilation, and yawning. The symptom of piloerection (bristling of hairs) or gooseflesh is the origin of the term *cold turkey* for the abstinence syndrome. Males may experience sweating and spontaneous ejaculations while awake.

Morphine, heroin, and methadone withdrawal syndrome begins 6 to 8 hours after the last dose following a period of at least a week of use. It reaches intensity during the second or third day and then subsides during the next week. Meperidine (Demerol) withdrawal begins within 8 to 12 hours from abstinence and lasts about 5 days.

See Box 22.1 for some signs and symptoms of intoxication and withdrawal.

Opioid withdrawal treatment. Methadone (Dolophine, Methadose) is a synthetic narcotic opioid. It is used to decrease the painful symptoms of opiate withdrawal. It also blocks the euphoric effects of opiate drugs such as heroin, morphine, and codeine, as well as semisynthetic opioids like oxycodone and hydrocodone. Methadone is only dispensed through an opioid treatment program certified by SAMHSA. Once-a-day dosing is adequate. Methadone, too, will eventually need to be

TABLE 22.2	Misuse of Opioids in Past Year by Demographics: Percentages, 2017 and 2018					
	AGES 12–17		AGES 18–25		AGES 26 OR OLDER	
	2017	2018	2017	2018	2017	2018
Total	3.1	2.8	7.3	5.6	3.8	3.6
Gender						
Male	2.7	2.4	7.4	5.8	4.5	3.9
Female	3.5	3.3	7.2	5.3	3.2	3.2
Hispanic/Race						
Non-Hispanic/Lat.	2.9	2.6	7.3	5.8	3.9	3.6
White	2.9	2.7	8.1	6.3	4.2	3.8
Black	3.6	2.6	6.3	4.7	3.0	3.6
AIAN[a]	2.6	0.9	6.6	7.4	6.5	6.2
Asian	1.9	2.3	2.7	3.0	1.8	1.0
2+ Races	3.3	2.3	9.2	6.9	4.2	4.3
Hispanic/Lat.	3.5	3.4	7.0	4.8	3.4	3.3
Education						
<High School	n/a	n/a	8.5	7.7	3.6	3.7
High School	n/a	n/a	7.6	5.9	3.8	3.9
Some College	n/a	n/a	7.6	5.3	4.8	4.5
College Graduate	n/a	n/a	4.6	3.6	3.1	2.5

[a]American Indian/Alaskan Native.
From Substance Abuse and Mental Health Services Administration. (2019). *Behavioral health trends in the United States: Results from the 2018 National Survey on Drug Use and Health.* Retrieved from NSDUHNationalFindingsReport2018 (2).pdf

BOX 22.1 Signs and Symptoms of Opioid Intoxication and Withdrawal

Opioid Intoxication	Opioid Withdrawal
Bradycardia (slow pulse)	Tachycardia (fast pulse)
Hypotension (low blood pressure)	Hypertension (high blood pressure)
Hypothermia (low body temperature)	Hyperthermia (high body temperature)
Sedation	Insomnia
Miosis (pinpoint pupils)	Mydriasis (enlarged pupils)
Hypokinesis (slowed movement)	Hyperreflexia (abnormally heightened reflexes)
Slurred speech	
Head nodding	Diaphoresis (sweating)
Euphoria	Piloerection (gooseflesh)
Analgesia (pain-killing effects)	Increased respiratory rate
Calmness	Lacrimation (tearing), yawning
	Rhinorrhea (runny nose)
	Muscle spasms
	Abdominal cramps, nausea, vomiting, diarrhea
	Bone and muscle pain
	Anxiety

From Substance Abuse and Mental Health Services Administration. (2006). *TIP 45 detoxification and substance abuse treatment* (DHHS Publication No. SMA 06-4224). Washington, DC: US Government Printing Office.

withdrawn via tapering or substituting another medication. In pregnant users, a low dose of methadone may be the safest course. Neonate withdrawal is usually mild and can be managed with paregoric.

Some serious side effects may occur while taking methadone. Patients should be instructed to seek medical care if they experience difficulty breathing or shallow breathing, feel light-headed or faint, or experience chest pain or a fast or pounding heartbeat. Hives, rash, or swelling of the face, lips, tongue, or throat could also be serious symptoms. Hallucinations or confusion should also be reported to a care provider.

Clonidine (Catapres), an alpha agonist antihypertensive, is often used to reduce the symptoms of opioid withdrawal. By blocking neurotransmitters that trigger sympathetic nervous system activity, clonidine eases sweating, hot flashes, watery eyes, and restlessness. This drug also decreases anxiety and may even shorten the detox process. Lofexidine (Lucemyra), another alpha agonist, has FDA approval for the mitigation of opioid withdrawal symptoms during abrupt discontinuation. It is marketed as enabling people to withdraw at home in a few days rather than a week. Lofexidine is cost prohibitive at $1,700 for a week's worth of treatment compared to $1 for clonidine (Brodwin, 2018).

Buprenorphine is also used to help people reduce or quit opiates. Buprenorphine is an opioid partial agonist. Like opioids, it produces effects such as euphoria or respiratory depression, but these effects are weaker than those of drugs such as heroin and methadone. The FDA has approved the following schedule III buprenorphine products, some of which contain naloxone:

- Subutex (buprenorphine) sublingual tablets
- Bunavail (buprenorphine and naloxone) buccal film

- Suboxone (buprenorphine and naloxone) sublingual tablets or sublingual film
- Zubsolv (buprenorphine and naloxone) sublingual tablets
- Sublocade (buprenorphine) is supplied as a prefilled syringe for subcutaneous administration once a month
- Probuphine (buprenorphine) is supplied by four 1-inch rods surgically implanted under the skin of the upper arm for 6 months

Side effects of buprenorphine include nausea, vomiting, constipation, muscle aches and cramps, insomnia, irritability, and fever. This drug is used only after abstaining from opioids for 12 to 24 hours and in the early stages of opioid withdrawal. It can bring on acute withdrawal for patients not in the early stages of withdrawal and who have other opioids in their bloodstream. Because buprenorphine is a long-acting drug, once patients have been stabilized, they can sometimes switch to an alternate-day oral, transmucosal formulation dosing instead of dosing every day.

Opioid maintenance therapy. Continued abstinence is the goal of maintenance therapy. Once sobriety has been achieved and detoxification is complete, pharmacotherapy and/or psychological interventions should be pursued. Buprenorphine/naloxone and methadone, as previously described, reduce cravings in maintenance therapy.

Naltrexone (ReVia), is an opioid antagonist that prevents intoxication. This FDA-approved drug works by blocking the activation of opioid receptors and prevents opioid drugs from producing rewarding effects such as euphoria. This medication-assisted treatment is typically dosed once a day.

An injectable long-acting form of naltrexone, Vivitrol, is given intramuscularly once a month. It has FDA approval for the prevention of relapse to opioid dependence following opioid detoxification. Because it lasts for weeks, it helps people with healthcare access problems and those who struggle with adherence. Side effects of naltrexone include GI distress, muscle cramps, dizziness, sedation, and appetite disturbances. Injection site reactions are common. About 70% of users experience reactions that range from pain, swelling, and bruising to more serious complications like cellulitis, induration, and, more rarely, abscess and necrosis.

Psychological treatment approaches. Individual therapy, behavioral therapy, cognitive behavioral therapy, family therapy, and social skills training may all be helpful in the management of opioid use disorder (Sadock et al., 2015). Support groups such as Narcotics Anonymous (NA), a 12-step program, are excellent sources of help. More structure is provided in residential treatment and therapeutic communities. They work best in cases of highly motivated individuals. Confrontation in the group environment and isolation from the outside world are emphasized in these settings.

Sedative, Hypnotic, and Antianxiety Medication Use Disorder

Drugs in this category include the benzodiazepines, benzodiazepine-like drugs (e.g., zolpidem, zaleplon), carbamates, barbiturates (e.g., secobarbital), and barbiturate-like hypnotics (e.g., methaqualone). This class includes all prescription

EVIDENCE-BASED PRACTICE

A Treatment for Addictions in Rats?

Problem

Opioid use disorder and its deadly consequences impact millions of people in the United States. Medication-assisted treatment and psychological approaches too often result in relapse and a return to taking the drugs.

Purpose of the Study

The purpose of the study is to find a new way to curb the opioid cravings that contribute to relapses. Researcher Fair Vassoler and her colleagues are exploring whether a new kind of deep brain stimulation can reduce drug-seeking behaviors.

Methods

The subjects in the study were rats who self-administered oxycodone. Researchers used an MRI to guide magnetic nanoparticles through the nasal cavity of addicted rats into the reward center of the brain. Externally, the particles were caused to oscillate, thereby stimulating adenosine that helps reduce cravings.

Key Findings

- The nanoparticles used in the study were determined to be the right size and structure to eliminate damage to the rats' brains.
- The technology appeared to decrease craving for the opioid drug.

Implications for Nursing Practice

As professionals, nurses are continually learning and keeping abreast of innovations in healthcare. The development of a non-pharmaceutical biological approach to addiction is an innovation with the potential to curb cravings and reduce deadly opioid use. Additional clinical rat trials may pave the way for future trials in humans.

Rajewski, G. (2020, March 12). Testing a new addiction therapy. *Tufts Now.* Retrieved from https://now.tufts.edu/articles/testing-new-addiction-therapy.

sleeping medications and almost all prescription antianxiety drugs. Craving is a typical feature. Use of these brain depressants negatively affects role performance and relationships. Significant tolerance and withdrawal can develop in anyone using these drugs, even for their intended indication. A use disorder diagnosis is only given in the presence of additional *DSM-5* criteria such as clinically significant maladaptive behavior or psychological changes.

The 12-month prevalence of this problem is about 0.2% in adults. It occurs in males slightly more often than in females. Sedative, hypnotic, and antianxiety medication use disorders are highest among 18- to 29-year-olds (0.5%) and lowest among individuals 65 and older (0.04%).

Sedative, hypnotic, and antianxiety medication intoxication. As a group of depressants, the criteria for intoxication make sense: slurred speech, incoordination, unsteady gait, nystagmus, and impaired thinking. Coma is a dangerous possibility with this class of drugs. Inappropriate aggression and sexual behavior, mood fluctuation, and impaired judgment may also be side effects.

Overdose treatment. Overdose treatment includes gastric lavage, activated charcoal, and careful vital sign monitoring. Patients who are awake after overdosing should be kept awake to prevent a loss of consciousness. If unconscious, an intravenous fluid line should be established. An endotracheal tube may be required to provide a patent airway, and mechanical ventilation can be used if necessary.

Sedative, hypnotic, and antianxiety medication withdrawal. Repeated depressing of the central nervous system, along with the body's daily attempt to return to homeostasis, results in rebound hyperactivity with the removal of the substance. Hence, we may see symptoms such as autonomic hyperactivity, tremor, insomnia, psychomotor agitation, anxiety, and grand mal seizures. The degree and timing of the withdrawal syndrome depends on the specific substance. Half-life is an important predictor of time.

Withdrawal treatment. Gradual reduction of benzodiazepines will prevent seizures and other withdrawal symptoms. Barbiturate withdrawal can be aided by using a long-acting barbiturate such as phenobarbital.

Stimulant Use Disorder

Amphetamine-type, cocaine, or other stimulant drugs are second only to cannabis as the most widely used illicit substances in the United States. They typically produce a euphoric feeling and high energy. Long-distance truckers, students studying for exams, soldiers in wartime, and athletes in competition use these drugs. As with all the use disorders, increased use, craving, and tolerance are accompanied by reduced ability to function in major roles. Stimulants represent a significant problem, as a use disorder pattern can occur in as little as 1 week.

The estimated 12-month prevalence for amphetamine-type stimulants is about 0.2% in adults. Both genders are affected equally. Intravenous stimulant use is greater in males, around 4:1. Cocaine use disorder is higher, 0.3%, with more male users.

Stimulant intoxication. People feel superhuman while using stimulants. They feel elated, euphoric, and sociable. Unfortunately, they are also hypervigilant, sensitive, anxious, tense, and angry. Physical symptoms include two or more of the following: chest pain, cardiac arrhythmias, high or low blood pressure, tachycardia or bradycardia, respiratory depression, dilated pupils, perspiration, chills, nausea or vomiting, weight loss, psychomotor agitation or retardation, weakness, confusion, seizures, or coma.

Stimulant withdrawal. Withdrawal symptoms begin within a few hours to several days. Symptoms include tiredness, vivid nightmares, increased appetite, insomnia or hypersomnia, and psychomotor retardation or agitation. Functionality is impaired during this withdrawal process. Depression and suicidal thoughts are the most serious side effects of stimulant withdrawal.

See Box 22.2 for some of the signs and symptoms of intoxication and withdrawal.

Withdrawal treatment. For amphetamines, an inpatient setting is usually necessary. Individual, family, and group therapy are helpful. Depending upon the amphetamine used, specific drugs may be used short term. Antipsychotics may be prescribed for a few days. If there is no psychosis, diazepam (Valium) is useful in treating agitation and hyperactivity. Once the patient has been withdrawn from the amphetamine, depression can be treated with antidepressants such as bupropion (Wellbutrin).

BOX 22.2 Signs and Symptoms of Stimulant Intoxication and Withdrawal

Stimulant Intoxication	Stimulant Withdrawal
Short Term	Depression
Increased energy	Hypersomnia (or insomnia)
Decreased appetite	Fatigue
Mental alertness	Anxiety
Increased heart rate/pressure	Irritability
Dilated pupils	Poor concentration
Long Term	Psychomotor retardation
Irregular heartbeat	Increased appetite
Chest pains	Paranoia
Increased risk of heart attack	Drug craving
Panic attacks	
Depression	
Delusions/hallucinations	
"Cocaine bugs" (skin sensation)	

From Substance Abuse and Mental Health Services Administration. (2006). *TIP 45 detoxification and substance abuse treatment* (DHHS Publication No. SMA 06-4224). Washington, DC: US Government Printing Office.

The 1- to 2-week cocaine withdrawal period is distinct because there are no physiological disturbances that require inpatient care. Outpatient settings may be tried as a first approach. Some patients experience fatigue, mood changes, disturbed sleep, craving, and depression. There are no drugs that reliably reduce the intensity of these symptoms. The intense craving associated with cocaine withdrawal may require hospitalization to remove the affected individual from the usual social settings and drug sources. Unscheduled urine drug testing is usually warranted.

Tobacco Use Disorder

Craving, persistent and recurrent use, and tolerance are all symptoms of tobacco use disorder. Dependence happens quickly. Cigarettes are the most commonly used tobacco product. The 12-month prevalence of tobacco use disorder is about 13% in adults. Rates are slightly higher in males as compared with females. Most people who use tobacco begin before the age of 18.

Tobacco withdrawal. Tobacco withdrawal is distressing. At least four of the following symptoms occur: irritability, anxiety, depression, difficulty concentrating, restlessness, and insomnia. Within days after smoking cessation, heart rates decrease by 5 to 12 beats/min. Within the first year after smoking cessation, people increase their weight by an average of 4 to 7 pounds.

Withdrawal treatment. Behavioral therapy is useful to teach the patient to recognize cravings and respond to them appropriately. Hypnosis has been used successfully to treat tobacco withdrawal. Nicotine replacement therapies in the form of gum, lozenges, nasal sprays, inhalers, and patches are highly successful treatments.

Two drugs have FDA approval for nicotine cessation. The antidepressant bupropion (Zyban) reduces the cravings for nicotine and withdrawal symptoms. Varenicline (Chantix) is a nicotinic receptor partial agonist that mimics the effects of nicotine, thereby reducing cravings and withdrawal. It also partially blocks the nicotine receptors, which blunts the effect of nicotine if smoking is resumed.

HEALTH POLICY

The Government's Response to Teenage Vaping

Electronic cigarettes, or e-cigarettes, are designed to deliver nicotine or related substances to users in the form of a vapor. These products can support cigarette addiction in adults. However, the United States had never experienced an epidemic of substance use arise as quickly as the current use of e-cigarettes in youth. Despite their harmless appearance, they are dangerous to young people. Concerns include the impact of nicotine on developing brains, inhaling harmful metals and carcinogens, vaping-induced lung injury, and potentially exploding devices.

In a recent cross-sectional survey with 19,018 participants, self-reported e-cigarette use was nearly 28% among high school students and nearly 11% among middle school students. Most of the students chose the flavored vaping products with fruit, menthol, or mint, with candy, desserts, or other sweets being the most commonly reported flavors.

How did this epidemic happen so fast? In part, it was most teenagers' perception that this product was safe. In larger part, it was due to manufacturers purposefully targeting young people. Targets included: offering scholarships to teenagers for essays describing the benefits of vaping, creating a buzz on social media, and sponsoring events such as rock concerts. Probably the best/worst marketing scheme was introducing flavors that appealed to kids, such as cotton candy and gummi bears.

In response to nearly universal condemnation of these practices, the US Food and Drug Administration banned a range of flavored e-cigarette products, with the exception of menthol and tobacco-flavored pods, in 2020. Companies such as Juul Labs, the largest producer of these products, are being investigated by the US government in preparation for legal action over their targeted marketing toward young people.

Cullen, K. A., Gentzke, A., Sawdey, M. D., Chang, J. T., Anic, G. M., Wang, T. W., et al. (2019). e-Cigarette use among youth in the United States, 2019. *JAMA 322*(21), 2095–2103.

Gambling Disorder

Gambling is a compulsive activity that causes economic problems and significant disturbances in personal, social, or occupational functioning. Individuals with this disorder are preoccupied with the behavior, experience an increasing desire to gamble, and lie to conceal the extent of the problem. They may try to control the behavior, cut back, or stop gambling. Otherwise honest people may commit illegal acts to finance their addiction. They may rely on others to help pay off debts and gamble to recoup losses.

The 1-year prevalence rate in females is about 0.2%, and for males it is about 0.6%. The lifetime prevalence of gambling disorder is about 0.4% to 1%. Early expression of gambling disorder is more common among males, although the progression is more rapid for females. This problem usually develops over the course of years. Gambling may be regular or episodic. Heavy gambling may be interspersed with abstinence. Stress and depression may increase this behavior.

Treatment. Legal problems, pressure from family, and other psychiatric problems may bring the person who gambles excessively into treatment. Gamblers Anonymous (GA) is a 12-step program modeled on Alcoholics Anonymous (AA). It involves public confession, peer pressure, and peer counselors who are reformed gamblers. Hospitalization may help by removing patients from gambling environments. Individual, group, and family therapy are useful in supporting the patient.

Medications such as selective serotonin reuptake inhibitors, bupropion (Wellbutrin), mood stabilizers (lithium), and anticonvulsants such as topiramate (Topamax) may be helpful. Second-generation antipsychotics have also been used in the treatment of gambling disorder. Naltrexone, an opioid antagonist, may be given to individuals with the most severe symptoms of gambling disorder.

CONSIDERING CULTURE

Female Gaming Addiction

Although gaming addiction is not included in the *DSM-5* (APA, 2013), it is recognized as a mental health disorder in the *International Classification of Disease,* 11th revision (World Health Organization, 2019). Gaming addiction is characterized by increasing priority given to gaming to the point of taking precedence over other interests and increasing gaming despite negative consequences.

Despite the fact that there is a growing number of gaming women, almost all research to date has been with males. This is especially a problem since women may be more vulnerable to online gaming addiction. Understanding the culture of women who game and their specific needs will be a priority as studies are conducted on this new disorder.

Adapted from World Health Organization. (2019). *International Classification of Disease* (11th revision). Retrieved from https://icd.who.int/browse11/l-m/en.

ALCOHOL USE DISORDER

Clinical Picture

Although alcohol is a sedative, it creates an initial feeling of euphoria. This is probably related to decreased inhibitions. A cluster of behavioral and physical symptoms characterizes alcohol use disorder. The full criteria for alcohol use disorder are listed in the *DSM-5* box. Severity is based on the number of symptoms: mild (two or three symptoms), moderate (four or five symptoms), and severe (presence of six or more symptoms).

DSM-5 CRITERIA FOR ALCOHOL USE DISORDER

A. A problematic pattern of alcohol use leading to clinically significant impairment or distress, as manifested by at least two of the following, occurring within a 12-month period:
   1. Alcohol is often taken in larger amounts or over a longer period than was intended.
   2. There is a persistent desire or unsuccessful efforts to cut down or control alcohol use.
   3. A great deal of time is spent in activities necessary to obtain alcohol, use alcohol, or recover from its effects.
   4. Craving or a strong desire or urge to use alcohol.
   5. Recurrent alcohol use resulting in a failure to fulfill major role obligations at work, school, or home.
   6. Continued alcohol use despite having persistent or recurrent social or interpersonal problems caused or exacerbated by the effects of alcohol.

Continued

7. Important social, occupational, or recreational activities are given up or reduced because of alcohol use.
8. Recurrent alcohol use in situations in which it is physically hazardous.
9. Alcohol use is continued despite knowledge of having a persistent or recurrent physical or psychological problem that is likely to have been caused or exacerbated by alcohol.
10. Tolerance, as defined by either of the following:
    a. A need for markedly increased amounts of alcohol to achieve intoxication or desired effect.
    b. A markedly diminished effect with continued use of the same amount of alcohol.
11. Withdrawal, as manifested by either of the following:
    c. The characteristic withdrawal syndrome for alcohol.
    d. Alcohol (or a closely related substance such as a benzodiazepine) is taken to relieve or avoid withdrawal problems.

Specify if:

In early remission: After full criteria for alcohol use disorder were previously met, none of the criteria for alcohol use disorder have been met for at least 3 months but for less than 12 months (with the exception that Criterion A4 may be met).

In sustained remission: After full criteria for alcohol use disorder were previously met, none of the criteria for alcohol use disorder have been met at any time during a period of 12 months or longer (with the exception that Criterion A4 may be met).

Specify if:

In a controlled environment: This additional specifier is used if the individual is in an environment where access to alcohol is restricted.

From the American Psychiatric Association. (2013). *Diagnostic and statistical manual of mental disorders* (5th ed.). Washington, DC: Author.

Epidemiology

Alcohol use disorder is far too common. In 2018, 14.8 million (5.4%) people in the United States were estimated to have alcohol use disorder (SAMHSA, 2019). About 401,000 (1.6%) adolescents aged 12 to 17 had a past-year alcohol use disorder. Young adults are particularly affected by alcohol use. About 3.4 million (10.1%) young adults aged 18 to 25 are estimated to have had this disorder. About 11.0 million (5.1%) adults 26 and older had an alcohol use disorder in the preceding year.

Rates of this disorder are higher, with almost twice the prevalence, among adult men versus adult women. In general, American Indians/Alaska Natives (12.1%) have the highest rates for alcohol use disorder and are disproportionately affected by alcohol problems (Vaeth, Wang-Schweig, & Caetano, 2017). Prevalence rates are higher in whites (8.9%), followed by Hispanics (7.5%), blacks (6.9%), and Asian Americans and Pacific Islanders (4.5%).

Comorbidity

Bipolar disorders, schizophrenia, and antisocial personality disorder are associated with an increase in rates of alcohol use disorder. Major depressive disorder is a risk factor for and a result of alcohol use disorder due to alcohol's depressant qualities. Alcohol may also reduce the immune response and predispose users to infection.

Risk Factors

Biological Factors

Genetic. Alcohol use disorder runs in families and about 40% to 60% of the risk comes from inheritance (APA, 2013). Monozygotic (identical) twins are more likely to share alcohol use problems than are dizygotic (fraternal) twins. Monozygotic male twins are more likely to share alcohol use disorder than are female twins. Up to a fourfold increase in risk occurs in children of affected individuals, even when the children are given up for adoption or raised in other homes.

There is some evidence to suggest that some genes may reduce the risk of alcohol consumption by impacting alcohol metabolism. For example, certain alleles of the alcohol dehydrogenase and aldehyde dehydrogenase genes can cause a buildup of acetaldehyde that creates the classic flushing response (Ebert, Finn, & Smoller, 2016).

Neurobiological. Individuals from families with a history of alcohol misuse have altered amygdalar, hippocampal, basal ganglia, and cerebellar volume (Cservenka, 2016). Functional magnetic resonance imaging studies show altered inhibitory control and working memory brain response in these individuals. There may be brain activity differences in areas involved in emotional and instinctual reward processing.

Environmental Factors

Social. Adolescents may be strongly influenced by their peers to engage in substance use. Alcohol, which has been referred to as a "social lubricant," may increase an adolescent's feeling of belonging. Using alcohol, tobacco, and marijuana at an early age is strongly associated with coming from a home with low parental supervision.

Cultural. Substance use may create a sense of community and belonging in otherwise isolated individuals. The lifestyle of individuals who use substances may even seem alluring and dramatic to vulnerable people.

In some cultures and religions, alcohol use is not accepted, and any use would be considered deviant. In other cultures, alcohol use is a regular part of everyday life, and the amount of consumption would be alarming to people outside the culture. Muslim-majority countries such as Pakistan, Libya, and Saudi Arabia have prohibitions against alcohol. In Afghanistan, it is illegal for citizens to purchase alcohol, but there are still places for foreigners to drink. In the United States, some Christian denominations such as Pentecostal, Baptist, and Mormon reject the use of alcohol.

Types of Problematic Drinking

Amounts of alcohol that are considered safe vary depending upon individual factors. Table 22.3 identifies the numbers of drinks that are considered acceptable, depending on the gender, age, and pregnancy.

Excessive drinking is described by two different terms. **Binge drinking** refers to drinking too much alcohol quickly. For women, this amount is four or more drinks within 2 hours; for men, this amount is five or more drinks within 2 hours. **Heavy drinking** is characterized by drinking too much, too often. Eight or more drinks in a week constitutes heavy drinking in

TABLE 22.3 Maximum Safe Number of Drinks Based on Population

	Men	Women	Pregnant	Adolescent	Older Adults
Day	4	3	0	0	3
Week	14	7	0	0	7

US Department of Health and Human Services. (2015). *2015–2020 dietary guidelines for Americans* (8th ed.). Retrieved from http://health.gov/dietaryguidelines/2015/guidelines/.

women. Men who drink more than 14 drinks in a week are considered heavy drinkers.

Alcohol Intoxication

The legal definition of intoxication in most states requires a blood concentration of 80 or 100 mg ethanol per deciliter of blood (mg/dL). This concentration may also be expressed as 0.08 to 0.10 g/dL. Signs and symptoms of alcohol intoxication based on blood alcohol are:

- 20 mg/dL (0.02 g/dL)—Two alcoholic drinks: Slower motor performance, decreased thinking ability, altered mood, and reduced ability to multitask.
- 50 mg/dL (0.05 g/dL)—Three alcoholic drinks: Impaired judgment, exaggerated behavior, euphoria, and lower alertness.
- 80 mg/dL (0.08 g/dL)—Four alcoholic drinks: Poor muscle coordination, altered speech and hearing, difficulty detecting danger, impaired judgment, poor self-control, and decreased reasoning.
- 100 mg/dL (0.10 g/dL)—Five alcoholic drinks: Slurred speech, poor coordination, and slowed thinking.
- 150 mg/dL (0.15 g/dL)—Six alcoholic drinks: Vomiting (unless high tolerance) and major loss of balance.
- 200 mg/dL (0.20 g/dL)—Eight to 10 alcoholic drinks: Memory blackouts, nausea, and vomiting.
- 300 mg/dL (0.30 g/dL)—More than 10 alcoholic drinks: Reduction of body temperature, blood pressure, respiratory rate, sleepiness, and amnesia.
- 400 mg/dL (0.40 mg/dL)—Impaired vital signs and possible death.

Intoxication is based on a number of factors, including how quickly the alcohol is consumed. Quicker ingestion results in higher levels of blood alcohol. In the United States, a standard drink is one that contains about 14 g of pure alcohol (National Institute on Alcohol Abuse and Alcoholism, n.d.). Fig. 22.2 illustrates the relative amount of alcohol in standard drinks.

Alcohol Withdrawal

Alcohol withdrawal occurs after reducing or quitting alcohol after heavy and prolonged use. The classic sign of alcohol withdrawal is tremulousness, commonly called the *shakes* or the *jitters*, which begins 6 to 8 hours after alcohol cessation (Sadock et al., 2015). Mild to moderate alcohol withdrawal includes agitation, lack of appetite, nausea, vomiting, insomnia, impaired cognition, and mild perceptual changes. Both systolic and diastolic blood pressure increases, as does pulse and body temperature. Chlordiazepoxide (Librium) is useful for tremulousness and mild to moderate agitation.

Psychotic and perceptual symptoms may begin in 8 to 10 hours. If your patient is undergoing withdrawal to the point of psychosis, it should be considered a medical emergency because of the risks of unconsciousness, seizures, and delirium. The benzodiazepines lorazepam (Ativan) or chlordiazepoxide (Librium) can be given either orally or intramuscularly and tapered over the following 5 to 7 days.

Withdrawal seizures may occur within 12 to 24 hours after alcohol cessation. These seizures are generalized and tonic-clonic. Additional seizures may occur within hours of the first seizure. Diazepam (Valium) given intravenously is a common treatment for withdrawal seizures.

Alcohol withdrawal delirium, also known as *delirium tremens (DTs)*, is a medical emergency that can result in the death in 20% of untreated patients, usually as a result of medical problems such as pneumonia, renal disease, hepatic insufficiency, or heart failure (Sadock et al., 2015). Alcohol withdrawal delirium may happen anytime in the first 72 hours. Autonomic hyperactivity may result in tachycardia, diaphoresis, fever, anxiety, insomnia, and hypertension. Delusions and visual and tactile hallucinations are common in alcohol withdrawal delirium.

Delusions and hallucinations may result in unpredictable behaviors as patients try to protect themselves from what they believe are genuine dangers. Patients on any medical floor are at risk for this condition after cessation of heavy drinking for 3 days and are a danger to themselves and others. Serious physical illness such as hepatitis or pancreatitis may increase the likelihood of alcohol withdrawal delirium. It is rare to see this syndrome in individuals in good physical health.

Prevention of alcohol withdrawal delirium is the goal. Oral diazepam (Valium) may be useful in the symptomatic relief of acute agitation, tremor, impending or acute DTs, and hallucinosis. Chlordiazepoxide (Librium) may keep your patient out of danger. However, once delirium appears, intravenous lorazepam (Ativan) is used to treat these severe symptoms. Seclusion may be necessary. Dehydration, often exacerbated by diaphoresis and fever, can be corrected with oral or intravenous fluids.

Cognitive Disturbances
Wernicke-Korsakoff Syndrome

People with a heavy use of alcohol for many years may suffer from short-term memory disturbances. One memory-reducing problem is Wernicke's (alcoholic) encephalopathy, an acute and reversible condition. Another problem is Korsakoff's syndrome, a chronic condition with a recovery rate of only about 20%. The pathophysiological connection between the two problems is a thiamine deficiency, which may be caused by poor nutrition associated with alcohol use or by the malabsorption of nutrients.

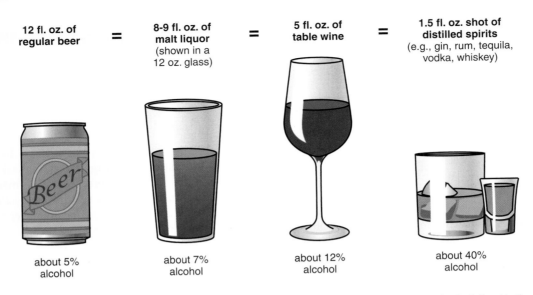

12 fl. oz. of regular beer = 8-9 fl. oz. of malt liquor (shown in a 12 oz. glass) = 5 fl. oz. of table wine = 1.5 fl. oz. shot of distilled spirits (e.g., gin, rum, tequila, vodka, whiskey)

about 5% alcohol   about 7% alcohol   about 12% alcohol   about 40% alcohol

Each beverage portrayed above represents one standard drink (or one alcohol drink equivalent), defined in the Unites States as any beverage containing .6 fl. oz. or 14 grams of pure alcohol. The percentage of pure alcohol, expressed here as alcohol by volume (alc/vol), varies within and across beverage types. Although the standard drink amounts are helpful for following health guidelines, they may not reflect customary serving sizes.

Fig. 22.2 What is a standard drink? (Adapted from National Institute on Alcohol Abuse and Alcoholism. [n.d.]. *What is a standard drink?* Retrieved from https://www.niaaa.nih.gov/what-standard-drink.)

Wernicke's encephalopathy is characterized by altered gait, vestibular dysfunction, confusion, and several ocular motility abnormalities (horizontal nystagmus, lateral orbital palsy, and gaze palsy). These eye-focused signs are bilateral but not necessarily symmetrical. Sluggish reaction to light and anisocoria (unequal pupil size) are also symptoms. Wernicke's encephalopathy may clear up within a few weeks or may progress into Korsakoff's syndrome, the more severe and chronic version of this problem.

Wernicke's encephalopathy responds rapidly to large doses of intravenous thiamine two to three times daily for 1 to 2 weeks. Treatment of Korsakoff's syndrome is also thiamine for 3 to 12 months. Most patients with Korsakoff's syndrome never fully recover, although cognitive improvement may occur with thiamine and nutritional support.

Blackouts

An extremely disturbing aspect of alcohol use is blackouts. Blackouts are caused by excessive consumption of alcohol followed by episodes of amnesia. During these periods of time, a person actively engages in behaviors, can perform complicated tasks, and appears normal. This phenomenon is due to alcohol's ability to block the consolidation of new memories into ones through the hippocampus and related temporal lobe structures.

Fetal Alcohol Syndrome

Fetal alcohol syndrome is a common cause of intellectual disability in the United States. Alcohol during pregnancy inhibits intrauterine growth and postnatal development, resulting in microcephaly, craniofacial malformations, and limb and heart defects. As adults, affected individuals tend to have a short stature. Women with alcohol-related disorders have a 35% risk of having a child with defects. Fig. 22.3 illustrates the facial features of fetal alcohol syndrome.

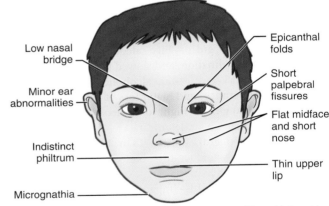

Low nasal bridge

Minor ear abnormalities

Indistinct philtrum

Micrognathia

Epicanthal folds

Short palpebral fissures

Flat midface and short nose

Thin upper lip

Fig. 22.3 Facial features of fetal alcohol syndrome. (From National Institute on Alcohol Abuse and Alcoholism. (2011). *Fetal alcohol spectrum disorders.* Retrieved from http://pubs.niaaa.nih.gov/publications/AA82/AA82.htm)

Systemic Effects

Peripheral Neuropathy

Chronic alcoholism leads to nutritional deficiencies, particularly thiamine, due to drinking rather than eating, leading to damage to the peripheral nervous system. The feeling of "pins and needles" in the lower extremities is a common symptom of peripheral neuropathy. Other symptoms include numbness, muscle weakness, sensitivity to touch, and burning. Discontinuation of alcohol will prevent further deterioration.

Alcoholic Myopathy

Binge drinking may cause a sudden acute alcoholic myopathy with muscle weakness and myonecrosis (muscle damage). Chronic alcoholic myopathy develops gradually. The characteristic symptom of this problem is a significant reduction in muscle mass and resulting muscle weakness. Recovery is possible if alcohol is avoided, but the time to recovery varies from rapid (days to weeks) with the acute form to lengthy (weeks to months) with the chronic form.

Alcoholic Cardiomyopathy

Direct toxic effects of alcohol can weaken and thin the muscles of the heart, leading to enlargement and eventual heart failure. Symptoms of alcoholic cardiomyopathy are similar to other types of heart failure, including fatigue, shortness of breath, and edema of the legs and feet.

Esophagitis

Inflammation of the esophagus is a direct result of the toxic effects of alcohol on the esophageal mucosa. The vomiting related to alcohol overuse is also contributory to this condition. Esophageal varices are distended veins within the esophagus or the upper part of the stomach that result from heavy drinking. These veins are at risk for bursting, which results in a medical emergency.

Gastritis

As a toxin, alcohol irritates and erodes the mucosal stomach lining. Symptoms of gastritis include nausea, vomiting, loss of appetite, belching, and bloating. Damage to the stomach lining may lead to ulcers and bleeding.

Pancreatitis

Prolonged and hazardous drinking may result in pancreatic damage. Excessive drinking, usually more than 5 years, may result in an acute attack of pancreatitis. Continued alcohol misuse eventually results in chronic pancreatitis in a minority of misusers. Abdominal pain, nausea, and vomiting are the major symptoms of acute pancreatitis. Withdrawal of alcohol in the early stages will reverse the condition. The chronic condition results in malnutrition, weight loss, and diabetes mellitus. Withdrawal of alcohol in the chronic condition may reduce inflammatory episodes and allow for better control of diabetes.

Alcoholic Hepatitis

Alcohol gets processed by the liver and produces highly toxic chemicals. Excessive alcohol over an extended period of time may result in a diseased and inflamed liver. Alcoholic hepatitis only occurs in a minority of heavy users. Genetic factors, such as how the body processes alcohol, other liver disorders (e.g., hepatitis C), malnutrition, and being female increase the risk of this disorder. Symptoms of alcoholic hepatitis include appetite changes, dry mouth, weight loss, nausea and vomiting, pain or swelling in the abdomen, jaundice, fever, confusion, and fatigue.

Cirrhosis of the Liver

Cirrhosis is a slowly progressing disease in which healthy liver tissue is replaced by scar tissue. Eventually, the liver can no longer function properly because the scar tissue blocks the flow of blood through the liver. This slows the processing of nutrients, hormones, drugs, and naturally produced toxins. Liver disease and cirrhosis was the tenth leading cause of death by disease in men in 2017 (Centers for Disease Control and Prevention, 2019). Symptoms of cirrhosis of the liver include easy bleeding and bruising, pruritus, jaundice, ascites, leg edema, weight loss, confusion, spider-like blood vessels on the skin (petechiae), and testicular atrophy. No treatment will cure cirrhosis or repair scarring. Liver transplantation may be necessary. Low-salt diets will reduce ascites.

Leukopenia

When there is liver damage, alcoholism may cause low white blood cells due to vitamin deficiencies and low protein intake. Low white blood cells predispose individuals to infection and disease. Symptoms of leukopenia include periodontitis and gingivitis, fatigue, weakness, fever, and abdominal pain. Improved nutrition and alcohol cessation are indicated for this condition.

Thrombocytopenia

Thrombocytopenia is a complication of liver cirrhosis characterized by a low platelet count. This is caused by platelet pooling in an enlarged spleen and decreased thromboprotein production in the liver. Symptoms of thrombocytopenia include excessive bruising (purpura), petechiae (particularly on lower legs), and prolonged bleeding from cuts. Platelet count begins to rise within 2 to 5 days of abstaining from alcohol.

Cancer

Alcohol consumption is a major risk factor for head and neck cancers, especially in the head and neck, esophagus, oral cavity, pharynx, and larynx (National Cancer Institute, 2018). Alcohol use is also associated with liver, breast, and colorectal cancers.

APPLICATION OF THE NURSING PROCESS

SCREENING

Alcohol is a major contributing factor in:
- Increased mortality and deaths
- Morbidity and disease
- Harm to others and injury
- Increased economic loss and disabilities

Alcohol can be fatal as a result of its severe withdrawal symptoms. Screening is essential to intervene early and provide treatment for people with substance use disorders and for those at risk of developing these disorders.

The Screening, Brief Intervention, and Referral to Treatment (SBIRT) program is a comprehensive, integrated, public health approach to the delivery of early intervention and treatment services for persons with substance use disorders as well as those who are at risk of developing these disorders. SBIRT identifies at-risk substance users for early intervention (SAMHSA, 2017) and consists of three major components:
- **Screening:** A nurse or other healthcare professional in any healthcare setting assesses the severity of substance use and identifies the appropriate level of treatment.
- **Brief Intervention:** A nurse or other healthcare professional focuses on increasing insight and awareness regarding substance use and motivation toward behavioral change.

- **Referral to Treatment:** A nurse or other healthcare professional provides those identified as needing more extensive treatment with access to specialty care.

A variety of other screening tools are available to assist healthcare practitioners in gaining important information on which to base plans of care. Additional screening tools are:

- AUDIT (The **A**lcohol **U**se **D**isorders **I**dentification **T**est)
- CAGE (Questions: Have you felt you needed to **c**ut down on your drinking? Are people **a**nnoyed by your drinking? Have you felt **g**uilty about your drinking? Have you ever had a drink in the morning (**e**ye-opener)? A score of 2 or more is significant, although a score of 1 requires further assessment.
- CAGE-AID (Questions are the same as CAGE but refers to **A**dapted to **I**nclude **D**rugs.)
- T-ACE (**T**olerance, **A**nnoyance, **C**ut down, **E**ye-opener)

Formalized alcohol screening is as simple as using the Alcohol Use Disorders Identification Test (AUDIT) developed for the World Health Organization. AUDIT has been effective for decades and continues to be used today (Babor et al., 2001; Table 22.4). The clinician can administer this tool or the patient can self-report.

During the screening process, instructions need to be clear and followed carefully. Nonjudgmental attitudes help with objectivity regardless of what the individual reveals. Several trends are important, such as the appearance of progression or loss of control and whether or not tolerance or withdrawal is present. Once the screening process identifies a potential problem, a more complete assessment is warranted.

ASSESSMENT

An alcohol use assessment is part of a more comprehensive assessment that evaluates the individual holistically. Ideally, this assessment involves an addiction professional with specialized knowledge and skills to make a diagnosis. The assessment will include a clinical examination of the background, pattern of substance use, and any mental health symptoms. The nurse will make special note of any history of trauma, a family history of substance use or mental health problems and any disabilities, as well as the individual's strengths and level of willingness to change. As a result of this assessment, the individual may be identified as having a substance-related disorder.

TABLE 22.4 The Alcohol Use Disorders Identification Test (AUDIT): Self-Report Version

Patient: Because alcohol use can affect your health and interfere with certain medications and treatments, it is important that we ask some questions about your use of alcohol. Be honest; confidentiality will be upheld.

Mark the frequency that best describes your answer to each question.

Questions	0	1	2	3	4	Score
1. How often do you have a drink containing alcohol?	Never	Monthly or less	2–4 times a month	2–3 times a week	4 or more times a week	
2. How many drinks containing alcohol do you have on a typical day when you are drinking?	1 or 2	3 or 4	5 or 6	7–9	10 or more	
3. How often do you have six or more drinks on one occasion?	Never	Less than monthly	Monthly	Weekly	Daily or almost daily	
4. How often during the last year have you found that you were not able to stop drinking once you had started?	Never	Less than monthly	Monthly	Weekly	Daily or almost daily	
5. How often during the last year have you failed to do what was normally expected of you because of drinking?	Never	Less than monthly	Monthly	Weekly	Daily or almost daily	
6. How often during the last year have you needed a first drink in the morning to get yourself going after a heavy drinking session?	Never	Less than monthly	Monthly	Weekly	Daily or almost daily	
7. How often during the last year have you had a feeling of guilt or remorse after drinking?	Never	Less than monthly	Monthly	Weekly	Daily or almost daily	
8. How often during the last year have you been unable to remember what happened the night before because of your drinking?	Never	Less than monthly	Monthly	Weekly	Daily or almost daily	
9. Have you or someone else been injured because of your drinking?	No		Yes, but not in the last year		Yes, during the last year	
10. Has a relative, friend, doctor, or other healthcare worker been concerned about your drinking or suggested you cut down?	No		Yes, but not in the last year		Yes, during the last year	
					Total	

Score: 8 or more in men; 7 or more in women needs further assessment.
Babor, T. F., Higgins-Biddle, J. C., Saunders, J. B., & Monteiro, M. (2001). *The alcohol use disorders identification test* (2nd ed.). Retrieved from http://apps.who.int/iris/bitstream/10665/67205/1/WHO_MSD_MSB_01.6a.pdf.

Family Assessment

Understanding the process of addiction from a holistic perspective requires careful attention to the family. Living with an individual who misuses alcohol or other substances is a source of stress and requires family system adjustments. Codependence is a cluster of behaviors originally identified through research involving the families of alcoholic patients. People who are codependent often exhibit overly responsible behavior—doing for others what others could just as well do for themselves. People who are codependent often define their self-worth in terms of caring for others to the exclusion of their own needs.

Self-Assessment

Alcohol use is self-inflicted. Carefully assessing personal thoughts, opinions, and feelings is the first step to remaining objective and establishing a therapeutic relationship with a person who misuses alcohol. Recognizing and dealing with our responses by practicing introspection is essential to the provision of patient-centered care protected from bias or countertransference.

You may be aware that registered nurses themselves might have personal substance use problems. For those nurses who become aware that they are engaging in risk-taking behaviors or that one of their colleagues may be experiencing difficulties, there are nonpunitive alternatives to discipline programs in the form of peer assistance. Many State Boards of Nursing have developed an alternative to discipline programs to help impaired nurses. To determine if your state has this model, check with your state's Board of Nursing.

NURSING DIAGNOSIS

Once the comprehensive substance use assessment has been completed in a thorough, objective manner, the data are analyzed and potential or actual problems and needs are identified. Clinical decision-making skills will be used to determine which of the identified problems requires a priority intervention.

OUTCOMES IDENTIFICATION

The goals for treatment planning arise from the preferred outcome for each problem. Outcome measures may include immediate detox and stabilization for individuals experiencing withdrawal, abstinence if individuals are actively drinking, motivation for treatment and engagement in early abstinence, and pursuit of a recovery lifestyle for after discharge. Table 22.5 identifies signs and symptoms commonly experienced with substance use disorders, offers potential nursing diagnoses, and suggests outcomes.

PLANNING

The treatment plan will be developed based on the assessment and diagnoses. For treatment to be successful, a patient-centered

TABLE 22.5 Signs and Symptoms, Nursing Diagnoses, and Outcomes for Substance-Related and Addictive Disorders

Signs and Symptoms	Nursing Diagnoses	Outcomes
Impulsiveness, loss of relationships and occupation due to focus on substances or gambling, legal problems, social isolation	Risk for suicide	Decreased suicide risk: Expresses feelings, verbalizes suicidal ideas, refrains from suicide attempts, plans for the future
Intoxication: Impaired cognition/judgment, impaired physical coordination, psychomotor agitation or retardation	Risk for injury	Remains free from injury while intoxicated
Depends on the overdosed substance (e.g., opiates—unresponsiveness, respiratory depression, pinpoint pupils, coma, hypothermia, hypotension, bradycardia)	Overdose	Overdose resolution: Returns to pre-overdose level of functioning, identifies mechanism of overdose
Depends on the substance of withdrawal (e.g., opiates—mood dysphoria, nausea, muscle aches, fever, insomnia, lacrimation, rhinorrhea, pupillary dilation, yawning, gooseflesh)	Withdrawal	Withdrawal cessation: Symptoms are controlled, returns to pre-withdrawal functioning
Reports not feeling well rested, decreased ability to function, reports awakening multiple times	Impaired sleep	Improved sleep: Minimal awakening, feels restored after sleep, sleeps recommended hours based on age
Substance use or gambling, decreased use of social support, destructive behavior toward self and others, difficulty organizing information, inadequate problem-solving, poor concentration, reports inability to cope	Impaired coping	Effective coping: Modifies lifestyle as needed to maintain sobriety, maintains abstinence from substances, engages in satisfying relationships
Does not perceive danger of substance use or gambling, minimizes symptoms, refuses healthcare attention, unable to admit impact of disease on life pattern	Denial	No denial: Accepts responsibility for behavior, maintains abstinence from substances
Substance use or gambling, lack of initiative, passivity, social isolation, reports no alternatives or personal control, anger, no meaning in life	Hopelessness	Expresses feelings of self-worth, verbalizes sense of personal identity, expresses meaning in life, sets goals, believes that actions impact outcomes
Blaming, broken promises, lying, enabling, manipulation, rationalization, projection, deterioration of family relationships	Dysfunctional family process	Improved family process: Identifies personal role in family dysfunction, honest communication, clear communication

International Council of Nursing Practice. (2019). *ICNP browser.* Retrieved from https://www.icn.ch/what-we-do/projects/ehealth/icnp-browser. ICNP® is owned and copyrighted by the International Council of Nurses (ICN). Reproduced with permission of the copyright holder.

approach includes the patient's goals. The plan should take into account the patient's ability to recognize the problem and readiness or motivation for change.

IMPLEMENTATION

Nursing Interventions

Basic nursing interventions are useful in providing a supportive environment for managing substance use disorders. Promoting safety and sleep are essential first-line interventions. Also, patients with alcohol use disorder may have severely compromised nutritional status due to choosing substance over sustenance. Gradually reintroducing healthy food and hydration helps support body systems and neurological functioning. Support and encouragement for self-care (hygiene) will help improve self-esteem in individuals who may have long neglected themselves.

The development of a therapeutic relationship sets the stage for exploring harmful thoughts, anxiety, hopelessness, and spiritual distress. An understanding of current coping skills along with the identification of new skills provides tools to test in a safe setting. Assistance in goal setting helps a patient to see beyond the current situation and instills hope and direction.

Nurses administer medications and provide ongoing assessment of their efficacy and side effects after administration. Nurses need to monitor vital signs frequently since an increase in pulse, blood pressure, and body temperatures are clear signs of withdrawal. The goal is to keep the patient safe and comfortable and stay ahead of withdrawal so the patient does not suffer.

Health Teaching and Health Promotion

If genetic vulnerability accounts for 40% to 60% of an individual's risk, prevention may be the best answer to addressing alcohol misuse (NIDA, 2018). Health teaching is a part of the school curriculum, and schools may offer classes on understanding addiction as a brain disorder, its risk factors, and ways to prevent or limit exposure to psychoactive substances. Promoting classes for developing healthy coping and stress management skills and activities for increasing self-confidence and self-efficacy would also lower the risks for use of psychoactive substances.

Social activities that increase supportive relationships reduce the impact of stressful life events and provide a venue for community activities that provide health education and promotion. Pay special attention to understanding the particular impact of trauma as a risk factor. Physical, sexual, or emotional abuse at any age; physical trauma from accidents; natural disasters; or acts of violence or war can all be predisposing factors for the use of psychoactive substances or processes.

EVALUATION

Evaluation occurs on several levels: assessing the effectiveness of the treatment plan, using objective data to check whether nursing actions addressed the patient's symptoms, and measuring the changes in the patient's behaviors for progress toward meeting stated goals. Problematic behaviors, patterns of expression,

or perceptions may improve or only undergo changes in small increments, requiring alterations in the action steps or even the goals of the treatment plan to meet the patient's needs.

During the treatment experience, conduct ongoing evaluation of the process to ensure that any transference or countertransference is managed and that the goals and outcomes of treatment remain patient centered. Evaluation will also make it possible to ensure that the patient acquires the necessary skills and competencies for continued reflection and maintenance of the new lifestyle identification.

TREATMENT MODALITIES

Biological Treatments
Pharmacotherapy

Previously in the chapter, we discussed medications used for other substances. Table 22.6 identifies medications used in the treatment of alcohol use disorder.

Psychological Therapies

Advanced practice nurses and other substance use and addiction treatment professionals use a number of psychotherapies. Cognitive behavioral therapy and motivational interviewing are commonly used evidence-based therapies.

Destructive and negative thinking patterns play into the development of maladaptive behavioral patterns like substance use disorders. **Cognitive behavioral therapy** helps patients explore thinking patterns so that the core belief system and any irrational core beliefs can be identified. Positive and negative consequences of alcohol use are explored. Patients learn to self-monitor their cravings and challenge these cravings realistically.

Motivational interviewing is an approach based on the transtheoretical or stages of change theory. It has gained popularity in its use as a brief, long-term, and supplementary intervention, particularly in the treatment of substance use disorders. It uses a person-centered approach to strengthen motivation for change (Tan, Lee, Lim, Leong, & Lee, 2015). The advanced practice nurse and patient usually meet for an hour at a time.

Individuals may be at stage one, *precontemplation*, and need assistance in admitting there is a problem. If they have acknowledged the problem, *contemplation*, they may still not be ready to commit to addressing it. The goal of treatment is to assist in the development of awareness and a commitment. *Preparation*, or getting ready, and *action*, or changing, take place in early treatment phases. The *maintenance* stage is the ongoing commitment to a recovery program. Without continuing action, the individual will likely return to previous behavior, *relapse*.

Care Continuum for Substance Use Disorders

Continuity of care occurs through a continuum starting with detoxification (detox), rehabilitation, halfway houses, partial programs, intensive outpatient (IOP), and outpatient settings (SAMHSA, 2015). Mutual support groups such as AA are strongly encouraged throughout the treatment process.

TABLE 22.6 Common Medications Used for Treatment of Alcohol Use Disorder

Generic (Brand Name)	Uses	Implications for the Therapeutic Process
Disulfiram (Antabuse)	Maintenance, relapse prevention, aversion therapy	Physical effects when alcohol is used: Intense nausea and vomiting, headache, diaphoresis (sweating), flushed skin, dyspnea (respiratory difficulties), and confusion. Avoid all alcohol and substances such as cough syrup and mouthwash containing alcohol.
Naltrexone (Vivitrol—injectable, ReVia, Depade—oral)	Withdrawal, relapse prevention, decreases pleasurable feelings and cravings	Oral or long-acting (once a month) injectable form. Nausea usually goes away after first month; headache, sedation. Pain at injection site, patient needs to be opiate free 10 days before initiation of medication.
Acamprosate calcium (Campral)	Relapse prevention	Begin taking on the fifth day of abstinence from alcohol. Tablets are taken three times a day. Side effects include diarrhea, gastrointestinal upset, appetite loss, dizziness, anxiety, and difficulty sleeping. Contraindicated in patients with renal impairment.
Benzodiazepines (lorazepam [Ativan], chlordiazepoxide [Librium], diazepam [Valium])	Withdrawal	Sedation, decreased anxiety, and blood pressure. Use CIWA-AR scale to assess dose according to agency policies. Assess for seizures that could lead to delirium tremens (DTs). If not treated, coma and ultimately death.
Anticonvulsants (Tegretol) Barbiturates (phenobarbital)	Withdrawal	Older treatments still used today. Other treatments have proven more effective and safer. Assess for seizures that could lead to delirium tremens if not treated, coma, and ultimately death.
Clonidine *(Catapres)*	Mild to moderate withdrawal	Alpha-agonist antihypertensive agent. Give every 4–6 h as needed. Side effects dizziness, hypotension, fatigue, and headache.

CIWA-AR, Clinical Institute Withdrawal Assessment for Alcohol.
Substance Abuse and Mental Health Services Administration and National Institute on Alcohol Abuse and Alcoholism. (2015). *Medication for the treatment of alcohol use disorder: A brief guide.* HHS Publication No. (SMA) 15-4907. Rockville, MD: Author.

CASE STUDY AND NURSING CARE PLAN

Alcohol Use Disorder

Mr. Stewart, aged 49 years, and his wife arrive in the emergency department. They are fearful that Mr. Stewart has had a stroke. His right hand is limp, and he is unable to hyperextend his right wrist and cannot feel his fingertips.

Ms. Winkler, the admitting nurse, begins the assessment. Mr. Stewart looks much older than his stated age. His complexion is ruddy and flushed. History taking is difficult. Mr. Stewart answers only what is asked, volunteering no additional information. He states that he took a nap that afternoon. When he woke up, he noticed the problems with his right arm.

Mr. Stewart has been unemployed for 4 years because the company he worked for went bankrupt. He has been unable to find a job but has an interview in 10 days. His wife is now working full time. They have two grown children who no longer live at home. As he talks about his children, his lips start to tremble and his eyes fill with tears.

Meanwhile, a nurse practitioner has examined Mr. Stewart. The diagnosis is radial nerve palsy. Mr. Stewart most likely passed out while lying on his arm. Because Mr. Stewart was intoxicated, he did not feel the signals (numbness and tingling) that his nerves sent out to warn him to move. He was in this position for so long that the resultant cutoff of circulation was sufficient to cause some temporary nerve damage.

Mr. Stewart's blood alcohol level is 0.31 mg/dL. This is three times the legal limit for intoxication in many states (0.1 mg/dL). Despite the high alcohol level, Mr. Stewart is alert and oriented, not slurring his speech or giving any other outward signs of intoxication. This incongruence is likely due to tolerance, a symptom of physical addiction.

Self-Assessment

Ms. Winkler has seen many patients with the disease of alcoholism make radical changes in their lives, and she has learned to view alcoholism as a treatable disease. She is aware also that it is the patient who makes the changes, and she no longer feels responsible when a patient is not ready to make that change.

Assessment

Subjective Data
- Complains of limpness in his right hand, inability to hyperextend his right wrist, and cannot feel his fingertips.
- Noticed the problems with his arm after a nap
- Unemployed for 4 years
- Upcoming job interview

Objective Data
- Appears older than age
- Complexion ruddy and flushed
- Short responses, volunteers little information
- Tearful when talking about children
- Blood alcohol level is 0.31 mg/dL
- Alert and oriented

Priority Diagnosis

Impaired coping related to alcohol use as evidenced by increased alcohol use and impairment in life functioning.

Continued

CASE STUDY AND NURSING CARE PLAN—cont'd

Outcomes Identification
Client will demonstrate mild to no change in health status and social functioning due to substance addiction.

Planning
Mr. Stewart's plan of care is personalized as follows:

Short-Term Goal	Intervention	Rationale	Evaluation
1. Client will acknowledge consequences associated with alcohol use.	1a. Identify with patient those factors (genetics, stress) that contribute to chemical addiction. 1b. Assist patient to identify negative effects of chemical dependency.	1a. Emphasis on alcoholism as a disease can lower guilt and increase self-esteem. 1b. Begins to decrease denial and increase problem-solving.	GOAL MET Client admits that he cannot find a new job when he is intoxicated.

Short-Term Goal	Intervention	Rationale	Evaluation
2. Client will commit to alcohol-use control strategies.	2a. Determine history of alcohol use. 2b. Identify support groups in community for long-term substance use treatment (for wife also).	2a. Identifies high-risk situations. 2b. Alcohol addiction requires long-term treatment; Alcoholics Anonymous (AA) is effective.	GOAL MET After 3 weeks, patient states that he attends AA every day. He is learning about his triggers and new coping skills. His wife attends Al-Anon.

Evaluation
See individual outcomes and evaluation in the care plan.

Detoxification (Detox)

Detox is warranted when the individual quits using a psychoactive substance known to cause withdrawal or when the individual is already in withdrawal. This is a medically managed inpatient program with 24-hour medical coverage while the patient's body clears itself of drugs. This process is accompanied by uncomfortable and even fatal side effects caused by withdrawal. Detox is also available as a medically monitored program with 24-hour professional supervision based on the severity of symptomatology and the presence of comorbid conditions.

Rehabilitation

Residential rehabilitation programs are available as medically managed and medically monitored inpatient programs. The medically managed programs usually employ 24-hour medical staff and provide intensive and specialized care for those individuals with either medical or psychiatric comorbid conditions. They offer professionally directed evaluation and treatment in short-term settings for those with acute distress and moderate impairment and long-term settings for those with chronic distress or severe impairment. Short-term rehabilitation offers rehabilitation (learning lost skills), while long-term rehabs offer habilitation (learning new skills).

Halfway Houses

Halfway houses offer residential treatment in a substance-free communal or family environment that provides opportunities for independent growth. Individuals continue the work started in other treatment programs, usually in a long- or short-term residential rehabilitation center. The focus is on extending the period of sobriety; getting case management assistance in addressing educational, economic, and social needs; and integrating new life skills into a solid modeled recovery program. Most residents live in these halfway houses but work outside.

Other Housing

Opportunities for community reintegration are also available in supportive housing units that are not part of treatment. Three-quarter-way houses, therapeutic communities, and housing programs offer drug-free living environments, peer support, and classes to assist or remediate the skills needed for daily living. Residents usually attend some type of outpatient substance use treatment to continue in their recovery program.

Partial Hospitalization Program

Partial hospitalization programs are an intensive form of outpatient programming for those individuals who do not need a 24-hour residential treatment, but who benefit from a structured treatment setting. Partial programs tend to run 5 days a week for about 6 hours a day with planned programming. This combination of psychotherapy and educational groups does not require the individual to have previous treatment experience. Participants may live in some type of supportive housing program or at an independent home. Medication management is available, but it is not usually medically monitored or managed in this setting.

Intensive Outpatient Programs

An alternative to a partial hospitalization program is an IOP program. This is a nonresidential program, highly structured with scheduled treatment groups and at least one individual session regularly. Medication management is usually available, but it will not be monitored. Participants attend at least 3 days a week for about 3 hours/day.

Outpatient Treatment

The least-intensive form of substance use treatment is outpatient. Treatment may be a mix of individual sessions and educational or psychotherapy groups as determined by the individual's needs and the treatment goals. It is structured, drug-free, and nonresidential. Programming consists of not more than 5 contact hours a week. Web-based interventions are also available for self-paced, anonymous collective participation in treatment efforts.

Alcoholics Anonymous

AA was founded in 1930 and is the oldest and best known of the 12-step programs. Anyone with the desire to quit drinking or using substances is welcome to attend meetings. Individuals learn how to be sober through the support of other members and the 12 steps. In most suburban and urban areas, meetings can be found every day and around the clock. Meetings are even available online and are structured for confidentiality and anonymity. Family members and other support are often welcome.

The 12-step model has been adopted worldwide. An internet search should reveal a 12-step program for any substance use problem and even specific populations, such as women, men, and certain groups. The size of meetings ranges from small (around 15) to large (more than 50). There are also meetings to address the special needs of family and significant others, such as Al-Anon for friends and family members and Alateen for teenage relatives.

Relapse Prevention

To maintain long-term sobriety, each individual must prepare for and anticipate the possibility of relapse. This includes identifying potential triggers to substance use, learning skills to regain abstinence in the event of use, and adopting healthy coping, identity, and stress management skills to address triggers before they threaten sobriety. Advances in technology have expanded options for maintaining long-term sobriety. Applications for smartphones, for example, offer a way to monitor behavioral patterns for relapse clues.

KEY POINTS TO REMEMBER

- Substance-related and addictive disorders are complex brain diseases characterized by craving, seeking, and using regardless of consequences.
- Most substance use disorders are characterized by addiction, intoxication, tolerance, and withdrawal.
- The cause of substance use is a combination of biological and environmental factors.
- Assessment of patients with substance use problems needs to be comprehensive and aimed at identifying common medical and psychiatric comorbidities.
- Individuals with a co-occurring diagnosis have more severe symptoms, experience more crises, and require longer treatment for successful outcomes.
- Substance use affects the family system of the patient and may lead to codependent behavior in family members.

- Relapse is an expected complication of substance use, and treatment includes a significant focus on teaching relapse prevention.
- Successful treatments include an integrated approach, self-help groups, psychotherapy, therapeutic communities, and pharmacotherapy.
- Nurses need to be aware of their own feelings about substance use so that they can provide empathy and hope to patients.
- Nurses are at higher risk for substance use disorders and should be vigilant for signs of impairment in colleagues to ensure patient safety and referral to treatment for the chemically dependent nurse.
- A variety of settings are helpful in meeting the needs of individuals who are trying to maintain recovery from alcohol.

CRITICAL THINKING

1. Write a paragraph describing your possible reactions to your patient who misuses substances.
   a. Would your response be different depending on the substance (e.g., alcohol versus heroin or marijuana versus cocaine)? Give reasons for your answers.
   b. Would your response be different if the person were a professional colleague? How?
2. Rosetta Seymour is a 15-year-old who has started using heroin nasally.
   a. Briefly discuss the trend in heroin use among teenagers.
   b. When Ms. Seymour asks you why she needs to take more and more to get "high," how would you explain to her the concept of tolerance?
   c. If she had just taken heroin, what would you find on assessment of physical and behavioral-psychological signs and symptoms?
   d. If she came into the emergency department with an overdose of heroin, what would be the emergency care? What might be effective long-term care?

3. Tony Mandala is a 45-year-old mechanic. He has a 20-year history of heavy drinking, and he says he wants to quit but needs help.
   a. Role-play an initial assessment with a classmate. Identify the kinds of information you would need to have to plan holistic care.
   b. Mr. Mandala tried stopping by himself but is in the emergency department in alcohol withdrawal. What are the dangers for Mr. Mandala? What are the likely medical interventions?
   c. What are some possible treatment alternatives for Mr. Mandala when he is safely detoxified? How would you explain to him the usefulness and function of AA? What are some additional treatment options that might be useful to Mr. Mandala? What community referrals for Mr. Mandala are available in your area?

CHAPTER REVIEW

1. Natalya, a patient with a history of alcohol use disorder, has been prescribed disulfiram (Antabuse). Which physical effects support the suspicion that the patient has relapsed? *Select all that apply.*
   a. Intense nausea
   b. Diaphoresis
   c. Acute paranoia
   d. Confusion
   e. Dyspnea

2. Which assessment data confirm the suspicion that a patient is experiencing opioid withdrawal? *Select all that apply.*
   a. Pupils are dilated
   b. Pulse rate is 62 beats/min
   c. Slow movements
   d. Extreme anxiety
   e. Sleepy

3. The nursing diagnosis *denial* is especially useful when working with substance use disorders and gambling. Which statements describe this diagnosis? *Select all that apply.*
   a. Reports inability to cope
   b. Does not perceive the danger of substance use or gambling
   c. Minimizes symptoms
   d. Refuses healthcare attention
   e. Unable to admit the impact of disease on life pattern

4. What action should you take when a female staff member is demonstrating behaviors associated with a substance use disorder?
   a. Accompany the staff member when she is giving patient care.
   b. Offer to attend rehabilitation counseling with her.
   c. Refer her to a peer assistance program.
   d. Confront her about your concerns and/or report your concerns to a supervisor immediately.

5. A patient diagnosed with opioid use disorder has expressed a desire to enter into a rehabilitation program. What initial nursing intervention during the early days after admission will help ensure the patient's success?
   a. Restrict visitors to family members only.
   b. Manage the patient's withdrawal symptoms well.
   c. Provide the patient a low-stimulus environment.
   d. Advocate for at least 3 months of treatment.

6. Lester and Alene have always enjoyed gambling. Lately, Alene has discovered that their savings account is down by $50,000. Alene insists that Lester undergo therapy for his gambling behavior. The nurse recognizes that Lester is making progress when he states:
   a. "I understand that I am a bad person for depleting our savings."
   b. "Gambling activates the reward pathways in my brain."
   c. "Gambling is the only thing that makes me feel alive."
   d. "We have always enjoyed gaming. I do not know why Alene is so upset."

7. Opioid use disorder is characterized by:
   a. Lack of withdrawal symptoms
   b. Intoxication symptoms of pupillary dilation, agitation, and insomnia
   c. Tolerance
   d. Requiring smaller amounts of the drug to achieve a high over time

8. Terry is a young male in a chemical dependency program. Recently, he has become increasingly distracted and disengaged. The nurse concludes that Terry is:
   a. Bored
   b. Depressed
   c. Bipolar
   d. Not ready to change

9. Max is a 30-year-old male who arrives at the emergency department stating, "I feel like I am having a stroke." During the intake assessment, the nurse discovers that Max has been working for 36 hours straight without eating and has consumed 8 double espresso drinks and 12 caffeinated sodas. The nurse suspects:
   a. Fluid overload
   b. Dehydration and caffeine overdose
   c. Benzodiazepine overdose
   d. Sleep deprivation syndrome

10. Donald, a 49-year-old male, is admitted for inpatient alcohol detoxification. The rationale for admission into this program is due to:
    a. Heavy use of a substance known to cause withdrawal
    b. A need for rehabilitation
    c. The potential for relapse
    d. CNS hypoactivity following cessation of alcohol consumption

1. **a, b, d, e;** 2. **a, d;** 3. **b, c, d, e;** 4. **d;** 5. **b;** 6. **b;** 7. **c;** 8. **d;** 9. **b;** 10. **a**

NGN CASE STUDY AND QUESTIONS

Kathy is a 61-year-old who is being admitted to a detoxification unit for long-term heavy alcohol use. Although she is technically a voluntary admission, the court gave her the choice of either inpatient detoxification or jail for driving while intoxicated. She is agitated and reports having "pins and needles" sensations and weakness in her lower extremities. She bounces her foot and knee constantly. The nurse has to repeat most questions. At one point she says, "You know, I would like to be free of this. I have a grandson now. I wish I could do it for him." She starts to cry. "I've tried to quit drinking before. I wish I could, but it can't. I'm useless to everyone! All the women in my mom's family are drunks." Kathy reports muscle weakness. She has had multiple treatments for major depressive disorder.

The nursing assessment is cut short as Kathy's agitation increases. She vomits during the interview and becomes confused. As she is helped to a bed, she calls out loudly, holding onto the nurse and begging "...please put me on Prozac. Please! They've given me that before for my depression, and honey, I am so depressed right now!"

She protests when her cough medicine is taken away, grabbing for it and crying, "I have allergies. I need my cough medicine. Please! I was in jail late last night and in court all morning and haven't had a drink in maybe 8 hours. I'm coming down off of something big!" She becomes incoherent with garbled speech. Bedside vitals show elevated pulse, systolic and diastolic blood pressure, and body temperature. She pushes the nurse away from her.

1. Choose the *most likely* options to complete the following statement.

   Based on the patient's current condition, the priority need will be to address the assessment findings indicating ____1____. Afterward, interventions should address ____2____ and ___3____.

Options for 1	Options for 2	Options for 3
a. Allergies	**a.** Family dysfunction	**a.** Allergies
b. Risk for suicide	**b.** Risk for suicide	**b.** Intravenous drug use
c. Alcohol withdrawal	**c.** Admission status	**c.** Alcohol withdrawal

Options for 1	Options for 2	Options for 3
d. Prozac withdrawal	**d.** Prozac withdrawal	**d.** Low blood pressure
e. Muscle weakness	**e.** Potential infant abuse	**e.** Muscle weakness

2. Once the patient's withdrawal is stabilized, which intervention will the nurse provide? *Select all that apply.*

   a. Reintroduce healthy food and hydration
   b. Discourage exploration of harmful thoughts
   c. Remind that relapses demonstrate lack of character
   d. Teach that cough medication is to be avoided
   e. Promote sleep and rest
   f. Teach about addiction being a brain disorder

NGN case study answers are on Evolve.

Visit the Evolve website for a posttest on the content in this chapter: http://evolve.elsevier.com/Varcarolis

REFERENCES

American Psychiatric Association. (2013). *Diagnostic and statistical manual of mental disorders* (5th ed.). Washington, DC: Author.

American Society of Addiction Medicine. (2019). *Definition of addiction.* Retrieved from https://www.asam.org/Quality-Science/definition-of-addiction.

Babor, T.F., Higgins-Biddle, J.C., Saunders, J.B., & Monteiro, M.G. (2001). *Alcohol Use Disorders Identification Test: Guidlines for use in primary care.* Retrieved from https://apps.who.int/iris/handle/10665/67205a.pdf.

Brodwin, E., & Gould, S. (2018, July 11). Doctors are calling out a new drug that helps people with addiction for costing more than $1,700 a week while a generic costs just $1. *Business Insider.* Retrieved from https://www.businessinsider.com/drug-for-opioid-withdrawal-costs-thousands-more-than-generic-2018-7.

Burke, J., & Gould, S. (2020, January 1). Legal marijuana just went on sale in Illinois. Here are all the states where cannabis is legal. *Business Insider.* Retrieved from https://www.businessinsider.com/legal-marijuana-states-201.

Centers for Disease Control and Prevention. (2019). Deaths: Leading causes for 2017. *National Vital Statistics Report. 68*(6). Retrieved from https://www.cdc.gov/nchs/data/nvsr/nvsr68/nvsr68_06-508.pdf.

Cservenka, A. (2016). Neurobiological phenotypes associated with a family history of alcoholism. *Drug and Alcohol Dependence, 158,* 8–21.

Ebert, D. H., Finn, C. T., & Smoller, J. W. (2016). Genetics and psychiatry. In T. A. Stern, M. Fava, T. E. Wilens, & J. F. Rosenbaum (Eds.), *Massachusetts General Hospital comprehensive clinical psychiatry* (2nd ed.) (pp. 677–701). St. Louis, MO: Elsevier.

Murray, A., & Traylor, J. (2019). Caffeine toxicity. *StatPearls.* Retrieved from https://www.ncbi.nlm.nih.gov/books/NBK532910/.

National Cancer Institute. (2018). *Alcohol and cancer risk.* Retrieved from http://www.cancer.gov/about-cancer/causes-prevention/risk/alcohol/alcohol-fact-sheet.

National Institute on Alcohol Abuse and Alcoholism. (n.d.). *A pocket guide for alcohol screening and brief intervention.* Retrieved from https://pubs.niaaa.nih.gov/publications/practitioner/pocketguide/pocket_guide2.htm.

National Institute on Drug Abuse. (2015). *Strategic plan 2016–2020.* Retrieved from http://www.drugabuse.gov/about-nida/strategic-plan.

National Institute on Drug Abuse. (2018). *Drugs, brains, and behavior: The science of addiction.* Retrieved from http://www.drugabuse.gov/publications/drugs-brains-behavior-science-addiction/introduction.

Nisavic, M., & Nejad, S. H. (2018). Patients with substance use disorders. In T. A. Stern, O. Freudenreich, F. A. Smith, G. L. Fricchione, & Jerrold F. Rosenbaum (Eds.), *Handbook of general hospital psychiatry* (7th ed.) (pp. 149–159). St. Louis, MO: Elsevier.

Sadock, B. J., Sadock, V. A., & Ruiz, P. (2015). *Kaplan & Sadock's synopsis of psychiatry* (11th ed.). Philadelphia, PA: Wolters Kluwer.

Stuyt, E. (2018). The problem with the current high potency THC marijuana from the perspective of an addiction psychiatrist. *Missouri Medicine, 115*(6), 482–486.

Substance Abuse and Mental Health Services Administration. (2015). *Prevention of substance abuse and mental illness: Continuum of care.* Retrieved from http://www.samhsa.gov/prevention.

Substance Abuse and Mental Health Services Administration. (2017). *Screening, Brief Intervention, and Referral to Treatment (SBIRT).* Retrieved from https://www.samhsa.gov/sbirt.

Substance Abuse and Mental Health Services Administration. (2018). *The SAMHSA strategic plan FY2019-FY2023.* Retrieved from https://www.samhsa.gov/about-us/strategic-plan.

Substance Abuse and Mental Health Services Administration. (2019). *Key substance use and mental health indicators in the United States: Results from the 2018 national survey on drug use and health.* Retrieved from https://www.samhsa.gov/data/.

Tan, S., Lee, M., Lim, G., Leong, J., & Lee, C. (2015). Motivational interviewing approach used by a community mental health team. *Journal of Psychosocial Nursing and Mental Health Services, 53*(12), 28–37.

US Food and Drug Administration. (2018). *FDA approves first drug comprised of an active ingredient derived from marijuana to treat rare, severe forms of epilepsy*. Retrieved from https://www.fda.gov/news-events/press-announcements/fda-approves-first-drug-comprised-active-ingredient-derived-marijuana-treat-rare-severe-forms.

Vaeth, P. A., & Wang-Schweig, M. , & Caetano, R. (2017). Drinking, alcohol use disorder, and treatment access and utilization among U.S. racial/ethnic groups. *Alcoholism, Clinical and Experimental Research, 41*(1), 6–19.

World Health Organization. (2019). *International Classification of Disease* (11th revision). Retrieved from. https://icd.who.int/browse11/l-m/en.

Neurocognitive Disorders

Jane Stein-Parbury

 Visit the Evolve website for a pretest on the content in this chapter: http://evolve.elsevier.com/Varcarolis

OBJECTIVES

1. Compare and contrast the clinical picture of delirium with that of dementia.
2. Discuss three critical needs of a person with delirium, stated in terms of nursing diagnosis.
3. Identify three outcomes for patients with delirium.
4. Summarize the essential nursing interventions for a patient with delirium.
5. Recognize the clinical picture of mild and major neurocognitive disorders.
6. Describe the clinical picture and progression of Alzheimer's disease.
7. Give an example of the following symptoms assessed during the progression of major neurocognitive disorders: (a) apraxia, (b) agnosia, and (c) aphasia.
8. Formulate three nursing diagnoses suitable for a patient with a major neurocognitive disorder and define two outcomes for each.
9. Formulate a teaching plan for a caregiver of a patient with major neurocognitive disorder, including interventions for (a) communication, (b) health maintenance, and (c) safe environment.
10. Compose a list of appropriate referrals in the community—including a support group, hotline for information, and respite services—for individuals with dementia and their caregivers.
11. Discuss pharmacological treatments for Alzheimer's disease.

KEY TERMS AND CONCEPTS

agnosia
agraphia
aphasia
apraxia
confabulation
delirium

dementia
executive function
hallucinations
hyperorality
hypervigilance
illusions

major neurocognitive disorder
mild neurocognitive disorder
perseveration
social cognition
sundowning

The clarity and purpose of an individual's personal journey through life depends on the ability to reflect on its meaning through cognitive processes. Disturbances in cognitive processing cloud or destroy the meaning of the journey. Cognition, the act of thinking through the knowledge and understanding that is acquired, represents a fundamental human feature that distinguishes living from existing. This mental capacity has a distinctive personalized impact on the individual's physical, psychological, social, and spiritual conduct of life. For example, the ability to remember the connections between related actions and how to initiate them depends on cognitive functioning.

Cognitive processes function on two hierarchical domains. Lower-level cognitive domains include the attention and orientation to the environment as well as the recognition of previously acquired information. Higher-level cognitive domains are more complex and include the following:

- Sustained attention and information processing.
- Planning, decision making, problem solving, and abstract thinking (executive function).
- Learning and memory, including retention, recall, and immediate and long-term memory.
- Using language, both expressive and receptive.
- Perceiving and navigating the environment through motor and visual senses (e.g., using a fork/spoon).
- Processing, storing, and applying information about other people and social situations (social cognition).

Neurocognitive disorders are manifested by alterations in cognitive functioning due to underlying physiological changes caused by brain pathology. These disorders are classified as delirium, mild neurocognitive disorders, and major neuro-cognitive disorders. Delirium affects lower-level functioning and is acute and reversible. In mild and major neurocognitive disorders, there is a decline in higher-level cognitive functioning. Mild neurocognitive disorders may or may not progress to being major. Major neurocognitive disorders, referred to as dementia, are progressive and irreversible (American Psychiatric Association [APA], 2013).

DELIRIUM

Clinical Picture

Delirium is an acute cognitive disturbance and often reversible condition that is common in hospitalized patients, especially older patients. It is characterized as a syndrome—that is, a constellation of symptoms rather than a disorder. The cardinal symptoms of delirium are an inability to direct, focus, sustain, and shift attention; an abrupt onset with clinical features that fluctuate with periods of lucidity; and disorganized thinking. Other characteristics include disorientation (often to time and place, but rarely to person), anxiety, agitation, poor memory, and delusional thinking. When hallucinations are present, they are usually visual. The *DSM-5* box identifies criteria for delirium.

DSM-5 CRITERIA FOR DELIRIUM

A. A disturbance in attention (i.e., reduced ability to direct, focus, sustain, and shift attention) and awareness (reduced orientation to the environment).

B. The disturbance develops over a short period of time (usually hours to a few days), represents a change from baseline attention and awareness, and tends to fluctuate in severity during the course of a day.

C. An additional disturbance in cognition (e.g., memory deficit, disorientation, language, visuospatial ability, or perception).

D. The disturbances in criteria A and C are not better explained by another preexisting, established, or evolving neurocognitive disorder and do not occur in the context of a severely reduced level of arousal such as coma.

E. There is evidence from the history, physical examination, or laboratory findings that the disturbance is a direct physiological consequence of another medical condition, substance intoxication or withdrawal (i.e., due to a drug of abuse or to a medication), or exposure to a toxin, or is due to multiple etiologies.

Specify whether there is:

Substance intoxication delirium. This diagnosis should be made instead of substance intoxication when the symptoms in criteria A and C predominate in the clinical picture and when they are sufficiently severe to warrant clinical attention.

From the American Psychiatric Association. (2013). *Diagnostic and statistical manual of mental disorders* (5th ed.). Washington, DC: Author.

Delirium is a medical emergency that requires immediate attention to prevent irreversible and serious damage (Dixon, 2018). Delirium is associated with increased morbidity and mortality and can have lasting long-term consequences, such as permanent cognitive decline (Inouye, 2018). In hospitalized patients, delirium is associated with longer hospital stays and increased complications (Moon & Park, 2018).

EVIDENCE-BASED PRACTICE

Do Nurses Detect Delirium?

Problem

Over half of older hospitalized patients experience delirium. This problem is not only costly but delirium is also associated with morbidity and mortality. Timely detection is essential to offset these negative outcomes, yet nurses often fail to recognize delirium.

Purpose of Study

The aims of the following study were to explore nurses' current practices in the assessment and identification of delirium and to inform educational programs.

Methods

Twenty-four registered nurses from a range of hospital units participated in semistructured group interviews that explored how they assessed delirium clinically. Qualitative methods were used in the analysis of interview data.

Key Findings

Three main themes emerged from the analysis:
- "It's not my job"

Participants reported that cognitive assessments were not part of their role, as these were formally conducted by allied health and medical staff or aged-care nurses. They considered that they could undertake delirium assessments if they had further training and education.
- "It's my job"

Conducting and reporting general observations were considered as part of their role. These included descriptions of the patients as "confused"; participants did not want to use the term *delirium* because they feared inappropriately stigmatizing and/or labeling patients.
- "It's complex"

There was a lack of understanding of the difference between delirium and dementia. Although participants recognized the role that family members could play in identifying delirium, they were concerned about confidentiality. Finally, they considered delirium to be emotionally distressing for patients and felt ill prepared to provide support.

Implications for Nursing Practice

Although they are in a prime position to notice delirium, nurses are not sufficiently skilled in its assessment. Any time a patient experiences an acute onset of confusion, delirium should be considered. Nurses must be aware of the nature of delirium, especially how it differs from dementia. Standardized assessment scales can improve the ability to detect delirium.

Coyle, M. A., Burns, P., & Traynor, V. (2017). Is it my job? The role of RNs in the assessment and identification of delirium in hospitalized older adults: An exploratory qualitative study. *Journal of Gerontological Nursing, 43*(4), 29–37.

Epidemiology

Delirium, often referred to as acute confusion, is an impairment of the lower-level cognitive domains of orientation, attention, and recognition. Most nurses will encounter delirium because it is a common complication of hospitalization. Ten percent to 30% of all general hospital patients develop delirium. In older frail patients, the prevalence of delirium can be as high as 60% (Moon & Park, 2018). In critically ill patients, the prevalence varies from 20% to 84% (Herling et al., 2018). The high degree of variability in the reported incidence of delirium is most likely due to its underrecognition by healthcare professionals.

Risk Factors

Delirium is always due to underlying physiological causes; these are usually multifactorial and involve a dynamic interplay of factors. There are underlying causes that place a patient at risk for developing delirium, and there are immediate factors that precipitate the syndrome. The interaction of the two results in delirium. The key known risk factors are cognitive impairment, immobilization, psychoactive medications, dehydration, infection, sleep deprivation, and vision or hearing impairment (Inouye, 2018). The risk factors listed in Box 23.1 are modifiable through nursing care.

The key to helping patients avoid the consequences of delirium is recognizing and investigating potential causes as soon as possible. Early recognition and diagnosis are challenging for clinicians owing to lack of knowledge about cognitive impairment and its clinical assessment and failure to interpret the signs and symptoms. The best evidence for the prevention and management of delirium in hospitalized patients is following clinical protocols for minimizing modifiable risk factors. Early detection of delirium may be improved by consultation with geriatric specialists.

APPLICATION OF THE NURSING PROCESS

ASSESSMENT

The nurse who suspects delirium should perform mental and neurological status examinations as well as a physical examination. If possible, additional information should be obtained from a person who knows the patient, such as a family member or friend. The patient's medication regimen should be reviewed carefully for drug interactions or toxicity profiles. Results of laboratory data, such as blood work and urinalysis, should be reviewed. If no recent laboratory information exists, the nurse can be instrumental in recommending an order for them.

Overall Assessment

The possibility of delirium should be considered when a patient abruptly demonstrates a reduced clarity of awareness of the environment as manifested by an impaired ability to direct, focus, sustain, or shift attention. You may have to repeat questions because the patient's attention wanders, goes off track, and needs to be refocused. Conversation is more difficult because irrelevant stimuli may easily distract the patient. An observation that the patient is no longer interacting meaningfully,

BOX 23.1 Risk Factors for Delirium

- Pain
- Infection
- Dehydration
- Hypoxia
- Immobilization
- Poor or inadequate nutrition
- Environment noise, lack of orienting material, movement to new area
- Sleep deprivation
- Sensory problems, especially hearing and vision
- Restraint use

staring straight through you, and not recalling who you are signals delirium.

A patient may have difficulty with orientation—first to time, then to place, and last to person. For example, a man with delirium may think that the year is 1972, that the hospital is home, and that the nurse is his wife. Orientation to person is usually intact. Disorientation and confusion are usually markedly worse at night and during the early morning. In fact, some patients may be confused or delirious only at night and may be lucid during the day.

Because nurses have the most frequent contact with hospitalized patients, they are in a prime position to be the first to detect the possibility of delirium. However, the fluctuating nature of delirium complicates assessments because the patient has periods of lucidity as well as confusion.

Cognitive and Perceptual Disturbances

It may be difficult to engage patients experiencing delirium in conversation because they are distracted, unable to focus, and exhibit memory impairment. In mild delirium, memory deficits are noticeable only on careful questioning. In more severe delirium, memory problems usually take the form of obvious difficulty in processing and remembering recent events. For example, the person might ask when a son is coming to visit even though the son left only an hour earlier.

Perceptual disturbances are also common. Perception is the processing of information about one's internal and external environment. Various misinterpretations of reality may take the form of illusions or hallucinations.

Illusions are errors in the perception of sensory stimuli. A confused person may mistake folds in the blanket for white rats or the cord of a window blind for a snake. The stimulus is a real object in the environment. However, the person misinterprets it, and it often becomes an object of fear. Unlike delusions or hallucinations, you can explain and clarify illusions for the individual.

Hallucinations are false sensory stimuli (refer to Chapter 12). Visual hallucinations are common in delirium, although tactile hallucinations may also be present. For example, persons experiencing delirium may become terrified when they see giant spiders crawling over the bedclothes or feel bugs crawling on or under their bodies. Auditory hallucinations are uncommon and occur more often in other psychiatric disorders, such as schizophrenia.

The person experiencing delirium can be aware that something is very wrong. Statements like "My thoughts are all jumbled" may signal cognitive problems. When perceptual disturbances are present, the emotional response is often one of fear and anxiety. When this happens, the person may show signs of psychomotor agitation.

Physical Needs

A patient with delirium becomes disoriented and may try to go home. Alternatively, a patient may think that the care facility *is* home. Wandering, pulling out intravenous lines and indwelling catheters, and falling out of bed are common dangers that require nursing interventions.

A person experiencing delirium has difficulty processing stimuli in the environment, and confusion magnifies the inability to recognize reality. Make the physical environment as simple and clear as possible. Objects such as clocks and calendars can maximize orientation to time. Eyeglasses, hearing aids, and adequate lighting without glare can maximize the person's ability to interpret more accurately what is going on in the environment. Interpersonally interacting with the patient when the patient is awake can help to reduce anxiety and misperceptions.

Self-care deficits, injury, or hyper-/hypoactivity may lead to skin breakdown and possible infection. Often this is compounded by poor nutrition, immobilization, and possible incontinence. These areas require nursing assessment and intervention.

Autonomic signs—such as tachycardia, sweating, flushed face, dilated pupils, and elevated blood pressure—are often present in delirium. Monitor and document these changes carefully, as they may require immediate medical attention.

You may also notice changes in the patient's sleep-wake cycle. In some cases, a complete reversal of the day and night sleep-wake cycle can occur. The patient's level of consciousness may range from lethargy to stupor or from semicoma to hypervigilance. In hypervigilance, patients are extraordinarily alert, and their eyes constantly scan the room. They may have difficulty falling asleep or may be actively disoriented and agitated throughout the night.

You should always suspect medications as a potential cause of delirium. This is especially true when there is polypharmacy and/or use of psychoactive agents. To recognize drug reactions or anticipate potential interactions before delirium actually occurs, it is important to assess all medications, prescriptions, *and* over-the-counter agents that the person is taking. Consultation with a pharmacist is recommended, especially when there is polypharmacy.

Moods and Behaviors

The individual's moods and physical behaviors may change dramatically within a short period. A person with delirium may display motor restlessness (agitation) or may be "quietly delirious" and appear calm and settled. When there is agitation, delirium is considered hyperactive; when there is no agitation, delirium is considered hypoactive. Moods may swing back and forth between fear, anger, anxiety, euphoria, depression, and apathy. A person may strike out from fear or anger or may cry, call for help, curse, moan, and tear off clothing one minute and become apathetic or laugh uncontrollably the next. In short, the patient's behavior and emotions are often erratic and fluctuating. The following vignette illustrates the fear and confusion a patient may experience during and after an episode of delirium.

> **VIGNETTE:** Peter Wright, age 43, survived numerous life-threatening complications after open-heart surgery to replace his mitral valve. He spent 3 weeks in an intensive care unit (ICU) and was then moved to a general medical unit.
>
> Peter became suspicious about his bed being moved. "Why are you taking me to another country?" He expressed concern that his organs would be removed and donated for transplantation. He began to yell for his wife. Peter "knew" that the very people who had saved his life were now out to get him.
>
> When he was sure nobody was looking, he climbed out of bed and attempted to leave the unit. The nurses responded by calling security personnel to escort him back to bed. Once he was safely in bed, the nurses applied mechanical restraints and sedated him.
>
> Peter's confusion disappeared the next day. Although he realized how distorted his thinking had been during the episode, the anxiety and fear he experienced remained with him for months after discharge from the hospital.

Self-Assessment

Because the behaviors exhibited by the patient with delirium can be directly attributed to temporary medical conditions, intense personal reactions in staff are less likely to arise. In fact, intense conflicting emotions are less likely to arise in nurses working with a patient with delirium than in nurses working with a patient with dementia. Nonetheless, it can be anxiety provoking to interact with these patients, especially given the unpredictability of their condition.

📄 ASSESSMENT GUIDELINES

Delirium

1. Do not assume that acute confusion in an older person is due to dementia.
2. Assess for acute onset and fluctuating levels of awareness.
3. Assess the person's ability to attend to the immediate environment, including responses to nursing care.
4. Establish the person's usual level of cognition by interviewing family or other caregivers.
5. Assess for past cognitive impairment—especially an existing dementia diagnosis—and other risk factors.
6. Identify disturbances in physiological status, especially infection, hypoxia, and pain.
7. Identify any physiological abnormalities documented in the patient's record.
8. Assess vital signs, level of consciousness, and neurological signs.
9. Assess potential for injury, especially in relation to potential for falls and wandering.
10. Maintain comfort measures, especially in relation to pain, cold, or positioning.
11. Monitor situational factors that worsen or improve symptoms.
12. Assess for availability of immediate medical interventions to help prevent irreversible brain damage.

NURSING DIAGNOSIS

Safety needs are a priority in nursing care. Patients with delirium often perceive the environment in a distorted way, and objects are often misperceived. For example, if feeling threatened or thinking that common medical equipment is harmful, the patient may pull off an oxygen mask, pull out an intravenous or nasogastric tube, or try to flee. In such a case, the person demonstrates a *risk for injury* as evidenced by sensory deficits or perceptual deficits (International Council of Nurses, 2019a).

Altered perception, *hallucinations*, and *disorientation*, and/or *restlessness* are major aspects of the clinical picture. *Fear* is one of the most common of all nursing diagnoses and may be related to illusions, delusions, or hallucinations as evidenced by verbal and nonverbal expressions of fearfulness. In addition, *agitation* may also be present. When some of these symptoms are present, *acute confusion* related to delirium is an appropriate nursing diagnosis.

If *fever* and *dehydration* (which are also nursing diagnoses) are present, you will address *risk for fluid imbalance* and *electrolyte imbalance*. If the underlying cause of the patient's delirium results in fever, decreased skin turgor, decreased urinary output or fluid intake, and dry skin or mucous membranes, then the nursing diagnosis of *impaired fluid intake* is appropriate. Fluid volume deficit may be related to fever, electrolyte imbalance, reduced intake, or infection.

Because disruption in the sleep-wake cycle may be present, the patient may be less responsive during the day and may become disruptively wakeful during the night. *Impaired sleep* related to impaired cerebral oxygenation or disruption in consciousness is a likely nursing diagnosis.

Engaging in communication with a delirious patient is difficult. An example of a nursing diagnosis addressing this problem is *impaired verbal communication* related to cerebral hypoxia or decreased cerebral blood flow as evidenced by confusion or clouding of consciousness.

OUTCOMES IDENTIFICATION

The overall outcome for the patient experiencing delirium is a return to a premorbid level of functioning. Appropriate outcomes include the following:

- Patient will remain safe and free from injury and falls.
- During periods of clarity, patient will be oriented to time, place, and person with the aid of nursing interventions such as the provision of clocks, calendars, maps, and other types of orienting information.
- Fluid balance and adequate nutrition will be maintained.
- Patient will feel comforted by a quiet, calm nursing presence.

PLANNING

Planning nursing care for a patient who is experiencing delirium involves special attention to the safety and security of the environment. You should address the following questions:

- Does the person have the necessary visual and auditory aids?
- Are there family members available to stay with the patient?
- Does the environment provide visual cues as to time of day and season of the year?
- Has the person experienced continuity of care providers?

IMPLEMENTATION

The priorities of treatment are to keep the patient safe while attempting to identify the cause. If the underlying disorder is corrected, complete recovery is possible. If, however, the underlying disorder is not corrected and persists, irreversible neuronal damage can occur. Nursing concerns therefore center on the following:

- Preventing physical harm due to confusion, aggression, or electrolyte and fluid imbalance
- Minimizing use of restraints because they increase confusion
- Assisting with identification and treatment of the underlying cause
- Using supportive measures to relieve distress

The *Nursing Interventions Statements* (International Council of Nurses, 2019b) can be used as a guide to develop

---

BOX 23.2 Interventions for the Management of Delirium

- *Assessing delirium and assessing orientation:* Initiate therapies to reduce or eliminate factors causing delirium.
  - Monitor neurological status on an ongoing basis. However, avoid frustrating the patient by quizzing with orientation questions that cannot be answered.
- Administer prn (as needed) medications for anxiety or agitation with caution.
- *Monitoring food and fluid intake:* Assist with needs related to nutrition, elimination, hydration, and personal hygiene.
- *Assessing safety and implementing safety regime:*
  - Physical restraints may increase symptoms and should be avoided if at all possible.
  - Family members can assist in maintaining safety to avoid restraint use.
  - Maintain a well-lit, hazard-free environment.
  - Encourage use of aids that increase sensory input (e.g., eyeglasses, hearing aids, and dentures).
- *Implementing comfort care* and *managing anxiety:*
  - Acknowledge patient's fears and feelings.
  - Provide optimistic but realistic reassurance.
  - Provide patient with information about what is happening and what can be expected.
  - Limit need for decision making, if frustrating or confusing to patient.
  - Accept patient's perceptions or interpretation of reality and respond to the theme or feeling tone.
  - Inform patient of person, place, and time, as needed.
  - Approach patient slowly and from the front and address patient by name.
  - Always introduce self to patient when approaching.
  - Communicate with simple, direct, and descriptive statements.
  - Encourage significant others to remain with patient.
  - Provide a consistent physical environment, daily routine, and caregivers.
  - Use environmental cues (e.g., signs, pictures, clocks, calendars, and color coding of environment) to stimulate memory, reorient, and promote appropriate behavior.
  - Provide a low-stimulation environment for patient in whom disorientation is increased by overstimulation.

From International Council of Nurses. (2019). *Nursing intervention statements: International Classification for Nursing Practice.* Geneva, Switzerland: Author.

---

interventions for a patient with delirium (Box 23.2). Medical management of delirium involves treating the underlying organic causes. If the underlying cause of delirium is not treated, permanent brain damage may ensue. Judicious use of antipsychotic or antianxiety agents may also be useful in controlling behavioral symptoms.

Never leave a patient in acute delirium alone. Because most hospitals and health facilities are unable to provide one-to-one supervision, you may have to encourage family members to stay with the patient.

EVALUATION

Outcome criteria for a person experiencing delirium include the following:

- Patient will remain safe.
- Patient will be oriented to time, place, and person by discharge.
- Underlying cause will be treated and ameliorated.

MILD AND MAJOR NEUROCOGNITIVE DISORDERS

Dementia is a broad term used to describe deterioration of cognitive functioning and global impairment of cognitive functioning. It is a term that does not refer to specific disease but rather to a collection of symptoms. The *DSM-5* (APA, 2013) incorporates forms of dementia into the diagnostic categories of mild and major neurocognitive disorders. These disorders are a result of actual brain pathology and are characterized by cognitive impairments that signal a decline from a person's previous functioning. When mild, the impairments do not interfere with activities of daily living, although the person may have to make extra efforts. Although a mild cognitive disorder is often considered to mark the beginning stages of dementia, this does not necessarily mean that it will progress to a major neurocognitive disorder (Alzheimer's Association, 2019). When progressive, these disorders become major neurocognitive disorders because they interfere with daily functioning and independence. Neurocognitive disorders are often characterized by memory deficits, but they also affect other higher levels of cognitive functioning such as problem solving (executive functioning) and complex attention. The *DSM-5* boxes describe the criteria for minor and major neurocognitive disorders.

TABLE 23.1	Common Types of Dementia
Type of Dementia	**Characteristics**
Alzheimer's disease ([AD] 60%–80% of dementias)	Early: Difficulty remembering recent conversations, names or events, apathy, and depression. Middle: Impaired communication, disorientation, confusion, poor judgment, and behavioral changes. Late: Difficulty speaking, swallowing, and walking.
Cerebrovascular disease (5%–10% of dementias)	One or more documented cerebrovascular events. Impaired judgment, poor decision making, planning and organizing, slow gait and poor balance.
Frontotemporal lobar degeneration (<10% of dementias)	Onset is usually between 45 and 60 years old (early onset). Marked changes in personality, disinhibition, difficulty with communication.
Lewy body disease (5%–10% of dementias)	Same as Alzheimer's disease but includes sleep disturbance, visual hallucinations, movement and visuospatial impairment.
Parkinson's disease (progression)	Problems with movement: slowness, rigidity, tremor, changes in gait.
Mixed pathologies	More than one cause, and more common than previously thought.

DSM-5 CRITERIA FOR MILD NEUROCOGNITIVE DISORDER

A. Evidence of modest cognitive decline from the previous level of performance in one or more cognitive domains (complex attention, executive function, learning and memory, language, perceptual-motor skills, or social cognition) based on concerns expressed by the person or a knowledgeable informant or clinician, and impairment in cognitive performance that is documented by standardized testing or quantifiable clinical assessment.

B. The cognitive deficits do not interfere with independence in everyday activities (i.e., at a minimum, requiring assistance with complex instrumental activities of daily living such as paying bills or managing medications), but these may require greater effort and compensatory strategies.

C. The cognitive deficits do not occur exclusively in the context of delirium.

D. The cognitive deficits are not better explained by another mental disorder (e.g., major depressive disorder, schizophrenia).

DSM-5 CRITERIA FOR MAJOR NEUROCOGNITIVE DISORDER

A. Evidence of significant cognitive decline from previous level of performance in one or more cognitive domains (complex attention, executive function, learning and memory, language, perceptual-motor skills, or social cognition) based on concerns expressed by the person, or a knowledgeable informant or clinician, and impairment in cognitive performance that is documented by standardized testing or quantifiable clinical assessment.

B. The cognitive deficits are sufficient to interfere with independence in everyday activities (i.e., at a minimum, requiring assistance with complex instrumental activities of daily living such as paying bills or managing medications).

C. The cognitive deficits do not occur exclusively in the context of delirium.

D. The cognitive deficits are not better explained by another mental disorder (e.g., major depressive disorder, schizophrenia).

From the American Psychiatric Association. (2013). *Diagnostic and statistical manual of mental disorders* (5th ed.). Washington, DC: Author.

The criteria for mild and major neurocognitive disorders are general descriptions of dementia without reference to an etiology. Specific etiologies of major disorders are listed in Table 23.1. Although the underlying etiology varies in neurocognitive disorders, nursing care is based on their behavioral manifestations. Therefore, approaches to care are not necessarily different for various etiologies. It is for this reason that the remainder of this chapter focuses on Alzheimer's disease (AD), the most frequently occurring major neurocognitive disorder.

ALZHEIMER'S DISEASE

Clinical Picture

AD, the most common cause of dementia, is a devastating disease that not only affects the person experiencing it but also places an enormous burden on the families and caregivers of those affected. As the population ages, it is likely that nurses practicing in any healthcare setting will encounter persons with AD; they must therefore be prepared to respond therapeutically.

TABLE 23.2 Memory Deficit: Normal Aging Versus Dementia

Typical Age-Related Changes	Signs of Alzheimer's Disease
Sometimes forgetting names or appointments, but remembering them later	Memory loss that disrupts daily life
Making occasional errors when balancing a checkbook	Challenges in planning or solving problems
Occasionally needing help to use the settings on a microwave or to record a television show	Difficulty completing familiar tasks
Forgetting the day of the week but figuring it out later	Confusion with time or place
Vision changes related to cataracts	Trouble understanding visual images or spatial relationships
Sometimes having difficulty finding the correct word	New problems with words in speaking or writing
Misplacing things from time to time and retracing steps to find them	Misplacing things and losing the ability to retrace steps
Making a bad decision once in a while	Decreased or poor judgment
Sometimes feeling weary of work, family, and social obligations	Withdrawal from social and work activities
Developing specific ways of doing things and becoming irritable when routine is disrupted	Changes in mood and personality

From Alzheimer's Association. (2019). *10 Early signs and symptoms of Alzheimer's disease*. Retrieved from https://www.alz.org/alzheimers-dementia/10_signs.

TABLE 23.3 Stages of Alzheimer's Disease

Stage	Hallmarks
Mild Alzheimer's disease ([AD] early stage)	The person and their loved ones notice memory lapses. The person may still be able to function independently but will experience: • Difficulties retrieving correct words or names • Trouble remembering names when introduced to new people • Challenges in performing tasks in social or work settings • Forgetting material that one has just read • Losing or misplacing a valuable object • Increasing trouble with planning or organizing
Moderate AD (middle stage)	The person confuses words, gets frustrated or angry, or acts in unexpected ways such as refusing to bathe. Symptoms become noticeable to others and such persons may • Forget events or their personal history • Become moody or withdrawn, especially in socially or mentally challenging situations • Be unable to recall their own address or telephone number or the high school/college from which they graduated • Become confused about where they are or what day it is • Need for help choosing proper clothing for the season or the occasion • Change sleep patterns, such as sleeping during the day and becoming restless at night • Be at risk of wandering and becoming lost • Become suspiciousness and delusional or compulsive, for example, repetitive behavior like hand wringing
Severe AD (late stage)	Patients lose the ability to respond to their environment, to carry on a conversation, and, eventually, to control movement. They may still say words or phrases, but communicating pain becomes difficult. Personality changes may take place and individuals need extensive help with daily activities. They may: • Require full-time, around-the-clock assistance with daily activities and personal care • Lose awareness of recent experiences and of their surroundings • Experience changes in physical abilities, including the ability to walk, sit, and eventually swallow • Have increasing difficulty communicating • Become vulnerable to infections, especially pneumonia

Adapted from Alzheimer's Association. (2019). *Stages of Alzheimer's*. Retrieved from https://www.alz.org/alzheimers-dementia/stages.

It is important to distinguish between normal forgetfulness and the memory deficit of AD and other dementias. Severe memory loss is *not* a normal part of growing older. Slight forgetfulness is a common phenomenon of the aging process (age-associated memory loss), but not memory loss that interferes with one's ability to function. Table 23.2 contrasts the memory changes that occur in typical aging and those seen in dementia.

Although dementia often begins with a worsening of the ability to remember new information, it is marked by progressive deterioration in other cognitive functions as well, such as problem solving and learning, along with a decline in the ability to perform activities of daily living. A person's declining intellect often leads to emotional changes such as anxiety, mood lability, and depression as well as neurological changes that produce hallucinations and delusions.

Progression of Alzheimer's Disease

AD is classified according to the stage of the degenerative process. Table 23.3 outlines the three stages—mild, moderate, and severe—which can be used as a guide to understanding the progressive deterioration seen in those diagnosed with AD. The first stage roughly corresponds to the *DSM-5* criteria for mild neurocognitive disorders, although this may not progress to outright dementia. Stages two and three relate to the *DSM-5* criteria for major neurocognitive disorder, which is considered to be dementia.

The loss of intellectual ability is insidious. The person with mild AD loses energy, drive, and initiative and has difficulty learning new things. Because personality and social behavior remain intact, others tend to minimize and underestimate the loss of the individual's abilities. The individual may continue to work, but the extent of the dementia becomes evident in new or demanding situations. Depression may occur early in the disease but usually resolves over time.

More severe symptoms appear as AD progresses. The person experiences **agnosia**, which is the inability to identify familiar objects or people, even a spouse. Apraxia is a common symptom, where a person so affected needs repeated instructions and directions to perform the simplest tasks: "Here is the face cloth. Pick up the soap. Now, put water on the face cloth, and rub the face cloth with soap."

Often, the person cannot remember the location of the toilet or is unaware of the process of urinating and defecating, resulting in incontinence. It is usually at this point that total care is necessary. For the family, this burden can be emotionally, financially, and physically devastating. For the person, the world becomes frightening and nothing makes sense. In response, agitation, paranoia, and delusions are common.

VIGNETTE: Mrs. White, 78 years old and a retired teacher, has always enjoyed an active life and good health other than an underactive thyroid, which has been successfully controlled. Remarkably, her only hospitalizations were for the births of her two children, now grown and married. She is a vibrant person who takes pride in her appearance and her beautiful home. She is beginning to forget things that she previously took for granted but jokes about her failing memory as "senior moments."

Her daughter recently found Mrs. White quite distressed as she attempted to make lasagna, her famous specialty. The ingredients were strewn all over the kitchen, and Mrs. White was frantically searching for a recipe. Her daughter was surprised, because neither of them had ever used a written recipe. Her daughter managed to help Mrs. White with step-by-step instructions in the construction of the lasagna. Her daughter was worried about her mother's failing memory, fearing that it was more than usual aging. She tried to broach the subject with her dad, a loving and loyal companion to Mrs. White. His reply was simply, "I don't know what you're talking about."

The situation reached a crisis point when her daughter discovered that Mrs. White was no longer taking her thyroid medication. Since Mrs. White had taken medication for her thyroid for 30 years and could not remember now, this signaled a progression in her condition.

It was painful, but her husband, too, began to realize that Mrs. White was not functioning properly. Her once clean house was in a state of disarray. She could no longer coordinate her clothing and usually wore the same outfit for a number of days. Often, her clothes were dirty and her makeup was applied in a disorganized manner.

Mrs. White would stare at both the newspaper and the television set, attempting to understand but unable to retain any information. She was often restless during the day, going from one random activity to another, often rearranging her favorite knickknacks in her curio cupboard. She would attempt to wash clothes but forget to put laundry detergent in the machine. She would empty half-filled drinking glasses onto the top of the gas range. If these mistakes were pointed out to her, she would become angry, stating, "I have always done it this way."

Eating became difficult as she did not seem to recognize food on her plate, and she was unable to use a knife and fork to cut her food. Sometimes, she would pick up a spoon and ask what it was. She began to lose weight.

Although Mrs. White had slept well throughout her adult life, she now began to wander at night, often waking her husband to ask questions. She would go to the kitchen and empty the cupboards. She would enter her wardrobe and rearrange her clothing, often leaving articles of clothing lying on the floor.

When she set kitchen paper towels on fire on the gas range, her husband and family realized that she could no longer function safely at home. Her husband was unable to leave her alone, even for short periods of time, as she would become extremely distressed, almost to the point of panic. She and her husband moved into an assisted living facility.

Epidemiology

AD attacks indiscriminately. It strikes men and women, people of various ethnicities, rich and poor, and individuals with varying degrees of intelligence. Although the disease can occur at a younger age (early onset), most of those with the disease are 65 years of age or older (late onset). It is estimated that 5.7 million Americans have AD (James & Bennett, 2019). The percentage of people who have dementia due to AD increases with age. One in ten people over the age of 65 has dementia due to AD. Two-thirds of people with dementia are women, since women tend to live longer.

Of the people with AD:
- 3% are between 65 and 75 years old
- 17% are between 75 and 84 years old
- 32% are 85 years old or older (Alzheimer's Association, 2019)

Risk Factors

Like most chronic illnesses, dementia results from multiple factors rather than a single cause. Of these factors, increasing age is the greatest risk factor. Many people who live to a very old age never experience significant memory loss or any other symptom of dementia. There are people in their 80s and 90s who lead active lives with their cognition intact. The slow, mild cognitive changes associated with aging do not necessarily impede daily functioning.

Biological Factors

Genetic. Some genetic mutations guarantee that a person will develop AD, although these account for less than 1% of all cases. These mutations lead to the devastating early-onset form of AD, which occurs before the age of 65 years and as young as age 30.

There is also a susceptibility gene; the e4 form of apolipoprotein E (*APOE*) has been identified for late-onset AD. This gene produces a protein that transports cholesterol in the bloodstream, which supports lipid transport and injury repair in the brain. Although this gene is associated with increased risk, results of research have been inconsistent. People with a family history of dementia are more likely to develop the disease, but their shared lifestyle also plays a role in addition to genetics (James & Bennett, 2019).

Cardiovascular disease. The health of the brain is closely linked to overall heart health, and there is evidence that people with cardiovascular disease are at greater risk of AD. Likewise, lifestyle factors associated with cardiovascular disease—such as inactivity, high levels of "bad" cholesterol, diabetes, and obesity—are risk factors for AD (Alzheimer's Association, 2019).

Head injury and traumatic brain injury. Brain injury and trauma are associated with a greater risk of developing AD and other dementias. People who suffer repeated head trauma, such as boxers and football players, may be at greater risk (James & Bennett, 2019).

Modifiable Risk Factors

Education and engaging in mentally stimulating activities are thought to increase cognitive reserve, or the ability to make use of neural networks, therefore reducing the risk of dementia. Other modifiable factors that reduce risk include physical exercise, social engagement, healthy diet, and sufficient sleep. Although promising, more research is needed in this area (Alzheimer's Association, 2019).

APPLICATION OF THE NURSING PROCESS

ASSESSMENT

Overall Assessment

AD is commonly characterized by the progressive deterioration of cognitive functioning. Initial deterioration may be so subtle and insidious that others may not notice it. In the early stages of the disease, the affected person may be able to compensate for and hide cognitive deficits. Family members may unconsciously deny that anything is wrong as a defense against the painful awareness that a loved one is deteriorating. As time goes on, symptoms become more obvious, and other protective mechanisms become evident.

Confabulation is the creation of stories or answers in place of actual memories to maintain self-esteem. For example, here the nurse addresses a patient who has remained in a hospital bed all weekend:

Nurse: Good morning, Ms. Jones. How was your weekend?

Patient: Wonderful. On Sunday I went to lunch with my family.

Confabulation is not lying. When people are lying, they are aware of making up an answer. Confabulation is an unconscious mechanism employed to protect the ego.

Perseveration is the persistent repetition of a word, phrase, or gesture that continues after the original stimulus has stopped. For example, a person may continue to repeat "hello" long after the initial greeting is over.

Agraphia occurs early in AD. It is the diminished ability and eventual inability to read or write.

Aphasia is the loss of language ability. Initially, the person has difficulty finding the correct word, then is reduced to a few words, and finally is reduced to babbling or mutism.

Apraxia is the loss of purposeful movement in the absence of motor or sensory impairment. This results in the inability to perform familiar and purposeful tasks. For example, in apraxia of dressing, the person is unable to put clothes on properly (e.g., putting arms in trousers).

Agnosia is the loss of sensory ability to recognize objects. For example, a person may lose the ability to recognize familiar sounds (auditory agnosia), such as a ringing telephone. This loss may extend to an inability to recognize a familiar object (visual or tactile agnosia), such as a magazine, pencil, or toothbrush.

Hyperorality refers to the tendency to put everything in the mouth and to taste and chew. **Sundowning**, or sundown syndrome, is the tendency for an individual's mood to deteriorate and agitation increase in the later part of the day, with the fading of light, or at night.

Other symptoms observed in AD include the following:

- Memory impairment. Initially, the person has difficulty remembering recent events. Gradually, deterioration progresses to include both recent and remote memory.
- Disturbances in executive functioning such as problem solving, planning, organizing, and abstract thinking.
- Diminution of emotional expression. At the most extreme end, there seems to be a complete absence of emotion. This is manifested in a flat affect and unresponsiveness.

Diagnostic Tests

A wide range of problems may be mistaken for AD. Major depressive disorder in older adults is frequently confused with the disease. Cognitive symptoms such as difficulty thinking clearly, problems concentrating, and difficulty making decisions that accompany depression are known as pseudodementia. On the other hand, many people with AD also meet the diagnostic criteria for a depressive disorder. In addition, dementia and depression or dementia and delirium *can* coexist. It is important that nurses be able to assess some of the important differences between depression, dementia, and delirium. Table 23.4 outlines important differences among these three phenomena.

Brain imaging—with computed tomography, positron emission tomography, and other developing scanning technologies—has diagnostic capabilities because these techniques can reveal brain atrophy and rule out other conditions such as neoplasms. The use of mental status questionnaires, such as the Mini-Mental State Examination and various other tests to identify deterioration in mental status and brain damage, is an important part of the assessment.

In addition to performing a complete physical and neurological examination, it is important to obtain a complete medical and psychiatric history, description of recent symptoms, review of medications used, and a nutritional evaluation. The observations and history provided by family members are invaluable to the assessment process.

Self-Assessment

Working with cognitively impaired people in any setting should make us aware of the enormous responsibility placed on caregivers. The behavioral problems these patients may display can cause tremendous stress for professionals and family caregivers alike. Caring for people unable to communicate and who have lost the ability to relate and respond to others is extremely difficult. Because stress is common when one is working with cognitively impaired individuals, it can be helpful to be proactive in minimizing the effects of stress by

- Understanding the nature of the disease so that expectations for the person can be realistic.
- Establishing attainable outcomes for the person and recognizing when they are achieved. These outcomes may be as minor as "patient feeds self with spoon."

🌐 CONSIDERING CULTURE

There are cultural differences in how dementia is conceptualized. Brooke and colleagues (2018) explored how a culturally diverse workforce approaches the care of the person with dementia. They found that in some cultures

- Dementia is regarded as a normal part of aging.
- Some languages do not even have a word for dementia.
- Families hide the fact that a family member has dementia because they feel shame.
- Filial piety, or the obligation to care for older family members, is a barrier to accessing services.

Person-centered dementia care requires an understanding of the cultural background of the person with dementia and caregivers. The cultural beliefs of care workers can hinder such care. Nurses are in a prime position to bring cultural understanding to the care of persons with dementia.

Adapted from Brooke, J., Cronin, C., Stiell, M., & Ojo, O. (2018). The intersection of culture in the provision of dementia care: A systematic review. *Journal of Clinical Nursing, 27*(17–18), 3241–3253.

TABLE 23.4	Comparison of Delirium, Dementia, and Depression		
	Delirium	**Dementia**	**Depression**
Onset	Sudden (over hours to days) and fluctuating during the course of the day	Slowly, over months and years	May have been gradual with exacerbation during crisis or stress
Cause or contributing factors	Underlying medical condition such as a urinary tract infection, substance intoxication, or effects of medications	Alzheimer's disease, vascular disease, human immunodeficiency virus infection, neurological disease, chronic alcoholism, head trauma	Lifelong history, losses, loneliness, crises, declining health, medical conditions
Cognition	Impaired attention span, memory deficit, disorientation, disturbances in perception, not related to other cognitive disorders or reduced level of arousal	Impaired memory, judgment, calculations, attention span, abstract thinking and agnosia	Difficulty concentrating, forgetfulness, inattention
Activity level	Can be increased or reduced; restlessness, behaviors may worsen in evening (sundowning); sleep-wake cycle may be reversed	Not altered; behaviors may worsen in evening (sundowning)	Usually decreased; lethargy, fatigue, lack of motivation; may sleep poorly and awaken in early morning
Emotional state	Rapid swings; can be fearful, anxious, suspicious, aggressive, have hallucinations and/or delusions	Flat; agitation	Extreme sadness, apathy, irritability, anxiety, paranoid ideation
Speech and language	Rapid, inappropriate, incoherent, rambling	Incoherent, slow (sometimes due to effort to find the right word), inappropriate, rambling, repetitious	Slow, flat, low
Prognosis	Reversible with proper and timely treatment	Not reversible; progressive	Reversible with proper and timely treatment

ASSESSMENT GUIDELINES

Alzheimer's Disease

1. Evaluate the person's current level of cognitive and daily functioning.
2. Identify any threats to the person's safety and security and arrange for their reduction.
3. Evaluate the safety of the person's home environment if possible (e.g., with regard to wandering, eating inedible objects, falling, engaging in provocative behaviors toward others).
4. Review the medications (including herbs, complementary agents) that the patient is taking.
5. Interview the family to gain a complete picture of the person's background and personality.
6. Explore how well the family is prepared for and informed about the progress of the person's dementia, depending on cause (if known).
7. Discuss with the family members how they are coping with the patient.
8. Review the resources available to the family. Determine if caregivers are aware of community support groups and resources.
9. Identify the needs of the family for teaching and guidance, such as understanding sundowning.

NURSING DIAGNOSIS

One of the most important areas of concern is the patient's safety. Many people with AD wander and can put themselves in danger. Injuries from falls and accidents can occur during any stage as confusion and disorientation progress. The potential for burns exists if the person is a smoker or is unattended while using the stove. The individual can take prescription drugs incorrectly or mistakenly drink from bottles of caustic fluids. *Risk for injury* is always a priority diagnosis in this population.

As the person's ability to recognize or name objects declines, *impaired verbal communication* becomes a problem. As memory diminishes and disorientation increases, *impaired cognition* and *confusion* occur.

Perhaps some of the most crucial aspects of the patient's care are support, education, and referrals for the family. Family members lose the love, function, support, companionship, and warmth that this person once provided. *Risk for caregiver stress* is always present, and planning with the family and offering community support is an integral part of appropriate care. It is also good to assess *family grief*, which may be an important target for intervention. Helping the family grieve can make the task ahead somewhat clearer and at times less painful. Review Table 23.5 for examples of the types of everyday problems faced by people with dementia, as these provide potential nursing diagnoses for such patients.

OUTCOMES IDENTIFICATION

Families who have a member with dementia face an exhaustive list of issues that must be addressed. Self-care needs, impaired environmental interpretation, chronic confusion, ineffective individual coping, and caregiver role strain are just a few of the areas that nurses and other healthcare members will have to target. Table 23.6 identifies signs and symptoms, nursing diagnoses, and associated outcomes for delirium and dementia.

PLANNING

Planning care for a person with dementia focuses on the person's immediate needs. Identifying the level of functioning and assessing caregivers' needs help focus planning.

IMPLEMENTATION

The attitude of unconditional positive regard is the nurse's single most effective tool in caring for people with dementia. It induces

TABLE 23.5 Problems That May Affect People With Dementia and Their Families

Problem	Examples	Problem	Examples
Memory impairment	Forgets appointments, visits, etc. Forgets to change clothes, wash, go to the toilet Forgets to eat, take medications Loses things	Repetitiveness	Repetition of questions or stories Repetition of actions
Disorientation	Time: Mixes night and day, mixes days of appointments, wears summer clothes in winter, forgets age Place: Loses way around house Person: Has difficulty recognizing visitors, family, spouse	Uncontrolled emotion	Distress Agitation Anger or aggression Demands for attention
		Uncontrolled behavior	Restlessness day or night Vulgar table or toilet habits Undressing Sexual disinhibition
Need for physical help	Dressing Washing, bathing Toileting Eating Performing housework Maintaining mobility	Incontinence	Urine Feces Urination or defecation in the wrong place
		Emotional reactions	Depression Anxiety Frustration and anger Embarrassment and withdrawal
Risks in the home	Falls Fire from cigarettes, cooking, heating Flooding Admission of strangers to home Wandering out	Other reactions	Suspiciousness Hoarding and hiding
		Mistaken beliefs	Still in paid work Parents or spouse still alive Hallucinations
Risks outside the home	Competence, judgment, and risks at work Driving, road sense Getting lost	Decision making	Indecisive Easily influenced Refuses help Makes unwise decisions
Apathy	Little conversation Lack of interest Poor self-care	Burden on family	Disruption of social life Distress, guilt, rejection Family discord
Poor communication	Dysphasia		

TABLE 23.6 Symptoms, Diagnoses, and Outcomes for Delirium and Dementia

Symptoms	Nursing Diagnoses	Outcomes
Wanders, has unsteady gait, acts out fear from hallucinations or illusions, forgets things (leaves stove on, doors open), falls	Risk for injury	No injury: Remains safe in hospital or at home
Awake and disoriented during the night (sundowning), frightened at night	Impaired sleep	Adequate sleep: Sleep pattern is regular, balances rest and activity
Unable to take care of basic needs, incontinence, imbalanced nutrition, insufficient fluid intake	Self-care deficit (bathing/hygiene, dressing, feeding, toileting)	Self-care needs are met with optimal participation by the patient
Sees frightening things that are not there (hallucinations), mistakes everyday objects for something frightening (illusions), may become paranoid and think that others are doing bad things (delusions)	Anxiety (severe/panic)	Reduced anxiety: Anxiety at a mild-moderate level, acknowledges the reality of an object or sound after it is pointed out
Does not recognize familiar people or places, has difficulty with short- and/or long-term memory, forgetful, confused	Acute/chronic confusion	Decreased confusion: Reports feeling safe, responds well to orientation interventions
Difficulty with communication, cannot find words, has difficulty in recognizing objects and/or people, incoherent	Impaired verbal communication	Able to communicate: Shares needs, connects with other patients, visitors, and staff at an optimal level with a variety of verbal and nonverbal methods
Devastated over losing place in life (during lucid moments), fearful and overwhelmed by what is happening	Hopelessness	Increased hope: Expresses feelings, demonstrates a decreased preoccupation with loss
Family and loved ones overburdened and overwhelmed, unable to care for patient's needs	Caregiver stress	Reduced caregiver stress: Caregivers express feelings in a supportive environment, have access to counseling and support groups, participate in care, utilize respite care

International Council of Nursing Practice. (2019). ICNP browser. Retrieved from https://www.icn.ch/what-we-do/projects/ehealth/icnp-browser. ICNP® is owned and copyrighted by the International Council of Nurses (ICN). Reproduced with permission of the copyright holder.

patients to cooperate with their care, reduces catastrophic out-breaks, and increases family members' satisfaction with care. Box 23.3 lists interventions related to the care of persons with dementia.

Person-Centered Care Approach

The conventional construction of dementia, based on a biolog-ical model and focusing on deficits, has been that the person is eventually lost to the disease. When they are viewed in this way, people with dementia can be isolated into a social death by being treated as if they were already dead.

These views are challenged by a model of care that focuses on the preservation of the personhood of people with demen-tia. **Patient-centered care** is based on an ethical position that personhood in dementia remains and should be honored. The patient-centered approach is focused on forming meaningful relationships with the person who has dementia and also the caregivers. Developing meaningful relationships maintains the unique identity of the person and promotes well-being. To achieve a person-centered approach to care, relationships must take priority over tasks. This can be challenging in many task-focused healthcare systems.

There is evidence that a person-centered approach to care can increase the quality of life for people with dementia living in residential care settings (Chenoweth et al., 2019). By approach-ing people with dementia in a manner that attempts to enter their world and provide care based on their unique life stories, they become calmer and more relaxed. The conclusion is that distressing behavior such as agitation is not simply a result of dementia but also of how they are being treated in their social-psychological world.

Health Teaching and Health Promotion

Educating families who have a cognitively impaired member is one of the most important health teaching duties that nurses encounter. Families who are caring for a member in the home must know about strategies for communicating and for struc-turing self-care activities (Table 23.7).

Referral to Community Supports

The Alzheimer's Association is a national agency that provides various forms of assistance to individuals with the disease and their families. The Alzheimer's Association has a Community Resource Finder that is useful in locating local resources. Additional resources that might be available in some commu-nities are in Table 23.8.

Some families manage the care of their loved one until death. Other families eventually find that they can no longer deal with the affected person's labile and aggressive behavior, incontinence, wandering, unsafe habits, or disruptive night-time activity. Family members must know where and how to place their loved one for care if this becomes necessary. Families need information, support, and legal and financial guidance at this time. When the nurse is unable to provide the relevant information, proper referrals by the social worker are needed. When you are counseling families, include informa-tion regarding advance directives, durable power of attorney, guardianship, and conservatorship in your communications. Useful guidelines for families in structuring a safe environ-ment and planning appropriate activities at home are listed in Table 23.9.

EVALUATION

Outcome criteria for people with cognitive impairments must be measurable, within the capabilities of the individual person, and evaluated frequently. As the person's condition continues to deteriorate, outcomes should reflect the person's diminished functioning. Frequent evaluation and reformulation of outcome criteria and short-term indicators can also help to reduce staff and family frustration and minimize the patient's anxiety by ensuring that tasks are not more complicated than the person can accomplish.

BOX 23.3   Interventions for Dementia Management

- *Supporting caregiver:* Include family members in planning, providing, and evaluating care, to the extent desired.
- *Assessing safety and implementing safety regime:* Identify and remove potential dangers in environment.
- *Assessing risk for falls*
- *Assessing tendency to wander*
- *Assessing discomfort*
- *Assessing pain*
- *Assessing cognition:* Determine and monitor cognitive deficit(s), using stan-dardized assessment tool.
- *Assessing self-care:* Identify usual patterns of behavior for such activities as sleep, medication use, elimination, food intake, and self-care.
- *Providing emotional support:* Ascertain what is important to these patients, their values and beliefs, as well as their life histories.
- *Assessing fatigue and facilitating rest:* Provide rest periods to prevent fatigue and reduce stress.
- *Monitoring food and fluid intake:* Monitor nutrition and weight. Provide fin-ger foods to maintain nutrition for patient who will not sit and eat.
- *Implementing comfort care and managing anxiety:*
  - Introduce self and address patient by name when initiating interaction and speak slowly.
  - Give one simple direction at a time in a respectful tone of voice.
  - Avoid frustrating patient by quizzing with orientation questions that can-not be answered.
  - Use distraction, rather than confrontation, to manage behavior.
  - Provide consistent caregivers, physical environment, and daily routine.
  - Provide a low-stimulation environment with adequate lighting.
  - Provide cues—such as current events, seasons, location, and names—to assist orientation.
  - Select television or radio programs based on cognitive processing abili-ties and interests.
  - Limit number of choices patient has to make so as not to cause anxiety.
  - Place patient's name in large block letters in room and on clothing, as needed.
  - Use symbols, rather than written signs, to assist patient in locating room, bathroom, or other area.

From International Council of Nurses. (2019). *Nursing intervention statements: International Classification for Nursing Practice.* Geneva, Switzerland: Author.

TABLE 23.7 Patient and Family Teaching: Guidelines for Self-Care in Dementia

Intervention	Rationale
Dressing and Bathing	
Have the person perform all tasks within his or her present capacity.	Maintains the person's self-esteem and uses muscle groups; impedes staff burnout; minimizes further regression.
Have the person wear own clothes, even if in the hospital.	Helps maintain the person's identity and dignity.
Use clothing with elastic and substitute fastening tape (Velcro) for buttons and zippers.	Minimizes the person's confusion and eases independence of functioning.
Label clothing items with the person's name and name of item.	Helps identify the person who may wander away and gives the person additional clues when aphasia or agnosia occurs.
Give step-by-step instructions whenever necessary (e.g., "Take this blouse. Put in one arm…now the other arm. Pull it together in front. Now….")	The person can focus on small pieces of information more easily; allows the person to perform at optimal level.
Make sure that water tank settings are low enough to prevent scalding.	Impaired judgment results in safety hazards.
If reluctant to perform self-care, ask again later.	Moods may be labile, and the person may forget but often complies after short interval.
Nutrition	
Monitor food and fluid intake.	Lack of appetite and confusion can impair intake.
Offer finger food that the person can take away from the dinner table.	Increases input throughout the day; the person may eat only small amounts at meals.
Weigh the person regularly (once a week)	Monitors fluid and nutritional status.
During periods of hyperorality, watch that the person does not eat nonfood items (e.g., ceramic fruit or food-shaped soaps).	The person puts everything into mouth; may be unable to differentiate inedible objects made in the shape and color of food.
Bowel and Bladder Function	
Begin bowel and bladder program early, beginning with bladder control.	Establishing same time of day for bowel movements and toileting—in early morning, after meals and snacks, and before bedtime—can help prevent incontinence.
Evaluate need for disposable diapers.	Prevents embarrassment and soiling.
Label doors to rooms, especially bathroom.	Environmental clues can maximize independent toileting.
Sleep	
Maintain a calm atmosphere during the day.	Reduces anxiety and promotes a calming night's sleep.
Expose the patient to morning light/sunlight.	Morning light/sunlight helps to reset circadian rhythms.
Avoid dosing cholinesterase inhibitors at bedtime.	Increased neural acetylcholine is associated with cortical arousal.
Nonmedication options to promote sleep should be tried before medication.	Medication may be dangerous in older adults (e.g., falling, hepatic and renal inefficiency).
Discontinue medication once sleep schedule is established.	Discontinuation reduces the likelihood of injury.
Avoid antipsychotic use.	Antipsychotic use in older adults is associated with strokes and death.
Avoid the use of restraints.	Can cause the person to become more terrified and fight against restraints until exhausted to a dangerous degree.

The overall outcomes for treatment are to promote the person's optimal level of functioning and delay further regression whenever possible. Working closely with family members and providing them with the names of available resources and support sources may help to increase the quality of life for both the family and the patient with AD (see the "Case Study and Nursing Care Plan").

TREATMENT MODALITIES

Biological Treatments

Pharmacotherapy

Medications for cognitive symptoms. Five medications have the US Food and Drug Administration's approval for the treatment of AD. Although these medications are used widely and have shown statistically significant effects in slowing the progression of the disease as compared with placebos, they produce only a clinically marginal improvement in cognition and functioning. The benefits of these medications wane after 1 to 2 years, so patients should weigh the potential side effects against the potential benefits.

Cholinesterase inhibitors. Because a deficiency of neural acetylcholine has been linked to AD, some medications aim to prevent its breakdown. These drugs function by inhibiting cholinesterase from breaking down acetylcholine into its components of acetate and choline. This allows for an increase in the availability and duration of action of acetylcholine, which leads to temporary improvement of some symptoms of AD.

The cholinesterase inhibitors produce small but short-lived improvements in cognitive functioning. Although they can

TABLE 23.8 Types of Services That May Be Available to People With Dementia

Type of Service	Services Provided
Family/caregiver Some people may live by themselves in the community; active case management is vital	Caregivers have a right to: Easy access to services Respite care Full involvement in decision making Assessment of the needs of both the caregiver and the person with dementia Information and referral Case management: Coordination of community resources and follow-up
Community services	Adult day care: Provides activities, socialization, supervision Physician services Protective services: Prevent, eliminate, and/or remedy effects of abuse or neglect Recreational services Transportation Mental health services Legal services
Home care	Meals on Wheels Home health aide services Homemaker services Hospice services Occupational therapy Paid companion or sitter services Physical therapy Skilled nursing Personal care services: assistance in basic self-care activities Social work services Telephone reassurance: regular telephone calls to individuals who are isolated and homebound[a] Personal emergency response systems: telephone-based systems to alert others that a person who is alone is in need of emergency assistance[a]

[a]Vital for those living alone.

delay the advancement of symptoms, there is little evidence that cholinesterase inhibitors slow the progression of dementia. There is minimal benefit after 1 year, and the risk of side effects doubles in people over 85 years of age.

The cholinesterase inhibitors include donepezil (Aricept), rivastigmine (Exelon), and galantamine (Razadyne). The cholinesterase inhibitors are indicated for mild to moderate stages of AD with the exception of donepezil, which is used for all stages, including severe AD. The most common side effects are gastrointestinal; these are usually temporary, and a decreased dose minimizes them. Patients should take these medications with food to reduce gastrointestinal side effects. In addition to common digestive system effects, they can rarely cause bradycardia due to their cholinergic-enhancing properties. They should be used with caution when patients are taking nonsteroidal antiinflammatory drugs (NSAIDs) due to the combined potential for gastrointestinal bleeding and ulceration.

The rivastigmine transdermal system (Exelon Patch) has FDA approval for all stages of AD. It is applied once a day, making it useful for people who have trouble swallowing pills. With this nonoral delivery method, there is no food requirement. It can cause skin irritation and should be discontinued if the irritation extends beyond the size of the patch.

N-methyl-D-aspartate receptor antagonist. Memantine (Namenda) is an N-methyl-D-aspartate (NMDA) receptor antagonist with FDA approval for moderate to severe dementia in AD. This medication is typically introduced after the cholinesterase inhibitors have been tried. Memantine regulates the activity of the neurotransmitter glutamate, which is present in higher levels with AD. Too much glutamate sticks to receptors, allowing too much calcium to move into neurons, which causes damage. Memantine occupies the same receptors, blocking glutamate, thereby preventing excessive calcium movement into the brain cells.

Patients may be given memantine and a cholinesterase inhibitor simultaneously. Once it has been established that this combination is tolerated, extended-release memantine and donepezil hydrochlorides (Namzaric) may be used (see Table 23.10).

Medications for behavioral symptoms. Most people with dementia will experience behavioral symptoms that reduce their quality of life, that are distressing to them and their caregivers, and that may lead to placement in a residential care facility. Some of the troubling behaviors are psychotic symptoms (hallucinations, paranoia), severe mood swings (depression is common), wandering, anxiety, agitation, and verbal or physical aggression (combativeness). These behaviors are not only distressing but may also lead to injuries from falls, infections, and incontinence.

Psychotropic medications may be prescribed, but these medications are associated with risk of mortality, mostly from cardiovascular and infectious causes. As a result, in 2008, the FDA emphasized that the use of antipsychotics for dementia-related psychosis is an unapproved indication. Therefore, any use of antipsychotics in this population is considered off label. Drug classifications that are used off label include antidepressants, antipsychotics, antianxiety agents, and anticonvulsants. Of these, antipsychotics have been used most often. These medications must be used with extreme caution.

A rule of thumb for older adults is to start low and go slow. Another is to use the smallest dose for the shortest duration possible and discontinue if they are not effective. In addition, because people with dementia are at high risk of developing delirium, additional medications should be used with caution. Because these medications are often prescribed on an as needed basis, it is a nursing judgment to administer them. They should be used as a last resort, after every other effort to manage the behavior has been exhausted.

TABLE 23.9 Patient and Family Teaching: Guidelines for Care at Home

Intervention	Rationale
Safe Environment	
Gradually restrict use of motor vehicles.	As judgment becomes impaired, the person may be dangerous to self and others.
Remove throw rugs and other objects in person's path.	Minimizes tripping and falling.
Minimize sensory stimulation.	Decreases sensory overload, which can increase anxiety and confusion.
If the person becomes verbally upset, listen and be supportive, allowing the person to be upset. Gradually try to redirect and change the topic.	Goal is to prevent escalation of anger. When attention span is short, the person can be distracted to more productive topics and activities.
Label all rooms and drawers. Label often-used objects (e.g., hairbrushes and toothbrushes).	May keep the person from wandering into other people's rooms. Increases environmental clues to familiar objects.
Install safety bars in bathroom.	Prevents falls.
Supervise the person while smoking.	Danger of burns is always present.
Wandering	
If the person wanders during the night, put mattress on the floor.	Prevents falls when the person is confused.
Have the person wear medical alert bracelet that cannot be removed (with name, address, and telephone number). Provide police department with recent pictures.	The person can easily be identified by police, neighbors, or hospital personnel.
Alert local police and neighbors about wandering.	May reduce time necessary to return the person to home or hospital.
If the person is in the hospital, have the person wear brightly colored vest with name, unit, and phone number printed on back.	Makes the person easily identifiable.
Put complex locks on door.	Reduces opportunity to wander.
Place locks at top of door.	In moderate and late Alzheimer-type dementia, ability to look up and reach upward is lost.
Encourage physical activity during the day.	Physical activity may decrease wandering at night.
Explore the feasibility of installing sensor devices.	Provides warning if the person wanders.
Useful Activities	
Provide picture magazines and children's books when the person's reading ability diminishes.	Allows continuation of usual activities that the person can still enjoy; provides focus.
Provide simple activities that allow exercise of large muscles.	Exercise groups, dance groups, and walking provide socialization, as well as increased circulation and maintenance of muscle tone.
Encourage group activities that are familiar and simple to perform.	Activities such as group singing, dancing, reminiscing, and working with clay and paint all help increase socialization and minimize feelings of alienation.

TABLE 23.10 FDA-Approved Drugs for Alzheimer's Disease

Generic (Trade)	Action	Indications	Side Effects
Cholinesterase Inhibitors			
Donepezil (Aricept, Aricept ODT[a])	Inhibits acetylcholinesterase, thereby increasing available acetylcholine	Mild, moderate, and severe Alzheimer's disease (AD)	Nausea, diarrhea, insomnia, muscle cramps, fatigue, anorexia
Rivastigmine (Exelon)		Mild to moderate AD	Nausea, vomiting, anorexia, indigestion, weakness
Rivastigmine transdermal system (Exelon Patch)		Mild, moderate, and severe AD	Nausea, vomiting, diarrhea
Galantamine (Razadyne, Razadyne ER)		Mild to moderate AD	Nausea, vomiting, diarrhea, dizziness, headache, decreased appetite, weight loss
N-methyl-D-aspartate (NMDA) Receptor Antagonist			
Memantine (Namenda, Namenda XR)	Regulates glutamate activity by blocking NMDA receptors, thereby decreasing excitatory neurotoxicity	Moderate to severe AD	Dizziness, headache, confusion, constipation
NMDA Receptor Antagonist/Cholinesterase Inhibitor			
Memantine/donepezil (Namzaric)	See memantine and donepezil.	Moderate to severe AD after a trial of donepezil	See side effects listed under memantine and donepezil

[a]Orally disintegrating tablet.
US Food and Drug Administration. (2016). *Drugs*. Retrieved from http://www.fda.gov/Drugs/.

▶ Neurobiology of Alzheimer's and the Effects of Medication

Two essential neurotransmitters implicated in Alzheimer's disease are acetylcholine and glutamate.

Acetylcholine is involved with learning, memory, and mood. As Alzheimer's disease progresses the brain produces less and less acetylcholine. What little acetylcholine is left is rapidly destroyed by the enzyme acetylcholinesterase.

　Cholinesterase inhibitors keep the acetylcholinesterase enzyme from breaking down acetylcholine, thereby increasing both the level and duration of action of the neurotransmitter acetylcholine.

Glutamate is involved with cell signaling, learning, and memory. Glutamate binds to cells at the N-methyl-d-aspartate (NMDA) receptor and allows calcium to enter the cell. In Alzheimer's disease, excess glutamate and chronic overexposure to calcium leads to damaged cells.

　NMDA antagonists helps reduce excess calcium by blocking some NMDA receptors.

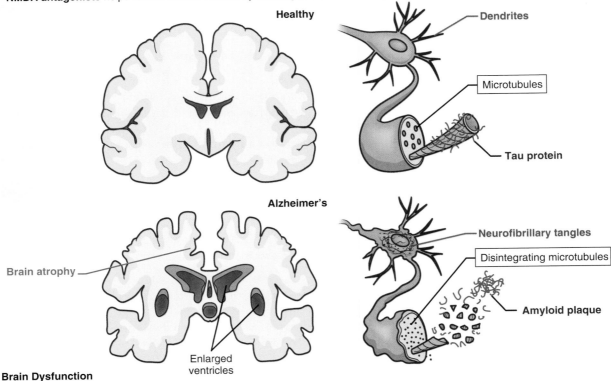

Brain Dysfunction

Amyloid plaques are sticky clumps found between nerve cells that may either cause or be the result of the disease. The clumps block communication at synapses that is normally protected by tau proteins and healthy microtubules. They may also activate immune system cells that trigger inflammation and devour disabled cells.

Neurofibrillary tangles are abnormal collections of protein threads inside nerve cells. They are comprised mainly of a protein called tau. Tangles disrupt the transport of food molecules, cell parts, and other key elements. This disruption results in cell death.

Brain atrophy is the cerebral cortex shriveling up, damaging areas involved in thinking, planning, and remembering. The hippocampus, an area of the cortex that is essential for memory, experiences severe shrinkage. Ventricles, the fluid-filled spaces within the brain, grow larger.

FDA-Approved Drugs for the Treatment of Alzheimer's Disease

Generic	Brand	Classification	Stage Approved For
Galantamine	Razadyne	Cholinesterase inhibitor	Mild to moderate
Donepezil	Aricept	Cholinesterase inhibitor	All stages
Rivastigmine Rivastigmine transdermal patch	Exelon Exelon patch	Cholinesterase inhibitor Cholinesterase inhibitor	Mild to moderate All stages
Memantine	Namenda	NMDA antagonist	Moderate to severe
Donepezil and memantine	Namzaric	Cholinesterase inhibitor and NMDA antagonist	Moderate to severe

Integrative Therapy

Nutrition may play a role in both the prevention and treatment of dementia. One such nutritional substance, omega-3 fatty acids, has been promoted as a means of modulating these diseases. Omega-3 fatty acids are essential for the body, but humans are unable to produce them. These acids must be obtained from food sources such as fatty fish, flaxseed, and canola oils.

Although some studies have drawn an association between omega-3 fatty acids and a lower incidence of dementia, the use of these substances in the treatment of dementia is controversial. In a systematic review of the literature, Canhada and colleagues (2018) concluded that omega-3 supplementation may be useful in improving mild cognitive disorders; however, there is insufficient evidence to support its use in more severe cases.

CASE STUDY AND NURSING CARE PLAN
Cognitive Impairment

For 4 years, Mr. Sloane has demonstrated progressive memory impairment, disorientation, and deterioration in functioning related to Alzheimer's disease. Now 67 years old, he retired at age 62 to spend some of his remaining "youth" with his wife and to do some of the things they had always wanted to do. At age 63, he was diagnosed with Alzheimer's disease.

Mr. Sloane is incontinent when he cannot find the bathroom. Despite close supervision, he wanders away from home. The police and neighbors bring him home an average of four times a week. He has fallen while getting out of bed at night, thinking that he is in a sleeping bag, camping out in the mountains. The family makes the painful decision to place him in a care facility for people with Alzheimer's disease.

Brian Jackson, a registered nurse, notices that Mr. Sloane becomes frustrated when he has difficulty finding the right words for things (aphasia). At one point Mr. Sloane asked, "Who is this woman?" pointing to his wife (agnosia).

Mrs. Sloane tells Brian that her husband can sometimes participate in dressing himself. At other times, he needs total assistance. At this point, Mrs. Sloane begins to sob, saying, "I can't bear to part with him ... but I can't do it anymore. I feel as if I've betrayed him."

Brian states, "This is a difficult decision for you." Brian suggests a support group, saying that "It might help you to feel that you are not alone." One of the groups he suggests is the Alzheimer's Association, a well-known self-help group.

Self-Assessment

Brian has worked on this unit for 4 years. He applied for this position shortly after his own father died of complications secondary to Alzheimer's disease. Brian refers to the process of living and dying with this disease as horrifying. His goal is to help others go through it with caring, dignity, and the highest level of functioning possible.

Caring for Mr. Sloane and his family is especially personal for Brian. Mr. Sloane is about the same age his father had been, looks somewhat like him, and has many of his mannerisms. Brian shared these feelings with his wife, and the two spent some time talking about his father and all they had been through together, good and bad. In the end, Brian sat back, breathed a deep sigh of relief, and thanked his wife for being there for him.

When Brian returned to work, he nearly walked right into Mr. Sloane. He was standing at the doorway wearing two shirts, a pair of pajama bottoms, and a baseball cap. "Are you the man who's taking me to pick up my car?" he asks. Brian smiles and says, "It looks like you have quite a day planned. Let's start with a cup of coffee," and redirects him to the day hall.

Assessment
Subjective Data

- Wanders away from home about four times a week.
- "I can't bear to part with him."
- "I feel as if I've betrayed him."

Objective Data

1. Incontinent
2. Aphasia
3. Agnosia
4. Difficulty dressing himself
5. Falls out of bed
6. Impaired memory
7. Frequently disoriented

Priority Diagnosis

- Risk for injury

Supporting Data

- Wandered away from home about four times a week
- Wanders despite supervision
- Falls out of bed at night

Outcome Criteria

Although Mr. Sloane has many unmet needs that require nursing interventions, Brian decides to focus on his physical safety. Criteria for a successful outcome are as follows:

- Highest level of functioning will be supported
- Optimal health will be maintained (nutrition, sleep, elimination).
- Patient will be free from fractures, bruises, contusions, burns, and falls.

Short-Term Goal	Intervention	Rationale	Evaluation
Mr. Sloane will remain free from injury	1. Minimize sensory stimulation. 2. Maximize meaningful stimulation that is personalized (e.g., favorite music). 3. If Mr. Sloane becomes upset, engage him first by attempting to understand the reason, then try distraction.	1. Decreased sensory stimulation offsets sensory overload, which increases anxiety and confusion. 2. Meaningful stimulation will help to maintain personhood and decrease anxiety. 3. Interpersonal engagement is necessary in order to attempt distraction or a change in topic.	**GOAL MET** During his first week in the facility, Mr. Sloane remained free from injury.

Continued

CASE STUDY AND NURSING CARE PLAN—cont'd

Short-Term Goal	Intervention	Rationale	Evaluation
	4. Label all rooms and drawers with pictures. Label often-used objects (e.g., hairbrushes and toothbrushes).	4. Labeling can keep the patient from wandering into other patients' rooms and increases environmental clues to familiar objects.	
	5. Encourage physical activity during the day.	5. Physical activity during the day might decrease wandering at night.	
	6. Provide a low bed.	6. This will prevent injuries in the case of falling out of the bed.	
	7. Provide adequate lighting in the bathroom at night.	7. Although darkness is important for sleep, light in the bathroom will decrease wandering and promote continence.	

Evaluation

Although Mr. Sloane continues to display wandering behaviors, his wandering has been contained within safe areas of the unit except for one instance when he wandered to the lobby. He was stopped by security and safely returned to the unit within 45 minutes. He has not fallen out of bed. Nursing interventions, such as placing his mattress on the floor and ensuring adequate lighting, have increased his safety while at the same time acknowledging that he continues to exhibit wandering behaviors.

KEY POINTS TO REMEMBER

- The term *neurocognitive disorder* refers to a disorder resulting from biological changes in the brain; it is marked by disturbances in orientation, memory, intellect, judgment, and affect.
- Delirium and dementia are discussed in this chapter because they are the neurocognitive disorders most frequently seen by healthcare workers.
- Delirium has an acute onset, it involves noticeable disturbances in consciousness and symptoms of disorientation and confusion that can change by the minute, hour, or time of day.
- Delirium is always secondary to an underlying condition. Therefore, it is usually temporary and transient; once the underlying cause has been treated, it may continue for hours to days. If the cause is not treated, permanent damage to the brain can result.
- Dementia usually has a more insidious onset than delirium. Global deterioration of cognitive functioning (e.g., memory, judgment, ability to think abstractly, and orientation) is often progressive and irreversible, depending on the underlying cause.

- All types of dementia are diagnosed as either mild or major neurocognitive disorders; they are differentiated by the person's functional ability.
- Signs and symptoms change according to the three stages of Alzheimer's disease: stage 1 (mild), stage 2 (moderate), and stage 3 (severe).
- Behavioral manifestations of Alzheimer's disease include confabulation, perseveration, agraphia, aphasia, apraxia, agnosia, hyperorality, touching things, and sundowning.
- No known cause or cure exists for Alzheimer's disease, although a number of drugs that increase the brain's supply of acetylcholine (a chemical that facilitates nerve communication) or regulate glutamate are helpful in slowing progression of the disease.
- People with Alzheimer's disease have many unmet needs and present numerous management challenges to both their families and healthcare workers.
- Specific nursing interventions for cognitively impaired individuals can improve communication, safety, and self-care. The need for family teaching and support is crucial.

CRITICAL THINKING

1. Martha Kendel, 82 years old, has AD. She lives with her husband, who has been trying to care for her in their home. Mrs. Kendel is having trouble dressing. She has put her blouse on backward and sometimes puts her bra on over her blouse. She often forgets where things are. She makes an effort to cook but has recently attempted to "put out" the electric burners of the stove with pitchers of water. Once in a while, she cannot find the bathroom in time, often mistaking it for a closet. Sometimes she cries because she is aware that she is losing her sense of her place in the world. She and her husband have always been loving companions, and he wants to keep her at home as long as possible.

a. Help Mr. Kendel by writing out a list of suggestions that he can try at home that might help facilitate (a) communication, (b) activities of daily living, and (c) maintenance of a safe home environment.

b. Identify at least three interventions appropriate to this situation for each of the areas previously cited.

c. Identify resources available for maintaining Ms. Kendel in her home for as long as possible. Provide the name of a self-help group that you would urge Mr. Kendel to join.

2. Share with your class or clinical group the name and function of at least three community agencies in your area that could be appropriate referrals for a family trying to cope with dementia.

CHAPTER REVIEW

1. Which statement made by the primary caregiver of a person with dementia demonstrates an accurate understanding of providing the person with a safe environment?
   a. "The local police know that he has wandered off before."
   b. "I keep the noise level low in the house."
   c. "We've installed locks on all the outside doors."
   d. "Our telephone number is always attached to the inside of his shirt pocket."

2. Which statement made by a family member tends to support a diagnosis of delirium rather than dementia?
   a. "She was fine last night but this morning she was confused."
   b. "Dad doesn't seem to recognize us anymore."
   c. "She's convinced that snakes come into her room at night."
   d. "He can't remember when to take his pills or whether he's bathed."

3. In terms of the pathophysiology responsible for both delirium and dementia, which intervention would be appropriate for delirium specifically?
   a. Assisting with needs related to nutrition, elimination, hydration, and personal hygiene
   b. Monitoring neurological status on an ongoing basis
   c. Placing an identification bracelet on patient
   d. Giving one simple direction at a time in a respectful tone of voice

4. What side effects should the nurse monitor for while caring for a patient taking donepezil (Aricept)? *Select all that apply.*
   a. Insomnia
   b. Constipation
   c. Bradycardia
   d. Signs of dizziness
   e. Reports of headache

5. What is the rationale for providing a patient diagnosed with dementia easily accessible finger foods thorough the day?
   a. It increases input throughout the day
   b. The person may be anorexic
   c. It helps with the monitoring of food intake
   d. It helps to prevent constipation

6. Ophelia, a 69-year-old retired nurse, attends a reunion of her former coworkers. Ophelia is concerned because she usually knows everyone, and she cannot recognize faces today. A registered nurse colleague recognizes Ophelia's distress and "introduces" Ophelia to those attending. The nurse practitioner understands that Ophelia seems to have a deficit in her
   a. Lower-level cognitive domain
   b. Delirium threshold
   c. Executive function
   d. Social cognition ability

7. After talking with her 85-year-old mother, Nancy became concerned enough to drive to her home and check on her. Her mother's appearance was disheveled, her words were nonsensical, she smelled strongly of urine, and there was a stain on her dressing gown. Because she is a nurse, Nancy recognizes that her mother's condition is likely due to
   a. Early-onset dementia
   b. A mild cognitive disorder
   c. A urinary tract infection
   d. Having skipped breakfast

8. Lucia, 70 years old, recently underwent a major orthopedic surgical procedure. On postoperative day 3, she responds to the nurse who has been caring for her with affection. At other times, however, she tells the nurse to leave because she does not recognize her and asks to have another nurse care for her, specifically naming the nurse as the "nice one." The most likely reason for Lucia's behavior is that she is
   a. Attention-seeking and manipulative
   b. Showing signs of early dementia
   c. Experiencing an acute delirium
   d. Playing one staff member off against another

9. Since his wife's death 2 months earlier, Aaron, 90 years of age and in good health, has begun to pay less attention to his hygiene and seems less alert to his surroundings. He complains of difficulty concentrating, disrupted sleep, and lacks energy. His family has to remind and encourage him to shower, take his medications, and eat, all of which he then does. Which of the following responses would be most appropriate?
   a. Reorient Mr. Smith by pointing out the day and date each time you have occasion to interact with him.
   b. Meet with the family and support them to accept, anticipate, and prepare for the progression of his stage 2 dementia.
   c. Avoid touch and proximity. These are likely to be uncomfortable for Mr. Smith and may provoke aggression when he is disoriented.
   d. Arrange for an appointment with a mental health professional for the evaluation and treatment of suspected major depressive disorder.

10. Nurses caring for patients who have neurocognitive disorders are exposed to stress on many levels. Specialized skills training and continuing education are helpful to diffuse stress, as well as which of the following? *Select all that apply.*
    a. Expressing emotions by journaling
    b. Describing stressful events on Facebook
    c. Engaging in exercise and relaxation activities
    d. Having realistic patient expectations
    e. Participating in a happy hour after work to blow off steam

1. c; 2. a; 3. b; 4. a, c, d, e; 5. a; 6. d; 7. c; 8. c; 9. d; 10. a, c, d

NGN CASE STUDY AND QUESTIONS

Ronald Cohen is a 76-year-old resident of a long-term care facility who is being admitted to a psychiatric unit in a general hospital after a series of incidents of combative behavior with staff. That morning, Mr. Cohen bit his nurse in response to the nurse's offer to help him while struggling with his shirt buttons. Shortly after, when the nurse was about to administer his blood pressure medication, he cursed and accused the nurse of trying to poison him. He slapped the nurse's arm out of the way, scattering the medication on the floor.

Mr. Cohen is unable to read the intake form or sign his name and does not remember his phone number, so the long-term care facility staff member assists. The staff member reports the patient's history of cardiovascular disease and recurrent sleeping difficulties and that he wandered off at night, saying he needed to get to football practice. Hospital staff observe the patient's unsteady gait and the use of stories to fill in memory gaps when asked basic questions.

When Mr. Cohen's daughter arrives, she apologizes for arriving an hour late. She expresses great concern about not being able to take care of her father since her mother died several years ago. She says, "I am an only child and don't know how I'm going to be able to support my dad much longer. I usually take him home every weekend from the long-term care facility, but he's becoming so unpredictable."

1. The nurse understands from the long-term care facility history and the daughter's statements that the patient has experienced a change in cognition.
   Identify the assessment findings that are consistent with cognitive changes in an older adult that require further evaluation. *Select all that apply.*
   a. Narcissism
   b. Agraphia
   c. Confabulation
   d. Aphasia
   e. Apraxia
   f. Sundowning
   g. Splitting
   h. Narcolepsy

2. Mr. Cohen is diagnosed with moderate Alzheimer's disease (middle stage) by an advanced healthcare provider. Which action will the nursing team implement when the patient is in their care? *Select all that apply.*

Actions	Implement
a. Minimize sensory stimulation	
b. Introduce simple exercises to enhance fine motor skills	
c. Avoid elastic and sticky fastening tapes (Velcro) on clothing; replace with simple buttons and zippers	
d. Offer two choices about when to perform self-care	
e. Expose to morning light/sunlight	
f. Provide picture magazines and children's books	
g. Provide a loosely structured environment to enhance the feeling of freedom	

NGN case study answers are on Evolve.

Visit the Evolve website for a posttest on the content in this chapter: http://evolve.elsevier.com/Varcarolis

REFERENCES

Alzheimer's Association. (2019). Alzheimer's Association Report: 2019 Alzheimer's disease facts and figures. *Alzheimer's & Dementia, 15,* 321–387.
American Psychiatric Association. (2013). *Diagnostic and statistical manual of mental disorders* (5th ed.). Washington, DC: Author.
Canhada, S., Castro, K., Schweigert Perry, I., & Luft, V. C. (2018). Omega-3 fatty acids' supplementation in Alzheimer's disease: A systematic review. *Nutritional Neuroscience, 21*(8), 529–538.
Chenoweth, L., Stein-Parbury, J., Lapkin, S., Wang, A., Liu, Z., & Williams, A. (2019). Effects of person-centered care at the organisational-level for people with dementia. A systematic review. *PLoS ONE, 14*(2), e0212686.
Dixon, M. (2018). Assessment and management of older patients with delirium in acute settings. *Nursing Older People, 30*(4), 35–42.
Herling, S. F., Greve, I. E., Vasilevskis, E. E., et al. (2018). Interventions for preventing intensive care unit delirium in adults. *Cochrane Database of Systematic Reviews, 11,* CD009783. https://doi.org/10.1002/14651858.CD009783.pub2.
Inouye, S. K. (2018). Delirium: A framework to improve acute care for older persons. *Journal of the American Geriatrics Society, 66*(3), 446–451.
International Council of Nurses. (2019a). *Nursing diagnosis and outcome statements: International Classification for Nursing Practice catalogue.* Geneva, Switzerland: Author.
International Council of Nurses. (2019b). *Nursing intervention statements: International classification for nursing practice catalogue.* Geneva, Switzerland: Author.
James, B. D., & Bennett, D. A. (2019). Causes and patterns of dementia: An update in the era of redefining Alzheimer's disease. *Annual Review of Public Health, 40,* 65–84.
Moon, K. J., & Park, H. (2018). Outcomes of patients with delirium in long-term care facilities: A prospective cohort study. *Journal of Gerontological Nursing, 44*(9), 41–50.
Rabinovici, G. D. (2019). Late-onset Alzheimer disease. *CONTINUUM: Lifelong Learning in Neurology, 25*(1), 14–33.
Siddiqi, N., Harrison, J. K., Clegg, A., et al. (2016). Interventions for preventing delirium in hospitalised non-ICU patients. *Cochrane Database of Systematic Reviews, 3,* CD005563. https://doi.org/10.1002/14651858.
US Food and Drug Administration. (2008). *FDA requests boxed warnings on older class of antipsychotic drugs.* Retrieved from https://www.fda.gov/NewsEvents/Newsroom/PressAnnouncements/2008/ucm116912.htm.

24

Personality Disorders

Margaret Jordan Halter and Christine A. Tackett

🌐 Visit the Evolve website for a pretest on the content in this chapter: http://evolve.elsevier.com/Varcarolis

OBJECTIVES

1. Identify characteristics of each of the 10 personality disorders.
2. Discuss guidelines for nursing care associated with each of the 10 personality disorders.
3. Analyze the interaction of biological determinants and other risk factors in the development of personality disorders.
4. Describe the emotional and clinical needs of nurses and other staff who work with patients who have personality disorders.

5. Formulate a nursing diagnosis for each of the personality disorders.
6. Discuss two nursing outcomes for patients with borderline and antisocial personality disorder.
7. Plan basic interventions for a patient with impulsive, aggressive, or manipulative behaviors.
8. Identify biological treatments and psychological therapies for each of the personality disorders.

KEY TERMS AND CONCEPTS

callousness
dialectical behavior therapy (DBT)
emotional dysregulation

emotional lability
impulsivity
personality

personality disorder
separation-individuation
splitting

We may often meet someone and think, "She's quite a dramatic person" or "What a detail-oriented character he is." When we make evaluations such as these about other individuals, we are reacting to their personalities. Personality comes from the Latin word *persona,* which means "mask," and it may refer to what other people see.

Personality is an individual's characteristic, relatively permanent pattern of thoughts, feelings, and behaviors that define her or his quality of experiences and relationships. A personality is considered unhealthy when an individual's interpersonal and social relationships and functioning are consistently maladaptive, complicated, or dysphoric. We know that personality can be protective for a person in times of difficulty, but it may also be a liability if it results in ongoing relationship problems or leads to emotional distress on a regular basis.

Until quite recently, we believed that personalities were fairly fixed entities. This belief was based on William James' (1892, p. 124) view, "By the age of 30, the character has set like plaster and will never soften again." More contemporary views challenge this notion. Rather than being set like plaster, the rate of personality change slows over time but does not cease. If personality traits evolve continually across the life span, we have an

opportunity to develop and support more adaptive functioning and social relationships.

OVERVIEW

Personality disorders are among the most challenging and complex group of disorders to treat. Individuals who meet the criteria for these disorders display significant challenges in self-identity or self-direction, and they have problems with empathy or intimacy within their relationships.

People with these disorders have difficulty recognizing or owning that their difficulties are problems of their personalities. They may truly believe that the problems originate outside of themselves. Still others may be unaware that their behavior is unusual, and they may not experience any distress.

Judgments about an individual's personality functioning should take into account the person's ethnic, cultural, and social backgrounds. Patients who differ from the majority culture or the culture of the clinician may be at risk for overdiagnosis of a personality disorder. Therefore, it is important to obtain additional information from others knowledgeable of the patient's particular cultural or ethnic norms before determining the presence of a personality disorder.

According to the American Psychiatric Association (APA, 2013), there are 10 personality disorders. They are grouped into clusters of similar behavior patterns and personality traits, as follows:

Cluster A: Behaviors described as odd or eccentric
   Paranoid personality disorder
   Schizoid personality disorder
   Schizotypal personality disorder
Cluster B: Behaviors described as dramatic, emotional, or erratic
   Borderline personality disorder
   Narcissistic personality disorder
   Histrionic personality disorder
   Antisocial personality disorder
Cluster C: Behaviors described as anxious or fearful
   Avoidant
   Dependent
   Obsessive-compulsive

This chapter begins with a discussion of eight personality disorders, including their prevalence, characteristics, nursing care guidelines, and treatment modalities. Each disorder is accompanied by a vignette for the purpose of illustration. Afterward, two of the most common and challenging personality disorders—borderline and antisocial—are described in more detail, along with an application of the nursing process.

CLUSTER A PERSONALITY DISORDERS

Paranoid Personality Disorder

Paranoid personality disorder is characterized by a longstanding distrust and suspiciousness of others based on the belief, unsupported by evidence, that others want to exploit, harm, or deceive the person. These individuals are hypervigilant, anticipate hostility, and may provoke hostile responses by initiating a counterattack.

The prevalence of paranoid personality disorder has been estimated at about 2% to 4% (APA, 2013). Slightly more men than women are diagnosed with this disorder. Relatives of patients with schizophrenia are more frequently affected with it. A diagnosis of paranoid personality disorder often precedes a schizophrenia diagnosis.

Symptoms may be apparent in childhood or adolescence. Parents may notice that their child doesn't have friends and experiences social anxiety. Young people with this disorder are frequently teased because of their odd behavior.

As adults, people with paranoid personality disorder tend to have difficult relationships due to their jealousy, controlling behaviors, and unwillingness to forgive. Projection, whereby people attribute their own unacknowledged feelings to others, is the dominant defense mechanism. For example, they may accuse their partners of being hypercritical when they themselves are constantly finding fault.

Guidelines for Nursing Care

- Considering the degree of mistrust felt by these individuals, all prearranged promises, appointments, and schedules should be strictly adhered to.
- Being too nice or friendly may be met with suspicion. Instead, clear and straightforward explanations of tests and procedures should be given before they are scheduled.
- It is best to use simple language and to project a neutral but kindly affect.
- When a patient exhibits threatening behaviors, it is essential to set limits.

Treatment Modalities

Individuals with paranoid personality disorder tend to reject treatment. If they somehow end up in a psychiatric treatment setting, they may appear puzzled and obviously suspicious about why this is happening. Paranoid people are difficult to interview because they are reluctant to share information about themselves for fear that the information will be used against them.

Psychotherapy is the first line of treatment for paranoid personality disorder. Individual therapy focuses on the development of a professional and trusting relationship. Because of their fears, patients may behave in a threatening manner. Therapists should respond by setting limits and dealing with delusional accusations in a realistic manner without humiliating the patients.

Group therapy is threatening to people with paranoid personality disorder. However, the group setting may be useful for improving social skills. Role playing and group feedback can help reduce suspiciousness. For example, if the patient says, "I think the therapist is singling me out," other group members may provide a reality check or describe similar feelings in the past.

An antianxiety agent such as diazepam (Valium) may be used to reduce a patient's anxiety and agitation. More severe agitation and delusions may be treated with an antipsychotic medication such as haloperidol (Haldol) in small doses for brief periods to manage mildly delusional thinking or severe agitation. The first-generation antipsychotic medication pimozide (Orap) may be useful in reducing paranoid ideation.

> **VIGNETTE:** Ms. Alonzo, 54 years old and unemployed, arrives at a mental health clinic complaining of depression and pain. She believes that her health maintenance organization has circulated her medical record to all healthcare providers to prevent her from being treated. She refuses to give any social history and is reluctant to share her telephone number. When the nurse indicates that the psychiatrist does not prescribe pain medications, she smiles bitterly and says, "So they already got to you."

Schizoid Personality Disorder

People with **schizoid personality disorder** exhibit a lifelong pattern of social withdrawal. They are somewhat expressionless and have a restricted range of emotional expression. Others tend to view them as odd or eccentric because of their discomfort with social interaction.

The prevalence rate of this disorder may be nearly 5% of the population (APA, 2013). Males are more often affected. Symptoms of schizoid personality disorder appear in childhood and adolescence. These young people tend to be loners, do poorly in school, and are the objects of ridicule from their peers because of their odd behavior. There is an increased prevalence of the disorder in families with a history of schizophrenia or schizotypal personality disorder. Abnormalities in the dopaminergic systems may underlie this problem.

Relationships are particularly affected because of the prominent feature of emotional detachment. People with this disorder do not seek out or enjoy close relationships. Neither approval nor rejection from others seems to have much effect. Friendships, dating, and sexual experiences are rare. If trust is established, the person may divulge numerous imaginary friends and fantasies.

The employment of persons with this disorder may be jeopardized if interpersonal interaction is required; however, they may be able to function well in a solitary occupation such as being a security guard on the night shift. They often endorse feelings of being an observer rather than a participant in life. They may describe feelings of depersonalization or detachment from self and the world.

Guidelines for Nursing Care

- Nurses should avoid being too "nice" or "friendly."
- Efforts to promote the patient's socialization are also to be avoided.
- Patients may be open to discussing topics such as coping and anxiety.
- Conduct a thorough assessment to identify symptoms that the patient is reluctant to discuss.
- Protect against ridicule from group members because of the patient's distinctive interests or ideas.

Treatment Modalities

Patients with schizoid personality disorder tend to be introspective. This trait may make them good, if distant, candidates for psychotherapy. As trust develops, these patients may describe a full fantasy life and fears, particularly of dependence. Psychotherapy can help improve their sensitivity to others' social cues.

Although group therapy is not a good first treatment choice, it may be helpful after individual work. Even though the patient may frequently be silent, group therapy provides valuable experience in practicing interactions and getting feedback from others. A noninvasive and supportive group can help individuals to overcome fears of closeness and feelings of isolation. Members may become quite important to the person with schizoid personality disorder, and this may be the person's dominant form of socialization.

As with other personality disorders, there is no medication to improve the patient's functioning. However, depressive symptoms may be treated with antidepressants such as bupropion (Wellbutrin), which can help increase the patient's pleasure in life. Second-generation antipsychotics, such as risperidone (Risperdal) or olanzapine (Zyprexa), are used to improve emotional expressiveness.

VIGNETTE: Mr. Gray, 30 years old and single, is a graduate student in mathematics at a large state university. He lives alone and has never been married. He works as a teaching assistant in a math classroom where the professor teaches the course remotely via the Internet. Mr. Gray wears thick glasses and his clothing is inconspicuous. He rarely smiles and seldom looks directly at the students even when he is answering questions. He does become somewhat animated when he writes lengthy solutions to math problems on the blackboard. He is content with his low-paying job and has never been in psychiatric treatment.

Schizotypal Personality Disorder

People with **schizotypal** (skit-sə-ˈtī-pəl) **personality disorder** do not blend in with the crowd. Their symptoms are strikingly strange and unusual. Magical thinking, odd beliefs, strange speech patterns, and inappropriate affect are hallmarks of this disorder.

Estimates on the prevalence of schizotypal personality disorder—which is more common in men than in women—vary from 0.6% to 4.6% (APA, 2013). As in the case of the other cluster A personality disorders, symptoms are evident in young people. People who have first-degree relatives with schizophrenia are at greater risk for this disorder. Abnormalities in brain structure, physiology, chemistry, and functioning are similar to those found in schizophrenia. For example, both disorders share reduced cortical volume.

The *Diagnostic and Statistical Manual of Mental Disorders,* 5th ed. ([*DSM-5*] APA, 2013) identifies this problem as both a personality disorder and also the first of the schizophrenia spectrum disorders. Chapter 12 discusses the schizophrenia spectrum disorders in greater detail.

As in the case of schizoid personality disorder, individuals with schizotypal personality disorder have severe social and interpersonal deficits. They experience extreme anxiety in social situations. Their contributions to conversations tend to ramble with lengthy, unclear, overly detailed, and abstract content. An additional feature of this disorder is paranoia. Individuals with schizotypal personality disorder are overly suspicious and anxious. They tend to misinterpret the motivations of others, suggesting that they are "out to get them," and they blame others for their social isolation. Odd beliefs (e.g., being overly superstitious) or magical thinking (e.g., "He caught a cold because I wished he would") are also common.

Psychotic symptoms seen in people with schizophrenia, such as hallucinations and delusions, can also exist with schizotypal personality disorder, but to a lesser degree and only briefly. A major difference between this disorder and schizophrenia is that people with schizotypal personality disorder can be made aware of their suspiciousness, magical thinking, and odd beliefs. Schizophrenia is characterized by far stronger delusions.

Guidelines for Nursing Care

- Respect the patient's need for social isolation.
- Nurses should be aware of the patient's suspiciousness and use appropriate interventions.
- Perform careful assessment as needed to uncover any other medical or psychological symptoms that may need intervention (e.g., suicidal thoughts).
- Be aware that strange beliefs and activities, such as strange religious practices or peculiar thoughts, may be part of the patient's life.

Treatment Modalities

Individuals with schizotypal personality disorder usually avoid treatment because they are socially anxious and somewhat paranoid. Sometimes, however, family members may be concerned enough by the individual's depressive or psychotic symptoms to suggest and foster treatment.

Because it is difficult to develop a therapeutic relationship or alliance with such an individual, the goal should be to provide supportive care. Helping to identify cognitive distortions may be useful. Clinicians should be aware that this population may be actively involved in groups that can complicate the clinical picture. These groups include unusual religious sects or occult-type societies.

Although there is no specific medication for schizotypal personality disorder, associated conditions may be treated. People with schizotypal personality disorder may benefit from low-dose antipsychotic agents such as risperidone (Risperdal) or olanzapine (Zyprexa) for psychotic-like symptoms and day-to-day functioning (Skodol, Bender, & Oldham, 2019). These agents help with symptoms such as ideas of reference or illusions. Major depressive disorder and anxiety disorders may be treated with antidepressants and antianxiety agents.

> **VIGNETTE:** Raymond, 55 years old and single, lives with his mother. He is the youngest of seven children raised in a farming community. Three of his siblings are deaf, and Raymond also has some hearing loss. Raymond started therapy with Jenny, an advanced practice psychiatric–mental health registered nurse, after sustaining a career-ending injury that left him completely disabled. Jenny and Raymond have been working together for several years.
>
> Raymond is distressed by his belief that everyone in his hometown greets him with sexual gestures. "They obviously think I'm gay." He thinks that truck drivers talk about his sexuality on their CB radios. These beliefs create great distress and anxiety for him. He occasionally yells at or gestures at the truck drivers. Jenny has been helping Raymond to understand that his perceptions may be faulty and that his hearing loss may be contributing to his perceptual difficulties and anxiety.

CLUSTER B PERSONALITY DISORDERS

Borderline Personality Disorder

A full description of borderline personality disorder follows the Cluster C disorders. The nursing process is described and illustrated with a case study and nursing care plan. Specific advanced practice biological and psychological treatment modalities for this disorder are provided.

Histrionic Personality Disorder

People with **histrionic personality disorder** are excitable and dramatic yet are often also high functioning. They may be referred to as "drama queens" or "drama majors." Classic characteristics of this population include extroversion, flamboyance, and colorful personalities. Despite this bold exterior, they tend to have limited abilities to develop meaningful relationships.

Histrionic personality disorder occurs at a rate of nearly 2% in community samples (APA, 2013). In clinical settings, it tends to be diagnosed more frequently in women than men. Symptoms begin by early adulthood. Inborn character traits such as emotional expressiveness and egocentricity have also been identified as predisposing an individual to this disorder.

This disorder is characterized by emotional attention-seeking behaviors, including self-centeredness, low frustration tolerance, and excessive emotionality. The person with histrionic personality disorder is often impulsive and may act flirtatiously or provocatively. Relationships do not last because the partner often feels smothered or reacts to the insensitivity of the histrionic person. The individual with histrionic personality disorder does not have insight into a personal role in breaking up relationships.

In general, individuals with this disorder do not think that they need psychiatric help. They may go into treatment for associated problems, such as major depressive disorder, which may be precipitated by losses, such as the end of a relationship.

Guidelines for Nursing Care

- Nursing care should reflect an understanding that seductive behavior is a response to distress.
- Communication and interactions should always be kept professional.
- Patients may exaggerate symptoms and have difficulty in functioning.
- Encourage and model the use of concrete and descriptive rather than vague and impressionistic language.
- Help patients to clarify their own feelings, as they often have difficulty identifying them.
- Teach and role model assertiveness.
- Assess for suicidal ideation. What was intended as a suicidal gesture may inadvertently result in the patient's death.

Treatment Modalities

Individuals with histrionic personality disorder have difficulty regulating their feelings and the expression of those feelings. Psychotherapy may promote the clarification of these feelings and their appropriate expression. Group therapy may be useful in this population, although distracting symptoms may be disruptive to group functioning.

There are no specific pharmacological treatments available for people with histrionic personality disorder. Medications such as antidepressants can be used for depressive or somatic symptoms. Antianxiety agents may be helpful in treating anxiety. Antipsychotics may be used if the patient exhibits derealization or illusions.

> **VIGNETTE:** Ms. Lombard, 35 years old and twice divorced, was admitted to an inpatient unit after an overdose of asthma medications and antibiotics. She took all her pills all at once after her primary care provider refused to order a sleeping pill for her. On the first night on the unit, she is withdrawn and tearful. By the next morning, she is neatly groomed, even wearing makeup, and is socializing with everyone. She denies thoughts of self-harm. Over the next 2 days, Ms. Lombard monopolizes the community meetings by talking about how unappreciated she is by her family. She seeks special attention from a male evening-shift registered nurse, asking if he can stay late after his shift to sit with her. When he refuses, she demands to be placed back on one-to-one precautions because she feels suicidal again.

Narcissistic Personality Disorder

Narcissistic personality disorder is characterized by feelings of entitlement, an exaggerated belief in one's own importance, and a lack of empathy. In reality, people with this disorder suffer from weak self-esteem and hypersensitivity to criticism. Narcissistic personality disorder is associated with less impairment in individual functioning and quality of life than the other personality-based disorders.

The prevalence of narcissistic personality disorder ranges from 0% to about 6% in community samples (APA, 2013). It tends to be more common in males than in females. Age of onset is difficult to determine because of the narcissistic traits that are typically found in adolescents. There may be a familial tendency for this disorder, as parents with narcissism may attribute an unrealistic sense of talent, importance, and beauty to their children. This puts the children at higher risk.

People with narcissistic personality disorder come across as arrogant and as having an inflated view of their importance. The individual with this disorder has a need for constant admiration along with a lack of empathy for others, a factor that strains most relationships over time. They are very sensitive to rejection and criticism and can be disparaging to others. A sense of personal entitlement paired with a lack of social empathy can result in the exploitation of others.

Underneath the surface of arrogance, people with narcissistic personality disorder feel intense shame and have a fear of abandonment. In keeping with these descriptions, the main pathological personality trait of narcissism is antagonism, represented by the grandiosity and attention-seeking behaviors. These individuals tend to tolerate rejection poorly. As a result, they may seek help for depression. They want therapists and/or their loved ones to appreciate their emotional pain and to value their efforts or special qualities.

Guidelines for Nursing Care

- Nurses should remain neutral and recognize the source of narcissistic behavior—shame and fear of abandonment.
- These patients can be helped to identify goals and to develop a stronger self-identity.
- Use the therapeutic nurse-patient relationship as an opportunity to practice how to engage in meaningful interaction.
- Avoid engaging in power struggles or becoming defensive in response to the patient's disparaging remarks.
- Do not directly challenge grandiose statements.
- Role model empathy.

Treatment Modalities

Because patients must confront their problem to make progress, treating people specifically for this disorder is difficult. Also, because they are not likely to seek help for their own problems, they are more likely to be involved in couples or family therapy than in individual treatment. In these family-oriented approaches, narcissistic individuals are likely to deflect suggestions that they contribute to family problems and will instead blame others.

If a person with narcissistic personality disorder somehow seeks treatment, individual cognitive behavioral therapy (CBT) can be helpful for deconstructing faulty thinking. Group therapy can also help the person in sharing with others, seeing their own qualities in others, and learning empathy.

Lithium (Eskalith, Lithobid) has been used in patients with narcissism who demonstrate mood swings. Antidepressants can also be used if the person has depressive symptoms.

> **VIGNETTE:** Dr. Donnelly is a 40-year-old attending psychiatrist at a university outpatient center. He is twice divorced and has no children. His grooming is impeccable, and he often describes his expensive shopping habits. He is usually late to staff meetings, and when he is not speaking, he yawns and shifts noisily in his seat. He has a reputation for angry outbursts directed at other therapists in the hallway for minor mistakes, such as a scheduling error. Dr. Donnelly becomes impatient when he must wait on line and often moves to the front of the line, which has led to confrontations.

Antisocial Personality Disorder

A full description of antisocial personality disorder is included after borderline personality disorder toward the end of the chapter. The nursing process is described and specific advanced practice biological and psychological treatment modalities for this disorder are discussed.

CLUSTER C PERSONALITY DISORDERS

Avoidant Personality Disorder

People with **avoidant personality disorder** are extremely sensitive to rejection, feel inadequate, and are socially inhibited. They avoid interpersonal contact owing to fears of rejection or criticism.

Avoidant personality disorder occurs in 2.4% of the US population (APA, 2013) and is found equally among men and women. Early symptoms of the disorder are often evident in infants and children. These symptoms include shyness and avoidance that, unlike common shyness, increase during adolescence and early adulthood.

The main pathological personality traits are low self-esteem associated with poor functioning in social situations, feelings of inferiority compared with peers, and a reluctance to engage in unfamiliar activities involving new people. Some can function in a protective environment. However, if their support system fails, they can suffer from depression, anxiety, and anger. They are especially sensitive to and preoccupied with rejection, humiliation, and failure. They often avoid new interpersonal relationships or activities because of their fears of criticism or disapproval (APA, 2013).

Guidelines for Nursing Care

- Nurses should use a friendly, accepting, and reassuring approach.
- Remember that being pushed into social situations can cause severe anxiety for these patients.
- Convey an attitude of acceptance toward patient fears.
- Provide the patient with exercises to enhance new social skills but use these with caution because any failure can increase the patient's feelings of poor self-worth.
- Assertiveness training can help the person learn to express needs.

Treatment Modalities

Individual and group therapy is useful in processing anxiety-provoking symptoms and in planning methods to approach and handle anxiety-provoking situations. Psychotherapy focuses on trust and assertiveness training.

Antianxiety agents can be helpful. Beta-adrenergic receptor antagonists (e.g., atenolol) help reduce autonomic nervous system hyperactivity. Antidepressant medications—including selective serotonin reuptake inhibitors (SSRIs) such as citalopram (Celexa) and serotonin norepinephrine reuptake inhibitors (SNRIs) such as venlafaxine (Effexor)—may reduce social anxiety (Ripoll et al., 2011). Serotonergic agents may help individuals with avoidant personalities feel less sensitive to rejection.

> **VIGNETTE:** Ms. Lowell, 35 years old and single, works for a computer repair company. As a child, she had few friends and never participated in extracurricular activities. She lives alone in her own apartment and has never had an adult intimate relationship. On the job, she rarely talks to coworkers and prefers to work alone. If she has any questions, she asks the supervisor and carefully follows directions. Although she has 7 years of experience and a good work record, she refused the offer of a promotion because it would require her to interact with customers.

Dependent Personality Disorder

Dependent personality disorder is characterized by a pattern of submissive and clinging behavior related to an overwhelming need to be cared for. This need results in intense fears of separation.

The prevalence rate of dependent personality disorder is fairly low with an estimate of about 0.5% (APA, 2013). Dependent personality disorder may be the result of chronic physical illness or punishment for independent behavior in childhood. The inherited trait of submissiveness may also be a factor.

People with dependent personality disorder have a great need to be taken care of. This can lead to patterns of submissiveness with fears of separation and abandonment by others. Because they lack confidence in their own ability or judgment, these individuals may manipulate others to assume responsibility for such activities as dealing with finances or child rearing. This may create problems by leaving them more vulnerable to exploitation by others because of their passive and submissive nature. Feelings of insecurity about their self-agency and lack of self-confidence may interfere with attempts at becoming more independent. They may experience intense anxiety when left alone for even brief periods of time (APA, 2013).

Guidelines for Nursing Care

- Nurses can help the patient identify and address current stressors.
- Be aware that strong countertransference may develop because of patient's demands for extra time and crisis states.

- The therapeutic nurse-patient relationship can provide a testing ground for increased assertiveness through role modeling and teaching of assertive skills.

Treatment Modalities

Psychotherapy is the treatment of choice for dependent personality disorder. CBT can help patients develop more healthy and accurate thinking by examining and challenging automatic thoughts that result in fearful behavior. This process can help in developing new perspectives and attitudes about the need for other people.

There are no specific medications indicated for this disorder, but symptoms of depression and anxiety may be treated with the appropriate antidepressant and antianxiety agents. Panic attacks can be helped with the tricyclic antidepressant imipramine (Tofranil).

> **VIGNETTE:** Ashley, 32 years old, is married and a former engineer. She is the mother to two young children, aged 3 years and 11 months. Ashley's depression and anxiety have been more severe since she stopped working. She feels inadequate and overwhelmed by her responsibilities, so her mother moved in with the young family at her daughter's request. Her therapist, an advanced practice psychiatric–mental health registered nurse, recommended that she receive brief treatment for depression and anxiety at the partial hospitalization program. Ashley quickly bonded with the advanced practice nurse, who is an older woman. She frequently asks her for reassurance that she is doing the right thing by coming to treatment and seeks her out frequently for extra individual sessions. Gradually, as the result of individual and group therapy, Ashley begins to realize that excessive dependence on her mother has contributed to her long-standing feelings of ineffectiveness, helplessness, and invalidation of her own parenting skills.

Obsessive-Compulsive Personality Disorder

Obsessive-compulsive personality disorder is characterized by limited emotional expression, stubbornness, perseverance, and indecisiveness. Preoccupation with orderliness, perfectionism, and control are the hallmarks of this disorder.

Obsessive-compulsive personality disorder is one of the most prevalent personality disorders. Prevalence rates range from about 2% to 8% (APA, 2013). It is more common in men than women. Oldest siblings tend to be affected more often than subsequent siblings. Risk factors for this disorder include a background of harsh discipline and having a first-degree relative with this disorder. Obsessive-compulsive personality disorder has been associated with increased relapse rates of depression and an increase in suicidal risks in people with co-occurring depression.

The main pathological personality traits of these individuals are rigidity and inflexible standards for self and others. They rehearse over and over how they will respond in social situations. They persist in goal-seeking behavior long after it is necessary, even if this is self-defeating or harms their relationships.

The preoccupation with persistence often results in losing the major point of the activity. Projects are often left incomplete because of these overly strict standards.

A distinction should be made between obsessive-compulsive disorder and obsessive-compulsive personality disorder. Obsessive-compulsive disorder is characterized by obsessive thoughts and repetition or adherence to rituals. People so affected are aware that these thoughts and actions are unreasonable. Obsessive-compulsive personality disorder is characterized more by an unhealthy focus on perfectionism. Such people "know" that their actions are right and feel comfortable with their self-imposed systems of rules.

People with obsessive-compulsive personality disorder often do feel genuine affection for friends and family. Yet leisure activities and friendships are dropped in favor of excessive devotion to work and productivity.

Guidelines for Nursing Care

- Nurses should guard against power struggles with these patients, as their need for control is very high.
- Patients with this disorder have difficulty dealing with unexpected changes.
- It is helpful to provide structure yet allow patients extra time to complete habitual behavior.
- Help patients to identify ineffective coping and to develop better coping techniques.

Treatment Modalities

Typically, patients seek help for obsessive-compulsive personality disorder, as they are aware of their own suffering. They may also seek treatment for anxiety or depression. The treatment course is often long and complicated. Both group therapy and behavioral therapy can be helpful, so that patients can learn new coping skills for their anxiety and see direct benefits for change from feedback within the group.

Clomipramine (Anafranil) may help reduce the obsessions, anxiety, and depression associated with this disorder. Other serotonergic agents such as fluoxetine (Prozac) may also be effective.

VIGNETTE: Mr. Wright is a 45-year-old single male postal worker in a small town. He lives alone and has never married. He is well groomed and wears a clean, neatly ironed uniform every day. He carefully follows all policies and procedures and is quite resistant whenever there is any update or change. He frequently challenges the supervisor about policy details and has been referred to the regional personnel office countless times for resolution of these conflicts. In staff meetings, he gives excessive circumstantial details and writes extra material on the back of any required report form. When he is dealing with the public, he sometimes gets into arguments with customers about postal rules or the schedule. The other staff members do not consider him to be a team player because he seldom volunteers to help others. Even if he is asked to help someone, he is quick to criticize his peer's performance. Although he has worked in the same office for 10 years, he has never advanced beyond the front-line position.

CONSIDERING CULTURE
Narcissistic Leadership in the Workplace

Narcissism has a negative connotation and we probably would not choose a friend based on that quality. But how about a leader? A group in China explored the effect of a narcissistic leader on team creativity. They found that leader narcissism had a positive impact on team creativity. This positive impact was especially marked when the team members were encouraged to participate in decision making.

It is worth considering whether US work groups would respond positively to a leader with narcissistic traits. Some general cultural differences may affect that response. For example, the Chinese workplace tends to be more hierarchical and respectful for those in positions of power. In addition, for the Chinese the group is the focus rather than the individual. Any success is considered a success for the team.

Adapted from Zhou, L., Li, J., Liu, Y., Tian, F., Zhang, X., & Qin, W. (2019). Exploring the relationship between leader narcissism and team creativity: evidence from R&D teams in Chinese high-technology enterprises. *Leadership & Organization Development Journal, 40,* 916–931.

BORDERLINE PERSONALITY DISORDER
Clinical Picture

As previously discussed, borderline personality disorder is a cluster B diagnosis. Cluster B diagnoses are described as dramatic, emotional, or erratic. This disorder is the best-known and most dramatic of the personality disorders. Borderline personality disorder is characterized by severe impairments in functioning. Its major features are patterns of marked instability, impulsivity, identity or self-image distortions, unstable mood, and unstable interpersonal relationships. It is marked by **emotional dysregulation**, a term that describes poorly modulated mood characterized by mood swings. Individuals with emotion regulatory problems have ongoing difficulty managing painful emotions in ways that are healthy and effective.

One of the primary features of borderline personality disorder is **emotional lability**, that is, rapidly moving from one emotional extreme to another. Typically, these emotional shifts include responding to situations with emotions that are out of proportion to the circumstances, pathological fear of separation, and intense sensitivity to perceived personal rejection.

Another disruptive trait common in people with borderline personality disorder is **impulsivity**, or acting quickly in response to emotions without considering the consequences. This results in damaged relationships and even in suicide attempts.

Self-destructive behaviors are prominent in this disorder. Ineffective and often harmful self-soothing habits such as cutting, promiscuous sexual behavior, and numbing with substances are common and may result in unintentional death. Chronic suicidal ideation is also a common feature of this disorder and influences the likelihood of accidental deaths. Co-occurring mood, anxiety, or substance disorders complicate the treatment and prognosis of the condition.

Borderline personality disorder is also characterized by feelings of antagonism, manifested in hostility, anger, and irritability in relationships. Physical violence toward intimate partners and nonintimate partners alike may occur. Rarely, a homicide of family members or others occurs. Violence is also manifested in destructive behaviors such as property damage.

An unusual feature of this disorder is the use of splitting as a primary defense mechanism or coping style. It involves an inability to view both positive and negative aspects of others as part of a whole, which results in viewing someone as either a wonderful person or a horrible person. This kind of dichotomous thinking and coping behavior is believed to be partly a result of the person's failed experiences with adult personality integration. It is likely influenced by exposure to earlier psychological, sexual, or physical trauma. For example, individuals with borderline personality disorder may idealize other people (e.g., friends, lovers, healthcare professionals) at the start of new relationships, hoping that these people will meet all of their needs. However, at the first disappointment or frustration, the individual's status quickly shifts to one of devaluation, and the other person is despised.

People with borderline personality disorder seek out treatment for depression, anxiety, suicidal and self-harming behaviors, and other impulsive behaviors, including substance use. The person with borderline personality disorder frequently seeks repeat hospitalizations. Although hospitalization may decrease self-destructive risk for such individuals, it is not regarded as an effective long-term solution. The following box, based on the *DSM-5*, lists the criteria for borderline personality disorder.

DSM-5 CRITERIA FOR BORDERLINE PERSONALITY DISORDER

A pervasive pattern of instability of interpersonal relationships, self-image, affects, and marked impulsivity, beginning in early adulthood and present in a variety of contexts as indicated by five (or more) of the following:

1. Frantic efforts to avoid real or imagined abandonment. (Note: Do not include suicidal or self-mutilating behavior covered in criterion 5.)
2. A pattern of unstable and intense interpersonal relationships characterized by alternating between extremes of idealization and devaluation.
3. Identity disturbances: Markedly and persistently unstable self-image or sense of self.
4. Impulsivity in at least two areas that are potentially self-damaging (e.g., spending, sex, substance abuse, reckless driving, binge eating). (Note: Do not include suicidal or self-mutilating behavior covered in criterion 5.)
5. Recurrent suicidal behavior, gestures, or threats, or self-mutilating behavior.
6. Affective instability due to a marked reactivity of mood (e.g., intense episodic dysphoria, irritability, or anxiety usually lasting a few hours and only rarely more than a few days).
7. Chronic feelings of emptiness.
8. Inappropriate, intense anger or difficulty controlling anger (e.g., frequent displays of temper, constant anger, recurrent physical fights).
9. Transient, stress-related paranoid ideations or severe dissociative symptoms.

From the American Psychiatric Association. (2013). *Diagnostic and statistical manual of disorders* (5th ed.). Washington, DC: Author.

Epidemiology

Borderline personality disorder occurs at a rate of about 1.6% in community studies (Skodol, Bender, & Oldham, 2019).

Although this disorder is more commonly diagnosed in women, it is likely that rates are about the same in men and women. About 70% of individuals in this population will attempt suicide and nearly 10% will complete the suicide.

This disorder results in extensive utilization of services from the healthcare system. Borderline symptoms seem to decrease with age. Over the course of a decade, people with borderline personality disorder experienced high rates of remission and low rates of relapse (Gunderson, 2011). Suicidal and self-harmful thoughts, in particular, tend to decrease with age (McMahon et al., 2019).

Comorbidity

Both physical and psychiatric disorders co-occur in individuals with borderline personality disorder. Psychiatric comorbidities include major depressive disorder, bipolar disorder, anxiety disorders, and sleep disorder (Shen et al., 2017). Substance use disorder is extremely common, with some studies suggesting that the rate of co-occurrence is above 50% (Pennay et al., 2011). Women with this disorder are more likely to have major depressive disorder, anxiety disorders, and posttraumatic stress disorder (Shen et al., 2017). Men are more likely to have substance use disorders or antisocial personality disorder.

Nonpsychiatric diagnoses are also associated with borderline personality disorder. They include diabetes, high blood pressure, fibromyalgia, and arthritis. Chronic pain is strongly associated with this personality disorder.

Etiology
Biological Factors

Genetic. Borderline personality disorder is about five times more common in first-degree biological relatives with the same disorder compared with the general population (APA, 2013). This disorder is highly associated with genetic factors such as hypersensitivity, impulsivity, and emotional dysregulation. A large-scale Swedish study of nearly 2 million health records identified that familial and twin studies support the potential role of genetic vulnerability at about 46% (Skoglund et al., 2019).

Neurobiological. There is evidence that serotonergic dysfunction may accompany the borderline trait of impulsivity. It may also contribute to the depression and aggression that commonly accompany this disorder. The serotonin transporter gene 5-HTT may have shorter alleles, which has been associated with lower levels of serotonin and increased impulsive aggression.

Structural and functional magnetic resonance imaging have revealed abnormalities in the prefrontal cortex and limbic regions. The frontal region is implicated in regulatory control processes and the limbic region is essential for emotional processing (Krause-Utz et al., 2014). Limbic hyperreactivity and diminished control by the frontal brain may explain poor processing of emotion, impulsivity, and interpersonal disturbances.

The neurobiology of borderline personality disorder feature provides more information about the neurobiology of this condition.

▶ Neurobiology of Borderline Personality Disorder

Borderline personality disorder is a serious and disabling brain disorder marked by impulsivity and emotional dysregultion. This dysregulation refers to emotional responses that are poorly modulated including angry outbursts, rage, marked fluctuation of mood, and self-harm that can shift within seconds.

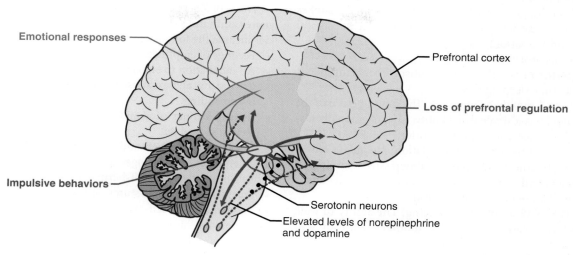

Brain Dysfunction

Prefrontal cortex is the command center of the brain and is involved in executive functioning. In times of stress the prefrontal cortex helps to regulate emotions and impulsive urges arising from the limbic system. In individuals with borderline personality disorder, the prefrontal cortex is less active during the processing of negative emotional stimuli.

Amygdala is responsible for the perception of emotions such as anger, fear, and sadness, as well as controlling aggression. People with borderline personality disorder have increased activity within the amygdala. A variety of other structures within the limbic system have also been implicated in borderline personality disorder.

Neurotransmitters are implicated in symptoms of borderline personality including dysregulated serotonin. Overactivation of norepinephrine may leave a person in a prolonged fight-or-flight response. Considering dopamine's role in thinking, mood regulation, and impulsive control, dopamine dysfunction is also likely a problem in borderline personality disorder.

Treatment Modalities to Support Emotional Regulation

Modality	What is Involved	Impact
Pharmacotherapy	Selective serotonin reuptake inhibitors (SSRIs), anticonvulsants, second-generation antipsychotics, lithium	Promotes mood regulation, reduces impulsivity, reduces anxiety, improves thinking
Dialectical behavioral therapy	Mindfulness, deep breathing, relaxation, distress tolerance, and interpersonal effectiveness training	Minimizes strong responses and improves ability to manage emotions

Cognitive Factors

Margaret Mahler (1895–1985), a Hungarian-born child psychologist who worked with emotionally disturbed children, developed a framework that is useful in considering borderline personality disorder. Mahler and colleagues (1975) suggest that such psychological problems are due to disruption of the normal separation-individuation between the child and the mother.

According to Mahler, an infant's development progresses from complete self-absorption—with an inability to see a difference between the infant and the primary caregiver—to an emotionally and physically differentiated toddler. Mahler emphasized the role of the significant other (traditionally the mother) in providing a secure emotional base of support that promotes enough confidence for the child to separate. This support is achieved through a balance of holding (emotionally and physically) a child enough for the child to feel safe while at the same time fostering and encouraging independence and natural exploration.

Problems may arise in this separation-individuation. If a toddler leaves her mother on the park bench and wanders off to the sandbox, ideally two things should happen. First, the child should be encouraged to go off into the world with smiles and reassurance: "Go on, honey, it's safe to go away a little." Second, the mother needs to be reliably present when the toddler returns, thereby rewarding her efforts. Clearly, parents are not perfect and are sometimes distracted and short tempered. Mahler notes that raising healthy children does not require that parents never make mistakes and that "good enough parenting" will promote successful separation-individuation.

Stages of this process are as follows:
- Stage 1 (birth to 1 month): Normal autism. The infant spends most of its time sleeping.
- Stage 2 (1 to 5 months): Symbiosis. The infant perceives the mother-infant as a single fused entity. Infants gradually distinguish the inner from the outer world.
- Stage 3 (5 to 10 months): Differentiation. The infant recognizes its distinctness from mother. Progressive neurological development and increased alertness draw the infant's attention away from self to the outer world.
- Stage 4 (11 to 18 months): Practicing. The ability to walk and explore greatly expands the toddler's sense of separateness.
- Stage 5 (18 to 24 months): Rapprochement. Toddlers move away from their mothers and come back for emotional refueling. Periods of helplessness and dependence alternate with the need for independence.
- Stage 6 (2 to 5 years): Object constancy, when children comprehend that objects (in this case, the object being the mother) are permanent even when they are not in the child's presence. At this point, the individuation process is complete.

Children who later develop borderline personality may have had this process disrupted. The rapprochement stage is particularly crucial and coincides with the "terrible twos," which are characterized by darting away and clinging and whining. Some experts suggest that this phase is not a desirable time for extended separation between parent and child.

Consider the previous ideal example of the child who wants to play in the sandbox. If the child wanders off to the sandbox and returns to a caregiver who is emotionally unavailable, perhaps hurt by the attempt at independence, the child feels unsafe to explore. Alternately, if the caregiver has personal issues related to dependency and abandonment, he may be threatened by the child's attempts at independence and respond with clinging and halting exploration. Thus, the child cannot safely move on to the next stage of development. A fear of abandonment by others, along with a sense of anger, carries over into adulthood.

APPLICATION OF THE NURSING PROCESS
ASSESSMENT
Assessment Tools

The preferred method for determining a diagnosis of borderline personality disorder is the semistructured interview obtained by clinicians. Self-report inventories, such as the well-known Minnesota Multiphasic Personality Inventory (MMPI), are useful because they have built-in validity and reliability scales for the clinician to refer to when test results are being interpreted.

Areas of assessment that are typically included on questionnaires and rating scales related to borderline personality disorder include the following:
- Feelings of emptiness
- An inclination to engage in risky behaviors, such as reckless driving, unsafe sex, substance use, binge eating, gambling, or overspending
- Intense feelings of abandonment that result in paranoia or feeling spaced out
- Idealization of others and becoming close quickly
- A tendency toward anger, sarcasm, and bitterness
- Self-mutilation and self-harm
- Suicidal behaviors, gestures, or threats
- Sudden shifts in self-evaluation that result in changing goals, values, and career focus
- Extreme mood shifts that occur in a matter of hours or days
- Intense, unstable romantic relationships

Patient History

Borderline personality disorder usually begins before adulthood. Important issues in assessment for borderline personality disorder include a history of suicidal or aggressive ideation or actions, treatment history, and medication (prescribed and illicit) use.

Significant areas about which further details must be obtained include current or past physical, sexual, or emotional abuse and level of current risk of harm from self or others. Information regarding prior use of any medication, including pharmacological agents, is important.

Self-Assessment

Because interpersonal difficulties are central to the problems faced by people diagnosed with borderline personality disorder, it is understandable that these problems surface in the treatment milieu and within the relationships between these patients and their caregivers. The therapeutic relationship often begins with an initial hesitancy on the part of the patient, then an upward curve of idealization by the patient toward the caregiver. This idealization is invariably followed by a devaluation of the caregiver when the patient is disappointed by unmet—frequently impossible—expectations.

For example, a female patient may briefly idealize her male nurse on the inpatient unit, telling staff and patients alike that she is "the luckiest patient because (she has) the best nurse in the hospital." The rest of the team understand that this comment is an exaggeration. After days of constant dramatic praise for the nurse, with subtle insults to the rest of the staff, some members of the team may start to become annoyed. A similar scenario can occur if the patient constantly complains about one staff member. Staff may be torn between defending and criticizing the targeted staff member.

EVIDENCE-BASED PRACTICE

Borderline Friends?

Problem

Intense and unstable interpersonal relationships are foundational in borderline personality disorder. Relationships are characterized by extremes of idealization to devaluation. A deficit in supportive and close friendships may serve to maintain the disorder.

Purpose of Study

To examine the nature of stability of social networks among women with borderline personality disorder.

Methods

Characteristics of relationships—satisfaction, support, closeness, conflict, and criticism—were assessed in 27 women with borderline personality disorder and 23 healthy controls over a 6-month period.

Key Findings

- Compared with healthy controls, people with borderline personality disorder had undergone significant changes in relationships and relationships that had been "cut off."
- Relationships of women in the borderline personality disorder group were perceived as more unstable than those of the control group.
- Women in the control group had more stability in relationships with frequent interactions and less stability in relationships with limited interactions.
- Women with borderline personality disorder had more instability in satisfaction in relationships with more interaction.

Implications for Nursing Practice

This study provides additional evidence that people with borderline personality disorder have problems with interpersonal relationships. An intervention that could be used is to review the characteristics used in the study as an exercise and discussion. The terms satisfaction, support, closeness, conflict, and criticism can be used to evaluate the quality of interactions with others.

Lazarus, S. A., Beeney, J. E., Howard, K. P., Strunk, D. R., Pilkonis, P. A., & Cheavens, J. S. (2019). Characterization of relationship instability in women with borderline personality disorder: A social network analysis. *Personality Disorders: Theory, Research, and Treatment, 11*(5), 312–320.

ASSESSMENT GUIDELINES

Borderline Personality Disorder

1. Assess for suicidal or violent thoughts toward others. If these are present, the patient will need immediate attention.
2. Determine whether the patient has a medical disorder or another psychiatric disorder (especially a substance use disorder) that may be responsible for the symptoms.
3. View the assessment about personality functioning from within the person's ethnic, cultural, and social background.
4. Has the patient experienced a recent important loss? Borderline personality disorder is often exacerbated after the loss of significant supporting people or in a disruptive social situation.
5. Evaluate for a change in personality in middle adulthood or later, which signals the need for a thorough medical workup or assessment for unrecognized substance use disorder.

Clinical supervision and additional education are helpful and supportive to staff on the front lines of care. Awareness and monitoring of one's own stress responses to patient behaviors facilitate more effective and therapeutic intervention regardless of the specific approach to patient care.

NURSING DIAGNOSIS

People with borderline personality disorder are usually admitted to psychiatric treatment programs because of symptoms of comorbid disorders or dangerous behavior. Emotions such as anxiety, rage, and depression and behaviors such as withdrawal, paranoia, and manipulation are among the most frequent problems that healthcare workers must address.

The nursing diagnosis *risk for self-mutilation* is most often associated with this disorder. Self-mutilation involves deliberate self-injurious behavior that causes tissue damage. The intent of this behavior is to attain relief of tension. Other nursing diagnoses directly relevant to borderline personality disorder are *risk for suicide, risk for violence, social isolation, impaired socialization, disturbed personal identity,* and *impaired coping.*

OUTCOMES IDENTIFICATION

Outcomes are established for individuals with borderline personality disorder based on the perspective that personality change occurs with one behavior change and one learned skill at a time. This can be expected to take a lot of time and repetition. In the acute-care setting, the focus is on the presenting problem, which may be depression or severe anxiety. Healthcare providers do not expect resolution of chronic behavior problems during an acute hospital stay.

Outcomes should address immediate problems based on reversing the problems identified in the nursing diagnosis. Therefore, *risk for self-mutilation* is accompanied by the outcome of *no mutilation* and *risk for suicide* is addressed with *no suicide.*

Table 24.1 lists common signs and symptoms associated with borderline personality disorder; it suggests nursing diagnoses and identifies potential outcomes.

PLANNING

A therapeutic relationship is essential with patients who have borderline personality disorder because most of them have experienced failed relationships, including therapeutic alliances. Their distrust and hostility can be a setup for failure. When patients blame and attack others, the nurse needs to understand the context of their complaints. These attacks originate from the feeling of being threatened. The more intense the complaints are, the greater the patient's fear of potential harm or loss. Be aware of manipulative behaviors such as flattery, seductiveness, and instilling guilt. The following case study presents a patient with borderline personality disorder.

TABLE 24.1 Signs and Symptoms, Nursing Diagnoses, and Outcomes for Borderline Personality Disorder

Signs and Symptoms	Nursing Diagnoses	Outcomes
History of suicide attempts, family history of self-destructive behavior, disturbed interpersonal relationships, isolation, impulsivity, manipulation to obtain nurturing relationships	Risk for suicide	No suicide: Patient remains free from harm, maintains healthy connections, maintains control without supervision, uses social support group, plans for the future
History of self-mutilation, impulsivity, biting, cuts on body, ingestion of harmful substances, inhalation of harmful substances, insertion of object into body orifice, picking at wounds, scratches on body, self-inflicted burns	Self-mutilation	No self-mutilation: Patient refrains from intentional self-inflicted injury, maintains self-control without supervision, obtains assistance as needed, uses support groups, follows treatment regimen
Impulsivity, history of other-directed violence, threats	Risk for violence	No violence: Expresses needs in a constructive manner, monitors anger, maintains self-control without supervision
Behavior unaccepted by dominant cultural group, hypersensitivity to negative evaluation, unstable relationships, reports feeling rejected, experiences feelings of difference from others, inability to achieve a sense of social engagement, intense and unstable relationships	Social isolation Impaired socialization	Exhibits receptiveness and sensitivity to others, cooperates with others, uses assertive behaviors as appropriate, interacts with others
Dependency, excessive emotional responses, attention-seeking behavior, reports feeling emptiness, uncertainty about goals, uncertain boundaries with others	Disturbed personal identity	Improved personal identity: Verbalizes clear sense of personal identity, performs social roles, challenges negative images of self, establishes personal boundaries, maintains awareness of thoughts and feelings
Difficulty in relationships, manipulation, destructive behavior toward others and self, inability to meet role expectations, inadequate problem solving, uses self-mutilation to calm self and summon nurturing	Difficulty coping	Improved coping: Uses effective coping strategies, expresses emotion, seeks emotional support, uses strategies to promote safety, takes responsibility for own actions, identifies community resources, obtains support, self-initiates goal-directed behavior

International Council of Nursing. (2019). ICNP browser. Retrieved from https://www.icn.ch/what-we-do/projects/ehealth/icnp-browser. ICNP is owned and copyrighted by the International Council of Nurses (ICN). Reproduced with permission of the copyright holder.

CASE STUDY AND NURSING CARE PLAN

Borderline Personality Disorder

Brianna Drake is a 24-year-old administrative assistant; she is single and lives alone. She has been seen in the emergency department several times for superficial suicide attempts. Now she has been admitted because she has cut her wrists, ankles, and labia with glass and has lost a lot of blood. This event was precipitated by her graduation from a community college. Brianna states, "I feel empty inside."

Upon admission, she is found to be sweet, serene, and grateful to all the nurses, calling them "angels of mercy." Within a week, she is angry at half of the nurses and demands a new primary nurse, saying that the one she has (to whom she had grown attached) hates her.

Brianna has a history of heavy drinking and has managed to sneak alcohol onto the unit. She has been found in bed with a young male patient. She continually breaks unit rules and then pleads to have the behavior forgiven and forgotten. When angry, she threatens to cut herself again. She appears restless and tense and often asks for antianxiety medication several times a shift. When asked what she is anxious about, she says, "Uh ... don't know... I feel so empty inside." Brianna frequently paces up and down the halls, looking angry.

Self-Assessment

Salma is a recent graduate and is Brianna's primary nurse. After the first week of working with Brianna, Salma is discouraged and dreads coming in to work. She confides to Nancy, a coworker with 20 years of experience, that Brianna "just knows how to get under my skin." The two nurses discuss the biological basis of borderline personality disorder and treatment principles. Nancy also suggests that a team meeting be held to evaluate the plan of care and to focus on consistent limit-setting among the staff.

Assessment

Subjective Data

- History of superficial suicide attempts
- History of heavy drinking
- Recent graduate from a community college
- States, "I feel empty inside"
- Calls nurses "angels of mercy"
- Requests a new primary nurse because current nurse hates her
- When angry threatens to cut herself
- Asks for antianxiety medication several times a shift

Objective Data

- Has cuts on wrists, ankles, and labia
- Was calm on admission
- Sneaked alcohol onto the unit
- Found in bed with a male patient
- Breaks unit rules
- Is restless and tense
- Paces with an angry expression

CASE STUDY AND NURSING CARE PLAN—cont'd
Borderline Personality Disorder

Priority Diagnosis
Difficulty coping related to inadequate psychological resources, as evidenced by self-destructive behaviors

Outcomes Identification
Patient will consistently demonstrate the use of effective coping strategies.

Planning
The initial plan is to maintain patient safety and to encourage verbalization of feelings and impulses instead of action.

Implementation
Brianna's plan of care is personalized as follows:
Outcome criteria: Patient will consistently demonstrate the use of effective coping strategies.

Short-Term Goal	Intervention	Rationale	Evaluation
Brianna will consistently demonstrate a decrease in stress as evidenced by talking about her feelings with staff every day and without acting-out behaviors.	1. Encourage verbalization of feelings, perceptions, and fears. 2. Support the use of appropriate defense mechanisms.	1. Discussing and understanding the dynamics of frustration can reduce frustration by helping the patient take positive action. 2. Discussing and understanding the meaning of defenses can help to reduce the potential for acting out.	**GOAL MET** Brianna was able to experience problems and deal with them appropriately. Acting out was minimal or absent. *Example:* Brianna had an appointment for a job interview. She wanted to stay in bed and avoid the interview, but instead she talked with the nurse about her fear of "growing up" and was able to get up and go to the interview.

Evaluation
See individual outcomes and evaluation in the care plan.

IMPLEMENTATION

People with borderline personality disorder are impulsive and may be suicidal, self-mutilating, aggressive, manipulative, and even psychotic during periods of stress. Provide clear and consistent boundaries and limits. Use straightforward communication. When behavioral problems emerge, calmly review the therapeutic goals.

A useful approach for patients with borderline personality disorder relates to the response to superficial self-destructive behaviors. Acting in accordance with unit policies, the nurse remains neutral and dresses the patient's self-inflicted wounds in a matter-of-fact manner. Then the patient is instructed to write down the sequence of events leading up to the injuries, as well as the consequences, before staff will discuss the event. This cognitive exercise encourages the patient to think independently about her behavior instead of merely ventilating her feelings. It facilitates the discussion with staff about alternative actions.

Teamwork and Safety

When individuals with borderline personality disorder are admitted to the hospital, partially hospitalized, or in day treatment settings, team management is a significant part of treatment. The primary goal is management of the patient's affect in a group context. Community meetings, coping skills groups, and socializing groups are all helpful for these patients. They have the opportunity to interact with peers and staff to discuss goals and learn problem-solving skills. Dealing with emotional issues that arise in the milieu requires a calm, united approach by the staff to maintain safety and to enhance self-control.

Common problems resulting from staff splitting can be minimized if the unit leaders hold weekly staff meetings in which staff members are allowed to ventilate their feelings about conflicts with patients and each other. Consistency and a team approach help to ensure productive use of therapeutic time and structure for the patient. Patient-centered approaches allow the patient to be part of the treatment planning.

EVALUATION

Evaluating treatment effectiveness in this patient population is difficult. Freedom from harm to self and others is a tangible and satisfying positive evaluation. Nurses may never know the real results of their intervention, particularly in acute-care settings. Even in long-term outpatient treatment, patients with borderline personality disorder experience too many disruptions to relationships to remain long enough for successful treatment. As noted earlier, however, some motivated patients may be able to learn to change their behavior, especially if positive experiences are repeated.

Each therapeutic experience offers an opportunity for self-observation during interactions with caregivers who consistently and reliably try to teach positive coping skills. Specific short-term outcomes may be achieved and, overall, the patient can be given the message of hope that the quality of one's life can always be improved.

TREATMENT MODALITIES

Biological Treatments

Pharmacotherapy

In the United States, there are no medications specifically approved by the FDA for treating borderline personality disorder. This means that prescribers must use the medications off-label until evidenced-based pharmacotherapies are proven to be safe and effective.

Psychotropic medications geared toward maintaining patients' cognitive function, symptom relief, and improved quality of life are available. People with borderline personality disorder often respond to antidepressants such as SSRIs, anti-convulsants, and lithium for symptoms of mood and emotional dysregulation. Naltrexone (Revia, Vivitrol), an opioid receptor antagonist, has been found to reduce self-injurious behaviors. Second-generation antipsychotics may control anger and brief episodes of psychosis.

Psychological Therapies

Advanced practice nurses are likely to interact with staff members regarding the treatment of individuals with borderline personality disorders as part of their practice and clinical supervision responsibilities. The advanced practice nurse may assist staff members in engaging these patients in a therapeutic relationship.

Advanced practice psychiatric–mental health registered nurses are often the clinical leaders in providing individual and group psychotherapy. There are three essential therapies for borderline personality disorder:

1. **Cognitive behavioral therapy (CBT):** CBT can help individuals to identify and change inaccurate core perceptions of themselves and others and relationship problems. CBT may result in a reduction of mood and anxiety symptoms and reduce the number of self-harming or suicidal behaviors.
2. **Dialectical behavior therapy (DBT):** DBT is an evidence-based therapy developed by Linehan (1993) to treat chronically suicidal individuals with borderline personality disorder. DBT combines cognitive and behavioral techniques with *mindfulness*, which emphasizes being aware of one's thoughts and actively shaping them.

   The goals of DBT are to increase the patient's ability to manage distress and improve interpersonal effectiveness skills. Treatment focuses on behavioral targets, beginning with the identification of and interventions for suicidal behaviors and then progressing to a focus on interrupting destructive behaviors (Fig. 24.1).
3. **Schema-focused therapy:** Schema-focused therapy combines parts of CBT with other forms of therapy that focus on the ways that individuals view themselves. This reframing of "schemas" is based on the notion that borderline personality disorder is the result of a dysfunctional self-image, probably brought about by a dysfunctional childhood. This dysfunctional self-image affects how individuals respond to stress, react to their environment, and interact with others.

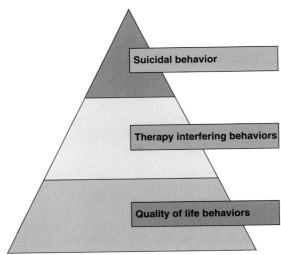

Fig. 24.1 Dialectical behavior therapy treatment targets.

ANTISOCIAL PERSONALITY DISORDER

Clinical Picture

This section focuses on a cluster B personality disorder that has a significant social impact. **Antisocial personality disorder** is a pattern of disregard for the rights of others and their frequent violation. People with this disorder may be more commonly referred to as sociopaths. This diagnosis is reserved for adults, but symptoms are evident by the midteens. Symptoms tend to peak during the late teenage years and into the mid-20s. By around 40 years of age, the symptoms may abate and improve even without treatment.

The main pathological traits that characterize antisocial personality disorder are antagonistic behaviors such as being deceitful and manipulative for personal gain or hostile if one's needs are blocked. The disorder is also characterized by disinhibited behaviors such as risk taking, disregard for responsibility, and impulsivity. Criminal misconduct and substance misuse are common in this population.

People with this disorder are mostly concerned with gaining personal power or pleasure; in relationships they focus on their own gratification to an extreme. They have little to no capacity for intimacy and, in relationships, will exploit others if it benefits them. One of the most disturbing qualities associated with antisocial personality disorder is a profound lack of empathy, also known as **callousness**. This results in a lack of concern about the feelings of others, the absence of remorse or guilt except in the face of punishment, and a disregard for meeting school, family, and other obligations.

These individuals tend to exhibit a shallow, unexpressive, and superficial affect. They may also be adept at portraying themselves as concerned and caring if these attributes help them to manipulate and exploit others. A person with antisocial personality disorder may be able to act witty and charming and be good at flattery and manipulating the emotions of others. The following box, based on the *DSM-5*, lists the criteria for antisocial personality disorder.

DSM-5 CRITERIA FOR ANTISOCIAL PERSONALITY DISORDER

A. A pervasive pattern of disregard for and violation of the rights of others, occurring since age 15 years, as indicated by three (or more) of the following:

1. Failure to conform to social norms with respect to lawful behaviors, as indicated by repeatedly performing acts that are grounds for arrest
2. Deceitfulness, as indicated by repeated lying, use of aliases, or conning others for personal profit or pleasure
3. Impulsivity or failure to plan ahead
4. Irritability and aggressiveness, as indicated by repeated physical fights or assaults.
5. Reckless disregard for safety of self or others
6. Consistent irresponsibility, as indicated by repeated failure to sustain consistent work behavior or honor financial obligations
7. Lack of remorse, as indicated by being indifferent to or rationalizing having hurt, mistreated, or stolen from another

B. The individual is at least 18 years of age.

C. There is evidence of conduct disorder with onset before age 15 years.

D. The features of antisocial behavior do not appear exclusively during the course of schizophrenia or bipolar disorder.

From the American Psychiatric Association. (2013). *Diagnostic and statistical manual of mental disorders* (5th ed.). Washington, DC: Author.

Epidemiology

Antisocial personality disorder is the most researched personality disorder, probably because of its marked impact on society in the form of criminal activity. The prevalence of antisocial personality disorder is between 0.2% and 3.3% (APA, 2013). The highest prevalence is among males with substance use disorders and in incarcerated individuals. Although the disorder is much more common in men, women may be underdiagnosed due to the traditional close association of this disorder with males.

Risk Factors

Biological Factors

Genetic. Antisocial personality disorder is genetically linked, and twin studies indicate a predisposition to this disorder. There are two main dimensions of genetic risk (Kendler et al., 2012). One is the trait of aggressive disregard, which refers to violent tendencies without concern for others; the other is the trait of disinhibition, which is a lack of concern for consequences.

Neurobiological. An alteration in serotonin transmission has been implicated with the aggression and impulsivity that frequently accompany this disorder. Levels of a metabolite of serotonin, 5-hydroxyindoleacetic acid, can be measured in urine and cerebrospinal fluid. It has been found to be lower in individuals with antisocial personality disorder. Lower levels of serotonin along with dopamine hyperfunction may contribute to aggression, disinhibition, and comorbid substance use (Seo et al., 2008).

Environmental Factors

It is likely that a genetic predisposition for characteristics of antisocial personality disorder such as a lack of empathy may be set into motion by childhood maltreatment. Inconsistent parenting and discipline, significant abuse, and extreme neglect are associated with this disorder. Children reflect parental attitudes and behaviors in the absence of more prosocial influences. Virtually all individuals who eventually develop this disorder have a history of impulse control and conduct problems as children and adolescents. Chapter 21 describes impulse control and conduct disorders in greater detail.

Cultural Factors

The assignment of a diagnosis of personality disorder cannot be entirely separated from the cultural context of both the individual and the person diagnosing. Cultural bias—including race, ethnicity, ageism, religion, and gender expectations—may unintentionally enter into the categorization. In a 2018 study, Hossain and colleagues found that the diagnosis of personality disorder was significantly less prevalent among blacks and other minority ethnic groups than among whites. They speculate that this underdiagnosis may be a form of reverse racism, where psychiatrists were reluctant to make a diagnosis of personality disorder owing to concerns that it might be perceived to be racist. Issues of access to care and treatment seeking were also cited as causes for low diagnosis among minorities.

> **VIGNETTE:** Richard is a 25-year-old divorced cab driver who was referred for psychiatric treatment by the court for competency evaluation after an assault charge. He told the arresting officer that he had bipolar disorder. He has a history of substance use and multiple arrests for disorderly conduct or assault. During his intake interview, he was polite and even flirtatious with the female psychiatric–mental health registered nurse. He insisted that he was not responsible for his behavior because he is manic. The only symptom he described was irritability. Richard pointed out that he cannot tolerate any psychotropic medications because of the side effects. He also noted that he had dropped out of three clinics after a few visits because "the staff don't understand me."

APPLICATION OF THE NURSING PROCESS

ASSESSMENT

People with antisocial personality disorder do not enter the healthcare system for treatment of their disorder unless they have been court ordered to do so. Psychiatric admissions may be initiated for anxiety and depression. Entering treatment may also be a way to avoid or address legal, financial, occupational, or other circumstances. Healthcare workers also encounter this population owing to the physical consequences of high-risk behaviors, such as acute injury and substance use. Questions asked during the assessment phase may not always result in accurate responses because the patient may become defensive or simply not tell the truth.

Self-Assessment

You may respond to a person with antisocial personality disorder in a variety of ways. Because these individuals have the capacity to be charming, you may want to defend the person as someone who is being unfairly treated and misunderstood. These feelings should be explored with your faculty or other experienced personnel. Conversely, if you are aware that your patient has a history of criminal acts, you may feel disdain or personally threatened. Again, share your concerns with individuals who are experienced in caring for this population. Awareness and monitoring of your own stress responses to patient behaviors facilitate more effective and therapeutic intervention.

📄 ASSESSMENT GUIDELINES

Antisocial Personality Disorder

1. Assess current life stressors
2. Assess for criminal history
3. Assess for suicidal, violent, and/or homicidal thoughts
4. Assess anxiety, aggression, and anger levels
5. Assess motivation for maintaining control
6. Assess for substance misuse (past and present)

NURSING DIAGNOSIS

Antisocial personality disorder presents a challenge for healthcare providers, who should consider the potential for disruption in psychiatric and medical-surgical settings. Diagnoses and nursing care plans should be geared toward maintaining safety and providing structure. Nursing diagnoses are focused on the protection of the patient and others from impulsive and premeditated acts and on improving coping skills.

The International Classification for Nursing Practice (International Council of Nurses, 2019) provides useful nursing diagnoses. The diagnoses with the most relevance to this disorder include *risk for violence, impaired impulse control*, and *impaired social interaction*.

OUTCOMES IDENTIFICATION

It is extremely difficult to achieve positive outcomes when one is working with a population with antisocial traits, but maintaining safety is the priority. Small incremental changes and progress will likely be the best outcomes. Outcomes will nullify or eliminate the problem described in the nursing diagnosis. Table 24.2 lists common signs and symptoms, nursing diagnoses, and outcomes for antisocial personality disorder.

PLANNING

Distrust, hostility, and a profound inability to connect with others will impair the usual process of developing a therapeutic relationship. In the context of antisocial personality disorder, the role of the nurse will be to provide consistency, support, boundaries, and limits. Providing realistic choices (e.g., selection of a particular group activity) may enhance adherence to treatment.

IMPLEMENTATION

People with antisocial personality disorder may be involuntarily admitted to psychiatric units for evaluation. With their freedom limited they tend to be angry, manipulative, aggressive, and impulsive. Try to prevent or reduce untoward effects of manipulation (flattery, seductiveness, instilling of guilt). Set clear and realistic boundaries and consequences and ensure that all staff follow limits. Carefully document behaviors and signs of manipulation. Be aware that antisocial patients can manipulate with feelings of guilt when they are not getting what they want.

Manipulative Behavior

Manipulation exists as an underlying current. Direct discussion of your concerns is the best approach. For example, you may address an undesirable behavior such as excessive flattery: "People enjoy hearing positive comments made by others about themselves. However, in the context of a nurse-patient relationship, these comments are not acceptable."

More severe sorts of manipulation, such as bullying the other patients and causing fear, should be addressed openly, along with consequences. This includes occurrences of undesired behavior or nonoccurrence of desired behavior. Depending on the setting, consequences can be in the form of rewards such as increased privileges or penalties such as the loss of privileges.

TABLE 24.2   Signs and Symptoms, Nursing Diagnoses, and Outcomes for Antisocial Personality Disorder

Signs and Symptoms	Nursing Diagnoses	Outcomes
Rigid posture, hyperactivity, pacing, history of child abuse, history of violence, violates rights of others, anger and aggression, impulsivity, substance misuse, negative role models	Risk for violence	No violence: Patient will not harm others, uses conflict resolution methods, controls impulses, expresses needs in a nondestructive manner, refrains from verbal outbursts, avoids violating others' personal space
Illegal behaviors, reckless behavior, acts before planning ahead, repeated fights, does not honor obligations	Impaired impulse control	Improved impulse control: Recognizes emotional cues to impulsivity, develops alternate coping strategies, takes responsibility for actions, obtains needed support, self-initiates goal-directed behavior
Unstable relationships, lacks empathy, projects hostility, shows behaviors unaccepted by dominant cultural group, grandiose, dysfunctional interactions, unaccepted social behavior	Impaired social interaction	Improved social interaction: Exhibits receptiveness, exhibits sensitivity to others, cooperates with others, interacts with others, exhibits consideration

International Council of Nursing Practice. (2019). *ICNP browser*. Retrieved from https://www.icn.ch/what-we-do/projects/ehealth/icnp-browser. ICNP® is owned and copyrighted by the International Council of Nurses (ICN). Reproduced with permission of the copyright holder.

Aggressive and Impulsive Behavior

Aggressive behavior usually has clues that it may be imminent; therefore, the best interventions are preventative. Assisting patients to recognize feelings of anger, their source, and identifying options for handling anger are a good first step. Seeking support from nursing staff provides external control and reassurance that staff will help keep the patient from losing control.

Therapeutic communication techniques are valuable tools for working with individuals with antisocial personality disorder. Simply being heard can defuse an emotionally charged situation. For example, the nurse can listen to a patient's emotional complaints about the staff and the hospital without correcting errors, simply noting that the patient truly feels hurt. Showing empathy may also decrease aggressive outbursts if the patient feels that staff members are trying to understand his feelings of frustration.

People with antisocial personality disorder can reduce their anxiety and anger through physical outlets. These outlets are typically limited in mental health facilities. In correctional settings there may be more options. In any case, walking is usually possible. Perhaps one-on-one interactions can be accomplished during a walk. Diversionary and therapeutic activities such as crafts and journal writing may be helpful in reducing impulsive angry responses. Chapter 27 more fully addresses the topics of anger, aggression, and violence.

Teamwork and Safety

The safety of patients and staff is a prime consideration in working with individuals in this population. To promote safety, the entire treatment team should follow a solid treatment plan that emphasizes realistic limits on specific behavior, consistency in responses, and consequences for actions. Careful documentation of behaviors will aid in providing effective interventions and in promoting teamwork.

EVALUATION

Evaluating treatment effectiveness in this patient population is difficult. Nurses may never know the real results of their interventions, particularly in acute-care settings. Even in long-term outpatient treatment, many patients with antisocial personality disorder find the relationship too intimate an experience to remain long enough for successful treatment. However, some motivated patients may be able to learn to change their behavior, especially if positive experiences are repeated.

Each therapeutic experience offers an opportunity for the patient to interact with caregivers, who consistently try to teach positive coping skills. Specific short-term outcomes may be accomplished, and overall, the patient can be given the message of hope that her quality of life can be improved.

TREATMENT MODALITIES

Biological Treatments

Pharmacotherapy

In the United States, there are no medications approved by the US Food and Drug Administration (FDA) specifically intended to treat antisocial personality disorder. This means that prescribers must use medications off label until evidence-based pharmacotherapies are proven to be safe and effective. People with antisocial personality disorder respond to mood-stabilizing medications such as lithium or valproic acid (Depakote) to help with aggression, depression, and impulsivity. SSRIs such as fluoxetine (Prozac) and sertraline (Zoloft) may be used to decrease irritability and help with anxiety and depression. Benzodiazepines may help with anxiety but should be used with caution because they are addictive. Methylphenidate (Ritalin) may help if there is a comorbidity of attention-deficit/hyperactivity disorder.

See Chapter 27 for a more detailed discussion of medications that target aggression.

Psychological Therapies

Psychotherapists, including advanced practice psychiatric–mental health registered nurses, encounter patients with antisocial personality disorders in a variety of inpatient and community settings. A more concentrated population of individuals with this disorder is obviously encountered by nurses who specialize in correctional nursing.

There is some evidence to suggest that people with antisocial traits do demonstrate an ability to bond with psychotherapists (Skodol, Bender, & Oldham, 2019). This bond can serve to improve their thinking and behaviors. Behavioral therapy is a basic approach that uses a system of rewards and punishment to promote positive behavior. CBT goes deeper and is useful in helping individuals to recognize sociopathic ways of thinking and then altering such behaviors. A specific form of CBT, mentalization behavioral therapy (MBT), is a long-term treatment that supports individuals' ability to recognize and understand their own and other people's mental states as well as to help them examine thoughts about themselves and others. Dialectical behavior therapy (DBT), which is similar to CBT, focuses on regulating emotions and being mindful; it is also useful in treating antisocial personality disorder.

Group therapy has the additional benefits of learning from others, supporting others, and feeling the camaraderie of working together. The therapies listed earlier can be delivered in a group format, either in person or online. There are specific groups, such as anger-management groups, that seek to support individuals with antisocial personality traits. Family therapy, both individual and group, is useful in supporting significant others and family members of people with antisocial personality disorder.

KEY POINTS TO REMEMBER

- All personality disorders share characteristics of inflexibility and difficulties in interpersonal relationships that impair social or occupational functioning.

- Personality disorders are most likely caused by a combination of biological and psychosocial factors.
- Patients with personality disorders often enter psychiatric treatment because of distress from a comorbid mental illness.

- Nurses may experience intense emotional reactions to patients with personality disorders and need to make use of clinical supervision to maintain objectivity.

- Despite the relatively fixed patterns of maladaptive behavior, some patients with personality disorders are able to change their behavior over time as a result of treatment.

CRITICAL THINKING

1. Mr. Beech is undergoing surgery for a broken leg. He is suspicious of the staff and believes that the intravenous medication he is receiving for hydration and preanesthesia will be used for harmful purposes. He keeps his eyes closed and refuses to answer or look at his family, who describe him as odd. He has schizotypal personality disorder.
   a. Explain how being friendly and outgoing may be threatening to Mr. Beech.
   b. Explain how being matter-of-fact and neutral and sticking to the facts would be effective to Mr. Beech.
   c. What could be done to give Mr. Beech some control over his situation as a hospitalized patient?
   d. How could you best handle his beliefs and lack of interpersonal comfort with caregivers so that both you and he would feel most comfortable?

2. Tiffany is brought to the emergency department after slashing her wrist with a razor. She has previously been in the emergency department for drug overdose and has a history of addictions. Tiffany can be sarcastic, belittling, and aggressive to those who try to care for her. When the psychiatric triage nurse comes in to see her, Tiffany is initially adoring and compliant, telling him, "You are the best nurse I've ever had, and I truly want to change." But when he refuses to support her request for diazepam (Valium) and meperidine (Demerol) for "pain," she yells at him, "You are a stupid excuse for a nurse. I want to see the doctor immediately." Tiffany has borderline personality disorder.
   a. What defense mechanism is Tiffany using?
   b. How could the nurse handle this situation while setting limits and demonstrating concern?

CHAPTER REVIEW

1. Which statement made by the psychiatric nurse demonstrates an accurate understanding of the factors that affect an individual's personality?
   a. "Therapy will help her identify that her problems are personality related."
   b. "I'll need to learn more about this patient's cultural beliefs."
   c. "It's encouraging to know that personality disorders respond well to treatment."
   d. "A person's personality is fluid and adjusts to current social situations."

2. When assessing a patient diagnosed with a borderline personality disorder, which statement by the patient warrants immediate attention?
   a. "My mother died ten years ago."
   b. "I haven't needed medication in weeks."
   c. "My dad never loved me."
   d. "I'd really like to hurt her for hurting me."

3. What is the current accepted professional view of the effect of culture on the development of a personality disorder?
   a. There are not enough studies to confirm the role that ethnicity and race have on the prevalence of personality disorders.
   b. The North American and Australian cultures produce higher incidences of personality disorders within their populations.
   c. Neither culture nor ethnic background is generally considered in the development of personality disorders.
   d. Personality disorders have been found to be primarily the products of genetic factors, not cultural factors.

4. Which personality disorders are generally associated with behaviors described as "odd or eccentric"? *Select all that apply.*
   a. Paranoid
   b. Schizoid
   c. Histrionic
   d. Obsessive-compulsive
   e. Avoidant

5. Which behaviors are examples of a primitive defense mechanism often relied upon by those diagnosed with a personality disorder? *Select all that apply.*
   a. Regularly attempts to split the staff
   b. Attempts to undo feelings of anger by offering to do favors
   c. Regresses to rocking and humming to sooth self when fearful
   d. Lashes out verbally when confronted with criticism
   e. Destroys another person's belongings when angry

6. Personality disorders often co-occur with mood and eating disorders. A young woman is undergoing treatment at an eating disorders clinic and her nurse suspects that she may also have a cluster B personality disorder because of her
   a. Desire to avoid eating
   b. Dramatic response to frustration
   c. Excessive exercise routine
   d. Morose personality traits

7. Larry is from a small town and began displaying aggressive and manipulative traits while still a teenager. Now 40 years old, Larry is serving a life sentence for the murders of his wife and her brother. John, the prison psychiatric nurse

practitioner, recognizes that Larry's treatment will most likely
a. Transform Larry to a model prisoner
b. Not improve Larry's coping skills
c. Reaffirm Larry's high-risk behaviors
d. Manifest as small incremental changes

8. Connor is a 28-year-old student, referred by his university for a psychiatric evaluation. He reports that he has no friends at the university and that people call him a loner. Connor has recently been "giving lectures" to pigeons at the university fountains. He is diagnosed as schizotypal, which differs from schizophrenia in that persons diagnosed as schizotypal
a. Can be made aware of their delusions
b. Are far more delusional than schizophrenics
c. Have a greater need for socialization
d. Do not usually respond to antipsychotic medications

9. Garret's wife of 8 years is divorcing him because their marriage never developed a warm or loving atmosphere. Garrett states in therapy, "I have always been a loner," and says that he was never concerned about what others think. The nurse practitioner suggests that Garrett try a trial of bupropion (Wellbutrin) to
a. Improve his flat emotions
b. Help him to get a good night's sleep
c. Increase the pleasure of living
d. Prepare Garrett for group therapy

10. Josie, a 27-year-old patient, complains that most of the staff do not like her. She says she can tell whether you are a caring person. Josie is unsure of what she wants to do with her life and her "mixed-up feelings" about relationships. When you tell her that you will be on vacation next week, she becomes very angry. Two hours later, she is found using a curling iron to burn her underarms and explains that it "makes the numbness stop." Given this presentation, which personality disorder would you suspect?
a. Obsessive-compulsive
b. Borderline
c. Antisocial
d. Schizotypal

1. **b**; 2. **d**; 3. **a**; 4. **a, b**; 5. **a, b, c**; 6. **b**; 7. **d**; 8. **a**; 9. **c**; 10. **b**

NGN CASE STUDY AND QUESTIONS

Natalie is a 33-year-old with borderline personality disorder who is being admitted to a psychiatric unit. She has a history of self-harm and most recently poured drain cleaner on her thighs. Other nonsuicidal self-injurious behavior includes cutting and

burning herself with cigarettes. She reports that her first psychiatric hospitalization was at the age of 8.

When asked about using the drain cleaner, Natalie asks for her partner to leave the room and tells the nurse, "Nobody listens. Nobody stays. I didn't want her to leave me." The patient also expresses "hating herself" and being "too ugly to love." She denies suicidal ideation and has no history of suicidal thoughts or actions.

Natalie is accompanied to the intake assessment by her partner, Lindsay, who pulls the registered nurse aside while Natalie is getting blood drawn. She said, "I think you should know that Natalie has been binge eating and engaging in risky behaviors such as thrill driving." Lindsay expresses her frustration, "One day she thinks I'm the best thing ever. The next day she despises me. I never know where I stand." The partner reports that Natalie has sudden outbursts of intense anger, disregard for personal boundaries, and extreme dependence on others. The partner says, "I can't be everything to her."

1. Choose the *most likely* options to complete the following statement.

In her relationship with her partner, Natalie displays ____1____ characterized by the ____2____ when she ____3____.

Options for 1	Options for 2	Options for 3
a. Grandiosity	a. Lack of empathy	a. Performs self-mutilation
b. Narcissism	b. Use of a defense mechanism	b. Expresses fear of abandonment
c. Avoidance	c. Sense of hopelessness	c. Sees her partner as all good or all bad
d. Splitting	d. Inflated sense of self	d. Engages in thrill-seeking behavior

2. The following are the nurse's own notes on today's observations. Identify the findings that support the diagnosis of borderline personality disorder. *Select all that apply.*
a. Idealizing and then hating the nurse
b. Unpredictable outbursts of frustration
c. Delusions of greatness
d. Auditory hallucinations
e. Swallowing nonfood substances
f. Chronic feelings of emptiness
g. History of unstable relationships

NGN case study answers are on Evolve.

Visit the Evolve website for a posttest on the content in this chapter: http://evolve.elsevier.com/Varcarolis

REFERENCES

American Psychiatric Association. (2013). *Diagnostic and statistical manual of mental disorders* (5th ed.). Washington, DC: Author.

Gunderson, J. G. (2011). Borderline personality disorder. *New England Journal of Medicine, 364*, 2037–2042.

Hossain, A., Malkov, M., Lee, T., & Bhui, K. (2018). Ethnic variation in personality disorder: Evaluation of 6 years of hospital admissions. *BJPsych Bulletin, 42*(4), 157–161.

International Council of Nurses. (2019). *International Classification for Nursing Practice catalog.* Retrieved from https://www.icn.ch/sites/default/files/inline-files/ICNP2019-DC.pdf.

James, W. (1892). *Psychology: The briefer course.* New York, NY: Henry Holt.

Kendler, K. S., Aggen, S. H., & Patrick, C. J. (2012). A multivariate twin study of the DSM-IV criteria for antisocial personality disorder. *Biological Psychiatry, 71*(3), 247–253.

Krause-Utz, A., Winter, D., Niedtfeld, I., & Schmah, C. (2014). The latest neuroimaging findings in borderline personality disorder. *Current Psychiatry Reports, 16*(438).

Linehan, M. M. (1993). *Cognitive behavioral treatment of borderline personality disorder.* New York, NY: Guilford.

Mahler, M. S., Pine, F., & Bergman, A. (1975). *The psychological birth of the human infant.* New York, NY: Basic Books.

McMahon, K., Hoertel, N., Peyre, H., Blanco, C., Fang, C., & Limosin, F. (2019). Age differences in DSM-IV borderline personality disorder symptom expression: Results from a national study using item response theory. *Journal of Psychiatric Research, 110*, 16–23.

Pennay, A., Cameron, J., Reichert, T., Strickland, H., Lee, N. K., Hall, K., et al. (2011). A systematic review of interventions for co-occurring substance use disorder and borderline personality disorder. *Journal of Substance Abuse Treatment, 41*, 363–373.

Ripoll, L. H., Triebwasser, J., & Siever, L. (2011). Evidence-based pharmacotherapy for personality disorders. *International Journal of Neuropsychopharmacology, 14*, 1257–1288.

Sansone, R. A., & Sansone, L. A. (2011). Gender patterns in borderline personality disorder. *Innovations in Clinical Neuroscience, 8*(5), 16–20.

Seo, D., Patrick, C. J., & Kennealy, P. J. (2008). Role of serotonin and dopamine system interactions in the neurobiology of impulsive aggression and its comorbidity with other clinical disorders. *Aggression and Violent Behavior, 13*(5), 383–395.

Shen, C. C., Hu, L. Y., & Hu, Y. H. (2017). Comorbidity study of borderline personality disorder: Applying association rule mining to the Taiwan national health insurance research database. *BMC Medical Informatics and Decision Making, 17*(1), 8.

Skodol, A. E., Bender, D. S., & Oldham, J. M. (2019). In L. W. Roberts (Ed.), Personality pathology and personality disorders. L.W. Roberts (Ed.), *Textbook of psychiatry* (6th ed.) (pp. 711–747). Washington, DC: American Psychiatric Association.

Skoglund, C., Tiger, A., Rück, C., Petrovic, P., Asherson, P., Hellner, & Kuja-Halkola, R. (2019). Familial risk and heritability of diagnosed borderline personality disorder: A register study of the Swedish population. *Molecular Psychiatry, 26*(3), 999–1008.

Volkert, J., Thorsten-Christian, G., & Rabung, S. (2018). Prevalence of personality disorders in the general adult population in Western countries: Systematic review and meta-analysis. *British Journal of Psychiatry, 26*(3), 999–1008.

25

Suicide and Nonsuicidal Self-Injury

Faye J. Grund

🌐 Visit the Evolve website for a pretest on the content in this chapter: http://evolve.elsevier.com/Varcarolis

OBJECTIVES

1. Define essential terms associated with suicide, including suicidal ideation, suicide attempt, suicide, and nonsuicidal self-injury.
2. Describe the growing problem of suicide in the United States.
3. Identify comorbid psychiatric disorders that accompany suicidality.
4. Discuss risk factors for the development of suicidal ideation and for suicide.
5. Identify evidence-based practice suicide risk assessment tools.
6. Discuss basic-level interventions to address suicidality in the hospital or in community settings.
7. Explain key elements of suicide precautions and environmental safety factors in the hospital.
8. Describe three expected reactions a nurse may experience when working with patients who have suicidal ideation.
9. Identify biological treatments and psychological therapies for patients with suicidal ideation.
10. Describe nonsuicidal self-injury in terms of the clinical picture, epidemiology, comorbidty, and risk factors.
11. Discuss nursing care for patients with nonsuicidal self-injury.
12. Identify biological treatments and psychological therapies for patients with nonsuicidal self-injury.

KEY TERMS AND CONCEPTS

cluster suicide
lethality
nonsuicidal self-injury (NSSI)
postvention

primary intervention
psychological autopsies
suicidal ideation
suicide

suicide attempt
suicide survivors

A tribute to Adam Hall on the first anniversary of his death from his loving mother, July 1, 2014:

Dearest Adam,

It's hard to believe that a year has gone by. The void created by your departure fills me with such emptiness... while echoes of your laughter linger... urging me and those whose lives you touched to press forward living life to the fullest, seizing and celebrating each moment.

I am so grateful to have been blessed with a son such as you. 26, almost 27 years were so fleeting a time. Over in what seems to have been a heartbeat. I purposed my life toward building your future, creating possibility in your life... 'living vicariously through you' (one of your favorite expressions).

So many questions remain. Golden moments flash across my mind, your warmth, your charm, the love you shared, the depth of your character, the contagious ardor with which you embraced your passions... impossible to capture in mere words.

You were loved, adored, and admired. You were so ardent and able. I was so proud of you and cherished you with all my being.

Love,

Mom

(Personal communication courtesy of Carolyn Bucklen)

SUICIDE

Suicide is devastating for those of us who lose a family member or friend. What brings a person to such a drastic and permanent solution to life's problems? As unimaginable as this act is to many of us, a human life ends by suicide every 11 minutes, leading to the loss of approximately 129 American lives daily (Centers for Disease Control and Prevention [CDC], 2019).

Suicide is largely preventable and should be considered a "never event." Yet too often, we direct efforts only toward individuals who are at immediate risk (Hogan & Grumet, 2016). In the year before their deaths, 83% of individuals were seen by a healthcare professional and 54% of those who died by suicide did not have a mental health diagnosis (Stone et al., 2018). Approximately 50% of patients who died by suicide made a healthcare visit within 1 month of their death. It is critical for healthcare providers to be advocates for this problem and to mobilize the community to reduce factors that may contribute to suicide.

Clinical Picture

An understanding of the clinical picture related to suicide can be achieved by first defining terminology that is used or not used to describe this topic. **Suicide** is death caused by self-directed injurious behavior with the intent to die as a result of the behavior (National Institute of Mental Health, 2019). In general, prior to taking any action, people contemplate the possibility of ending their lives. **Suicidal ideation** is thinking about death, including the wish to be dead, considering methods of accomplishing death, and formulating plans to carry the act out. A **suicide attempt**, also referred to as a suicidal act, is engaging in potentially self-injurious behavior with the intention of death. These attempts may result in death, injuries, or no injuries. Suicide is the intentional act of ending one's life by any means. A term with which most of us are familiar is "commit suicide." However, the use of that term is generally discouraged due to concerns of stigmatizing people with an association to a criminal act, such as committing a robbery or homicide.

The American Psychiatric Association's *Diagnostic and Statistical Manual of Mental Disorders*, 5th edition (DSM-5, 2013) provides clinicians with criteria to diagnose psychiatric disorders. A new condition, suicidal behavior disorder, was proposed for the DSM-5 in 2013. This proposal was controversial. Supporters for its inclusion believed that such a diagnosis would be a better way to identify and track individuals who are at greatest risk for suicide. Opponents argued that such a label was unnecessary since diagnosing associated conditions such as major depressive disorder already provided a way to identify and track risk. In the end, suicidal behavior disorder was voted down but was added to the manual in a section called conditions for further study.

The main criterion for suicidal behavior disorder is a suicide attempt within the last 24 months. Individuals with suicidal acts remain at higher risk for subsequent suicide attempts and death. The period after 12 months, but before 24 months, is considered to be in early remission. The DSM-5 (APA, 2013) specifies that the act could not be better identified as nonsuicidal self-injury, which will be discussed later. Suicidal behavior disorder does not include suicidal ideation or preparatory acts for suicide. Further, this condition is not diagnosed when suicidal behaviors occur as part of delirium, confusion, or for political or religious purposes.

In this chapter, we review facts about suicide, discuss assessment and care of patients who may be suicidal, and address the needs of patient's families. Another disorder that is also included in the conditions for further study in the DSM-5 (APA, 2013), nonsuicidal self-injury, is also discussed in this chapter.

Epidemiology

According to the CDC (2018) over 47,000 people died by suicide in 2017, making it the 10th leading cause of death in the United States. In 2017, suicide was the second leading cause of death for 10- to 34-year-olds, the fourth leading cause of death in 35- to 54-year-olds, and the eighth leading cause of death among 55- to 64-year-olds (CDC, 2017). However, the age-adjusted suicide rate from 1999 through 2017 has increased 33% (Hedegaard, Curtin, & Warner, 2018). Suicide rates among veterans were 1.5 times greater than among the US general population, after adjusting for age and gender (US Department of Veterans' Affairs, 2018). Box 25.1 provides some facts about suicide, including data for specific age groups.

The number of suicides may actually be double or triple to those reported due to underreporting. Purposefully crashing a car into a bridge abutment or overdosing on opioids may appear to be accidental. However, many reported accidents, poisonings, and deaths ruled on autopsy as undetermined are actually suicides.

Comorbidity

Psychiatric disorders are risk factors for suicide. Approximately 46% of people who die by suicide had previously been diagnosed with a mental illness (CDC, 2018). Major depressive disorder, substance use, and psychosis are the diagnoses most commonly associated with suicide. Approximately 50% of those who complete suicide are experiencing a major depressive episode at the time of death (Bradvik, 2018). Individuals diagnosed with anxiety, personality, eating, and trauma-related disorders are also at greater risk for suicide. Loss of relationships, financial difficulty, and impulsivity are also common precursors to suicide.

Ten years after diagnosis, about 10% of individuals diagnosed with schizophrenia die by suicide. By 30 years after diagnosis, the incidence of suicide increases to 15% (Goldberg, 2019). Suicidal ideation is often seen during the first few years of the illness. It is the leading cause of early death in this population. Twenty percent of patients diagnosed with schizophrenia will attempt suicide at least once. Individuals with a diagnosis of schizophrenia attempt suicide related to the depressive, negative symptoms rather than to command hallucinations or delusions.

Patients with substance use disorders, who use both legal and illicit substances, have a higher suicide risk. Many individuals who die by suicide have alcohol or other substances in their blood at the time of death and have used an illicit substance in the days before their death. Alcohol, a depressant, reduces inhibitions. Individuals who are otherwise ambivalent about whether to end their lives may act on suicidal thoughts. Opiates, including heroine and prescription painkillers, are present in 27% of deaths by suicide, and alcohol is present in 41% of deaths by suicide (CDC Morbidity and Mortality, 2018).

Risk Factors
Biological Factors
Genetic. Suicidal behavior may run in families. Margaux Hemingway's death in 1996 was the fifth suicide among four generations of writer Ernest Hemingway's (1899–1961) family. Twin and adoption studies suggest genetic factors in suicide. Concordance rates are higher among monozygotic (identical) twins than among dizygotic (fraternal) twins.

Studies stress the importance of both genetic and epigenetic (external gene altering) factors. Coon et al. (2018) found

BOX 25.1 Suicide Facts: 2017

General
- Suicide is the 10th leading cause of death for all ages.
- Substances are often associated with suicide. Toxicology tests of individuals who committed suicide in 16 states found that nearly 33% tested positive for alcohol, 10.2% for marijuana, 4.6% for cocaine, and 20% for opiates or prescription painkillers.
- Firearms were the most common method of death by suicide, accounting for a little more than half (50.57%) of all suicide deaths. The next most common methods were suffocation (including hangings) at 27.72% and poisoning at 13.89%.

Gender Statistics
- Men died by suicide 3.54 times more often than women. White males accounted for almost 70% of all suicide deaths.
- During their lifetime, women reported a suicide attempt 1.4 times as often as men.
- For males, the suicide rate increased by 26% between 1999 and 2017. Of significance, for females, the rate increased by 53% during the same time frame.

Racial and Ethnic Statistics
- Suicide rates increased from 1999 to 2017 for all race and ethnicity groups except for non-Hispanic Asian and Pacific Islander groups.
- Non-Hispanic American Indian or Alaska Natives had the highest suicide rates for both males and females in age groups from 15 to 44 years old in 2017.
- In 2017, the highest US age-adjusted suicide rate was among Whites (15.85 per 100,000).
- Hispanics and Latinos have the lowest suicide rates among all racial/ethnic groups in the United States.

Age Statistics
- In 2017, the highest suicide rate (20.2 per 100,000) was among adults between the ages of 45–54; the second highest rate occurred in individuals 85 years and over (20.1 per 100,000).
- Suicide is the second-leading cause of death among 10- to 14-year-olds, 15- to 24-year-olds, and 25- to 34-year-olds.
- Men ages 85 and older have the highest suicide rate of any age group in the United States.

Attempted Suicide
- Estimates indicate that in 2017 nearly 1.4 million adults aged 18 and older made a suicide attempt.
- In 2015, approximately 575,000 people were treated in emergency departments for self-inflicted injuries.
- Approximately 7.4% of youths in grades 9–12 reported a suicide attempt in the last 12 months.
- There is one suicide for every 25 attempted suicides.

Centers for Disease Control and Prevention. (2017). *Data and Statistics Fatal Injury Report for 2017*. Retrieved from https://webappa.cdc.gov/cgi-bin/broker.exe.

four genetic variants associated with suicide (*SP110*, *AGBL2*, *SUCLA2*, and *APH1B*).

Neurobiological. Low serotonin levels are related to depressed mood. Studies have found low levels of serotonin or its metabolites in the cerebrospinal fluid of patients who are suicidal. Postmortem examinations of individuals who die by suicide also reveal low levels of serotonin in the brainstem and/or the frontal cortex.

Cognitive Factors
Sigmund Freud originally theorized that suicide resulted from unacceptable aggression toward another person that is turned inward. Karl Menninger added to Freud's work by describing three aspects of suicidal hostility: the wish to kill (revenge), the wish to be killed (guilt), and the wish to die (hopelessness). Aaron Beck identified a central emotional factor underlying suicide intent: hopelessness. Cognitive styles that contribute to higher risk are rigid all-or-nothing thinking, inability to see different options, and perfectionism.

Environmental Factors
Family characteristics have been identified that increase the likelihood of suicide ideation and attempts in young children (Deville et al., 2020). Conflict within the family and neglect through low parental monitoring are associated with childhood suicidality. Adverse childhood experiences—including physical, sexual, and emotional abuse; parents in prison; and family history of suicidality—increase the risk for suicidal ideation and suicide attempts in adulthood by up to 2.7 times (Thompson et al., 2019).

The suicide of a relative, peer, idol, or public figure may result in cluster suicides, sometimes referred to as *contagion suicides* or *copycat suicides*. Clusters occur closer together in time and space than would normally be expected in a given community. They spiked even more among men and those who ended their lives, like Robin Williams, by suffocation (Fink et al., 2018). Adolescents are at especially high risk due to their immature prefrontal cortex, the portion of the brain that controls the executive functions involving judgment, frustration tolerance, and impulse control.

Cultural Factors
Cultural factors, including religious beliefs, family values, sexual orientation, gender identity, bullying behavior, and attitude toward death, have an impact on suicide rates. In the United States, between 1999 and 2017, age-adjusted suicide rates increased for all race and ethnicity groups except for non-Hispanic Asian or Pacific Islander groups. The largest increase was among non-Hispanic American Indian or Alaska Native, where since 1999 the incidence in women rose significantly more than for men (139% vs. 71%). In 100,000 people, the age-adjusted suicide rate was highest among whites (15.85), followed by American Indians and Alaska Natives (13.42), blacks (6.61), and Asians and Pacific Islanders (6.59) (Coon et al., 2018).

In the United States, black men die by suicide more often than black women, with a peak rate in young adulthood and middle age. Black students report a higher rate of suicide attempts (9.8%) compared to white students (6.1%). Protective factors include religion and the role of the extended family.

Among Hispanics, Catholicism, in which suicide is considered a sin, and the importance of the extended family decrease the risk for suicide. There is also the philosophy of *fatalismo*, a belief that divine providence regulates the world. This philosophy removes blame from the individual who is unable to control adverse events. Suicidal risk for recent Hispanic immigrants

CONSIDERING CULTURE

Underreported Death by Suicide in South Korea

Suicide rates in South Korea are reportedly the 10th highest in the world, but this ranking may actually be higher. This is partly due to the common practice of family members reporting cause of death and signing death certificates rather than medical providers or coroners. While noble motivations for suicide such as preserving one's honor and integrity or sending a political message are acceptable, purely personally motivated suicide is considered shameful. The cultural norm of *filial piety* is strongly held by South Korean families and children are taught to respect parents and ancestors. Suicide breaks the sacred cultural rule of familism, usurping the authority of parents and desecrating ancestors. Thus, stigma extends beyond the one who died to the family due to their inability to foster appropriate values to their child.

The government may soon require that death certificates be completed by medical personnel or the coroner. This will help to more accurately identify the prevalence of suicide, the methods used in suicide, and support the implementation of suicide reduction initiatives. At the same time, the government needs to respect the cultural norms associated with familism. A stigma reduction program may be foundational as South Korea addresses this problem.

Adapted from Im, S. J., Ben Park, B., & Ratcliff, K. (2018). Cultural stigma manifested in official suicide death in South Korea. *Journal of Death and Dying, 77*(4), 386–403.

TABLE 25.1   Factors Contributing to Deaths by Suicide

Factors Contributing to Deaths by Suicide	Percentage Present Upon Review (%)
Relationship problem	42
Crisis in the past or upcoming 2 weeks	29
Problematic substance use	28
Physical health problem	22
Job/financial problem	16
Criminal legal problem	9
Loss of housing	4

From CDC's National Violent Death Reporting System. (2018). *Many factors contribute to suicide among those with and without mental health conditions.* Retrieved from https://www.cdc.gov/vitalsigns/suicide/infographic.html#graphic3.

includes not understanding the US healthcare system, fear of being deported, and language barriers. The risk for immigrants to the United States becomes higher the longer they live in the States (CDC, 2017).

Protective factors among Asians include adherence to religions that emphasize interdependence between the individual and society, making self-destruction disrespectful to the group and selfish. However, suicide may be preferable if it prevents bringing shame to the family. Death by suicide may be viewed as a potentially honorable solution to life problems, such as financial difficulty, for older adults in this population.

Social Factors

Humans are social beings that have evolved by banding together, yet we are increasingly isolated. Texting has replaced talking on the phone. People drive to work alone. Suburbanites frequently do not know their neighbors. Urban dwellers know that making eye contact or talking to strangers is a taboo. Isolation sets the stage for loneliness and despair. Table 25.1 identifies social factors that contribute to deaths by suicide.

Social media have led to the rapid spread of messages about suicide, both positive and negative. Stories regarding individuals who overcame a suicidal crisis can be inspirational and instill hope. On the negative side, social media groups can be harmful and even deadly. For example, the Blue Whale suicide game moderators ask young people to take on a series of challenges that end with them eventually killing themselves. An Instagram post with specific references to suicide, suicide methods, emotional states, and death wishes using explicit pictures spread rapidly (Arendt, 2019). Following the post, suicides increased in several countries.

The impact of social media on suicide prevention is worthy of further study. Some media outlets allow you to report suicidal content and to offer help for the person who posted it. Many of the sites utilize analytical capabilities to identify and help report suicidal posts. The Crisis Text Line (2019) allows individuals in crisis to directly text a counselor for help. The group collects data and provides open access of aggregate data from texters. This data includes:

- About 75% of the texters are younger than 25
- 9% of texts come from the 10% lowest-income zip codes
- 6% of texters report they are Native American and 14% are Latino/Hispanic
- 21% who text about anxiety and stress also identify thoughts of suicide

In a more formal way, society regulates a specific suicide, namely, assisted suicide. In the United States, individual states have the authority to regulate, allow, or prohibit assisted suicide. Six states currently have laws in place, including California, Colorado, Montana, Oregon, Vermont, and Washington State. Increasingly, states are considering cases to determine the legality of assisted suicide. Other countries, including the Netherlands, Belgium, Switzerland, Columbia, and Canada, have laws in place allowing physician-assisted suicide. The ethical and moral dilemmas in this evolving trend are clear.

Another societal concern is suicide bombing, which has grown exponentially since September 11, 2001. Academic researchers and policy makers have identified that suicide terror results from interactive factors at the individual, organizational, and societal levels (Harmon et al., 2018).

Other Risk Factors

Risk factors for suicide include the following (CDC Violence Prevention, 2019):

- Family history of suicide
- Family history of child maltreatment (adverse childhood events)
- Previous suicide attempt(s)
- History of mental disorders, particularly clinical depression
- History of alcohol and substance use disorders

- Feelings of hopelessness
- Impulsive or aggressive tendencies
- Cultural and religious beliefs (e.g., belief that suicide is a noble resolution of a personal dilemma)
- Local epidemics of suicide
- Isolation, a feeling of being cut off from other people
- Barriers to accessing mental health treatment
- Loss (relational, social, work, or financial)
- Physical illness; those individuals who have chronic illnesses are at increased risk of suicide. Loss of mobility, disfigurement, and chronic pain are especially associated with suicide.
- Easy access to lethal methods
- Unwillingness to seek help because of the stigma attached to mental health and substance use disorders or to suicidal thoughts

Extensive data are available about risk factors for suicide based on epidemiological studies and psychological autopsies (i.e., retrospective reviews of the deceased person's life within several months of death to establish likely diagnoses at the time of death). There is also evidence concerning protective factors (those that tend to reduce risk). Box 25.2 provides a description of significant psychosocial risk and protective factors for suicide.

APPLICATION OF THE NURSING PROCESS

Suicide risk assessment is based on identifying specific risk and protective factors, taking a psychosocial and health history, and establishing a therapeutic relationship with the patient during the interview. The nurse usually completes this assessment in conjunction with other clinicians because comparison of data and impressions from two or more interviewers can result in a more comprehensive evaluation.

ASSESSMENT

Assessment tools are helpful in providing a baseline evaluation that can be compared over time. One assessment tool that encompasses both risk and protective factors, provides the clinician with a tool to benchmark risk, and suggests interventions is the Suicide Assessment Five-Step Evaluation and Triage (SAFE-T). This tool was established based on sponsored research outcomes from the Substance Abuse and Mental Health Services Administration. A free pocket guide can be downloaded from http://store.samhsa.gov/product/SMA09-4432. The tool allows the clinician to benchmark relative risk (high, moderate, low) and to develop a treatment plan, in consultation with the patient, to reduce current risk. Another tool that has proven useful for assessment and widely utilized is the Columbia-Suicide Severity Rating Scale (C-SSRS) (Substance Abuse and Mental Health Services Administration, 2014).

Verbal and Nonverbal Clues

Individuals considering suicide usually provide some clues to their intent, especially to people who are supportive of them,

---

BOX 25.2 Suicide Warning Factors, Risk Factors, and Protective Factors

Warning Factors (immediate risk of suicide)
- Often talking or writing about death, dying, or suicide
- Making comments about being hopeless, helpless, or worthless
- Expressions of having no reason for living; no sense of purpose in life; saying things like "It would be better if I wasn't here" or "I want out"
- Increased alcohol and/or drug misuse
- Withdrawal from friends, family, and community
- Reckless behavior or more risky activities, seemingly without thinking
- Dramatic mood changes
- Talking about feeling trapped or being a burden to others

Risk Factors (characteristics that make it more likely that an individual will consider, attempt, or die by suicide)
- Previous suicide attempt(s)
- A history of suicide in the family
- Substance use
- Mood disorders (depression, bipolar disorder)
- Access to lethal means (e.g., keeping firearms in the home)
- Losses and other events (e.g., the breakup of a relationship or a death, academic failures, legal difficulties, financial difficulties, bullying)
- History of trauma or abuse
- Chronic physical illness including chronic pain
- Exposure to the suicidal behavior of others

Protective Factors (characteristics that make it less likely that individuals will consider, attempt, or die by suicide)
- Effective mental healthcare; easy access to a variety of clinical interventions
- Strong connections to individuals, family, community, and social institutions
- Marriage, having children
- Problem-solving and conflict resolution skills
- Contact with providers (e.g., follow-up phone call from healthcare professional)

American Psychiatric Association. (2018). *Suicide prevention.* Retrieved from http://www.psychiatry.org/patients-families/suicide-prevention.

---

such as nurses. These clues come in the form of open messages, also known as overt statements, or in a concealed manner, known as covert statements. Additionally, the nurse should teach family members and other support people in the community regarding these statements that may indicate risk. Examples include the following:

Overt Statements
- "I can't take it anymore."
- "Life isn't worth living anymore."
- "I wish I were dead."
- "Everyone would be better off if I died."

Covert Statements and Nonverbal Clues
- "It's okay now. Soon everything will be fine."
- "Things will never work out."
- "I won't be a problem much longer."
- "Nothing feels good to me anymore and probably never will."
- "How can I give my body to medical science?"

Most often, it is a relief for people contemplating suicide to finally talk to someone about their despair and loneliness. Asking about suicidal thoughts does not give people the idea to end their life by suicide. Asking is, in fact, a professional responsibility similar to asking about chest pain in cardiac conditions. Talking openly leads to a decrease in isolation and can increase problem-solving alternatives for living. People who contemplate suicide, attempt suicide, and even those who regret the failure of their attempt are often extremely receptive to talking about their suicide crisis. Specific questions to ask about suicidal ideation include the following:

- Have you ever felt that life was not worth living?
- Have you been thinking about death recently?
- Do you ever think about suicide?
- Have you ever attempted suicide?
- Do you have a plan for ending your life?
- If so, what is your plan for suicide?

The following dialogue illustrates how the nurse can make covert messages more open:

Nurse: You haven't eaten or slept well for the past few days, Theresa.

Theresa: No, I feel pretty low lately.

Nurse: How low are you feeling?

Theresa: Oh, I don't know. Nothing seems to matter to me anymore. It's all so meaningless…

Nurse: Tell me about it, Theresa. I want to understand how you're feeling. What is meaningless?

Theresa: Life…the whole thing…nothingness. Life is a bad joke.

Nurse: Are you saying you don't think life is worth living?

Theresa: Well…yes. It's all so hopeless anyway.

Nurse: Are you thinking of ending your life?

Theresa: Oh, I don't know. Well, sometimes I think about it. I probably would never go through with it.

Nurse: Theresa, let's talk more about what you're thinking and feeling. This is important. I'll need to share your thoughts with other members of the staff.

The nurse should be alert for nonverbal behavioral clues, including showing a sudden brightening of mood with more energy (especially after recently being prescribed an antidepressant medication), giving away possessions, writing letters, or organizing financial affairs. Individuals may be at greater risk as their mood lifts because they have enough energy to act on their feelings of ambivalence regarding suicide.

Establishing a therapeutic relationship with the patient and asking directly about suicidal feelings are essential elements of the nurse-patient relationship. Asking about suicidal ideation is the single most important assessment (and intervention). Possible reasons for hesitancy in screening include lack of personal comfort, lack of professional confidence, and time constraints. Crisis intervention techniques involve listening for the emotional feeling message underlying the verbal message, especially when the patient presents as angry, hostile, and overwhelmed. The therapeutic alliance established with a patient is a dynamic, changeable interaction. Thus, you should be constantly assessing and documenting it.

Lethality of Suicide Plan

The evaluation of a suicide plan is extremely important in determining the degree of suicidal risk. There are three main elements to consider when evaluating lethality: (1) Is there a specific plan with details? (2) How lethal is the proposed method? (3) Is there access to the planned method? People who have definite plans for the time, place, and means are at highest risk.

Based on the lethality of a method, which indicates how quickly a person would die by that mode, you can classify the method as higher or lower risk. Higher-risk methods, also referred to as *hard methods*, include:

- Using a gun
- Jumping off a high place
- Hanging
- Poisoning with carbon monoxide
- Staging a car crash

Examples of lower-risk methods, also referred to as *soft methods*, include:

- Cutting wrists
- Inhaling natural gas
- Ingesting pills

When the patient confirms access to the proposed method, the situation is more serious. A man who has access to a high building and states that he will jump from it or a woman who has a gun and says that she will shoot herself is at serious risk for suicide. When people are experiencing psychotic episodes, they are also at high risk—regardless of the specificity of details—because impulse control and judgment are grossly impaired. A person suffering psychosis is particularly vulnerable when depressed or having command hallucinations.

Self-Assessment

Healthcare professionals working with individuals who have suicidal ideation need collaboration with other clinicians. Fear, grief, anger, puzzlement, and condemnation of suicidal feelings and intent are common emotions experienced. If these intense emotional responses are not acknowledged, countertransference may limit effective intervention. Understanding the patient with suicidal behavior disorder,

📄 ASSESSMENT GUIDELINES

Suicide

1. Assess risk factors, including history of suicide (in family, friends), degree of hopelessness and helplessness, and lethality of plan.
2. Assess protective factors that may be built upon.
3. If there is a history of suicide attempt, assess intent, lethality, and injury; determine whether the patient's age, medical condition, psychiatric diagnosis, or current medications put the patient at higher risk.
4. A change from sad or depressed to happy and peaceful may be a red flag. Often, an individual's decision to end their life by suicide gives a feeling of relief and calm.
5. Always assess social supports and helpfulness of significant others, particularly if you need to manage the patient on an outpatient basis.

TABLE 25.2   Signs and Symptoms, Nursing Diagnoses, and Outcomes for a Patient With Suicidal Ideation

Signs and Symptoms	Potential Nursing Diagnoses	Outcomes
Gives overt or covert clues (e.g., "I can't stand the pain"), has a plan (gun), is in high-risk category on assessment (elderly or teenager, isolated, depressed, had a recent loss), has a psychiatric diagnosis (substance use, depression, borderline personality disorder, anorexia nervosa, or psychosis)	*Risk for suicide*	Remains free from injury, expresses will to live, discloses plan for suicide if present, refrains from attempting suicide
Overwhelmed with situational crises, relies heavily on drugs or alcohol, has few supportive systems, shows poor problem-solving skills	*Impaired coping*	Identifies coping mechanisms to assist with situational crisis; identifies social support within community
Lacks hope for the future, believes nothing can change intolerable situation, intense feelings of isolation, no control over the future	*Hopelessness*	Expresses willingness to call on others for help, identifies one support system within community
Feels worthless, ineffective, a burden to others, cannot do anything right	*Chronic low self-esteem*	Describes feelings of self-worth

International Council of Nursing Practice. (2019). *ICNP browser.* Retrieved from https://www.icn.ch/what-we-do/projects/ehealth/icnp-browser. ICNP® is owned and copyrighted by the International Council of Nurses (ICN). Reproduced with permission of the copyright holder.

as well as acknowledging, understanding, and accepting the emotions that arise from working with and caring for these patients, is essential.

NURSING DIAGNOSIS

The nursing diagnosis with the highest priority is *risk for suicide.* Feelings of hopelessness, anger, frustration, abandonment, and rejection are common among people who have suicidal ideation. Nursing diagnoses that address problems related to depressed mood, anxiety, mania, or disturbed thought include *self-care deficit, impaired sleep, impaired nutritional intake,* and *anxiety.* See the clinical chapters focusing on depressive disorders, bipolar disorders, and schizophrenia spectrum disorders for more information.

OUTCOMES IDENTIFICATION

Relevant outcomes will address and reduce or reverse the problems identified in the nursing diagnoses. According to the International Council of Nurses (2019), the outcome for the diagnosis of *risk for suicide* is *decreased risk for suicide.* Table 25.2 describes signs and symptoms, potential nursing diagnoses, and outcomes for suicidal behavior.

PLANNING

The plan of care for the patient with suicidal ideation is based on risk and protective factors. When there is a comorbid psychiatric disorder, the treatment plan includes appropriate nursing approaches (e.g., care for patients with depression or schizophrenia). The patient's significant others need to be involved because the patient's perception of isolation is a significant cause of hopelessness.

IMPLEMENTATION

Nursing interventions for patients with suicidal ideation and suicide attempts focus on prevention, treatment, and postvention. Improving overall community mental health services may reduce the incidence of suicide more effectively than extensive efforts directed at identifying individuals who are contemplating suicide. Therefore, more attention focused on prevention that involves community-wide participation will lead to improved outcomes.

Prevention is a **primary intervention** and includes activities that provide support, information, and education to prevent suicide (Box 25.3). Primary intervention is practiced in a wide variety of community settings, such as schools, homes, churches, clinics, hospitals, and work settings. Elementary school children are screened using evidence-based tools that focus on both risk factors and warning signs. High schools are adopting suicide prevention curricula that involve elements of education, peer support, discussions about risk and prevention factors, and warning signs.

Nurses can learn about suicide prevention through the Question, Persuade, Refer (QPR) model (Quinnett, 2007). This model, originally developed in 1995, is a simple educational "train the trainer" program that provides education about how to recognize a mental health emergency, get individuals at risk the help they need, and provide hope through the process. The Case Study and Nursing Care Plan represents the case of a young woman with suicidal ideation treated in an outpatient setting.

Psychosocial Interventions

The key element is establishing a therapeutic alliance to encourage the patient to engage in more realistic problem solving. Helpful staff characteristics include warmth, sensitivity, interest, and consistency. After hospitalization, nurses may work with

CASE STUDY AND NURSING CARE PLAN

A Patient With Suicidal Ideation in the Outpatient Setting

Olivia is a 23-year-old single waitress who arrives at the emergency department by ambulance after a first suicide attempt. Her live-in boyfriend had narrowly prevented her from fatally shooting herself with their gun. She sustained a minor scalp wound and is under observation. She stares at the ground, talks softly, and looks profoundly sad. The psychiatric nurse and psychiatrist on call interview her.

She states that she has been under increasing stress for the past 2 months since entering a management-training program at work. Olivia ultimately failed at the program and lost her job. She states, "I have tons of bills and Christmas is coming." She admits to keeping her feelings to herself. "I don't want my family to find out what a mess I've made of things...again." She denies having a social network. Olivia reports she self-medicates with drugs and alcohol. She states that she feels "like a total loser."

Because Olivia continues to state that she wants to end her life, she is hospitalized. After careful assessment, the psychiatrist prescribes an antidepressant. Problems relating to her depressive state, such as poor appetite, insomnia, self-care deficit, and anxiety, are assessed and monitored. After 3 days on suicide precautions, she is no longer acutely suicidal and agrees to continue treatment in the outpatient division of the hospital.

Self-Assessment

Mrs. Ruiz is a registered nurse with 5 years' experience. Mrs. Ruiz feels empathy for Olivia's attempt to end her life. Yet, she also feels conflicted because she believes, as a Catholic, that attempting to take your life is a sin. Mrs. Ruiz recognizes her own feelings and knows that Olivia has problems with which she can help.

Assessment

Subjective Data

- Reported first suicide attempt in a 23-year-old female

- Self-medicating with alcohol and substances
- Lacks a social support system
- Recent failure at work and subsequent loss of job
- No history of bipolar disorder or related behaviors
- "I have tons of bills and Christmas is coming."
- "I don't want my family to find out what a mess I've made of things...again."

Objective Data

- Minor scalp wound
- Stares at the ground
- Talks softly
- Looks sad

Priority Diagnosis

Risk for suicide as evidenced by suicide attempt, substance use, job loss, debt, and lack of social support.

Outcomes Identification

Patient will experience a decreased suicide risk by consistently using suicide prevention resources and social support groups within the community.

Planning

The initial plan is to establish a working relationship with Olivia, involving her in planning her own treatment and identifying alternative actions for suicidal ideation in the future.

Implementation

Ms. Ruiz develops the following nursing care plan.

Short-Term Goal	Intervention	Rationale	Evaluation
1. Olivia will seek help when feeling self-destructive.	1a. Assess suicidal ideation status. 1b. Even if Olivia denies suicidal ideas, develop a future plan. 1c. Monitor effectiveness of antidepressant therapy and assess for side effects.	1a. Suicide attempts increase the rate of subsequent attempts. Ongoing periodic checks provide support and external boundaries. 1b. Demonstrates concern and offers alternatives if suicidal thoughts return. 1c. Important to assess for agitation and increase in suicidal feelings and to monitor for lifting of depressive state.	**GOAL MET** Olivia agrees to talk to the nurse about suicidal feelings, which she denied during checks. Once discharged, if clinic is closed, she will call the crisis hotline. Olivia agreed to a session that included her boyfriend, and he removed the gun from her apartment. No adverse side effects. Increase in socialization, improved hygiene, reported improvement in sleep and appetite. States her mood is improving, and she feels more hopeful.
2. Olivia will talk about painful feelings by the end of the first week.	2a. Listen attentively and provide feedback. 2b. Refocus attention back to Olivia and the emotions underlying her anger. 2c. Give frequent opportunities for discussion of feelings through verbal invitation and stated concern.	2a. Support and feedback make patients feel stronger and better able to handle stress. 2b. Arguments and power struggles keep attention away from important issues. 2c. Aggressive, hostile communications cover painful feelings. When patient can express feelings in words, there is less need to act them out.	**GOAL MET** During the initial sessions, angry communication is constant. By the end of the first week, Olivia states, "You really want to understand." Olivia talks of feeling like a failure as a daughter, girlfriend, and employee.
3. Olivia will explore other employment opportunities by the end of the second week.	3. Alternative solutions can be explored once feelings and problems are identified.	3. Acceptable alternatives increase a future orientation and decrease hopelessness. Patient can experience feelings of control over situation.	**GOAL MET** By the end of the second week, Olivia talks about attending a job fair. She accepted a referral to social services for registering for unemployment benefits and debt management.

Evaluation

See individual outcomes and evaluation within the care plan.

BOX 25.3 Goals of the National Strategy for Suicide Prevention

- Integrate and coordinate suicide prevention activities across multiple sectors and settings.
- Implement research-informed communication efforts designed to prevent suicide by changing knowledge, attitudes, and behaviors.
- Increase knowledge of the factors that offer protection from suicidal behaviors and that promote wellness and recovery.
- Promote responsible media reporting of suicide, accurate portrayals of suicide and mental illnesses in the entertainment industry, and the safety of online content related to suicide.
- Develop, implement, and monitor effective programs that promote wellness and prevent suicide and related behaviors.
- Promote efforts to reduce access to lethal means of suicide among individuals with identified suicide risk.
- Provide training to community and clinical service providers on the prevention of suicide and related behaviors.
- Promote suicide prevention as a core component of healthcare services.
- Promote and implement effective clinical and professional practices for assessing and treating those identified as being at risk for suicidal behaviors.
- Provide care and support to individuals affected by suicide deaths and attempts to promote healing and implement community strategies to help prevent further suicides.
- Increase the timeliness and usefulness of national surveillance systems relevant to suicide prevention and improve the ability to collect, analyze, and use this information for action.
- Promote and support research on suicide prevention.
- Evaluate the impact and effectiveness of suicide prevention interventions and systems and synthesize and disseminate findings.

US Department of Health and Human Services, Office of the Surgeon General, & National Action Alliance for Suicide Prevention. (2012). *National Strategy for Suicide Prevention: Goals and objectives for action.* Washington, DC: Author.

these patients in the clinic, in a partial hospitalization program (PHP), or in home care.

One particular aspect of counseling is the use of a patient safety plan. This is a written six-step plan that includes identification of warning signs, internal coping strategies, social settings, and people who provide distraction. It also provides instructions to patients on whom they can ask for help, professionals or agencies where they can find help during a crisis, and how to make the environment safe (Fig. 25.1). Additionally, this written safety plan asks patients to identify what is worth living for in their lives.

A significant nursing intervention to assist the patient with suicidal ideation in regaining self-control is the careful administration of medication. Medications prescribed to high-risk patients are monitored carefully. Lethal overdose is nearly impossible with the newer antidepressants such as selective serotonin reuptake inhibitors (SSRIs). Overdose remains a concern with tricyclic antidepressants and monoamine oxidase inhibitors. Mouth checks may be used to be sure that patients are not saving (hoarding) medications in the hospital. In the community, provision of a limited-day supply or family supervision is required.

Health Teaching and Health Promotion

The nurse teaches the patient about psychiatric diagnoses, medications and complementary therapies, and age-related developmental crises. Teaching is also important regarding community resources, coping skills, stress management, and communication skills. Additionally, teaching regarding the development of a safety plan is important in the prevention of suicide. When possible, include the family or significant others to strengthen the patient's support system.

Case Management

Case management and care coordination are important aspects of nursing care for the patient with suicidal ideation. The patient's perception of being alone without supports often blinds the patient to the real support figures who are present. Reconnecting the patient with family and friends is a major focus, whether in the hospital or the community. Aftercare referrals may include information on the following resources: treatment providers, substance treatment centers, crisis hotlines, support groups for patients or families, and recreational activities to enhance socialization and self-esteem. Encouraging the patient to get reacquainted with a previous spiritual support system may also be beneficial.

Milieu Therapy

Nurses play an important role in the treatment of patients who are at risk, those who have suicidal ideation, and those who have made a suicide attempt. In the hospital or community setting, the registered nurse utilizes psychosocial and psychobiological interventions, safety and teamwork, health teaching, case management, and care coordination to provide care to patients who have suicidal ideation or have attempted suicide.

An interprofessional approach that emphasizes communication involving clinicians, nurses, social workers, therapists, counselors, and support persons is essential for reducing the number of suicides. This collaborative approach maximizes patient safety and improves outcomes through timely communication and improved coordination of care.

For patients with acute suicidal intentions, suicide precautions, in accordance with hospital policy, are part of the plan of care. Nursing staff must continuously observe patients who are suicidal. Table 25.3 provides a general description of suicide precautions. This intense attention from the nurse provides for safety and allows for constant reassessment of risk.

Monitoring flow sheets for suicide precautions is more clinically useful if they include a description of the patient's affect and behavior. For example, instead of noting "Patient watching television," the nurse will describe the patient's affect (e.g., hostile, fearful, calm) at each observation. Flow sheets should also indicate clear accountability for staff starting and ending their periods of observation. In addition to observing the patient, the nurse is responsible for monitoring the environment for safety hazards. Review Box 25.4 for guidelines on how to minimize physical risks in the environment.

Studies show that acute care of patients who are suicidal is usually effective. Suicide risk is highest in the first few days of hospital admission and during times of staff rotation. Assessment of suicidal risk must be an ongoing process. You should perform an assessment particularly before a change in level of observation or upon sudden improvement or worsening of symptoms.

Patient Safety Plan Template

Step 1:   Warning signs (thoughts, images, mood, situation, behavior) that a crisis may be developing:

1. _____
2. _____
3. _____

Step 2:   Internal coping strategies—Things I can do to take my mind off my problems without contacting another person (relaxation technique, physical activity):

1. _____
2. _____
3. _____

Step 3:   People and social settings that provide distractions:

1. Name _____ Phone _____
2. Name _____ Phone _____
3. Place _____ 4. Place_____

Step 4:   People whom I can ask for help:

1. Name _____ Phone _____
2. Name _____ Phone _____
3. Name _____ Phone _____

Step 5:   Professionals or agencies I can contact during a crisis:

1. Clinician Name_____ Phone _____
   Clinician Pager or Emergency Contact #_____
2. Clinician Name_____ Phone _____
   Clinician Pager or Emergency Contact #_____
3. Local Urgent Care Services_____
   Urgent Care Services Address_____
   Urgent Care Services Phone_____
4. Suicide Prevention Lifeline Phone: 1-800-273-TALK (8255)

Step 6:   Making the environment safe:

1. _____
2. _____

The one thing that is most important to me and worth living for is:

_____

Fig. 25.1 Patient safety plan template. (From Stanley, B., & Brown, G. [2008]. *How can a safety plan help?* National Suicide Prevention Lifeline. Retrieved from http://suicidepreventionlifeline.org/wp-content/uploads/2016/08/Brown_StanleySafetyPlanTemplate.pdf.)

TABLE 25.3	Suicide Precautions With Constant One-to-One Observation	
Staff Assessment	**Possible Patient Symptoms**	**Nursing Responsibilities**
Patient with suicidal ideation or delusions of self-mutilation who, according to assessment by unit staff, presents clinical symptoms that suggest a clear intent to follow through with the plan or delusion	1. Patient is currently verbalizing a clear intent to harm self. 2. Patient shows no insight into existing problems. 3. Patient has poor impulse control. 4. Patient has already attempted suicide in the recent past by a particularly lethal method (e.g., hanging, gun, carbon monoxide poisoning).	1. One-to-one nursing observation and interaction 24 h a day (never let patient out of staff's sight). 2. Chart patient's whereabouts and record mood, verbatim statements, and behavior every 15–30 min per protocol. 3. Ensure that meal trays contain no glass or metal silverware. 4. When patient is sleeping, hands should always be in view, not under the covers. 5. Observe patient swallow each dose of medication.

Documentation of Care

As for documentation, you must ensure that the record is complete and identify any late entries. Courts require that the patient be periodically evaluated for suicidal risk, that the treatment plan provide for high-level security, and that staff members follow the individual treatment plan. Despite following institution protocols, treatment plans, and the appropriate standards of practice, suicides do still happen. This is especially the case for patients in the community. Human behavior is simply not predictable.

HEALTH POLICY

Establishing a Three-Digit Suicide Crisis Line

In August 2018, a historic piece of legislation known as the National Suicide Hotline Improvement Act was signed into law. This act was passed with unanimous support of Congress due to concern for the increasing numbers of suicides among the general population and among military personnel. The Substance Abuse and Mental Health Services Administration (SAMHSA), the Federal Communications Commission (FCC), and the United States Department of Veterans Affairs (VA) worked together to produce a report on the potential impact of the designation of an N11 dialing code for a suicide prevention and mental health crisis hotline system and possible recommendations for improving the National Suicide Prevention Lifeline.

This report was finalized in February 2019 https://docs.fcc.gov/public/attachments/DOC-359095A1.pdf. It outlined the context and background of prior legislation, the history, development, and structure of the national lifeline, the effectiveness and challenges of the lifeline, the potential impact of the N11 suicide crisis line, the effectiveness of other three-digit numbers, including "911" and "211" in the country, and how the current lifeline could be improved to reach more people in crisis.

In July of 2020, the FCC announced that 9-8-8 will be the new universal number for the National Suicide Prevention Hotline. This easy to use number will be operational in July of 2022. 9-8-8 will improve public access to mental health care and suicide prevention resources, support help-seeking, and help to establish an entry point for crisis care.

American Foundation for Suicide Prevention. (2020). *Nation's largest suicide organization celebrates National Suicide Hotline Designation Act (S.2661) becoming law.* Retrieved from https://www.prnewswire.com/news-releases/nations-largest-suicide-prevention-organization-celebrates-national-suicide-hotline-designation-act-s2661-becoming-law-301154888.html.

BOX 25.4 Environmental Guidelines for Minimizing Suicidal Behavior on the Psychiatric Unit

- Use plastic utensils and count utensils when the tray is collected.
- Do not assign patient to a private room, and ensure the door remains open at all times.
- Jump-proof and hang-proof the bathrooms by installing breakaway shower rods and recessed shower nozzles.
- Keep electrical cords to a minimal length.
- Install unbreakable glass in windows. Install tamper-proof screens or partitions too small to pass through. Keep all windows locked.
- Lock all utility rooms, kitchens, adjacent stairwells, and offices. All nonclinical staff (e.g., housekeepers, maintenance workers) should receive instructions to keep doors locked.
- Take all potentially harmful gifts (e.g., flowers in glass vases) from visitors before allowing them to see patients. Search all items brought to patients by visitors.
- Go through personal belongings with patient present, and remove all potentially harmful objects (e.g., belts, shoelaces, metal nail files, tweezers, matches, razors, perfume, and shampoo).
- Ensure that visitors do not bring in or leave potentially harmful objects in patient's room (e.g., matches, nail files).
- Search patient for harmful objects (e.g., drugs, sharp objects, cords) if allowed to leave unit on pass.

Suicide Survivors

Suicide survivors, the circle of survivors of a person who has completed suicide, are the largest group of mental health casualties related to suicide. It is estimated that for every suicide there are 60 survivors. Surviving family and friends may experience overwhelming guilt and shame compounded by the difficulty of discussing the frequently taboo subject of suicide, sadness, loneliness, abandonment, and disbelief.

While parental death in childhood from any cause increases the risk of suicidality in adult offspring, the risk of suicidality is greater with exposure to suicide than other deaths (Hua et al., 2019). Compared with a nonexposed control group, offspring who are exposed to parental suicide have been found to be nearly four times more likely to die by suicide (Lee et al., 2018). The death of a child also impacts the surviving parents. Suicide puts parents at greater risk of psychological morbidity and physical health problems compared to other causes of death (Ross et al., 2018).

One survivor wrote a personal account several years after the suicide of her daughter:

If only I hadn't responded with anger and frustration during our last phone call…she was angry with herself and seemed to want to pick a fight with me—which was the pattern. If I could have looked past her angry words and instead tuned into the desperation behind them, maybe I could have gotten her to open up to me. Now I can only look back and consider the many, many times I should have picked up on the severity of her illness and how she struggled. If I have any advice for others based on my experience, it is to get connected, listen, and be a real part of the lives of those you love. That's the only way you'll know when something is just not right and understand their deep despair. This also applies to friends and family of survivors. Please don't treat us like we're 'contagious.' And please do talk about our loss. The worst thing possible is to avoid mention of our lost loved one.

Healthcare providers are often involved in providing mental healthcare and support to survivors, which is referred to as **postvention**. Survivors recommend the following suggestions to healthcare professionals:

- If being a survivor is the main reason an individual seeks treatment, remember that the survivor, not the deceased, is the patient. Focus on the patient's thoughts and feelings, and do a thorough assessment as you usually would.
- If you are a friend or relative of a suicide survivor, remember that the most difficult time for these survivors is not so much in the immediate aftermath of the suicide. Rather, it is in the weeks, months, and *years* following their loss. Make frequent efforts to reach out to these individuals, especially on the most difficult anniversary dates. Do not be afraid of talking about the deceased person. In fact, speak of them often. While this may seem counterintuitive and uncomfortable for most, survivors of suicide want their loved one to be remembered in this way. Talking reduces the hurt, isolation, and stigma.

Is a Loss Due to Suicide a Risk Factor for Suicide?

Problem

Most mental health professionals agree that losing a relative or a friend to suicide is in itself a risk factor for suicide. We do not know, however, if that risk is just like any other sudden loss by death or if the risk increases when applied to relative or peer suicide.

Purpose of Study

This study was conducted to test the hypothesis that young adults bereaved by suicide have an increased risk of suicidal ideation and suicide attempts as compared with other young adults bereaved by other sudden deaths.

Methods

There were 3432 respondents aged 18 to 40 who studied or worked at higher education institutions in the United Kingdom recruited for this online survey. To be included in the study, inclusion criteria were that participants experienced the natural, unnatural, or suicide loss of a close friend or relative since the age of 10. Two key questions were, "Have you ever thought about taking your life?" and "Have you ever made an attempt to take your life?"

Key Findings

- Adults who were bereaved by suicide had a higher probability of attempting suicide than those bereaved by sudden natural causes.
- The effect of suicide bereavement was similar whether participants were blood related to the deceased or not.

Implications for Nursing Practice

Bereavement by suicide is a specific risk factor for suicide attempts. Nursing assessments should always involve a screening for a history of suicide in blood relatives, nonblood relatives, and friends.

Pitman, A. L., Osborn, D. P. J., Rantell, K., & King, M. B. (2016). Bereavement by suicide as a risk factor for suicide attempt: A cross-sectional national UK-wide study of 3432 young bereaved adults. *British Medical Journal Open, 6*(1).

- If being a survivor comes out as an incidental finding during an assessment, ask open-ended questions and evaluate how much the survivor has resolved the loss.
- Recommend community resources and survivor support groups and show empathy about the loss of someone to suicide. Know about local SOS support groups in your area and refer the survivors and their families as soon as possible following the suicide.

Staff members who provided care for a patient who ended one's life by suicide within the treatment facility are similarly traumatized by suicide. Staff may also experience symptoms of posttraumatic stress disorder with guilt, shock, anger, shame, and decreased self-esteem. Group support is essential as the inpatient treatment team conducts a thorough psychological postmortem assessment. The team will carefully review the event to identify the potential overlooked clues, faulty judgments, or changes that are needed in agency protocols.

Most facilities have a clear policy about communication with families after suicide. Although some lawyers advise having no contact except through them, others recommend designating a spokesperson that can address the feelings of the family without discussing the details of the patient's care. Give referrals to family members to assist them in dealing with their grief and to address any emotional problems that develop, especially in adolescents.

EVALUATION

Evaluation of a patient with suicidal ideation is ongoing. The nurse must be constantly alert to changes in mood, thinking, and behavior. The nurse also looks for indications that the patient is communicating thoughts and feelings more readily and that the patient's social network is widening. If the person is able to talk about feelings and engage in problem solving with you, this is a positive sign.

Suicidal behavior is the result of interpersonal turmoil. If an episode of major depressive disorder is the main admitting diagnosis and a serious suicidal gesture resulted from this depression, both problems are initially assessed and treated. When the patient is no longer an acute suicide risk, treating the suicidal ideation and depressive disorder becomes the main focus of care. Essentially, the nurse evaluates each short-term goal and establishes new ones as the patient progresses toward the long-term goal of resolving suicidal ideation.

Once stabilized, the patient may be admitted to a PHP. PHPs tend to be 6 hours a day, 5 days a week. An intensive outpatient (IOP) treatment program is another slightly shorter option, usually 3 hours a day, 3 days a week. Both the PHP and IOP allow patients to go home in the evening to practice new coping skills. Community-based support groups are also available that are effective and financially affordable for the patient. Nurses should be knowledgeable about, and proactive in, referring patients to these support groups.

TREATMENT MODALITIES

Biological Treatments

Pharmacotherapy

Pharmacological interventions are used to alleviate symptoms of comorbid disorders. Antidepressants are used for patients who have a depressive disorder or an anxiety disorder. Close monitoring must occur, especially when patients begin medication and when the dosage changes. Strong nursing care involves careful patient (and family, if appropriate) teaching about the benefits and risks of antidepressant therapy.

There is clear evidence that long-term lithium treatment for bipolar disorder and major depressive disorder significantly reduces suicide and suicide attempts. Because lithium frequently causes serious side effects and necessitates periodic blood work to test for therapeutic levels, patient and family education is important to support adherence.

For patients experiencing psychotic or bipolar manic episodes, antipsychotic medication is usually ordered. Second-generation antipsychotics are preferable to first-generation antipsychotics because they have fewer adverse effects. Some studies have shown a reduced overall mortality rate among patients with schizophrenia receiving clozapine (Clozaril) (Vermeulen et al., 2019). Monitor the use of clozapine closely due to the risk of severe side effects, including agranulocytosis, myocarditis, and altered glucose metabolism.

Antianxiety medication may help treat risk factors such as severe anxiety, panic, and agitation for those who struggle with suicidal ideation. Anxiety is often comorbid with depression, dysthymia, bipolar, and personality disorders.

Intravenous and nasal ketamine, a rapid-acting antidepressant which is believed to act on glutamate, may reduce suicidal ideation within the first three treatments by potentially increasing the amount of glutamate in the spaces between neurons (Ballard et al., 2018). Intravenous administration is not approved by the US Food and Drug Administration (FDA). However, the FDA recently approved esketamine, a nasal spray formulation, for treatment-resistant depression.

Brain Stimulation Therapy

An alternative somatic treatment for acute suicidal risk is electroconvulsive therapy (ECT). Evidence suggests that ECT decreases acute suicidal ideation. This treatment is useful for patients with depression or psychosis whose behavior is considered life threatening and for whom waiting for medication to take effect is not feasible. It is also safe and effective for pregnant patients, patients with certain medical conditions who cannot tolerate medication, and patients who do not respond to multiple trials of medication. Refer to Chapter 14 for further discussion of ECT.

Psychological Therapies

The psychiatric-mental health advanced practice registered nurse may treat patients with suicidal ideation directly with psychotherapy, psychobiological interventions, clinical supervision for direct care staff, or consultation in nonpsychiatric settings (e.g., healthcare unit, nursing home, or forensic site). Following hospitalization, the advanced practice nurse may provide aftercare for the patient who has coexisting psychiatric disorders. This care includes individual and family therapy and medication management.

NONSUICIDAL SELF-INJURY

Clinical Picture

A condition related to suicidal behavior is **nonsuicidal self-injury (NSSI)**. This type of injury is the intentional damage to one's own body tissue, without conscious suicidal intent, and for purposes not socially or culturally sanctioned (International Society for the Study of Self-Injury, 2018). These self-injuries are deliberate and are direct attempts to inflict painful injuries to the surface of the body without intending to die. The behavior most commonly consists of cutting, burning, scraping/scratching skin, biting, hitting, skin picking, and interfering with wound healing. Minor behaviors such as picking off a scab or biting nails are not considered self-injury. Often, people who self-injure report multiple methods of physical damage, with the methods varying across cultures.

Like suicidal behavior disorder, NSSI is not an official disorder in the DSM-5 (APA, 2013) but is a condition that needs further study. Proposed criteria identify a minimum of 5 days within the last year of self-inflicting damage in the absence of suicidal intent. The source of these damaging behaviors includes a desire to feel relief from negative thoughts or feelings such as anxiety, anger, and distress. Self-loathing and a belief that they are bad, defective, or deserving of punishment is common in this population. Impaired interpersonal relationships may also be the impetus for self-injury. Like other obsessive problems, a preoccupation with self-injury is usually present, even when it is not acted on.

Another reason given for these behaviors is to achieve a short, but intense, state of euphoria during or after the injurious act. This euphoria may be the result of the release of endogenous opiates in response to tissue damage. There is a term for these good feelings—pain offset relief. Self-injuring people and non–self-injuring people alike experience this relief when pain ends. People with NSSI seem to tap into this phenomenon.

Other criteria for NSSI include that the behavior is not socially sanctioned, such as part of a religious ritual. Individuals with this disorder experience a significant level of distress. This distress, along with preoccupation, interferes with the individual's ability to function interpersonally, academically, occupationally, and other areas of functioning. This diagnosis is made in the absence of other explanations for the self-injuries. Other explanations involve foreign substances that result in delirium, substance intoxication, or substance withdrawals. Self-injurious behaviors in conditions such as autism, psychotic episodes, and intellectual disabilities would not result in a diagnosis of NSSI. Trichotillomania (hair-pulling) disorder and excoriation (skin-picking) disorder also do not meet the criteria for NSSI.

Despite the less ominous sounding name of NSSI compared to suicidal behavior disorder, outcomes for people who self-injure can eventually become fatal. Chesin et al. (2017) found that adults with a history of youth NSSI were twice as likely to attempt suicide. The younger the age of onset, the more likely suicide attempts will occur (Muehlenkamp & Brausch, 2019).

Epidemiology

The lifetime prevalence of nonsuicidal self-injury is difficult to accurately determine due to attempts to conceal the behavior. However, approximately two million cases are reported annually in the United States. Between 6% and 23% of the US population engage in these behaviors at some time in their life. About 15% of adolescents and 17% to 35% of college students engage in self-injurious behaviors (Mahoney, 2018). NSSI peaks between 20 and 29 years of age, and declines in early adulthood. The ratio of females to males with this disorder is about 3:1 or 4:1.

Comorbidity

Self-harm in the absence of suicidal ideation, which does not meet the criteria for the disorder, often occurs with other mental health disorders. These disorders include major depressive disorder, anxiety, eating disorders, and substance use disorders.

Seventy percent of females with borderline personality and thirty percent with eating disorders are affected by NSSI (Mahoney, 2018). Eating disorders co-occur in 55% of individuals with NSSI behaviors.

Risk Factors
Biological Factors
Several neurochemical pathways in the brain may play a role in the development of these behaviors. Although studies are inconclusive, the neurotransmitter group of monoamines—including serotonin, dopamine, and the opioid system, as well as the hypothalamic-pituitary-adrenal (HPA) axis—lead to an increased level of stress vulnerability. When stress occurs, the patient may use NSSI to restore an opioid homeostasis.

Another area that is being explored in regard to NSSI is brain activation in response to negative images. In one study, compared to healthy control participants, the NSSI group showed decreased amygdala activity to negative images of such items as razor blades and knives (Hooley et al., 2020). This finding suggests that individuals with NSSI have diminished aversion in regard to those items.

Cognitive Factors
From a behavioral standpoint, NSSI may be a form of self-punishment. Painful actions are employed as a way to make up for acts that caused harm or distress to others. Positive reinforcement, in the form of a reward, may support self-injurious acts. For example, cutting may result in reduced anxiety and, perhaps, the help of a significant other. Negative reinforcement is also evidenced in NSSI. Negative reinforcement involves eliminating something that is unpleasant or uncomfortable in response to an action.

Environmental Factors
Individuals with NSSI tend to come from families with adverse events such as parental divorce, socioeconomic challenges, and interparental violence. This disorder is associated with parental harsh punishment, limited monitoring by the parents, and poor quality of attachment. Paternal maltreatment is associated with greater addictive qualities of self-injuring.

Societal Factors
Youth who self-injure may feel isolated from their peers. They may have frequent peer victimization and negative social self-worth. Self-injurious behaviors such as cutting may also be viewed as a social phenomenon. Individuals often learn about these behaviors from peers who engage in self-injury. Subsequently, they begin using the behaviors to alleviate personal discomfort. A common environment for self-injury contagion is the psychiatric inpatient unit. Frequently, after an individual who engages in NSSI is admitted, others on the unit begin to engage in the behaviors as well.

Social contagion through the media may be increasing NSSI through pictures and communication about the disorder. Instagram, for example, once housed thousands of photos of injuries varying from mild to severe (Brown et al., 2018). The more severe the injury, the more comments that are generated.

Instagram subsequently developed a policy that prohibits content concerning self-harm or suicide.

APPLICATION OF THE NURSING PROCESS

There is limited research on the effectiveness of nursing care for patients who engage in NSSI. However, holistic interdisciplinary approaches to care where patients are included in planning their care will likely lead to best outcomes. Identifying the individual's comorbid conditions and providing nursing care based on these conditions is important.

ASSESSMENT

Initial assessment includes open discussion of the incidence, prevalence, and factors associated with the NSSI with the individual. This will help decrease the stigma that is associated with the behavior. Since traumatic events may be a trigger for self-injury, assessing whether there were traumatic events in the individual's life is important for ongoing management (Young et al., 2016).

A thorough history from the patient regarding the self-injurious behavior includes types of self-injury, triggers for the behavior, frequency of the behavior, and motivation for engaging in the behavior. Additionally, ask the patient what has worked effectively in stopping the behaviors in the past. Appropriate physical assessment to determine the condition of wounds, if present, allows you to plan appropriate interventions.

Self-Assessment
Nurses caring for patients who engage in self-injury report that they are emotionally affected by caring for these patients. Emotions experienced include feeling defeated by relapses, discouragement, and powerlessness. Additionally, nurses need to be aware that transference may occur through projection of the patient's emotions onto the nurse. Establishing appropriate professional boundaries with the patient is important for self-care, as is collaboration with other clinicians.

NURSING DIAGNOSIS

The nursing diagnoses with the highest priorities are *risk for self-mutilation* and *self-mutilation*. Patients may be experiencing feelings of anxiety, tension, and self-loathing. Consider any nursing diagnosis that is appropriate for underlying comorbid psychiatric conditions, such as major depressive disorder, bipolar disorder, and borderline personality disorder. See the specific clinical chapters for further information.

OUTCOMES IDENTIFICATION

Outcomes will be aimed at removing the risk of self-injury and self-mutilation itself. Therefore, an overall outcome is that the patient will experience no mutilation. Goals to assist in meeting this outcome include:
- Refrains from obtaining tools for self-injury
- Requests assistance from the staff as needed

- Uses available support groups
- Uses medication as prescribed
- Identifies alternate coping strategies

PLANNING

The plan of care for individuals who engage in self-injury includes demonstration of a caring attitude toward the patient, bearing hope for recovery, observing for signs of self-harm, evaluating the need for medication, and providing appropriate interventions for patients' wounds and injuries. Engage patients in their recovery plan, which encompasses a six-step approach to recovery, including (1) limiting setting for safety, (2) developing self-esteem, (3) discovery of the motive for self-injury and the role it served for the patient, (4) learning that self-injury can be self-controlled, (5) replacing the self-injury with coping skills, and (6) entering a maintenance phase.

IMPLEMENTATION

Basic nursing interventions for patients with NSSI include caring for the patient's wounds and injuries, establishing a therapeutic alliance, and teaching coping skills to replace the self-injurious behaviors. A therapeutic relationship will provide support and an alternative to self-injury when anxiety increases.

EVALUATION

Similar to suicidal behavior, the evaluation of patients with NSSI behaviors is ongoing. The development of a therapeutic alliance

with the patient allows for the patient to trust the care provider. The nurse must continue to evaluate whether the patient is communicating thoughts and feelings accurately and whether the patient's perception is that engagement in the behaviors is declining while being replaced with appropriate coping skills.

TREATMENT MODALITIES
Biological Treatments
Pharmacotherapy

It is usually necessary to treat comorbid conditions such as major depressive disorder, bipolar disorder, and anxiety disorders before targeting self-injury behaviors. There is some evidence to support the use of medications targeting the serotonergic, dopaminergic, and opioid systems (Turner et al., 2014). They include SSRIs (e.g., fluoxetine [Prozac]), second-generation antipsychotics (e.g., aripiprazole [Abilify] and ziprasidone [Geodon]), serotonin norepinephrine reuptake inhibitors (e.g., venlafaxine [Effexor]), opioids (buprenorphine), and opioid antagonists (naltrexone).

Psychological Therapies

Advanced practice psychiatric-mental health registered nurses may work with patients who use self-injury to cope. Specific therapies that are used include cognitive behavioral therapy, dialectical behavior therapy, and group therapy. Dialectical behavioral therapy is utilized to reduce emotional dysregulation and increase stimulus control. Access to lethal means is important as suicidal ideation often accompanies NSSI. Individuals are encouraged to learn skill building to replace destructive behaviors.

KEY POINTS TO REMEMBER

- Suicide is a significant public health problem in the United States and should be approached as a "never event."
- Specific biological, psychosocial, and cultural factors increase the risk of suicide.
- Treating the coexisting psychiatric disorder may help most patients with suicidal ideation.
- Certain health conditions and psychiatric diagnoses are associated with increased risk for suicide.
- Every suicide attempt must be taken seriously even if the person has a history of multiple attempts.
- Nursing care of the patient who is suicidal is challenging but rewarding. Patients' desperate feelings evoke intense reactions in staff, but most people with suicidal behaviors respond to treatment and do not end their life by suicide.
- If a patient dies by suicide, family, friends, and healthcare workers are traumatized and need postvention, including support, understanding, and possibly including referrals for psychiatric treatment.
- NSSI is a problem that is becoming increasingly important, especially among young people.
- Social contagion of NSSI is a serious implication in the spread of this compulsive behavior.
- Treatment for self-injurious behaviors includes a supportive therapeutic relationship, adopting alternate coping methods, medication, and psychotherapy, such as dialectical behavior therapy.

CRITICAL THINKING

1. Locate and review the suicide protocol at your hospital unit or community center. Are there any steps you anticipate having difficulty carrying out? Discuss these difficulties with your peers or clinical group.
2. How would you respond to another staff member who expresses guilt over the suicide of a patient on your unit?
3. Identify three common and expected emotional reactions that a nurse might have when initially working with persons who manifest suicidal behavior disorder.
   a. How do you think you might react?
   b. What actions could you take to deal with the event and obtain support?

CHAPTER REVIEW

1. Which patient statement does not demonstrate an understanding of a suicide safety plan?
   a. "Going for a really long, hard run helps clear my mind and stops the suicidal thoughts."
   b. "I will take extra medication if I start getting those self-destructive feelings."
   c. "My sister is always there for me when I start getting suicidal."
   d. "I keep the suicide prevention phone number in my wallet."

2. Which interventions will help make the environment on the unit safer for patients with suicidal ideation? *Select all that apply.*
   a. All windows are kept locked.
   b. Every shower has a breakaway shower rod.
   c. Eating utensils are counted when trays are collected.
   d. Patient doors are kept open.
   e. Staying within listening distance of the patient.

3. What are the nursing responsibilities to a patient expressing suicidal thoughts? *Select all that apply.*
   a. Instituting one-to-one observation.
   b. Documenting the patient's whereabouts and mood every 15 to 30 minutes.
   c. Ensuring that the patient has no contact with glass or metal utensils.
   d. Ensuring that patient has swallowed each individual dose of medication.
   e. Discussing triggers of depression.

4. When considering community suicide prevention programs, what population should the nurse plan to service with regular suicide screenings? *Select all that apply.*
   a. 10- to 34-year-olds
   b. Males
   c. College-educated adults
   d. Rural population
   e. Native American

5. Research supports that which intervention implemented on a long-term basis significantly reduces the incidence of suicide and suicide attempts in a patient diagnosed with bipolar disorder?
   a. An antipsychotic medication
   b. Electroconvulsive therapy (ECT)
   c. One-on-one observation
   d. Lithium

6. Gladys is seeing a therapist because her husband died by suicide 6 months ago. Gladys tells her therapist, "I know he was in pain, but why didn't he leave me a note?" The therapist's best response would be:
   a. "He probably acted quickly on his impulse to kill himself."
   b. "He did not want to think about the pain he would cause you."
   c. "He was not able to think clearly due to his emotional pain."
   d. "He thought you may think it was an accident if there was no note."

7. Martin is a 23-year-old male with a new diagnosis of schizophrenia, and his family is receiving information from a home health nurse. The topic of education is suicide prevention, and the nurse recognizes effective teaching when the mother says:
   a. "Persons with schizophrenia rarely die by suicide."
   b. "Suicide risk is greatest in the first few years after diagnosis."
   c. "Suicide is not common in schizophrenia due to confusion."
   d. "Most persons diagnosed with schizophrenia die of suicide."

8. Sigmund Freud, Karl Menninger, and Aaron Beck theorized that hopelessness was an integral part of why a person ends one's life by suicide. A more recent theory suggests suicide results from:
   a. Elevated serotonin levels
   b. The diathesis-stress model
   c. Outward aggression turned inward
   d. A lack of perfectionism

9. Which person is at the highest risk for suicide?
   a. A 50-year-old married white male with major depressive disorder who has a plan to overdose if circumstances at work do not improve.
   b. A 45-year-old married white female who recently lost her parents, suffers from bipolar disorder, and attempted suicide once as a teenager.
   c. A young single white male who misuses alcohol, is hopeless, impulsive, has just been rejected by his girlfriend, and has ready access to a gun he has hidden.
   d. An older Hispanic male who is Catholic, living with a debilitating chronic illness, recently widowed, and who states, "I wish that God would take me too."

10. Kara is a 23-year-old patient admitted with major depressive disorder and suicidal ideation. Which intervention(s) would be therapeutic for Kara? *Select all that apply.*
    a. Focus primarily on developing solutions to the problems that lead the patient to feel suicidal.
    b. Assess the patient thoroughly and reassess the patient at regular intervals as levels of risk fluctuate.
    c. Avoid talking about the suicidal ideation as this may increase the patient's risk for suicidal behavior.
    d. Meet regularly with the patient to provide opportunities for the patient to express and explore feelings.
    e. Administer antidepressant medications cautiously and conservatively because of their potential to increase the suicide risk in Kara's age group.
    f. Help the patient to identify positive self-attributes and to question negative self-perceptions that are unrealistic.

1. b; 2. a, b, c, d; 3. a, b, c, d; 4. a, b, e; 5. d; 6. c; 7. b; 8. b; 9. c; 10. b, d, e, f

Visit the Evolve website for a posttest on the content in this chapter: http://evolve.elsevier.com/Varcarolis

REFERENCES

American Psychiatric Association. (2013). *Diagnostic and statistical manual of mental disorders* (5th ed.). Washington, DC: Author.

Arendt, F. (2019). Suicide on Instagram: Content analysis of a German suicide-related hashtag. *Crisis, 40*(1), 36–41.

Ballard, E., Yarrington, J., Farmer, C., et al. (2018). Characterizing the course of suicidal ideation response to ketamine. *Journal of Affective Disorders, 241,* 86–93.

Bradvik, L. (2018). Suicide risk and mental disorders. *International Journal of Environmental Research and Public Health, 15*(9), 2028.

Brown, R.C., Fischer, T., Goldwich, A.D., Keller, R., Young, R., & Plener, P.L. (2018). #Cutting: Non-suicidal self-injury (NSSI) on Instagram. *Psychological Medicine, 48*(2), 337–346.

Centers for Disease Control and Prevention. (2017). *Data and Statistics Fatal Injury Report for 2017.* Retrieved from https://webappa.cdc.gov/cgi-bin/broker.exe.

Centers for Disease Control and Prevention. (2018). *10 Leading causes of death by age group: United States 2017.* Retrieved from https://www.cdc.gov/injury/wisqars/pdf/leading_causes_of_death_by_age_group_2017-508.pdf.

Centers for Disease Control and Prevention. (2018). *Suicide rising across the US: More than a mental health concern.* Retrieved from https://cdc.gov/vitalsigns/suicide.

Centers for Disease Control and Prevention. (2019). *Preventing suicide.* Retrieved from https://www.cdc.gov/violenceprevention/suicide/fastfact.html.

Centers for Disease Control National Violent Death Reporting System. (2018). *Many factors contribute to suicide among those with and without mental health conditions.* Retrieved from https://www.cdc.gov/vitalsigns/suicide/infographic.html#graphic3.

Centers for Disease Control Violence Prevention. (2019). *Risk and protective factors.* Retrieved from https://www.cdc.gov/violenceprevention/suicide/riskprotectivefactors.html.

Chesin, M. S., Galfavy, H., Sonmez, C. C., et al. (2017). Nonsuicidal self-injury is predictive of suicide attempts among individuals with mood disorders. *Suicide & Life-Threatening Behavior, 47*(5), 567–579.

Coon, H., Darlington, T., DiBlasi, E., et al. (2018). Genome-wide significant regions in 43 Utah high-risk families implicate multiple genes involved in risk for completed suicide. *Molecular Psychiatry.* https://doi.org/10.1038/s41380-018-0282-3.

Crisis Text Line. (2019). *Crisis trends: March 2018.* Retrieved from on https://crisistrends.org/.

Curtin, S. C., & Hedegaard, H. (2019). Suicide rates for females and males by race and ethnicity: United States, 1999-2017. *National Center for Health Statistics: Health E-Stats.* Retrieved from https://stacks.cdc.gov/view/cdc/79168.

DeVille, D. C., Whalen, D., Breslin, F. J., et al. (2020). Prevalence and family-related factors associated with suicidal ideation, suicide attempts, and self-injury in children aged 9 to 10 years. *Journal of the American Medical Association, 3*(2), e1920956.

Federal Communications Commission. (2019). *Report on the National Suicide Hotline Improvement Act of 2018.* Retrieved from https://docs.fcc.gov/public/attachments/DOC-359095A1.pdf.

Fink, D.S., Santaella-Tenorio, J., & Keyes, K.M. (2018). *Increase in suicides the months after the death of Robin Williams in the US.* Retrieved from https://doi.org/10.1371/journal.pone.0191405.

Goldberg, J. (2019). What's the prognosis for someone with schizophrenia? *Web MD.* Retrieved from https://www.webmd.com/schizophrenia/schizophrenia-outlook.

Harmon, V., Mujkic, E., Kaukinen, C., & Weir, H. (2018). Causes and explanations of suicide terrorism: A systematic review. *Homeland Security Affairs, 14,* article 9. Retrieved from https://www.hsaj.org/articles/14749.

Hedegaard, H., Curtin, S., & Warner, M. (2018). *Suicide mortality in the United States, 1999-2017.* National Center for Health Statistics. data brief no. 330. Retrieved from https://www.cdc.gov/nchs/products/databriefs/db330.htm.

Hogan, M., & Grumet, J. G. (2016). Suicide prevention: An emerging priority for health care. *Health Affairs, 35*(6), 1084–1090.

Hooley, J. M., Dahlgren, M. K., Best, S. G., Gonenc, A., & Gruber, S. A. (2020). Decreased amygdalar activation to NSSI-stimuli in people who engage in NSSI: A neuroimaging pilot study. *Frontiers in Psychiatry, 11,* 238.

Hua, P., Bugeja, L., & Maple, M. (2019). A systematic review on the relationship between childhood exposure to external cause parental death, including suicide, on subsequent suicidal behaviour. *Journal of Affective Disorders, 257,* 723–734.

International Council of Nurses. (2019). *International Classification for Nursing Practice catalog.* Retrieved from https://www.icn.ch/sites/default/files/inline-files/ICNP2019-DC.pdf.

International Society for the Study of Self-Injury. (2018). *What is self-injury?* Retrieved from https://itriples.org/about-self-injury/what-is-self-injury.

Lee, K.Y. , Li, C.Y., Chang, K.C., Lu, T.H., & Chen, Y.Y. (2018). Age at exposure to parental suicide and the subsequent risk of suicide in young people. *Crisis, 39,* 27–36.

Mahoney, B. (2018). *Self-Injury Awareness Day March 1, 2018.* Retrieved from https://discoverymood.com/blog/self-injury-awareness-day-march-1-2018/.

Mosseri, A. (2019). *Taking more steps to keep the people who use Instagram safe.* Retrieved from https://about.instagram.com/blog/announcements/more-steps-to-keep-instagram-users-safe.

Muehlenkamp, J.J., & Brausch, A.M. (2019). Protective factors do not moderate risk for past-year suicide attempts conferred by recent NSSI. *Journal of Affective Disorders, 245,* 321–324.

National Institute of Mental Health. (2019). *Suicide in America: Frequently asked questions.* NIH Publication No. TR18-6389. Retrieved from https://www.nimh.nih.gov/health/publications/suicide-faq/index.shtml.

National Institute of Mental Health. (2021). *Suicide.* Retrieved from https://www.nimh.nih.gov/health/statistics/suicide.shtml#:~:text=on%20the%20rise.-,Definitions,might%20not%20result%20in%20injury.

Quinnett, P. (2007). *QPR gatekeeper training for suicide prevention: The model, rationale, and theory.* Unpublished manuscript. Retrieved from http://www.uwlax.edu/conted/pdf/2012QPRtheoryPaper.pdf.

Ross, V., Kõlves, K., , Kunde, L., & De LeoParents, D. (2018). Experiences of suicide-bereavement: A qualitative study at 6 and 12 Months after loss. *International Journal of Environmental Research in Public Health, 15*(4), 618.

Stanley, B., & Brown, G. (2008). *How can a safety plan help?* National Suicide Prevention Lifeline. Retrieved from http://suicidepreventionlifeline.org/wp-content/uploads/2016/08/Brown_StanleySafetyPlanTemplate.pdf.

Stone, D., Simon, T., Fowler, K., et al. (2018). Vital signs: Trends in state suicide rates, United States, 1999-2016 and circumstances contributing to suicide, 27 states, 2015. *Morbidity and Mortality Weekly Report, (67)*22.

Substance Abuse and Mental Health Services Administration (SAMHSA). (2014). *Columbia-Suicide Severity Rating Scale (C-SSRS): Risk assessment (Lifeline crisis center version).* Retrieved from https://suicidepreventionlifeline.org/wp-content/uploads/2016/09/Suicide-Risk-Assessment-C-SSRS-Lifeline-Version-2014.pdf.

Thompson, M. P., Kingree, J. B., & Lamis, D. (2019). Associations of adverse childhood experiences and suicidal behaviors in adulthood in a US nationally representative sample. *Child: Care, Health, and Development, 45*(1), 121–128.

Turner, B. J., Austin, S. B., & Chapman, A. L. (2014). Treating nonsuicidal self-injury: A systematic review of psychological and pharmacological interventions. *Canadian Journal of Psychiatry, 59*(11), 576–585.

US Department of Health and Human Services (HHS), Office of the Surgeon General, & National Action Alliance for Suicide Prevention. (2012). *National Strategy for Suicide Prevention: Goals and objectives for action.* Washington, DC: Author.

US Department of Veterans Affairs. (2018). *VA National Suicide Data Report 2005-2016: Office of Mental Health and Suicide Prevention.* Washington, DC: Author.

Vermeulen, J. M., VanRooijen, G., van de Kerkhof, M. P., Sutterland, A. L., Correll, C. U., & deHaan, L. (2019). Clozapine and long-term mortality risk in patients with schizophrenia: A systematic review and meta-analysis of studies lasting 1.1–12.5 years. *Schizophrenia Bulletin, 45*(2), 315–329.

Young, C., Simonton, A., Key, S., Barczyk, A., & Lawson, K. (2016). Closing in on crisis. *Informing Clinical Practice Regarding Nonsuicidal Self-Injury in Youth, 31*(3), 334–341.

26

Crisis and Disaster

Margaret Jordan Halter

 Visit the Evolve website for a pretest on the content in this chapter: http://evolve.elsevier.com/Varcarolis

OBJECTIVES

1. Analyze a critical or crucial time in your life in terms of your perception of the event, situational support, and coping mechanisms.
2. Identify the three types of crises—maturational, situational, and adventitious—and provide an example of each.
3. Identify at least two nursing diagnoses that have relevance to individuals who are experiencing a crisis.
4. Provide concrete examples of interventions to minimize crisis situations.
5. Compare and contrast the differences among primary, secondary, and tertiary prevention, and identify appropriate intervention strategies.
6. List at least five resources in the community that could be used as referrals for a patient in crisis.
7. Recognize disaster occurrences and management as global concerns.
8. Describe the potential roles of nurses in disaster situations.

KEY TERMS AND CONCEPTS

adventitious crisis
crisis
crisis intervention
disaster

equilibrium
homeostasis
maturational crisis
mitigation

primary prevention
secondary prevention
situational crisis
tertiary prevention

This edition of *Foundations of Psychiatric-Mental Health Nursing* was revised while in quarantine during the biggest global pandemic of the past century. Any nursing student reading this chapter has experienced this crisis firsthand, watching the reports of the rising number of fatalities due to the coronavirus. Most of us were afraid, if not for ourselves, for loved ones who were older or had pre-existing conditions. Anxiety levels ran high as the country and states wrestled with the accompanying economic disaster. For some vulnerable people, the stress of the coronavirus pandemic caused an emergence or exacerbation (i.e., worsening) of psychiatric symptoms.

In this chapter, we will discuss characteristics of crisis, theoretical models regarding crisis, types of crises, and phases of crisis. Nursing care for people experiencing crises is discussed along with levels of prevention that are commonly used to structure crisis care. Finally, this chapter addresses crises that may impact communities at the local, regional, national, and global level.

CRISIS CHARACTERISTICS

The human organism's internal environment maintains a relatively stable state while interacting with external forces. This stable state is referred to as **homeostasis** or **equilibrium**. A **crisis**, which is a major disturbance caused by a stressful event or threat, disrupts this homeostasis. In a crisis, normal coping mechanisms fail, resulting in an inability to function as usual. Equilibrium is replaced by disequilibrium.

A successful outcome for a crisis depends on (1) the realistic perception of the event, (2) adequate situational supports, and (3) adequate coping mechanisms.

Perception of the Event

An important concept associated with crisis is that of individual perception, which may range from realistic to distorted. The perception of threat is based on a person's unique perspective and coping abilities.

People vary in the way they absorb, process, and use information from the environment. Some people may respond to a minor event as if it were life threatening. Conversely, others may assess a life-threatening event and carefully consider options. For example, 10-year-old twins Amy and Annie's parents are divorcing. Amy's grades plummet, she becomes despondent, and has trouble sleeping. Annie, on the other hand, announces to her friends, "We get to move, I'll have a new bedroom that I can paint, and we will be able to walk to school."

Situational Support

Situational support includes all the people who are available that can be depended upon to help during the time of a crisis. Nurses and other health professionals who use crisis intervention are providing situational support.

Coping Mechanisms

Coping mechanisms and skills are acquired through a variety of sources, such as cultural responses, modeling behaviors of others, and life opportunities that broaden experience and promote the adaptive development of new coping responses. Many factors compromise a person's ability to cope with a crisis event. These may include the number of other stressful life events with which the person is currently coping, other unresolved losses, concurrent psychiatric disorders or medical problems, excessive fatigue or pain, and the quality and quantity of a person's usual coping skills.

A depiction of two potential responses to a stressful event is illustrated in Fig. 26.1

A crisis may pose a threat to personality organization; however, it also presents an opportunity for personal growth, development, and change. Successful crisis resolution results from the development of adaptive coping mechanisms, reflects ego

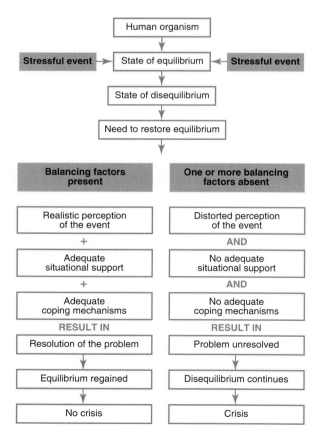

Fig. 26.1 Paradigm: The effect of balancing factors in a stressful event. (From Aguilera, D. C. [1998]. *Crisis intervention: Theory and methodology* [8th ed.]. St. Louis, MO: Mosby.)

development, and suggests the employment of physiological, psychological, and social resources.

CRISIS THEORY

On November 28, 1942, one of the deadliest single-building fires in history occurred. A nightclub—the Cocoanut Grove in Boston—was filled beyond capacity with more than 1,000 people. When a fire broke out, people ran to the main entrance, which was a single revolving door. The door quickly became jammed with people and unusable. Other inward swinging exit doors trapped crowds as they desperately tried to escape. Laws requiring outward swinging exit doors were enacted as a result of this fire.

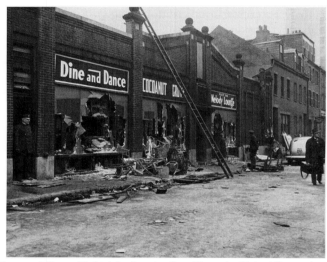

Cocoanut Grove Nightclub after the fire. (Photo by United States Army Signal Corps on November 30, 1942. Courtesy of the Trustees of the Boston Public Library/Print Department at http://www.bpl.org [CC-BY-NC-ND 2.0].)

Erick Lindemann, a Boston psychiatrist, conducted a classic study of the close relatives and friends of the 492 victims of the fire. This study formed the foundation of crisis theory and clinical intervention. He concluded that immediate behavioral responses to crisis were not abnormal or pathological. Rather, they were predictable and normal grief behaviors that consisted of:

- Preoccupation with the lost one
- Identification with the lost one
- Expressions of guilt and hostility
- Disorganization in daily routine
- Somatic complaints

Lindemann (1944) proposed that interventions could eliminate or decrease potential serious personality disorganization in the immediate aftermath of the crisis. He believed that the same interventions that were helpful in bereavement—brief therapy and grief work—would prove just as helpful in dealing with other types of stressful events.

Gerald Caplan (1964) expanded crisis theory to all traumatic events and outlined crisis intervention strategies. His theory is grounded in the concept of homeostasis and returning the individual to a state of equilibrium. He noticed that psychiatric patients dealt with crises in a maladaptive manner and ended up less healthy than before the crisis. Caplan believed that personal and social resources were the key to preventing deterioration after a time of crisis.

Numerous contemporary clinicians and theorists continue to redefine and enhance our understanding of crisis and effective intervention continues. The 1961 report of the Joint Commission on Mental Illness and Health addressed the need for community mental health centers throughout the country. This report stimulated the establishment of crisis services, which are now an important part of mental health programs in hospitals and communities.

Roberts's seven-stage model of crisis interventions (Fig. 26.2) is a useful model in helping individuals who have suffered from an acute crisis. It is also used with people who are diagnosed with acute stress disorder.

TYPES OF CRISES

An understanding of the types of crises lays the groundwork for the application of the nursing process. There are a variety of systems used to classify types of crises in the literature. No matter the names or number of categories, these systems tend to cover and include the same stressors. In this textbook, we identify three basic types of crisis situations: (1) maturational (or developmental) crises, (2) situational crises, and (3) adventitious crises. Identifying which type of crisis the individual is experiencing or has experienced supports the development of a patient-centered plan of care.

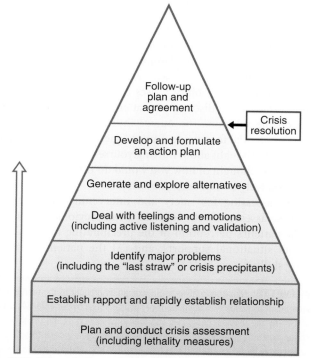

Fig. 26.2 Roberts's Seven-Stage Model of Crisis Intervention. (From Roberts, A. R., & Ottens, A. J. [2005]. The seven-stage crisis intervention model: A road map to goal attainment, problem solving, and crisis resolution. *Brief Treatment and Crisis Intervention, 5*[4], 329–339.)

Maturational Crisis

Erik Erikson (1902–1994) conceptualized development as occurring in eight predetermined and consecutive life stages (psychosocial crises), each of which results in a positive or negative outcome (refer to Table 2.6 in Chapter 2). Each developmental stage represents a developmental, or **maturational crisis**.

When a person reaches a new stage, former coping methods may no longer be effective, and new coping mechanisms have yet to be developed. Thus, for a time, the person is without sufficient defenses. This often leads to feelings of lack of control, resulting in increased tension and anxiety. Examples of events that can precipitate a maturational crisis include leaving home for the first time, marriage, the birth of a child, retirement, and the death of a parent.

Erikson believed that the way these crises are resolved at one stage affects the person's ability to pass through subsequent stages. Each crisis provides the starting point for movement toward the next stage. If a person lacks support systems and adequate role models, successful resolution may be difficult or may not occur. Unresolved problems in the past and inadequate coping mechanisms adversely affect what is learned in each developmental stage. When a person experiences severe difficulty during a maturational crisis, professional intervention may be indicated.

Factors may disrupt individuals' progression through the maturational stages. For example, alcohol and drug addiction disrupts progression through the maturational stages. Unfortunately, this interruption often occurs among adolescents. When control over addictive behavior is achieved, the young person's growth and development may be delayed. For example, when a 22-year-old recovers from addiction after 8 years of use, he may have limited psychosocial and problem-solving skills for a person his age.

Situational Crisis

A **situational crisis** arises from events that are unusually distressing and often unanticipated. Examples of situations that may precipitate a crisis include a job loss or change, the death of a loved one, a change in financial status, divorce, and psychiatric or physical illness.

Whether or not these events precipitate a crisis, again, depends on factors such as the degree of support available from friends, family members, and others. General emotional and physical status also impacts our ability to tolerate stressful events.

Adventitious Crisis

The term adventitious comes from the Latin *adventicius*, meaning coming from outside, and *advenire*, meaning chance happening. An **adventitious crisis**, then, is a traumatic and external event that happens unexpectedly. This type of crisis may be natural, human, and accidental. Natural disasters may be the result of such events as epidemics, floods, fires, and earthquakes. Humans may be the source of adventitious crises through one-on-one violence—such as rape and murder—acts of terrorism, wars, riots, shootings, and bombings. Accidents are another source of adventitious crises and include such events as airline crashes, structural collapses, and nuclear power plant failures.

Adventitious crises can result in serious post-trauma psychiatric conditions, including acute stress disorder and posttraumatic stress disorder. Pre-existing conditions, such as major depressive disorder, panic disorder, and bipolar disorder, may be exacerbated due to the trauma of all types of crises.

It is possible to experience more than one type of crisis situation simultaneously. As you might expect, the presence of more than one crisis further taxes individual coping skills. Consider a 51-year-old woman who may be going through menopause (maturational) when her husband dies suddenly of cancer (situational).

PHASES OF CRISIS

Through extensive study of individuals experiencing crisis, Caplan (1964) identified behaviors that followed a fairly distinct path. These behaviors are categorized in four phases of crisis response.

Phase 1

A person is exposed to a serious stressor or problem, which results in increased anxiety. The increase in anxiety stimulates the use of usual coping methods and defense mechanisms in an effort to address the problem and decrease anxiety.

Phase 2

If the usual coping methods and defense mechanisms fail and the threat persists, anxiety will continue to rise, producing increased discomfort. Individual functioning becomes disorganized. Trial-and-error attempts at problem-solving and restoring balance begin.

Phase 3

If the trial-and-error attempts fail, anxiety can escalate to severe and panic levels. The person mobilizes automatic relief behaviors, such as withdrawal and flight. Resolution may occur at this stage. Resolution may be achieved by compromising needs or redefining the situation to reach an acceptable solution.

Phase 4

If the problem is not solved and new coping skills are ineffective, anxiety can overwhelm the person and lead to serious personality disorganization, depression, confusion, violence against others, or suicidal behavior.

APPLICATION OF THE NURSING PROCESS

Nurses, perhaps more than any other group of healthcare professionals, care for people who are experiencing disruptions in their lives. Because people typically experience increased stress and anxiety in medical, surgical, and psychiatric settings, nurses, as 24/7 direct-care professionals, are positioned to provide care. This nursing care is based on the principle of crisis intervention, a directive, time-limited, and goal-directed strategy designed to assist individuals who are experiencing a crisis. It has been shown to be effective in helping people adaptively cope with stressful events. Knowledge of crisis intervention

BOX 26.1   Foundation for Crisis Intervention

- A crisis has a limited duration and usually resolves within 4–6 weeks.
- Once a crisis is resolved, individuals will emerge at one of three different functional levels:
  - A higher level of functioning.
  - The same level of functioning.
  - A lower level of functioning.
- The goal of crisis intervention is to return the patient to at least the pre-crisis level of functioning.
- The form of crisis resolution depends on the person's perceptions, actions, and the support of others.
- During a crisis, people are often more receptive than usual to outside intervention. With intervention, new and adaptive means of problem solving may be adopted.
- Crisis intervention is here-and-now oriented, with a focus on the person's present problem and resolution of the immediate crisis.
- Due to the disequilibrium of crisis and accompanying anxiety, the nurse takes a more active and directive role in intervention than during non-crisis states.
- Early intervention increases the chance for a positive outcome.

techniques is an important skill of all nurses no matter the practice specialty or clinical setting.

Crisis theory defines aspects of crisis that are basic to crisis intervention and relevant for nurses (Box 26.1).

ASSESSMENT

General Assessment

Components of crisis assessment come from established crisis theory and constitute a sound knowledge base for the application of the nursing process. Data gained from the assessment guide both the nurse and the patient in setting realistic and meaningful goals and in planning possible solutions to the problem situation.

Self-harm is a possibility. Crises may result in such serious disorganization and discomfort that ending the pain may seem a reasonable solution. The nurse's initial task is to assess the patient's potential for suicide. Sample questions to ask include:
- Have you thought about hurting yourself?
- Have you thought of how you would do this?
- Do you feel you can keep yourself safe?

After assessing for safety and intervening appropriately, the nurse assesses the three main areas previously discussed: (1) the patient's perception of the precipitating event, (2) the patient's situational supports, and (3) the patient's personal coping skills.

VIGNETTE: Madison, a 25-year-old woman, is brought to the emergency department by police with allegations of spousal abuse by her wife. Madison is seen by the medical personnel and then interviewed by the psychiatric-mental health registered nurse working in the emergency department. The nurse calmly introduces herself and tells Madison she would like to talk with her. The nurse says, "It looks as if things are overwhelming. Is that how you're feeling?" Madison is slumped in the chair, her hands in her lap, head hanging down, and has tears in her eyes. She nods.

Assessing Perception of the Precipitating Event

The nurse's task is now to assess the individual's perception of the problem. The more clearly the person can define the problem, the more likely the person will identify effective solutions. Sample questions and comments that facilitate the assessment include the following:

- What leads you to seek help now?
- Has anything upsetting happened to you within the past few days or weeks?
- Describe how you are feeling right now.
- How does this situation affect your life?
- How do you see this event affecting your future?
- What do you hope to get out of this treatment?

> **VIGNETTE: Nurse:** "Madison, tell me what happened."
> **Madison:** "I can't go home…, I am so afraid…, No one believes me…, I can't go through it again."
> **Nurse:** "Tell me what you can't go through again."
> (Madison starts to cry, shaking with sobs. The nurse sits quietly for a moment and then speaks.)
> **Nurse:** "Tell me what is so terrible. Let's look at it together."
> After a while, Madison tells the nurse that her wife has always had a bad temper. Recently, she began to hit her and the abuse becomes particularly brutal when she drinks. The beatings have become much worse over time. Madison states, "I'm afraid that she'll eventually kill me."

Assessing Situational Supports

Next, the nurse determines resources by assessing the patient's support systems. When available, family and friends can be involved by offering emotional or material support. If these resources are unavailable, the nurse acts as a temporary support person while assisting the patient to establish relationships with individuals or groups in the community. Sample questions include the following:

- Is there anyone—family or friends—you would like to have involved in your care?
- Have you ever used a community agency for support?
- Do you have a religious affiliation?
- Are you active in a religious group?

> **VIGNETTE: Nurse:** "Madison, what are your options? Do you have any family who can support you?"
> **Madison:** "No. My family is in another state."
> **Nurse:** "How about friends?"
> **Madison:** "I really don't have any friends. My wife's control and jealousy has made it impossible for me to have friends. She finds fault with everyone."
> **Nurse:** "What about your co-workers?"
> **Madison:** "My co-workers are nice, but I can't tell them things like this."
> The nurse learns that Madison does well at work. Madison explains that her job helps her forget her problems for a little while. Getting good job reviews also has another reward: it is the only time her spouse says anything nice about her.

Assessing Coping Skills

Finally, the nurse assesses the patient's coping skills. Common positive coping mechanisms may be seeking out someone to talk to, writing feelings in a journal, or engaging in other physical activity. Ineffective coping includes overeating, drinking, smoking, withdrawing, yelling, and fighting. Sample questions to ask include the following:

- What have you been doing to relieve the anxiety you have been feeling?
- What has helped in the past to relieve stress?
- Did you try it this time? If so, what was different?
- What helped you through difficult times in the past?

> **VIGNETTE: Nurse:** "You've been through an emotionally painful time. Your anxiety is understandable. What has helped you in the past to make you feel calmer?"
> **Madison:** "I don't know. Probably talking."
> **Nurse:** "Okay. While you're here, we will talk for at least 30 minutes each day. In group therapy, you will have the chance to share what you've been going through and hear about how others cope."
> **Madison:** "Thanks. I don't want to be in an abusive marriage. I just don't know where to turn."
> **Nurse:** "I understand. We will work together to come up with a plan."

ASSESSMENT GUIDELINES

Crisis

1. Determine whether the patient is able to identify the *precipitating event*.
2. Assess the patient's understanding of *situational supports*.
3. Identify the patient's usual *coping styles* and determine what coping mechanisms may help the present situation.
4. Determine whether there are certain religious or cultural beliefs that need to be considered in assessing and intervening in this patient's crisis.
5. Assess whether this situation is one in which the patient needs primary prevention (education, environmental manipulation, or new coping skills), secondary prevention (crisis intervention), or tertiary prevention (rehabilitation).

Self-Assessment

Nurses are most effective when they monitor and acknowledge personal feelings and thoughts when caring for patients in crisis. Addressing maturational crises that you have experienced, such as becoming an empty nester, or situational crises, such as the loss of a parent, may be triggers for personal feelings, memories, and fears. Recognizing these triggers and your responses to them increases your ability to be therapeutic and to maintain focus on the patient.

Adventitious crises can be overwhelming for anyone. Even experienced nurses become overwhelmed when witnessing and intervening with catastrophic situations. Natural disasters and accidents are horrific while they are occurring and in their aftermath. The violence perpetrated on others may be unfathomable. Mental healthcare providers experience psychological distress from working with traumatized populations and may even develop posttraumatic stress disorder.

Debriefing is an important step for staff in coming to terms with overwhelmingly violent or otherwise disastrous situations. Such an intervention helps staff put the crisis in perspective and begin their own recovery. Debriefing is discussed in detail later in the chapter.

NURSING DIAGNOSIS

The International Classification for Nursing Practice (International Council of Nurses, 2019) provides nursing diagnoses to consider for a person who may experience a crisis. The most logical choice for individuals who are experiencing anxiety, inefficient communication, problem-solving difficulty, and inability to recognize or access resources is *crisis*. When this diagnosis is applied to the tension in family functioning and communicaiton, it becomes *family crisis*. A diagnosis of *risk for impaired coping* provides structure for addressing and improving coping skills. The nursing diagnosis of *impaired coping* is useful once ineffective behaviors are apparent. *Impaired coping* may be evidenced by an inability to meet basic needs or role expectations. While crises may be experienced individually (such as you totaling your car), events may be severe or widespread enough to impact whole families and communities. Therefore, *risk for* (or actual) *impaired family coping* and *risk for* (or actual) *impaired community coping* become essential diagnoses.

Anxiety is a universal response to a crisis and is an essential nursing diagnosis. *Anxiety* may be linked to a maturational, situational, or adventitious crisis. The diagnostic label specifies the level as mild, moderate, severe, or panic level (e.g., *moderate anxiety*). The level may fluctuate over time and the care plan will require modification to reflect this fluctuation. Severe- and panic-level anxiety are prioritized and need to be addressed and the anxiety reduced before learning more effective coping skills.

OUTCOMES IDENTIFICATION

The outcome for a crisis or a family crisis nursing diagnosis is crisis resolution. Overall outcomes for coping are aimed at effective coping for the individual, family, and community. The overall outcome for anxiety is reduced anxiety. Table 26.1 identifies signs and symptoms commonly experienced in crises, offers potential nursing diagnoses, and suggests outcomes.

PLANNING

Nurses are called upon to plan and intervene through a variety of crisis-intervention modalities. These modalities include disaster nursing, mobile crisis units, group work, health education and crisis prevention, victim outreach programs, and telephone hotlines. You may be involved in planning and intervention for an individual (e.g., cases of physical abuse), for a group (e.g., students after a classmate's suicide or shooting), or for a community (e.g., disaster nursing after tornadoes, shootings, and airplane crashes).

VIGNETTE: In a group meeting with the nurse and a social worker, Madison announces that she has decided to leave her wife and not return home. Madison, the nurse, and the social worker establish goals:
- Madison will return to her pre-crisis state within 2 weeks.
- Madison will find a safe environment.
- Madison will identify at least two outside supports within 24 h.

⊕ CONSIDERING CULTURE

Religion in the Coronavirus Culture War

During times of crisis, people with religious convictions, and even people who formerly had religious convictions, turn to their faith and religious leaders for support and comfort. However, in March of 2020 in the early days of the US response to the coronavirus outbreak, leaders called for bans on all large gatherings. This ban included sporting events, graduations, conferences, and religious services. Religious services were not specifically targeted nor were they specifically exempted. Justice Antonin Scalia provided a 1990 Supreme Court decision as justification for applying general rules to religious groups: We have never held that an individual's religious beliefs excuse him from compliance with an otherwise valid law prohibiting conduct that the State is free to regulate.

Banning religious services resulted in challenges of being anti-constitutional. Opponents noted that it was okay to go to grocery stores and pharmacies, but visiting churches was not. Still, most religious groups complied with the restrictions. Muslims were urged by their leaders to celebrate the holy month at home rather than in mosques. Catholic churches also suspended public mass. At Easter, cellphone records indicate that a large majority of Christians observed this occasion at home.

Creative approaches to receiving the support of the religious community rapidly sprang up. Almost immediately, religious services began to be livestreamed into homes. Seders were celebrated on Zoom. Some out-of-the-box thinkers came up with drive-in theaters as a way to maintain social distancing guidelines while congregating together.

Creative approaches to receiving the support of the religious community rapidly sprang up. Almost immediately, religious services began to be livestreamed into homes. Seders were celebrated on Zoom. Some out-of-the-box thinkers came up with drive-in theaters as a way to maintain social distancing guidelines while congregating together.

Adapted from Frum, D. (2020, May 1). Trump brings religion into the coronavirus culture war. *The Atlantic.* Retrieved from https://www.the-atlantic.com/ideas/archive/2020/05/trump-brings-religion-coronavirus-culture-war/611044/.

TABLE 26.1 Signs and Symptoms, Diagnoses, and Outcomes for Crisis Intervention		
Signs and Symptoms	**Nursing Diagnoses**	**Outcomes**
Severe-panic anxiety, inefficient communication, problem solving difficulty, inability or decreased ability to recognize or access resources	*Crisis*	Crisis resolution: mild-moderate anxiety, effective communication, restored problem-solving ability, accesses resources
Inability to meet basic needs, decreased use of social support, inadequate problem solving, inability to attend to information, isolation	*Impaired coping*	Effective coping: modifies lifestyle as needed, uses effective coping strategies, reports decrease in physical symptoms of stress, reports decrease in negative feelings
Changes in family relationships and functioning, difficulty performing family caregiver role	*Impaired family coping*	Effective family coping: manages family problems, expresses feelings openly among family members, respite for caregiver, caregiver feels a sense of control
Unsatisfactory pattern of community responses, not meeting community needs, ineffective guidance, unresponsive to cultural needs, sustained community anxiety	*Impaired community coping*	Effective community coping: meets community safety needs, provides mental health support, supports cultural differences
Excessive fear, obsessively monitoring (e.g., news, social media, health), feels a loss of control	*Anxiety* (identify level)	Reduced anxiety: realistic appraisal of the threat, limits monitoring of anxiety-provoking stimuli, focuses on aspects within personal control

International Council of Nursing Practice. (2019). *ICNP browser.* Retrieved from https://www.icn.ch/what-we-do/projects/ehealth/icnp-browser. ICNP® is owned and copyrighted by the International Council of Nurses (ICN). Reproduced with permission of the copyright holder.

IMPLEMENTATION

Psychosocial Interventions

Crisis intervention is a function of the psychiatric-mental health registered nurse. The focus is on the present problem only and has two initial goals:

1. **Patient safety.** You can apply external controls for protection of the patient in crisis if the patient is suicidal or homicidal.
2. **Anxiety reduction.** Use anxiety-reduction techniques so the patient can mobilize inner resources.

During the initial interview, the patient in crisis needs to experience feelings of safety. Feelings of support and hope will temporarily diminish anxiety. The nurse needs to play an active role by indicating that help is available by using crisis-intervention skills competently and showing genuine interest and support.

The nurse may act as educator, advisor, and role model, always keeping in mind that it is the patient who solves the problem, not the nurse. The following are important assumptions when working with a patient in crisis:

- The patient is ultimately in charge for life direction.
- The patient is able to make decisions.
- The crisis counseling relationship is one between partners.

The nurse helps the patient to gain new perspectives on the situation. The nurse supports the patient during the process of finding constructive ways to solve or cope with the problem. It is important for the nurse to be mindful of how difficult it is for the patient to change behavior. Table 26.2 offers guidelines for nursing interventions and corresponding rationales.

Levels of Prevention

Crisis interventions are directed toward three levels of prevention: (1) primary, (2) secondary, and (3) tertiary.

Primary Prevention

Primary prevention promotes mental health and reduces mental illness to decrease the incidence of crisis. On this level the nurse can:

- Work with a patient to recognize potential problems by evaluating the patient's experience of stressful life events.
- Teach the patient specific coping skills, such as decision making, problem solving, assertiveness skills, meditation, and relaxation skills.
- Assist the patient in evaluating the timing or reduction of life changes to decrease the negative effects of stress as much as possible. This may involve working with a patient to plan environmental changes, make important interpersonal decisions, and rethink changes in occupational roles.

Secondary Prevention

Secondary prevention establishes intervention during an acute crisis to *prevent* prolonged anxiety from diminishing personal effectiveness and personality organization. The nurse's focus is to ensure the safety of the patient. After safety issues have been addressed, the nurse works with the patient to assess the patient's problem, support systems, and coping styles. Desired goals are explored and interventions planned. Secondary care lessens the time a patient is mentally disabled during a crisis. Secondary care occurs in hospital units, emergency departments, clinics, or mental health centers, usually during daytime hours.

Tertiary Prevention

Tertiary prevention programs and services provide long-term support for those who have experienced a crisis. Social and community facilities that offer tertiary prevention include rehabilitation centers, sheltered workshops, day hospitals, and outpatient clinics. Goals are to facilitate optimal levels of functioning and prevent further emotional disruptions. People with severe and persistent mental problems are often

TABLE 26.2 Guidelines for Crisis Intervention	
Intervention	**Rationale**
Assess for suicidal or homicidal thoughts or plans.	Physical safety is always the first consideration.
Take initial steps to make patient feel safe and less anxious.	A person who feels safe and less anxious is able to more effectively problem solve solutions with the nurse.
Listen carefully (e.g., make eye contact, give frequent feedback to verify and convey understanding, summarize what patient says).	People who believe others are really listening are more likely to believe that someone cares about their situation and that help may be available, which offers hope.
Crisis intervention calls for directive and creative approaches. Initially, the nurse may make phone calls to arrange babysitters, schedule a visiting nurse, find shelter, or contact a social worker.	A person who is confused, frightened, or overwhelmed may be temporarily unable to perform usual tasks.
Identify needed social supports (with patient's input) and mobilize the priority.	Determine a person's need for shelter, help with care for children or elders, medical workup, emergency medical attention, hospitalization, food, safe housing, and self-help groups.
Identify needed coping skills (e.g., problem solving, relaxation, assertiveness, job training, newborn care, self-esteem building).	Increasing coping skills and learning new ones can help with the current crisis and help minimize future crises.
Involve patient in identifying realistic, acceptable interventions.	The person's involvement in planning increases a sense of control, self-esteem, and adherence to plan.
Plan regular follow-up (e.g., phone calls, clinic visits, home visits) to assess patient's progress.	Evaluate the plan to see what works and what does not.

extremely susceptible to crisis, and community facilities provide the structured environment that can help prevent problem situations.

Online forums and support groups are available for virtually every type of crisis that can be experienced. While locating this type of support may seem natural and intuitive to many of us, some people would benefit by suggestions. A thoughtful and beneficial intervention is doing a search for appropriate and reputable e-based support and providing your patient with this information.

Critical incident stress debriefing. **Critical incident stress debriefing (CISD)** is an example of tertiary prevention directed toward a group that has experienced a crisis. CISD consists of a seven-phase group meeting that offers individuals the opportunity to share their thoughts and feelings in a safe and controlled environment. It is used to debrief staff on an inpatient unit following a patient suicide or an incident of violence, to debrief crisis hotline volunteers, to debrief schoolchildren and school personnel after multiple school shootings, and to debrief rescue and healthcare workers who have responded to a natural disaster or a terrorist attack such as that on the World Trade Center in New York City.

The phases of CISD are:

- *Introductory phase*—Meeting purpose is explained; an overview of the debriefing process is provided; confidentiality is ensured; guidelines are explained; team members are identified; and questions are answered.
- *Fact phase*—Participants discuss the facts of the incident; participants introduce themselves, tell their involvement in the incident, and describe the event from their perspective.
- *Thought phase*—Participants discuss their first thoughts of the incident.
- *Reaction phase*—Participants talk about the worst thing about the incident—what they would like to forget, what was most painful.
- *Symptom phase*—Participants describe their cognitive, physical, emotional, or behavioral experiences at the incident scene and describe any symptoms they felt following the initial experience.
- *Teaching phase*—The normalcy of the expressed symptoms is acknowledged and affirmed; anticipatory guidance is offered regarding future symptoms; the group is involved in stress-management techniques.
- *Reentry phase*—Participants review material discussed, introduce new topics, ask questions, and discuss how they would like to bring closure to the debriefing. Debriefing team members answer questions, inform, and reassure; provide written material; provide information on referral sources; and summarize the debriefing with encouragement, support, and appreciation.

VIGNETTE: After talking with the nurse and the social worker, Madison seems open to going to a safe house for battered women. She also agrees to talk to a counselor at a mental health facility. The nurse sets up an appointment at which she, Madison, and the counselor will meet.

EVALUATION

As previously discussed, the goal of crisis intervention is to return people to their pre-crisis level of functioning. Evaluation of this goal is the single best indicator of successful crisis intervention.

EVIDENCE-BASED PRACTICE

Do Crisis Lines Reduce Suicide Risk?

Problem
Crisis hotlines have traditionally been used to address immediate problems, de-escalate the caller, and link people with services. The hotlines could do more by providing outreach, follow-up, and actually intervening to reduce future risk.

Purpose of the Study
This study explored the feasibility and effectiveness of using the Safety Planning Intervention (SPI), which is a brief intervention designed to help manage suicidal crises. The SPI is a list of coping strategies that includes monitoring for warning signs of a suicidal crisis, using internal coping strategies, reaching out to family and friends, seeking community support, and restricting access to lethal means of suicide.

Methods
Counselors ($N = 271$) at five centers in the National Suicide Prevention Lifeline network were trained to use SPI. The counselors provided self-report surveys three times: immediately after the training time, at the end of the study, and 9 months later.

Key Findings
- Counselors reported that SPI was feasible and helpful, and was used on both incoming and follow-up calls.
- SPI may be a promising intervention for reducing callers' future suicide risk.

Implications for Nursing Practice
Nurses in all settings work with patients who are experiencing healthcare crises due to pain, fear, and uncertainty. During these traumatic periods, suicidal thoughts are far too common. Tools such as the SPI provide a base for nursing interventions for patients and families.

Labouliere, C. D., Stanley, B., Lake, A. M., & Gould, M. S. (2019). Safety planning on crisis lines: feasibility, acceptability, and perceived helpfulness of a brief intervention to mitigate future suicide risk. *Suicide and Life-Threatening Behavior*. https://doi.org/10.1111/sltb.12554.

TREATMENT MODALITIES

Crisis intervention can happen in almost any setting. Traditionally, people seeking emergency services go to hospitals. Unfortunately, not only are emergency rooms expensive, but they may also lack the time and staff with specialized training necessary to address patients' needs.

Models of providing emergency care are referred to, not surprisingly, as crisis care. The Substance Abuse and Mental Health Service Administration provides national guidelines for behavioral health crisis care (Substance Abuse and Mental Health Service Administration, 2020). The evidence base for these services is growing, and research has shown that these services can have an impact on healthcare costs as well as quality of life.

Crisis Call Lines

The National Suicide Prevention Lifeline is available for suicide prevention and crisis assistance at 1-800-273-8255 (1-800-273-TALK) and online chats. Veteran-specific care is also available through this number by pressing 1 once connected. In 2020 the US Federal Communication Commission (FCC) adopted rules to establish the number 988 as the new, nationwide, 3-digit phone number for Americans in crisis to connect with the national lifeline (FCC, 2021). 988 will be available for consumer use by July 16, 2022.

Crisis call lines are essential first-line support for people in acute crises. They provide 24/7/365 immediate responses from a variety of people—from professionals to trained volunteers. An assessment for suicidal ideation along with an assessment for potential violence to others are vital. These confidential services do not require insurance and can link people with other community services. Ideally, programs will also offer text and chat options to better engage virtual communities.

Warm Lines

Similar to crisis hotlines, warm lines provide confidential telephone support. Unlike crisis hotlines, warm lines are not designed for crisis situations, but to prevent escalation of distress. This support service is provided by trained consumers, people who have lived experience using mental health services. These consumers provide emotional support, comfort, and information.

Crisis Intervention Teams

Crisis intervention teams are available to reach any person where they are, including home, workplace, or any other community-based location. A licensed and/or credentialed clinician, such as a psychiatric nurse practitioner, who is qualified to conduct assessments is an integral part of the team. Peers, who have a first-person understanding of crisis care, are incorporated into these teams. Essential services include:

- Triage and screening, including a suicidality assessment
- De-escalation
- Peer support
- Coordination with medical and behavioral health services
- Crisis planning and follow-up

One of the main goals of crisis teams is to reduce unnecessary trips to the emergency department and avoid subsequent hospitalizations. Diversion from incarceration is another goal of crisis teams. The Crisis Intervention Team (CIT) program is a partnership of law enforcement, mental health and addiction professionals, individuals who live with mental illness and/or addiction disorders, their families, and other advocates (CIT International, 2017). Because law enforcement officers are the first responders in most crises, specialized police-based training helps them recognize mental illness-related behaviors. This training also improves communication, identifies mental health resources for those in crisis, and supports officer and community safety. Ultimately, individuals with mental illness are kept out of jail and gain access to treatment.

Crisis Stabilization Facilities

The goal of crisis stabilization facilities is to provide short-term care (under 24 hours) and to quickly de-escalate crisis situations and avoid unnecessary and costly hospitalizations. The goal is to eliminate or reduce acute symptoms of psychiatric disorders. Participants are provided with a range of community-based resources and a safe environment for care and recovery.

All referrals, walk-ins, and first responder drop-offs are accepted. Patients are provided with specific connections for outpatient care, such as residential substance treatment or partial hospitalization programs.

Psychiatrists or psychiatric nurse practitioners serve as clinical leaders of the multi-disciplinary crisis team. Some facilities use telehealth to satisfy this requirement. Licensed and/or credentialed clinicians work in conjunction with peers with lived experience similar to the experience of the population served. Suicide and potential for violence screens are conducted when they are clinically indicated.

Psychiatric Advance Directive Plan

A psychiatric advance directive plan is a proactive method of addressing a crisis situation before it occurs. Usually, advance directives are used in end-of-life situations. In psychiatry, these plans take the form of a document that is developed by the consumer to be used in crisis situations where the consumer is unable to make decisions. It stipulates wishes such as treatment choices, treatment facilities, and providers, and designates a support person who can be involved in decision making.

DISASTER RESPONSE

There is a growing awareness of interdependencies that exist among all members of the global community. Each successive large-scale earthquake, tsunami, hurricane, flood, or wildfire has ripple effects regardless of where in the world it occurs. The coronavirus pandemic that began in 2019 significantly increased our understanding of the magnitude of disasters. Directly or remotely, we experience some element of the far-reaching depletion of human, economic, and natural resources.

A decade of 21st-century disaster literature supports disaster preparedness by developing resilient communities and assessing disaster risks on a local level. Considering the unique forms of devastation connected with any disaster, reducing risk within local communities should be expedient, eventually extending into networking communities, then to larger societal and national programs.

Professional nurses regularly provide strong and dynamic core contributions to the multiple facets of disaster and recovery relief efforts around the world. Professional nurses are experienced care providers and managers of care who are adaptable with critical thinking and problem-solving expertise. Also, professional nurses are visibly emerging around the world both as

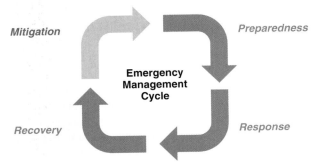

Fig. 26.3 Emergency Management Cycle. (From Federal Emergency Management Agency. [2019]. Unit 4: FEMA training. Retrieved from https://training.fema.gov/emiweb/downloads/is111_unit%204.pdf.)

disaster researchers and authors, and as pivotal spokespeople in disaster management planning arenas.

The Federal Emergency Management Agency [FEMA] (2018) outlines a four-phase disaster management continuum (Fig. 26.3).

1. Mitigation: Attempt to limit a disaster's impact on human health and community function. This phase includes actions taken to prevent or reduce the cause, impact, and consequences of disasters.
2. Preparedness: The protective plan designed before the event takes place to structure the response, assess risk, and evaluate damage. This phase includes such activities as constructing warning systems, developing emergency operating plans, and planning for communication with the public.
3. Response: The response phase occurs in the immediate aftermath of a disaster. During the response phase, business and other operations do not function normally. Personal safety and well-being in an emergency and the duration of the response phase depend on the level of preparedness. Examples of responses include the activation of emergency plans and systems, sending out messages to the public, providing shelter, evacuation, and search and rescue.
4. Recovery: During the recovery period, restoration efforts occur concurrently with regular operations and activities. The recovery period from a disaster can be prolonged.

Evaluation may be the sixth phase of the disaster management continuum. Looking back provides greater clarity and helps to refine and improve future mitigation, preparation, response, and recovery strategies.

Disaster Management Context

On November 25, 2002, the events of 9/11 prompted the creation of a government cabinet, the Department of Homeland Security (DHS). Its charge was to coordinate responses to US disasters, particularly in situations where local and state

CASE STUDY AND NURSING CARE PLAN

Crisis

Sandy Gregg, an advanced practice psychiatric-mental health registered nurse, is called to the neurological unit to see Ahiga Begay, a 43-year-old man with Guillain-Barré syndrome. He has severe muscle weakness and is not yet able to breathe on his own.

The nurse manager reports that Mr. Begay makes sexually suggestive remarks, uses abusive language, and has angry outbursts. The nurses state that they have tried to be patient and understanding. However, nothing seems to get through to him.

Mr. Begay, a Native American, was employed as a taxi driver. His fiancée visits him every day. He needs assistance with every aspect of his activities of daily living. Because of his severe muscle weakness, he has to be turned and positioned every 2 hours and fed through a gastrostomy tube.

Assessment

Ms. Gregg gathers data from Mr. Begay, the nursing staff, and Mr. Begay's fiancée.

Perception of the Precipitating Event

Mr. Begay expresses anger about needing a nurse to "scratch my head and help me blow my nose." He still cannot figure out how his illness developed. He says the doctors told him that it was too early to know for sure if he would recover completely but that the prognosis was hopeful.

Support System

Ms. Gregg speaks with Mr. Begay's fiancée. She learns that Mr. Begay has been angry and impatient with her, too. However, she intends to stand by him. Mr. Begay strongly identifies with his Native American cultural group. With minimal ties outside their reservation, neither Mr. Begay nor his fiancée has much knowledge of community support.

Personal Coping Skills

Mr. Begay comes from a male-dominated subculture where men are expected to be strong leaders. His ability to be an independent person with the power to affect the direction of his life is central to his perception of being a man.

Mr. Begay feels powerless, out of control, and enraged. He is handling his anxiety by displacing these feelings onto the environment, namely, the staff and his fiancée. This redirection of anger temporarily lowers his anxiety and distracts him from painful feelings. His behavior leads others to minimize interactions with him, which increases his sense of isolation and helplessness.

Self-Assessment

Ms. Gregg meets with the staff twice. The staff discuss feelings of helplessness and lack of control stemming from their feelings of rejection by Mr. Begay. They talk about their anger about Mr. Begay's behavior and frustration about the situation. Ms. Gregg points out to the staff that Mr. Begay's feelings of helplessness, lack of control, and anger at his situation are the same feelings the staff are experiencing.

The nurses develop a plan to focus more on the patient, less on personal reactions, and decide on two approaches they can try as a group. First, they will not take Mr. Begay's behavior personally. Second, Mr. Begay's displaced feelings will be refocused back to him.

Priority Diagnosis

Impaired coping related to inadequate coping methods as evidenced by inappropriate use of defense mechanisms (displacement), anger, isolation, and continued escalation of anxiety.

Outcomes Identification

Mr. Begay will experience improved coping and will state that he feels more comfortable discussing difficult feelings by discharge.

Implementation

Mr. Begay's care plan is personalized as follows:

CASE STUDY AND NURSING CARE PLAN—cont'd

Short-Term Goal	Intervention	Rationale	Evaluation
1. By the end of the week, Mr. Begay will be able to name and discuss at least two feelings about his illness and lack of mobility.	a. Nurse will meet with patient daily for 15 min at 7:30 a.m. b. When patient lashes out, nurse will remain calm. c. Nurse will consistently redirect and refocus anger from environment back to patient (e.g., "It must be difficult to be in this situation"). d. Nurse will come on time each day and stay for allotted time.	a. Night is usually the most frightening for patient; in early morning, feelings are closer to surface. b. Patient perceives that nurse is in control of her feelings. This can reassure patient and increase patient's sense of security. c. Refocusing feelings offers patient opportunity to cope effectively with his anxiety and decreases need to act out. d. Consistency sets stage for trust and reinforces that patient's anger will not drive nurse away.	**GOAL MET** Within 7 days, Mr. Begay speaks to nurse more openly about feelings.

Dialogue	Therapeutic Tool/Comment
Nurse: "Mr. Begay, I'm here as we discussed. I'll be spending 15 minutes with you every morning. We could use this time to talk about some of your concerns."	Nurse offers herself as a resource, gives information, and clarifies her role and patient expectations. Night is Mr. Begay's most difficult time. In the early morning, he will be the most vulnerable and open for therapeutic intervention and support.
Mr. Begay: "Listen, sweetheart, my only concern is how to get a little sexual relief, get it?"	
Nurse: "Being hospitalized and partially paralyzed can be overwhelming for anyone. Perhaps you wish you could find some relief from your situation."	Nurse focuses on the process "need for relief," not the sexual content, and encourages discussion of feelings.
Mr. Begay: "What do you know, Miss Know-it-all? I can't even scratch my nose without getting one of those fools to do it for me..."	
Nurse: "It must be difficult to have to ask people to do everything for you."	Nurse restates what the patient says in terms of his feelings and continues to refocus away from the environment back to the patient.
Mr. Begay: "Yeah... The other night a fly kept landing on my face. I had to yell for 5 minutes before one of those stupid aides came in."	
Nurse: "Having to rely on others for everything can be a terrifying experience for anyone. It sounds extremely frustrating for you."	Nurse acknowledges that frustration and anger would be a natural response for anyone in this situation. This encourages the patient to talk about these feelings instead of acting them out.
Mr. Begay: "Yeah... It's a bitch...like a living hell."	

Evaluation

After 6 weeks, Mr. Begay is able to get around with assistance, and his ability to perform his activities of daily living is increasing. Although Mr. Begay still feels angry and overwhelmed, he is able to identify his feelings and acts them out less often. He is able to talk to his fiancée about his feelings, and he lashes out at her less. He is looking forward to going home, and his boss is holding his old job. He contacted the Guillain-Barré Society to attend a support group.

Staff feel more comfortable and competent in their relationships with Mr. Begay. The goals have been met. Mr. Begay and Ms. Gregg agree that the crisis is over and terminate their visits. Mr. Begay is given a crisis line number and encouraged to call if he has questions or feels the need to talk. He is also provided with the Guillain-Barré syndrome website for education and support.

resources were inadequate to the presenting challenges. As a result, the DHS has ultimate governmental responsibility for the safety of US citizens and territories while ensuring that adequate preparedness, response, and recovery protocols are immediately available.

To achieve its objectives, the DHS uses civilian first responders, local emergency response professionals who prepare for and respond to natural disasters or terrorist threats or any other large-scale event. In 2004, DHS furthered its agenda and created the National Incident Management System (NIMS) to help first responders from different disciplines and areas to effectively work together when a community exhausts its available resources in addressing a large-scale occurrence.

To understand NIMS operations, incident command system training (ICS) is required. ICS provides a common organizational structure facilitating an immediate response to occurrences by establishing a clear chain of command that supports the coordination of personnel and equipment at the event site. The DHS has developed minimal core competencies for individuals expected to participate in an event and has included these in established training programs (FEMA, 2012).

KEY POINTS TO REMEMBER

- Crises not only can lead to personality disorganization but also can offer opportunities for emotional growth.
- There are three types of crises: maturational, situational, and adventitious.
- Crises are usually resolved within 4 to 6 weeks.
- Crisis intervention therapy is short term, from 1 to 6 weeks, and focuses on the present problem only.
- Resolution of a crisis takes three forms: a patient emerges at a higher level, at the pre-crisis level, or at a lower level of functioning.
- Social support and intervention can promote successful resolution.
- Nurses take an active and directive approach with the patient in crisis.
- Whenever possible, the patient is an active participant in setting goals and planning possible solutions.

- Crisis intervention is usually aimed at the mentally healthy patient who generally is functioning well but is temporarily overwhelmed and unable to function.
- The crisis model can be adapted to meet the needs of patients in crisis who have long-term and persistent mental problems.
- Specific qualities in the nurse that can facilitate effective intervention are a caring attitude, flexibility in planning care, an ability to listen, and an active approach.
- The basic goals of crisis intervention are to reduce the individual's anxiety level and to support the effort to return to the patient's pre-crisis level of functioning.
- Disaster occurrences and management are global concerns that involve nurses.
- Disaster-preparedness training can optimize nursing contributions to disaster planning and management.

CRITICAL THINKING

1. List the three important areas of the crisis assessment once safety concerns have been identified. Give examples of two questions in each area that need to be answered before planning can take place.
2. Taylor is 21 years old and a junior in nursing school. She tells her nursing instructor that her 45-year-old father has been drinking heavily for years and recently lost his job. Adding to the family's stress is that her mother has multiple sclerosis with worsening symptoms. Taylor plans to quit school to take care of her.
   a. How many different types of crises are going on in this family? Discuss the crises from the viewpoint of each family member.
   b. If this family came for crisis counseling, what areas would you assess? What kinds of questions would you ask to evaluate each member's individual needs and the needs of the family as a unit (perception of events, social supports, coping styles)?
   c. Formulate some tentative goals you might set in conjunction with the family during this crisis period.
   d. Identify specific referral agencies in your area that would be helpful if members of this family were willing to expand their use of outside resources and to stabilize the situation.
   e. How would you set up follow-up visits for this family? Would you see the family members together, alone, or in a combination during the crisis period (4 to 6 weeks)? How would you decide whether follow-up counseling was indicated?

CHAPTER REVIEW

1. Which patient statement indicates the helpfulness of the nurse-patient relationship?
   a. "I appreciate the time you spent with me. I have a better understanding of what I can do to manage my problem."
   b. "I really need to talk with you. You always give me good advice about how to address my anger issues."
   c. "If it wasn't for you and the hours we've spent talking, I don't think I would be on my way to getting my anxiety under control."
   d. "You always showed me sympathy when I was at my lowest point after the sexual assault. Knowing you had been there too was such a help."
2. A female nurse had been sexually assaulted as a teenager. She finds it difficult to work with patients who have undergone the same trauma. What is the most helpful response?
   a. Discussing these feelings with the nurse supervisor.
   b. Requesting that these patients not be a part of her patient assignment.
   c. Discussing these feelings with a mental health professional.
   d. Accepting her role in providing unbiased, respectful, and professional care to all patients.

3. A patient whose history includes experiences with abusive partners is being treated for major depressive disorder. The patient's care plan includes *rape-trauma syndrome* among its nursing diagnoses. What goal is directly associated with this diagnosis?
   a. Remains free from self-harm
   b. Wears appropriate clothing
   c. Reports feeling stronger and having a sense of hopefulness
   d. Demonstrates appropriate affect for both positive and negative emotions
4. The nurse is engaged in crisis intervention with a female patient who states, "I have no reason to keep on living." What is the nurse's initial intervention?
   a. Advise the patient about the services available to help her.
   b. Ask the patient, "Have you ever been this depressed before?"
   c. Ask the patient, "Do you have any plan to hurt yourself or anyone else?"
   d. Assure the patient that she is in a safe place and will be well cared for.

5. Which statement concerning a crisis experience is true and should be used as a guideline for crisis management care? *Select all that apply.*
   a. A crisis is self-limiting and usually resolves within 4 to 6 weeks.
   b. The earlier the interventions are implemented, the better the expected prognosis.
   c. The nurse should maintain a nondirective role.
   d. The patient in crisis is assumed to be mentally unhealthy and in an extreme state of disequilibrium.
   e. The goal of crisis management is to return the patient to at least the pre-crisis level of functioning.

6. Which statement about crisis theory will provide a basis for nursing intervention?
   a. A crisis is an acute time-limited phenomenon experienced as an overwhelming emotional reaction to a problem perceived as unsolvable.
   b. A person in crisis has always had adjustment problems and has coped inadequately in the usual life situations.
   c. Crisis is precipitated by an event that enhances a person's self-concept and self-esteem.
   d. Nursing intervention in crisis situations rarely has the effect of stopping the crisis.

7. Lilly, a single mother of four, comes to the crisis center 24 hours after a fire in which all the houses within a one-block area were wiped out. All of Lilly's household goods and clothing were lost. Lilly has no other family in the area. Her efforts to mobilize assistance have been disorganized, and she is still without shelter. She is distraught and confused. You assess the situation as:
   a. A maturational crisis.
   b. An adventitious crisis.
   c. A crisis of confidence.
   d. An existential crisis.

8. When responding to the patient in question 7, the intervention that takes priority is to:
   a. Reduce anxiety.
   b. Arrange shelter.
   c. Contact out-of-area family.
   d. Hospitalize and place the patient on suicide precautions.

9. Which belief would be least helpful for a nurse working in crisis intervention?
   a. A person in crisis is incapable of responding to instruction.
   b. The crisis counseling relationship is one between partners.
   c. Crisis counseling helps the patient refocus to gain new perspectives on the situation.
   d. Anxiety-reduction techniques are used so the patient's inner resources can be accessed.

10. The highest-priority goal of crisis intervention is:
    a. Anxiety reduction.
    b. Identification of situational supports.
    c. Teaching specific coping skills that are lacking.
    d. Patient safety.

1. **a**; 2. **c**; 3. **c**; 4. **c**; 5. **a, b, e**; 6. **a**; 7. **b**; 8. **a**; 9. **a**; 10. **d**

Visit the Evolve website for a posttest on the content in this chapter: http://evolve.elsevier.com/Varcarolis

REFERENCES

Caplan, G. (1964). *Principles of preventive psychiatry.* New York, NY: Basic Books.
CIT International. (2017). *Learn about CIT programs.* Retrieved from https://www.citinternational.org/Learn-About-CIT.
Federal Communications Commission. (2021). *Suicide prevention hotline.* Retrieved from https://www.fcc.gov/suicide-prevention-hotline.
International Council of Nurses. (2019). *International Classification for Nursing Practice catalog.* Retrieved from https://www.icn.ch/sites/default/files/inline-files/ICNP2019-DC.pdf.
Joint Commission on Mental Illness and Health. (1961). *Action for mental health: Final report, 1961.* New York, NY: Basic Books.
Lindemann, E. (1944). Symptomatology and acute grief. *American Journal of Psychiatry, 101,* 141–148.
Substance Abuse and Mental Health Service Administration. (2020). *National guidelines for behavioral health crisis care.* Retrieved from https://www.samhsa.gov/sites/default/files/national-guidelines-for-behavioral-health-crisis-care-02242020.pdf.

27

Anger, Aggression, and Violence

Lorann Murphy

Visit the Evolve website for a pretest on the content in this chapter: http://evolve.elsevier.com/Varcarolis

OBJECTIVES

1. Define anger, aggression, and violence.
2. Identify biological and cognitive risk factors for increased angry, aggressive, or violent feelings and behaviors.
3. Discuss three types of assessment questions and their value in the nursing process.
4. Compare and contrast interventions for a patient with healthy coping skills with those for a patient with marginal coping behaviors.
5. Apply at least four principles of deescalation with a moderately angry patient.
6. Describe two criteria that make the use of seclusion or restraint more appropriate than verbal intervention.
7. Role-play with classmates using understandable but unhelpful responses to anger and aggression in patients.
8. Role-play with classmates using helpful responses to anger and aggression in patients.

KEY TERMS AND CONCEPTS

aggression
anger
critical incident debriefing

deescalation techniques
restraint
seclusion

trauma-informed care
validation therapy
violence

Anger, aggression, and violence are the subjects of daily news headlines. Child abuse, youth violence, suicide, elder abuse, sexual abuse, and intimate partner abuse are concerns nationwide. A more recent form of violence is found with the use of communication technologies. The Centers for Disease Control and Prevention (2018) has a website dedicated to violence prevention. Nurses are in a unique position to help prevent violence and intervene to decrease harm.

CLINICAL PICTURE

Anger is an emotional response to frustration of desires, a threat to one's needs (emotional or physical), or a challenge. It is a normal emotion that can even be positive when it is expressed in a healthy way. Once anger is acknowledged, channeling anger into productive pursuits such as exercise, art, or cleaning out a closet is healthy. Anger can also be a motivator to try harder or an aid in survival when fighting is the last and only resort.

Aggression is an action or behavior that results in a verbal or physical attack. Aggression tends to be used synonymously with violence. However, aggression is not always inappropriate and is sometimes necessary for self-protection. On the other hand, **violence** is always an objectionable act that involves intentional use of force that results in, or has the potential to result in, injury to another person.

Coping with a patient's anger is a challenge. Effective nursing intervention becomes more difficult when the anger becomes personal and is directed at the nurse or nursing student. Nursing interventions should, ideally, begin before anger and aggression become a problem. Violence is often associated with psychiatric disorders. You may find that there is impulsive violence in psychosis, borderline personality disorder, posttraumatic stress disorder (PTSD), and intermittent explosive disorder. Anxiety is often the precipitant for negative feelings and behaviors. Assessing and responding to this anxiety can have extremely positive returns. Refer to Chapter 15 for interventions to reduce anxiety before it becomes a crisis.

EPIDEMIOLOGY

The Centers for Disease Control and Prevention (2019) reports that seven people die every hour in the United States from violence. It is likely that you will need to manage violent behavior at some point in your career. Nurses are frequent targets of violence because they have the most direct patient contact. Violence can occur anywhere in the hospital, but it is most frequent in the emergency rooms; however, psychiatric units, geriatric units, and intensive care units are also overrepresented in patient and patients' significant other attacks.

Examples of violence involving healthcare workers include:

- Two emergency medical technicians (EMTs) were taking a woman with psychiatric issues to Massachusetts General Hospital when the woman stabbed an EMT in the body and legs at least seven times. One wound to the abdomen was 4 inches deep (CBS Boston, 2019).
- A nurse in Louisiana died after getting into an altercation with a patient on a mental health floor while she was trying to assist a coworker who was being attacked (Brusie, 2019).
- As an emergency room nurse in Wisconsin attempted to medicate a patient, the patient hit her in the face, grabbed her stethoscope, and choked her (Staudinger, 2019).

COMORBIDITY

A great deal of research has been done on aggression and violence in people with PTSD and substance use disorders. Nearly 11% of patients with a first bipolar I psychotic episode demonstrate aggressive behavior (Khalsa et al., 2018).

Anger and hostility have effects on physical well-being. Anger and hostility may be predictive of hospitalizations for multiple chronic illnesses (Keith et al., 2017). They are risk factors for hypertension and cardiovascular disease. Anger and hostility in older adults are related to a higher prevalence of inflammation and chronic illness (Barlow et al., 2019).

RISK FACTORS

Biological Factors

Genetic

Anger and aggression were once necessary for survival. As a result, some individuals may be more biologically predisposed to respond to life events with irritability, easy frustration, and anger. Researchers have identified a modification of the monoamine oxidase A (MAOA) gene that is associated with aggressive tendencies (Klasen et al., 2019). This genetic tendency coupled with various environmental factors may lead to a person having more violent tendencies.

Neurobiological

Neurological conditions are associated with anger and aggression. Brain tumors, Alzheimer disease, temporal lobe epilepsy, and traumatic injury to certain parts of the brain result in changes to personality that could include increased violence. Many patients with brain injury have severe behavior disorders, including aggressiveness, that disrupt their lives.

Neural circuits in various regions of the brain are related to aggression. One area of the brain associated with aggression is the limbic system. It is located just beneath the cerebrum on both sides of the thalamus. It is responsible for combining higher mental functions and primitive emotions into one system, learning, and the formation of memories. Important structures within this system include the amygdala, hippocampus, and hypothalamus. The amygdala helps the brain to recognize potential threats and whether to activate the

fight-or-flight response. Research supports that various subdivisions of the amygdala are responsible for different types of aggression (Haller, 2018). The size of the amygdala is inversely related to aggressive responses (Matthies et al., 2012). That is, the smaller the amygdala, the more likely are aggressive responses and vice versa.

The hippocampus lies in close proximity to the amygdala and connects to it. This seahorse-shaped structure is essential to the formation of memories. Animal studies suggest that neurons in the hippocampus are associated with social aggression (Leroy et al., 2018).

The hypothalamus is located in the center of the brain below the thalamus. It has a function in endocrine and neurological pathways. The hypothalamus is associated with aggressive behavior, especially the ventrolateral portion is the key area (Hashikawa et al., 2017).

The large prefrontal cortex in humans also plays an important role in aggressive behavior. This area of the brain is responsible for executive function. Executive function allows us to distinguish between good and bad, consequences of actions, goal-directed behavior, and suppressing socially unacceptable activities. Structural abnormalities of the prefrontal cortex have been associated with aggression in individuals with schizophrenia (Leclerc et al., 2018). Bertsch et al. (2019) found that deficits in the prefrontal cortex were connected to anger-related aggression in males with borderline personality disorder.

Neurotransmitters

Neurotransmitters, especially serotonin, dopamine, and gamma-aminobutyric acid (GABA), play a role in anger and aggression. Serotonin can both inhibit and stimulate aggressive behavior depending on the part of the brain being affected. Dopamine's impact on reward-seeking behavior may increase aggression. Like serotonin, dopamine can both enhance aggression and also reduce impulsivity that leads to aggression. GABA, the main inhibitory neurotransmitter, may reduce aggressiveness. Reduced GABA may increase impulsivity and aggressive responses. Glutamate levels are associated with aggression in antisocial personality disorder (Smaragdi et al., 2019).

Cognitive Factors

In *Civilization and Its Discontents,* Freud (1930) asserted that conflict between sexual needs and societal norms was the source of dissatisfaction, aggression, hostility, and ultimately violence. Menninger (2007) suggested that the struggle for control over our lives is a fundamental drive in every person. If that control is threatened, we experience trauma, and it is from that trauma that anger, aggression, and violence may originate.

Early behaviorists believed that emotions, including anger, were learned responses to environmental stimuli (Skinner, 1953). The stimulus is often a perceived threat, and this perception leads to the emotional and physiological arousal necessary to act. Although the threat is usually understood as an alert to physical danger, Beck (1976) noted that other threats to areas such as values, beliefs, and moral code could also lead to anger. For example, clinic patients kept waiting for long periods of time without explanation may perceive this wait as a lack of respect. When the initial appraisal is followed by thoughts such as, "They have no right to treat me this way. I am a person too," anger may escalate and violence is possible. Patients less predisposed to anger might interpret the wait as a sign that the clinic is busy. These patients might be frustrated by the situation. However, in the absence of anger they might be proactive and ask how much longer the wait is likely to be, find distractions in the environment, or reschedule the appointment.

Social learning researchers demonstrated that children learn aggression by observing and imitating behaviors of others, especially if that behavior is rewarded (Bandura, 1973). Thus, children who watch television violence or experience violence in the home learn aggressive ways of resolving problems. Not only is television violence portrayed as an option for resolving conflict, but most of those violent acts do not result in negative consequences. Bullying is another less extreme form of violence that is far more prevalent and has significant consequences. Bullying is any negative activity, including teasing, kicking, hitting, and spitting, intended to bother or harm someone else.

CONSIDERING CULTURE

Male Victims of Domestic Violence

Intimate partner violence (IPV) against men is a common, yet underresearched, phenomenon. Approximately 1 in 10 men report experiencing IPV. Most of the time (97%), the perpetrator was female. Men have unique barriers to seeking help and reporting IPV. Men experience fear of exposure, challenges to their masculinity, and diminished confidence. Men are afraid of being accused of being the actual perpetrator. They may also believe that there is nowhere to turn for help. Furthermore, men may be committed to the relationship and worry about disrupting the status quo.

During the course of assessment and care, nurses may discover abusive situations in male patients. When this happens, it is important for nurses to be sensitive and supportive. Assure the patient that the interaction will be confidential. Open-ended questions encourage the patient to express his feelings. Abused male patients should be connected with social services such as domestic violence support services and legal aid.

Adapted from Huntley, A. L., Potter, L., Williamson, E., Malpass, A., Szilassy, E., & Feder, G. (2019). Help-seeking by male victims of domestic violence and abuse (DVA): A systematic review and qualitative evidence synthesis. *BMJ Open, 9,* e021960.

APPLICATION OF THE NURSING PROCESS

ASSESSMENT

General Assessment

When patients are experiencing anger, you often see it manifested behaviorally. Increased demands, irritability, frowning, redness of the face, pacing, twisting of the hands, or clenching and unclenching of the fists are all signs of irritation. Speech may either be increased in rate and volume or may be slowed, pointed, and quiet. You should address any change in behavior from what is typical for that patient. Box 27.1 identifies signs and symptoms that indicate the risk of escalating anger leading to aggressive behavior.

BOX 27.1 Predictors of Violence

Signs and symptoms that usually (*but not always*) precede violence:
- Hyperactivity: most important predictor of imminent violence (e.g., pacing, restlessness)
- Increasing anxiety and tension: clenched jaw or fist, rigid posture, fixed or tense facial expression, mumbling to self (patient may have shortness of breath, sweating, and rapid pulse)
- Verbal abuse: profanity, argumentativeness
- Loud voice, change of pitch; or very soft voice, forcing others to strain to hear
- Stone silence
- Intense eye contact or avoidance of eye contact
- Recent acts of violence, including property violence
- Alcohol or drug intoxication
- Possession of a weapon or object that may be used as a weapon (e.g., fork, knife, rock)
- Isolation that is uncharacteristic
- Milieu characteristics conducive to violence:
  - Overcrowding
  - Staff inexperience
  - Provocative or controlling staff
  - Poor limit setting
  - Arbitrary revocation of privileges

It is also important to assess the patient's history of aggression or violence. Most of our reactions to stimuli come from our previous experiences; therefore, identifying patients' triggers is essential. Initial and ongoing assessment of the patient can reveal problems before they escalate to anger and aggression. Such assessment also leads directly to the appropriate nursing diagnosis and intervention.

Some hospitals use the electronic medical record (EMR) to assist in the potential for violence. The violence assessment starts in the emergency department or nursing unit and continues every shift. If the patient is considered to be at risk of violence, an electronic flag is shown both on the EMR and in the patient's room (Burkoski et al., 2019).

HEALTH POLICY

Workplace Violence

The California Occupational Safety and Health Administration (CAL/OSHA) adopted a regulation that requires hospitals to identify risk factors for violence and train staff in responding to threats. Healthcare providers are required to log and report all incidents whether or not an injury occurred. Hospitals are mandated to develop a workplace violence prevention plan and an effective response plan for actual or potential events.

Gooch, P. P. (2018). Hospital workplace violence prevention in California: New regulations. *Workplace Health & Safety, 66*(3), 115–119.

Trauma-informed care is an older concept of providing care that has recently been reintroduced. It is based on the notion that disruptive patients often have histories that include violence and victimization. These traumatic histories can impede patients' ability to self-soothe, result in negative coping responses, and create a vulnerability to coercive interventions (e.g., restraint) by staff. Trauma-informed care focuses on the patient's past experiences of violence or trauma and on the role these experiences currently play in their lives.

EVIDENCE-BASED PRACTICE

Nurse Bullying

Problem
Up to 80% of nurses have reported some form of bullying over their career. The consequences of bullied nurses include disturbed communication, absenteeism, and staff turnover. All of these consequences negatively impact patient care.

Purpose of Study
The purpose of the study was to identify the prevalence of bullying, describe the relationship of bullying on mental and physical health, and explore the role of resilience as a mediator.

Methods
An online survey was emailed to 2250 registered nurses in one state. The respondents (N = 345) were asked to complete surveys that measured bullying, health, and resilience.

Key Findings
- Approximately 40% of the nurses had experienced bullying.
- Bullying at work was witnessed by 68% of respondents.
- Nurses who experienced bullying had significantly lower than average physical and mental health scores and a higher level of perceived stress.
- Overall, nurses had a higher than average resilience score.
- Bullied nurses had significantly lower resilience scores.

Implications for Nursing Practice
This study provides more evidence that bullying is a common problem among nurses. These findings can be extended to other areas, such as education (students and faculty) and administration. Speaking up, either by sharing with others or by directly confronting the bully, can change the culture from one of bullying to one of safety.

Sauer, P. A., & McCoy, T. P. (2017). Nurse bullying: Impact on nurses' health. *Western Journal of Nursing Research, 39*(2), 1533–1546.

ASSESSMENT GUIDELINES

Anger and Aggression

General risk identification includes assessing for the following:
1. A history of violence is the single best predictor of future violence.
2. Patients who are delusional, hyperactive, impulsive, or predisposed to irritability are at higher risk for violence.
3. Major factors associated with violence can be assessed with these questions:
   - Does the patient have a wish or intent to harm?
   - Does the patient have a plan?
   - Does the patient have the means available to carry out the plan?
   - Does the patient have demographic risk factors: male gender, aged 14 to 24 years, low socioeconomic status, inadequate support system, and prison time?
4. Aggression by patients occurs most often in the context of limit-setting by the nurse.
5. History of limited coping skills, including lack of assertiveness or use of intimidation, indicates a higher risk of using violence.

Self-Assessment

Like patients, nurses have their own histories. The nurse's ability to intervene effectively depends on self-awareness of strengths, needs, concerns, and vulnerabilities. Without this awareness, nursing interventions can end up being impulsive or emotion-based responses. Self-awareness includes recognizing choice of words and tone of voice, as well as nonverbal communication through body posture and facial expressions.

NURSING DIAGNOSIS

Patients may have coping skills that are adequate for day-to-day events but may be overwhelmed by the stresses of illness or hospitalization. Other patients may have a pattern of maladaptive coping that is marginally effective and coping strategies that may increase the possibility of anger and aggression. When the nursing assessment identifies potential for anger or aggression, *risk for violence* is a logical choice. Sometimes, patients may turn their anger inward. Therefore, *risk for suicide* should be addressed. Anger and aggression may be related to poor methods of coping; *impaired coping* is the nursing diagnosis used to address this problem. *Stress overload* and *impaired impulse control* are also important nursing diagnoses to consider for this population (International Council of Nurses, 2019).

OUTCOMES IDENTIFICATION

Clearly defined outcome criteria are important for identifying the behaviors that staff can encourage if their interventions have been successful. Table 27.1 identifies signs and symptoms commonly experienced with anger and aggression, offers potential nursing diagnoses, and suggests outcomes.

PLANNING

Planning interventions requires a sound assessment, including patient history (e.g., previous acts of violence, comorbid disorders, and past triggers) and present coping skills. Patients need to be willing and able to learn alternative and nonviolent ways of handling angry feelings.

IMPLEMENTATION

Ideally, intervention begins before any sign of escalation. It is important to develop a relationship of trust with the patient by having numerous brief, nonthreatening, nondirective interactions (e.g., talking about the weather, sports, or something of interest to the patient).

General Interventions

If you can attempt to determine what the patient is feeling, you have already begun to intervene. Frequently, you can accomplish this by telling the patient that you are concerned and want to listen. It is essential to acknowledge the patient's needs, regardless of whether the expressed needs are rational or possible to meet. It is equally as important to clearly state your expectations for the patient's behavior: "I expect that you will stay in control."

TABLE 27.1	Signs and Symptoms, Nursing Diagnoses, and Outcomes for Aggression	
Signs and Symptoms	**Nursing Diagnoses**	**Outcomes**
Body language (rigid posture, clenching of fists and jaw, hyperactivity, pacing), history of violence, history of family violence, history of substance use	*Risk for violence*	No violence: Identifies angry feelings, identifies alternatives to aggression, refrains from verbal outbursts, avoids violating others' space, maintains self-control
Impulsivity, suicidal ideation, overt or covert statements regarding killing self, feelings of worthlessness, hopelessness, helplessness	*Risk for suicide*	No suicide: Expresses feelings, verbalizes suicidal ideas, refrains from suicide attempts, plans for the future
Difficulty with simple tasks, inability to function at previous level, poor problem solving, poor cognitive functioning, verbalizations of inability to cope	*Impaired coping*	Effective coping: Identifies current coping methods, uses support system, uses new coping strategies, engages in personal actions to manage stressors effectively
Demonstrates feelings of anger, impatience, reports feelings of pressure, tension, difficulty in functioning, anger, impatience, reports problems with decision making	*Stress overload*	Stress management: Expresses feelings constructively, reports feelings of calmness and acceptance, physical symptoms of stress are reduced or absent, decision making is optimal

International Council of Nursing Practice. (2019). *ICNP browser.* Retrieved from https://www.icn.ch/what-we-do/projects/ehealth/icnp-browser. ICNP® is owned and copyrighted by the International Council of Nurses (ICN). Reproduced with permission of the copyright holder.

However, patient behavior may escalate quickly, or the patient may mask early signs of distress. Nurses may be distracted and miss those early signs. Some agitated patients may be so acutely upset that they do not respond to early nursing interventions. In these situations, the problem with anger may not be resolved before the risk for violence arises. Pharmacological intervention, seclusion, or restraint may be necessary to ensure the safety of patients and staff.

Approach the patient in a controlled, nonthreatening, and caring manner. If you are experiencing fear, you may find that this is quite challenging. Maintaining a calm exterior while your interior is in an upheaval requires considerable self-discipline and will come with experience.

Patients who are at risk for violence need much more personal space than those who are not. Allow the patient enough space so that you are perceived as less of a threat. Always stay approximately 1 foot farther than the patient can reach with arms or legs. Be sure you have left yourself an escape route if necessary; that is, make sure that the patient is not between you and the door.

When anger is escalating, a patient's ability to process decreases. It is important to speak to the patient slowly and in short sentences using a low and calm voice. Never yell but continue to model controlled behavior.

Use open-ended statements and questions such as "You think people are treating you unfairly?" rather than challenging statements such as "What is going on right now?" Avoid ending statements with "Okay?" because it may give the impression that choices exist. Find out what is behind the angry feelings and behaviors. Identify the patient's options, and encourage the individual to assume responsibility for choices made. You may want to give two options, such as "Do you want to go to your room or to the quiet room for a while?" This approach decreases the sense of powerlessness that often precipitates violence.

Pay close attention to the environment. Choose a quiet place to talk to the patient but one that is visible to staff. This is most beneficial in helping a patient regain control. Staff should know you are working with the patient, keep an eye on the interaction, and be prepared to intervene if the situation escalates.

BOX 27.2   Deescalation Techniques: Practice Principles

- Maintain the patient's self-esteem and dignity
- Maintain calmness (your own and the patient's)
- Assess the patient and the situation
- Identify stressors and stress indicators
- Respond as early as possible
- Use a calm clear tone of voice
- Invest time
- Remain honest
- Determine what the patient considers to be needed
- Identify goals
- Avoid invading personal space; in times of high anxiety, personal space increases
- Avoid arguing
- Give several clear options
- Use genuineness and empathy
- Be assertive (not aggressive)
- Do not take chances; maintain personal safety

From Mason, T., & Chandley, M. (1999). *Management of violence and aggression* (p. 73). Philadelphia, PA: Churchill Livingstone.

Medication may be helpful or even essential. It is the nurse's role to assess for appropriateness of as-needed medications. The nurse also educates the patient about the medication, the reason it is being given, and the potential side effects of the medication, even if the patient is out of control. Pharmacotherapy for acute management of violence and for the long-term management of chronic aggression is discussed following the application of the nursing process.

Box 27.2 lists some principles underlying deescalation techniques.

Health Teaching and Health Promotion

One of the most important roles a nurse plays in a patient's recovery is that of role model and educator. You can model appropriate responses and ways to cope with anger, teach patients a variety of methods to appropriately express anger, and educate patients regarding coping mechanisms, deescalation techniques, and self-soothing skills to manage behavior. It is also helpful to assist the patient in identifying triggers for angry or aggressive behavior. One method that can be used if the patient is not out of control is a "do over." The patient who responds inappropriately can try again to respond in a more appropriate way while being coached by the nurse.

Interest in using alternative interventions such as mindful living in healthy patients has been gaining interest (Chenneville et al., 2020). Nurses may introduce these concepts and educate the patient on how to incorporate them into their lives.

Teamwork and Safety

A multidisciplinary approach is important for all patients but especially for a patient with behavioral issues. All team members must implement a plan of care and execute that plan. During team meetings, staff should discuss intervention strategies. The plan for discharge with appropriate follow-up, possibly with an anger-management course, must be put into place. The consistency of intervention among all team members is key to the patient's success.

A thorough consideration of the environment is important when considering anger and aggression on the unit. It is important to be proactive and not reactive. It is hard to imagine how the stimulation of a psychiatric unit might be experienced by someone whose anxiety is extremely high or who is delusional or confused. If the patient has enough control, sometimes simply taking a timeout to the patient's room is sufficient. A multi-sensory room is another form of timeout. It is also known as a *Snoezelen*, named partly from the Dutch word for "dozing." This quiet room is partially lit, has relaxing music available, and has comfortable furniture and soft pillows. It promotes feelings of security and safety.

Realize that behavior rarely occurs in a vacuum. The nurse must examine the milieu as a whole and identify the stressors patients have to deal with, especially patients who have an antisocial personality disorder. These individuals tend to create havoc and make it appear that another patient is at fault, either for their own pleasure or for their own purposes (e.g., escaping the unit or getting into the medication room). So even while dealing with an incident, staff must be aware of what could be happening in the surrounding environment.

There are six basic considerations for ensuring safety:

1. Avoid wearing dangling earrings, necklaces, and scarves in acute care environments. The patient may become focused on these and grab at them, causing serious injury.
2. Ensure that there is enough staff for backup. Only one person should talk to the patient, but staff need to maintain an unobtrusive presence in case the situation escalates.
3. Always know the layout of the area. Correct placement of furniture and elimination of obstacles or hazards are important to prevent injury if the patient requires physical interventions.
4. Do not stand directly in front of the patient or in front of the doorway. The patient may consider this position as confrontational. It is better to stand off to the side and encourage the patient to have a seat.

5. If a patient's behavior begins to escalate, provide feedback: "You seem to be very upset." Such an observation allows exploration of the patient's feelings and may lead to deescalation of the situation.
6. Avoid confrontation with the patient, either through verbal means or through a "show of support" with security guards. Verbal confrontation and discussion of the incident must occur when the patient is calm. A show of force by security guards may serve to escalate the patient's behavior. Security personnel are better kept in the background until they are needed to assist.

Use of Seclusion or Restraints

Despite strong interventions, patients may progress to violence and require seclusion or restraint. When this happens, it is essential to have an organized approach to the seclusion or restraint. Legally, seclusion and restraint are implemented only when a patient creates a risk of harm to self or others and no less restrictive alternative is available. These measures should never be used for punishment or for the convenience of staff. Seclusion or physical restraint is used only after alternative interventions have been tried. These interventions include verbal interventions, offering an as needed medication, decreasing sensory stimulation, presence of a significant other, frequent observation, or one-on-one observation of the patient.

According to the US Department of Health & Human Services (HHS), Centers for Medicare and Medicaid Services (2008), seclusion refers to "the involuntary confinement of a patient alone in a room, or area from which the patient is physically prevented from leaving" (p. 96). The goal of seclusion is never punitive. Rather, the goal of seclusion is safety of the patient and others. Seclusion is less restrictive than restraint and may be helpful in reducing sensory overstimulation.

Restraint is defined as "any manual method, physical or mechanical device, material, or equipment that immobilizes or reduces the ability of a patient to move his or her arms, legs, body, or head freely" (HHS, 2008, p. 90).

There are several contraindications for the use of seclusion and restraint (Sadock et al., 2017). Patients who have extremely unstable medical and psychiatric conditions are not considered safe candidates for these treatments. Chronic obstructive pulmonary disease, spinal injury, seizure disorder, and pregnancy are examples of contraindicated problems. Delirium or dementia may make seclusion and restraint intolerable due to the absence of stimulation. These restrictive measures should be avoided in patients who are overtly suicidal and those who require monitoring for severe drug reactions or overdoses.

A patient may not be held in seclusion or restraint without an order from a licensed practitioner, although in emergency situations, the order may be received after the fact. Once in restraint, a patient must be directly observed and formally assessed at frequent regular intervals for level of awareness, level of activity, safety within the restraints, hydration, toileting needs, nutrition, and comfort. Licensing and accreditation agencies mandate how frequently you need to observe patients in seclusion and restraint.

Each team member is trained in the correct use of seclusion and restraint. The team should be organized before approaching the patient so that there is a clear leader and each team member has a role. The team leader is the only person talking to the patient to decrease stimuli. The patient must be given every opportunity to regain control so that the least restrictive method can be used. If restraints are to be used, the patient is informed at this point of the team's intent and the reason for the actions. The team remains calm and acts as quickly as possible.

Once the patient is placed in seclusion or restrained, the nurse must get an order from the appropriate healthcare provider. The nurse may also get an order for medication and administer it to the patient. The team leader continues to communicate with the patient in a calm, steady voice indicating decisiveness, consistency, and control. Guidelines for the use of mechanical restraints are in Box 27.3.

While the patient is in seclusion or restraint, close monitoring to determine the patient's ability to reintegrate into unit activities is mandatory. Reintegration should be gradual and geared toward the patient's ability to handle increasing amounts of stimulation. If the reintegration proves to be too much for the patient and results in increased agitation, the individual is returned to the room or another quiet area. Patients must be able to follow commands and control behaviors before reintegration can occur.

In general, a structured reintegration is the best approach. Once the patient no longer requires the locked seclusion room or restraints and is able to exercise self-control, the patient can be returned to the unit. Afterward, the patient should be observed carefully to maintain safety. In some cases, the patient may require further seclusion or restraint for which you would have to obtain another order.

Critical Incident Debriefing

Immediately after the seclusion or restraint episode, the staff must engage in debriefing with one another. Staff analysis of the episode of violence, referred to as **critical incident debriefing**, is crucial for a number of reasons. First, a review is necessary to ensure that quality care was provided to the patient. Staff members need to critically examine their response to the patient. Questions to be answered include the following:

- Could we have done anything that would have prevented the episode? If yes, then what could have been done, and why was it not done in this situation?
- Did the team respond as a team? Were team members acting according to the policies and procedures of the unit? If not, why not?
- How do staff members feel about this patient? About this situation? Feelings of fear and anger are discussed and handled. Employee morale, productivity, use of sick leave time, transfer requests, and absenteeism are all affected by patient violence, especially if a staff member has been injured. Staff members must feel supported by their peers and by the organizational policies and procedures established to maintain a safe environment.
- Is there a need for additional staff education regarding how to respond to violent patients?

BOX 27.3   Guidelines for Use of Mechanical Restraint

Indications for Use
- To protect the patient from self-harm
- To prevent the patient from assaulting others

Legal Requirements
- Multidisciplinary involvement
- Appropriate healthcare provider's signature according to state law
- Patient advocate or relative notification
- Seclusion/restraint discontinued as soon as possible

Documentation
- Patient's behavior leading to restraint/seclusion
- Least-restrictive measures used before restraint
- Interventions used and patient's response to interventions
- Plan of care for restraint/seclusion use implemented
- Ongoing evaluations by nursing staff and appropriate healthcare providers

Clinical Assessments
- Patient's mental state at time of restraint
- Physical examination for medical problems possibly causing behavioral changes
- Need for restraints

Observation
- Staff in constant attendance
- Complete written record every 15 min
- Monitor vital signs
- Assess range of movement
- Observe blood flow in hands/feet
- Observe that restraint is not rubbing
- Provide for nutrition, hydration, and elimination

Release Procedure
- Patient must be able to follow instructions and stay in control
- Termination of restraints
- Debrief with patient

Restraint Tips
- Physical holding of a patient against will is a restraint
- Four side rails up is a restraint except in seizure precautions
- Keeping patients in their room by physical intervention is seclusion
- Tucking sheets in so tightly patient cannot move is a restraint
- Orders for seclusion/restraint cannot be prn ("as needed")

- How did the actual restraining process go? What could have been done differently? Do not focus only on whether staff members were acting like a team.
- If injury occurred, has it been reported and cared for? It has been shown that there is vast underreporting of violence against healthcare staff.

When the patient is reintegrated into the unit, discussion with the patient is an important part of the therapeutic process. Going over what occurred allows the patient to learn from the situation, to identify the stressors that precipitated the out-of-control behavior, and to plan alternative ways of responding to these stressors in the future.

The nurse must provide documentation in situations in which violence was either averted or actually occurred, including the following:

- Behaviors that occurred as the patient was escalating
- Nursing interventions and the patient's responses
- Evaluation of the interventions used
- Detailed description of the patient's behaviors during the assaultive stage
- All nursing interventions used to defuse the crisis
- Patient's response to those interventions
- Observations of the patient and interventions performed while the patient was in restraints and/or seclusion
- The way the patient was reintegrated into the unit milieu

EVALUATION

Ultimately, the most important outcome when working with patients who respond with anger, aggression, and violence is the safety of everyone concerned. Therefore, no violence and no suicide are the basic measures. Beyond safety, patients with poor coping and stress overload will demonstrate improved coping and improved stress management.

> **VIGNETTE:** A 19-year-old man has been a quadriplegic for 2 years. He also has a history of illicit drug use that began in grade school, an inability to set or work toward long-term goals, and a primary coping style of anger and intimidation. The patient is admitted to an inpatient psychiatric unit because of increasing suicidal ideation. He states that his preferred means of coping with anger is to "cuss people out" and run into them with his wheelchair.
>
> The nurse sets aside time to discuss triggers for his anger. He identifies several triggers, such as feeling unheard and controlled by the staff. Together, the nurse and patient examine alternative ways for him to deal with these situations. Two coping strategies are telling the staff he doesn't feel they are listening to him and letting them know he needs to be involved in planning his care.
>
> The patient and nurse also role-play a situation in which the staff member tells the patient that he must attend a group session. Such a situation would usually result in the patient's becoming angry and aggressive. In the role-play, he is willing to "try out" alternative responses to communicate his feelings and thus to handle his anger. In addition, the patient is willing to enter into a behavioral contract with the nurse, stating that he will not curse at staff or assault anyone with his wheelchair. Instead, he will let the staff know when he is feeling angry and what the triggering issue is so that he can find a non-aggressive resolution.
>
> Because the patient is motivated to gain personal control, he responds positively to these suggestions. In addition, once it becomes clear that feeling unheard and out of control underlie most episodes of anger, the patient is able to target these issues for problem solving. He develops effective and appropriate ways to make himself heard and understood. The patient's suicidal impulses, which occur when he is frustrated, also diminish.

TREATMENT MODALITIES

Biological Treatments
Pharmacotherapy
When a patient is showing increased signs or symptoms of anxiety or agitation, it is appropriate to offer the patient an as-needed medication to alleviate symptoms. When used in conjunction

with psychosocial interventions and deescalation techniques, this can prevent an aggressive or violent incident.

Antipsychotics and antianxiety agents are used in the treatment of acute symptoms of anger and aggression. These agents, their form of delivery, and considerations are in Table 27.2. Haloperidol (Haldol) has historically been the most widely used first-generation antipsychotic. An inhaled first-generation antipsychotic, loxapine (Adasuve), has been approved for use in limited settings due to the potential for a fatal bronchospasm. Second-generation antipsychotics such as olanzapine (Zyprexa) and ziprasidone (Geodon) have gained popularity due to reduced side effects compared with first-generation drugs. Orally disintegrating tablet versions of second-generation antipsychotics such as olanzapine (Zyprexa Zydis) are alternatives to injectable medication. The tablets disintegrate in saliva almost immediately and effects occur rapidly.

Antianxiety benzodiazepines such as lorazepam (Ativan) may reduce the amount of antipsychotic that is needed to control agitation. A combination of an antipsychotic such as haloperidol (Haldol) and a benzodiazepine such as lorazepam (Ativan) is also used intramuscularly. Diphenhydramine (Benadryl) or benztropine (Cogentin) added to the injection reduces extrapyramidal side effects.

The long-term treatment of anger, aggression, and violence is based on treating the underlying psychiatric disorder. Selective serotonin reuptake inhibitors (SSRIs), lithium, anticonvulsants, benzodiazepines, second-generation antipsychotics, and beta-blockers are all used successfully for specific patient populations. Anger and aggression related to attention-deficit/hyperactivity disorder may be reduced through the use of psychostimulants. Table 27.3 gives an overview of the drugs used to manage chronic aggression.

ANGER, AGGRESSION, AND VIOLENCE IN GENERAL HOSPITAL SETTINGS

Unique circumstances of patients require a more customized approach to care. In the following, we take a closer look at intervening in various settings and with patients who have cognitive deficits.

Patients With Healthy Coping Skills Who Are Overwhelmed

A patient loses autonomy and control when hospitalized, which can cause a great deal of related distress. When this stress is combined with the uncertainty of illness, a patient may respond in ways that are not usual for him or her. A careful nursing assessment, with history and information from family members, helps to evaluate whether a patient's anger is a usual or an unusual way of managing stress.

Interventions for patients whose usual coping strategies are healthy involve finding ways to reestablish or substitute similar means of dealing with the hospitalization. This problem solving occurs in collaboration with the patient in interactions that demonstrate the nurse acknowledges the patient's distress, validates it as understandable under the circumstances,

TABLE 27.2 Drugs Used for Acute Management of Violent Behavior

Generic (Trade)	Forms	Considerations
Antianxiety Agents (Benzodiazepines)		
Lorazepam (Ativan)	PO, SL, IM, IV	Drug of choice in this class Use with caution with hepatic dysfunction
Alprazolam (Xanax)	PO	Paradoxical (opposite response) with personality disorders and older adults
Diazepam (Valium)	PO, IM, IV	Rapid onset of calming and sedating Long half-life; use with caution in older adults
First-Generation Antipsychotics		
Haloperidol (Haldol)	PO, IM, IV	Favorable side-effect profile. Due to risk of neuroleptic malignant syndrome, keep hydrated, check vital signs, and test for muscle rigidity Cardiac monitoring required for IV use
Perphenazine	PO	Risk of neuroleptic malignant syndrome increases, keep hydrated. Frequent vital sign checks and testing for muscular rigidity are recommended.
Chlorpromazine (Thorazine)	PO, PR, IM	Very sedating Injections can cause pain; watch for hypotension
Loxapine (Adasuve)	Inhalation	Rapid systemic delivery. Available only through a restricted program. Risk for fatal bronchospasm—contraindicated for individuals with breathing disorders.
Second-Generation Antipsychotics		
Risperidone (Risperdal)	PO, orally disintegrating tablet	Calms while treating underlying condition Monitor for hypotension with reflex tachycardia
Olanzapine (Zyprexa, Zyprexa Zydis)	PO, IM, orally disintegrating tablet	Useful in patients unresponsive to haloperidol Calms while treating underlying condition Monitor for hypotension Avoid IM combination with lorazepam
Ziprasidone (Geodon)	PO, IM	Use cautiously with QT prolongation Less sedating
Combinations		
Haloperidol (Haldol), lorazepam (Ativan), and diphenhydramine (Benadryl) or benztropine (Cogentin)	IM	Commonly used in the acute setting Men who are young and athletic are at increased risk of dystonia If agitation increases, it may be akathisia caused by the drug
Lorazepam (Ativan) and diphenhydramine (Benadryl), or benztropine (Cogentin)	IM	Consider this combination if patient has difficulty taking haloperidol

From Gerken, A. T., Gross, A. F., & Sanders, K. M. (2016). Aggression and violence. In T. A. Stern, M. Fava, T. E. Wilens, & J. F. Rosenbaum (Eds.). *Massachusetts General Hospital comprehensive clinical psychiatry* (2nd ed., p. 716). St. Louis, MO: Elsevier.

and indicates a willingness to search for solutions. Validation includes making an apology to the patient when appropriate, such as when a promised intervention (e.g., changing a dressing by a certain time) has not been delivered, or sympathizing with the patient about the "horrible food" by assisting with menu selections.

Patients who have become angry may be unable to moderate this emotion enough to problem solve with their nurses. Others may be unable to communicate the source of their anger. Often, the nurse—knowing the patient and the context of the anger—can make an accurate guess at what feeling is behind the anger. Naming this feeling can lead to a dissipation of the anger, help the patient to feel understood, and lead to a calmer discussion of the distress. Some of the feelings that can precipitate anger are listed in Box 27.4. The following vignette provides an example of nursing interventions that are helpful in dissipating anger in a hospital situation.

> **VIGNETTE:** Rachel, a 41-year-old woman with a history of peripheral vascular disease, vascular grafts, and repair of graft occlusions, is admitted to the hospital with severe pain in her left foot. Tests show that vessels to the foot are occluded. Additional surgery is ruled out, and medication is prescribed. Unfortunately, the medication is ineffective, and the tissue of the foot begins to necrotize.
>
> The physician recommends amputation. Rachel refuses the surgery, demands unproven therapies, and is extremely angry with the hospital staff. The treatment team is concerned about the spread of tissue death and signs of systemic infection. This concern increases the patient's feeling of being out of control and feelings of competence in her own care.
>
> Rachel's anger and unwillingness to discuss her condition end when the nurse empathizes with her feelings of fear and being out of control. Once the anger is reduced, the nurse is able to help Rachel negotiate more time for the final decision. This allows her time to process anticipatory grieving, including stages of denial, anger, and bargaining. In this interval, the patient's wish to explore alternative therapies is addressed through second and third medical opinions. Rachel is also able to spend more time discussing her concerns with her family.

TABLE 27.3 Drugs Used for Long-Term Management of Chronic Aggression

Class	Population	Considerations
Selective serotonin reuptake inhibitors (SSRIs)	Depression, anxiety, personality disorder, dementia, and intellectual disability	Reduces irritability, impulsivity, and aggression Stabilizes mood Use cautiously with bipolar disorder
Lithium	Intellectual disability, conduct disorder, antisocial personality, bipolar disorder, and prison inmates	TSH and renal panels before treatment Due to antiaggressive properties, blood levels can be lower than those necessary to treat bipolar mania
Anticonvulsants	Schizophrenia, prison inmates, antisocial/borderline personality, conduct disorders, and bipolar disorders	Significantly reduces impulsive aggression Similar doses with bipolar disorder Multiple drug interactions Periodic blood levels Monitor CBC and liver function
Gabapentin	Patients with co-existing anxiety disorder and personality disorders	No interactions with other anticonvulsants Monitor renal functioning Potential for misuse
Benzodiazepines	Should have underlying component of anxiety	Potential for abuse, dependence, and withdrawal May cause paradoxical aggression
Second-generation antipsychotics	Schizophrenia, psychosis, and mania	Clozapine superior to other second-generation drugs but must monitor absolute neutrophil count (ANC) monthly Less extrapyramidal symptoms and better adherence than first-generation antipsychotics
Beta-blockers	Organic brain disease, brain injury, intellectual disability	Propranolol contraindicated with asthma, COPD, and type 1 diabetes Sedation side effects may explain antiaggressive effects
Psychostimulants	ADHD in children and adults	Potential for addiction and misuse

From Gerken, A. T., Gross, A. F., & Sanders, K. M. (2016). Aggression and violence. In T. A. Stern, M. Fava, T. E. Wilens, & J. F. Rosenbaum (Eds.), *Massachusetts General Hospital comprehensive clinical psychiatry* (2nd ed., p. 716). St. Louis, MO: Elsevier.

BOX 27.4 Feelings That May Precipitate Anger

- Discounted
- Embarrassed
- Frightened
- Found out guilty
- Humiliated
- Hurt
- Ignored
- Inadequate
- Insecure
- Unheard
- Out of control of the situation
- Rejected
- Threatened
- Tired
- Vulnerable

Patients With Marginal Coping Skills

Patients whose coping skills were marginal before hospitalization need a different set of interventions than those with basically healthy ways of coping. Patients with maladaptive coping are poorly equipped to use alternatives when their initial attempts to cope are unsuccessful or are inappropriate. Such patients frequently manifest anger that moves quickly from anxiety to aggression. For some people, anger and intimidation are primary strategies used to obtain their short-term goals of feelings of control or mastery. For others, the anger occurs when limited or primitive attempts at coping are unsuccessful and alternatives are unknown. For these patients, anger and violence are particular risks in inpatient settings.

This is especially true for hospitalized patients with chemical dependence who may be anxious about being cut off from their substance of choice. They may have well-founded concerns that any physical pain will be inadequately addressed. Many patients with marginal coping also have personality styles that externalize blame. That is, they see the source of their discomfort and anxiety as being outside themselves. Relief must therefore also come from an outside source (e.g., the nurse, medication).

Interventions begin with attempts to understand and meet the patient's needs. For instance, you can moderate baseline anxiety by providing comfort items before they are requested (e.g., decaffeinated coffee, deck of cards). This can build rapport and acts symbolically to reassure. Reducing ambiguity or uncertainty can also help to minimize anxiety. This strategy includes clear and concrete communication. Nurses should be clear about what is within the nurse's power to provide, such as "I can't order Vicodin for you, but I will talk with your nurse practitioner about what we can do."

Interventions for anxiety might also include the use of distractions such as magazines, action comics, and video games. In general, distractions that are colorful and do not require sustained attention work best, although this varies according to the patient's interests and abilities. Finally, patients with a high level of baseline anxiety and limited coping skills are helped when their interactions with the treatment team are predictable. This may include speaking with the physician at a specific time each day and consistency in nursing assignments. Individuals from outside the unit such as a chaplain or a volunteer may help by giving the patient more attention.

Because these patients have limited coping skills, once anxiety is moderated, nursing interventions include teaching alternative behaviors and strategies. For patients who externalize blame, it is best to precede such teaching by a gentle challenge. The challenge serves to engage the patient's interest in teaching that might otherwise be seen as irrelevant. This intervention is also important in that the nurse has (1) avoided a punitive or demeaning response that might have fueled escalation of the patient's anger, (2) taught a number of strategies, and (3) provided the patient with choices and thus with more control.

Often, people communicate anger verbally. If attempts to teach alternatives have not been successful, you can use three interventions:

1. The first is to leave the room at the point that verbal abuse begins. The patient can be told that you will return in a specific amount of time (e.g., 20 minutes). A matter-of-fact, neutral manner is important because fear, indignation, and arguing are gratifying to many patients who verbally abuse. Alternatively, if the nurse is in the middle of a procedure and cannot leave immediately, the nurse can break off conversation and eye contact, completing the procedure quickly and matter-of-factly before leaving the room. The nurse avoids arguing, threatening, or responding negatively to the patient.
2. Withdrawal of attention of verbal abuse is successful only if a second intervention is also used. This step requires attending positively to, and thus reinforcing, appropriate communication. Interventions can include discussing non–illness-related topics, responding to requests, and providing emotional support.
3. A predictable routine such as scheduled contacts with the nurse (e.g., every 30 or 60 minutes) may reduce anxiety. This routine provides nursing that is not contingent on the patient's behavior and therefore does not reinforce anger and aggressive responses. Of course, the patient's illness or injury may require assessment or intervention outside the scheduled contact times. These visits can be carried out in a calm, brief, matter-of-fact manner.

> **VIGNETTE:** A 21-year-old man who was in an automobile accident is bedridden with a pelvic fracture. During his first day of admission, he yells and uses expletives demanding the nurses to come into his room.
>
> The nurse who is assigned to the patient for the evening stops in his doorway after he yells at her and asks in mild disbelief, "Is this working for you? Do nurses really come in here when you yell at them that way?" The patient responds sullenly, justifying his behavior by complaining about his care. However, the nurse's challenge has caught his attention, and she goes on to suggest alternative strategies for contacting her and other nurses. The patient gradually adopts these strategies.

Patients With Cognitive Deficits

Patients with cognitive deficits are particularly at risk for acting aggressively. Such deficits may result from delirium, dementias (e.g., Alzheimer disease, multiinfarct dementia), or brain injury (see Chapter 23). Traditional approaches to disorientation and to the agitation it can cause have relied heavily on reality orientation and medication. Reality orientation consists of providing the correct information to the patient about place, date, and current life circumstances. For many patients, this is comforting

because it reminds them of pertinent information and helps them to feel grounded. For others, reality orientation does not work. Because of their cognitive disorder, they can no longer "enter into our reality." They become frightened and more agitated and may become aggressive.

Orientation aids, such as a calendar and a clock, can provide easy reference and increased autonomy. Such aids must be prominent and easily read by patients with diminished eyesight. Sedating medication may calm agitation, but the risks often outweigh the benefits. Sedation further clouds a patient's sensorium, which makes disorientation worse and increases the risk of falls and injuries. It is better to examine alternative interventions.

Typically, patients experiencing delirium will be in and out of reality. At times they will appear perfectly fine, and at others they will have a clouded sensorium. They will sometimes fall asleep as you are talking to them. Often, patients with delirium have visual hallucinations, commonly of children, animals, or bugs. Occasionally, they will show periods of paranoia. The best intervention for delirium is to find and treat the medical cause. The next choice is to medicate the symptoms with a low-dose antipsychotic and discontinue it as the delirium clears.

Patients with any clouding of the sensorium have difficulty interpreting environmental stimuli. Another set of interventions involves making the environment as simple, predictable, and comfortable as possible. Simplicity includes decreasing sensory stimuli. In the hospital, this might include placing the patient's bed away from doorways that enter onto the hall and choosing not to turn on the television. Establishing a routine of activities for each day and displaying the day's schedule prominently in the patient's room can provide predictability. You can enhance the comfort of the patient by providing familiar photographs and objects from home. The availability of a rocking chair can provide a rhythmic source of self-soothing.

Sometimes, the patient with a cognitive disorder experiences such severe agitation and aggression that it is referred to as a *catastrophic reaction*. The patient may scream, strike out, or cry because of overwhelming fear. Calm and unhurried care is the best approach to take with such a patient. To respond effectively to episodes of agitation, it is crucial to identify the antecedents (i.e., what preceded the episode) and the consequences of such episodes. Once antecedents are understood, interventions are often obvious.

Patients who misperceive their setting or life situation can use validation therapy to calm themselves. Some disoriented older patients believe that they are young and feel the need to return to important tasks that were a significant part of those earlier years. For example, a woman may insist that she must go home to take care of her babies. Telling the patient that her babies have grown up and there is no home to return to is not only cruel but nontherapeutic and will result in increased agitation. It is often more helpful to reflect back to the patient the feelings behind her demand and to show understanding and concern for her worry.

Rather than attempting to reorient the patient, the nurse should ask the patient to further describe the setting or situation reported to be a problem (e.g., the need to return home). During the conversation, the nurse can comment on what appears to be underlying the patient's distress, thus validating it. In the earlier example, the woman who believes that she needs to return home to care for her children is asked to tell the nurse more about her children. The nurse may note that the patient misses her children and that the current setting gets lonely at times:

Nurse: "Mrs. Green, you miss your children, and this can be a lonely place."

As the nurse shows interest in aspects of the patient's life, the nurse establishes himself or herself as a safe understanding person. In turn, the patient often becomes calmer and more open to redirection. As patients reminisce in this fashion, they often bring themselves into the present:

Patient: "Of course, they're all grown and doing well on their own now."

Refer to Chapter 23 for a more detailed discussion of interventions for people with cognitive impairments. Refer to Chapter 31 for a more detailed discussion of the use of validation and reminiscent therapeutic modalities for older adults.

KEY POINTS TO REMEMBER

- Violence in the United States is widespread. Nurses are particularly likely to come across anger, aggression, and violence if they work in the emergency department, psychiatric units, geriatric units, and intensive care units.
- Understanding patient cues to escalating aggression, appropriate goals for intervention for individuals in a variety of situations, and helpful nursing interventions is important for nurses in any setting.
- The expression of anger can lead to increased anger and to negative physiological changes.
- Biological factors and cognitive factors provide explanations for anger, aggression, and violence.
- It is helpful for providers of care to know what cues to look for and what to assess verbally and nonverbally when a patient's anger is escalating.
- A patient's past aggressive behavior is the most important indicator of future aggressive episodes.
- Working with angry and aggressive patients is a challenge for all nurses, and a careful understanding and recognition of one's personal responses to angry or threatening patients can be crucial.
- Many approaches are effective in helping patients deescalate and maintain control.
- Seclusion and restraint may be necessary to ensure the safety of the patient, other patients, and the staff. They should be used only when other less restrictive measures such as verbal intervention, offering as-needed medication, and reducing stimuli have failed.
- Each unit should have a protocol for the safe use of restraints and for the humane management of care during the time the patient is restrained and clear guidelines for understanding and protecting the patient's legal rights.
- Medications such as antianxiety agents, antipsychotics, antidepressants, and mood stabilizers may be useful in treating acute violence and chronic aggression.
- Patients who are overwhelmed, possess marginal coping skills, or have cognitive deficits require special attention to reduce and prevent episodes of anger, aggression, and violence.

CRITICAL THINKING

1. Jenea admits a 24-year-old man with mania to an inpatient unit. She notes that the patient is irritable, has trouble sitting during the interview, and has a history of assault.
   a. Identify appropriate responses the nurse can make to the patient.
   b. What interventions should be built into the care plan?
   c. Identify at least three long-term outcomes to consider when planning care.
2. What are the two indications for the use of seclusion and restraint rather than verbal interventions? Provide rationales for your answers.

3. Discuss the use of restraint and seclusion with your clinical group or in class. Choose a side and defend it (even if you do not necessarily believe it) regarding the following:
   a. There are always better alternatives to seclusion and restraint.
   b. Seclusion and restraint are underutilized, and people who have tried to limit their use have gone too far.

CHAPTER REVIEW

1. Which individuals are most at risk for displaying aggressive behavior? *Select all that apply.*
   a. An adolescent embarrassed in front of friends.
   b. A young male who feels rejected by the social group.
   c. A young adult depressed after the death of a friend.
   d. A middle-aged adult who feels that concerns are going unheard.
   e. A patient who was discovered telling a lie.

2. A newly admitted male patient has a long history of aggressive behavior toward staff. Which statement by the nurse demonstrates the need for more information about the use of restraint?
   a. "If his behavior warrants restraints, someone will stay with him the entire time he's restrained."
   b. "I'll call the primary provider and get an as-needed (prn) seclusion/restraint order."

c. "If he is restrained, be sure he is offered food and fluids regularly."

d. "Remember that physical restraints are our last resort."

3. Which intervention(s) should the nurse implement when helping a patient who expresses anger in an inappropriate manner? *Select all that apply.*

a. Approach the patient in a calm, reassuring manner.

b. Provide suggestions regarding acceptable ways of communicating anger.

c. Warn the patient that being angry is not a healthy emotional state.

d. Set limits on the angry behavior that will be tolerated.

e. Allow any expression of anger as long as no one is hurt.

4. Which guidelines should direct nursing care when deescalating an angry patient? *Select all that apply.*

a. Intervene as quickly as possible.

b. Identify the trigger for the anger.

c. Behave calmly and respectfully.

d. Recognize the patient's need for increased personal space.

e. Demands are agreed to as long as they will not result in harm to anyone.

5. Which comorbid condition would result in cautious use of an SSRI for a patient with chronic aggression?

a. Asthma

b. Anxiety disorder

c. Glaucoma

d. Bipolar disorder

6. Patrick is a widower with four daughters. He enjoyed a healthy relationship with each of them until they reached puberty. As the girls began to mature physically, he acted in an aggressive manner, often beating them without provocation. Patrick is most likely acting on:

a. Self-protective measures

b. Stress of raising four daughters

c. Frustration of unhealthy desire

d. Motivating his daughters to be chaste

7. A nurse named Darryl has been hired to work in a psychiatric intensive care unit. He has undergone training on recognizing escalating anger. Which statement indicates that he understands danger signs in regard to aggression?

a. "I need to be aware of patients who are withdrawn and sitting alone."

b. "An obvious change in behavior is a risk factor for aggression."

c. "Patients who seek constant attention are more likely to be violent."

d. "Patients who talk to themselves are the most dangerous."

8. An effective method of preventing escalation in an environment with violent offenders is to develop a level of trust through:

a. A casual authoritative demeanor

b. Keeping patients busy

c. Brief, frequent, nonthreatening encounters

d. Threats of seclusion or punishment

9. A 24-hour observation is a good choice for restraint in which of the following patients?

a. An inmate with suicidal ideation on hospice care

b. A sex offender in the psychiatric intensive care unit

c. An aggressive female with antisocial personality disorder

d. An inmate diagnosed with paranoid schizophrenia

10. Chronic obstructive pulmonary disease, spinal injury, seizure disorder, and pregnancy are conditions that:

a. Frequently result in out of control behavior.

b. Respond well to therapeutic holding.

c. Necessitate the use of only two-point restraint.

d. Contraindicate restraint and seclusion.

1. **a, b, d, e**; 2. **b**; 3. **a, b, d**; 4. **a, b, c, d**; 5. **d**; 6. **c**; 7. **b**; 8. **c**; 9. **a**; 10. **d**

Visit the Evolve website for a posttest on the content in this chapter: http://evolve.elsevier.com/Varcarolis

REFERENCES

Bandura, A. (1973). *Aggression: A social learning analysis.* New York, NY: Prentice Hall.

Barlow, M. A., Wrosch, C., Gouin, J. P., & Kunzmann, U. (2019). Is anger, but not sadness, associated with chronic inflammation and illness in older adulthood? *Psychology and Aging, 34*(3), 330–340.

Beck, A. (1976). *Cognitive therapy and the emotional disorders.* New York, NY: International Universities Press.

Bertsch, K., Krauch, M., Roelofs, K., Cackowski, S., Herpertz, S. C., & Volman, I. (2019). Out of control? Acting out anger is associated with deficient prefrontal emotional action control in male patients with borderline personality disorder. *Neuropharmacology, 156,* 107463.

Brusie, C. (2019, April 18). *Nurse dies after being attacked by mental health patient—Manslaughter charges.* Retrieved from https://nurse.org/articles/nurse-attacked-by-patient-dies-manslaughter/.

Burkoski, V., Farshait, N., Yoon, J., Clancy, P. V., Fernandes, K., & Howell, M. R., et al. (2019). Violence prevention: Technology-enabled therapeutic intervention. *Nursing Leadership, 32*(SP), 58–70.

CBS Boston. (2019, July 11). *Mass. lawmakers push to increase penalties in health care worker attacks.* Retrieved from https://boston.cbslocal.com/2019/07/11/emt-stabbing-boston-massachusetts-health-care-worker-attacks-legislation/.

Centers for Disease Control and Prevention. (2018). *Violence prevention.* Retrieved from https://www.cdc.gov/violenceprevention/index.html.

Centers for Disease Control and Prevention. (2019). *National violent death reporting system.* Retrieved from https://www.cdc.gov/violenceprevention/datasources/nvdrs/index.html.

Chenneville, T., Machacek, M., Little, T., & Aguila, E. (2020). Effects of a mindful rational living intervention on the experience of destructive emotions. *Journal of Cognitive Psychotherapy, 31*(2), 101–117.

Freud, S. (1930). *Civilization and its discontents.* Austria: Internationaler Psychoanalytischer Verlag Wien.

Haller, J. (2018). The role of central and medial amygdala in normal and abnormal aggression: A review of classical approaches. *Neuroscience and Biobehavioral Reviews, 85*, 34–43.

Hashikawa, Y., Hashikawa, K., Falkner, A. L., & Lin, D. (2017). Ventromedial hypothalamus and the generation of aggression. *Frontiers in Systems Neuroscience, 11*, 94.

International Council of Nurses. (2019). *International Classification for Nursing Practice catalog.* Retrieved from https://www.icn.ch/sites/default/files/inline-files/ICNP2019-DC.pdf.

Keith, F., Krantz, D. S., Chen, R., Harris, K. M., Ware, C. M., & Lee, A. K., et al. (2017). Anger, hostility, and hospitalizations in patients with heart failure. *Health Psychology, 36*(9), 829–838.

Khalsa, H. K., Baldessarini, R. J., Tohen, M., & Salvatore, P. (2018). Aggression among 216 patients with a first-psychotic episode of bipolar I disorder. *International Journal of Bipolar Disorders, 6*(1), 18.

Klasen, M., Wolf, D., Eisner, P. D., Eggermann, T., Zerres, K., & Zepf, F. D., et al. (2019). Serotonergic contributions to human brain aggression networks. *Frontiers in Neuroscience, 13*, 42.

Leclerc, M. P., Regenbogen, C., Hamilton, R. H., & Habel, U. (2018). Some neuroanatomical insights to impulsive aggression in schizophrenia. *Schizophrenia Research, 201*, 27–34.

Leroy, F., Park, J., Asok, A., Brann, D. H., Meira, T., & Boyle, L. M., et al. (2018). A circuit from hippocampal CA2 to lateral septum disinhibits social aggression. *Nature, 564*, 213–218.

Matthies, S., Rusch, N., Weber, M., Lieb, K., Philipsen, A., & Tuescher, O., et al. (2012). Small amygdala—High aggression? The role of the amygdala in modulating aggression in healthy subjects. *World Journal of Biological Psychiatry, 13*, 75–81.

Menninger, W. W. (2007). Uncontained rage: A psychoanalytic perspective on violence. *Bulletin of the Menninger Clinic, 71*(2), 115–131.

Sadock, B. J., Sadock, V. A., & Ruiz, P. (2017). *Kaplan and Sadock's synopsis of psychiatry* (11th ed.). Philadelphia, PA: Wolters Kluwer.

Skinner, B. (1953). *Science and human behavior.* New York, NY: Macmillan.

Smaragdi, A., Chavez, S., Lobaugh, N. J., Meyer, J. H., & Kolla, N. J. (2019). Differential levels of prefrontal cortex glutamate+glutamine in adults with antisocial personality disorder and bipolar disorder: A proton magnetic resonance spectroscopy study. *Progress in Neuro-Psychopharmacology & Biological Psychiatry, 93*, 250–255.

Staudinger, S. (2019). Racine man charged after allegedly choking nurse with stethoscope. *WDJT Milwaukee.* Retrieved from https://www.cbs58.com/news/racine-man-charged-after-allegedly-choking-nurse-with-stethoscope.

US Department of Health and Human Services, Centers for Medicare and Medicaid Services. (2008). *Revised interpretive guidelines for seclusion and restraint.* Retrieved from https://www.cms.gov/Medicare/Provider-Enrollment-and-Certification/SurveyCertification-GenInfo/Downloads/SCLetter08-18.pdf.

28

Child, Older Adult, and Intimate Partner Violence

Margaret Jordan Halter

 Visit the Evolve website for a pretest on the content in this chapter: http://evolve.elsevier.com/Varcarolis

OBJECTIVES

1. Identify the nature and scope of family violence and factors contributing to its occurrence.
2. Describe risk factors for both victimization and perpetration of family violence.
3. Identify three indicators of (a) physical abuse, (b) sexual abuse, (c) neglect, and (d) emotional abuse.
4. Describe four areas to assess when interviewing a person who has experienced abuse.
5. Identify two common emotional responses the nurse might experience when faced with a person who has been abused.
6. Formulate four nursing diagnoses for the survivor of abuse and list supporting data from the assessment.
7. Write out a safety plan for a victim of intimate partner abuse.
8. Discuss the legal and ethical responsibilities of nurses when working with families experiencing violence.
9. Compare and contrast primary, secondary, and tertiary levels of prevention, giving two examples of intervention for each level.
10. Describe at least three possible referrals for an abusive family, including the telephone numbers of appropriate agencies in the community.
11. Discuss three therapeutic modalities useful in working with abusive families.

KEY TERMS AND CONCEPTS

act of commission
act of omission
crisis situation
economic abuse
emotional abuse
family violence

neglect
perpetrator
physical abuse
primary prevention
safety plan
secondary prevention

sexual abuse
shelters or safe houses
survivor
tertiary prevention
vulnerable person

There's no place like home. This is a statement familiar to most of us, and home is a source of refuge and peace for many. Yet for some children, adults, and older adults, the home is a dangerous place where family members or intimate partners demonstrate disregard for the rights of others. **Family violence**, also called domestic violence, is among the most important public health issues in the United States. Nurses are in a unique position to respond to family violence and are educated to identify, evaluate, and treat both victims and perpetrators of violence.

TYPES OF ABUSE

Legal definitions of family or domestic violence vary from state to state. Thirty-eight states place domestic violence and definitions within the criminal code. Generally speaking, the major types of abuse include the following:

- **Physical abuse** is the infliction of physical pain or bodily harm such as slapping, punching, hitting, choking, pushing, restraining, biting, throwing, and burning.
- **Sexual abuse** is any form of sexual contact or exposure without consent or in circumstances in which the victim is incapable of giving consent. Sexual abuse is also referred to as *sexual assault* or *rape* and is discussed in Chapter 29.
- **Emotional abuse** is the undermining of a person's self-worth. This may include constant criticism, humiliating, diminishing one's abilities, name-calling, intimidating, isolating, and damaging relationships with others.
- **Neglect** is the failure to provide for physical, emotional, educational, and medical needs.
- **Economic abuse** is controlling a person's access to economic resources, making an individual financially dependent. Forbidding school attendance or employment keeps a person dependent.

CRISIS SITUATION

Anyone may be at risk for abuse in a **crisis situation**, or a situation that puts stress on a family with a violent member. A person with effective impulse control, problem-solving skills, and a healthy support system is less likely to resort to violence. However, stressful life events tax coping skills, leaving the perpetrator incapable of dealing with the situation. Social isolation caused by frequent moves or an inability to make friends contributes to ineffective coping during crisis situations.

THE PERPETRATOR AND THE VULNERABLE PERSON

The term **perpetrator** applies to any member of a household who is violent toward another member, such as parents, partners, siblings, and extended family members. Perpetrators often consider their own needs to be more important than anyone else's and look toward others to meet their needs. Both male and female perpetrators perceive themselves as having poor social skills. They describe their relationships with their partners as being the closest they have ever known, and they typically lack supportive relationships outside the relationship.

The **vulnerable person** is the family member upon whom abuse is perpetrated. This individual is variously referred to as the *victim, survivor,* or *victim/survivor*. Using the term **survivor** recognizes the recovery and healing process that follows victimization and does not have the connotation of passivity that *victim* has.

CHILD ABUSE

Child abuse can take the form of something improper that is done to a child, which is an act of commission. Acts of commission are deliberate and intentional. They include physical, sexual, and emotional abuse. An **act of omission**, or neglect, occurs when a child's basic physical, emotional, or educational needs are not met or when a child is not protected from harm. Acts of omission include physical neglect, emotional neglect, medical and dental neglect, educational neglect, inadequate supervision, and exposure to violence.

Epidemiology

In 2018, there were 2.4 million referrals for child abuse and neglect (Administration for Children and Families [ACF], 2020). The most common form of abuse was neglect (73%), followed by physical abuse (46%), and medical neglect (8%). Almost 85% of victims suffer from a single maltreatment type and about 16% have two or more maltreatment types, usually neglect and physical abuse. Of the 1,770 children who died from abuse, about 73% suffered from neglect and about 46% suffered physical abuse alone or combined with some other maltreatment type.

The youngest children are the most vulnerable for mistreatment. An astonishing 28% of abused children are younger than three years old and 15% are less than one year old (Fig. 28.1) (ACF, 2020). Approximately 78% of children who die are younger than 4 years of age. Boys die at a slightly higher rate than girls.

The prevalence of sexual abuse in children is difficult to determine due to the fact that children are often unable to describe their experience. About 40% do not exhibit clear symptoms of sexual abuse (American Psychological Association, 2014). Relatively uncommon in infants, sexual abuse increases with age. By age 17, sexual abuse and sexual assault occur in nearly 27% of all girls and about 5% of all boys (Finkelhor, Shattuck, Turner, & Hamby, 2014). Adults are responsible for these cases of abuse and assault about 11% of the time for girls and about 2% for boys. Females are at most risk in late adolescence.

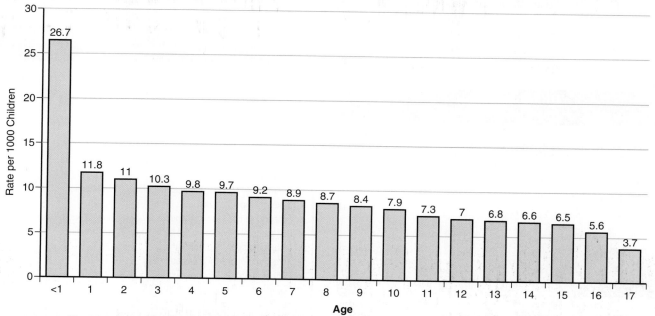

Fig. 28.1 Child and adolescent victims of violence by age. (From Administration for Children and Families. (2020). *Child maltreatment 2018.* Retrieved from https://www.acf.hhs.gov/cb/resource/child-maltreatment-2018.)

About 92% of child abuse perpetrators are the victim's parents (ACF, 2020). Females are somewhat more likely to abuse children. Nearly 40% of victims are maltreated by a mother acting alone and about 22% of victims are maltreated by a father acting alone.

The prevalence of child abuse varies based on race and ethnicity. Table 28.1 provides childhood maltreatment rates based on race and ethnicity.

Comorbidity

The occurrence of one type of abuse is a fairly strong predictor of the occurrence of another type. The secondary effects of abuse, such as anxiety, depression, and suicidal ideation, are healthcare issues that can last a lifetime. Major depressive disorder and posttraumatic stress disorder (PTSD) are two of the most prevalent disorders resulting from childhood trauma.

Family violence is common in the childhood histories of juvenile offenders, runaways, violent criminals, prostitutes, and those who in turn are violent toward others. Exposure to abuse can adversely affect a child's development because the energy needed to successfully accomplish developmental is instead devoted to coping with abuse.

Abused adolescents exhibit more psychopathological changes, poorer coping and social skills, a higher incidence of dissociative identity disorder, and poorer impulse control than do other adolescents. Women who are victims of prolonged childhood sexual abuse are more likely to develop major psychiatric distress.

Risk Factors

Risk factors for child abuse include being perceived as being different due to temperamental traits, congenital abnormalities, or chronic disease. Perhaps the child reminds the parents of someone they do not like, such as an ex-spouse. Children who do not live up to the parents' fantasy of what the child should be like are at risk. Children who are the result of unwanted pregnancies are at higher risk.

Interference with emotional bonding between parents and child, which can occur because of a premature birth or prolonged illness requiring hospitalization, has also been found to increase the risk for future abuse. Adolescents are abused at least as frequently as younger children. However, such abuse is often overlooked, perhaps because society views adolescents as capable of defending themselves.

Box 28.1 identifies characteristics of parents who abuse their children.

INTIMATE PARTNER VIOLENCE

Intimate partner violence is abuse within the context of an intimate partner relationship, where one partner asserts power and control over the other. Intimate partner violence includes physical violence, rape, stalking, and psychological aggression by a current or former intimate partner. The intimate partner may be a spouse, boyfriend/girlfriend, dating partner, or ongoing sexual partner.

Epidemiology

About 25% of women and 10% of men have experienced intimate partner violence during their lifetime (CDC, 2019). A subgroup, teen dating violence, is experienced by nearly 1 in 11 females and about 1 in 15 male high school students. About 10% of women and 2% of men report having been stalked by an intimate partner. Females between the ages of 18 and 34 experience the highest rate of intimate partner violence.

Nearly half of married couples have instances of abuse. Evidence suggests that intimate partner violence affects same-sex relationships at about the same rates as heterosexual relationships (Stephenson, Rentsch, Salazar, & Sullivan, 2011). One out of 10 homicides is due to spousal murder. More than half of women who are murdered are or were in an intimate relationship with their killer.

Risk Factors

Men who abuse may believe in male dominance and need to be in charge. Physically acting out makes them feel more in control, more masculine, and more powerful. Parent–child interactions,

TABLE 28.1   Childhood Abuse and Fatalities Rates by Race and Ethnicities: 2018

Race or Ethnicity	Abuse Cases per 1000 Victims	Fatalities per 100,000 Victims
African American	14	5.48
American Indian or Alaska Native	15.2	3.12
Asian	1.6	0.44
Hispanic	8.1	1.63
Pacific Islander	9.3	2.22
White	8.2	1.94
Children of multiple races	11.0	3.50

Data from the Administration for Children and Families. (2020). *Child maltreatment 2018*. Retrieved from https://www.acf.hhs.gov/cb/resource/child-maltreatment-2018.

BOX 28.1   Characteristics of Abusive Parents

- A history of abuse, neglect, or emotional deprivation as a child
- Family authoritarianism
- Low self-esteem, feelings of worthlessness, depression
- Poor coping skills
- Social isolation (may be suspicious of others)
- Involvement in a crisis situation
- Unrealistic expectations of child's behavior
- Frequent use of harsh punishment
- History of severe mental illness, such as schizophrenia
- Violent temper outbursts
- Expects the child to satisfy needs for love, support, and reassurance
- Projection of blame onto the child for parents' "troubles"
- Inability to seek help from others
- Perception of the child as bad or evil
- History of drug or alcohol misuse
- Feeling of little or no control over life
- Low tolerance for frustration
- Poor impulse control

peer group experiences, observations of the partner dyad, and the influence of the media (television, comics, video games, movies) support the same message: Males can expect to be in a position of power in relationships and may use physical aggression to maintain that position.

Pathological jealousy is a characteristic of an intimate partner abuser. Many perpetrators refuse to allow their partners to work outside the home. Some demand that their partners work in the same place as they do so that they can monitor activities and friendships. It is common for abusers to accompany their partners to and from activities. They may forbid the victim from having personal friends or to participate in activities outside the home. Perpetrators may restrict mobility by monitoring an odometer and keeping stopwatches. Even after imposing such restrictions, abusers often accuse their partners of infidelity or other acts of betrayal. Controlling finances and expenditures is an additional means of limiting the freedom of the abused.

Individuals are more likely to engage in family violence when they use substances. Alcohol and other drugs (illicit or prescribed) tend to weaken inhibitions and lead to a disregard of social rules prohibiting violence. The victim may rationalize that alcohol and drugs cause the abuse, saying, "He was drunk and didn't know what he was doing." However, even when drug and alcohol use is reduced or eliminated, family violence usually still occurs.

Pregnancy may trigger or increase violence. The partner may resent the added responsibility of a baby or may resent the relationship the baby will have with its mother. Violence also escalates when the woman makes a move toward independence, such as visiting friends without permission, getting a job, or going back to school. Victims are at greatest risk for violence when they threaten to or actually leave the relationship.

Cycle of Violence

Walker (1979) describes a pattern of behavior that perpetrators of violence may use to control their partners. This cycle consists of three stages: the tension-building stage, the acute battering stage, and the honeymoon stage.

- The **tension-building stage** begins with minor incidents, such as pushing, shoving, and verbal abuse. During this time, the victim often ignores or accepts the behavior due to fear of escalation. Abusers then rationalize that their behavior is acceptable. As the tension builds, both participants may try to reduce it. The abuser may try to reduce the tension with the use of alcohol or drugs, and the victim may try to reduce the tension by minimizing the importance of the incidents ("I should have had the house neater…dinner ready").
- The **acute battering stage** occurs when the tension peaks. It is usually triggered by an external event or by the abuser's emotional state. Some experts believe that the victim may actually provoke the incident to remove the tension and fear and to move on to the honeymoon phase.
- After the abuse occurs, the abuser and victim enter a period of calm known as the **honeymoon stage**. During this stage, the abuser usually demonstrates kindness and loving behaviors. The abuser, at least initially, feels remorseful and apologetic and may bring presents, make promises, and tell the

victim how much she is loved and needed. The victim usually feels needed and loved and hopes for change. Legal proceedings or plans to leave initiated during the acute battering stage may be abandoned.

Unfortunately, without intervention, the cycle will repeat itself. Over time, the periods of calmness and safety become briefer, and the periods of anger and fear are more intense. Each repeat of the pattern erodes the victim's self-esteem. The victim either believes the violence was deserved or accepts the blame for it. This can lead to feelings of depression, hopelessness, immobilization, and self-deprecation. Fig. 28.2 illustrates the cycle of violence

> **VIGNETTE:** The nurse in a walk-in clinic assesses Janet for bilateral corneal abrasions. The nurse becomes suspicious as she notes the patient's vague responses to history questions and her unrelenting checking of the clock, followed by the urgent statement, "I've got to get home." On further questioning, Janet reveals that she is often quite fatigued due to caring for her five children, all under the age of 7. Her husband, who works until 2 a.m., expects her to be awake when he comes home from work and have a warm meal ready. "He hits me if I'm asleep." She had taped her eyes open so that even if she were lying down when he came home, she would look awake. "I didn't even think about taking my contacts out."

OLDER ADULT ABUSE

For many older adults, the golden years are anything but golden. It can be a sad, stressful time filled with pain, anxiety, and poverty. Older adult mistreatment is defined as intentional actions that cause harm or creates a risk of harm to a vulnerable person. This mistreatment includes failure to provide for the older adults' basic needs or to protect them from harm. Family member, custodians, and care facility personnel may inflict physical abuse and sexual abuse. Financial abuse is an additional problem in this population. Caretakers may steal cash or credit cards or coerce the older person to transfer property or accounts. Victims also lose personal belongings, vehicles, medication, and food stamps. All 50 states have enacted laws to prosecute older adult abuse.

Abuse of older adults is too commonly found in the news. Recent examples include:

- An 87-year-old woman in Missouri died 2 days after being found naked and lying in a bed soaked with urine and fecal matter (Farley, 2017). Her daughter was charged in the incident. She said she'd have taken better care of her, but she was too tired.
- New Jersey healthcare workers wearing floral scrubs were caught on camera as they lashed out, striking helpless patients (Sullivan, 2016). Workers were seen roughly force-feeding a 91-year-old Alzheimer patient and ignoring a woman who fell to the floor.
- A Cleveland man used surveillance cameras to catch nursing home employees abusing his 78-year-old mother (Shea, 2020). Footage revealed she was being abused and neglected. The man is now pushing for a state law that would allow cameras in all nursing homes.

Epidemiology

The Centers for Disease Control and Prevention (CDC, 2017) estimate that about 1 out of every 10 adults older than age 60

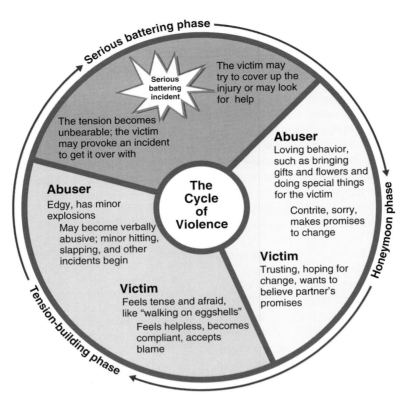

Fig. 28.2 The cycle of violence. (Redrawn from YWCA of Annapolis and Anne Arundel County, 1517 Ritchie Highway, Arnold, MD 21012.)

who live at home are victims of abuse. This number may be far higher in that for every case reported, five go unreported. This lack of reporting may be due to isolation, dependency, and fear of retaliation. Further complicating the picture is that the older adult may be caring for him- or herself, which creates the potential for self-neglect. Abuse occurs in both institutional and family settings. Family members are often the perpetrators in most of the incidents.

> **VIGNETTE:** Walter, a 73-year-old man, came to the ambulatory care clinic looking very fatigued and complaining of pain in his left shoulder "since last night." Holding his left arm close to his side, Walter averted his eyes from those of the receptionist, nurse, and doctor. When asked if anything had occurred that might have caused the pain, he answered, "I fell." When asked why he did not seek care the previous night, Walter stated, "I...I...thought it would go away overnight." X-rays revealed a fractured clavicle. After additional direct, supportive questioning, the patient admitted his son had shoved him to the floor.

Risk Factors

Older adults may become vulnerable because they are in poor mental or physical health or are disruptive due to disorders such as Alzheimer disease. The dependency needs of older adults are usually what put them at risk for abuse. The typical victim is female, over 75 years of age, white, living with a relative, and experiencing a physical and/or mental impairment.

Caring for older adults can be stressful in the best of cases, but in families in which violence is a coping strategy, the

potential for abuse is high. Parents who abuse their own children are more likely to end up as targets for abuse by their offspring. A spouse who is abused may retaliate in later years by responding with violence to failing physical or cognitive health.

> **VIGNETTE:** Ms. Randall, 83-years-old, is admitted from an adult foster home for evaluation of deterioration in her mental status. She is confused and disoriented as to time and place and is unable to give a coherent history. Blood and urine are collected for diagnostic evaluation. The laboratory report notes semen in the urine. Adult Protective Services is called to begin an investigation into the adult family home.

APPLICATION OF THE NURSING PROCESS

ASSESSMENT

General Assessment

You will encounter victims of violence in every healthcare setting. Therefore, you should screen all patients for possible abuse. Symptoms may be vague and can include chronic pain, insomnia, hyperventilation, or gynecological problems. Attention to the interview process and setting are important to facilitate accurate assessment of physical and behavioral indicators of family violence. All assessments should include questions to elicit a history of sexual abuse, family violence, and drug use or abuse. Any assessment should be completed with the victim alone, and it is helpful to have an institutional policy that facilitates screening in private.

Interview Process and Setting

You can gather important and relevant information about the family situation by conducting a routine assessment with tact, understanding, and a relaxed attitude. When interviewing, sit near the patient and spend some time establishing trust and rapport before focusing on the details of the violent experience. Establishing trust is crucial if the patient is to feel comfortable enough to self-disclose. The interview should be nonthreatening and supportive.

It is better to ask about ways of solving disagreements or methods of disciplining children rather than to use the words abuse or violence. It is also important not to assume a person's sexual orientation. Use the term partner when asking about the relationship. Key interviewing guidelines are listed in Box 28.2.

The person who experienced the violence should be allowed to tell the story without interruption. Verbal approaches may include the following:

- Tell me about what happened to you.
- Who takes care of you? (for children and dependent older adults)
- What happens when you do something wrong? (for children) *or* How do you and your partner/caregiver resolve disagreements? (for women and dependent older adults)
- What do you do for fun?
- Who helps you with your child(ren)/parent?
- What time do you have for yourself?

Questions that are open-ended and require a descriptive response can be less threatening and elicit more relevant information than questions that are direct or can be answered with *yes* or *no*:

- What arrangements do you make when you have to leave your child alone?

- How do you discipline your child?
- When your infant cries for a long time, how do you get him/her to stop?
- What is it about your child's behavior that bothers you the most?

When trust has been established, openness and directness about the situation can strengthen the relationship with those experiencing or perpetrating violence. A five-question assessment tool developed by Soeken, McFarlane, Parker, & Lominack, 1998 has been used extensively to assist in the routine identification of intimate partner abuse (Fig. 28.3).

VIGNETTE: Charlene Peters is a 42-year-old married woman in a relationship she describes as "bad for a long time." She is brought to the emergency department by ambulance with swollen eyes, lips, and nose, and lacerations to her face. She tells the nurse that her husband had been asleep for an hour before she joined him. When she got into bed, Charlene tried to redistribute the blankets. Suddenly he leaped from the bed and began pummeling her face with his fists. He screamed, "Don't you ever wake me up again" and threw her against the wall. She cried out to her 11-year-old son to call 911. The police arrived, called an ambulance, and took Mr. Peters to jail.

The nurse takes Charlene to a private examination room for a full assessment. Mrs. Peters states that her relationship with her husband has always been stormy. The beatings began 5 years earlier when she was pregnant with their second child. The beatings had increased in intensity, and this emergency department visit is the fifth in a year. Tonight was the first time she ever called the police.

Charlene is shaken. Periods of crying alternate with periods of silence. She appears apathetic and in a moderate level of anxiety. The nurse explores alternatives designed to help her reduce the danger when she is discharged. "I'm concerned that you will be hurt again if you go home. What options do you have?" Charlene agrees that she is in danger. Along with the nurse, Charlene makes plans to move to a women's shelter with her two children. She also plans to file for a restraining order.

The nurse charts the abuse referrals. Keeping careful and complete records helps to ensure that Charlene will receive proper follow-up care and will assist her when and if she pursues legal action.

BOX 28.2 Interview Guidelines

Do

- Conduct the interview in private.
- Be direct, honest, and professional.
- Use language the patient understands.
- Ask the patient to clarify words not understood.
- Be understanding.
- Be attentive.
- Inform the patient if you must make a referral to Children's or Adult Protective Services, and explain the process.
- Assess safety and help reduce danger (at discharge).

Do Not

- Try to "prove" abuse by accusations or demands.
- Display horror, anger, shock, or disapproval of the perpetrator or situation.
- Place blame or make judgments.
- Allow the patient to feel "at fault" or "in trouble."
- Probe or press for answers the patient is not willing to give.
- Conduct the interview with a group of interviewers.

Assessing Types of Abuse
Physical Abuse

A series of minor complaints, such as headaches, back trouble, dizziness, and accidents (especially falls), may be a covert indicator of violence. Overt signs of battering include bruises, scars, burns, and other wounds in various stages of healing, particularly around the head, face, chest, arms, abdomen, back, buttocks, and genitalia. Injuries that should arouse the nurse's suspicion are listed in Box 28.3.

If the explanation does not match the injury seen or if the patient minimizes the seriousness of the injury, you should suspect abuse. Ask patients directly in a nonthreatening manner if someone close to them has caused the injury. Observe the nonverbal response, such as hesitation or lack of eye contact. Then ask specific questions such as: "When was the last time it happened? How often does it happen? In what ways are you hurt?" Inconsistent explanations serve as a warning that further investigation is necessary. Vague explanations should also alert

ABUSE ASSESSMENT SCREEN

1. Within the last year, have you been hit, slapped, kicked, or otherwise physically hurt by someone?

☐ Yes ☐ No

If yes, by whom? _____

Total number of times: _____

2. Since you've been pregnant, have you been hit, slapped, kicked, or otherwise physically hurt by someone?

☐ Yes ☐ No

If yes, by whom? _____

Total number of times: _____

Mark the area of injury on the body map below.

3. Within the last year, has anyone forced you to have sexual activities?

☐ Yes ☐ No

If yes, who? _____

Total number of times: _____

4. Have you ever been emotionally or physically abused by your partner or someone important to you?

☐ Yes ☐ No

If yes, by whom? _____

Total number of times: _____

5. Are you afraid of your partner or anyone listed above?

☐ Yes ☐ No

Score each incident according to the following scale:

1 = Threats of abuse including use of a weapon

2 = Slapping, pushing; no injuries and/or continuing pain

3 = Punching, kicking, bruises, cuts, and/or continuing pain

4 = Beating up, severe contusions, burns, broken bones

5 = Head injury, internal injury, permanent injury

6 = Use of weapon, wound from weapon

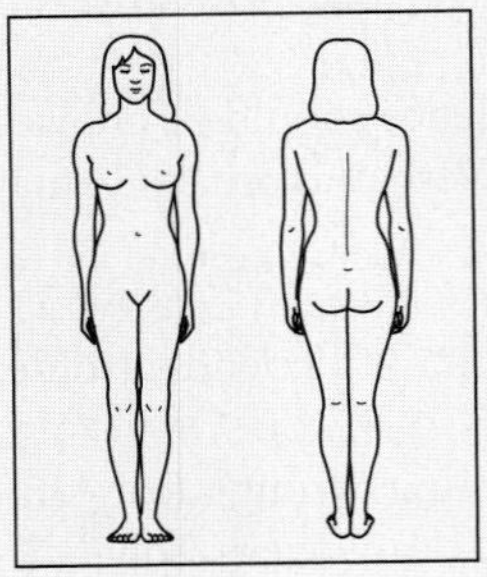

SCORE

Fig. 28.3 Abuse assessment screen. (From Soeken, K., McFarlane, J., Parker, B., & Lominack, M. (1998). The abuse assessment screen: A clinical instrument to measure frequency, severity and perpetrator of abuse against women. In J. Campbell [Ed.], *Empowering survivors of abuse: Health care for battered women and their children* [pp. 575–579]. New Brunswick, NJ: Transaction.)

BOX 28.3 Common Presenting Problems of Victims of Abuse

Emergency Department
- Bleeding injuries, especially to head and face
- Internal injuries, concussions, perforated eardrum, abdominal injuries, severe bruising, eye injuries, strangulation marks on neck
- Back injuries
- Broken or fractured jaw, arms, pelvis, ribs, clavicle, legs
- Burns from cigarettes, appliances, scalding liquids, acids
- Psychological trauma, anxiety, attacks of hyperventilation, heart palpitations, severe crying spells, suicidal tendencies
- Miscarriage

Ambulatory Care Settings
- Perforated eardrum, twisted or stiff neck and shoulder muscles, headache
- Depression, stress-related conditions (e.g., insomnia, violent nightmares, anxiety, extreme fatigue, eczema, loss of hair)
- Talk of having "problems" with husband or son, describing person as very jealous, impulsive, or an alcohol or substance user
- Repeated visits with new complaints
- Bruises of various ages and specific shapes (fingers, belt)

Any Setting
- Signs of stress due to family violence: emotional, behavioral, school, or sleep problems and increase in aggressive behavior
- Injuries in a pregnant woman
- Recurrent visits for injuries attributed to being "accident-prone"

the nurse to possible abuse. "She fell from a chair [from a lap, down the stairs]." "He was running away." "The hot water was turned on by mistake."

Nonspecific bruising in older children is common. Any bruises on an infant younger than 6 months of age should be considered suspicious. **Shaken baby syndrome**, the leading cause of death as a result of physical abuse, usually occurs in children younger than 2 years old. Injuries are a result of the brain moving in the opposite direction as the baby's head. A baby who has been shaken may have respiratory problems, bulging fontanels, retinal hemorrhages, and central nervous system damage resulting in seizures, vomiting, and coma.

Physical abuse can occur prior to birth. Assessment of mothers should include alcohol and substance use patterns. Infants with prenatal alcohol exposure may experience fetal alcohol spectrum disorders, which results in brain damage and growth problems. Other substance use should also be assessed. In 2018, there were 27,709 referrals to child protective services for infantile prenatal substance exposure (IPSE) (ACF, 2020). IPSE results in neonatal abstinence syndrome (NAS) withdrawal. NAS is characterized by symptoms that lasts for days to weeks. Symptoms include irritability in infants and difficulty soothing and long-term health and developmental problems, such as hearing, vision, and learning difficulties.

HEALTH POLICY

Intimate Terrorism in the Time of the Pandemic

The coronavirus pandemic resulted in global panic and lockdowns. People were asked by their governments and health authorities to shelter at home to prevent the spread of the virus. After the novelty of being in shared crisis and baking bread wore off, even under the best of circumstances family members felt the strain of being in close quarters with one another.

Another opportunistic infection was spreading during the time of limited social movement: intimate terrorism (Taub, 2020). Domestic violence became more intense, frequent, and dangerous. Research supports that abuse surges during times of family togetherness, such as holidays and vacations. It is not surprising that intense months of family isolation would drive the rates of abuse up, particularly among women, children, and pets.

Task forces across the United States were charged with increasing protection for vulnerable individuals. The government maintains a strong system of support for victims of violence. For emergency situations, 911 is the best option. Local and national hotlines provide verbal support, while chat hotlines provide anonymous and less noticeable by the perpetrator support.

Sexual Abuse

Sexualized behavior is one of the most common symptoms of sexual abuse in children. Younger children may have precocious sexual knowledge, may draw sexually explicit images, or demonstrate sexual aggression. One telling clue is when a child acts out sexual interactions in play, for example, with dolls. Masturbation may be predominant in sexually abused children. In older children, sexual promiscuity is one of the most common symptoms of sexual abuse.

Symptoms of PTSD, such as nightmares, somatic complaints, and feelings of guilt, are also common in children who are sexually abused. In adults who were sexually abused as children, there are a variety of emotional, behavioral, and physical consequences, with depression being the most commonly reported symptom. Other consequences include anxiety, suicide, aggression, chronic low self-esteem, chronic pain, obesity, substance misuse, self-mutilation, and PTSD.

Emotional Abuse

Emotional abuse may exist on its own or in conjunction with physical or sexual abuse. Although it is less obvious and more difficult to assess than physical violence, you can identify it through indicators such as low self-esteem, reported feelings of inadequacy, anxiety and withdrawal, learning difficulties, and poor impulse control.

Neglect

Neglected children and older adults often appear undernourished, dirty, and poorly clothed. Neglect is also manifested by inadequate medical care, such as lack of immunizations and untreated medical or dental conditions.

Economic Abuse

Economic abuse may take the form of failure to provide for the needs of the victim when adequate funds are available. Bills may be left unpaid by the person in charge of finances, which may result in disconnection of the heat or electricity. In the case of spousal abuse, the perpetrator may prevent the victim from pursuing education or finding a job, thereby ensuring dependency.

Assessment Variables

Anxiety

Nonverbal responses to the assessment interview may indicate the victim's anxiety level. Agitation and anxiety bordering on panic are often present in victims experiencing violence. Because they live in fear, abused individuals remain vigilant and unable to relax or sleep. Signs and somatic symptoms of living with chronic stress and severe levels of anxiety include hypertension, irritability, and gastrointestinal disturbances. Hesitation, lack of eye contact, and use of vague statements such as "It's been rough lately" indicate that the situation is difficult to talk about.

Coping Mechanisms

Coping mechanisms used by many individuals in order to endure living in violent and terrifying situations often prevent the termination of the relationship. These coping mechanisms may take the form of flawed beliefs or myths (Table 28.2). Because of feelings of confusion, shame, despair, and powerlessness, victims may withdraw from interaction with others, increasing their isolation.

Coping mechanisms also can be viewed in the context of the family. Assessing parents regarding early family relationships can provide additional information about attitudes in the home and the way they might influence coping. Asking parents about how they were disciplined as children may provide insight into their child-rearing attitudes and practices.

Living with and caring for children and older adults can cause frustration, stress, and anger. Unless there are appropriate outlets for stress, abuse can occur. Box 28.4 is a useful guide for assessing the risk of child and/or older adult abuse in the home.

Support Systems

The person experiencing abuse is usually in a dependent position, relying on the perpetrator for basic needs. This dependence, along with the isolation the perpetrator imposes on the person, limits the victim's access to support systems. Children's options are especially limited, as are those of the physically and mentally disabled. Assessing for support should focus on intrapersonal, interpersonal, and community resources.

Suicide Potential

A person experiencing violence may feel desperate to leave yet be trapped in an abusive relationship. Suicide may seem like the only option. In fact, victims of intimate partner violence are twice as likely to attempt suicide (Clay, 2014). Horrifying cases of murder–suicide are most likely to occur in the context of this type of abuse. Older adult abuse and neglect are strongly associated with cases of suicide in the older adult population.

Children who were subjected to abuse are at increased risk for suicide as adults. Sexual abuse and, to a lesser degree, physical abuse create this risk. The identity of the abuser and the frequency of the abuse influence the degree of suicide risk. When

TABLE 28.2   Abuse: Myth Versus Fact

Myth	Fact
The victim's behavior causes violence.	The victim's behavior is not the cause of the violence. Violence is the abuser's pattern of behavior.
Men have the right to keep their wives and/or children in line.	No person has the right to beat or hurt another person.
Intimate partner abuse is a minor problem.	There is a real danger that abusive partners may kill victims.
Battered women are masochistic and like to be beaten. They could leave if they really wanted to.	Women do not like, ask, or deserve to be abused. Factors influencing a decision to leave include fear of injury or death, financial dependence, and welfare of children.
Family abuse occurs in poorly educated people from poor, working-class backgrounds.	Abuse can happen in a tenement or a mansion in families of all socioeconomic, religious, cultural, and educational backgrounds.
Family matters are private, and families should be allowed to take care of their own problems.	Intervention in family abuse is justified; abuse always escalates in frequency and intensity, can end in death, and is passed on to future generations.
Myths victims commonly believe: "I can't live without him/her." "If I hadn't done _____, it wouldn't have happened." "She/he will change." "I stay for the sake of the children." "He's jealous because he loves me."	These myths are coping mechanisms used to allay panic in a situation of random and brutal violence. They give the illusion of control and rationality.
Alcohol and stress are the causes of physical and verbal abuse.	There are no excuses, and abuse is not acceptable behavior. People are abusive because they believe that violence and aggression are acceptable and effective responses to real or imagined threats.
Violence occurs only between heterosexual partners.	All partners, no matter the sexual orientation, experience violence for reasons similar to those in heterosexual relationships.
Pregnancy protects a woman from battering.	Battering frequently begins or escalates during pregnancy.

the abuser is an immediate family member and when the abuse is repeated, the risk is increased.

A suicide attempt may be the presenting problem in the emergency department. With sensitive questions conducted in a caring manner, the nurse can elicit the history of violence. Often, the means of attempted suicide is overdose with a combination of alcohol and other central nervous system depressants or sleeping medications.

When the crisis of the immediate suicide attempt has been resolved, careful questioning to determine lethality is in order. For example, if the patient still feels that life is not worth living, has a suicide plan, and has the means to carry it out, you must consider admission to an inpatient psychiatric unit. On the other hand, if the patient is talking about future plans and about staying "for the sake of the children," outpatient referrals are appropriate.

Homicide Potential

When working with an abused spouse, ask whether the patient feels safe going home and, if so, whether a safety plan is in place for when the violence recurs. Always assess the potential for lethality. Certain factors place a vulnerable person at greater risk for homicide, including the following:

- The presence of a gun in the home
- Alcohol and drug misuse
- History of violence on the part of the perpetrator in other situations
- Extreme jealousy and obsessiveness on the part of the perpetrator

The perpetrator of violence may eventually become the victim. Therefore, always ask individuals victimized by violence if they have ever felt like killing the perpetrator. If yes, ask whether they have the means to do so. If the answer is yes, intervention is required.

Drug and Alcohol Use

A person experiencing violence may self-medicate with alcohol or other drugs as a way of escaping an intolerable situation. The drugs are usually central nervous system depressants, such as benzodiazepines, prescribed by physicians for stress-related symptoms (e.g., insomnia, gastrointestinal upsets, anxiety, and difficulty concentrating). Assess for a chronic alcohol or drug problem (refer to Chapter 22) and provide appropriate treatment referrals. The patient should not be discharged to the abuser. Treatment choices can include both inpatient and outpatient options.

Assessment Documentation

Because of the possibility of future legal action, it is essential that the healthcare record contain an accurate and detailed description of the victim's medical history, the psychosocial history of the family, and observations of the family interactions during the interviews. Especially important in documentation of findings from the initial assessment are:

1. Verbatim statements of who caused the injury and when it occurred.
2. A body map to indicate size, color, shape, areas, and types of injuries, with explanations (see Fig. 28.3).
3. Physical evidence of sexual abuse, when possible.

Follow procedures for evidence collection carefully as this can impact legal action. If the abuse has just occurred, ask the patient to return in a day or two for more photographs, as bruises

BOX 28.4 Factors to Assess During a Home Visit

For a Child

- Responsiveness to infant's signals
- Caregiver's facial expressions in response to infant
- Playfulness of caregiver with infant
- Nature of physical contact during feeding and other caretaking activities
- Temperament of infant
- Caregiver's history of harsh discipline or abuse as a child
- Parental attitudes:
  - Feelings of inadequacy as a parent
  - Unrealistic expectations of child
  - Fear of "doing something wrong"
  - Attribution of negative qualities to newborn
  - Misdirected anger
  - Continued evidence of isolation, apathy, anger, frustration, projection
  - Adult conflict
- Environmental conditions:
  - Sleeping arrangements
  - Child management
  - Home management
  - Use of supports (formal and informal)
- Need for immediate services for situational (economics, child care), emotional, or educational information:
  - Information about hotlines, babysitters, homemakers, parent groups
  - Information about child development
  - Information about child care and home management services

For an Older Adult

- Absence of or lack of access to basic necessities (food, water, medications)
- Unsafe housing
- Lack of or inadequate utilities, ventilation, space
- Poor physical hygiene
- Lack of assistive devices, such as hearing aids, eyeglasses, wheelchair
- Medication mismanagement (outdated prescriptions, unmarked bottles)

---

may be more evident at that time. You must assure the patient of the confidentiality of the record and of its power should legal action be initiated. Even if intervention does not occur at this time, begin the record. The next provider will be aware of the problem and will be in a better position to offer support.

📋 ASSESSMENT GUIDELINES

Family Violence

Assess:
1. Signs and symptoms of victims of abuse
2. Potential for abuse in vulnerable families, for example, some indicators of vulnerable parents who might benefit from education and instruction in effective coping techniques
3. Physical, sexual, and/or emotional abuse, and neglect and economic maltreatment of older adults
4. Family coping patterns
5. Patient's support system
6. Drug or alcohol use
7. Suicidal or homicidal ideas
8. Posttrauma syndrome

Self-Assessment

Working with those who experience violence may arouse intense and overwhelming feelings. Strong negative feelings toward abuse may cloud your judgment and interfere with objective assessment and intervention, no matter how you try to cover or deny personal bias. Common responses of healthcare professionals to violence are listed in Table 28.3.

A personal history of abuse may cause you to identify too closely with the victim, and personal issues connected with the abuse may surface, further clouding judgment. Sharing perceptions and feelings with other professionals can help reduce feelings of isolation and discomfort.

NURSING DIAGNOSIS

The International Classification for Nursing Practice (ICNP) (International Council of Nurses, 2019) provides a variety of useful nursing diagnoses for abusive situations. While many of the diagnoses are directed toward protecting vulnerable family members, you can also include the perpetrator in plans of care. Safety is the number one concern and is addressed in *risk for violence, risk to be victim of child abuse, risk to be victim of intimate partner violence, risk to be victim of older adult violence,* and *risk for suicide. Rape-trauma syndrome* is addressed in Chapter 29.

Living in a situation where vulnerable individuals feel unsafe and helpless results in additional nursing diagnoses. *Anxiety, fear, hopelessness,* and *powerlessness* are significant considerations in abusive situations. Perpetual negative messages and being treated in a disrespectful manner suggest the diagnoses of *chronic low self-esteem* and *situational low self-esteem.* Deficits in managing day-to-day household and role responsibilities are addressed in *impaired coping.*

The family as patient may be the focus. Like individuals, families may experience difficulties managing responsibilities and

TABLE 28.3 Common Responses of Healthcare Professionals to Violence

Response	Source
Anger	Anger may be felt toward the person responsible for the abuse, toward those who allowed it to happen, and toward society for condoning its occurrence through attitudes, traditions, and laws
Embarrassment	The victim is a symbol of something close to home: the stress and strain of family life unleashed as uncontrollable anger
Confusion	The view of the family as a haven of safety and privacy is challenged
Fear	A small percentage of perpetrators are dangerous to others
Anguish	The nurse may have experienced abuse
Helplessness	The nurse may want to do more, eliminate the problem, or cure the victim and/or perpetrator
Discouragement	Discouragement may result if no long-term solution is achieved
"Blame the victim" mentality	Healthcare workers can get caught up in blaming the victim for behaviors they see as provoking the abuse

stressors, resulting in a nursing diagnosis of *impaired family coping*. The inability to achieve family functions and tasks and to handle tensions and stress is addressed with *impaired family process*. Parents who are unwilling or unable to raise children in a safe environment with consistent and appropriate expectations will benefit from a diagnosis of *impaired parenting*. Tending to children, adolescents, and aging individuals can result in frustration for anyone, but even more so in vulnerable individuals. *Caregiver stress* provides a basis for planning outcomes and targeting interventions.

OUTCOMES IDENTIFICATION

Outcomes are developed to reduce or reverse the problem addressed in the nursing diagnosis. Coping diagnoses, for example, employ outcomes that seek to improve coping. Other outcomes are aimed at eliminating abuse where the individual is free from being hurt or exploited. Simply put, outcomes regarding abuse would read no [specify type].

You should make the identification of desired outcomes patient-centered and therefore developed in conjunction with the survivor and primary support person. Continually reassess these outcomes and revise them as new information about the survivor's needs emerges.

Table 28.4 identifies signs and symptoms, potential nursing diagnoses, and outcomes for victims of child, intimate partner, and older adult abuse, as well as for individuals who abuse.

PLANNING

Nurses and other healthcare workers encounter abuse frequently, not only in healthcare settings but also in their communities and families. The nurse is often the first point of contact for people experiencing abuse and thus is in an ideal position to contribute to prevention, detection, and effective intervention. The Joint Commission requires staff education in family violence and abuse, as well as the development of standards of care to guide clinical practice.

Most hospitals and community centers provide protocols for dealing with child, intimate partner, or older adult abuse. Unless it is a case of child abuse in which the child has been removed from the home, most interventions performed after necessary emergency care will take place within the community. Plans should center on the patient's safety first. Whenever it is possible or in the best interests of the patient, plans should be discussed with the patient. Planning should also take into consideration the needs of the abuser(s) (e.g., parents, caretakers, spouse, or partner) if they are motivated to learn alternatives to abuse and violence.

IMPLEMENTATION

Reporting Abuse

Nurses are legally mandated to report suspected or actual cases of child and vulnerable adult abuse. The appropriate agency may be the state or county child welfare agency, law enforcement agency, juvenile court, or county health department. Each state has specific guidelines for reporting, including whether the report can be oral, written, or both, and within what time period the suspected abuse or neglect must be reported (immediately, within 24 hours, or within 48 hours). Every abused person is a crime victim, and assault with a weapon is reportable in most states. All 50 states have marital rape statutes. The following vignette gives an example of a child-abuse case that requires reporting.

TABLE 28.4　Signs and Symptoms, Nursing Diagnoses, and Outcomes for Family Violence		
Signs and Symptoms	**Potential Nursing Diagnoses**	**Outcomes**
History of abuse, history of violence, substance use, poor coping skills, limited impulse control	*Risk for violence* *Risk to be victim of child abuse* *Risk to be victim of intimate partner violence* *Risk to be victim of older adult violence*	No violence: Family members remain free of harm
Desperate to leave situation, feeling trapped, hopelessness, history of abuse as a child, suicide attempt	*Risk for suicide*	Decreased suicide risk: No suicidal thoughts, plans for the future, living in a safe environment
Feels endangered, distressed, scanning the environment, vigilance, uncertainty, isolation, feelings of helplessness, decreased control over environment, abuse	*Anxiety* *Fear*	Reduced anxiety and fear: Behavioral manifestations of anxiety absent, reports a decrease in anxiety, reports feeling safe, expresses expectations of a positive future, sets goals
Poor eye contact and body posture, lack of respect from significant others, traumatic situation, neglect, feelings of shame and low self-esteem, feelings of worthlessness	*Chronic low self-esteem*	Improved self-esteem: Maintains eye contact and erect posture, describes positive level of confidence, expects positive responses from others, describes feelings of success and self-worth
Poor coping skills, hostility, impulsivity, inadequate problem solving, substance use	*Impaired coping Impaired family coping*	Improved coping: Discusses the abusive behavior, obtains needed treatment, controls impulses, refrains from substance use

International Council of Nurses. (2019). *ICNP browser.* Retrieved from https://www.icn.ch/what-we-do/projects/ehealth/icnp-browser. ICNP is owned and copyrighted by the International Council of Nurses (ICN). Reproduced with permission of the copyright holder.

VIGNETTE: Two nurses who work in a family practice clinic are suspicious of child abuse. Hannah, 12 years old, has recurrent urinary tract infections. Her father, who accompanies her into the bathroom when she is providing urine samples, always brings her to clinic visits. He answers all questions for Hannah even when providers direct the questions to her.

After pressure by the nurses, the physician agrees to ask Hannah some questions in private. The nurses think the physician has minimized the problem, asked superficial questions, and dismissed their concerns. They decide to report their concerns to Children's Protective Services. They inform the father, who becomes outraged at their accusations and threatens to change doctors.

Subsequent investigation confirms the likelihood of sexual abuse, and Hannah is placed in temporary foster care with follow-up counseling. The father refuses treatment and threatens to sue the nurses. Four months later, the father leaves the family.

The case in the preceding vignette illustrates that a reasonable basis for suspecting abuse, not proof, is all that is required to report. Nurses must attempt to maintain both an appropriate level of suspicion and a neutral, objective attitude. One can be too concerned and jump to conclusions, which is what the physician in this case thought the nurses were doing. On the other hand, too little concern can result in an incomplete examination to avoid confrontation, which is what the nurses thought the physician was doing. Given these opposing stances, the case was reported as required by law and ethical standards, and Children's Protective Services was given the opportunity to investigate.

Culture

Culture is important because it is central to how people organize their experience. Even the most acculturated people have a tendency to revert to their cultural past in organizing coping strategies after a stressful event. If there is a language barrier, the nurse should speak slowly and clearly in English, without using jargon, and allow time for the response. If the patient speaks no English, provide a trained medical interpreter. A family member should *not* be used as an interpreter to ensure confidentiality and to protect the person from future retaliation.

Counseling

Counseling includes crisis intervention measures. It is important to emphasize that people have a right to live without fear of violence, physical harm, or assault. Telling an abused person that "no one deserves to be hit" can be a powerful statement in and of itself. The role of the nurse is to support the victim, counsel about safety, and facilitate access to other resources as appropriate.

You should counsel individuals experiencing intimate partner violence about developing a safety plan, a plan for a rapid escape when abuse recurs. Ask patients to identify the signs of escalation of violence and to pick a particular sign that will tell them that "now is the time to leave." If children are present, they can all agree on a code word that, when spoken by the parent, means "It is time to go." If the individual plans ahead, it may be possible to leave before the violence occurs. It is important that the plan include a destination and transportation. The nurse should suggest packing the items listed in Box 28.5 ahead of time. The person should keep the packed bag in a place where the perpetrator will not find it.

BOX 28.5   Personalized Safety Guide

Suggestions for Increasing Safety While in the Relationship
- I will have important phone numbers available to my children and myself.
- I can tell _____ and _____ about the violence and ask them to call the police if they hear suspicious noises coming from my home.
- If I leave my home, I can go to (list four places) _____, _____, _____, or _____.
- I can leave extra money, car keys, clothes, and copies of documents with _____.
- If I leave, I will bring _____ (see checklist).
- To ensure safety and independence, I will open my own savings account, rehearse my escape route with a support person, and review safety plan on _____ (date).

Suggestions for Increasing Safety When the Relationship Is Over
- I can change the locks; install steel or metal doors, a security system, smoke detectors, and an outside lighting system.
- I will inform _____ and _____ that my partner no longer lives with me and ask them to call the police if the perpetrator is observed near my home or my children.
- I will tell people who take care of my children the names of those who have permission to pick them up. The people who have permission are _____, _____, and _____.
- I can tell _____ at work about my situation and ask _____ to screen my calls.
- I can avoid stores, banks, and _____ that I used when living with my battering partner.
- I can obtain a protective order from _____. I can keep it on or near me at all times, as well as have a copy with _____.

- If I feel down and ready to return to a potentially abusive situation, I can call _____ for support or attend workshops and support groups to gain support and strengthen my relationships with other people.

Important Phone Numbers
- Police _____
- Hotline _____
- Friends _____
- Shelter _____

Checklist of Items to Take
- Identification
- Birth certificates for me and my children
- Social Security card
- School and medical records
- Money, bank books, credit cards
- Keys to house, car, office
- Driver's license and registration
- Medications
- Change of clothes
- Welfare identification
- Passport(s), green card, work permit
- Divorce papers
- Lease or rental agreement, house deed
- Mortgage payment book, current unpaid bills
- Insurance papers
- Address book
- Pictures, jewelry, items of sentimental value
- Children's favorite toys and/or blankets

If a survivor of intimate partner violence chooses to leave, shelters or safe houses (for both sexes) are available in most communities. They are open 24 hours a day and can be reached through hotline information numbers, hospital emergency departments, YWCAs, or the local office of the National Organization for Women. The address of the house is usually kept secret to protect abused individuals from attack by the perpetrator. Besides offering protection, many of these shelters and safe houses serve important educational and consciousness-raising functions. Patients should be given the number of the nearest available shelter even if they decide for the present to stay with their partners.

Case Management

Community mental health centers are becoming increasingly involved in the delivery of services to victims and perpetrators of abuse. Nurses working in these settings have the opportunity to coordinate community, medical, criminal justice, and social services to provide comprehensive assistance to families in crisis.

Promotion of Community Support

An important intervention is to support help seeking. You may provide referral numbers and even stand by as the patient makes a phone call for an appointment. Make specific referrals regarding emergency financial assistance and legal counseling available to each patient. Vocational counseling is another referral that may be appropriate. Give patients referrals to parenting resources that enable them to explore alternative approaches to discipline (e.g., no hitting, slapping, or other expressions of violence).

Health Teaching and Health Promotion

In families at risk for abuse, health teaching and health promotion include meeting with both the individual and the family to help them learn to recognize behaviors and situations that might trigger violence.

Explain normal developmental and physiological changes to enable family members to gain a more positive view of the victim and the crisis situation. Gaining a more complete understanding can help family members broaden their insight and thus increase their compassion. They may then begin to anticipate new stress situations and be able to prepare for them before a crisis occurs.

Nurses who work on a maternity unit are often in a position to identify risk factors for abuse between new parents and initiate appropriate interventions, including education about effective parenting and coping techniques. Share information about these interventions with the patient's healthcare team for appropriate monitoring and follow-up. Parents who are candidates for special attention include the following:

- New parents whose behavior toward the infant is rejecting, hostile, or indifferent.
- Teenage parents who require special help in handling the baby and discussing their expectations of the baby and their support systems.

- Parents with cognitive deficits for whom careful, explicit, and repeated instructions on caring for the child and recognizing the infant's needs are indicated.
- Parents who grew up watching their mothers be abused. This is a significant risk factor for perpetuation of family violence.

Nurses can also recognize when children are at risk and make referrals to community resources, including emergency child care facilities, emergency telephone numbers, numbers of 24-hour crisis centers or hotlines, and respite programs in which volunteers take the child for an occasional weekend so that parents can get some relief. Community health nurses can make home visits to identify risk factors for abuse in the crucial first few months of life during which the style of parent-child interactions is established. See Box 28.4 for important factors for the community health nurse to assess during a home care visit. Such observations made by nurses in clinic and public health settings are fundamental in case findings and evaluation.

Prevention of Abuse
Primary Prevention

Primary prevention consists of measures taken to prevent the occurrence of abuse. Identifying individuals and families at high risk, providing health teaching, and coordinating supportive services to prevent crises are examples of primary prevention. Specific strategies include:

1. Reducing stress
2. Reducing the influence of risk factors
3. Increasing social support
4. Increasing coping skills
5. Increasing self-esteem

Community health nurses are in a unique position to assess family functioning in the home during visits for other medical problems. In addition, the community health nurse and clinic nurse maintain contact with the family over time, which allows for assessment of changes. They are also in an excellent position to connect parents to appropriate resources in the community that can meet their needs. All nurses can work to reduce society's acceptance of violence by working toward social policy change.

Secondary Prevention

Secondary prevention involves early intervention in abusive situations to minimize their disabling or long-term effects. Nurses can establish screening programs for individuals at risk, participate in the medical treatment of injuries resulting from violent episodes, and coordinate community services to provide continuity of care. Healthcare professionals can help reduce stress and depression by providing supportive therapy, support groups, pharmacotherapy, and contact information for community resources. Social dysfunction or lack of information can be addressed by counseling and education. You can reduce caregiver burden by arranging assistance in caring for the family member, housekeeping, or, in cases in which caregiving needs exceed even optimal caregiver capacity, by placing the patient in a more appropriate setting. The following vignette illustrates a successful secondary prevention effort.

VIGNETTE: Six-year-old Gavin is brought to the school nurse by his teacher, who says he had complained of an upset stomach. When the nurse examines Gavin, she notices bruises on his arms and abdomen. Gavin appears frightened and hesitant to speak.

Nurse: "How did you hurt yourself, Gavin?" *(Gavin looks down and starts to cry.)* "It's OK if you don't want to talk about it."

Gavin: *(Does not look at the nurse and speaks softly.)* "My mom hit me."

Nurse: "Tell me what happened before that."

Gavin: "Mom was mad because I didn't put my toys away."

Nurse: "What does your mom usually do when she gets mad?"

Gavin: "She yells mostly. Sometimes she hits me."

Nurse: "Tell me about the hitting."

Gavin: "Mom hits me a lot since my dad left." *(Gavin starts to cry to himself.)*

Gavin appears well nourished and properly dressed. He is at his approximate developmental age except for some language delay; however, because of the physical evidence and history, the nurse notifies Children's Protective Services, and the family situation is evaluated for possible placement of Gavin in protective custody. The initial evaluation concludes that there is no indication of serious potential harm to the child and that Gavin should return home. The mother, who is initially defensive, starts to cry and states, "I can't cope with being alone, and I don't know where to turn."

Nursing interventions center on caring for Gavin's immediate health needs, finding supports for the mother to help her cope with crises, providing a counseling referral for the mother to learn alternative ways of expressing anger and frustration, and informing the mother of parents' groups.

Tertiary Prevention

Tertiary prevention, which often occurs in mental health settings, involves nurses facilitating the healing and rehabilitative process by counseling individuals and families, providing support for groups of survivors, and assisting survivors of violence to achieve their optimal level of safety, health, and well-being. Legal advocacy programs for survivors of intimate partner violence are an example of tertiary prevention. Complementary therapies, such as mindfulness-based stress reduction, can also assist survivors in the healing process.

EVALUATION

Failures of interventions with abusive families often are due to problems within the social, economic, and political systems in which we live. Nurses can direct their interventions to the social environment. Questions that nurses should consider are:

- Is corporal punishment an acceptable technique for guiding behavior in children?
- How do we address the unequal burden of caregiving responsibilities placed on women?
- Why is a low priority given to education and preparation for parenthood?
- How can we change the belief that older adults have little social value?

TREATMENT MODALITIES

Psychological Therapies

Nurse who are educated at the master's or doctoral level and certified in advanced practice psychiatric nursing are qualified to conduct specialized therapy. This type of therapy is most effective after crisis intervention, when the situation is less chaotic and tumultuous. A variety of therapeutic modalities are available for the treatment of people who are abused and people who abuse.

Individual Therapy

The goals of individual therapy for a survivor are empowerment, the ability to recognize and choose productive life options, and the development of a solid sense of self. People who have experienced abuse as a child or have left a violent relationship may choose individual therapy to address symptoms of depression, anxiety, somatization, or PTSD.

Many of the psychological symptoms shown by women who have been abused can be understood as complex survival strategies and responses to violence. Nurses must address the guilt, shame, and stigmatization experienced by survivors of abuse. It is helpful for nurses to understand that the individual's feelings and behaviors may be reflective of the grieving process due to numerous losses as a result of the abusive relationship. Helping the survivor work through the stages of grieving can promote healing.

Individual therapy is often indicated for the perpetrator, particularly when an individual psychopathological process is identified. Therapy for the perpetrator is most effective when it is court mandated because the perpetrator is more likely to complete the course of treatment. Nurses engaged in therapy with perpetrators have a duty to warn potential victims if they conclude that the perpetrator is a danger. Refer to Chapter 6 for a more detailed discussion of the duty to warn and duty to protect.

Family Therapy

Because abuse is a symptom of a family in crisis, each part of the family system needs attention. Also, because change in one member of the family system affects the whole system, all members need support and understanding. Interventions may maximize positive interactions among all family members. Couples therapy can put the abused partner at increased risk of harm or even death. Conjoint therapy should take place *only* if the perpetrator has had individual therapy and has demonstrated change as a result, and if both parties agree to participate.

Expected outcomes are that the perpetrator will recognize destructive patterns of behavior, learn alternative responses, control impulses, and refrain from abusive behavior. Intermediate goals are that members of the family will openly communicate and learn to listen to one another. Refer to Chapter 35 for a more detailed discussion of family therapy.

Group Therapy

Participation in therapy groups provides assurances that one is not alone and that change is possible. Because many survivors of abuse have been isolated, they have been deprived of validation and positive feedback from others. Working in a group can help diminish feelings of isolation, strengthen feelings of self-esteem and self-worth, and increase the potential for realistic problem solving in a supportive atmosphere.

Groups often use cognitive behavioral techniques to help the abuser see abusive actions as behavioral patterns that they can change. In therapy groups, perpetrators learn to recognize the thoughts preceding an abusive incident, the responses to the thoughts, and how to interrupt negative feelings about their partners. Perpetrators who have never discussed problems with anyone before are encouraged to discuss their thoughts and feelings. Group therapy can help create a community of healing and restoration. Refer to Chapter 34 for a more detailed discussion of group therapy.

CASE STUDY AND NURSING CARE PLAN

Family Violence

Helen Duff is a recently widowed 84-year-old woman. She had been living in a third-floor walk-up in the city. Due to her son John's concerns over the level of crime in the neighborhood and her declining health, Ms. Duff moved in with him. He and his wife, Judy, have been married for 20 years and have three children 6 to 18 years of age, all living in a rather cramped three-bedroom house.

Chrissy Green, a visiting nurse, monitors Ms. Duff's blood pressure. Over a series of visits, the nurse notices that her patient is looking unkempt, pale, and withdrawn. While taking her blood pressure, Chrissy observes bruises on her arms that look like her arms have been grabbed. When asked about the bruises, Ms. Duff says that she slipped in the bathroom. Ms. Duff stiffens in her chair when her daughter-in-law, Judy, enters the room. The nurse notices that Judy avoids eye contact with Ms. Duff.

When the nurse asks about the injuries, Judy responds angrily, blaming Ms. Duff for causing so many problems. She will not explain the reason for the change in Ms. Duff's behavior or the origin of the bruises. She merely comments, "I have had to give up my job since my mother-in-law came here. It's been difficult and crowded. The kids are complaining. We are having trouble making ends meet since I gave up my job, and my husband is no help at all."

Self-Assessment

This is the first time that Chrissy Green has encountered the potential mistreatment of an older adult. She discusses her reactions with other team members of the visiting nurse service. Although she understands the daughter-in-law's frustration, she feels anger toward her. There is no justification for inflicting harm on another person. The team agrees that this family could use support. If the suspected abuse does not stop, they will need to take more drastic measures and contact legal services.

Assessment
Subjective Data
- Stressful crowded living conditions
- Economic hardships leading to stress
- No support for the daughter-in-law from the rest of the family for the care of Ms. Duff
- Ms. Duff states she slipped in the bathroom, but physical findings do not support this explanation.
- Judy states, "It's been difficult and crowded."

Objective Data
- Physical symptoms of abuse (bruises) and neglect (unkempt appearance)
- Withdrawn and apprehensive behavior
- No eye contact between Ms. Duff and her daughter-in-law

Nursing Diagnosis
On the basis of the data, the nurse formulates the following nursing diagnosis:
- *Risk to be victim of older adult violence related* to increased family stress as evidenced by signs of violence

Outcomes Identification
Overall outcome: No violence
Short-term indicators:
- Evidence that physical violence has ceased
- Evidence that emotional abuse has ceased

Planning
Chrissy Green discusses several possible outcomes with members of her team, giving attention to the priority of outcomes and to whether they are realistic in this situation. She also plans to report the abuse to Adult Protective Services and to work with Ms. Duff, Judy, and the rest of the family to improve this situation.

Implementation
Ms. Duff's plan of care is personalized as follows:

Short-Term Goal	Intervention	Rationale	Evaluation
1. On each visit made by the nurse, the patient will state that abuse has ceased.	1a. Assess severity of signs and symptoms of abuse. 1b. Do a careful home assessment to identify other areas of abuse and neglect. 1c. Discuss with patient factors leading to abuse and concern for safety.	1a. Accurate charting (body map, pictures with permission, verbatim statements) helps follow progress and provides legal data. 1b. Check for inadequacy of food, blocked stairways, medication safety issues. All indicate abuse and neglect. Determine the kinds of problems in the home, and plan intervention. Identify community resources that could help the patient and her caregivers. 1c. Allows family stressors and potential areas for intervention to be identified. Validates that situation is serious and increases patient's knowledge base.	**GOAL MET** Patient states that after family talked to the nurse and planned strategies, physical abuse no longer occurs.
2. Within 2 weeks, patient will be able to identify at least two supportive services to deal with emergency situations.	2. Discuss with patient supportive services such as hotlines and crisis units to call in case of emergency situations and develop a written list.	2. Maximizes patient's safety through use of support services.	**GOAL MET** Patient has a list with important phone numbers. She has called the hotline once to get information on transportation to the senior center in town.

CASE STUDY AND NURSING CARE PLAN—cont'd

Family Violence

Short-Term Goal	Intervention	Rationale	Evaluation
3. Within 3 weeks, family members will identify difficult issues that increase their stress levels.	3. Discuss with family members their feelings, and identify at least four areas that are most difficult for the various family members.	3. Listening to each family member and identifying unmet needs helps both family and nurse identify areas that require changing and appropriate interventions.	**GOAL MET** Family members identify areas such as overwork, lack of free time, lack of privacy, and financial difficulties, all of which increase their stress levels.
4. Within 3 weeks, family will seek out community resources to help with anger management, need for home-maker support, and other needs.	4. Identify potential community supports, skills training, respite places, homemakers, financial aids, etc., that might help meet family's unmet needs.	4. When stressed, individuals solve problems poorly and do not know about or cannot manage to organize outside help. Finances are often a problem.	**GOAL MET** Judy is responding well to anger management groups. Both Judy and her husband are attending a support group for caregivers.

Evaluation

Eight weeks after Chrissy Green's initial visit, Ms. Duff appears well groomed, friendly, and more spontaneous in her conversation. She comments, "Things are better with my daughter-in-law." No bruises or other signs of physical violence are noticeable. She is considerably more outgoing and has even taken the initiative to contact an old friend. Ms. Duff has talked openly to her son and daughter-in-law about stress in the family. Ms. Duff says that she went for a walk when her daughter-in-law Judy appeared tense and returned to find that the tension had lessened. Neither Ms. Duff nor her family has initiated plans for alternative housing.

■ KEY POINTS TO REMEMBER

- Abuse can occur in any family and can be predicted with some accuracy by examining the characteristics of perpetrators and vulnerable people in which violence is likely.
- Abuse can be physical, sexual, emotional, economic, or can be caused by neglect.
- The most common form of child abuse is neglect.
- Risk factors for child abuse include being younger than 4, being a child who is somehow different, and an impairment in the emotional bond between parent and child.
- Intimate partner violence tends to become progressively worse and can end in death.
- A cycle of violence with tension-building, acute battering, and honeymoon stages is commonly present in cases of intimate partner violence.
- Older adult abuse is far too common and is often difficult to uncover due to dependency.
- Family members and custodial healthcare workers are most often implicated in abuse of older adults.
- Assessment includes identifying indicators of abuse, levels of anxiety, coping mechanisms, support systems, suicide and homicide potential, and alcohol and drug misuse.
- Registered nurses are legally mandated to report suspected or actual abuse in the case of children and vulnerable adults.
- Community referral and support are essential in helping individuals and families with abusive situations.

■ CRITICAL THINKING

1. A colleague who has witnessed a child being abused states, "I don't think it's any of our business what people do in the privacy of their own homes."
   a. What would you be legally required to do?
   b. What are your ethical responsibilities?
2. You successfully convinced your colleagues to assess routinely for abuse, and now they want to know how to do it. How would you go about teaching them to assess for child abuse? Intimate partner abuse? Older adult abuse?
3. Your health maintenance organization's routine health screening form for adolescents, adults, and older adults has just been changed to include questions about family abuse. How would you respond to patients who indicate on this form that abuse occurs in their home?
4. Identify at least four referrals in your community for a victim of family violence.
5. Identify two referrals in your community for a perpetrator of family violence.

CHAPTER REVIEW

1. Which statement made by a new mother should be explored further by the nurse?
   a. "I have three children, that's enough."
   b. "I think the baby cries just to make me angry."
   c. "I wish my husband could help more with the baby."
   d. "Babies are a blessing, but they are a lot of work."
2. Which problem is observed in children who regularly witness acts of violence in their family? *Select all that apply.*
   a. Phobias
   b. Low self-esteem
   c. Major depressive disorder
   d. Narcissistic personality disorder
   e. Posttraumatic stress disorder
3. What situation associated with a caregiver presents the greatest risk that an older adult will experience abuse by that caregiver?
   a. The caregiver is a single male relative.
   b. The caregiver was neglected as a child.
   c. The caregiver is under the age of 30.
   d. The caregiver has little experience with older adults.
4. What safety-related responsibility does the nurse have in any situation of suspected abuse?
   a. Protect the patient from future abuse by the abuser.
   b. Inform the suspected abuser that the authorities have been notified.
   c. Arrange for counseling for all involved parties, but especially the patient.
   d. Report suspected abuse to the proper authorities.
5. The nurse is assisting a patient to identify safety issues that may occur now that she has left an abusive partner. What telephone numbers should be available to the patient? *Select all that apply.*
   a. The police department
   b. An abuse hotline
   c. A responsible friend or family member
   d. A domestic violence shelter
   e. The hospital emergency department
6. Secondary effects of abuse often manifest as arrested development in children due to the fact that:
   a. Coping is easier than emotional growth
   b. Energy for development is diverted to coping
   c. Children cannot differentiate love from abuse
   d. Abuse fosters a sense of belonging, even if dysfunctional
7. The use of a patient-centered interview technique works well for gathering information about abusive situations. It is a good use of clinical time to sit near the patient and:
   a. Establish trust and rapport
   b. Ask lots of questions
   c. Interrupt the patients' story to allow for decompression
   d. Utilize closed-ended questions
8. The abused person is often in a dependent position, relying on the abuser for basic needs. At particular risk are children and older adults due to:
   a. The love they have for parents or children.
   b. Their limited options.
   c. The need to feel safe at home.
   d. Other relatives do not want them.
9. An appropriate expected outcome in individual therapy regarding the perpetrator of abuse would be:
   a. A decrease in family interaction so there are fewer opportunities for abuse to occur.
   b. The perpetrator will recognize destructive patterns of behavior and learn alternate responses.
   c. The perpetrator will no longer live with the family but have supervised contact while undergoing intensive inpatient therapy.
   d. A triad of treatment modalities, including medication, counseling, and role-playing opportunities.
10. Perpetrators of domestic violence tend to: *Select all that apply.*
   a. Have relatively poor social skills and have grown up with poor role models.
   b. Believe they, if male, should be dominant and in charge in relationships.
   c. Force their mates to work and expect them to handle the financial decisions.
   d. Be controlling and willing to use force to maintain their power in relationships.
   e. Prevent their mates from having relationships and activities outside the family.

1. **b**; 2. **a, b, c, e**; 3. **b**; 4. **d**; 5. **a, b, c, d**; 6. **b**; 7. **a**; 8. **b**; 9. **b**; 10. **a, b, d, e**

Visit the Evolve website for a posttest on the content in this chapter: http://evolve.elsevier.com/Varcarolis

REFERENCES

Administration for Children and Families. (2020). *Child maltreatment 2018.* Retrieved from https://www.acf.hhs.gov/cb/resource/child-maltreatment-2018.

American Psychological Association. (2014). *Child sexual abuse: What parents should know.* Retrieved from http://www.apa.org/pi/families/resources/child-sexual-abuse.aspx.

Centers for Disease Control and Prevention. (2017). *Elder abuse prevention.* Retrieved from https://www.cdc.gov/features/elderabuse/index.htmlphysical.

Centers for Disease Control and Prevention. (2019). *Preventing intimate partner violence.* Retrieved from https://www.cdc.gov/violenceprevention/intimatepartnerviolence/fastfact.html.

Clay, R. A. (2014). *Suicide and intimate partner violence.* Retrieved from http://www.apa.org/monitor/2014/11/suicide-violence.aspx.

Farley, D. (2017). *Victim of suspected elderly abuse dies.* Retrieved from http://www.semissourian.com/story/2373464.html.

Finkelhor, D., Shattuck, A., Turner, H. A., & Hamby, S. L. (2014). The lifetime prevalence of child sexual abuse and sexual assault assessed in late adolescence. *Journal of Adolescent Health, 55*(3), 329–333.

International Council of Nurses. (2019). *ICNP browser*. Retrieved from https://www.icn.ch/what-we-do/projects/ehealth-icnptm/icnp-browser.

Shea, J. (2020). Man whose mother was abused by aides pushes for state law to allow cameras in all nursing homes. *Fox8*. Retrieved from https://fox8.com/news/man-whose-mother-was-abused-by-aides-pushes-for-state-law-to-allow-cameras-in-all-nursing-homes/.

Soeken, K., McFarlane, J., Parker, B., & Lominack, M. (1998). The abuse assessment screen: A clinical instrument to measure frequency, severity and perpetrator of abuse against women. In J. Campbell (Ed.), *Empowering survivors of abuse: Health care for battered women and their children* (pp. 575–579). New Brunswick, NJ: Transaction.

Stephenson, R., Rentsch, C., Salazar, L., & Sullivan, P. (2011). Dyadic characteristics and intimate partner violence among men who have had sex with men. *Western Journal of Emergency Medicine*, *12*(3), 324–332.

Sullivan, S. P. (2016, December 22). *Elder abuse caught on video*. Retrieved from http://www.nj.com/news/index.ssf/2016/12/elder_abuse_caught_on_video_ag_announces_free_home.html.

Taub, A. (2020, April 6). A new Covid-19 crisis: Domestic abuse rises worldwide. *New York Times*. Retrieved from https://www.nytimes.com/2020/04/06/world/coronavirus-domestic-violence.html.

Walker, L. E. (1979). *The battered woman* (2nd ed.). New York, NY: Springer.

29

Sexual Assault

Margaret Jordan Halter and Jodie Flynn

Visit the Evolve website for a pretest on the content in this chapter: http://evolve.elsevier.com/Varcarolis

OBJECTIVES

1. Define sexual assault, sexual violence, rape, attempted rape, and completed rape.
2. Identify potential relationships between sexual offenders and victims, including marital rape, statutory rape, date rape, and drug-facilitated sexual assault.
3. Discuss the epidemiology of rape, stalking, and sexual assault.
4. Describe the role of the sexual assault nurse examiner to a colleague.
5. Describe common reactions to rape and sexual assault.
6. Identify five areas to assess when you are working with a person who has been sexually assaulted.

7. Analyze your personal thoughts and feelings regarding rape and its impact on survivors.
8. Identify priority nursing diagnoses to address responses to sexual assault.
9. Formulate two long-term outcomes and two short-term goals for the nursing diagnosis rape-trauma.
10. Identify five overall guidelines for nursing interventions related to sexual assault in emergency settings.
11. Discuss three evaluation criteria that would indicate improvement of responses or resolution for a person who has suffered a sexual assault.
12. Identify psychological therapies that are useful in treating individuals who have experienced sexual assault.

KEY TERMS AND CONCEPTS

date (or acquaintance) rape
attempted rape
completed rape
drug facilitated sexual assault
rape-trauma

rape-trauma response
revictimization
sexual assault nurse examiner (SANE)
sexual assault
sexual violence

spousal (marital) rape
survivor
statutory rape
victim

In 2008, Elisabeth Fritzl, a 42-year-old Austrian woman, reported to police that she had been imprisoned in the soundproofed, windowless cellar of her family home since the age of 18. Her own father, Josef Fritzl, lured her there, locked her in, and raped her repeatedly for the next 24 years. This abuse resulted in seven children, one of whom died shortly after birth. Three of the surviving children were taken upstairs to be raised by Fritzl and his wife. He explained to his wife that their daughter, Elisabeth, had run away to join a cult and had left the children on the doorstep. The other three children remained in the cellar with their mother, never seeing the light of day. They were forced to witness the continual rape of their mother by their father/grandfather.

When the moldy, dark conditions caused the eldest daughter, Kersten, 19, to become gravely ill, Elisabeth begged Fritzl to get her treatment. Fritzl relented and took her to a hospital where Elisabeth would later be taken to visit. It was there that Elisabeth revealed the nature of her daughter's illness and her own abuse on the condition that she would never have to see her father

again. Elisabeth was reunited with all of her children. Fritzl was sentenced to life in prison for the criminally insane.

SEXUAL ASSAULT AND SEXUAL VIOLENCE

This story is horrific and demonstrates some of the most contemptible violations that can be perpetrated by one human being on another. This chapter further explores these types of violations, which often go unreported. Sexual assault and sexual violence are broad terms that encompass unwanted sexual advances and sexual harassment to rape. Some definitions of sexual assault do not include rape, treating rape specifically as its own category. Incest, human sex trafficking, and female genital mutilation are other examples of sexual assault.

Although sexual assault generally involves adult males assaulting adult females, it includes any combination of females, males, adults, and children. Vulnerable individuals, such as the disabled and older adults, are often targeted. Sexual violence also includes denying emergency contraception or measures to prevent sexually transmitted infections and organized rape during conflict or war. Sexual homicide is a particularly chilling form of sexual assault. Also known as erotophonophilia, sexual homicide is sexual activity performed before, during, or after the commission of a murder.

Rape

According to the Federal Bureau of Investigation (FBI) (2019a), rape is the third most common violent crime in the United States after aggravated assault and robbery (Fig. 29.1). Victims are traumatized, both physically and emotionally, and are often seen in healthcare settings. Nurses are instrumental in providing holistic care for those who have been sexually assaulted and also in helping to preserve evidence. Preservation of evidence can lead to the prosecution of a crime or the exoneration of an innocent person of interest. Therefore, it is essential that nurses be adequately informed about their roles and responsibilities with regard to providing both medical and legal care.

Rape is classified into two categories: attempted rape and completed rape.

Attempted Rape

Threats of rape or intention to rape that is unsuccessful are referred to an **attempted rape**. Examples of rape attempts include the following:

- A man attacked a woman on the street, knocked her down, and attempted to rape her. A pedestrian frightened the man away before he could complete the attack.
- At a local bar, a man slipped gamma-hydroxybutyric acid (GHB), a drug sometimes used to facilitate sexual assault, into his date's drink. Her friends would not allow her to leave

with him. After an investigation, detectives concluded that the man intended to rape the woman.

Completed Rape

Completed rape is defined as "penetration, no matter how slight, of the vagina or anus with any body part or object, or oral penetration by a sex organ of another person, without the consent of the victim" (FBI, 2019b). This revised definition is expected to lead to more uniform statistical reporting of rape. It replaces a decades-old definition that did not account for crimes against men, threats of violence, and all rapes in which the victim is a child and unable to consent. The term *forcible rape* was removed because the term rape clearly implies force. Examples of completed rape include the following:

- A female high school student was drinking with a male classmate at her house. The male gave her a pill that he said would make her feel "really good." Later, the woman could not recall what happened after she took the pill. A rape kit indicated semen from sexual penetration.
- A man working in a residential facility led a woman with a severe mental disability to the woods behind the facility. There, he fondled her and sexually penetrated her. Because of the woman's disability, she was unable to understand and consent to the sexual act.
- One night a woman's husband, who was very drunk, accused her of sleeping around. He became enraged, pushed her onto the bed, and penetrated her with an object. She was too afraid to fight back.

Sexual Offenders and Relationships With Victims

Although we often think of a stranger lurking in the shadows of a parking lot as the typical sexual offender, this is not true. **Spousal (marital) rape** is penetration of one's partner, spouse, or significant other without consent. Historically, sexual intercourse was considered a marital right. Owing in large part to the feminist movement, marital rape was outlawed in 50 states by the early 1990s. It took longer for laws to be enacted that allowed perpetrators of marital rape to be sentenced in the same way. One US state still requires that violence or the threat of violence must have existed in order for the act to be considered a case of rape.

Statutory rape is a legally recognized category in the United States. This type of rape assumes that minors do not have the capacity to consent to sexual activity even if they agree to it or initiate it. In most states, the age of consent is between 16 and 18 years.

Date rape and **acquaintance rape** are terms that refer to nondomestic relationships where the perpetrator is known to the victim. Date rape and acquaintance rape are common, with as many as one in four college women reporting such an occurrence.

Drug-facilitated sexual assault involves drug or alcohol intoxication resulting in the inability to give consent. Victims lose the ability to fight off attackers, develop amnesia, and become unreliable witnesses. Most perpetrators are known to their victims. This type of crime typically involves female victims, although male-to-male assaults also occur.

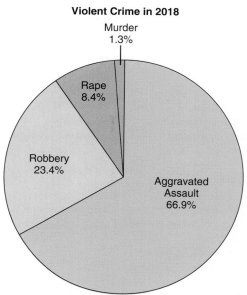

Violent Crime in 2018

Murder 1.3%
Rape 8.4%
Robbery 23.4%
Aggravated Assault 66.9%

Fig. 29.1 Violent crime in 2018. (From Federal Bureau of Investigation. [2019]. 2018 crime statistics released. Retrieved from https://www.fbi.gov/news/stories/2018-crime-statistics-released-093019.)

The increase in the prevalence and incidence of drug-assisted rape led to the passage of the Drug-Induced Rape Prevention and Punishment Act in 1996. This law allows up to 20 years' imprisonment and fines for anyone who intends to commit a violent crime by administering a controlled substance to an unknowing individual (US Department of Justice, 1997). Table 29.1 provides information about date-rape drugs.

Laws and Sexual Assault

Because state laws vary with regard to sexual assault, it is important to identify how sexual acts are medically and legally defined within your community. Based on your jurisdiction and legal mandates, healthcare providers may be required to report a sexual assault to law enforcement. All states require mandatory reporting if the victim is a child as defined by state law. Most states require reporting if the victim is a dependent adult, again, as defined by state law. Identification may be withheld if the individual wishes to remain anonymous. Evidence can be stored until the individual decides whether or not to report the assault.

Regardless of whether individuals report the sexual assault to police, states and tribal governments are required to pay or reimburse for sexual assault examinations. This requirement came about with the enactment of the Violence Against Women Act (VAWA) of 1994. Failure to comply with this reimbursement mandate results in loss of funding from the VAWA grant initiatives. This mandate is person-centered and gives control back to those individuals who should be the primary decision makers in personal health and legal matters.

In this chapter, individuals who have been sexually assaulted are referred to using the female pronoun because far more women experience this crime. However, the principles discussed apply to any gender. Terms used to refer to this population vary. People who have been sexually assaulted are referred to as **survivors** by advocacy groups and as **victims** by the legal system. In this chapter, individuals are often referred to as *patients* because they are being cared for in healthcare settings.

EPIDEMIOLOGY

Rape

In the United States, an estimated 19.3% of females and 1.7% of males have been raped at some time in their lives (Breiding et al., 2014). The 12-month prevalence is estimated at 1.6% in females. For females, the first rape experience occurs before age 25 years in nearly 79% of cases and before age 18 years in about 40%. Both males and females are more likely to be raped by a male. The lifetime and 12-month prevalence of intimate partner rape is estimated at nearly 9% and around 1%, respectively.

Almost half of female victims have been raped by an acquaintance. Intimate partners accounted for about 45% of female victims (Breiding et al., 2014). Nearly 60% of females who experience alcohol/drug facilitated penetration were victims of acquaintances. About 45% of male victims were raped by an acquaintance, and intimate partners raped 29% of male victims.

TABLE 29.1	**Drugs Associated With Date Rape**		
Drug, Alternate Names, and Status in the United States	**Form, Mechanism of Action, and Onset**	**Effect on Victim**	**Overdose Symptoms and Treatment**
GHB (gamma-hydroxybutyric acid) Also known as *G, Georgia home boy, liquid ecstasy, salty water, scoop, and many* others. Legal in the United States for narcolepsy Schedule III; central nervous system depressant. Often made in home labs.	Liquid, white powder, or pill with a salty taste; newer pills are oval and green-gray in color. A dye in these commercial pills makes clear liquids turn bright blue and dark drinks turn cloudy. A metabolite of gamma-aminobutyric acid. Onset is within 5–20 min; duration is dose related and ranges from 1–12 h.	Produces relaxation, euphoria, and disinhibition. Incoordination, confusion, deep sedation, and amnesia. Tolerance and dependence exhibited by agitation, tachycardia, insomnia, anxiety, tremors, and sweating.	Respiratory depression, seizures, nausea, vomiting, bradycardia, hypothermia, agitation, delirium, unconsciousness, and coma. Intubation for severe respiratory distress; atropine for bradycardia, and benzodiazepines for seizure activity. Vomiting should be induced when possible.
Rohypnol (flunitrazepam)[a] Also known as *forget-me pill, roofies, club drug, roachies, R2, and rophies.* Schedule IV potent benzodiazepine. Not legal in the United States.	Pill that dissolves in liquids. Ten times stronger than diazepam. Onset is within 10–30 min and lasts 2–12 h.	More potent when combined with alcohol; causes sedation, psychomotor slowing, muscle relaxation, and amnesia. Dependence and tolerance may develop.	Overdose unlikely. Airway protection and gastrointestinal decontamination.
Ketamine Also known as *black hole, bump, K, kit kat, purple, and Special K.* Legal in the United States for anesthesia, mainly in animals.	Comes as a liquid or a white powder. An anesthetic frequently used in veterinary practice; also a hallucinogenic substance related to phencyclidine (PCP). Onset is within 30 s intravenously and 20 min orally; duration is only 30–60 min; amnesia effects may last longer.	Causes dissociative reaction, with a dreamlike state leading to deep amnesia and analgesia and complete compliance of the victim. Victim may become confused, paranoid, delirious, and/or combative, with drooling and hallucinations.	Airway maintenance and use of anticholinergics such as atropine and benzodiazepines.

[a]Two other benzodiazepines, clonazepam (Klonopin) and alprazolam (Xanax), are also used.
Data from Office of Women's Health. (2012). *Date rape drugs fact sheet.* Retrieved from http://womenshealth.gov/publications/our-publications/fact-sheet/date-rape-drugs.html.

A male who is raped is more likely to experience physical trauma and to have been victimized by several assailants. Reports of male-to-male rape occur primarily in locked institutions, such as prisons and maximum security hospitals. Males experience the same devastation, physical injury, and emotional consequences as females. Although they may cover their responses, they too benefit from care and treatment.

Race and ethnicity are associated with rape. Females who identify as multiracial are the most likely to be raped, followed by American Indian/Alaskan Native and black non-Hispanic females.

Stalking

About 15% of females and nearly 6% of males have been victims of stalking at some point in their lives (Breiding et al., 2014). The 12-month prevalence of stalking is about 4% of females and 2% of males. Most female victims (about 54%) and nearly half of male victims (nearly 50%) were first stalked before 25 years of age.

Sexual Assault

All types of unwanted sexual behavior are referred to sexual assault. Precise estimates of sexual assault cannot be determined because this crime is greatly underreported, particularly less violent assaults such as grabbing, fondling, and verbal threats.

Table 29.2 summarizes the lifetime prevalence of rape, stalking, and sexual assault.

Specialized Sexual Assault Services

Facilities may have trained sexual assault nurse examiners (SANEs) or other specially trained clinicians to provide care to patients who have been sexually assaulted. A SANE is a registered nurse who has specialized training in caring for sexual assault patients, has demonstrated competency in conducting medical and legal evaluations, and has the ability to be an expert witness in court.

The SANE uses the nursing process with a patient-centered approach during the examination process. A SANE is a member of the Sexual Assault Response Team (SART), a multidisciplinary team approach to caring for victims of sexual assault. Members include nurses, physicians, attorneys, social service workers, advocates, mental health professionals, forensic laboratory personnel, and other collaborative agencies that provide services for sexual assault patients. If a SANE or specially trained clinician is not available in your facility, nurses should be prepared to provide both the medical and legal aspects of care.

CLINICAL PICTURE

Just as there is no typical patient presentation after a sexual assault, emotional responses will vary from person to person. However, many survivors experience criteria for the diagnoses of acute stress disorder and posttraumatic stress disorder (PTSD) following this type of crime. Chapter 16 provides a complete description of these disorders.

Most people who are raped suffer severe and long-lasting emotional trauma. Long-term effects of sexual assault may include major depressive disorder, anxiety, fear, and even suicide. Other consequences of this horrific offense include difficulties with daily functioning, low self-esteem, sexual dysfunction, and somatic (physical) complaints. Individuals may experience recurrent and intrusive memories, dreams, flashbacks, and psychological or physiological distress in response to cues that remind the individual of the assault. Dissociative symptoms may alter the sense of reality and result in the inability to remember (amnesia) parts of the traumatic event. Avoidance of situations, places, events, or objects that remind them of the experience is common. Hyperalertness, being easily startled, anxiety, and angry outbursts accompany the emotional dysregulation from the traumatic event.

Some people experience depersonalization, or feeling detached from their mental process or their bodies. This depersonalization feels like living in a dream. Derealization is a similar concept associated with trauma. This is characterized by feeling like the world is dreamlike, distant, or distorted.

Victims of incest may experience a negative self-image, depression, eating disorders, personality disorders, self-destructive behavior, and substance misuse. A history of sexual abuse in psychiatric patients is associated with a characteristic pattern of symptoms that may include depression, anxiety disorders, substance use disorders, suicide attempts, self-mutilation, compulsive sexual behavior, and psychosis-like symptoms.

TABLE 29.2　Lifetime Prevalence of Rape, Stalking, and Sexual Assault by Sex and Race/Ethnicity of Victim

	RAPE		STALKING		SEXUAL ASSAULT[a]	
	Females	Males	Females	Males	Females	Males
All races, non-Hispanic, Hispanic	19.3	1.7	15.2	5.7	—	—
White, non-Hispanic	20.5	1.6	15.9	4.7	46.9	22.2
Black, non-Hispanic	21.2	—	13.9	9.1	38.2	24.4
Hispanic	13.6	—	14.2	8.2	35.6	26.6
American Indian/Alaskan Native	27.5	—	24.5	—	55.0	24.5
Asian or Pacific Islander	—	—	—	—	31.9	15.8
Multiracial	32.3	—	22.4	9.3	64.1	39.5

[a]Includes being made to penetrate a perpetrator, sexual coercion, unwanted sexual contact, and noncontact unwanted sexual experiences.
Data from Breiding, M. J., Smith, S. G., Basile, K. C., Walters, M. L., Chen, J., & Merrick, M. T. (2014). Prevalence and characteristics of sexual violence, stalking, and intimate partner violence victimization: National Intimate Partner and Sexual Violence Survey, United States, 2011. *Morbidity and Mortality Weekly Report*. Retrieved from https://www.cdc.gov/mmwr/preview/mmwrhtml/ss6308a1.htm.

APPLICATION OF THE NURSING PROCESS

ASSESSMENT

General Assessment

Initial evaluations may be extremely stressful to already traumatized individuals A police interview, repeated questioning by health professionals, and the physical examination itself may add to the trauma of the patient. Advocacy in the form of a careful patient-centered assessment on the part of the nurse supports the patient during this process. The nurse should talk with the patient, the family, or friends who accompany the patient to gather as much objective data as possible for assessing the crisis. The nurse then assesses the patient's (1) level of anxiety, (2) coping mechanisms, (3) available support systems, (4) signs and symptoms of emotional trauma, and (5) signs and symptoms of physical trauma. Information obtained from the assessment is then analyzed, and nursing diagnoses are formulated.

Level of Anxiety

Patients experiencing severe-to-panic levels of anxiety will not be able to solve problems or process information. Support, reassurance, and appropriate therapeutic techniques can lower the patient's anxiety and facilitate mutual goal setting and the assimilation of information. Refer to Chapters 10 and 15 for more detailed discussions of the levels of anxiety and therapeutic interventions.

Coping Mechanisms

The same coping skills that have helped the survivor through other difficult problems in her life will be useful in adjusting to the rape. In addition, new ways of getting through the difficult times may be developed for both the short- and long-term adjustment. Behavioral responses include crying, withdrawing, smoking, using alcohol and drugs, talking about the event, becoming extremely agitated, confused, disoriented, incoherent, and even laughing or joking.

Cognitive coping mechanisms are the thoughts people have that help them deal with high anxiety levels. A positive cognitive response might be "At least I am alive and will get to see my children again." Not-so-positive responses may become generalized as a way to sum up the situation: "It's my fault this happened; my mother warned me about working in such a trashy place" may develop into an ego-damaging refrain. If such thoughts are verbalized, the nurse will know what the patient is thinking. If not, the nurse can ask questions such as "What are you thinking and feeling?" "What can I do to help you in this difficult situation?" or "What has helped in the past?"

Available Support Systems

The availability, size, and usefulness of a patient's social support system should be assessed. Often, partners or family members do not understand the survivor's feelings about the sexual assault, and they may not be the best supports available. Pay careful attention to verbal and nonverbal cues from the patient that may communicate the strength of her social network.

Involve the patient, family, or friends accompanying the patient or other healthcare providers in collaborative holistic data collection. Obtaining information from others is particularly important if the patient is unable to provide details surrounding the sexual assault (i.e., the patient is unconscious, nonverbal, or has a disability). If interpreter services are needed, a certified medical interpreter should be contacted.

VIGNETTE: Celia, a home care provider, brings Ms. Smith, a 64-year-old woman with a history of schizophrenia, to the emergency department. Celia tells the triage nurse that Ms. Smith, who is also a paraplegic, has been reclusive for the past few days and behaving strangely. According to Celia, Ms. Smith does not eat, sleeps all day, and repeatedly says that she is pregnant.

The triage nurse asks Ms. Smith, "Can you tell me why you are here?" She begins to sob, stares at the floor, rocks back and forth in her wheelchair, and mutters, "Someone is hurting me, and I am pregnant." A physical assessment reveals bruises on her upper thighs and breasts. The triage nurse has been trained as a sexual assault nurse examiner and immediately recognizes that Ms. Smith needs a sexual assault evaluation. She states, "I believe you, and I will help you. You are safe here." Ms. Smith responds quietly, "Thank you."

Signs and Symptoms of Emotional Trauma

The first challenge for any healthcare provider is to identify if the patient is a forensic patient. A forensic patient is anyone who seeks treatment and also needs to interact with the legal system or has the potential to interact with the legal system. Patients may disclose a history of sexual assault or report a history that is inconsistent with physical findings. Others may demonstrate a behavioral change that causes a concern for family, friends, caregivers, or other healthcare providers. Patients may seek help at a healthcare facility after a sexual assault occurs, visit their primary care provider, or contact law enforcement.

A nursing history should be obtained and carefully recorded. When you are taking a history, you should determine only the details of the assault that will be helpful in addressing the patient's immediate physical and psychological needs. You allow the patient to talk at a comfortable pace and pose questions in nonjudgmental descriptive terms. Always avoid asking "why" questions, because they are inherently evaluative. For example, "Why did you walk home alone?" or "Why didn't you run?"

Suicidal ideation may be present and should be assessed. Ask direct questions such as, "Are you thinking of harming yourself?" or "Have you ever tried to kill yourself before or after this attack occurred?" If the answer is yes, the nurse conducts a thorough suicide assessment (i.e., plan, means to carry it out), as described in Chapter 25.

Signs and Symptoms of Physical Trauma

It is essential that nurses provide psychological support while collecting and preserving legal evidence. The nurse should be aware of the patient's reactions during the physical examination and advise her to report any signs of pain or discomfort immediately.

During the examination, the nurse will inspect and palpate for any signs of injury. Recent injuries may not show visible bruising. Palpating the skin and finding tender spots can improve evidence collection and further the documentation of an injured site. Physical signs of injury after sexual assault can include injuries to the face, head, neck, extremities, and anogenital areas. Physical injuries should be carefully documented (i.e., size, color, description, and location of injury), both in narrative and pictorial form, using preprinted body maps, hand-drawn copies, or photographs. If an injury is present, ask the patient if she knows how that injury occurred. It is important to recognize that many reported cases of sexual assault do not include physical signs of injury.

The nurse will collect and preserve legal evidence such as blood; hair samples; oral swabs; nail swabs or scrapings; and anal, genital, or penile swabs. Facilities may have standardized sexual assault evidence collection kits that provide direction on how to collect and preserve evidence. This can be helpful to nurses and other clinicians who do not have specialized training in evidence collection and preservation.

The nurse takes a gynecological history, including the date of the last menstrual period and the likelihood of current pregnancy, and assesses for a history of sexually transmitted infections. A detailed genital examination, with a speculum, is needed to observe for signs of injury for the female patient. If the patient has never undergone a genital examination, the steps of the examination will have to be explained. The nurse plays a crucial role in reducing **revictimization**, which refers to the trauma of the examination itself, because the patient may experience it as another violation of her body. Recognizing this, the nurse can explain the examination procedure in a way that will be reassuring and supportive.

Best Practice Guidelines

The examination involves the following five steps:
1. Head-to-toe physical assessment, observing for signs of injury
2. Detailed genital examination, observing for signs of injury
3. Evidence collection and preservation
4. Documentation of physical findings (both written and photographic)
5. Treatment, discharge planning, and follow-up care

The patient has the right to decline parts of the legal or medical examination. Informed consent must be provided and consent forms signed before taking photographs, doing a physical examination, and proceeding with any other procedures that might be needed to collect evidence and provide treatment. A shower and change of clothing should be made available to the patient as soon as possible after the examination and collection of evidence.

According to guidelines from the Centers for Disease Control and Prevention (CDC, 2015), providing prophylactic treatment for sexually transmitted diseases is common practice. Sexually transmitted diseases, including HIV and hepatitis exposure, are often a concern of patients who are sexually assaulted. This worry should always be addressed and the patient given the information needed to evaluate the likelihood of risk and need for follow-up care. With this information, the patient and her sexual partner or partners can make educated choices about testing and safer sex practices until further testing can be done and results communicated.

Almost 3 million females in the United States have experienced a rape-related pregnancy (CDC, 2020). Those who are raped by a former or current intimate partner are more likely to become pregnant than those who are raped by an acquaintance or stranger. This may be due to reproductive coercion on the part of the intimate partner who wants the victim to become pregnant.

Pregnancy prevention is offered in the emergency department once pregnancy tests establish that the patient was not already pregnant before the assault. Emergency contraception or morning-after pills are contraceptives that do not cause abortion. They act on follicular development and inhibit ovulation. If no egg is available to the sperm, then pregnancy cannot occur.

Assessment data are carefully documented, including verbatim statements by the patient, detailed observations of emotional and physical status, and results of the physical examination. Laboratory tests are noted and findings recorded as soon as they are available.

Self-Assessment

Nurses' attitudes influence the physical and psychological care received by rape survivors. Knowing the myths and facts surrounding sexual assault can increase your awareness of your personal beliefs and feelings regarding rape. If you examine your personal feelings and reactions *before* encountering a patient who has been sexually assaulted, you will be better prepared to give empathetic and effective care. Examining your feelings about abortion is also important because a patient might choose an abortion if a pregnancy results from rape. Table 29.3 compares rape myths and facts.

NURSING DIAGNOSIS

Addressing the broad category of sexual offenses is accomplished by using *victim of sexual assault* as a priority diagnosis. The nursing diagnosis that focuses on the immediate consequences of rape is **rape-trauma** (International Council of Nurses [ICN], 2019). This diagnosis is defined as the "physical and psychological condition after forced participation in sexual relations or intercourse." Another diagnosis, **rape-trauma response**, addresses longer-term reactions. It is defined as a "maladaptive response that occurs to the victim after a rape associated with disorganizing lifestyle and long-term process of reorganization of lifestyle" (ICN, 2019). Defining characteristics of rape-trauma response are listed in Box 29.1.

A variety of diagnoses would also apply to the victim of sexual assault. They include, but are not limited to, the following:
- Disturbed personal identity
- Situational low self-esteem
- Interrupted family process
- Impaired sexual functioning
- Anxiety
- Fear
- Social isolation

TABLE 29.3 Myth Versus Fact: Rape

Myth	Fact
Many women really want to be raped.	Women do not ask to be raped—no matter how they are dressed, what their behavior is, or where they are at any given time. Studies show that depictions of violence toward women in the media lead to attitudes that foster tolerance of rape.
Most rapes occur for the purpose of sex.	Sex is used as an instrument of violence in rape. Rape is an act of aggression, anger, or power.
In most cases, it is strangers who rape women.	The majority (69%) of rape victims are raped by someone they know.
An unarmed man cannot rape a healthy adult woman who resists.	Most men can overpower most women because of differences in body build. Also, the victim may panic, which makes her actions less effective than usual.
Most charges of rape are unfounded.	There is no evidence to show that there are more false reports for rape than for other crimes. Most rape victims do not even report the rape.
Rapes usually occur in dark alleys.	Over 50% of all rapes occur in the home.
Rape is usually an impulsive act.	Most rapes are planned; over 50% involve a weapon.
Nice girls don't get raped.	Any woman is a potential rape victim. Victims range in age from 6 months to 90 years.
There was not enough time for a rape to occur.	There is no minimal time limit that characterizes rape. It can happen very quickly.
Only females are raped.	There are a growing number of male rape victims.

BOX 29.1 Defining Characteristics of Rape-Trauma and Rape-Trauma Response

Shame	Mood swings	Anxiety	Dissociation
Guilt	Aggression	Fear	Disorganization
Helplessness	Anger	Disturbed sleep	Shock
Powerlessness	Agitation	Nightmares	Confusion
Dependence	Revenge	Sexual dysfunction	Phobias
Low self-esteem	Substance misuse	Muscle tension	Paranoia
Depression	Suicide attempts	Hyperalertness	

OUTCOMES IDENTIFICATION

Overall, the expected outcome for *victim of sexual assault, rape-trauma,* and *rape-trauma response* would be improved responses to the traumatic experience. Improvement that may be indicated prior to leaving acute care settings includes verbalizing details of the experience, expressing feelings, understanding the common responses to assault, identifying a short-term plan to deal with the immediate situation, and connecting with a community-based rape victims' advocate. Longer-term goals include physical healing, emotional healing of intrusive memories and nightmares, reduction in fear and anxiety, and improved social interactions.

PLANNING

Unless the patient has sustained serious physical or psychological injury, treatment is provided and the patient is released. Because the ramifications of rape are experienced for an extended time after the acute phase, the plan of care includes information for follow-up care. The patient needs information about available community supports and how to access them. Nurses may also encounter rape survivors in other settings when they are no longer in acute distress but still dealing with the aftermath of rape. Such settings include inpatient facilities, the community, and the home. A comprehensive plan of care addresses the continuing needs of the rape survivor in any setting.

IMPLEMENTATION

Timely intervention can reduce the aftermath of rape. The occurrence of rape can be the most devastating experience in a person's life and constitutes an acute situational (unexpected) crisis. Typical crisis reactions reflect cognitive, affective, and behavioral disruptions. For survivors to return to their previous level of functioning, it is necessary for them to fully mourn their losses, experience anger, and work through their fears. Box 29.2 provides a summary of care for sexual assault and rape victims in the emergency setting.

Counseling

The sexual assault patient may be too traumatized, ashamed, or afraid to go to the hospital. Cultural definitions of what constitutes rape may also affect the decision to seek treatment. For these reasons, 24-hour telephone and chat lines—such as the Rape, Abuse, and Incest National Network (RAINN)—provide direct communication with volunteers trained in rape crisis support. These types of support services focus on helping the person through the period of acute distress by assessing what has happened and determining what kind of assistance is needed. Counselors provide empathetic listening, the survivor is encouraged to go to the emergency department, and the main focus is on the immediate steps the person may take.

The most effective approach for counseling in the emergency department or crisis center is to provide nonjudgmental care and optimal emotional support. Conveying the confidential nature of the visit is crucial. Simply listening and letting the patient talk is a powerful intervention. A patient who feels listened to and understood is no longer alone and feels more in control of the situation.

It is especially important to help the survivor and significant others to separate issues of vulnerability from blame. Although the person may have made choices that made her more vulnerable, she is not to blame for the rape. She may, however, decide to avoid some of those choices in the future (e.g., walking alone late at night or excessive use of alcohol). Focusing on her behavior (which is controllable) allows the survivor to believe that similar experiences can be avoided in the future.

BOX 29.2 Care for Rape and Sexual Assault Victims

1. Sexual assault patients are provided a safe and private environment upon arrival in an emergency care setting, with access to a community-based advocate.
2. Emergency nurses use a trauma-informed approach throughout the sexual assault patient's complex plan of care.
3. Sexual assault patients receive consistent, objective, immediate medical care as well as options for the collection of evidence by emergency nurses and physicians who know the protocols for evidence collection.
4. Whenever possible, forensic nurses with specific training as SANEs are consulted or assigned to care for this patient population.
5. Sexual assault patients receive medically appropriate sexually transmitted disease prophylaxis and emergency contraception.

From the Emergency Nurses Association & International Association of Forensic Nurses. (2016). *Adult and adolescent sexual assault patients in the emergency care setting.* Retrieved from https://www.ena.org/docs/default-source/resource-library/practice-resources/position-statements/joint-statements/adultandadolescentsexualassaultpatientser.pdf?sfvrsn=234258f1_6.

VIGNETTE: Ms. Smith comes to see that it was not her fault that she was raped and feels comfortable that she is believed. Ms. Smith is now verbal and able to recall the events of the sexual assault to the healthcare providers and SANE before discharge.

With the patient's consent, the nurse involves her support system, which includes her family, friends, and group home providers. The nurse discusses with them the nature and trauma of sexual assault and possible delayed reactions that may occur. Ms. Smith expressed the aftermath of her assault, "It takes a few days to hit you. It was bad. It was really rough for my mom. I needed to be reassured. I needed to be told that there was nothing I could have done to prevent it. Understanding helps."

Social support is tremendously beneficial. The survivor who is able to confide comfortably in one or two friends or family members, especially immediately after the assault, is likely to experience fewer somatic manifestations of stress. In many cases, family and friends need support and reassurance as much as the survivor does. This is especially true for those from traditional cultures, particularly those cultures that believe that sexual assault brings shame to the entire family. The long-standing cultural myth that women are the property of men still prevents some people from empathizing with the woman's severe emotional wound and from being supportive. Instead, in these cases, the woman is devalued.

Promotion of Self-Care Activities

When you are preparing a patient for discharge, you should provide all referral information and printed follow-up instructions. Printed instructions include potential physical concerns and emotional reactions, legal matters, victim compensation (state financial assistance paid through perpetrators' fines and fees), and online resources (e.g., support groups) can help. This is important because the amount of verbal information the patient can retain likely will be limited due to her high levels of anxiety. Written material can be referred to repeatedly over time. Healthcare referrals are provided for continuity of care, and information regarding victim assistance programs can also be given.

Case Management

The emotional state and other psychological needs of the patient should be reassessed by telephone or personal contact within 24 to 48 hours of discharge from the hospital. Make sure you discuss this with the patient before discharge. Also, the most up-to-date contact information should be on file in the medical record. Referrals should be made for resources or support services. Effective crisis intervention and continuity of care require outreach activities and services beyond the emergency medical setting.

Survivors may avoid seeking treatment from psychiatric–mental healthcare providers owing to stigma. Therefore, the outpatient nurse should make a more focused assessment of stress-related symptoms and/or depression and ascertain the need for mental health referral. Reporting symptoms and seeking medical treatment are adaptive coping behaviors and can be reinforced.

Follow-up visits should occur at least 2, 4, and 6 weeks after the initial evaluation. At each visit, the patient should be assessed for psychological progress, the presence of sexually transmitted diseases, and pregnancy. Follow-up examinations provide an opportunity to (1) detect new infections acquired during or after the assault, (2) complete hepatitis B vaccination if indicated, (3) complete counseling and treatment for other STDs, and (4) monitor side effects and adherence to postexposure prophylactic medication if prescribed.

EVALUATION

We consider sexual assault survivors to be in recovery if they are relatively free of any signs or symptoms of acute stress disorder and PTSD. Signs of recovery include the following:

- Sleeping well with few instances of episodic nightmares or broken sleep
- Eating as they did before the rape
- Being calm and relaxed or only mildly suspicious, fearful, or restless
- Getting support from family and friends
- Generally positive self-regard
- The absence or only mild instances of somatic reactions
- Returning to prerape sexual functioning and interest

In general, the closer the survivor's lifestyle is to the pattern that was present before the rape, the more complete the recovery has been.

Nurses need to review hospital-based policy and procedure manuals to determine if protocols have been established in how to care for a sexual assault patient. If your facility does not have a policy, consider establishing one for your area.

The International Association of Forensic Nurses (IAFN, 2015) provides SANE Education Guidelines for the evaluation of adult/adolescent and pediatric patients. Certification is provided by the IAFN for nurse providers (i.e., SANE-A, SANE-P).

TREATMENT MODALITIES

Psychological Therapies

Psychiatric–mental health advanced practice registered nurses and other advanced practice professionals may provide individual or group psychotherapy. These therapies may be designed for survivors of sexual assault or perpetrators of sexual assault.

Survivors

Most of those who have been raped are eventually able to resume their previous lifestyle and level of functioning after supportive services and crisis counseling. However, many continue to experience emotional trauma, including flashbacks, nightmares, fear, phobias, and other symptoms associated with PTSD (refer to Chapter 16). Major depressive disorder

---

CASE STUDY AND NURSING CARE PLAN

Rape

Kayla is a 36-year-old single mother of two. One evening she and her friends go bowling. Kayla is tired and decides to go home before her friends leave their game. A man at the bowling alley offers to take her home. Not in the habit of going home alone with men she does not know, she hesitates. A friend whom she trusts encourages her to go with John and says "he's a good guy."

John drives Kayla home. He asks if he can use the bathroom before driving home. She hesitantly agrees. After using the bathroom, John approaches Kayla and forcibly kisses her. As she protests, John becomes more aggressive. She manages to get away from him briefly, but he catches her and begins to pummel her with his fists and to bite her. He says, angrily, "If you don't do what I say, I'll break your neck" and proceeds to rape her. A neighbor hears the commotion and calls the police. When the police arrive, John is gone and they take Kayla to the emergency department. The neighbor meets them there.

In the emergency department, Kayla is visibly shaken. She keeps saying over and over, "I shouldn't have let him take me home. I should have fought harder. I shouldn't have let him do this."

The nurse takes Kayla to a quiet room and then notifies the advanced practice registered nurse practitioner and the rape victim advocate. When the nurse comes back, she tells Kayla that she would like to talk to her before the doctor comes. Kayla glances at her neighbor and then stares at the floor. The nurse asks the neighbor to wait outside.

Kayla: "It was horrible. I feel so dirty."

Nurse: "You have had a traumatic experience."

Kayla: "I feel so ashamed. I never should have let that man take me home."

Nurse: "You think that if you hadn't gone home with a stranger, this wouldn't have happened?"

Kayla: "Yes ... I shouldn't have let him do it; I shouldn't have let him rape me."

Nurse: "You mentioned that he said he would break your neck if you didn't do as he said."

Kayla: "Yes, he said that ... he was going to kill me. It was awful."

Nurse: "It seems you did the right thing to stay alive."

As the nurse continues to talk with Kayla, her anxiety level seems to decrease. The nurse talks to Kayla about the kinds of symptoms rape victims often have after a rape and explains that the reactions she might have 2 or 3 weeks from now are normal.

The nurse says that the nurse practitioner will want to examine her and explains the procedure. Kayla signs a consent form. While Kayla is being prepared for her examination, the nurse notices bite marks and bruising on both breasts. She also notes Kayla's lower lip, which is cut and bleeding. The nurse keeps detailed notes of her observations and draws a body map depicting the injuries. After the examination, Kayla is given clean clothes and a place to shower.

Self-Assessment

The nurse has worked with rape survivors before and has helped develop the hospital's protocol for sexual assault victims. It took a while for her to be able to remain both neutral and responsive because of her own anger at this type of violence. She recalls a time when a woman came in stating that she was raped but was so calm, smiling, and polite that the nurse initially did not believe her story. She had not, at that point, examined her own feelings or dealt with the popular societal myths regarding rape. It was only later, when she had spoken with more experienced healthcare personnel, that she learned that crisis reactions could seem bizarre, confusing, and contradictory.

Assessment
Subjective Data
- "It was horrible. I feel so dirty."
- "I shouldn't have let him rape me."
- "He said that he was going to kill me."
- Guilt
- Self-blame

Objective Data
- Crying
- Staring at the floor
- Bruises and bite marks on breasts
- Lip cut and bleeding
- Rape reported to the police

Priority Nursing Diagnosis
Rape-trauma due to sexual assault.

Outcomes Identification
Patient will experience an improved rape-trauma response.

Planning
The nurse plans to provide emotional and physical support to Kayla while she receives care in the emergency setting and to make sure that Kayla is aware of the importance of follow-up care.

Implementation
Kayla's plan of care is personalized as follows:

CASE STUDY AND NURSING CARE PLAN—cont'd

Rape

Short-Term Goal	Intervention	Rationale	Evaluation
1. Patient will begin to express reactions and feelings about the assault before leaving the emergency department.	1a. Remain neutral and nonjudgmental and assure patient of confidentiality. 1b. Do not leave patient alone. 1c. Allow the patient negative expressions and behavioral self-blame while using reflective techniques. 1d. Assure patient she did the right thing to save her life. 1e. When the patient's anxiety level decreases to moderate, encourage problem solving. 1f. Teach common reactions experienced by people in the long-term reorganization phase (e.g., phobias, flashbacks, insomnia, increased motor activity).	1a. Lessens feelings of shame and guilt and encourages sharing of painful feelings. 1b. Deters feelings of isolation and escalation of anxiety. 1c. Fosters feelings of control. 1d. Decreases burden of guilt and shame. 1e. Increases survivor's feeling of control in her own life. (When in severe anxiety, a person cannot solve problems) 1f. Helps survivor to anticipate reactions and understand them as part of the recovery process.	**GOAL MET** Patient was able to share her feelings and express guilt. She realizes that she is not to blame. Anxiety was reduced to mild-moderate.
2. Patient will receive appropriate interventions to protect her physical status and support future legal proceedings.	2a. Explain rape protocol procedures and why they are being done. 2b. Provide as much privacy as possible during the examination. Have as few people as necessary present to provide care. 2c. Document physical injuries, collect evidence, and record verbatim statements by the patient. 2d. Provide prophylactic treatment for sexually transmitted diseases, assess for pregnancy, and offer pregnancy prevention.	2a. To decrease anticipatory anxiety and reduce revictimization. 2b. Posttrauma patients are extremely vulnerable. Additional people in the environment will increase anxiety. 2c. Careful documentation and data collection will support the patient in pursuing legal action. 2d. Sexually transmitted diseases and pregnancy are to be considered as possibilities after a rape.	**GOAL MET** Patient underwent a thorough physical examination, received prophylactic treatment to prevent sexually transmitted diseases and pregnancy, and will have the evidence she needs for legal proceedings.

Evaluation

Kayla is able to express her feelings in the emergency department and talk about the possible reactions she might experience as she moves through the reorganization phase. Her anxiety level is reduced to mild-moderate.

and suicidal ideation often follow a sexual assault. Some people who survive rape may be susceptible to a psychotic episode or an emotional disturbance so severe that hospitalization is required. Others whose emotional lives may be overburdened with multiple internal and external pressures may require individual psychotherapy.

Rape victims benefit from group therapy or support groups. Group therapy can make the difference between a person's coming out of the crisis at a lower level of functioning or gradually adapting to the experience with an increase in coping skills. Support groups are available locally or online. There are support groups specific to rape, acquaintance rape, date rape, and incest. Blogs may provide a useful outlook and a source of support.

Perpetrators

Psychotherapy is essential for perpetrators of sexual assault if behavioral change is to occur. Unfortunately, most perpetrators do not acknowledge the need for behavioral change, and no single method or program of treatment has been found to be totally effective. The nurse's awareness of personal feelings and reactions will be crucial to avoid interference with the therapeutic process.

KEY POINTS TO REMEMBER

- Sexual assault is a common and often underreported crime of violence.
- Females are far more likely to be victims of sexual assault and tend to know their perpetrators. Sexual assault of males tends to be underreported due to the humiliation and stigma attached to such victimization.
- Psychoactive substances play a major role in sexual assault, and alcohol is the most commonly used date-rape drug.

Other disinhibiting and amnestic substances play a role in forcible sex acts.
- A rape survivor experiences a wide range of feelings, which may or may not be exhibited to others.
- Sexual assault is often followed by feelings of fear, degradation, anger, and rage. Helplessness, anxiety, sleep disturbances, disturbed relationships, flashbacks, depression, and somatic complaints are also common.

- The initial medical evaluation may be frightening and stressful. A police interview, repeated questioning by health professionals, and the physical examination itself all have the potential to add to the trauma and revictimization of the sexual assault.
- Nurses can minimize repetition of questions and support the patient as she goes through the medical and legal evaluation.

- Survivors require long-term healthcare that can include counseling to minimize long-term effects of the rape and assisting in a return to a normal living pattern.
- Telephone and online resources are available to assist sexual assault and rape survivors.

CRITICAL THINKING

1. Jonah, 18 years of age, is brutally beaten and sexually assaulted by an unidentified male as he makes his way home from a party in an unfamiliar part of town. He is found semiconscious by a passerby and taken to the emergency department. Jonah has bite marks on his neck; extensive bruises around his head, chest, and buttocks; and has sustained a cracked rib and anal tears.

   Ms. Santinez, a nurse and rape counselor in the emergency department, works with Jonah using the hospital's sexual assault protocol and evidence collection kit. Jonah appears stunned and confused and has difficulty focusing on what the nurse says. He states repeatedly, "This is crazy, this can't be happening … I can't believe this has happened to me … Oh, my God, I can't believe this."

   a. What areas of Jonah's assessment should be given highest priority by Ms. Santinez and her staff while he is in the emergency department?

   b. Chart the signs and symptoms of Jonah's physical and emotional trauma and verbatim statements in as much detail as you can.

   c. Identify the short-term outcome criteria for Jonah that ideally would be met before he leaves the emergency department.

   d. What information does Jonah need to have regarding potential signs and symptoms that may occur in the near future? Why is this important for him to understand?

   e. Identify what Jonah's recovery might look like as a survivor of sexual assault. What resources are available to him?

   f. If Jonah does not wish to report the sexual assault to police, would you still complete the examination?

CHAPTER REVIEW

1. Which statement made by a sexually assaulted patient strongly suggests the drug gamma-hydroxybutyric acid (GHB) was involved in the attack?
   a. "I remember everything that happened but felt too tired to fight back."
   b. "The drink I was given had a salty taste to it."
   c. "They tell me I was unconscious for 24 hours."
   d. "I heard that I was fighting the nursing staff and saying that they were trying to kill me."

2. Considering the guilt that women feel after being sexually assaulted, which nursing assessment question has priority?
   a. "Do you want the police to be called?"
   b. "Did you recognize the person who assaulted you?"
   c. "Do you have someone you trust that can stay with you?"
   d. "Do you have any thoughts about harming yourself?"

3. Which statement is an accurate depiction of sexual assault?
   a. Rape is a sexual act.
   b. Most rapes occur in the home.
   c. Rape is usually an impulsive act.
   d. Women are usually raped by strangers.

4. Which signs and symptoms are associated with rape-trauma and rape-trauma response? *Select all that apply.*
   a. Outbursts of anger
   b. Major depressive disorder
   c. Auditory hallucinations

   d. Flashbacks
   e. Amnesia for the event

5. Which racial identification places a woman at the greatest risk of being sexually assaulted in her lifetime?
   a. Multiracial
   b. American Indian
   c. Black non-Hispanic
   d. White

6. The stress of being raped often results in suffering similar to people who have witnessed a murder or had a physiological reaction to trauma, resulting in which of the following?
   a. Posttraumatic stress disorder
   b. Anxiety
   c. Depression
   d. All of the above

7. A young woman named Carly was raped after closing shift behind the restaurant where she works. Six months have passed and Carly has not been able to return to work, refuses to go out to eat, and feels that she has less value as a woman now that she has been raped. Carly's clinical presentation suggests:
   a. Reexperiencing
   b. Hyperalertness
   c. Avoidance
   d. Physical effects

8. Ron is a victim of assault and has revealed to his family and friends the fact that he was raped. The family reacts with horror and disgust, and the nurse caring for Ron recognizes that
   a. Ron's family is being judgmental.
   b. Ron's family should leave the hospital.
   c. Ron's family will also need support.
   d. Ron's family's dynamics are dysfunctional.

9. Perpetrators of sexual assault are often incarcerated but frequently do not undergo therapy. Samuel, convicted of rape and sentenced to 15 years in prison, has asked to see a therapist. The psychiatric nurse practitioner is surprised to learn of the request, as many perpetrators
   a. Boast of their assault history.
   b. Feel regret and remorse.
   c. Do not acknowledge the need for change.
   d. Are unable to recognize rape as a crime.

10. You are working at a telephone hotline center when Abby, a rape victim, calls. Abby states she is afraid to go to the hospital. What is your best response?
    a. "I'm here to listen, and we can talk about your feelings."
    b. "You don't need to go to the hospital if you don't want to."
    c. "If you don't go to the hospital, we can't collect evidence to help convict your rapist."
    d. "Why are you afraid to seek medical attention?"

1. **b**; 2. **d**; 3. **b**; 4. **a, b, d, e**; 5. **a**; 6. **d**; 7. **c**; 8. **c**; 9. **c**; 10. **a**

Visit the Evolve website for a posttest on the content in this chapter: http://evolve.elsevier.com/Varcarolis

REFERENCES

Breiding, M. J., Smith, S. G., Basile, K. C., et al. (2014). Prevalence and characteristics of sexual violence, stalking, and intimate partner violence victimization: National Intimate Partner and Sexual Violence Survey, United States, 2011. *Morbidity and Mortality Weekly Report*. Retrieved from https://www.cdc.gov/mmwr/preview/mmwrhtml/ss6308a1.htm.

Centers for Disease Control and Prevention. (2015). *Sexually transmitted diseases treatment guidelines*. Retrieved from http://www.cdc.gov/std/tg2015/sexual-assault.htm.

Centers for Disease Control and Prevention. (2020). *Understanding pregnancies resulting from rape in the United States*. Retrieved from https://www.cdc.gov/violenceprevention/datasources/nisvs/understanding-RRP-inUS.html.

Drug-Induced Rape Prevention and Punishment Act, 21 U.S.C. § 841(b)(7). (1996).

Federal Bureau of Investigation (FBI). (2019a). *2018 crime statistics released*. Retrieved from https://www.fbi.gov/news/stories/2018-crime-statistics-released-093019.

Federal Bureau of Investigation (FBI). (2019b). *2018 crime in the United States*. Retrieved from https://ucr.fbi.gov/crime-in-the-u.s/2018/crime-in-the-u.s.-2018/topic-pages/rape.

International Association of Forensic Nurses. (2015). *Sexual assault nurse examiner (SANE) education guidelines*. Retrieved from http://c.ymcdn.com/sites/www.forensicnurses.org/resource/resmgr/2015_SANE_ED_GUIDELINES.pdf.

International Council of Nurses. (2019). *ICNP browser*. Retrieved from https://www.icn.ch/what-we-do/projects/ehealth-icnptm/icnp-browser.

US Department of Justice, Office of the Attorney General. (1997). *September 23 memorandum for all United States attorneys*. Retrieved from http://www.usdoj.gov/ag/readingroom/drugcrime.htm.

30

Dying, Death, and Grieving

Sandra S. Yaklin

 Visit the Evolve website for a pretest on the content in this chapter: http://evolve.elsevier.com/Varcarolis

OBJECTIVES

1. Describe the evolution of life-saving measures and their impact on end-of-life issues.
2. Discuss the role of palliative care and hospice in supporting patients and families facing chronic diseases and terminal illnesses.
3. Identify stages of the dying process as described by Kübler-Ross.
4. Discuss the following topics regarding death: artificial nutrition and hydration, euthanasia, and legally assisted suicide.
5. Describe the components of advance care planning for death.
6. Distinguish nursing care at the end of life, including communication, presence, and symptom management.
7. Discuss the process of death and associated care for the patient and the family.
8. Explain the distinction between grief, bereavement, and mourning.
9. Differentiate grieving, persistent complex bereavement disorder, and disenfranchised grief.
10. Describe nursing care for individuals who are grieving and are experiencing complicated grieving.

KEY TERMS AND CONCEPTS

advance directives
anticipatory grief
artificial nutrition and hydration
bereavement
disenfranchised grief

durable power of attorney for healthcare
euthanasia
grieving
hospice
legally assisted death

living will
mourning
palliative care
persistent complex bereavement disorder

"...even if I'm dying, until I actually die, I am still living."...
Kalanithi (2016)

Caring for another human as death approaches challenges and rewards nurses in profound and personal ways. Nurses support dignity in the dying process. Nurses can also facilitate enduring and positive memories for family members and caregivers. In this chapter, we will explore one of the most intimate of subjects that any of us will face: grief and end of life. We will begin by discussing the process of dying and death and then turn our attention to the grieving process.

DEATH AND DYING

In 1900, the primary cause of death in the United States was infectious diseases and the average adult only lived to the age of 47 (Centers for Disease Control and Prevention, 2006). Most of those diseases have been eradicated. Currently, chronic health problems such as heart disease, cancer, stroke, Alzheimer's disease, and kidney disease are the primary causes of death. Despite these chronic health problems, expectancy has soared to nearly 79 years (Murphy et al., 2018).

In the early 1900s, death commonly occurred at home and people who were dying were surrounded by family and community. Today, death tends to occur in hospitals and nursing homes, resulting in most people being unfamiliar with the act of dying and death.

We are accustomed to having tools such as surgery, medications, and diagnostic technologies to combat life-threatening conditions. Advances in technology have blurred the line between life and death. We can artificially feed those who cannot eat. We can breathe for those who cannot breathe. We can filter blood when kidneys fail. We can restart hearts, kill cancers, and transplant organs. Despite our skills and technology, we all still die.

In some ways, dying has become more complex precisely because there is so much we can do to sustain and prolong life. In fact, the medical model is based on the prolongation of life. When does one more surgery, one more round of chemotherapy, or seeing one more doctor end? These are profound issues for individuals facing the prospect of death and their families.

An Aging Population

The United States experienced an unprecedented birth rate in the 18 years after the end of World War II (1946–64). This generation became known as the baby boomers. The 79 million baby boomers account for a staggering 26% of the total US population. The number of individuals over the age of 65 will nearly double from 43.1 million in 2012 to 83.7 million by 2050. Every day for the next 19 years, 10,000 baby boomers will turn 65. By 2034, for the first time in history, the number of older adults will surpass the number of children: People age 65 and over are expected to number 77 million, while children under age 18 will number 76.5 million (Vespa, 2018) (Fig. 30.1).

This growing sector of the population will place unprecedented strains on a healthcare system where health spending is growing faster than the overall economy. In 2017, the United States spent almost twice as much on healthcare as other high-income countries (Papanicolas et al., 2018). For this reason, there are concerns regarding how the US healthcare system will pay for the burgeoning healthcare needs of the baby boomer generation.

Medicare is the federal government's national program that provides health insurance for older adults. Medicare is a fee-for-service system, which means that more medical services result in more reimbursement for healthcare providers. One frequently cited statistic is that the 5% of Medicare patients who die annually account for approximately 25% of all Medicare dollars spent (Riley & Lubitz, 2010). Thus, those concerned about the overall cost of healthcare spending have been concerned that futile and unnecessarily aggressive medical care at the end of life is the cause. Even trained professionals may find it difficult to distinguish between the certain-to-die and the likely-to-die. More recent analyses regarding the high cost of end-of-life care resulted in different conclusions. Healthcare expenditures in the last 3 years of life were attributable to the cost of chronic conditions and functional limitations rather than to the cost of aggressive end-of-life medical care (Einav et al., 2018; French et al., 2017).

> There is no good death. It always hurts, both the dying and the left behind. But there is a good enough death.
> Neuman (2017)

Models for End-of-Life Care
Hospice

In the 1960s, as people approached death, they were routinely shifted into hospital rooms with phrases like "We're sorry, there's nothing more we can do for you." Despite the care of health professionals and visits from helpless relatives, mortally ill people were often neglected, isolated, and left to die in pain. In 1967, Cicely Saunders established St. Christopher's Hospice in London to address this state of neglect (Stolberg, 1999). At

St. Christopher's, patients' physical comfort was aggressively pursued with around-the-clock pain medication that allowed these patients to experience a higher quality of life. Effective pain management enabled them to take care of legal and financial matters, engage in normal activities, such as shopping, say goodbyes, restore damaged relationships, and prepare spiritually for death. Hospice is now a standard model of care that supports and cares for patients who are facing death. This service is available to everyone, regardless of age, diagnosis, or the ability to pay. To qualify, a physician or advanced practice nurse certifies that life expectancy is 6 months or less. In addition, the patient must choose hospice care rather than curative treatments.

Hospice care begins after treatment of the disease or condition is stopped, when it is clear that survival is not possible. Hospice care involves a multidisciplinary team approach that focuses on patient care and symptom reduction rather than on cure. This approach meshes well with values in nursing. Physicians, nurses, chaplains, and social workers collaborate to navigate the questions, concerns, and decisions faced by those who are dying. Hospice care goes beyond caring for the patient to include caring for the family. Hospice services are delivered in the following places (National Hospice and Palliative Care Organization, 2019):

- Routine hospice care, the most common level of care, is provided at individual residences.
- Continuous home care is provided between 8 and 24 hours a day to manage pain and other acute medical symptoms in terminally ill patients. This care is mainly nursing care along with caregiver and aide services.
- Inpatient respite care provides temporary relief to the patient's primary caregiver. Respite care can be provided in hospitals, hospice facilities, or long-term care facilities that have 24-hour nursing presence.
- General inpatient care provides pain control or other acute symptom management that cannot easily be provided in other settings. Inpatient care can be provided in hospitals, hospice inpatient facilities, or other nursing facilities with 24-hour registered nursing care available.

Nonprofit and for-profit hospice organizations have proliferated, and there are currently over 4515 hospice agencies in the United States (NHPCO, 2019). This number represents a nearly 10% increase since 2014. Medicare covers almost all aspects of hospice care with little expense to patients or families, as long as a Medicare-approved hospice program is used. The number of older Americans who died in a hospital rather than at home or community hospice setting decreased from 2000 to 2015 (Teno et al., 2018).

Many people cite the 6-month rule to determine eligibility for hospice care. Six months or less is thought to be the amount of time that physicians, nurse practitioners, or physician assistants must certify that a person has to live. This misconception can be traced back to Medicare, which provides financial assistance in benefit periods of 90 days (Edwards, 2015). Medicare estimates that most people using hospice require two of these benefit periods. If, however, patients experience improved health, they can leave and return to hospice, or if care is required for a longer period of time, they can stay in hospice longer.

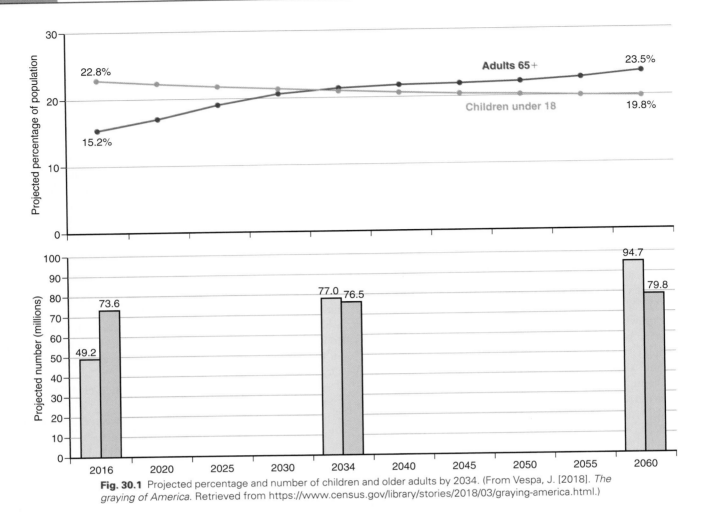

Fig. 30.1 Projected percentage and number of children and older adults by 2034. (From Vespa, J. [2018]. *The graying of America*. Retrieved from https://www.census.gov/library/stories/2018/03/graying-america.html.)

At the time of entry to hospice, medications and other treatments are evaluated. Medications used to treat the underlying illness are commonly discontinued. Are other medications necessary, beneficial, and not harmful are questions that should be asked. The goal is quality of life. For example, a person with diabetes may decide to give up a strict schedule of blood sugar testing and begin enjoying sweets again. An additional consideration is to the cost. Palliative medications related to a patient's terminal illness are covered by Medicare's hospice benefit. Other medications may continue to be covered by the patient's insurer or the patient may not have other insurance.

Palliative Care

Like hospice care, palliative care promotes comfort. Unlike hospice care, palliative care can begin at the time of diagnosis and continue throughout the treatment of the illness. Palliative care is specialized medical and nursing care for people living with serious illness. People may or may not be terminally ill to benefit from this type. Caring for those with incurable chronic diseases such as diabetes, heart disease, and dementia requires long-term palliative support. Palliative care is patient- and family-centered care that optimizes quality of life anticipating, preventing, and treating suffering. Palliative care addresses physical, intellectual, emotional, social, and spiritual needs.

Palliative caregivers promote patient autonomy, access to information, and choice.

Key components of both hospice and palliative care philosophy include:
- Honoring the experiences of the patient and family
- Respecting autonomy and informed choice
- Allowing care to be directed by the patient (and family)
- Honoring the dignity of the patient and family.

The National Hospice Organization was founded in 1978 with a mission of leading social change for improved care at the end of life. In 2000, the National Hospice Organization was renamed the National Hospice and Palliative Care Organization to reflect the inclusion of palliative care. The Hospice Nurses Association was formed in 1986 and renamed Hospice and Palliative Association in 1998 to provide a network for nurses working in this specialty.

Death and Dying Theory

Dr. Elisabeth Kübler-Ross, a Swiss-American psychiatrist, began actively listening to the terminally ill. Her groundbreaking work has provided a powerful conceptualization of the human response to death and loss. Kübler-Ross (1973) identified distinctive phases, or cycles, in people's responses to terminal illness:

- **Denial and Isolation:** Denial is typically a brief reaction, in which the patient is in disbelief or shock about the situation. This phase functions as a buffer after receiving shocking news and allows the patient to regroup. This phase can also result in "doctor shopping," in which the patient will seek advice from other specialists in hopes that the diagnosis will indeed be a mistake. Examples of expressions in this phase include, "There has been a mix-up with my test results," or "No, it can't be true. That's impossible."
- **Anger:** This phase typically surfaces when patients are ready to acknowledge their illness, when they come to terms with the fact that they are, in fact, seriously ill. The patient becomes pessimistic and unhappy. An example of a question in this phase is, "Why me? Why not someone else?" This phase is particularly difficult for the family and medical personnel to deal with because the anger is often projected unpredictably on to others. The most important things the angry patient needs are respect, understanding, attention, and time.
- **Bargaining:** As the patient attempts to deal with overwhelming feelings of vulnerability and helplessness, the individual may secretly try to make deals with a higher power to prolong life. Examples of this include, "I'll stop smoking if I can just stay alive long enough to attend my daughter's wedding."
- **Depression:** This phase arises when patients can no longer avoid a sense of great loss. They can feel guilty because of the strain they feel they're putting on their family and a deep sadness for experiences they may miss out on. Kübler-Ross defines two phases of depression: preparatory and reactive. Preparatory refers to patients preparing themselves for their final separation from this world, while reactive encompasses the unrealistic guilt or shame patients feel about their illness. In this phase, it is imperative that patients are allowed to express their justified sadness.
- **Acceptance:** Although this phase should not be confused with happiness, it does warrant a quiet peacefulness in the end of life. It is a final time for resting, free of pain and struggle. The patient may wish for solitude and may not be as talkative. Times of silence during visits may be the most meaningful mode of communication for these patients. This phase can be notably difficult for loved ones of the patient, as they may not have accepted the impending loss and view the patient's ambivalence with death as "giving up."

Kübler-Ross also realized that personal growth did not necessarily cease in the last stages of life. On the contrary, it often accelerated (Kübler-Ross, 1973).

FACILITATING DEATH

As previously discussed, there is much we can do to sustain and prolong life. How far is going too far? Are we ever obligated to end the suffering of people who are in agony due to tremendous pain or who are unable to end their own lives due to muscle-wasting conditions such as Lou Gehrig disease (amyotrophic lateral sclerosis)?

For most of human history, death was defined by the almost simultaneous cessation of cardiac, respiratory, and neurologic function. Technology has changed this, and the ability to maintain cardiac and respiratory function has radically altered who can be kept alive. The burden of defining death has shifted to the brain and has resulted in numerous hotly contested legal battles.

Beginning in the 1970s, complex medical legal cases began to emerge concerning who is really alive. Brain death is the loss of function of the entire cerebrum and brainstem, resulting in coma, no spontaneous respiration, and loss of all brainstem reflexes (Maiese, 2019). Vegetative states can occur when respiratory and cardiac function is returned, usually through medical intervention, but brain function remains significantly and usually permanently impaired. This neurological dysfunction results in the patient's loss of self-awareness and environmental awareness. Recovery does not generally occur. Cases of persistent vegetative states (duration > 1 month) have resulted in protracted legal battles between families and caregiving institutions.

A precedent-setting case occurred in 1976, when 21-year-old Karen Anne Quinlan suffered a severe anoxic brain injury after mixing alcohol and diazepam (Valium). Due to respiratory failure, she was intubated and placed on a ventilator. The Quinlan family drama unfolded before the American public. They petitioned the State of New Jersey for the right to remove the ventilator because Karen had previously informed her family that she would not want to be kept alive artificially. The court ultimately ruled in favor of the Quinlan family, citing the right to privacy. The ruling supported the autonomy of Karen's family to choose to withhold medical treatment even if it resulted in death. By the time the judge ruled in favor of the family, however, Karen had stabilized and was able to breath on her own. She remained alive in a vegetative state for 10 more years.

This legal case began a national discussion about what constitutes a "good death." Do we wish to die hooked up to machines in an ICU? How far does the right of privacy extend when making life and death decisions? Can families stop treatment or remove life-sustaining treatment? Does this right extend to assisting a suffering loved one to die? Conversely, what if a family continues to insist their loved one receive futile care? Doctors and nurses suffer deep trauma when faced with aggressive efforts to sustain life when death appears unavoidable. Each of these questions have been the source of professional and legal interest. Medical ethicists espouse the principles of autonomy and choice and thus support decisions to eliminate or forgo medical treatment.

Artificial Nutrition and Hydration

The provisions of food and water are emotionally charged activities. Disagreements about the best course of action can result in deep fractures within families. On the one hand, is disinterest in eating and drinking a sign of impending death? On the other hand, would sustenance and hydration increase the quality of life and chance of remaining alive? Does withholding food or water inflict suffering on the dying? Doctors, nurses, and legal institutions have attempted to wrestle with these penetrating questions. High-profile legal battles continue regarding artificial food and hydration.

Laws have also been created to help both families and medical institutions determine the circumstances under which nutrition and artificial hydration may be removed from patients.

According to the US Patient Self Determination Act (1990), an individual patient or designated surrogate can decide whether or not to refuse life-sustaining or life-prolonging treatments. The act also affirms the right to withhold artificial nutrition or hydration, as well as the right to withdraw these support measures.

Artificial nutrition and hydration through feeding tubes or intravenous fluids is legally considered a medical intervention and not a comfort measure. Supplementation of food and water is therefore not a component of basic care for people who are actively dying. It does not generally benefit people who are dying. In fact, providing artificial hydration by such means as intravenous fluids can increase edema, pulmonary congestion, ascites, nausea, and vomiting. Generally, the unwillingness or inability to eat and drink is caused by the impending death of the patient.

National medical and nursing organizations have crafted position papers to define evidence-supported practices on artificial nutrition and hydration at the end of life. The Hospice and Palliative Nurses Association suggests that the decision to use artificial nutrition and hydration be made on a case-by-case basis. The American Nurses Association (ANA, 2017) has also published a policy statement of artificial nutrition and hydration at the end of life (Box 30.1).

Nurses caring for the dying can encourage families to offer water orally as often as their actively dying loved one desires and is able to swallow. Listening to patients and their family members and including the interdisciplinary team in this decision is vitally important. One distinction to keep in mind is that the patient is not dying of dehydration or lack of food, but rather from their illness.

Euthanasia

Often called mercy killing, euthanasia is the act of putting someone to death. Euthanasia means that someone other than the patient commits an action with the intent of ending the patient's life. Three types of euthanasia exist:

- Voluntary euthanasia is requested by the patient and is typically performed when a person is suffering from a terminal illness and is in great pain.
- Passive euthanasia is the omission of acts (i.e., withdrawing or withholding) that would keep a patient alive who is unable to participate in decision making. Examples of passive euthanasia include discontinuing a medication that is keeping a patient alive or not performing a life-saving procedure on a person.
- Involuntary euthanasia is actively ending the life of a person who is able to perform consent, typically by the injection of a lethal drug. This active form of euthanasia may result in charges of homicide.

Legally Assisted Death

Traditionally, assisting in the death of another person has been an emotionally charged issue with negative and pejorative language used to describe it. Particularly problematic was the word "suicide" within the label, as in physician-assisted suicide. Patients are already dying and not choosing to die through suicide but choosing one form of death over another. In this chapter, we refer to assisted death as legally assisted death.

BOX 30.1   American Nurses Association Position Statement on Artificial Nutrition and Hydration

Adults with decision-making capacity, and surrogate decision-makers for patients who lack capacity, are in the best position to weigh the risks, benefits, and burdens of nutrition and hydration at the end of life, in collaboration with the health care team. The acceptance or refusal of clinically appropriate food and fluids, whether delivered by oral or artificial means, must be respected, provided the decision is based on accurate information and represents patient preferences. If a patient chooses food, even if that intake may cause harm (e.g., oral feedings in people who are at risk of aspirating), the nurse is responsible for minimizing risk (i.e., using both positional changes and slow, assisted feedings). This is consistent with ANA's values and goals of respect for autonomy, relief of suffering, and expert care at the end of life.

Other neutral terms you may hear that describe assisted death include:

- Death with dignity
- Assisted dying
- Assisted death
- Physician-assisted death
- Physician-assisted dying
- Aid in dying
- Physician aid in dying
- Medical aid in dying

Unlike euthanasia, in assisted death, someone else makes the means of death available, but does not act as the direct agent of death. The federal government allows each state to legislate its own laws about the legality of legally assisted death. Typically, the laws allow terminally ill patients with a life expectancy of no more than 6 months to request medication from a licensed prescriber that is taken to hasten death.

Individuals in Montana and California do not have statutes that allow assisted death, but individuals may pursue this option through the courts. The following states allow legally assisted death (ProCon.org, 2019):

- Oregon—1997
- Washington—2009
- Vermont—2013
- District of Columbia—2015
- Colorado—2016
- Hawaii—2019
- New Jersey—2019
- Maine—2019

The most well-known name associated with euthanasia and assisted death is Jack Kevorkian (1928–2011). Kevorkian was a Michigan physician-pathologist who claimed to have assisted at least 130 terminally ill patients to die. Janet Adkins, a 54-year-old woman with early-onset Alzheimer's disease was his first public assisted death in 1990. She self-administered a lethal injection. He was charged with murder, but those charges were dropped because there were no state laws outlawing assisting in someone's death.

Subsequently, juries acquitted Kevorkian three times on charges of assisted suicide. He was finally convicted of second-degree murder after filming and broadcasting his administration of a lethal dose of medication to a terminally ill patient with Lou Gehrig disease. He served 8 years in prison.

Kevorkian's death-related research was unsettling to nurses. They referred to Kevorkian's research as "doctor death's death rounds" (McClellan, 2014). This description eventually led to the nickname that was used for him decades later—Dr. Death.

In the last few years, nursing and medical associations have revised their position statements on PAS. The ANA revised its position statement regarding the nurse's role in legally assisted death (Box 30.2) to reflect evolving values regarding end-of-life choices. This evolution is a move from direct opposition to a more neutral stance and represents a substantive shift (Sulmasy et al., 2018).

Arguments Pertaining to Legally Assisted Death

Advocates of legally assisted death believe that misuse of this practice can be prevented through state regulations that ensure informed, competent, and freely made decisions. Opponents believe that opening the door to assisted death will result in a slippery slope where people may be coerced into this act by heirs or a profit-driven healthcare system.

Individual liberty. One argument concerns individual liberty compared with the state's responsibility to protect its citizens. Under the law, individuals have the right to refuse or withdraw treatment. However, this is counterbalanced by the notion that the government has a constitutional power to override certain rights to protect citizens from irrevocable acts.

Autonomy. A primary value of citizens of the United States is individualism. The ethical concept of autonomy supports self-determination. Every competent person has the right to make momentous decisions based on personal convictions. An opposing argument notes that human beings are the stewards but not the absolute masters of the gift of life.

Quality of care. Removal of legal bans on assisted death would likely enhance the opportunity for excellent end-of-life care for all patients. Legislation could be enacted to require that patients receive the best in palliative care. Opponents of this position cite that the aim of medicine should be to facilitate a death that is pain-free, but one that is also a human experience. A good natural death contributes to a strong society.

Nonmaleficence. Another ethical concept relevant to euthanasia is that of nonmaleficence or doing no harm. Is helping to end life harmful? From the patient's perspective, there may be no difference between ending life by providing a lethal injection and by stopping treatment that prolongs life. On the other hand, as nurses, we have been taught that the role of the nurse is to promote, preserve, and protect human life. Assisted death violates the oath to do no harm and may be considered the ultimate betrayal of trust between the patient and the nurse.

Beneficence. Beneficence is the other side of the coin of nonmaleficence and means to do good. Patients could benefit from relief that is now legally available to people who have physicians who are willing to risk assisting them to die. On the other hand, a misdiagnosis of the illness, inadequate assessment of competence, or pressure from the family or the physician might place the patient in jeopardy. Doing good means to preserve and support life.

ADVANCE CARE PLANNING

Advance care planning helps patients and their families discuss values, preferences, and end-of-life goals (Zwakman et al., 2018). Families and unpaid caregivers provide the "overwhelming majority of care" for those at the end of life (Ornstein et al., 2017). As a result, including them in advance care planning is important and valuable.

Caregivers facing the prospect of making end-of-life decisions for a loved one without the benefit of these conversations are more likely to suffer from depression, anxiety, and stress in the months after the death. Encouraging patients to talk about end-of-life issues and complete paperwork to support their wishes is an important intervention for basic-level registered nurses. Nurse practitioners and physicians are now able to bill Medicare for advance care planning services, including time spent in end-of-life conversations (Centers for Medicare and Medicaid Services, 2020).

Advance Directives

Since the 1960s, people have increasingly sought to participate in decision making about healthcare. In 1990, Congress passed the **Patient Self-Determination Act (PSDA)** (1990) requiring that healthcare facilities provide clearly written information for every patient, including legal rights to make healthcare decisions, especially the right to accept or refuse treatment.

The PSDA also establishes the right of a person to provide directions, or advance directives, for clinicians to follow in the event of a serious illness. Such a directive indicates preferences for the types and amount of medical care desired. The directive comes into effect should physical or mental incapacitation prevent the patient from making healthcare decisions.

Every healthcare facility receiving federal funds is required to have written policies, procedures, and protocols in compliance with the PSDA. The law does not specify who talks with patients about treatment decisions, but nurses often discuss these issues with patients. If the advance directive of a patient is not being followed, the nurse is required to intervene on the patient's behalf. Although nurses may discuss options with their patients, they may not assist patients in writing advance directives because this is considered a conflict of interest.

An advance directive is composed of two elements, a durable power of attorney for healthcare and a living will. Both of these documents can be developed by forms available from each US state. These documents must be in writing, and the patient's signature must be witnessed. Depending on state and institutional provisions, signatures may need to be documented by a notary.

Durable Power of Attorney

The **durable power of attorney for healthcare** is the designation of a person to act as the patient's medical decision maker. The patient must be competent when making the appointment and must also be competent to revoke the power. Individuals do not have to be terminally ill or incompetent to allow the empowered individual to act on their behalf.

Living Will

A **living will** is a personal statement of how and where one wishes to die. This living will provides guidance or instructions for making healthcare decisions. It is activated only when the person is terminally ill and incapacitated, and a competent patient may alter a living will at any time. The question of whether an incompetent person can change a living will is addressed on a state-by-state basis. Developing a living will does not always guarantee its application.

Provider Orders for Life-Sustaining Treatment

Provider/physician orders for life-sustaining treatment (POLST) and medical orders for life-sustaining treatment (MOLST) are terms that are used interchangeably. For the sake of this discussion, we are using the nurse-inclusive language of POLST. Physicians and advanced practice registered nurses write these orders based on the patient's preferred code status in the case of cardiopulmonary arrest where heartbeat and respirations have stopped.

As with most issues related to health and medical care, each state develops specific definitions, guidelines, and forms. For example, Florida uses either a full code or do not resuscitate (DNR), while Ohio uses a full code along with DNR/comfort care designations. You can become familiar with your state's requirements through a simple internet search.

Despite differences between states, most use some form of the following terms and approaches to care:

1. **Full code:** All life-saving measures are initiated. Chest compressions are used to resuscitate the heart, electric defibrillation may be used to treat arrhythmias, and intubation will be initiated to provide oxygen.
2. **Do not resuscitate:** Cardiopulmonary resuscitation will not be initiated in the event of cardiopulmonary arrest.
3. **Do not resuscitate–comfort care arrest (DNR–CCA):** Permits the use of all life-saving measures prior to cardiopulmonary arrest. Only comfort care is provided after the cessation of heartbeats and respirations. Comfort care includes airway suctioning, oxygen administration, positioning, and pain medications.

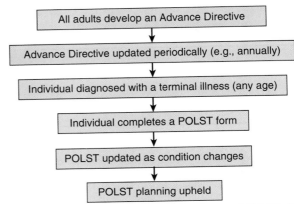

Fig. 30.2 Timeline for use of advance directives and POLST. *POLST,* Physician orders for life-sustaining treatment. (Modified from Polst California. [n.d.]. *POLST for patients and loved ones.* Retrieved from https://capolst.org/polst-for-patients-loved-ones/.)

4. **Do not resuscitate–comfort care only (DNR–CCO):** Care focuses on providing pain-free quality of life and comfort free of invasive procedures and intubation. This order is generally reserved for people with a terminal illness, short life expectancy, or little chance of surviving cardiopulmonary resuscitation.

A POLST order is signed by the patient or legally recognized healthcare agent and the healthcare provider. For hospitalized patients, skilled care patients, and residents of custodial or long-term care, a POLST is written and becomes part of the chart. For non-hospitalized patients, most states provide wallet-size ID cards and DNR jewelry, such as bracelets or necklaces. Family members should be made aware of the patient's wishes.

Ethical dilemmas can occur in regard to these life or death decisions. For example, when a patient has a feeding tube and a DNR–CCO status is later initiated, do we remove the feeding tube? What happens when family members are not informed about the existence of a DNR, the patient goes into cardiopulmonary arrest, and the family demands CPR? Careful planning, documentation, and communication reduce the chances for these dilemmas to occur.

Fig. 30.2 illustrates a timeline for developing advance directives and POLST.

NURSING CARE AT THE END OF LIFE

For patients and family members to make informed choices and goals, conversations between healthcare providers, patients, and families need to occur. The focus should be on supporting patients' informed choices and goals of care. According to the American Nurses Association's *Code of Ethics* (2015), nurses have a moral duty to help patients determine these preferences and goals at the end of life.

Communication

Despite being trained to discuss difficult and sensitive issues with patients and families, nurses are often afraid to talk about death. Talking about death is difficult because of the emotions involved, including our own fear, uncertainty, lack of control, lack of information, and conflict. To minimize the role of these emotions, it is important for the nurse to establish a therapeutic relationship before asking patients or families to make difficult decisions at the end of life.

Art of Presence

Caring for patients who are terminally ill requires some shifts in professional expectations. Whole-person care involves seeing the patient first and foremost as a human being and being attentive to all aspects of suffering. As front-line caregivers, nurses usually help patients get better, stronger, and more independent. Patients who are terminally ill are going to grow weaker, sicker, and ultimately die. There are often ways nurses can take action to make a patient feel better, such as pain medication, bathing, and turning. Sometimes, however, the best action is simply being present with people who are dying and their families.

Two essential skills associated with the art of presence are listening and observing. Reflect back to the speaker by restating or summarizing the message. Ask the patient and family open-ended questions, such as:

- Would you tell me what this is like for you?
- How do you see your condition right now?
- Where do you see things going?
- Are you worried about anything?
- What are you hoping for?

Sometimes saying little or nothing is also a good approach. You can practice staying silent and giving the patient or family member time to respond. The presence of a caring nurse can invite and permit the patient to discover new dimensions of personal experiences, bringing greater wholeness.

Symptom Management

Excellent symptom management is a hallmark of palliative nursing. The patient and/or the patient's advance directives and medical proxy determine the goals of care. Palliative care offers a wide spectrum of interventions to alleviate symptoms guided by patients' own reports and careful assessment. Some of the most commonly reported end-of-life symptoms are constipation, dyspnea, fatigue, depression, and delirium. Each symptom must be assessed individually.

It is easy to confuse treatable, reversible, and temporary conditions by attributing them to the terminal diagnosis. For example, if a patient reports feeling depressed, it is important to not assume that symptoms are due to the dying process. Depression, pain, or other treatable problems must be addressed and treated. If a patient becomes confused or lethargic, it is essential to rule out such things as medication effects, dehydration, delirium, urinary tract infections, or constipation.

Addressing pain symptoms is one of the most important quality of life concerns. Pain involves the whole person with physical, spiritual, and emotional components. According to The Joint Commission, a hospital accrediting agency, pain is the fifth vital sign along with heart rate, respiratory rate, blood pressure, and temperature (Morone & Weiner, 2013). Unlike the other vital signs, clinicians have no way of verifying or validating a patient's subjective pain. Nurses have an ethical responsibility to treat pain by providing respectful, individualized care to all patients experiencing pain regardless of the person's personal characteristics, values, or beliefs (ANA, 2018). Treating pain is complex and requires detailed assessment of the site, character, onset, duration, frequency, intensity, exacerbating/palliating factors, physical examination, and rating of pain using a pain scale.

Patients and family members may wonder about the dangers of opioid use to treat pain. Most people are aware of the serious opioid epidemic in the United States even if they do not know exact statistics. In fact, there were more than 70,200 opioid-related overdose deaths in 2017 (Centers for Disease Control and Prevention [CDC], 2018). Nurses can emphasize that addiction is not a concern for patients who are dying. Keeping patients as pain free as possible is the overriding goal.

> **VIGNETTE:** You are caring for a 42-year-old man dying of lung cancer. The patient is agitated, grimacing, and clutching the bed sheets. When you ask him if he needs pain medication, he averts his gaze and looks out the window. His wife says, "I think he's worried that the medication will make him so sleepy that he will miss the visit of my daughter and me." You respond, "Perhaps we can use the lower dose of morphine that's been ordered for now, and give him more after your visit." The wife gratefully replies, "Yes, let's try that."

Families are often concerned that pain medication might shorten their loved one's life. Patients and families look to the nurse to help address this concern. The Hospice and Palliative Nurses Association (2017) provides a position statement on this topic. They believe that nurses and other healthcare providers must advocate for effective, efficient, and safe pain and symptom management. Alleviating suffering for every patient receiving end-of-life care should be the goal regardless of age, diseases, history of substance misuse, or site of care.

Anticipatory Grief

Once a life-threatening diagnosis has been received or curative efforts are stopped, people begin a period of grieving called anticipatory grief (International Council of Nurses, 2019), sometimes referred to as anticipatory mourning. This type of grief is anticipatory in the sense that a future loss is being mourned in the present. It happens as people acknowledge the importance of the dying person, adjust their lives to accommodate the intervening time, and foresee how their futures will be altered by the loss.

The experience of anticipatory grief varies by individual, family, and culture. Aspects of finalizing the connection include spending time together, talking, making memories, life review, saying goodbye (often indirectly or metaphorically), touch, communication, taking care of business, and detaching from one another. A common emotional experience is anger—at the disease, the medical community, others, life—in addition to sadness, hurt, fear, anxiety, and hidden grief.

Palliative Care for Patients With Dementia

According to the World Health Organization (2019), there are 50 million people diagnosed with dementia in the world with 10 million people diagnosed annually. Therefore, all caregivers should receive education on the unique elements of palliative dementia care to increase comfort and enhance quality of life. Individuals with advanced dementia experience significant impairments in insight, language, and judgment, which limit their ability to communicate unmet needs and desires. Imagine that you were a patient and could not communicate when you felt pain or discomfort. Difficult behaviors in dementia patients, such as irritability or refusal to cooperate with care, are often forms of communication indicating discomfort in body, mind, or spirit. Anticipating a patient's needs can help prevent or reduce behaviors arising from an inability to communicate needs.

It helps if caregivers can focus on the person rather than the disease. We can recognize the numerous opportunities to affirm the meaning of the patient's life, uphold dignity, and provide pleasurable sensory and spiritual experiences. The goal is to create meaningful connections for these patients.

It is also important to address healthcare decisions for advanced dementia, such as resuscitation, hospitalization, antibiotics, and nutrition/hydration. Healthcare providers should: (1) identify the patient's goals for care and consider educating the family to minimize aggressive medical interventions, (2) eliminate medications that may detract from safety or quality of life, and (3) proactively manage issues such as pain and depression.

Families and friends spend a significant amount of time, finances, and emotions caring for a loved one with dementia. It is important to recognize and support the role of family caregivers as they navigate the day-to-day challenges and cope with losses. The Marwit-Meuser Caregiver Grief Inventory is a tool that identifies the unique forms of grief experienced by caregivers of individuals with dementia. High scores may indicate a need for intervention and formal support. Low scores indicate either denial of distress or positive adaptation. This inventory is found is Fig. 30.3.

Developmental Tasks in Dying

Ira Byock (1997), an American palliative care physician, believes that the final stage of life has its own developmental tasks. Human beings are social beings with individual and shared dreams, pasts, and future hopes. The process of dying remains filled with opportunities for growth, reconciliation, and meaning. Task work at the end of life is not just a *to do* list, it is the

ANSWER KEY						
1 = **Strongly Disagree** // 2 = Disagree // 3 = Somewhat Agree // 4 = Agree // 5 = **Strongly Agree**						
1	I've had to give up a great deal to be a caregiver.	1 2 3 4 5				A
2	I feel I am losing my freedom.	1 2 3 4 5				A
3	I have nobody to communicate with.	1 2 3 4 5				C
4	I have this empty, sick feeling knowing that my loved one is "gone".	1 2 3 4 5				B
5	I spend a lot of time worrying about the bad things to come.	1 2 3 4 5				C
6	Dementia is like a double loss... I've lost the closeness with my loved one and connectedness with my family.	1 2 3 4 5				C
7	My friends simply don't understand what I'm going through.	1 2 3 4 5				C
8	I long for what was, what we had and shared in the past.	1 2 3 4 5				B
9	I could deal with other serious disabilities better than this.	1 2 3 4 5				B
10	I will be tied up with this for who knows how long.	1 2 3 4 5				A
11	It hurts to put her/him to bed at night and realize that she/he is "gone."	1 2 3 4 5				B
12	I feel very sad about what this disease has done.	1 2 3 4 5				B
13	I lay awake most nights worrying about what's happening and how I'll manage tomorrow.	1 2 3 4 5				C
14	The people closest to me do not understand what I'm going through.	1 2 3 4 5				C
15	I've lost other people close to me, but the losses I'm experiencing now are much more troubling.	1 2 3 4 5				B
16	Independence is what I've lost... I don't have the freedom to go and do what I want.	1 2 3 4 5				A
17	I wish I had an hour or two to myself each day to pursue personal interests.	1 2 3 4 5				A
18	I'm stuck in this caregiving world and there's nothing I can do about it.	1 2 3 4 5				A

Self-Scoring Procedure: Add the numbers you circled to derive the following sub-scale and total grief scores. Use the letters to the right of each score to guide you.

Personal Sacrifice Burden (*A Items*)   = _____

Heartfelt Sadness & Longing (*B Items*)   = _____

Worry & Felt Isolation (*C Items*)   = _____

Total Grief Level (Sum A + B + C)   = _____

Fig. 30.3 Marwit-Meuser Caregiver Grief Inventory—Short Form. (From Marwit, S. J., & Meuser, T. M. [2005]. Development of a short form inventory to assess grief in caregivers of dementia patients. *Death Studies, 29*[3], 191–205.)

TABLE 30.1 Developmental Landmarks and Tasks for the End of Life

Sense of completion with worldly affairs	Transfer of fiscal, legal, and formal social responsibilities
Sense of completion in relationships with community	Closure of multiple social relationships (employment, commerce, organizational, congregational). Components include expressions of regret, expressions of forgiveness, acceptance of gratitude and appreciation
	Leave taking; the saying of goodbye
Sense of meaning about one's individual life	Life review
	The telling of "one's stories"
	Transmission of knowledge and wisdom
Experienced love of self	Self-acknowledgement
	Self-forgiveness
Experienced love of others	Acceptance of worthiness
Sense of completion in relationships with family and friends	Reconciliation, fullness of communication and closure in each of one's important relationships. Component tasks include expressions of regret, expressions of forgiveness and acceptance, expressions of gratitude and appreciation, acceptance of gratitude and appreciation, expressions of affection.
	Leave taking; the saying of goodbye
Acceptance of the finality of life and of one's existence as an individual	Acknowledgement of the totality of personal loss represented by one's dying and experience of personal pain of existential loss
	Expression of the depth of personal tragedy that dying represents
	Decathexis (emotional withdrawal) from worldly affairs and cathexis (emotional connection) with an enduring construct or acceptance of dependency
Sense of a new self (personhood) beyond personal loss	
Sense of meaning about life in general	Achieving a sense of awe
	Recognition of a transcendent realm
	Developing/achieving a sense of comfort with chaos
Surrender to the transcendent, to the unknown; "letting go"	

From Byock, I. R. (1996). The nature of suffering and the nature of opportunity at the end-of-life. *Clinics in Geriatric Medicine, 12*(2), 237–252.

person's choice to do—or not to do. See Table 30.1 for a list of some of the tasks a patient may move through at the end of life.

THE DYING PROCESS

The process of dying varies based upon the underlying cause. Some general signs of approaching death include:

- Growing weakness (asthenia)
- Loss of appetite
- Increasing drowsiness

- Change in mentation (shortening attention span, difficulty processing information)
- Circulatory changes (increased heart rate, decreased blood pressure)
- Mottling of skin (grayish-blue splotches on knees, ankles, feet)
- Decrease in urine production
- Breathing changes (Cheyne-Stokes respirations)

Agitation and delirium are not uncommon at the end of life. One of the more disturbing changes that sometimes accompanies the dying process is the presence of a death rattle, which is caused by pooling of saliva in the upper airway.

Hospice and palliative care nurses must provide families with information about what to do when their loved one dies. When the patient dies at home, the family should telephone their hospice provider. After the phone call is received by hospice, a registered nurse will be sent to the home. Upon arrival, the nurse will enter the home respectfully and guide the family members.

Family members are invited to remain at the bedside if they desire. The identity of the patient is confirmed by the nurse. The nurse will then use a stethoscope to listen for a heartbeat for 2 minutes while feeling for a pulse and watching for respirations. After 2 minutes without a heartbeat or breath, the nurse will pronounce the time of death, stating, "I am pronouncing the time of death at (time/date)." Sometimes, family members are confused by the fact that the official time of death is the pronouncement time rather than the time that the patient stopped breathing. It might be important to clarify for family members that this is the time that is used for the death certificate.

Each facility or hospice program will have a policy regarding the kind of postmortem care that is provided. Families will remember the actions of the nurse, so take care to communicate deep respect for both the dead and for the bereaved. The nurse should also offer to contact a social worker or chaplain, if desired. Family members should be invited to participate in this care if they desire. Care may vary according to culture but may include bathing, combing hair, or dressing in a special outfit.

The nurse may call the medical examiner to see if an autopsy is necessary. The laws regarding notification vary from state to state. Typically, autopsies are only required if the death is unexpected, unusual, or there is suspected abuse (e.g., broken bones or falls). Once the medical examiner releases the patient, the nurse will then contact the funeral home to come and pick the body up.

GRIEVING

Loss is part of the human experience, and grieving is the response that enables people to accept and reconcile with the loss and adapt to change. Grieving is a normal and complex process in response to loss. We grieve the commonplace losses in our lives—loss of a relationship (e.g., divorce, separation, death, abortion), health (e.g., a body function or part, mental or physical capacity), a friendship, status or prestige, security (e.g., occupational, financial, social, cultural), or a dream. Other normal losses include changes in circumstances such as retirement, promotion, marriage, and aging. These losses can promote growth through adaptation or may result in apathy, anger, and resentment.

Losing a significant person through death is a major life crisis. Long-term relationships bond us to each other deeply, shaping our world and our identity in it. The loss of a loved one can diminish aspects of our own self-concept. Grief is experienced holistically, affecting us emotionally, cognitively, spiritually, and physically. Those who grieve sometimes describe the death of a loved one as feeling like an amputation.

While grief is a reaction to a loss, bereavement, derived from the Old English word *berafian*, meaning "to rob," is the period of grieving after a death. Mourning refers to things people do to cope with grief, including shared social expressions of grief such as viewing hours, funerals, and bereavement groups. Everyone grieves but not everyone engages in the work of mourning. The length of time, degree, and ritual for mourning are often typically determined by cultural, religious, and familial factors.

The goals of mourning have evolved from doing the grief work, getting over it, and moving on with life. Mourning is a complex, individual, culturally embedded process of accepting the death. It involves confronting the painful experience of grief, constructing an identity and a life in a transformed environment, and finding an enduring relationship with the deceased based not on physical presence but on accurate memory.

Depending on many factors, this process can take months to a number of years. Losses transform lives, and we are never quite the same person again. Over time, people move from pain defining who they are and constant preoccupation with their loss to living with the residual pain and forever carrying the memory of the loved one.

Grieving Theories

A variety of theories exist to explain the process of grieving. Freud (1957) introduced the concept of "grief work," which referred to the process of looking at the past, reliving memories, and detaching from the deceased. Freud believed that grief needs to be confronted; this concept continued to be useful for later theory and therapy.

Most early theories are based on stages such as described by Kübler-Ross (1973) and Bowlby (1973) by which individuals progress toward the resolution of the loss. Later theorists such as Worden (2018) took a more dynamic approach by viewing the grieving process as tasks. All stage theories follow a similar pattern and are similarly useful.

As previously discussed, Kübler-Ross's groundbreaking work provides a framework for understanding reactions to dying. Her stage theory was eventually applied to the grieving process as well. Denial, anger, bargaining, depression, and acceptance are used to explain responses to loss (Kübler-Ross, 1973).

John Bowlby (1973), a British psychologist, relied on childhood attachment experiences to explain bereavement reactions in adulthood. He believed that grief is an instinctive universal response to separation. According to Bowlby, grief evolves through a sequence of four overlapping and flexible phases: shock and numbness, yearning and protest, despair and disorganization, and reorganization and recovery.

Worden (2018) identifies tasks that have to be worked through if grief is to be resolved. His model emphasizes moves from passive phases of grief to four active tasks of mourning.

- **Task 1**: Accepting the reality of loss.
- **Task 2**: Working through and experiencing the pain of grief.
- **Task 3**: Adjusting to an environment without the deceased person. The bereaved person must embrace new roles and adjust to the changing dynamics of the environment. Often, the full extent of what this involves, and what has been lost, is not realized until sometime after the loss.
- **Task 4**: Withdrawing emotionally from or relocating the deceased and moving on. Relocation requires that the bereaved person form an ongoing relationship with memories of the deceased while beginning to engage in activities that bring pleasure, such as new relationships.

Worden notes that every loss must be assessed in the context of mediating factors. These factors include the nature of the person who died, the nature of the attachment, the circumstances of the death, personality factors, family history, social circumstances, and life changes resulting from the death. His model can help to empower the mourner and serve as a specific guide for the nurse providing counseling.

While viewing the grieving process as linear—from denial to eventual acceptance—is attractive, grieving is just not that neat. In reality, these stages overlap and may be non-sequential. Stroebe and Schut (1999) suggest a dual process model of coping and bereavement. It incorporates the stage/phase models of loss-oriented processes with the restoration of a new lifestyle. The restoration process involves coping with everyday life, building a new identity, and developing new relationships. Table 30.2 summarizes the dual process model.

Grief and Technology

As minute details of our lives emerge in social media, so does grief. During or after the loss of a loved one, social media can serve as an outlet for a grieving person to express thoughts and feelings and get positive supportive feedback. In one study, Facebook profiles of deceased individuals were reviewed for the posts made by loved ones. Results indicate a potential for loved ones to continue a bond with the deceased by sharing memories, expressing sorrow, and gaining social support (Getty et al., 2011). Social networking technologies can help people make sense of death and maintain the legacy of the deceased (Brubaker et al., 2014).

TABLE 30.2	**Dual Process Model of Coping**
Loss-Oriented Processes	**Restoration-Oriented Process**
Grief work	Attending to life changes
Intrusion of grief	Distraction from grief
Denial/avoidance of restoration changes	Doing new things
Breaking bonds/ties	Establishing new roles/ identities/relationships

TABLE 30.3 Symptoms of Grief Versus Major Depressive Disorder

Symptom	Grief	Major Depressive Disorder
Feelings	Emptiness and loss	Depressed mood and anhedonia (inability to experience pleasure)
Physical	Insomnia, poor appetite, weight loss, decreased energy that gradually improves	Insomnia, poor appetite, weight loss, decreased energy
Intensity	Intense sadness and anger that occurs in waves and gradually subsides	Depressed mood is constant, most of the day, nearly every day
Thoughts	Focused on the deceased and reminders of the deceased	Self-critical, pessimistic ruminations, accompanied by thoughts of death
Mood	Depressed mood intermittent; increasingly positive emotions such as humor	Pervasive unhappiness and misery
Guilt	May experience guilt over failing the deceased (e.g., not visiting enough, not expressing love enough)	Continual, excessive, and inappropriate guilt
Self-esteem	Intact; reorganization tasks may impact sense of self (e.g., "Who am I without him?")	Worthlessness and self-loathing
Thoughts of death	May focus on someday reuniting with the deceased	Focused on ending the pain of depression; may develop a plan for death

Data from American Psychiatric Association. (2013). *Diagnostic and statistical manual of mental disorders* (5th ed.). Washington, DC: Author.

Grief Versus Major Depressive Disorder

An individual who is grieving is clinically different from a person who has major depressive disorder. The previous edition of the American Psychiatric Association's (APA) *Diagnostic and Statistical Manual of Psychiatry, Fourth Edition Text Revision (DSM-IV-TR)* discouraged clinicians from diagnosing an individual with major depressive disorder within 2 months of the loss of a loved one. This clinical guideline was referred to as the bereavement exclusion. The fifth edition of the manual, the *DSM-5*, however, removed this exclusion. Table 30.3 clarifies the difference between symptoms in grief and major depressive disorder.

Types of Grieving and Associated Nursing Care
Grieving

Grieving, also known as acute grieving, is the painful experience after a loss. The International Council of Nurses (2019) defines the nursing diagnosis of *grief* as feelings of sorrow associated with anticipatory or actual significant loss and death. There is no clear ending for grieving. Gradually the sadness diminishes, the pain subsides, and the individual moves on.

Nursing care for individuals who are grieving supports positive expectations for the future and re-engaging in activities and interests. As discussed previously in the dying and death section, the art of presence will reduce isolation in the grieving individual. Eye contact, the suitable use of touch, and a posture of attentiveness express warmth and provide comfort.

Listening is the absolute best nursing intervention that a nurse can use. People need to tell their stories, usually over and over, and move through the storyline in their own time. Sincere expression of sympathy, such as "I am so sorry for your loss. You must be devastated," shows engagement, interest, and empathy. Avoid clichés and minimizing expressions, which may actually be damaging. Saying "Have you considered having another child?" or "She is no longer suffering" suggest that the patient replace the deceased loved one or wanted the loved one to suffer. Table 30.4 describes some examples of communication to avoid and communication to use with grieving individuals.

Spiritual care is important to people with spiritual convictions and religious beliefs. Assess the role of faith in your patient's life and the perspective of death that accompanies religious beliefs. Offer support and referrals to pastoral counseling (when available) or community resources.

Grief support groups are available for every type of loss (e.g., spouse, child, pet), age group, and special conditions (e.g., disease, suicide, casualty of war). Hearing from others in various levels of grief, sharing the story of loss with others and receiving feedback, and being part of a group that really understands are powerful tools for healing. People may choose to attend local groups or online support groups depending on what works best and feels most comfortable.

Successful grieving is suggested by the following attributes:
- Accepting that the loved one has died.
- Experiencing adaptive appraisals of oneself in relation to the deceased.
- Avoidance of reminders of the loss is no longer present.
- Belief that life is worth living without the deceased.
- Increased sense of identity apart from the lost relationship.
- Engaging in activities, pursuing relationships, or planning for the future.
- Distressing memories of the deceased are under control.
- Anger over the loss is no longer present.

Persistent Complex Bereavement Disorder

The APA (2013) has proposed a diagnosis to account for and address prolonged grieving. While not yet an official disorder, **persistent complex bereavement disorder** is included in the *DSM-5* as a condition for further study. This medical diagnosis attempts to better understand the nature and clinical course of grief that becomes unshakeable. In addition to the timing, this persistent grief may be debilitating to relationships, impair occupational and academic performance, and significantly impact day-to-day functioning. Persistent complex bereavement disorder would apply to individuals whose acute grief persists beyond 12 months in adults

TABLE 30.4   Communication and Grief

What Not To Say	What To Say	Rationale
"I know how you feel."	"Your loss must be devastating. I can't imagine how you must be feeling right now."	Unfortunately, you cannot really know how that person feels.
"When my mother died, I cried for months and could hardly eat… (…*and proceed with long story*)."	"When I lost my mother, I was in a fog for days. This must be difficult for you right now."	While it is helpful to know that others have experienced loss, during the acute grief period the focus should be on the griever. Sharing lengthy stories is not helpful.
After a sudden and unexpected death: "At least he didn't suffer."	"It must have been so shocking to lose your husband so suddenly. Did he have any symptoms?"	No one wants suffering for a loved one, yet sudden deaths are also highly traumatizing. Chances to prepare and say goodbye are lost.
"Have you thought about getting another ____ (wife, pet, job)?"	"Your loved one was irreplaceably special."	Grievers are not interested in a replacement; they want their loved one back.
"She is with God now."	"I can only imagine how much you are missing her now."	Implying that the loss is God's doing may make the griever feel betrayed or punished by God. This statement also assumes that the griever believes in God.
"You can be grateful for the time you had together."	"You were married for 36 years."	This implies that the griever is ungracious. The griever is probably gracious but still wants the loved one back.
"Let me know if there is anything I can do for you."	"I would like to take the flowers from the funeral home to your house."	The grieving person is overwhelmed. Suggesting that they find something for you to do is an additional burden. Make a concrete offer of assistance.

and 6 months in children. Suicidal ideation and disinterest in living make this type of bereavement particularly dangerous.

Days with symptoms of complex bereavement disorder are experienced more often than not. The symptoms include:

1. Persistent longing for the deceased (children may express this yearning in play and behavior)
2. Intense sorrow and pain
3. Preoccupation with the deceased
4. Preoccupation with the circumstances of the death

Six of the following symptoms are experienced daily more often than not:

A. Reactive distress
   1. Difficulty accepting the death
   2. Experiencing disbelief or emotional numbness
   3. Difficulty with positive memories of the deceased
   4. Anger related to the loss
   5. Maladaptive views about oneself, such as self-blame
   6. Excessive avoidance of reminders of the loss
B. Social and identity disruption
   1. A desire to die to be with the deceased
   2. Difficulty trusting others
   3. Feeling alone or detached from others
   4. Feeling that life is meaningless
   5. Confusion about one's role in life
   6. Difficulty or reluctance to purse interests

The prevalence of this problem is about 2.4% to 4.8% (APA, 2013). It is more common in females than in males, perhaps because females tend to outlive their spouses. High degrees of dependency on the deceased person and the death of a child are risk factors.

Care for the individual who is experiencing dysfunctional grieving begins with an ICN (2019) nursing diagnosis of *risk for dysfunctional grieving* if risk factors exist. *Dysfunctional grieving* is the diagnosis to use if the problem has already occurred. An overall outcome for both diagnoses is improved grieving.

Nursing care for **persistent complex bereavement disorder** includes the care previously discussed for grieving. Protection from self-harm is an additional nursing intervention for this population. See Chapter 25 for care associated with suicidal ideation. Encouraging the patient to talk and helping to integrate the good and bad aspects of the deceased into a unified whole is an important aspect of care. Assisting with functioning in everyday life, such as encouraging adequate nutrition and hydration, monitoring sleep, and encouraging physical activity, may be required.

Disenfranchised Grief

Sometimes, an individual experiences an intense loss that is not congruent with a socially recognized relationship. Examples are a lover, a divorced spouse, a caregiver, an abortion, or a pet. We call this disenfranchised grief. This could also include the grief felt by healthcare workers over the loss of a patient. Typically, these mourners do not have the opportunity to publicly grieve the loss. Expressing grief would be viewed as unacceptable. To acknowledge and recognize such losses can help the griever begin the work of mourning.

When taking care of a patient who has experienced an unconventional loss, it is important to provide support and guidance. Seeking individual psychotherapy may be instrumental in working through conflicting feelings and issues. Local support groups may be of benefit, but there is always concern about anonymity and disclosure outside the group. Another good source of support is an anonymous virtual support group. There are actually many online support groups for disenfranchised grief.

Grief Caused by Public Tragedy

Public tragedies can cause another kind of loss. Public or collective tragedies involve a loss whose impact is felt broadly across a community or the general public. Even if we are not directly involved, these public tragedies affect our sense of security and alter our worldview. Entire communities and nations are shocked by genocide, war, assassinations, natural disasters, and school shootings. Most recently, the coronavirus pandemic thrust the entire world into a tragedy where millions of lives were lost. The 24-hour cycle of media coverage gives us all constant access to this and other tragedies across the world. It is important to explore the impact of public tragedies. As with other losses, acknowledging and validating the personal impact of the loss is therapeutic.

SELF-CARE

Nurses are on the forefront of caring for the sick and dying. Nurses should model good self-care because daily exposure to grief and dying can lead to increased vulnerability to emotional attachments and compassion fatigue. Nurses often grow attached to some patients and may experience both anticipatory grieving and bereavement. To maintain emotional balance and health, it is essential to rely on the support of others and practice good self-care. This is a journey that promotes greater self-understanding, wisdom, and compassion.

Nurses should practice conscious self-care in both their professional and private lives. The ANA *Code of Ethics* Provision 5.2 (2017a) states that nurses should model the same care for their own health that they teach to their patients (Box 30.3).

> **BOX 30.3 Guidelines for Self-Care When Caring for the Dying**
>
> 1. Remind yourself that what is happening to your patients and their families is not happening to you. This is their life circumstance right now but not your own.
> 2. When you notice that you are having a particularly strong emotional reaction, either positive or negative (countertransference), take it as a signal to explore your deeper issues or needs by talking with a trusted friend, counselor, or colleague.
> 3. Protect your private life by practicing time management, avoiding working outside of normal hours, protecting your pager or home telephone number, and taking regular days off and vacations.
> 4. Clearly state what you can and cannot do for your patients so your human and professional limitations are known upfront.
> 5. Practice humility. There is much you can do, but there is also much that is unknown and unknowable.
> 6. Do your own mourning when your heart is touched and you need to acknowledge the importance of others in your life. Even after a person has died, you can honor the relationship you had in your memory. Attend funerals or create grieving rituals when this happens.
> 7. Create a healthy, balanced private life by exercising regularly, eating a balanced diet, sleeping adequately, and leaving time for vacations and nurturing friendships.

KEY POINTS TO REMEMBER

- The hospice movement offers compassionate care for those who are dying, generally during the last 6 months of life. Hospice care focuses on patients' physical and emotional comfort and offers holistic support for dying people and their families.
- Like hospice care, palliative care promotes comfort for the patient and the patient's family. Palliative care may begin at the time of diagnosis and continue throughout the course of the disease or disorder.
- Kubler-Ross provides a strong conceptualization through a five-stage cycle that includes denial and isolation, anger, bargaining, depression, and acceptance.
- Increasingly sophisticated medical interventions have resulted in new legal, moral, and ethical issues pertaining to end-of-life issues, such as artificial nutrition and hydration, euthanasia, and legally assisted death.
- Nurses assist patients and families to understand advanced care planning, including advance directives (i.e., durable power of attorney, living will) and orders for life-sustaining treatment.
- When providing end-of-life care to people with dementia, challenging behaviors may communicate discomfort in mind, body, or spirit. Care should focus on providing meaningful connections with patients and between family members and their loved one.
- Providing timely and ongoing information about the disease and its effects and about physical and psychological signs of death can help the family deal with anticipatory mourning.
- Grief, bereavement, and mourning are distinct processes and normal reactions to a loss, real or perceived, including the loss of a person, loss of security, loss of self-confidence, and loss of a dream.
- Indicators of the potential for dysfunctional grieving include social isolation, extensive dependency on the deceased person, unresolved interpersonal conflicts, loss of a child, violent and senseless death, and/or a catastrophic loss.
- Grief work is successful when the relationship to the deceased person has been restructured, energy is available for new relationships and life pursuits, and the mourner can remember realistically both the pleasures and the disappointments of the lost relationship.
- Nurses are often exposed to individuals who are dying and their families. Self-evaluation and recognition of personal feelings is essential to promote self-care.

CRITICAL THINKING

1. George is dying of pancreatic cancer. His wife and adult children are asking about using hospice. Help George's family make an informed decision by describing hospice care.
2. What are some concrete ways in which you can help another to cope with loss? Identify specific components in the following areas:
   a. How can you let George tell his story, and what is the potential therapeutic value of doing so?
   b. What are some things you might say that could offer comfort?

CHAPTER REVIEW

1. Which statement made to the grieving patient demonstrates effective therapeutic communication? *Select all that apply.*
   a. "Your loved one was irreplaceably special."
   b. "It must be comforting to know that he is with God now."
   c. "You can be very grateful for the time you had together."
   d. "I would like to take the flowers from the funeral home to your house."
   e. "Your loss must be devastating. I can't imagine how you must be feeling right now."

2. Considering the subject of medically assisted death, which statements identify the pros and cons of the argument associated with the issue of nonmaleficence? *Select all that apply.*
   a. From the patient's perspective, there is no difference between ending life by providing a lethal prescription and by stopping treatment that prolongs life.
   b. Assisted death violates the oath to "do no harm" and destroys trust between patient and nurse.
   c. There is equal protection under the law that allows the right to refuse or withdraw treatment and to commit suicide.
   d. Every competent person has the right to make decisions based on personal convictions.
   e. Human beings are the stewards but not the absolute masters of the gift of life.

3. Which statement made by a patient demonstrates acceptance of criteria required of hospice care?
   a. "I want my family to be with me."
   b. "There is no cure for my illness. I've accepted that."
   c. "It's important to me that I die in my own home."
   d. "I don't want my family to bear the burden of caring for me."

4. Which statement made by a widow demonstrates that her grief work has been effective? *Select all that apply.*
   a. "I can remember how much my deceased husband loved chocolate chip ice cream."
   b. "Painting is my new passion, and I really enjoy learning the various strokes."
   c. "Jim could be very stubborn when he thought he was right."
   d. "I don't know why he had to die."
   e. "I just can't believe he's gone."

5. Which factor has the greatest influence on the hospice nurse's ability to provide respectful professional care?
   a. Acceptance that death is a natural part of life.
   b. Possession of excellent caregiving nursing skills.
   c. The existence of a healthy, well-balanced personal life.
   d. The desire to work with both the patient and the family.

6. There is conflict surrounding the dying experience in modern medicine. The medical model of treatment in the United States has traditionally been focused on the prolongation of life. What intrinsic factor plays into this medical model?
   a. Healthcare workers do not want their patients to die.
   b. Medicare is a fee-for-service model.
   c. Palliative care is expensive to administer.
   d. Keeping people alive as long as possible is the ethical thing to do.

7. Holly is a 53-year-old female with terminal breast cancer. Holly's nurse in the hospital brings up the subject of hospice care. Holly becomes upset and states, "I am not ready to give up and die." You respond that hospice is:
   a. A model of healthcare that emphasizes quality of life for you and your family.
   b. The end of curative treatments and pain management.
   c. A multidisciplinary team providing curative and therapeutic treatment.
   d. An aggressive medical plan to end suffering and hasten death.

8. Guadalupe is the matriarch of a large family. She is terminally ill and none of her family members know her end-of-life wishes. The best action for the nurse is to:
   a. Discuss a durable power of attorney.
   b. Organize a family meeting with Guadalupe's permission to discuss her goals and wishes.
   c. Have a family meeting without Guadalupe so as not to upset her.
   d. Ask the doctor to tell Guadalupe that she is dying.

9. A bereavement group run by a local hospice includes a woman who is distraught over her supervisor's death. The woman appears severely distressed. She has trouble functioning with activities of daily living and making the simplest of decisions. The group facilitator recognizes that this woman is suffering from disenfranchised grief after learning:
   a. The woman was in love with her married supervisor.
   b. She has not taken enough time off work to grieve properly.
   c. The supervisor died over a year ago.
   d. Her family is not involved enough to support her.

10. Dying patients with a neurocognitive disorder such as Alzheimer's disease are especially challenging to provide care for. They may have symptoms or pain that they are unable to adequately describe or define. What is a reversible condition that could respond to an intervention and improve anxiety, or agitation?
    a. Inability to communicate
    b. Distended bladder, constipation, or nausea
    c. Reduced urinary output
    d. Weakness due to the dying process

1. **a, d, e**; 2. **a, b**; 3. **b**; 4. **a, b, c**; 5. **c**; 6. **d**; 7. **a**; 8. **b**; 9. **a**; 10. **b**

🌐 Visit the Evolve website for a posttest on the content in this chapter: http://evolve.elsevier.com/Varcarolis

REFERENCES

American Nurses Association. (2015). *Code of ethics with interpretative statements* (2nd ed.). Silver Spring, MD: Author.

American Nurses Association. (2017). *Nutrition and hydration at the end of life*. Retrieved from https://www.nursingworld.org/practice-policy/nursing-excellence/official-position-statements/id/nutrition-and-hydration-at-the-end-of-life/.

American Nurses Association. (2018). *The ethical responsibility to manage pain and the suffering it causes*. Retrieved from https://www.nursingworld.org/~495e9b/globalassets/docs/ana/ethics/theethicalresponsibilitytomanagepainandthesufferingitcauses2018.pdf.

American Psychiatric Association. (2013). *Diagnostic and statistical manual of mental disorders* (5th ed.). Washington, DC: Author.

Bowlby, E. (1973). *Attachment and loss: Separation, anxiety and anger* (vol. 2). New York: Basic Books.

Brubaker, J. R., Dombrowski, L. S., Gilbert, A. M., Kusumakaulika, N., & Hayes, G. R. (2014). *Stewarding a legacy: Responsibilities and relationships in the management of post-mortem data*. Paper presented at the Proceedings of the SIGCHI Conference on Human Factors in Computing Systems. Toronto, Canada.

Byock, I., & Byock, A. (1997). *Dying well: The prospect for growth at the end of life*. New York: Riverhead Books.

Centers for Disease Control and Prevention. (2018). *Understanding the epidemic*. Retrieved from https://www.cdc.gov/drugoverdose/epidemic/index.html.

Centers for Medicare and Medicaid Services. (2020). *Advance care planning*. Retrieved from https://www.cms.gov/Outreach-and-Education/Medicare-Learning-Network-MLN/MLNProducts/Downloads/AdvanceCarePlanning.pdf.

Edwards, J. (2015, Feb. 25). *Common myths of hospice care debunked*. Forbes. Retrieved from https://www.forbes.com/sites/nextavenue/2015/02/25/common-myths-of-hospice-care-debunked/#3010b7574527.

Einav, L., Finkelstein, A., Mullainathan, S., & Obermeyer, Z. (2018). Predictive modeling of US health care spending in late life. *Science*, *360*(6396), 1462–1465.

French, E. B., McCauley, J., Aragon, M., Bakx, P., Chalkley, M., Chen, S. H., et al. (2017). End-of-life medical spending in last twelve months of life is lower than previously reported. *Health Affairs*, *36*(7), 1211–1217.

Freud, S. (1957). *The standard edition of the complete works of Sigmund Freud* (vol. XIV). London, UK: Hogarth.

Getty, E., Cobb, J., Gabeler, M., Nelson, C., Weng, E., & Hancock, J. (2011). *I said your name in an empty room: Grieving and continuing bonds on Facebook*. Paper presented at the Proceedings of the SIGCHI Conference on Human Factors in Computing Systems, Toronto, Canada.

Hospice and Palliative Nurses Association. (2017). *HPNA position statement on pain management at the end of life*. Retrieved from https://advancingexpertcare.org/position-statements.

International Council of Nurses. (2019). *International Classification for Nursing Practice catalog*. Retrieved from https://www.icn.ch/sites/default/files/inline-files/ICNP2019-DC.pdf.

Kalanithi, P. (2016). *When breath becomes air*. New York, NY: Random House.

Kübler-Ross, E. (1973). *On death and dying*. Routledge.

Maiese, K. (2019). *Vegetative state and minimally conscious state*. Routledge. Retrieved from https://www.merckmanuals.com/professional/neurologic-disorders/coma-and-impaired-consciousness/vegetative-state-and-minimally-conscious-state.

McClellan, D. (2014, March 16). Dr. Jack Kevorkian dies at 83; "Dr. Death" was advocate, practitioner of physician-assisted suicide. *Los Angeles Times*. Retrieved from https://www.latimes.com/local/obituaries/la-me-jack-kevorkian-20110604-story.html.

Morone, N. E., & Weiner, D. K. (2013). Pain as the fifth vital sign: Exposing the vital need for pain education. *Clinical Therapeutics*, *35*(11), 1728–1732.

Murphy, S. L., Xu, J., Kochanek, K. D., & Arias, E. (2018). Mortality in the United States, 2017. *Los Angeles Times*. Retrieved from https://pubmed.ncbi.nlm.nih.gov/30500322/.

National Hospice and Palliative Care Organization. (2019). *NHPCO facts and figures*. Retrieved from https://39k5cm1a9u1968hg74aj3x51-wpengine.netdna-ssl.com/wp-content/uploads/2019/07/2018_NHPCO_Facts_Figures.pdf.

Neuman, A. (2017). *The good death: An exploration of dying in America-*. Boston, MA: Beacon.

Ornstein, K. A., Kelley, A. S., Bollens-Lund, E., & Wolff, J. L. (2017). A national profile of end-of-life caregiving in the United States. *Health Affairs*, *36*(7), 1184–1192.

Papanicolas, I., Woskie, L. R., & Jha, A. K. (2018). Health care spending in the United States and other high-income countries. *JAMA*, *319*(10), 1024–1039.

ProCon.org. (2019). *States with legal physician-assisted suicide*. Retrieved from https://euthanasia.procon.org/states-with-legal-physician-assisted-suicide/.

Riley, G. F., & Lubitz, J. D. (2010). Long-term trends in Medicare payments in the last year of life. *Health Services Research*, *45*(2), 565–576.

Stolberg, S. G. (1999). Reflecting on a life of treating the dying. *New York Times*, F7.

Stroebe, M., & Schut, H. (1999). The dual process model of coping with bereavement: Rationale and description. *Death Studies*, *23*(3), 197–224.

Sulmasy, D. P., Finlay, I., Fitzgerald, F., Foley, K., Payne, R., & Siegler, M. (2018). Physician-assisted suicide: Why neutrality by organized medicine is neither neutral nor appropriate. *Journal of General Internal Medicine*, *33*(8), 1394–1399.

Teno, J. M., Gozalo, P., Trivedi, A. N., Bunker, J., Lima, J., Ogarek, J., & Mor, V. (2018). Site of death, place of care, and health care transitions among US Medicare beneficiaries, 2000-2015. *JAMA*, *320*(3), 264–271.

US Patient Self Determination Act. (1990). HR 4449 C.F.R. Retrieved from https://www.congress.gov/bill/101st-congress/house-bill/4449.

Vespa, J. (2018). *The U.S. joins other countries with large aging populations*. Retrieved from https://www.census.gov/library/stories/2018/03/graying-america.html.

World Health Organization. (2019). *Dementia*. Retrieved from https://www.who.int/news-room/fact-sheets/detail/dementia.

Worden, J. W. ((2018). *Grief counseling and grief therapy: A handbook for the mental health practitioner*. New York, NY: Springer Publishing Company.

Zwakman, M., Jabbarian, L., van Delden, J., van der Heide, A., Korfage, I., Pollock, K., et al. (2018). Advance care planning: A systematic review about experiences of patients with a life-threatening or life-limiting illness. *Palliative medicine*, *32*(8), 1305–1321.

31

Older Adults

Margaret Jordan Halter and Leslie A. Briscoe

 Visit the Evolve website for a pretest on the content in this chapter: http://evolve.elsevier.com/Varcarolis

OBJECTIVES

1. Identify statistics related to aging in the United States.
2. Describe mental health disorders that may occur in older adults.
3. Discuss the importance of pain assessment and tools used to assess pain in older adults.
4. Explain the negative impact of ageism that is evident in discriminatory labels, public policy, and research.
5. Explain the importance of a comprehensive assessment in older adults.
6. Recognize the significance of healthcare costs for older adults.
7. Compare the facts and myths about aging.
8. Analyze how ageism may affect attitudes and willingness to care for older adults.
9. Apply the nursing process to the care of older adults.
10. Identify at least four priority nursing diagnoses in the care of older adults.
11. Discuss basic nursing interventions in the care of older adults.
12. Identify psychological therapies used in the treatment of older adults.
13. Identify treatment settings for the care of older adults.

KEY TERMS AND CONCEPTS

ageism
agnosia
aphasia
apraxia

delirium
guardianship
late-life mental illness
medication reconciliation

Patient Self-Determination Act (PSDA)
polypharmacy
prescribing cascade

The focus of this chapter is on addressing the mental health needs of a specific population—older adults. People with mental illness prior to age 65 usually continue to experience symptoms and continue to need care later in life. In addition, mental health prior to age 65 does not provide older adults with immunity from subsequent psychiatric conditions. Too often, disorders are left untreated. Many older adults do not recognize symptoms; some deny there is a problem; others feel shame and concern related to stigma; and others dismiss symptoms as part of getting older. As nurses, we can help address these problems and the unique needs of older people with mental illness.

STATISTICS ON AGING

An aging population is a global phenomenon that is occurring at a record-breaking rate, especially in developing countries. This increase in the proportion of older adults impacts the economy, health, and social services. Globally, there were 703 million older people in 2019 (United Nations, 2019). This number represents an increase of individuals aged 65 years or more from 6% in 1990 to 9% in 2019 (United Nations, 2019). That proportion is expected to rise to a stunning 16% by 2050, resulting in one in six people of the world's population being 65 years or over.

The United States as a whole is growing older. The median age for all races and ethnicities increased from 37.2 years in 2010 to 38.2 years in 2018 (US Census Bureau, 2019a). This statistic means that more than half of the population is older than 38.2 years of age. This upward shift is due in large part to the baby boomers—born after World War II from 1946 to 1964—who are passing the 65-year mark. The share of the population 65 years and older was 16% in 2018, a number that grew by about 3% since 2017. The growth in this age group is on par with the approximate 30% increase since 2010. At the same time, the under 18 population decreased by about 1%.

Life expectancy has also been increasing. Life expectancy in the United States is projected to increase by about 6 years, from 79.7 in 2017 to 85.6 in 2060 (US Census Bureau, 2020). While women will continue to live longer than men, men will experience greater increases in life expectancy than women. The greatest gains in life expectancy will be among U.S. born non-Hispanic black men and non-Hispanic American Indians and Alaskan natives. The number of centenarians, those individuals 100 years and older, has increased from 54,410 in 2010 to 93,927 in 2018 (US Census Bureau, 2019a).

During the first half of 2020, US life expectancy actually decreased a staggering full year in response to the first wave of

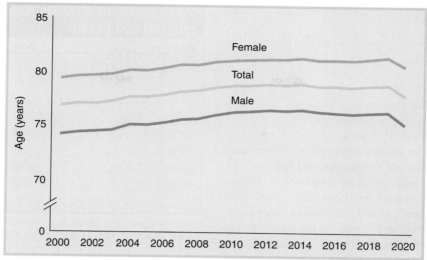

Fig. 31.1 Life expectancy at birth, by sex: United States 2000-2020. (Source: National Center for Health Statistics. [2021]. *Vital statistics rapid release report no. 010: Provisional life expectancy estimates for January through June, 2020.* Retrieved from https://www.cdc.gov/nchs/data/vsrr/VSRR010-508.pdf.)

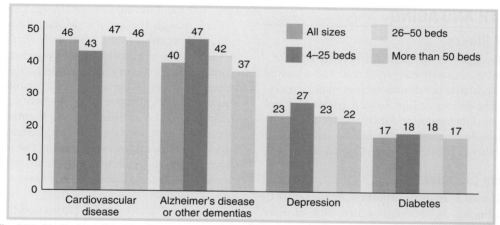

Fig. 31.2 Medical conditions among residential care residents by community size. (From Centers for Disease Control and Prevention. [2015]. *Variation in residential care community resident characteristics.* Retrieved from http://www.cdc.gov/nchs/products/databriefs/db223.htm.)

the coronavirus pandemic (National Center for Health Statistics, 2021) (Fig. 31.1). In the first half of 2020, life expectancy at birth for the total US population was 77.8 years, declining by 1.0 year from 78.8 in 2019. Minorities were disproportionately impacted by the outbreak, with Black Americans losing almost 3 years and Hispanics almost 2 years. The year 2020 was the deadliest in US history, with deaths topping 3 million, the most deaths the country had ever seen. A comparable, yet significantly less deadly, decline in life expectancy occurred during World War II in the 1940s, with 405,399 deaths (Congressional Research Service, 2020). As statistics become available for subsequent waves of the illness through 2021, the numbers are likely to get worse.

As people live longer, they are more likely to face chronic illness and disability. At least 80% of older adults have at least one chronic disease, and 77% have at least two (National Council on Aging, n.d.). The most common chronic illnesses are heart disease, cancer, stroke, and diabetes, which are responsible for almost two-thirds of all deaths each year.

The risk of developing a chronic illness dramatically increases with age. Individuals 75 and older are the most prone to chronic illnesses and functional disabilities. After age 85, there is a one in three chance of developing dementia, immobility, incontinence, or another age-related disability. Fig. 31.2 illustrates selected medical conditions in residential care residents based on facility size.

Women generally outlive men. This has significant ramifications for society at large and for the healthcare system in particular. Not only do women make up the largest proportion of older adults, they also use healthcare services more frequently than men and seek services earlier, even for minor conditions.

Chronological age is an arbitrary indicator of function, because there are significant variables that contribute to the health and functioning of older adults. For example, individuals who live beyond 100 years old are generally healthier (Ailshire et al., 2015). About 23% of centenarians reach age 100 with no major chronic disease and 18% have no disability. More than half (55%) reach this milestone without cognitive impairment.

Common classifications for people 65 years and older is:

- **Young-old:** 65 to 74 years
- **Middle-old:** 75 to 84 years
- **Old-old:** 85 to 100 years
- **Centenarians:** 100 to 104 years
- **Semisupercentenarians:** 105 to 109 years
- **Supercentenarians:** 110 to 119 years

Aging is accompanied by limited regenerative abilities and increased susceptibility to disease, syndromes, and sickness. The last years of life are often punctuated by losses, some obvious and some subtler. While retirement may be welcome, it still represents the loss of a career and possibly self-identity. Losses may be people—a spouse, children, and friends. As the ability to care for themselves becomes more difficult, familiar surroundings and independence may be lost in favor of assisted living or residential care. Older adults experience diminished senses—taste, smell, hearing, and sight. Cognitive decline and physical health problems weigh on an individual's day-to-day functioning.

MENTAL HEALTH AND AGING

Late-Life Mental Illness

Older adults who develop late-life mental illness are less likely than young adults to be accurately diagnosed and receive mental health treatment. Psychiatric conditions such as major depressive disorder, cognitive deficits, and prolonged grieving are not a normal part of aging. Diagnosing and treating psychiatric disorders prolongs the individual's ability to remain independent and increases the ability to take the lead in personal choices.

Major Depressive Disorder

Major depressive disorder is more common in people with chronic health conditions. As previously stated, 80% of older adults have at least one chronic health condition. Estimates of major depressive disorder vary depending on the setting. In the community the range is about 1% to 5%, in hospitalized patients it is 11.5%, and in individuals receiving home healthcare it is 13.5% (Centers for Disease Control [CDC], 2017).

Major depressive disorder is quite common after cardiac events and strokes, but care providers can confuse it with dementia or delirium. A careful, systematic assessment is necessary to properly distinguish among the three. Depression and the nonagitated form of delirium—hypoactive delirium—may result in the common symptoms of apathy, withdrawal, and tearfulness. Onset is a key assessment finding. While delirium occurs suddenly over a matter of hours or days, depression grows and persists over at least 2 weeks. Dementia results in profound memory disturbances that impact day-to-day functioning with a slow and insidious onset.

See Chapter 14 for an in-depth discussion on major depressive disorder.

Suicide

From 2009 to 2018, the age-adjusted suicide death rate increased from 11.76 to 14.24 per 100,000 people (CDC, 2020a). Older

TABLE 31.1   Suicide Rates by Age Group per 100,000 People

Age	Rate
85+	19.07
75–84	18.71
65–74	16.31
55–64	20.2
45–54	20.04
35–44	18.22
25–34	17.53
15–24	14.46
<15	0.99

From Hedegaard, H., Curtin, S. C., & Warner, M. (2020). *Increase in suicide mortality in the United States, 1999–2018.* Retrieved from https://www.cdc.gov/nchs/products/databriefs/db362.htm.

adults take their own lives at a high rate. Men 65 and older face a high risk of suicide, while adults 85 and older, regardless of gender, are the third most likely group to die from suicide. Table 31.1 identifies suicide rates by age group.

Even though the known suicide rate among older adults is high, especially among white non-Hispanic males, suicide in this group is probably underreported. The CDC (2015) estimates that for every one completed suicide, there are four suicide attempts in the older adult population. The numbers also do not reflect those who passively or indirectly commit suicide by alcohol misuse, starving themselves, overdosing or mixing medications, stopping life-sustaining drugs, getting into auto accidents, or simply losing the will to live. Treating depression is cost-effective, saves lives, and decreases healthcare expenditures. Chapter 25 provides an in-depth discussion of suicide.

Early identification of risk factors and treatment for depression are key measures for suicide prevention. Risks for suicide include:

- Diagnosable psychiatric illness (psychosis, anxiety, substance use, previous suicide attempts)
- Psychological alterations (personality, emotional reactivity, impulsiveness)
- Stressful life events

Other risk factors include access to weapons, access to large doses of medications, and chronic or terminal illness. Some protective factors include spiritual beliefs, being married, personal resilience, perception of social/family support, and having children.

Selective serotonin reuptake inhibitors (SSRIs) are a first line of treatment for major depressive disorder. This category is often helpful if anxiety, worry, or rumination is problematic. If pain or diabetic neuropathy is a comorbid condition, serotonin norepinephrine reuptake inhibitors (SNRIs) are often prescribed. Treatment-resistant depression can be treated with psychostimulants such as methylphenidate. Electroconvulsive therapy is also a highly effective and safe approach for depression, particularly in older adults who may not tolerate medication or fail to improve.

Anxiety Disorders

In older adults, anxiety disorders are often undiagnosed and prevalence estimates vary greatly. The most common anxiety disorder in this age group is generalized anxiety disorder. This disorder is often associated with pain, with both problems increasing the other. That is, increased pain increases anxiety and increased anxiety results in increased perception of pain. It becomes difficult to tease out the source and symptoms to target.

One unique anxiety-related problem in older adults is the fear of falling. This problem even has its own acronym: FOF. Its impact on keeping individuals homebound is similar to agoraphobia because FOF results in activity restriction resulting in increased muscle weakness and impaired balance. A Falls Efficacy Scale is included in Table 31.2 to assess the extent of fear of falling.

Risk factors for anxiety include childlessness, low socioeconomic status, and having experienced trauma. Other risk factors include being female, single, and having multiple medical conditions. Protective factors include social support, spiritual beliefs, physical activity, cognitive stimulation, and having coping strategies.

First-line treatment for anxiety disorders in all age groups, including older adults, is SSRIs along with cognitive behavioral therapy. Benzodiazepines such as lorazepam (Ativan), alprazolam (Xanax), or diazepam (Valium) are also used to treat anxiety but are often prescribed inappropriately in older adults. Using this class of drugs may result in increased falls, fractures, mental decline, and delirium. When used in low doses, these problems are less likely, but it is better to avoid the drugs in this class if at all possible. One meta-analysis by He et al. (2019) found that benzodiazepines were associated with a significant increase risk for dementia, particularly with medications that have longer half-lives such as diazepam (Valium) and that are taken for more than 3 years.

Chapter 15 discusses anxiety disorders in greater detail.

Delirium

Delirium is a time-limited medical condition caused by physiological changes usually due to an identifiable underlying pathology. Fluctuations in consciousness and changes in cognition develop over a short period of time (hours to days). Unfortunately, disorientation in older adults may be labeled as dementia and disregarded. It is crucial to obtain data from family or caregivers about a baseline level of functioning. A patient who is newly confused, falling, disrobing, and fighting with staff should be assessed for delirium. Asking family members questions such as "Has your mother been shopping and cooking for herself?"; "Does she pay her own bills?"; or "Does she ever get lost when driving?" may give subtle clues about whether changes are acute or have been coming on slowly.

Treatment of delirium begins with identifying the cause. You may ask, "Is your father taking any new medication?" or "Has your father fallen or hit his head recently?" The delirium may be due to drug reactions or toxicity, infections, electrolyte or metabolic imbalances, anemia, thyroid dysfunction, vitamin

TABLE 31.2 Falls Efficacy Scale

On a scale from 1 to 10, with 1 being very confident and 10 being not confident at all, how confident are you that you do the following activities without falling?

Activity	1 = Very Confident; 10 = Not Confident at All
Take a bath or shower	
Reach into cabinets or closets	
Walk around the house	
Prepare meals not requiring carrying heavy or hot objects	
Get in and out of bed	
Answer the door or telephone	
Get in and out of a chair	
Getting dressed and groomed	
Total Score	

Source: Tinetti, M. E., Richman, D., & Powell, L. (1990). Falls efficacy as a measure of fear of falling. *Journal of Gerontology, 45*(6), 239–243.

deficiencies, stroke, and a multitude of other problems. A multidisciplinary approach is often helpful to identify causation. Pharmacists are helpful in identifying possible drug-related effects. Geriatricians provide a comprehensive approach to physical assessment. Psychiatric consultation can provide mental status evaluation and recommendations for treatment of behaviors.

Chapter 23 provides more information about delirium.

Neurocognitive Disorders

The most common neurocognitive disorders are Alzheimer's disease and vascular disease. Both are characterized by a functional decline, aphasia (difficulty finding words), apraxia (difficulty carrying out motor functions), agnosia (failure to recognize objects), and disturbances in executive functioning (organizing, planning, abstracting, insight, judgment). Changes in executive functioning may result in forgetting how to make old family recipes or the inability to pay bills. Tragically, limited insight and judgment often lead to increased vulnerability to exploitation. Chapter 23 presents a more complete picture of delirium and dementia and associated care.

Alcohol Use Disorder

Alcohol is the most commonly misused substance among individuals 65 and older (Substance Abuse and Mental Health Services Administration, 2019). Alcohol misuse often goes unrecognized, unreported, and untreated. The precursors to late-onset alcohol use problems are often related to environmental conditions and may include retirement, widowhood, and loneliness. Previously, work, family responsibilities, and marriage may have been protective in keeping a person with vulnerability from drinking too much. Once these demands are gone and the structure of daily life is removed, there may be little impetus to stay sober.

Risk factors for heavy drinking in older adults are being male and single, having less than a high school education, low income, and cigarette smoking. Additionally, depression often plays a role in increased alcohol consumption in the older adult. Identifying alcohol and substance use problems is often difficult because the personality and behavioral changes frequently go unrecognized. Whenever there is a suspicion or indication that an older adult is misusing alcohol, the healthcare provider should conduct a screening test. The Michigan Alcoholism Screening Test–Geriatric version (MAST-G; Box 31.1) is an instrument commonly used to assess older adults' alcohol use.

The older person who misuses alcohol may be confused, malnourished, unkempt, thin, depressed, and unsteady. Diarrhea, urinary incontinence, decreased functional status, and failure to thrive may also be present. Long-term excessive alcohol use can lead to alcohol-induced dementia. Symptoms include impaired executive functioning and significant lack of insight. This is in contrast to the memory or language problems of Alzheimer's disease.

EVIDENCE-BASED PRACTICE

Why Do Older Adults Attempt Suicide?

Problem
Suicide rates increase with age, particularly in white males. There is limited understanding regarding the reasons older people attempt suicide.

Purpose of the Study
The purpose of this study was to gain an understanding about the reasons for late-life suicide.

Methods
Researchers interviewed 103 participants age 70 years and older. Subjects were older adults who were seen in emergency rooms after a suicide attempt in Sweden over a 3-year period. Multiple tools were used to measure cognition, illness rating, psychiatric symptoms, and depression. In addition, there was a clinical interview and medical record review. Participants were followed for 1 year through continued review of their records.

Key Findings
- The most common method for suicide attempt was overdose ($N = 73$).
- Approximately one-third of participants had previous suicide attempts.
- Approximately 70% lived alone.
- Reasons for the attempt included: To escape (29%), reduced functioning and autonomy (24%), psychological problems (24%), somatic problems and physical pain (16%), feeling like a burden (13%), social problems and family conflict (13%), and a lack of meaning in life (8%).
- Lethal means of suicide attempt and reattempts were associated with a sense of not belonging.

Implications for Nursing Practice
It is important to understand and recognize potential risk factors for suicide in the older adult. Nurses have the ability to screen for and identify those who may be at greatest risk. Targeting those at greater risk may guide interventions such as increasing socialization, interpersonal therapy, or an environmental change.

From Van Orden, K., Wiktorsson, S., Duberstein, P., Berg, A., & Waern, M. (2015). Reasons for attempted suicide in later life. *American Journal of Geriatric Psychiatry, 23*(5), 536–544.

BOX 31.1 Michigan Alcoholism Screening Test—Geriatric Version (Mast-G)

Please answer "Yes" or "No" to each question by marking the line next to the question. When you finish answering the questions, please add up how many "Yes" responses you checked and put that number in the space provided at the end.

1. After drinking, have you ever noticed an increase in your heart rate or beating in your chest? _____ Yes _____ No
2. When talking to others, do you ever underestimate how much you actually drank? _____ Yes _____ No
3. Does alcohol make you sleepy so that you often fall asleep in your chair? _____ Yes _____ No
4. After a few drinks, have you sometimes not eaten or been able to skip a meal because you didn't feel hungry? _____ Yes _____ No
5. Does having a few drinks help you decrease your shakiness or tremors? _____ Yes _____ No
6. Does alcohol sometimes make it hard for you to remember parts of the day or night? _____ Yes _____ No
7. Do you have rules for yourself that you won't drink before a certain time of the day? _____ Yes _____ No
8. Have you lost interest in hobbies or activities you used to enjoy? _____ Yes _____ No
9. When you wake up in the morning, do you ever have trouble remembering part of the night before? _____ Yes _____ No
10. Does having a drink help you sleep? _____ Yes _____ No
11. Do you hide your alcohol bottles from family members? _____ Yes _____ No
12. After a social gathering, have you ever felt embarrassed because you drank too much? _____ Yes _____ No
13. Have you ever been concerned that drinking might be harmful to your health? _____ Yes _____ No
14. Do you like to end an evening with a nightcap? _____ Yes _____ No
15. Did you find your drinking increased after someone close to you died? _____ Yes _____ No
16. In general, would you prefer to have a few drinks at home rather than go out to social events? _____ Yes _____ No
17. Are you drinking more now than in the past? _____ Yes _____ No
18. Do you usually take a drink to relax or calm your nerves? _____ Yes _____ No
19. Do you drink to take your mind off your problems? _____ Yes _____ No
20. Have you ever increased your drinking after experiencing a loss in your life? _____ Yes _____ No
21. Do you sometimes drive when you have had too much to drink? _____ Yes _____ No
22. Has a doctor or nurse ever said he or she was worried or concerned about your drinking? _____ Yes _____ No
23. Have you ever made rules to manage your drinking? _____ Yes _____ No
24. When you feel lonely, does having a drink help? _____ Yes _____ No

TOTALS: _____ **Yes** _____ **No**

Scoring: A score of 3 points or less is considered to indicate no alcoholism; a score of 4 points is suggestive of alcohol use disorder; a score of 5 points or more indicates alcohol use disorder.

From Blow, F. C., Brower, K. J., et al.: The Michigan Alcoholism Screening Test-Geriatric Version (MAST-G): A new elderly specific screening instrument. *Alcoholism: Clinical and Experimental Research 16,* 372, 1992.

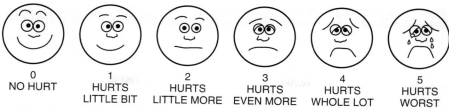

Fig. 31.3 Wong-Baker FACES Pain Rating Scale. Explain to the patient that the first face represents a person who feels happy because he has no pain, and that the other faces represent people who have pain, ranging from a little to a lot. Explain that face 10 represents a person who hurts as much as you can imagine, but you don't have to be crying to be in that much pain. Ask the patient to choose the face that best reflects how he or she is feeling. (From Hockenberry, M., & Wilson, D. [2013]. *Wong's essentials of pediatric nursing* [9th ed.]. St. Louis, MO: Mosby.)

Pain

Pain is common among older adults and affects their sense of well-being and quality of life. Conditions that result in pain include arthritis, peripheral vascular disease, and diabetic neuropathy. Major depressive disorder may cause or increase the perception of pain. Pain can affect the older adult's functioning and ability to perform activities of daily living (ADLs) such as walking, toileting, and bathing, especially if the pain is from musculoskeletal disease. Pain can lead to increased stress, delayed healing, decreased mobility, disturbances in sleep, decreased appetite, and agitation with accompanying aggressive behaviors. Chronic pain is linked to depression, low self-esteem, social isolation, and feelings of hopelessness.

Barriers to Accurate Pain Assessment

The appropriate assessment and treatment of pain in older adults may have complications. They may believe that pain is an inevitable part of aging, an indication of impending death, too expensive to test and diagnose, or a sign of weakness. External obstacles to pain management include inadequate assessment by healthcare professionals, complicated clinical presentation, assumptions by healthcare professionals that pain is part of aging, and communication deficits due to cognitive impairment.

The use of open-ended questions such as "Tell me about your [pain, aches, soreness, or discomfort]" adds significantly more information. Assess changes in behavior that indicate pain, especially in patients who have language impairment due to conditions such as dementia or strokes. Unlike younger adults, older adults may understate pain using milder words such as *discomfort, hurting,* or *aching.* Multiple painful problems may occur together, making differentiation of new pain from pre-existing pain difficult. Sensory impairments, memory loss, dementia, and depression can add to the difficulty of obtaining an accurate pain assessment. Interviews with family members, caregivers, or friends may be helpful.

Assessment Tools

When pain is suspected, the nurse begins with a physical assessment for medical origins of the pain and assesses the level of pain. The Wong-Baker FACES Pain Rating Scale (Fig. 31.3) is an active assessment instrument. The FACES scale shows facial expressions on a scale from 0 (a smile) to 5 (crying grimace). Respondents choose the face that depicts the pain they feel.

People with cognitive deficits often act out due to pain. The Pain Assessment in Advanced Dementia (PAINAD) scale evaluates the presence and severity of pain in patients with advanced neurocognitive disorders who no longer have the ability to communicate verbally. The scale evaluates five domains: breathing, negative vocalization, facial expression, body language, and consolability (Box 31.2). The score assists the caregiver in the development of appropriate pain intervention.

Pain Management

Pharmacotherapy. Pain can be managed with pharmacotherapy and alternative measures. Pharmacotherapy pain management relies on the use of nonprescription and prescription medications, which are frequently based on the recommendation of the healthcare provider. Persistent pain is common among older individuals. However, older adults may experience adverse drug reactions due to age- and disease-related changes in pharmacodynamics and pharmacokinetics. Careful monitoring of medication effects will aid in avoiding overmedication or undermedication. Hepatic and renal functioning should be evaluated periodically.

Nonopioids. Nonopioids are useful for mild-to-moderate pain. Acetaminophen is the preferred nonopioid medication. However, while it relieves pain, it does nothing to reduce inflammation. Acetaminophen can be toxic to the liver. The maximum dose should be reduced to 50% to 75% in adults with a history of alcohol use problems or reduced hepatic function.

Nonselective nonsteroidal antiinflammatory drugs (NSAIDs) work by inhibiting one or both of two enzymes involved in the production of inflammation, pain, and fever—cyclooxygenase-1 and cyclooxygenase-2 (COX-1 and COX-2). COX-1 functions to protect the lining of the stomach and intestines from the damaging effects of acid, promote blood clotting, and regulate normal kidney function. When these enzymes are inhibited, gastrointestinal bleeding and nephrotoxicity are potentially dangerous side effects of nonselective NSAIDs. Nonselective NSAIDs include drugs such as ibuprofen (e.g., Motrin, Advil), naproxen sodium (e.g., Aleve), diclofenac sodium (e.g., Voltaren), and aspirin.

A newer group of NSAIDs that selectively inhibits only one COX enzyme is called a COX-2 inhibitor. Because this classification of drugs does not block COX-1, they do not cause ulcers or increase the bleeding risk to the extent of the older NSAIDs.

BOX 31.2   Pain Assessment in Advanced Dementia Scale

Instructions: Observe the patient for 5 minutes before scoring his or her behaviors. Score the behaviors according to the following chart. The patient can be observed under different conditions (e.g., at rest, during a pleasant activity, during caregiving, after the administration of pain medication).

Behavior	0	1	2	Score
Breathing Independent of vocalization	Normal	Occasional labored breathing Short period of hyperventilation	Noisy labored breathing Long period of hyperventilation Cheyne-Stokes respirations	
Negative vocalization	None	Occasional moan or groan Low-level speech with a negative or disapproving quality	Repeated troubled calling out Loud moaning or groaning Crying	
Facial expression	Smiling or inexpressive	Sad Frightened Frown	Facial grimacing	
Body language	Relaxed	Tense Distressed pacing Fidgeting	Rigid Fists clenched Knees pulled up Pulling or pushing away Striking out	
Consolability	No need to console	Distracted or reassured by voice or touch	Unable to console, distract, or reassure	
			TOTAL SCORE	

Scoring: The total score ranges from 0 to 10 points. A possible interpretation of the scores is: 1–3 = mild pain; 4–6 = moderate pain; 7–10 = severe pain. These ranges are based on a standard 0–10 scale of pain, but have not been substantiated in the literature for this tool.
Warden V, Hurley A. C., & Volicer L. (2003). Development and psychometric evaluation of the Pain Assessment in Advanced Dementia (PAINAD) scale. *Journal of the American Medical Directors Association, 4*(1), 9–15.

Celecoxib (Celebrex) is the only selective COX-2 inhibitor available in the United States.

In 2015, the US Food and Drug Administration (FDA) strengthened an existing warning in prescription and over-the-counter drug labels. This warning indicates that nonaspirin NSAIDs can increase the chance of a heart attack and stroke. These serious side effects can occur as early as the first week of using these drugs. The risk may increase the longer NSAIDs are used and increase with higher doses. Upper and lower gastrointestinal bleeding is also a risk with NSAIDs, particularly in people over 65.

Neuropathic pain may be treated with pain modulators such as gabapentin (Neurontin), pregabalin (Lyrica), SNRIs, and tricyclic antidepressants. Chronic pain may be treated with duloxetine (Cymbalta). Consultation with a pain-management specialist is often helpful with chronic pain syndromes. Some considerations in pharmacological pain management in older adults are listed in Box 31.3.

Opioids. Opioids may be indicated for treating moderate-to-severe acute pain. Opioids are metabolized in the liver and excreted by the kidneys either unchanged or as metabolites. As the result of normal aging, renal insufficiency often occurs, making older adults susceptible to drug effects and metabolite accumulation. Initial doses of opioids should be reduced in older patients, and longer dosing intervals should be scheduled.

The trend is to avoid opioids for non–cancer-related chronic pain due to evidence that the risks are significant, including increased risk of fractures, hospitalization, and mortality. Furthermore, they may not even be beneficial for long-term pain. Prescribers also reported concern about misuse of opioids by family and friends.

BOX 31.3   Tips for Pharmacological Pain Management in Older Adults

- Remember that older adults often receive pain medication less often than younger adults, which results in inadequate pain relief. Compensate for this.
- Safe administration of analgesics is complicated because of possible interactions with drugs used to treat multiple chronic disorders, nutritional alterations, and altered pharmacokinetics in older adults.
- Analgesics reach a higher peak and have a longer duration of action in older adults than in younger individuals. Start with one-fourth to one-half the adult dose and titrate up carefully.
- Give oral analgesics around the clock when initiating pain management. Administer on an as-needed basis later on as indicated by the patient's pain status.
- If acute confusion occurs, assess for other contributing factors before changing the medication or stopping analgesic use. Confusion in postoperative patients is associated with unrelieved pain rather than with opiate use.
- Acetaminophen is an effective analgesic in older adults, although it is ineffective in reducing inflammation. There is an increased risk of end-stage renal disease with long-term use. It does not produce the increased stroke and myocardial infarction risk or gastrointestinal bleeding seen with nonsteroidal anti-inflammatory drugs (NSAIDs). *Acetaminophen*
- Opioids have a greater analgesic effect and longer duration of action for moderate-to-severe pain than non-opioid analgesics. Opioids should be avoided for non-cancer-related chronic pain due to evidence that risks may outweigh the benefits. Risks include increased risk of fractures, hospitalization, and mortality.
- Assess bowel function daily because constipation can be a frequent side effect of opioid use.

Data from Davis, M., & Srivastava, M. (2003). Demographics, assessment and management of pain in the older adult. *Drugs and Aging, 20*(1), 23–35.

Older adults' response to pain treatment is improved when the patient actively participates in treatment decisions. A trusting and mutually respectful relationship with providers reduces anxiety and associated pain. Being understood supports the goal of patient-centered care.

Nonpharmacological pain treatments. Nonpharmacological treatments for pain include physical therapy, vagal nerve stimulation, exercise, hydrotherapy, heat and cold packs, chiropractic, and transcutaneous electrical nerve stimulation (TENS). Yoga, biofeedback, hypnosis, acupuncture, massage, Reiki, guided imagery, reflexology, and therapeutic touch are integrative therapies for managing pain. Herbal remedies include cayenne, capsaicin, ginger extract, echinacea, kava, and willow bark. It is important to ask older adults if they are utilizing any alternative treatments for pain relief. Pain-management education is important for both the patient and caregivers. Refer to Chapter 36 for a full discussion of integrative therapies.

It is critical for nurses to evaluate the effectiveness of pain interventions at regular intervals and to be attentive to behavioral changes or verbal responses that indicate the patient is experiencing pain. It is a common misconception to assume that the ability to perceive pain decreases with aging. No physiological changes in pain perception in older adults have been demonstrated.

HEALTHCARE CONCERNS OF OLDER ADULTS

Financial Burden

Healthcare expenses for older adults are nearly four times higher than the expenses for the rest of the population. With the predicted growth in this population, illness prevention and maintenance of functional ability must be priorities. According to the US Census Bureau (2019b), approximately 10% of people 65 and older live below the poverty level ($12,140).

Medicare Part D has reduced the financial burden of paying for medications. In 2020, Medicare Part D paid 75% of total drug costs after a deductible of up to $435 and a monthly premium are paid (Medicare.gov, 2020). Depending upon the plan chosen by the individual, co-payments (e.g., $10 per prescription) or coinsurance (e.g., 10% of the drug cost) is required. Once out-of-pocket and covered medication expenses reach $4020, the coverage gap, or so-called "donut hole," starts. People are still required to pay monthly premiums during the coverage gap period. Once expenses reach $6350 (not including monthly premiums), catastrophic coverage kicks in. After that point, the insured pays only a small coinsurance amount or copayment for covered drugs the rest of the year.

Nurses need to be aware of these financial burdens that impact health practices and help seeking. Education for older adults regarding availability and use of other resources, such as patient assistance programs for expensive medications, is crucial. Encourage your patients to ask their physicians and pharmacists about financial assistance for medications. Local advocacy agencies such as the American Association of Retired Persons (AARP) or Area Agency on Aging often have free assistance in selecting a Medicare insurance plan that will best cover their specific medications.

Caregiver Burden

Another phenomenon with an aging population is the increase in caregiver burden. Caregiver burden is the amount of physical, emotional, financial, and psychosocial support provided to a loved one with a chronic illness. One common scenario is a two-income family in the middle of raising children and planning for retirement who are faced with assisting parents. This family is sometimes referred to as a sandwich family—sandwiched between two generations. Another is one older adult spouse taking care of the other. Dwindling healthcare benefits, shorter hospital stays, limited home-care options, greater life expectancy, and complicated procedures to access care have increased the need for adult children and aging spouses to provide uncompensated care to loved ones. Due to the stress of this burden, caregivers are at risk for depression and caregiver burnout.

Agencies and associations provide helpful and up-to-date information, including medication information, resources, and support groups. These rich resources can be found online. They include:

- AARP
- Alzheimer's Association
- U.S. National Library of Medicine
- Family Caregiver Alliance
- U.S. Department of Veterans Affairs
- Caregiver Action Network
- National Institute on Aging
- Administration on Aging

Unfortunately, having family caregivers may not be an option for older adults who have chronic psychiatric disorders. Schizophrenia and bipolar disorders often take a toll on family members and intimate relationships, and it is not uncommon for those with severe mental illness to have no family available for support as they age. Grown children may be estranged because of a parent's frequent hospitalization, poor parenting ability, or paranoid symptoms. The support system of those aging with chronic mental illness often becomes case managers, community nurses, and mental health providers.

Ageism

Western cultures do not generally view growing older as a privilege, and old age does not tend to confer a revered social status upon those who have attained it. Ageism is discrimination against older people due to negative and inaccurate stereotypes (Lundebjerg et al., 2017). This bias differs from other forms of discrimination in that it cuts across gender, race, religion, and socioeconomic status. Ageism is notable in the language we use, public policy, and research.

Language

Certain terms in healthcare related to older people have been rejected for being stereotypical and pejorative (i.e., negative connotations or disapproving) such as demented, senile, or aged. One term that is still widely used has come under criticism, namely, the word "elderly." Referring to people as elderly is considered ageist and diminishes older adults as sick, frail, and physically dependent. Furthermore, elderly has no equal term for young people (pederly?). Senior citizen is another bothersome term that has, again, no opposite in describing young people (junior citizens?) and is generally considered an inappropriate title.

President John F. Kennedy designated May 1963 as Senior Citizens Month, which was celebrated for 17 years (U.S. Census Bureau, 2017). In 1980, President Jimmy Carter issued a proclamation changing the name of this observance to Older Americans Month. More recently, in response to public sentiment and following the American Medical Association's *Manual of Style*, the *Journal of the American Geriatric Society* (Lundebjerg et al., 2017) released guidelines for referring to people 65 years of age and older. Words that writers are asked not use in this journal's articles are aged, elder, elderly, and seniors. Instead, writers are instructed to use the term older adult in describing people older than 65. In addition, contributors are asked to identify a specific age range (e.g., "older adults aged 75 to 84") when discussing their research or making recommendations about patient care or the health of a population.

In this chapter specifically, and in this textbook as a whole, the term elderly has been eliminated. Instead, we are using the term older adult exclusively to refer to the over-65 population.

Public Policy

You can observe the results of ageism in every level of society. Financial and political support for programs geared toward older adults are difficult to obtain. However, groups such as the Gray Panthers and the AARP are powerful governmental lobbying groups that fight to change this disturbing attitude.

Research

Traditionally, researchers have used subjects between the ages of 18 and 65 when developing treatments. Older adults have been excluded from clinical trials for medication being tested due to concerns over polypharmacy or the presence of a chronic illness. Information about medications obtained from a younger, healthier population may not be generalizable to older, sicker adults. In 2012, the FDA issued guidelines that recommended the geriatric population be included in clinical trials of medications. The rationale for this recommendation included:

- Trial participants should represent the patient population receiving the therapy.
- People over age 65 make up the majority of patients being treated for chronic conditions.
- This population has age-related physiological changes that can affect the pharmacokinetics and pharmacodynamics of medications, which may influence dosing recommendations.

HEALTHCARE DECISION-MAKING

Advance Directives and Portable Medical Orders

A written document stating how you want medical decisions to be made if you lose the ability to make them for yourself is called an advance directive. It may also be called a living will. This document spells out what sort of life-prolonging measures should be taken if there's no hope for recovery. Another document, a portable medical order abbreviated POLST, delineates what sort of action should be taken in the event of a cardiopulmonary arrest. These topics are addressed in more depth in Chapter 30.

Guardianship

A **guardianship** is a court-ordered relationship in which one party, the guardian, acts on behalf of an individual, the ward. For a guardianship to be enacted, the ward must be lacking capacity to manage personal and/or financial affairs. After an evaluation, usually by a physician or psychologist, probate court determines if guardianship is necessary. Many people with mental illness, mental retardation, traumatic brain injuries, and organic brain disorders, such as dementia, have guardians. It is important that healthcare workers identify patients who have guardians and communicate with the guardians when healthcare decisions are being made.

APPLICATION OF THE NURSING PROCESS

Nurses work with and provide care for older adults in a variety of settings. In each of these settings, the nurse is responsible for applying the nursing process in a patient-centered way. Some nursing students are not given adequate information and are not exposed to older patients, and they may hold ageist views when beginning nursing careers (Chippendale, 2015). It is vital for nurses to provide respect to older patients and appreciate their wisdom and life experience. Positive attitudes toward older adults and their care can be promoted and instilled during basic nursing education.

There are many theories about the process of aging from biological, genetic, psychological, and psychosocial perspectives (Box 31.4). Substantial literature is available regarding what shortens life expectancy and on behaviors that predispose humans to disease. Current trends center on the concept of aging well and how aging well can be accomplished. Nursing is about maintenance of health, prevention of illness, and helping individuals with their response to disease. There is a growing focus on healthy eating, exercise, socialization, spirituality, effective coping skills, avoiding alcohol/tobacco, and healthy relationships as a basis for aging well. Nurses can play a vital role in this movement as educators and advocates for health.

Box 31.5 provides some facts and myths about aging that influence how society perceives the older adult.

BOX 31.4 Major Theories of Aging

Biological

- **Cellular functioning:** Cells accumulate damage, resulting in errors of replication.
- **Error theory:** Error in protein synthesis results in impaired cellular function.
- **Oxidative stress theory:** Production of free radicals increases and the body's ability to remove them decreases, resulting in DNA damage.
- **Wear-and-tear theory:** Internal and external stressors harm cells.
- **Programmed aging theory:** Biological or genetic clock plays out on genes.
- **Neuroendocrine theory:** A programmed decline in the functioning of the nervous, endocrine, and immune systems where cells lose their ability to reproduce.
- **Immunity theory:** An accumulation of damage and decline in the immune system.

Developmental

- **Jung's theory of personality:** Individuals move from outward achievement to self-acceptance.
- **Erikson:** Integrity is built on morality and ethics.
- **Peck:** Redefining self, letting go of occupational identity, rising above body discomforts, and establishing meaning accompanies successful aging.
- **Maslow:** Self-actualization and the evolution of developmental needs occur as the individual ages.
- **Tornstam:** Disengagement with the world can be a time of introspection, leading to wisdom.

Psychosocial

- **Role theory:** The ability of an individual to adapt to changing roles predicts adjustment to aging.
- **Activity theory:** Actions, roles, and social pursuits are important for satisfactory aging.
- **Disengagement theory:** Mutual withdrawal occurs between the aging person and others.
- **Continuity theory:** Life satisfaction and activity are expressions of enduring personality traits.
- **Age-stratification theory:** Individuals are viewed as members of an age group (e.g., young, middle-age, old) with similarities to others in the group.
- **Modernization theory:** Modern society devalues the contributions of elders and elders themselves.

Data from Jett, K. (2015). Theories of aging. In E. A. Touhy & K. Jett (Eds.). *Ebersole & Hess' toward healthy aging: Human needs and nursing response* (9th ed., pp. 31–39). St. Louis, MO: Elsevier.

BOX 31.5 Facts and Myths About Aging

Facts

- The senses of vision, hearing, touch, taste, and smell decline with age.
- Muscular strength decreases with age. Muscle fibers atrophy and decrease in number.
- Regular sexual expressions are important to maintain sexual capacity and effective sexual performance.
- At least 50% of restorative sleep is lost as a result of the aging process.
- Older adults are major consumers of prescription drugs because of the high incidence of chronic diseases in this population.
- Older adults have a high incidence of depression.
- Many individuals experience difficulty when they retire.
- Older adults are prone to becoming victims of crime.
- Older widows appear to adjust better than younger ones.

Myths

- Most adults past the age of 65 have dementia.
- Older adults are unable to learn new tasks.
- As individuals age, they become more rigid in their thinking and set in their ways.
- Older adults are well off and no longer impoverished.
- Most older adults are infirm and require help with daily activities.
- Most older adults are socially isolated and lonely.

ASSESSMENT

Nurses who work with older adults need specific knowledge about normal aging, drug interactions, and chronic disease. Those who work with older patients who have mental health problems or cognitive deficits need to have additional skills in effective communication, behavioral intervention, and recognition of how the care setting affects the older individual. The National Institutes of Health recommends a comprehensive geriatric assessment. This comprehensive assessment includes a focus on physical and mental health; functional, economic, and social status; and environmental factors that might impinge on the person's well-being. Fig. 31.4 provides an example of a comprehensive geriatric assessment.

Assessment Strategies With Older Adults

An examination and interview of an older adult conducted in unfamiliar surroundings can produce anxiety. Unlike younger patients who may be comfortable discussing personal issues—family conflicts, feelings of sadness, sexual practices, finances, and bodily functions—older adults may view these topics as private or taboo. As a result, they may be uncomfortable discussing them. It is important to respect these feelings while reviewing essential history by:

- Conducting the interview in a private area.
- Introducing oneself and asking patients what they would like to be called (unless you are an older adult, the use of the first name is rarely appropriate unless you are asked to do so).
- Establishing rapport and putting the patient at ease by sitting or standing at the same level as the patient.
- Ensuring that lighting is adequate and noise level is low in recognition of the fact that hearing and vision may be impaired.
- Using touch (with permission) to convey warmth while at the same time respecting the patient's comfort level with personal touch.
- Summarizing the interaction, inviting feedback and questions, and thanking patients for giving their time and information.

Physical Assessment

A thorough assessment, including a physical assessment and diagnostic testing, must precede any treatment and/or diagnosis of a mental illness in older adults. Common tests include thyroid, kidney, and liver function; complete blood count; comprehensive metabolic panel; vitamin B_{12}, folic acid, and therapeutic drug levels; urinalysis; serology (RPR); β-type natriuretic peptide (BNP); HIV testing; and computed tomography (CT) of the head when indicated.

Medication Reconciliation

In older adults, it is important to perform a systematic review of current medication use known as medication reconciliation. Medication reconciliation is the process of developing the most accurate list possible of all medications a patient is taking. This list should include prescription, non-prescription, vitamin, and herbal drug name, dose, frequency, and route. The purpose of this process is to reduce adverse incidents, side effects, and potentially lethal combinations.

Assessing the use of multiple medications for the same condition (polypharmacy) includes prescription, over-the-counter drugs, and herbal agents. Adverse drug reactions, or

COMPREHENSIVE GERIATRIC ASSESSMENT						
Name:		Date of birth:			Gender:	
Physical Health						
Chronic disorder						
Vision	Adequate	Inadequate	Eyeglasses: Y N		Needs evaluation	
Hearing	Adequate	Inadequate	Hearing aids: Y N			
Mobility	Ambulatory: Y N		Assistive device:			
	Falls: Y N				Needs evaluation	
Nutrition	Albumin:	TLC:	HCT:			
	Weight:	Weight loss or gain: Y N			Needs evaluation	
Incontinence	Y N	Treatment:	Y N		Needs evaluation	
Medications	Total number:	Reviewed & revised: Y N				
	Adverse effects/allergy:					
Screening	Cholesterol:	TSH:	B_{12}:		Folate:	
	Colonoscopy: Date:		N/A			
	Mammogram: Date:		N/A			
	Osteoporosis: Date:		N/A			
	Pap smear: Date:		N/A			
	PSA: Date:		N/A			
Immunization	Influenza: Date:					
	Pneumonia: Date:					
	Tetanus: Date:		Booster:			
Counseling	Diet	Exercise	Calcium	Vitamin D		
	Smoking	Alcohol	Driving	Injury prevention		
Mental Health						
Dementia	Y N	MMSE score:	Date:	Cause (if known):		
Depression	Y N	GDS score:	Date:	Treatment: Y N		
Functional Status						
ADL	Bathing: I D		Dressing: I D		Toileting: I D	
	Transferring: I D		Feeding: I D		Continence: Y N	

Fig. 31.4 Comprehensive geriatric assessment. *ADL*, Activities of daily living; B_{12}, vitamin B^{12}; *D*, dependent; *GDS*, Geriatric Depression Scale; *HCT*, hematocrit; *I*, independent; *MMSE*, Mini-Mental State Examination; *N*, no; *PSA*, prostate-specific antigen; *TLC*, total lymphocyte count; *TSH*, thyroid-stimulating hormone; *Y*, yes.

negative responses to drugs, are common among the older adult. Older adults are at greater risk for these events due to multiple medical problems and memory issues that may result in taking too little or too much medication. Renal and liver impairment affect excretion and are associated with dose-related adverse reactions.

Metabolic changes and decreased drug clearance compound the risk of drug-drug interactions. The risk of adverse drug interactions doubles for people taking five to seven medications as compared with those taking fewer than five medications. For people taking eight or more medications, the risk of adverse drug reactions increases fourfold. The American Geriatrics Society (2019) recently updated the criteria for and list of potentially inappropriate medications for older adults. The list now includes 30 medications or medication classes that should be avoided in older adults, and 40 medications or medication classes that should be used with caution. Two criteria were added due to the opioid crisis—not prescribing opioids along with benzodiazepines or gabapentinoids.

Prescribing cascades happen when drug-induced symptoms are treated with another drug. The provider may assess the side effect of the first drug as part of the original medical problem or a new one. Prescribing cascades are particularly problematic and complicated. One of the most common examples is when a person begins antiparkinson therapy for symptoms brought about by antipsychotics. Antiparkinson drugs may bring about new and dangerous symptoms, such as delirium and orthostatic hypotension. Cholinesterase inhibitor drugs used to treat dementia (e.g., donepezil, rivastigmine, and galantamine) may cause urinary incontinence and diarrhea. These symptoms may result in a prescribing cascade with use of an anticholinergic such as oxybutynin, which can cause cognitive dulling and confusion.

Pharmacists have begun to play a critical role in reviewing and advising on matters of prescribing for the older adult. Maher et al. (2014) identify how polypharmacy affects the older adult. They cite nine negative clinical consequences of inappropriate drug use:

1. Increased healthcare costs
2. Adverse drug reactions
3. Drug interactions
4. Nonadherence
5. Decline in functional status
6. Increased cognitive impairment
7. Increased falls
8. Increased urinary incontinence
9. Increased risk of malnutrition

Common problems associated with medication include confusion, which can be caused by anticholinergics, antihistamines, benzodiazepines, and benzodiazepine withdrawal. Psychosis has been linked to the use of levodopa, steroids, and even cholesterol-lowering medications. Depressive symptoms have been linked with alpha-adrenergics and opiates.

Mental Status Exam

Assessment of the cognitive, behavioral, and emotional status of the older adult is important in managing the nursing care

of the patient. The periodic repetition of screening tools serves to evaluate the effectiveness of interventions targeting mood problems. The Geriatric Depression Scale (Short Form) (Box 31.6) is a subjective yes/no questionnaire. The Cornell Scale for Depression in Dementia is an objective behavioral checklist for caregivers to help identify the presence of depressive symptoms (Alexopoulos, 1988). It is also important to recognize that having thoughts or wishes of death may occur during times of acute medical illness or emotional distress, so it is essential to further assess for suicidal intent and/or plans by asking questions such as:

- Have you ever thought about ending your life or wish you didn't wake up?
- Have you ever felt that life is not worth living?
- Have you ever tried to hurt yourself in the past?
- Have you considered specific methods to harm yourself?
- What methods have you considered to harm yourself?
- Do you have the means to harm yourself, such as firearms? (This question may be addressed to family members and/or caregivers as appropriate.)

When individuals—older adults included—are sick or are in significant pain, they may verbalize "I just wish I would die" or "If I had a gun, I'd shoot myself." These comments should never be ignored, but rather explored. Often, people may simply feel frustrated, desperate, ignored, unheard, or disrespected, and unable to articulate these emotions. Encourage patients to say more about what they are experiencing, get more information, actively listen, and offer support. These types of statements and data are always documented and reported to the care provider. If there are active suicidal thoughts and intent, the individual

---

BOX 31.6 Geriatric Depression Scale (Short Form)

Geriatric Depression Scale: Short Form: Choose the best answer for how you have felt over the past week:

1. Are you basically satisfied with your life? YES / **NO**
2. Have you dropped many of your activities and interests? **YES** / NO
3. Do you feel that your life is empty? **YES** / NO
4. Do you often get bored? YES / **NO**
5. Are you in good spirits most of the time? YES / **NO**
6. Are you afraid that something bad is going to happen to you? **YES** / NO
7. Do you feel happy most of the time? YES / **NO**
8. Do you often feel helpless? **YES** / NO
9. Do you prefer to stay at home, rather than going out and doing new things? **YES** / NO
10. Do you feel you have more problems with memory than most? **YES** / NO
11. Do you think it is wonderful to be alive now? YES / **NO**
12. Do you feel pretty worthless the way you are now? **YES** / NO
13. Do you feel full of energy? YES / **NO**
14. Do you feel that your situation is hopeless? **YES** / NO
15. Do you think that most people are better off than you are? **YES** / NO

Answers in bold indicate depression. Score 1 point for each bolded answer. A score >5 points is suggestive of depression. A score ≥10 points is almost always indicative of depression. A score >5 points should warrant a follow-up comprehensive assessment.

From Greenberg, S. H. (2012). *Geriatric Depression Scale (GDS)*. Hartford Institute for Geriatric Nursing, NYU College of Nursing. Retrieved from https://consultgeri.org/try-this/general-assessment/issue-4.pdf.

should not be left alone. Notify other staff and the mental health team and develop a plan to keep the patient safe.

Interventions for the prevention of suicide in older adults are discussed in greater depth later in this chapter. Also refer to Chapter 25 for a more detailed discussion of suicide assessment and intervention.

Older Adult Drivers

In general, older adults engage in safer driving behaviors than other age groups, including more frequently wearing seat belts, driving when conditions are safest, and not drinking and driving (CDC, 2020b). However, older adults—particularly those age 75 or more and male—have higher crash rate deaths than middle-age (35 to 54) drivers (Cicchino, 2015). These deaths are mainly due to increased vulnerability in the event of a crash. In addition, age-related declines in vision and cognitive functioning might affect driving abilities.

If there is evidence an older adult can no longer safely drive a vehicle or if there have been occurrences of frequent small collisions or getting lost, it is appropriate to consult with medical providers for assessment. It may be appropriate to contact the state bureau of motor vehicles for a driving evaluation to determine the older adult's ability for safe operation of a vehicle. Other times, in the best interest of public safety, family can be encouraged to facilitate having older adults give up the keys to the car or disable a car so it will not run.

⊕ CONSIDERING CULTURE

Keeping Jose at Home

Jose is a 75-year-old married man born and raised in Puerto Rico. He came to the United States in his 20s, served in the military, and worked in the steel industry until retirement. Jose was active in his church and served as the treasurer for many years. He was head of a family with five daughters in a traditional patriarchal home. Jose's wife never worked outside the home, did not drive, and spoke little English, despite having been in the United States most of her adult life.

The family began to notice significant changes in Jose's behavior and function. His primary care provider ruled out physical illness, and Jose was referred for Alzheimer's disease evaluation.

His wife and his oldest daughter, Maria, accompanied him for the evaluation. Jose was pleasant and cooperative. His daughter helped to interpret when necessary.

Jose's wife and Maria were most alarmed by Jose's withdrawal from church activities after experiencing an inability to manage his treasurer duties. He also lost interest in activities, had difficulty organizing his day, and needed reminders to shave and shower. Evaluation revealed a moderate to severe cognitive impairment.

Despite being instructed not to drive, his daughters were not willing to take the keys as this would be disrespectful. Eventually, Jose was pulled over by police due to erratic driving. He was agitated at the time and was briefly hospitalized.

Recognizing the potential danger in driving, his family devised a solution. They disabled the car. This allowed Jose to maintain his authority, keep the keys, yet prevented him from driving.

Jose's wife and daughters made sure Jose took his medication, had proper nutrition, and was able to maintain his daily routine. Jose eventually stopped speaking English and reverted to his primary language. Although the dementia progressed over the next 5 years, he was never placed in long-term care. His family continued to care for him until the end.

Older Adult Abuse

Abuse or exploitation is another area to explore during a nursing assessment. Questions about being hit, pushed, kicked, and slapped are important. It is also imperative to inquire about care being withheld. Not being fed, cleaned, helped, or cared for is also abuse. Asking "How are you being treated at home?" or "Are you afraid of anyone?" may encourage further exploration. Financial exploitation is another issue that is difficult to uncover. Older adults may feel ashamed or embarrassed to admit they have been taken advantage of by family, friends, or strangers. Box 31.7 provides helpful interview techniques to use with older adults. The topic of older adult violence is discussed in depth in Chapter 28.

NURSING DIAGNOSIS

The *International Classification for Nursing Practice* (ICNP) (International Council of Nurses, 2019) provides nursing diagnoses that are useful for older adults. Most of the nursing diagnoses identified can also be written in terms of *risk for.* Maslow's Hierarchy of Needs (see Chapter 2) provides a useful framework for prioritizing nursing care. Therefore, *acute/chronic pain, impaired low nutrition intake, impaired fluid intake, constipation,* and *impaired sleep* are essential diagnoses to consider in the older adult population.

Safety needs are the next level of priority. Some essential safety diagnoses include *risk for injury, risk for falls, impaired ability to manage medication regime, victim of older adult abuse,* and *confusion.* Higher level needs fall under Maslow's categories of love and belonging needs and esteem. Specific ICNP nursing diagnoses address those higher-level needs such as *loneliness,*

BOX 31.7 Helpful Techniques for Interviewing Older Adults

- Gather preliminary data before the session and keep questionnaires relatively short.
- Ask about often-overlooked problems, such as difficulty sleeping, incontinence, falling, depression, dizziness, or loss of energy.
- Pace the interview to allow the patient to formulate answers; resist the tendency to interrupt prematurely.
- Use yes-or-no or simple-choice questions if the older patient has trouble coping with open-ended questions.
- Begin with general questions such as, "How can I help you most at this visit?" or "What's been happening?"
- Be alert for information on the patient's relationships with others, thoughts about families or co-workers, typical responses to stress, and attitudes toward aging, illness, occupation, and death.
- A request such as, "Tell me about how you spend your days" often provides important information.
- Assess mental status for deficits in recent or remote memory and determine if confusion exists.
- Be aware of all medications the patient is taking, and assess for side effects, efficacy, and possible drug interactions.
- Determine how fast the condition of the patient has been changing to assess the extent of the patient's concerns.
- Include the family or significant other in the interview process for added input, clarification, support, and reinforcement.

hopelessness, impaired role performance, chronic low self-esteem, and *disturbed personal identity.*

The family/caregivers' role in the lives of older adults may be the focus of nursing care, particularly if the patient becomes incapacitated. Identifying problems such as *caregiver stress* and *impaired family process* support the provision of meaningful nursing interventions.

OUTCOMES IDENTIFICATION

Shared decision making promotes goal attainment and effective nursing care. Including the patient and caregivers (when appropriate) supports the goals and care. Outcome criteria are realistic and attainable. As with any nursing care plan, outcomes should seek to improve the nursing diagnoses, resulting in such outcomes as improved fluid intake, no injury, and improved role performance.

IMPLEMENTATION

The trend for patient-centered care, relationship-based care, and the patient as a participant in care may be foreign concepts to the older adult. Most have experienced medical care as "listening to the doctor" regardless of whether or not they agree. This shift in approach may need much reinforcement with the older adult who has been socialized as a passive recipient of healthcare.

Certain psychotherapeutic methods are especially useful for older adults:

- Providing empathetic understanding and active listening
- Encouraging ventilation of feelings and normalizing emotional responses
- Reestablishing emotional equilibrium when anxiety is moderate to severe
- Providing health education, discussing alternative solutions, and encouraging questions
- Assisting in the use of problem-solving approaches
- Allowing adequate time to process information
- Ensuring hearing aids are working or using an amplifier to facilitate good communication
- Providing written information in large print

The nurse uses counseling skills to assist the patient with exploring the present situation, looking at alternatives, and planning for the future. Sometimes, counseling is provided in a group setting. This approach helps build relationships, provides focus on the here and now, and reduces feelings of isolation.

There is growing evidence that physical and mental exercise helps maintain and improve cognitive function. Nurses can encourage this activity with cognitive stimulation activities, which may be conducted individually or in groups of five to eight people. This evidence-based approach may result in significant improvement in language skills. Examples of cognitively stimulating activities are word games, puzzles, music, and discussion of past events.

Reminiscence is a cognitive stimulation activity that engages individuals in socialization and rapport building. In groups or individually, the nurse can encourage discussion about past pleasant events or memories such as first car, favorite memory from school, favorite band or song, or seasonal activities growing up. Assisting to evoke pleasant feelings or memories is an

BOX 31.8 Patient and Family Teaching: Drug Safety

- Learn about your medicines: Read medicine labels and package inserts and follow the directions.
- If you have questions, ask your nurse, pharmacist, or primary care provider.
- Talk to your team of healthcare professionals about your medical conditions, health concerns, and all the medicines you take (prescription and over-the-counter medicines), as well as dietary supplements, vitamins, and herbal supplements. The more they know, the more they can help.
- Keep track of side effects or possible drug interactions, and let your doctor know right away about any unexpected symptoms or changes in the way you feel.
- Be sure to keep all care provider appointments.
- Use a calendar, pillbox, or something to help you remember what medications you need to take and when.
- Write down information your healthcare provider gives you about your medicines or your health condition.
- Take a friend or relative to your doctor's appointments if you think you need help to understand or remember what the doctor tells you.
- Have a "medicine check-up" at least once a year. Go through your medicine cabinet to get rid of old or expired medicines.
- Ask your healthcare provider or pharmacist to go over all the medicines you now take. Remember to tell them about all the over-the-counter medicines, vitamins, dietary supplements, and herbal supplements you take.

effective method to improve mood, particularly in those with memory impairment.

Evidence about the biology of mental illness and the discovery of new psychotropic medications has expanded the role of nurses who work with older adults. Nurses play a vital role in monitoring, reporting, and managing medication side effects such as acute dystonia, akathisia, pseudoparkinsonism, neuroleptic malignant syndrome (NMS), serotonin syndrome, and anticholinergic effects. Physical assessment of response to medication is also important; this includes monitoring vital signs, pain, laboratory work, elimination (bowel and bladder), changes in gait, prevention of falls, and neurological checks when appropriate. Teaching patients and/or family about management of medications is a vital part of nursing care (Box 31.8).

EVALUATION

Evaluation of nursing care for older adults, as with any population, is ongoing. You may find that outcomes are only partially met, and plans may need to be revised to reflect realistic outcomes. Also, priorities may often change when caring for older adults, and the plan of care is revised to reflect those changes.

TREATMENT MODALITIES
Psychological Therapies

Advanced practice professionals such as psychiatric nurse practitioners may provide individual and/or group psychotherapy to older adults. Individual modalities, such as cognitive behavioral therapy, motivational interviewing, interpersonal therapy, and psychodynamic therapy, are commonly used. Group therapy focuses on instilling hope by diminishing social isolation and loneliness. Group members can learn creative ways to improve mood and increase quality of life.

TREATMENT SETTINGS FOR OLDER ADULTS

Hospital-Based Care

Care for older adults with psychiatric conditions may become unmanageable at home.

Medical providers are responsible for determining an appropriate level of care. This may range from acute outpatient options to residential care and hospitalization. These and other treatment options follow.

Partial Hospitalization

Partial hospitalization programs are recommended for ambulatory patients who do not need 24-hour psychiatric nursing care. These programs are often used as a bridge from inpatient care to community living. They provide structured activities along with nursing and medical supervision, intervention, and treatment. These programs tend to be located within general hospitals, in psychiatric hospitals, or as part of the community mental health system.

Inpatient

An older adult may require inpatient psychiatric care for conditions such as acute mental status changes with agitation, psychotic symptoms, major depressive disorder, suicidal ideation, bipolar disorder, and schizophrenia. Inpatient treatment is recommended when the patient is at risk of self-harm, whether intentional or unintentional, or poses a risk of harm to other people.

Hospitalization also may be an opportunity for the patient to receive much-needed physical assessment of the skin, feet, hair, mouth, and perineal areas. These assessments can uncover hidden infections, unhealed wounds, and growths that may otherwise have been missed and can lead to needed medical attention.

Specialized geropsychiatric units provide a comprehensive and specialized approach to care. These units utilize a multidisciplinary approach to assessment, treatment planning, implementation, and evaluation of care. Ideally, the team consists of registered nurses, geriatric psychiatrists, geriatricians, social workers, pharmacists, psychologists, dietitians, occupational therapists, and physical therapists.

One of the major roles of the nurse is milieu management. This involves assisting in adjustment to the environment, keeping the unit safe by making sure roommates are compatible, call lights are within reach, and patients at risk for falling are close to the nurses' station.

Recognizing the tone of the unit and making modifications when needed, such as reducing noise levels and decluttering areas, are critical roles of the staff nurse. Another vital aspect of nursing is the prevention and reduction of agitation by maintaining a visible presence on the unit and anticipating the patient's needs. Crisis intervention techniques may be necessary if an agitated patient does not respond to redirection or verbal attempts to deescalate agitation. As a crisis situation unfolds, staff response will largely determine the outcome, and a well-trained crisis team improves these outcomes. The crisis team leader is usually a nurse for several reasons:

1. Nurses provide professional care 24 hours a day, 7 days a week, and have detailed knowledge of patients and the milieu.
2. The nurse is aware of the patient's medical condition.
3. The nurse is able to guide the team and help prevent injury to patients who may need physical restraint.

After the crisis has been deescalated, the team leader, the team, and other patients (as indicated) need to discuss the situation; this will help restore a sense of safety and calm. As the agitated patient gains control, it is important to help the individual ease back into the milieu with dignity.

Home-Based Services

Day Care Programs

Multipurpose centers provide a broad range of services, including (1) health promotion and wellness programs; (2) health screening; (3) social, educational, and recreational activities; (4) meals; and (5) information and referral services. For those in need of mostly custodial care services, adult day care is an appropriate choice. Older adults are cared for during the day and stay in a home environment at night. The programs allow older adults to continue their present living arrangements and maintain their social ties to the community; they also relieve families of the burden of 24-hour-a-day care for older adult dependents.

Home Healthcare

Home healthcare assists the homebound older adult to adjust to and manage illness and disability either before or after hospitalization. It is often the role of the home healthcare nurse to help a person affected by a cognitive disorder, medical illness, or a severe and persistent mental illness to remain in the home. The National Association of Area Agencies on Aging assists in providing local home care services, such as housekeeping, meal preparation, and assistance with ADLs, to increase the older adult's ability to live independently. Chapter 4 discusses home psychiatric-mental healthcare in greater detail.

Community Support Services

Community support services are an alternative to promote the older adult's independent functioning and reduce the stress on the family system. These programs provide specialized case management services that assist older adults with coordination of care and other supports, such as Meals on Wheels and transportation.

Respite Care

Family caregivers are at great risk for burnout. Respite care is designed to allow caregivers to have a break for a specific number of days. During this time, the patient is admitted to a nursing facility for a planned number of days. Family can then go on vacation, travel, or just have a needed break from caregiving. Respite care also can be provided in the home.

Residential Care

As discussed in Chapter 4, the psychiatric care system has increasingly become focused on the goal of community living rather than institutional living, but resources necessary to meet this goal have been chronically underfunded. Individuals who would benefit from residential care are often moved from the most structured environment (inpatient care) to unstructured environments. These settings vary greatly and families and guardians should be educated to investigate what specific services will be provided.

Assisted Living

Assisted living can provide care for people who are managing chronic mental illness such as major depressive disorder or anxiety, or have complex medication management needs. This setting is utilized when a resident needs minimal assistance with ADLs. Meals are provided as well as 24-hour assistance as needed. Care is tailored to the needs of the resident, and care is paid for based on needs. This level of care is usually not covered by insurance and can be quite expensive. There are waiver programs in some states that provide for Medicaid reimbursement.

Skilled Nursing Facilities

As acute hospital care of older adults with psychiatric illnesses is decreasing, the use of long-term skilled nursing facilities is increasing. The use of these facilities to treat older adults with mental illness is controversial. Opponents fear that skilled nursing facilities will become the psychiatric institutions of the 21st century, providing little more than custodial care.

Whereas some long-term care settings provide specialized psychiatric-mental healthcare or behavioral units, most do not. There may be little consistency in the education of nurses and nursing assistants in appropriate psychiatric assessment and intervention. Staff may believe that patients who refuse personal hygiene, medication, or wound care are exercising their rights to refuse care rather than recognizing the negative symptoms of schizophrenia or major depressive disorder. Nurses who repeatedly accept these refusals without further evaluation may inadvertently contribute to a patient's deterioration.

Federal legislation has had a significant impact on the treatment of older adults in extended-care facilities. The Patient Self-Determination Act (PSDA) of 1990 encourages all people to engage in decisions about the types and extent of medical care they want to accept or refuse should they become unable to make those decisions due to illness. This Act requires all healthcare agencies (hospitals, long-term care facilities, and home health agencies) receiving Medicare and Medicaid reimbursement to recognize the living will and power of attorney for healthcare as advance directives.

Nurses can play an important role in advocating for psychiatric evaluation and intervention to assist with (1) medication management, (2) monitoring and documenting behavioral issues, (3) notifying the physician of behavioral changes, and (4) planning care for the needs of those residents with mental illness.

Due to past inappropriate use of restraints, which led to injuries and deaths, federal legislation regarding their safe use was put into place. The requirements governing the use of restraints include the following:

1. Consultation with a physical and/or occupational therapist.
2. The least restrictive measures must be considered and documented.
3. A physician's order is required.
4. Consent of the resident or family must be obtained.
5. Documentation must be provided that the restraint enables the resident to maintain maximum functional and psychological well-being.

KEY POINTS TO REMEMBER

- The older adult population is increasing exponentially.
- The increase in the number of older adults poses a challenge not only to nurses but also to the entire healthcare system to respond to the special needs of this population.
- Attitudes toward older adults are often negative, reflecting ageism—a bias against older adults based solely on age. Ageism occurs at all levels of society and even among healthcare providers, which affects the way we render care to our older patients.
- Maintaining a positive regard that demonstrates respect will improve interactions with older adults.
- Nurses who care for older adults in various settings may function at different levels. All should be knowledgeable about the process of aging and be aware of the differences between normal and abnormal aging changes.

- The PSDA established guidelines and a philosophy of care that call for patients to be free from unnecessary use of drugs and physical restraints.
- The use of more than five medications doubles the risk of an adverse reaction.
- Accurate pain assessment is important, and the nurse must remember that older adults tend to understate their pain.
- Nurses working with older adult patients with psychiatric conditions should be knowledgeable about psychotherapeutic approaches relevant for the older adult.
- A variety of treatment settings are available to older adults. The level of disability, cognitive abilities, and psychiatric disorders influence the choice of setting.

CRITICAL THINKING

1. Mr. Jackson, a 70-year-old African American, has received treatment for alcohol withdrawal. He is quiet, refuses to eat, does not sleep at night, and admits to wishing he would die. He also confides that he attempted suicide when his wife died 5 years earlier, and that is when he started drinking heavily.
   a. Culturally, what may be helpful to know about older African Americans' response to major depressive disorder?

   b. Which depression assessment tool is appropriate to use in assessing the severity of Mr. Jackson's condition? Explain your answer.
2. Mrs. Duff is 75 years old and lives with her daughter's family. She has moderate-advanced Alzheimer's disease. Although Mrs. Duff's family wants to keep her at home for as long as possible, they are overwhelmed by her needs and unable to leave her alone. What community supports might be best for Mrs. Duff? Explain your answer.

CHAPTER REVIEW

1. During an interview with a patient, which question asked of an older adult is associated with the Patient Self-Determination Act?
   a. "Who besides yourself may have access to your medical information?"
   b. "Have you discussed your end-of-life choices with your family or designated surrogate?"
   c. "Do you have the information you need to make an informed decision about your treatment?"
   d. "How can I help you feel comfortable about this interview and any decisions you need to make?"

2. Which statement made by a nurse requires immediate correction by the supervisor?
   a. "Many older patients are depressed."
   b. "Retirement is a difficult time for older patients."
   c. "Cognitive decline is normal in patients who are 65 and older."
   d. "Sleep-related problems are often reported by older adults."

3. Considering psychosocial role theory, which patient demonstrates healthy adjustment to aging?
   a. The 70-year-old who is training for a 5-mile running race
   b. The older adult who controls diabetes with diet and exercise
   c. The retiree who volunteers 3 days a week at the local library
   d. The 80-year-old who is upbeat and hopeful during chemotherapy for lung cancer

4. The older patient is discussing chronic pain and asks the primary care provider for a prescription. Which medication should the nurse anticipate being ordered rather than an opioid?
   a. Gabapentin
   b. Acetaminophen
   c. Morphine
   d. Fentanyl

5. Which statement by an older patient with a mild neurocognitive disorder demonstrates a safe response to beginning a new medication?
   a. "I read the information the pharmacist gave me when I got the prescription filled."
   b. "My daughter comes with me to appointments so that we get all the information we need."
   c. "I know I can call my doctor if I think of any questions later."
   d. "I always follow the instructions on the medication bottle."

6. Anxiety problems in older adults can manifest as a fear of falling, greatly influencing an older adult's personal freedom. A home health nurse checking on a patient with mild dementia and anxiety related to falling should question which new order?
   a. Yoga and tai-chi
   b. Xanax
   c. Relaxation techniques
   d. Electric wheelchair

7. Fred is an older adult with spinal stenosis and who is being treated with a short-term prescription of opioids for an acute episode of back pain. His nurse recognizes additional teaching is necessary when Fred states:
   a. "Sitting up straight seems to reduce the pain."
   b. "Sometimes I use a heating pad on my back."
   c. "Once I get moving for the day my pain gets better."
   d. "My wife and I share my Norco for our aches and pains."

8. Ling works as a registered nurse in an Alzheimer's care home. Ling has a specialized rapport-building technique she uses called reminiscence. She uses this technique by:
   a. Telling the residents stories about her grandparents' lives.
   b. Playing music from the residents' formative years.
   c. Reviewing movies that the residents enjoy.
   d. Encouraging the residents to talk about pleasurable past events.

9. Marco, age 83, has dementia and difficulty feeding himself despite the fact that there is nothing wrong with his motor functions. Which term should the nurse use to document this finding?
   a. Aphasia
   b. Apraxia
   c. Agnosia
   d. Anergia

10. Programs recommended for ambulatory patients who do not need 24-hour nursing care with structured activities along with nursing and medical supervision, intervention, and treatment are called:
    a. Respite programs
    b. Inpatient care units
    c. Hospice
    d. Partial hospitalization programs

1. **b**; 2. **c**; 3. **c**; 4. **a**; 5. **b**; 6. **b**; 7. **d**; 8. **d**; 9. **b**; 10. **d**

🌐 Visit the Evolve website for a posttest on the content in this chapter: http://evolve.elsevier.com/Varcarolis

REFERENCES

Ailshire, J. A., Beltrán-Sánchez, H., & Crimmins, E. M. (2015). Becoming centenarians: Disease and functioning trajectories of older US adults as they survive to 100. *Journals of Gerontology, 70*(2), 193–201.

Alexopoulos, G. S. (1988). Cornell scale for depression in dementia. *Biological Psychiatry, 23*(3), 271–284.

American Geriatrics Society. (2019). American Geriatrics Society 2019 updated AGS Beers Criteria® for potentially inappropriate medication use in older adults. *Journal of American Geriatric Society, 63*, 2227–2246.

Centers for Disease Control and Prevention. (2015). *Suicide: Facts at a glance.* Retrieved from http://www.cdc.gov/violenceprevention/pdf/suicide-datasheet-a.PDF.

Centers for Disease Control and Prevention. (2017). *Depression is not a normal part of growing older.* Retrieved from https://www.cdc.gov/aging/mentalhealth/depression.htm.

Centers for Disease Control and Prevention. (2020a). *1999-2018 Wide ranging online data for epidemiological research, multiple cause of death files.* Retrieved from http://wonder.cdc.gov/ucd-icd10.html.

Centers for Disease Control and Prevention. (2020b). *Older adult drivers.* Retrieved from https://www.cdc.gov/motorvehiclesafety/older_adult_drivers/index.html.

Chippendale, T. (2015). Factors associated with interest in working with older adults: Implications for educational practices. *Journal of Nursing Education, 54*(9), S89–93.

Cicchino, J. B. (2015). Why have fatality rates among older drivers declined? The relative contributions of changes in survivability and crash involvement. *Accident Analysis & Prevention, 83,* 67–73.

Congressional Research Service. (2020). *American war and military casualties: Lists and statistics.* Retrieved from https://fas.org/sgp/crs/natsec/RL32492.pdf.

He, Q., Chen, X., Wu, T., Li, L., & Fei, X. (2019). Risk of dementia in long-term benzodiazepine users: Evidence from a meta-analysis of observational studies. *Journal of Clinical Neurology, 15*(1), 9–19.

International Council of Nurses. (2019). *ICNP browser.* Retrieved from https://www.icn.ch/what-we-do/projects/ehealth-icnptm/icnp-browser.

Lundebjerg, N. E., Trucil, D. E., Hammond, E. C., & Applegate, W. B. (2017). *When it comes to older adults, language matters:* Journal of the American Geriatrics Society *adopts modified American Medical Association style.* Retrieved from https://onlinelibrary.wiley.com/doi/pdf/10.1111/jgs.14941.

Maher, R., Hanlon, J., & Hajjar, E. (2014). Clinical consequences of polypharmacy in elderly. *Expert Opinion on Drug Safety, 13*(1), 57–65.

Medicare.gov. (2020). *What medicare Part D drug plans cover.* Retrieved from Medicare.gov.

National Center for Health Statistics. (2021). *Provisional life expectancy estimates for January through June, 2020.* Retrieved from https://www.cdc.gov/nchs/data/vsrr/VSRR10-508.pdf.

National Council on Aging. (n.d.). *Facts about aging.* Retrieved from https://www.ncoa.org/news/resources-for-reporters/get-the-facts/healthy-aging-facts/.

National Institute of Mental Health. (2015). *Suicide statistics, anxiety statistics.* Retrieved from https://www.nimh.nih.gov/health/topics/suicide-prevention/index.shtml.

National Institute on Aging. (2015). *Alcohol use in older adults.* Retrieved from https://www.nia.nih.gov/health/publication/alcohol-use-older-people.

Substance Abuse and Mental Health Services Administration. (2019). *Key substance use and mental health indicators in the United States. Results from the 2018 National Survey on Drug Use and Health.* Retrieved from https://www.samhsa.gov/data/report/2018-nsduh-annual-national-report.

United Nations. (2019). *World population ageing 2019.* Retrieved from https://www.un.org/en/development/desa/population/publications/pdf/ageing/WorldPopulationAgeing2019-Highlights.pdf.

US Census Bureau. (2017). *Facts for features: Older Americans month—May 2017.* Retrieved from https://www.census.gov/newsroom/facts-for-features/2017/cb17-ff08.html.

US Census Bureau. (2019a). *National population by characteristics, 2010-2019.* Retrieved from https://www.census.gov/data/tables/time-series/demo/popest/2010s-national-detail.html.

US Census Bureau. (2019b). *Income and poverty in the United States—2018.* Retrieved from https://www.census.gov/library/publications/2019/demo/p60-266.html.

US Census Bureau. (2020). *Historical and projected life expectancy in the United States.* Retrieved from https://www.census.gov/content/dam/Census/library/publications/2020/demo/p25-1145.pdf.

United States Food and Drug Administration. (2012). *Guidance for industry E7 studies in support of special populations: Geriatrics.* Retrieved from http://www.fda.gov/downloads/Drugs/GuidanceComplianceRegulatoryInformation/Guidances/UCM189544.pdf.

United States Food and Drug Administration. (2015). *FDA drug safety communication: Nonsteroidal anti-inflammatory drugs can cause heart attacks and strokes.* Retrieved from http://www.fda.gov/Drugs/DrugSafety/ucm451800.htm.

32

Serious Mental Illness

Kathryn Witner and Edward A. Herzog

Visit the Evolve website for a pretest on the content in this chapter: http://evolve.elsevier.com/Varcarolis

OBJECTIVES

1. Discuss the effects of serious mental illness on daily functioning, interpersonal relationships, and quality of life.
2. Describe three common problems associated with serious mental illness.
3. Define anosognosia and its impact on accessing treatment and maintaining treatment adherence.
4. Discuss five evidence-based practices for the care of individuals with serious mental illness.
5. Explain the role of the nurse in the care of people with a serious mental illness.
6. Develop a nursing care plan for an individual with serious mental illness.
7. Discuss the causes of treatment nonadherence and plan interventions to promote treatment adherence.
8. Identify current issues affecting individuals with serious mental illness, such as outpatient commitment and incarceration.

KEY TERMS AND CONCEPTS

anosognosia
assertive community treatment (ACT)
deinstitutionalization
guardianship
insurance parity
National Alliance on Mental Illness

outpatient commitment
peer support specialist
psychoeducation
psychiatric advance directives
recovery model
serious mental illness (SMI)

social skills training
stigma
supported employment
transinstitutionalization
vocational rehabilitation

The term **serious mental illness (SMI)** refers to a group of psychiatric conditions, most of which tend to be biological in origin, that can significantly affect one's level of functioning and quality of life, especially when untreated. Leaders in mental health and illness use two terms—serious and severe—interchangeably, with one word often defining the other. US organizations, including the National Institute of Mental Health (NIMH, 2021), the Substance Abuse and Mental Health Services Administration (SAMHSA, 2020), and the National Alliance on Mental Illness (NAMI, n.d.), use the term serious mental illness, abbreviated as SMI. The World Health Organization (WHO, 2018) refers to the same group of illnesses as severe mental disorders.

SMIs include disorders that can be part of a group, such as mood disorders, personality disorders, psychotic disorders, as well as the different subtypes of schizophrenia. In 2017, almost 11.4 million adults (about 4.6% of all adults) in the United States lived with an SMI (NIMH, 2021). Fig. 32.1 illustrates the prevalence of SMI based on demographic characteristics.

SMIs can be lifelong disorders that oftentimes have an early onset during the late teenage years. Many patients can experience successful recovery and function at high levels with minimal to no symptoms of their disorder. Other times, the chronicity of the disorder can create cycles of recovery and decompensation in which the symptoms wax and wane. The degree to which individuals experience residual symptoms can depend on a variety of things, such as the type of illness, access to treatment, and coexisting medical or substance use disorders.

SMIs can be devastating and difficult to manage. Individuals with SMI are more likely to be victims of crime, have coexisting medical illnesses that are typically undertreated, and have shorter life expectancies. Individuals with SMIs are also more likely to experience homelessness, incarceration, be unemployed or underemployed, live in poverty, and have little to no advocacy for their needs.

Day-to-day functioning is impacted for people with SMIs. Activities of daily living (ADLs), functioning at work or school, maintaining relationships, and interacting socially may be a struggle. Other impairments are related to leisure activities, health maintenance, being safe in the community, and managing finances. They can experience difficulty exercising sound judgment, controlling impulses, concentrating, and coping with

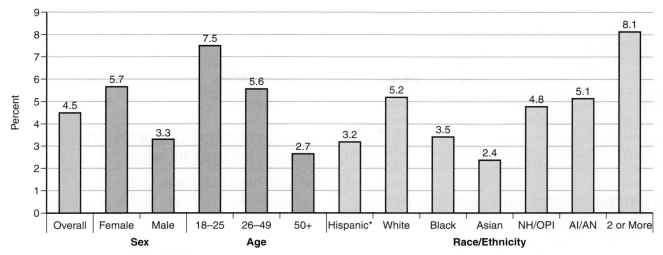

*All other groups are non-Hispanic or Latino
NH/OPI = Native Hawaiian / Other Pacific Islander
AI/AN = American Indian / Alaskan Native

Fig. 32.1 Prevalence of serious mental illness in the United States. (National Institute of Mental Health. [2018]. *Serious mental illness among US adults.* Retrieved from http://www.nimh.nih.gov/health/statistics/prevalence/serious-mental-illness-smi-among-us-adults.shtml.)

everyday stressors. Unfortunately, with all of these struggles, the path to recovery can be an uphill battle.

Reduced access to healthcare services significantly impacts one's ability to achieve and maintain a state of recovery from SMIs. Homelessness decreases quality of life and consistency of care coordination, while limited resources minimize the potential for successful engagement in treatment. Often, individuals with SMIs feel that they live in a world different than everyone else around them, making them feel alienated within their own communities.

Social stigma and lack of awareness by the general public creates a negative image against those with SMIs, which unfortunately contributes to the healthcare disparity seen within this population.

In this chapter, the primary term we will use for people with SMI is *clients*, which is a term commonly used in outpatient treatment settings. The term *client* refers to people who seek services and actively participate in their treatment and path to recovery and wellness. Other terms used to refer to individuals with SMI are *people with mental health conditions* and *people with serious mental health conditions*. In the context of a caregiver relationship, particularly outpatient clients who become hospitalized, they are usually referred to as *patients*.

SERIOUS MENTAL ILLNESS ACROSS THE LIFESPAN

SMI can affect individuals of any age, demographic, or background. Treatment for SMIs has changed drastically over the past several decades, transitioning from an institutionalization method of treatment, to more outpatient, community-based services and promoting independence. Typically, older adults are more accustomed to the institutionalization form of treatment with extended hospitalizations. Younger adults still may experience hospitalizations; however, this tends to be shorter in

length, with more of an emphasis on receiving treatment within the community.

Older Adults

Older adults with SMIs have likely received their care within state mental hospitals. Typically, these individuals lived within the hospital and were cared for by a variety of staff members. Even though the overall percentage of the population who suffered from SMIs was minimal, they posed an incredible burden on the community and social policy in regard to placement and demand for care. Oftentimes, treatment was strictly regimented and quality of care was suboptimal. Human rights were not a top priority, and therefore, many violations of basic rights occurred. These patients generally had little input into the course of their treatment.

This institutional inpatient care model was widely accepted, as many families struggled to care for and provide consistent housing for individuals with SMIs. As a result, older adults may have become *institutionalized* or adapted to life in institutions where decisions were often made for them with disregard for any of their own input. Transitioning to independence in the community has been difficult after years of institutionalization.

Years of poor health maintenance, inadequate diet and housing, and substance use takes a toll on older adults physically. In addition, older adults tend to require more care for medication-induced medical conditions such as diabetes or metabolic syndrome (refer to Chapter 12). Due to their complex medical and psychiatric needs, older adults tend to live in assisted living or nursing home facilities where they are cared for, rather than being in the community with support and resources designed to assist them in maintaining their level of independent functioning.

Younger Adults

People without a history of institutionalization can sometimes have less of an issue with passivity and dependency. Instead, most experience hospitalizations that are typically shorter in length, followed by being referred to care on an outpatient basis. Unfortunately, these hospital stays can stabilize the illness but may fail to overcome not recognizing the need for treatment. This lack of recognition leads to poor treatment adherence, which contributes to a cycle of treatment, brief recovery, nonadherence, and relapse. Intermittent treatment puts young adults with SMI at particular risk for additional problems. These problems include increased frequency of relapse and hospitalizations, arrest and incarceration, homelessness, substance use, unemployment, and poorer long-term prognosis.

DEVELOPMENT OF SERIOUS MENTAL ILLNESS

SMI has much in common with chronic physical illness: the original problem increasingly overwhelms and erodes the ability to cope, which results in new problems. For example, in chronic congestive heart failure, the lungs and kidneys deteriorate due to cardiac insufficiency. Similarly, a person with schizophrenia may experience paranoia and a loss of social skills, causing interactions to become more anxiety provoking. The person begins to withdraw and experiences avoidance by others. This results in increased isolation and lack of support when support is most needed. As a result, coping abilities and functioning continue to deteriorate.

REHABILITATION VERSUS RECOVERY: TWO MODELS OF CARE

For many years, the concept of **rehabilitation**, which focused on managing patients' deficits and helping them learn to live with their illnesses, was the forefront of psychiatric care. Staff directed the treatment and focused on helping patients to function in their daily roles. The goal was to stabilize the disability, with little focus on the idea of recovery.

Advocacy movements in mental health produced sweeping change. First, individuals with SMI began to refer to themselves as clients to emphasize the choices they have regarding their care and course of treatment. This movement challenged the rehabilitation model as being paternalistic and focused on living with disability rather than on improving quality of life and achieving recovery. The recovery model, which has its roots in the substance use community, developed as a result.

The recovery model is supported by the National Alliance on Mental Illness (NAMI), the leading mental health consumer support and advocacy organization in the United States. Many other mental health organizations also support the recovery model.

The recovery model:
- Is patient/client-centered.
- Is hopeful and empowering.
- Emphasizes the person and the future rather than the illness and the present.
- Involves an active partnership between patient and care providers.
- Focuses on strengths and abilities rather than dysfunction and disability.
- Encourages independence and self-determination.

- Focuses on achieving goals of the patient's choosing (not the staff's).
- Emphasizes staff working collaboratively with clients, building on strengths to help consumers achieve the highest possible quality of life.
- Aims for increasingly productive and meaningful lives for those with SMI.

ISSUES CONFRONTING INDIVIDUALS WITH SERIOUS MENTAL ILLNESS

Establishing a Meaningful Life

Finding meaning in life and establishing goals can be difficult for people living with SMI, particularly if they also experience poor self-esteem. Patients struggle with the possibility that they may never be the person they once expected to be. It is helpful to find ways to reset goals so that meaning can be found in new directions, such as helping others, volunteering, or even successfully managing their illness. This reset is important to achieve a satisfactory quality of life and to avoid despair.

If a person cannot work or attend school, there is a significant amount of free time to fill. This free time can result in boredom and stagnation. Options for constructive use of leisure time are limited if a person does not have transportation or lacks financial means. Helping the patient discover affordable options to structure free time and bring pleasure to life is important to recovery and wellness. Helpful options include renting books/movies from the local library, volunteering, and going for walks to nearby parks. Joining a clubhouse or day program can counter social withdrawal, increase social skills, and build support systems.

Comorbid Conditions
Physical Disorders

People with SMI are at greater risk of co-occurring physical illnesses, such as hypertension, obesity, cardiovascular disease, and diabetes. The risk of premature death is more than three times greater than the general population and, on average, patients with SMI have a shortened lifespan of 10 to 20 years (John et al., 2018). Contributing factors include poor understanding of medical conditions, medication nonadherence, missed appointments and follow-up, and limited financial and community resources.

A mental illness can distract healthcare staff from the patient's presenting medical needs. Persons with SMI may feel or be told that they are unwelcome in clinic waiting rooms because of their behaviors, appearance, or hygiene. Also, expressing health concerns in an eccentric or unclear manner can skew the quality of care received.

One patient with schizophrenia was experiencing priapism—a medically dangerous extended period of erection—as a medication side effect. Due to psychotic thinking, he interpreted the pain to the staff as "demons sticking needles in my [penis]." The resident did not assess for priapism partly because of the bizarre description, his assumption that the patient's distress was due to his mental illness, and possibly his own discomfort working with this population.

There is strong support for integrating mental and physical healthcare in a single setting to enhance access, improve coordination, and facilitate staff understanding and communication. One example is for mental health centers partnering with primary care providers so that their clients can receive both forms of care in a single coordinated delivery setting.

Suicide

Suicide occurs 12 times more frequently in people with SMI. For example, half of those with schizophrenia attempt suicide, and one in 10 succeeds. Consider a successful premed student who develops SMI, then 3 years later finds herself unemployed and living in a group home. There is a significant disconnect between her former life path and her current situation. The loss of what might have been can lead to acute or chronic grief that, along with the chronicity of the illness and its demands and impact on daily life, can contribute to despair, depression, and risk of suicide. Helping the patient find meaning and strong support systems can help prevent suicidal thoughts and attempts.

Substance Use

Nearly 30% of adults diagnosed with a mental illness also abuse drugs and/or alcohol (HelpGuide, 2019). Substance use in this population can largely involve alcohol, marijuana, and illegal drugs such as methamphetamines and cocaine. It can be a maladaptive response to boredom or a form of self-medication, countering the dysphoria, anxiety, or other symptoms caused by illness or its treatment. Substance use significantly increases the risk of relapse and impairs judgment and impulse control.

While cigarette smoking has declined among the general population over the past decade, there has been little change among people with SMI. For example, those with mental illnesses account for 40% of cigarettes sold in the United States, even though they represent a small portion of the overall population (Lipari & Van Horn, 2017). The prevailing belief that nicotine is a form of self-medication that improves cognitive ability has not been supported by research. Nicotine can, however, reduce the effectiveness of certain psychotropic medications. In fact, nicotine raises blood pressure and heart rate, therefore physiologically causing anxiety, contrary to the belief that nicotine helps reduce anxiety as reported by individuals with SMIs.

Social Problems
Stigma

Stigma is the perception that an individual is flawed. The perception is covertly or overtly linked to some personal defect in the person being stigmatized. A lack of understanding and incorrect beliefs about mental illness result in stigma about SMI. For example, some may believe that people with SMI are violent when in fact violence is rare. Nonetheless, the result of this stigmatizing belief is fear and avoidance of people with SMI, particularly those who have psychotic disorders. Stigma can cause shame, anger, and isolation in individuals and can lead to discrimination in healthcare, housing, and employment.

It is often hard to grasp that individuals can recover from mental illness. This is mostly due to stereotypical images of mental illness and limited corrective contact with people with SMIs. Initiatives such as NAMI's StigmaFree program seeks to improve understanding and acceptance through public education and campaigning for the reduction and elimination of stigma (NAMI, 2019a).

Isolation and Loneliness

Social isolation and loneliness are concerns with SMIs. Stigma, poor self-image, passivity, impaired hygiene, and similar factors reduce social interaction and interfere with relationships. Romantic relationships may be difficult to maintain and some may never experience a romantic relationship. Clubhouse programs and support groups can be an alternative way for individuals with SMI to meet others that not only share a similar lifestyle but can also empathize with their struggles and recovery process. As a result, a network of friendship can be built and even a romantic relationship can develop as well, while developing social skills and comfort.

Victimization

Stereotypes suggest that people with SMI are more likely to be violent than people without mental illness, but the reverse is actually true. People with mental illness are more likely to be *victims* of violence than *perpetrators* (Ghiasi et al., 2019). Sexual assault or coerced sexual activity also occurs in this vulnerable population. Impaired judgment, impaired interpersonal skills, impaired emotional recognition, poor self-esteem, dependency, and appearing more vulnerable to criminals may contribute to victimization. Drug use and poor living conditions in high-crime neighborhoods increase the risk of victimization and can worsen psychiatric conditions.

Economic Challenges
Unemployment and Poverty

Work and career tend to be a significant part of our personal identity. Lower levels of cognitive functioning, psychotic symptoms, and disorganized thinking can interfere with one's ability to work and maintain employment. More than 60% of people with SMI are unemployed, and disability benefits generally do not provide adequate income for personal and living expenses (Sherman et al., 2017). Finding an employer open to hiring a person with SMI can be difficult, and antidiscrimination laws do not guarantee a job. Some mental health treatment facilities offer employment-based programs. Fig. 32.2 illustrates employment services offered in mental health treatment facilities.

Medications for psychiatric symptoms can be quite costly. Copays or Medicaid spend-downs (the monthly need to exhaust personal funds to continue Medicaid eligibility) are obstacles to treatment and obtaining prescription medication. Even with insurance, individuals may find that upfront costs are too high, there are limits to mental health coverage, or that coverage does not include any mental healthcare.

Providing mental healthcare coverage equal to that for physical healthcare, or insurance parity, was required under the Affordable Care Act of 2010. Yet many insurers still treat mental illness differently, for instance, requiring preauthorization

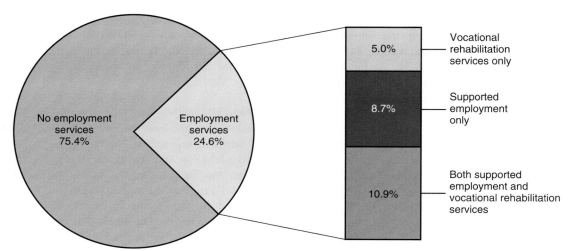

Fig. 32.2 Employment services in mental health facilities. (Hudock, W. J., Lynch, S. E., Sherman, L. J., & Teich, J. (2017). *Availability of supported employment in specialty mental health treatment facilities and facility characteristics: 2014.* Substance Abuse and Mental Health Services Administration. Retrieved from https://www.samhsa.gov/data/sites/default/files/report_3071/ShortReport-3071.html.)

for care when preauthorization is not required for comparable physical healthcare. Obtaining preauthorization can be a lengthy and time-consuming process, at times with no success. Short-term, limited-duration insurance coverage, enacted in 2017, is not required to comply with the Federal Parity Law.

Housing Instability

People with SMI often have limited funds and housing options. Affordable housing may require living far from resources such as stores, healthcare, and support people or living in unsafe neighborhoods. For an adult who expects autonomy, living with parents can be challenging and may result in conflict. Nonadherence with treatment, impaired self-care, and household disruption often result in individuals being asked or being told to leave the shared housing.

For people with SMI who have attained housing apart from family members, an episode of erratic or threatening behavior may lead to eviction. Eviction leads to a negative reputation among landlords, which may close doors to future housing. If police are involved, they may not recognize symptoms of mental illness, leading to arrest. Imagine a client who is experiencing hallucinations in public. She becomes disruptive and is arrested, instead of the police de-escalating the situation accordingly. This arrest can potentially leave the woman ineligible for housing subsidies or public housing. Even with a subsidy, waiting lists might be several years long. Even then, the cost of living has risen substantially in many areas, making housing unaffordable even with subsidies. Finding and maintaining housing can be challenging. Clients can also lose housing due to extended hospitalization.

Fortunately, options such as "no reject, no eject" housing are becoming common. These are group homes that hold the client's room even if hospitalized for extended periods of time. Some states have been granted waivers to allow the use of Medicaid-based funding for housing-related services (Abrams, 2019). This is a tremendous offering, since adequate housing is a social determinant of health.

Caregiver Burden

Caregivers, particularly family members, are challenged to cope with the persistent needs of individuals with SMI and may find themselves unable to shoulder the burden. They report that navigating the mental health system is challenging and stressful. Due to stigma or isolation, caregivers often carry this burden with little support, emotionally and financially.

Ensuring that caregivers are connected with resources and connecting the patient with services that will increase independence, such as vocational and housing support, are essential nursing interventions (NAMI, 2019b). Caregivers also age, become ill, and require care themselves, which often poses a difficult adjustment when a caregiver can no longer provide care or housing. Planning for the transition from family caregivers to other caregivers or independence before a crisis occurs and planning for financial support such as living trusts can preserve stability and help avoid relapse.

Treatment Issues
Anosognosia

Anosognosia (uh-no-sog-NOH-zee-uh), the inability to recognize one's illness due to illness itself, affects most people with SMI. In SMI, the illness affects the one organ needed to have insight and make good decisions: the brain. As a result, it can take months or years for a person with SMI to recognize, acknowledge, and accept a mental illness. Anosognosia may seem like the person is in denial. While this can happen, anosognosia is much more likely in SMI. Lack of awareness of one's mental illness is a significant obstacle to treatment. Table 12.3 in Chapter 12 includes interventions for anosognosia.

Nonadherence

Nonadherence to treatment can quadruple the likelihood of relapse. Anosognosia, medication side effects, medication costs, lack of trust in providers, poor access to care, and the stigma of mental illness also cause nonadherence. Factors that promote adherence, such as establishing a trusting therapeutic relationship, can be overlooked. Healthcare providers often respond primarily with medication education and pointing out the consequences of nonadherence, but patients faced with repetitive medication groups and exhortations to take medications may become *more* resistant rather than insightful. Box 32.1 describes nursing interventions that promote adherence.

Medication Side Effects

Psychotropic medications can produce a range of distressing side effects, from involuntary movements to increased risk of diabetes. Some side effects (e.g., dystonias) are treatable. Others may be temporary and diminish over time, or the individual can compensate for these through behavioral changes. For example, many psychotropic medications can cause drowsiness. If appropriate, clients can take these medications in the evening, usually before bedtime, to avoid daytime drowsiness. Addressing side effects is essential to promote adherence and maximize quality

---

BOX 32.1 Interventions to Improve Adherence to Treatment

- Encourage careful selections of medications that are most likely to be effective, well tolerated, and acceptable to the patient.
- Actively help the patient to manage side effects to avert/minimize distress that could cause nonadherence.
- Simplify treatment regimens to make them more acceptable and understandable to the patient (e.g., once-a-day dosing instead of twice).
- Tie treatment adherence to achieving the *patient's* goals (not staff's or society's) to increase motivation. Reinforce improvements (e.g., living in the community without rehospitalization), connecting them to treatment adherence.
- Assign consistently committed caregivers skilled at building trusting therapeutic relationships and who will be able to work with the patient for extended periods of time.
- To improve patient insight and motivation, educate the patient and family about SMI and the role of treatment in recovery. However, education alone will not lead to adherence, particularly for people with anosognosia.
- Minimize obstacles to treatment by aiding with treatment costs and access.
- Involve the patient and family in support groups with members who have greater insight and firsthand experience with illness and treatment—people whose viewpoints the patient may be more likely to appreciate and accept. Peer support specialists could be especially helpful here.
- Provide culturally sensitive care. Not attending to cultural beliefs and practices (e.g., mistrust of healthcare and authority figures or valuing self-sufficiency or privacy above healthcare) can result in rejection of treatment.
- When other interventions have not been successful, use medication monitoring and long-acting forms of medication (depot injections or sustained-release forms) to increase the likelihood that needed medication will be in the patient's system. Note: Mouth checks may not find pills hidden in the patient's mouth; engaging the patient in conversation for several minutes after he takes the pills is also of limited benefit. For people on oral medications, fast-dissolving or liquid forms are the best options for ensuring their ingestion.
- Never reject, blame, or shame the patient when nonadherence occurs. Instead, label it as simply an issue for continuing focus, and accept that achieving adherence often requires numerous tries. Remind yourself that nonadherence is common and often is due to anosognosia from the illness itself.

---

of life. Chapter 3 provides a detailed discussion of drugs used in the treatment of SMI, as do chapters on specific disorders.

Treatment Inadequacy

NAMI evaluates services provided to those with SMI and finds most states lacking adequate services to reach the majority of those with SMIs. There were several barriers to individuals finding a psychiatric provider or therapist. NAMI cited the following top three barriers (2017):

- Not accepting new patients
- Not accepting insurance plans
- Not close enough to work or home

Although standards of care exist for most SMIs, the level and quality of care can vary between different providers and treatment centers. An essential goal for providers is to continually update programs and practices (NAMI, 2017).

Residual Symptoms

Residual symptoms are symptoms that do not improve completely with consistent treatment. For example, a client being treated for schizophrenia may have strange beliefs, social withdrawal, or low energy even after psychosis has disappeared. These residual symptoms may occur even with consistent treatment and taking medication as prescribed. This can be frustrating, and clients may feel that these symptoms mean that treatments are not effective. This leads to helplessness and despair, and the patient may discontinue treatment as a result, worsening the illness.

Since residual symptoms tend to occur in older patients, comorbid physical symptoms may be responsible and should be explored (Khan et al., 2017). Once they have been ruled out, novel pharmacological treatment options should be considered for addressing symptoms such as lack of energy or social interest. Psychosocial interventions such as individual therapy and group therapy may improve mood. Addressing social isolation by expanding social outlets and physical inactivity by increasing regular exercise will result in a reduction of residual symptoms.

Relapse, Chronicity, and Loss

The majority of patients with an SMI face the possibility of relapse even when adhering to treatment, which may contribute to hopelessness and helplessness. Living with an SMI paradoxically requires *more* effort and emotional resources from people *less* able to cope with such demands. Each relapse can cause loss of relationships, employment, and housing, adding that much more loss to the patient's life and making discharge planning significantly more complicated. For many clients, each relapse can be more severe in regard to the level of decompensation, and longer hospitalization stays.

SERIOUS MENTAL ILLNESS RESOURCES

Our understanding of mental illness in general and SMI specifically has increased dramatically since the days of institutionalization. Research and educational support are available through governmental and grassroots organizations. Documentaries are also excellent sources of information for both healthcare providers and consumers. Box 32.2 highlights organizations and documentaries that address issues related to SMI.

Comprehensive Community Treatment

Ideally, the community-based mental healthcare system provides comprehensive, coordinated, and cost-effective care for the client with mental illness. However, services—particularly for SMI—are fragmented and inefficient, with blurring of responsibility among agencies, programs, and levels of government. Many clients "fall through the cracks," and those who receive treatment have difficulty achieving financial independence because of limited job opportunities and the fear of losing health insurance in the workplace. Now, many can opt into the Medicaid Buy-In program, which is a state Medicaid benefit group that allows individuals coverage who would otherwise be ineligible due to their earnings (Centers for Medicare and Medicaid Services, 2018).

The goal of community psychiatric treatment is to improve the client's ability to function independently and achieve a satisfying quality of life. Community mental health centers, private providers (psychiatrists, psychologists, counselors, social workers, and advanced practice registered nurses [APRNs]), and other private, public, and governmental agencies provide outpatient care. Community services vary with local needs and resources.

Rural communities or those with limited finances may provide only mandated services (and limited access to them), whereas other communities may have a broad array of accessible services. Needed services may be unavailable or have long waiting lists due to funding cutbacks, and clients may have difficulty finding the services they need amid the maze of agencies and services.

Community Services and Programs

The public healthcare system provides most care to those with SMIs. This system uses tax support to provide services even to those who are indigent and without adequate (or any) health insurance. Community mental health centers typically provide psychiatric or medical-somatic services and prescribe and monitor medications. Psychiatrists, advanced practice psychiatric-mental health registered nurses, and sometimes physician assistants provide these services along with support from registered nurses, therapists, counselors, and mental health workers.

Case management helps patients with day-to-day needs, treatment coordination, and access to services. Paraprofessional staff (people trained to assist professionals) usually provide this care. They work in the patient's home, school, and vocational

---

BOX 32.2   Resources

Organizational Resources

Mental Health America is a nonprofit organization of advocates, consumers, and significant others who work to strengthen mental health services and educate the nation about mental health issues. Its website provides resources pertaining to recovery, wellness, and severe/serious mental illness.

The **National Alliance on Mental Illness** (NAMI) is a support and advocacy organization for people with SMI and those who care about them. It has national, state, and local chapters and provides a wealth of educational materials and services. NAMI provides a variety of support groups and educational programs, including:

Family-to-Family is a free eight-session class for families and friends of people with mental illness. Taught by NAMI-trained family members, it helps participants understand mental illness, increase coping skills, and become advocates for their loved ones.

Peer-to-Peer is a free eight-session educational program for adults with SMI who want to understand their illness and move toward recovery. It is taught by trained peers who themselves are recovering from SMI.

The **National Institute of Mental Health** (NIMH) is an offshoot of the National Institutes of Health and is the main national research organization for mental illness. Its website contains information about research findings, proposals, and grants, as well as a variety of educational resources on mental illness.

The **Substance Abuse and Mental Health Services Administration** (SAMHSA) seeks to reduce the impact of substance misuse and mental illness and works to move research findings into practice. Its website offers much useful information, including a mental health services locator to help consumers find local services.

Video Resources

Bedlam (2020). Examines the mental health crisis through intimate stories of people in emergency departments, jails, and homeless camps. Getting well cannot happen in a cell. Explores the reality of replacing mental healthcare with detention.

Definition of Insanity (2020). Follows a team public servants of working through the courts to steer people with mental illness with court cases on a path from incarceration to recovery.

Frontline: The New Asylums (2005). Details the societal factors that led to the incarceration of hundreds of thousands of people with severe mental illness in American jails and prisons. The video chronicles the financial and human consequences of this unintended and disastrous policy.

Frontline: The Released (2009). This companion video to *The New Asylums* follows inmates with mental illness as they are released to the community. The inadequacies and strengths of the community mental health system become apparent as the inmates struggle to establish a life outside of institutions.

Kings Park: Stories from an American Mental Institution (2011). Follows a group of former patients as they visit the now-closed state hospital where they spent months or years of their lives. Interviews chronicle the lives and experiences of those deinstitutionalized from the state hospital system, sometimes only to experience still sadder fates.

Minds on the Edge: Facing Mental Illness (2011). Features a discussion of issues facing individuals with severe mental illness. Using hypothetical situations and featuring mental health professionals, advocates, policy makers, and consumers, looks at the problems in the mental health system and offers insights into ways that this population could be helped more effectively.

Right to Fail (2019). A series that explores the struggles and complex debate behind independent living for people with severe mental illness. It chronicles the potential for people to succeed on their own terms with the right support, and also the right to fail.

The Soloist (2009). Based on a true story, this film chronicles the life of a man whose promising musical career was interrupted by schizophrenia. It accurately portrays severe mental illness and many of the issues experienced by consumers and those who attempt to help them.

settings and coordinate overall care, facilitating access to services while providing basic education, guidance, and support. Case managers may provide **medication monitoring**, observing and facilitating the patient's use of medications to promote adherence. One evidence-based model of case management for patients with SMIs is **assertive community treatment (ACT)**, discussed later in this chapter.

Day programs provide structure and therapeutic activities to patients who attend the program one or more days a week. Services often include education regarding social skills, ADLs, and prevocational skills (the fundamentals needed before one can be successfully employed [e.g., interviewing, dressing for work]). Day programs also provide social contact and peer support. Staff monitor the patient's status so that they can detect and address concerns quickly. A variety of staff, and sometimes clients themselves, provide day program services. **Peer support specialists** (i.e., other clients who are in recovery) may provide some of the services.

Individual and group psychotherapy includes counseling and therapy based on a variety of models, usually provided by independently licensed mental health professionals (e.g., licensed independent social workers). Psychotherapy approaches for SMI include (1) family therapy (helping family members function more effectively by providing skills and knowledge necessary to support loved ones with mental illnesses), (2) **psychoeducation** groups (educating about mental health topics [e.g., psychotropic drugs] and skills [e.g., conflict resolution]), and (3) support groups (providing support related to daily challenges of living with chronic illness).

The following services may be provided by community mental health centers or through other public and private agencies:

Crisis intervention services focus on helping patients regain their ability to cope when facing overwhelming stress, such as psychological trauma or relapse. Impaired cognition and problem-solving increase the risk of crisis in people with SMI. Stressors, such as changes in routines at home or work, physical or financial problems, victimization, or anniversaries of traumatic events, may overwhelm coping and result in crises. A person with SMI and limited coping abilities may respond to a small stressor first by seeking hospitalization. Crisis intervention seeks to help that person manage the stressor in less-restrictive settings and avoid more-disruptive inpatient care.

Crisis intervention emphasizes finding new support or calling on existing resources for additional support. Crisis services range from staff on call who provide direct support 24 hours a day by phone or in person, to support lines (or "warm" lines, for lower levels of distress) or hotlines (for crises and high levels of distress) providing phone-based screening, support, crisis intervention, and referral services. Crisis residential or stabilization programs in some communities typically provide a stay of several days to 2 weeks when acuity is too great to remain in a community residence but not high enough to require hospitalization.

Emergency psychiatric services provide emergency assessments, crisis intervention, and sometimes emergency medications or adjustments. Individuals with SMI may be unable to recognize that their illness is worsening or that they are becoming unsafe. Therefore, most communities provide a 24-hour emergency psychiatric evaluation program that can initiate emergency inpatient admissions on an involuntary basis. An additional emergency service is a **mobile crisis team.** It is composed of mental health professionals who go to residences, jails, or even street corners. In some communities, law-enforcement officers are responsible for initiating involuntary emergency psychiatric evaluations. Local probate courts can also order such evaluations upon petition by family members or other interested parties.

Housing services help people progress toward independent living and to maintain stability and avoid homelessness. Settings include supervised or unsupervised group homes and independent community housing. Board-and-care homes provide room, board, and limited supervision by laypeople in their homes. Programming may target special populations such as individuals with a forensic history. This group includes criminal offenders who may have been found not guilty by reason of insanity who no longer require inpatient care, but require special or intensive monitoring and programming in the community.

Partial hospitalization programs (PHPs), often affiliated with inpatient programs, typically provide most of the services available to inpatients but on an outpatient basis. Patients usually attend PHPs Monday through Friday for most of the day. Inpatients may be stepped down to PHP programs from inpatient units for further stabilization before being released to other community services. Outpatients may use PHP services to control symptoms in order to avoid inpatient care. **Intensive outpatient programs (IOPs)** are similar but tend to be less lengthy.

Community outreach programs often focus on homeless individuals or people who do not seek care on their own. Professional or paraprofessional teams work in the community to engage people with mental illness who need services and to provide patient advocacy. Often, these patients can be difficult to reach and connect with; therefore, continuous outreach is needed before even minimal contact is made. **Multiservice centers** collaborate with outreach programs to supply hot meals, laundry, and shower facilities. They can also provide clothing, social activities, and transportation to and from services. For SMI people who are homeless or living in drop-in shelters, these centers provide access to phones and a mailing address, usually essential when seeking work or benefits.

Substance Use Treatment

A variety of services exist for those who have a dual diagnosis of SMI and alcohol-related or drug-related problems. Substance disorder clinics provide therapeutic and rehabilitative services and medication-assisted treatments such as detoxification or methadone. They also provide psychosocial interventions and psychotherapy. Help for families is also available. Most clinicians endorse integrated treatment that is delivered by a single provider rather than split between a mental health agency and a drug/alcohol agency. Refer to Chapter 22 for a detailed discussion of treatment settings for patients with substance use disorders.

> **VIGNETTE:** Christopher, who has a history of SMI, is causing a disturbance in the public library. He is arrested when he refuses a police officer's order to leave. Charged with disorderly conduct, he is subsequently found to be "guilty but insane" and conditionally released to mandatory psychiatric treatment. At a local clinic, he receives a long-acting intramuscular antipsychotic medication due to his history of nonadherence. He also joins a day program and is assigned to a case manager, who helps him apply for Supplemental Security Income. When his aging parents state that he can no longer live with them, he moves to a group home. Because Christopher wants to work, he is referred to Goodwill Industries, where he receives job training and coaching, leading to a job unloading trucks. The stable housing and the requirements of his conditional release lead to consistent treatment and prevent nonadherence. He remains stable and employed for the next 5 years.

EVIDENCE-BASED TREATMENT APPROACHES

Assertive Community Treatment

Assertive community treatment (ACT) involves consumers working with a multidisciplinary team that provides a comprehensive array of services. This team approach eliminates the need for multiple departments or agencies to provide services. Research supports this model for improving the quality of life and reducing inpatient admissions, incarceration, and homelessness among people with SMI (Mueser, 2019). At least one member of the team is available 24 hours a day for crisis care, though this may not be available depending on resources. The emphasis is on treating patients within their own environment. Although ACT programs cost more to operate, proponents believe those costs are offset by reduced care costs elsewhere.

Cognitive Behavioral Therapy

Cognitive behavioral therapy (CBT) has been effective in helping individuals with SMI reduce and cope with symptoms such as delusions and impaired social functioning (Provincial System Support Program, 2017). The cognitive component of CBT focuses on patterns of thinking and "self-talk" (i.e., what one says to oneself internally). It identifies distorted thinking and negative self-talk and guides patients to substitute more effective ways of thinking. The behavioral component of CBT uses natural consequences and positive reinforcers (rewards) to shape the person's behavior in a more positive or adaptive manner. Refer to Chapter 2 for a more detailed discussion of CBT.

> **VIGNETTE:** Christopher has done well in a group home and decides to move to his own apartment. Over the next 2 months, his mental status remains stable. However, his nurse, who weighs him monthly, notices that he has lost 12 pounds. Christopher denies any change in his eating habits, and he doesn't follow up with the primary care provider to whom he's been referred. During the next 6 weeks, he loses another 10 pounds. Christopher's work supervisor noticed that Christopher is talking out loud to himself, is more isolated, and today, smelled of alcohol. The supervisor dismisses him for the day and requires him to get treatment before returning to work. At his appointment, the psychiatrist, nurse, and nurse-therapist discuss these changes and recommend that Christopher go into the PHP for support and medication reevaluation. Although he denies that he has a problem, Christopher reluctantly agrees.

Cognitive Enhancement Therapy

Cognitive enhancement therapy (CET) is based on the principle of neuroplasticity—that healthier areas of the brain can assume neurological functions for the compromised areas of the brain. CET is a lengthy process of structured computer-based drills and group exercises (e.g., 60 or more) that incrementally challenge and strengthen functions such as focusing attention and processing and recalling information. It can also help with interpreting social and emotional information, such as judging a person's mood from expression or tone of voice. Research has shown that CET leads to sustained improvement in cognition and improves social and vocational functioning (Wojtalik et al., 2017).

Family Support and Partnerships

Families and significant others can face significant stresses related to the mental illness of a loved one, and both may suffer from insufficiencies in empathy and understanding. Sound **family support** is one of the strongest predictors of recovery. When treatment providers work as empathic partners with patients and significant others, this enhances treatment and reduces conflict. NAMI's Family-to-Family program focuses on understanding SMI, coping skills, and the recovery process (NAMI, 2019b). NAMI meetings and support groups are specific to various SMIs. For example, the Depression and Bipolar Support Alliance serves as an excellent source of support and practical guidance for primary consumers (patients) and secondary consumers (their significant others).

Social Skills Training

Social skills training is an evidence-based practice that focuses on teaching a wide variety of social and ADL skills, largely with the focus of making progress in small increments. People with SMI often have social deficits that cause functional impairment. For example, a person may not realize that standing too close to others can cause discomfort for others, which can lead to negative outcomes such as rejection or a poor job evaluation. Care providers break down complex interpersonal skills, such as resolving a conflict, into more manageable subcomponents. They then teach them how to manage the problem step by step. They also use role-playing and group interaction to practice skills.

> **VIGNETTE:** Christopher is admitted to the PHP. He attends groups on medication, living with SMI, substance use, and symptom management. The clinicians notice odd behavior. Christopher will only eat or drink out of unopened containers and seems guarded. He discloses that he has not taken any medication since he moved out of his group home. The psychiatrist changes his prescription to a quick-dissolving oral and a long-acting injectable medication. He begins to eat normally and gains 4 pounds in 2 weeks.
>
> He is discharged from the PHP a month later. He again attends the day program at the community mental health center. There, he is provided with structure, supportive group therapy, socialization, case management, and medication management. His case manager finds him a room in a family care home with a supportive caregiver. Over the next 3 months, Christopher gradually returns to his baseline functioning. He returns to work 2 days a week and also attends the day program 2 days a week.

Vocational Rehabilitation and Related Services

Clients with SMI who are employed experience improved socialization, confidence, organizational abilities, income, and quality of life. Vocational services, or **vocational rehabilitation**, typically include training skills to enhance employment and financial support for attaining employment. Day programs may use a **clubhouse model** in which clients run the programming for peers. Client-run businesses, such as a coffee shop or housekeeping service, teach all members to perform a job in the business as well as different aspects of running a business. Such programs have led to the **supported employment** model, which has been shown to be more effective in helping individuals with SMI achieve employment (McKay et al., 2018). Elements of this approach include:

1. Financial incentives to employers to employ people with SMI
2. Rapid placement in a competitive job preferred by the patient
3. Continuing individualized support on the job
4. Integration of mental health and employment services

EVIDENCE-BASED PRACTICE

What Is the Link Between Antipsychotic Medication and Diabetes?

Problem
Individuals with SMI are at a higher risk for developing diabetes. This risk is associated with the use of antipsychotic medications.

Purpose of This Study
The purpose of this study was to review recent studies that link diabetes with antipsychotic medication and to identify methods for decreasing this risk.

Methods
Publications including literature reviews, meta-analyses, and randomized controlled trials from the last 5 years were reviewed.

Key Findings
- Second-generation antipsychotic medications, which are more widely used and effective than first-generation antipsychotics, increased the risk of developing diabetes, especially in adolescents and young adults.
- Clozapine and olanzapine use are associated with a higher risk of developing diabetes compared with other antipsychotic medications.
- Antipsychotics directly affect insulin sensitivity and secretion.

Implications for Nursing Practice
Antipsychotic medications are highly effective. However, understanding the risk of diabetes and strategies to prevent diabetes is crucial for nurses who advocate for and educate patients. Early screening and lifestyle changes are effective ways to prevent and manage diabetes, especially when initiated at the start of antipsychotic therapy.

Holt, R. (2019). Association between antipsychotic medication use and diabetes. *Current Diabetes Reports, 19*(10), 96.

OTHER TREATMENT APPROACHES

Court-Involved Intervention

Psychiatric advance directives are legal documents that allow an individual whose disorder is in remission to direct how to manage treatment if judgment becomes impaired during a relapse. For example, a client can agree to accept hospitalization or medications, should a relapse occur. This proactive plan helps the consumer maintain control over treatment and avoid the need for involuntary admission and court involvement. These directives do vary by state, so it is important to understand how laws by state mandate this.

Guardianship involves the appointment of a person (guardian) to make decisions for the consumer during times when judgment is impaired or is disabled with anosognosia. Guardians may be family members, significant others, or attorneys. They are typically appointed during a court process addressing the issue of whether or not a patient is competent to provide for personal needs and make appropriate decisions regarding psychiatric care.

Individuals who have been appointed a guardian typically may not enter into contracts or authorize their own treatment. All of those actions require the guardian's approval. In some cases, the guardian's authority is limited to the person's finances, as when a client is functional in most respects but unable to manage money, placing basic needs for food and shelter at risk. The guardian is responsible for using the client's funds to meet such needs. An alternative is the use of a **payee**, often a volunteer or staff member at a community agency or center, whom the consumer agrees to allow to manage the finances, usually via a contract. Payees can be very beneficial for clients, as they can work together to create a budget and ensure the client is learning about managing the finances.

Consumer-Run Programs

As previously discussed with vocational rehabilitation, **client-run programs** may be informal clubhouses, which can offer socialization, recreation, group classes, as well as types of services. They may also be competitive businesses, such as snack bars or janitorial services, which provide needed services and client employment while encouraging independence and building vocational skills. In Cincinnati, Ohio, for example, clients working with a food service professional run a restaurant open to the public, while both learning skills and developing experience in the food-service industry. Community mental health centers typically have client-run programming as part of day programs that are very successful and meaningful for clients and staff alike.

Peer Support

Peer support involves receiving support from one's peers. This can be from untrained peers in a peer support group or by specially trained and sometimes certified **peer support specialists**. NAMI and other programs offer training that enables consumers to assist peers effectively in their recovery process. Peer support specialists may work in hospitals or day programs to encourage and help their peers, and act as an advocate for clients. They draw on firsthand experience with SMI to enhance their effectiveness. People with SMI are often more open to accepting support from people who have experienced what they are going through, which can improve coping skills.

Technology

Technology can reduce healthcare-associated costs, and improve treatment access and client outcomes. Electronic records available in multiple locations can assist in assessments or promote continuity of care anywhere in the community. Those who cannot afford electronic access often have, or can be provided with, a cell phone, allowing for improved monitoring and faster response if, for example, a patient misses an appointment. Smartphone applications can help clients manage stress, prevent weight gain through exercise or dietary means, and remember scheduled treatments or appointments. Text reminders can promote treatment adherence by tracking medications or appointments. Medication dispensers that track when medications are taken are also helpful. Personnel in remote locations are now able to speak with clients by telephone or internet-based video when patients cannot otherwise access distant services or specialists. Telemedicine is becoming more widespread in an attempt to reach more clients and deliver care to a bigger population of individuals suffering with SMIs.

Exercise

Exercise holds benefits for people with SMI, including improved coping with symptoms, reduced anxiety and depression, and enhanced self-esteem. Exercise helps with weight control, which is essential for people with weight-related comorbidities such as diabetes and hypertension. Exercise is a cost-effective intervention that can be done almost anywhere. While SMI symptoms such as avolition are obstacles to exercise, motivational and group interventions can improve exercise participation (Wang et al., 2018). Many community recreational centers provide discounted passes or memberships for individuals with SMIs, creating more incentive for them to participate in an active lifestyle. Day centers and clubhouses can also offer exercise classes, such as yoga and outdoor hiking groups.

NURSING CARE OF PATIENTS WITH SERIOUS MENTAL ILLNESS

Nurses encounter patients with SMI in a variety of medical and psychiatric settings. All roles and techniques used by psychiatric-mental health nurses in inpatient psychiatric settings also apply in the community and other outpatient healthcare settings.

Assessment Strategies

Important aspects of assessment include:

- Intentional risk to self or others: Suicidality or homicidality
- Unintentional risk: Inadequate nutrition, clothing inadequate for the weather, neglect of medical needs, or carelessness while driving, smoking, or cooking
- Depression or hopelessness
- Anxiety
- Signs of impending relapse: Decreased sleep, increased impulsivity or paranoia, diminished reality testing, increased delusional thinking, or command hallucinations
- Physical health problems that can cause psychiatric symptoms and be mistaken for mental illness or relapse (e.g., brain tumors or drug toxicity)
- Comorbid illnesses: To ensure that the patient provides appropriate self-care and receives adequate healthcare

- Treatment nonadherence: Signs such as worsening of symptoms, unused medications, missed appointments, illicit drug use, or reluctance to discuss these issues

Table 32.1 lists selected signs and symptoms of problems associated with SMI, potential nursing diagnoses that apply to the patient with SMI, and examples of specific nursing outcomes.

Intervention Strategies

Box 32.3 outlines relevant nursing interventions for the management of SMI. Basic nursing interventions for patients with SMI are listed in the following text. Additional interventions are in Table 12.3 in Chapter 12 and in other chapters covering individual mental illnesses.

- Involve the patient in goal setting and treatment planning. This increases treatment adherence and improves treatment outcomes.
- Emphasize quality of life rather than simply focusing on symptoms, as this conveys an interest in the person rather than the illness and promotes recovery.
- Maintain sustained therapeutic relationships; trust in providers is key to overcoming anosognosia and achieving treatment adherence. People with SMI often require extended periods to form these connections.
- Focus on coping with current issues rather than past difficulties.
- Encourage reality testing to enable clients to recognize and counter hallucinations and delusional thinking. For instance, if a person experiences frightening hallucinations while in public, the person can learn to scan the room and determine if others seem frightened. If not, the client can learn techniques about how to cope with hallucinations to prevent a possible negative event occurring in public.
- Enable clients to recognize and respond to stigma. Stigma predisposes SMI people to isolation and social discomfort. The resulting isolation contributes to loneliness and reduces access to support, thus creating a repetitive cycle of isolation and disengagement of treatment.
- Promote social skills and provide opportunities for socialization, especially with positive role models, such as other clients who are further along in recovery.
- Involve clients in support groups such as NAMI that expose members to those who can truly empathize. Such groups provide support, socialization opportunities, and practical suggestions for issues and problems facing clients and significant others. Peer support specialists are another excellent resource for this purpose.
- Educate clients about their illness and recovery. Understanding the illness enhances coping, treatment adherence, and quality of life.
- Care for the whole person. SMI patients have more physical illness; poorer hygiene and health practices; less access to effective medical treatment; and increased risk for victimization, STDs, and undesired pregnancies. They also have more premature mortality than the general population. Avoiding obesity through exercise and good nutritional practices can reduce the risk of comorbidities such as metabolic syndrome. Sound physical health conserves energy and resources for use

TABLE 32.1 Signs and Symptoms, Nursing Diagnoses, and Outcomes for Serious Mental Illness

Signs and Symptoms	Nursing Diagnoses	Outcomes
Absence of eye contact, difficulty expressing thoughts, difficulty in comprehending usual communication pattern, inappropriate verbalization	Impaired verbal communication	Improved verbal communication: Exchanges messages accurately with others, uncompromised spoken language, accurately interprets messages received
Withdrawal, inappropriate interpersonal behavior, social discomfort, lack of belonging	Impaired socialization	Improved socialization: Engages others, appears relaxed, cooperates with others, uses assertive behaviors as appropriate, exhibits sensitivity to others
Absence of supportive significant other(s), preoccupation with own thoughts, shows behaviors unaccepted by dominant cultural group, withdrawn, reports feeling alone, feels different from others, feels rejected	Social isolation	Decreased social isolation: Interacts with others (e.g., family, friends, neighbors, mental health consumers), participates in community activities (e.g., church, volunteer work, clubs), participates in leisure activities with others
Failure to keep appointments, missing medication dosages, evidence of exacerbation of symptoms, failure to progress	Nonadherence to [medication regime, treatment regime]	Adherence to [medication regime, treatment regime]: Discusses prescribed treatment regimen with health professional, performs treatment regimen as prescribed, keeps appointments with health professionals, monitors own treatment response
Self-negating verbalization, lacks success in life events, hesitant to try new situations, indecisive behavior, lack of eye contract, nonassertive behavior	Chronic low self-esteem	Improved self-esteem: Describes feelings of self-worth, fulfills personally significant roles, maintains eye contact, accepts compliments from others
Apprehension about care receiver's care if caregiver is unable to provide care, apprehension about possible institutionalization of care receiver, lack of time to meet personal needs, anger, stress, frustration, impatience, limited social life	Caregiver stress	Reduced caregiver stress: Caregiver receives adequate respite, social support, opportunities for leisure activities, supplemental services to assist with care; caregiver reports sense of control and certainty about future

International Council of Nursing Practice. (2019). *ICNP browser.* Retrieved from https://www.icn.ch/what-we-do/projects/ehealth/icnp-browser. ICNP® is owned and copyrighted by the International Council of Nurses (ICN). Reproduced with permission of the copyright holder.

BOX 32.3 Interventions for Serious Mental Illness

Self-Care Assistance: ADLs[a]

- Teach the appropriate and safe storage of medications.
- Assist with the use of public transportation (e.g., buses and bus schedules, taxis, city, or county transportation for disabled people).
- Assist in establishing safe methods and routines for cooking, cleaning, and shopping.

Family Support

- Encourage family to share concerns, feelings, and questions.
- Accept the family's values in a nonjudgmental manner.
- Provide emotional support and connect to support resources such as NAMI and respite services.
- Promote congruence among patient, family, and staff expectations.

[a] Partial list.
ADLs, Activities of daily living; *NAMI,* National Alliance on Mental Illness. From Bekhet, A. K., Zauszniewski, J. A., Matel-Anderson, J., Suresky, M. J., & Stonehouse, M. (2018). Evidence for psychiatric and mental health nursing interventions. *Online Journal of Issues in Nursing, 23*(2). Retrieved from http://ojin.nursingworld.org/MainMenu-Categories/ANAMarketplace/ANAPeriodicals/OJIN/TableofContents/Vol-23-2018/No2-May-2018/Evidence-Psychiatric-Mental-Health-Interventions.html.

in coping with SMI. Case management plays a significant role in assisting clients to connect with medical care providers.

- Involving individuals with co-occurring substance use disorders in Alcoholics Anonymous and Narcotics Anonymous (AA/NA) and other dual-diagnosis services. Substance use disorder rates are high in SMI populations. These disorders

increase relapse, foster disengagement with treatment, and interfere with recovery. Achieving sobriety is most associated with AA and integrated treatment programs.

Evaluation

Evaluation is ongoing. Psychiatric nurses evaluate the degree to which the outcomes have been met. At this point in the nursing process, care may be re-prioritized based on the patient's progress.

CURRENT ISSUES AFFECTING INDIVIDUALS WITH SERIOUS MENTAL ILLNESS

Outpatient Commitment

Involuntary inpatient care has long been used to treat those who are unable to recognize their illness (anosognosia) and the need for treatment. Outpatient commitment, which provides mandatory treatment in the community, is relatively new. Typically ordered by a court when a patient leaves a hospital or prison, it is for people who would otherwise be unlikely to continue treatment, resulting in their becoming a danger to self or society.

The practice of outpatient commitment is controversial. On the one hand, individuals who do not recognize having a mental illness are provided with healthcare and, potentially, a better quality of life. They are allowed maximum freedom and are able to live in the community and avoid institutionalization. On the other hand, this approach is paternalistic and at odds with the recovery model of mental healthcare. Research on the effectiveness of outpatient commitment has demonstrated results that both support and reject this approach. Clients may struggle with the inability to make their own decisions with participation in treatment, and the consequences can be severe should they not engage in treatment. They may feel forced into treatment, which may have little to no benefit on their recovery if it is not on their terms.

Criminal Offenses and Incarceration

People with SMIs may commit crimes due to desperation, impaired judgment, or impulsivity. Most often, they are nonviolent crimes such as petty theft or disorderly conduct. Police may also become involved with people who seem unable to care for themselves, have become a public nuisance, or cannot be persuaded to accept treatment but do not meet criteria for involuntary treatment (usually imminent danger to self or others). For example, a client with impaired judgment without shelter in cold weather may stay in a laundromat for warmth. The presence of unkempt persons talking to themselves and not using appropriate personal space will cause others to feel uncomfortable. If expelled, they are at risk of hypothermia. In such a case, the risk to self may not be "imminent," and emergency hospitalization is not a legal option. Significant others or police may then seek their arrest simply for their own safety.

Most mental illness advocates believe that incarceration is harmful. Imprisonment can lead to victimization, despair, relapse due to stress or overstimulation, loss of housing or employment, and inadequate treatment. Criminal convictions may make consumers ineligible for most housing or employment, trapping them in a cycle of release and reincarceration.

Advocates support diversion from jail to clinical care. Many communities have adopted interventions to achieve diversion. Police are receiving education that helps them identify behaviors associated with mental illness, distinguish these behaviors from criminal intent, and connect people with services rather than jailing them. Special mental health courts are designed to intercept people whose crimes are secondary to mental illness. These courts employ specially trained officials with authority to order treatment in lieu of conviction, thereby avoiding the stigma and the consequences of conviction and incarceration.

Deinstitutionalization and Transinstitutionalization

Prior to the 1960s, people often lived long term in state psychiatric hospitals (refer to Chapter 4). The newer treatments available in the 1960s improved many patients' conditions enough that they no longer needed to be institutionalized and could live instead in the community. Deinstitutionalization, the mass shift of patients from state hospitals into the community, began in the 1960s and has continued since. However, planned systems of community care needed by individuals with SMI did not always materialize, leaving them to fend for themselves without access to the services they needed. It was also common for patients to experience difficulty in adjusting to independence after years of being institutionalized.

As a result, former patients ended up being readmitted to state hospitals or cared for in other kinds of institutions. Transinstitutionalization is the shifting of a person or population from one kind of institution to another, such as a state hospital, jail, prison, nursing home, or shelter. For example, people who were discharged from state hospitals ended up homeless and subsequently were arrested for a variety of crimes. Now there are more people with SMI in jails and prisons than in hospitals.

Inadequate Access to Care

SMI often makes it difficult for individuals to work or find well-paying jobs and jobs with health insurance benefits. As a result, people with SMI tend to rely on the public mental health system, which is run by state and local governments, with services delivered largely by state hospitals and community mental health centers. One consequence of deinstitutionalization was that 90% of state hospital beds were eliminated, making it difficult to provide hospital care to many who continue to need inpatient care. Further, most public mental health services rely on state and local funding, and the economic recession that began in 2007 has resulted in funding cutbacks that have reduced already-overwhelmed mental health and related services.

Inpatient and outpatient services for children and adolescents are in especially short supply. The result is that delayed admissions and waiting lists for outpatient care are now commonplace. The Affordable Care Act and Medicaid expansion have resulted in dramatically more people with SMI having health insurance (Guth, Garfield, & Rudowitz, 2020). However, even those with insurance, who can use private care providers, often find that there are still barriers to getting needed care, such as burdensome preauthorization requirements (required for psychiatric care but not for medical care) that discourage or delay access to needed services. Even with the expansion of Medicaid and insuring many who were previously uninsured, many clinicians and care providers are overwhelmed more than ever with rising patient-to-provider ratios, contributing to the disparity that is long overdue to be rectified.

KEY POINTS TO REMEMBER

- Patients with SMI often suffer from multiple impairments in thinking, emotions, perception, and interaction with others.
- The recovery model stresses hope, strengths, quality of life, patient involvement as an active partner in treatment, and eventual recovery.

- The course of SMI involves exacerbations and remissions; these can be discouraging and lead a patient to believe recovery is not possible.
- People with SMI often suffer complications due to comorbid conditions such as physical disorders, suicide, and substance use.

- Social problems related to SMI include stigmatization, isolation, and victimization.
- Economic challenges for people with SMIs include unemployment, poverty, and housing instability.
- One of the most difficult symptoms of SMI is anosognosia, the inability to recognize one's illness due to the illness itself.

- Coordinated comprehensive community services help people with SMI to function at an optimal level, but such services may not be available or accessible to those who need them.
- The family and support systems play a major part in the care of many people with SMI, so they should be included as much as possible in planning, education, and treatment activities.

CRITICAL THINKING

1. John Yang, 42, dually diagnosed with schizophrenia and cannabis (marijuana) use disorder, is brought to the clinic by his mother, Mrs. Yang. Because they are new in town, she does not know what is available in the community. John takes haloperidol (Haldol), but Mrs. Yang says he often refuses it because of muscle rigidity and sexual side effects. They have tried several first-generation antipsychotic drugs without success.
   a. What areas of John's life might you want to explore in your assessment? Consider relationships, employment history, cognitive abilities, coping, and behavior. How would you use this information for long-term planning?
   b. As a patient advocate, how might you respond to John's medication nonadherence with first-generation antipsychotics?
   c. What obstacles to adherence exist for a dually diagnosed patient? What approach or change in treatment would offer John the best chance of success?
   d. Which resources mentioned in this chapter might be appropriate for John?
   e. Identify three areas of psychoeducation you'd provide for John and his mother.

CHAPTER REVIEW

1. Which statement made by a patient diagnosed with an SMI reflects a common situation associated with this disorder in *today's* healthcare system? *Select all that apply.*
   a. "I have been in a state institution most of my life."
   b. "I've been homeless for years."
   c. "Once a care provider knows my psychiatric history, my physical problems are not taken seriously."
   d. "No one wants to hire a person with mental issues."
   e. "My family doesn't want to be around me because I hear voices."
2. What is the primary reason the nurse should include the family of a patient with an SMI in treatment planning?
   a. They know the patient better than anyone.
   b. The patient is likely willing to listen to them.
   c. They are likely the patient's support system.
   d. The patient will turn to them first when needing help.
3. A 73-year-old man was diagnosed with an SMI at age 20. Subsequently, he was frequently hospitalized. Two years ago, he was transferred to a group home. When considering the effects of institutionalization, which behavior demonstrates adaptation to the new environment?
   a. Willingly takes his medications
   b. Keeps his room neat and clean
   c. Makes himself lunch when he is hungry
   d. Enjoys spending the afternoon watching television
4. Due to the need to self-medicate for anxiety, a patient diagnosed with schizophrenia smokes two packs of cigarettes a day. What unique risk does nicotine pose to this patient's health?
   a. Lung cancer
   b. Cardiovascular constriction
   c. Impaired psychotropic medication therapy
   d. Increased incidence of lung-reacted disorders

5. Which functions are often simultaneously impaired when a patient is experiencing an SMI? *Select all that apply.*
   a. Cognition
   b. Emotions
   c. Perceptions
   d. Social interactions
   e. Self-care
6. Charlie is coping well with an SMI diagnosis. He and his 91-year-old father live together on the family farm. This stable and secluded life has allowed Charlie to live with minimal stimulation, and his relapses have been few. Charlie's caseworker makes a visit to open up a conversation on where Charlie will live when his father can no longer care for him. By bringing up the topic now, the caseworker is hoping to:
   a. Arrange housing for Charlie for when his father dies.
   b. Avert a relapse and preserve stability in Charlie's life.
   c. Rescue Charlie when the crisis occurs.
   d. Make Charlie realize he will soon live independently.
7. Jimmy has been hospitalized three times for schizophrenia. Typically, he is very disorganized, spends his money irresponsibly, and loses his housing when he does not pay the rent. In turn, Jimmy cannot be located by his case manager, which leads to treatment nonadherence and relapse. Which response would be most therapeutic? *Select all that apply.*
   a. Advise Jimmy that if he does not pay his rent, he will be placed in a group home instead of independent housing.
   b. Discuss with Jimmy the option of having a guardian who will ensure that the rent is paid and that his money is managed to meet his basic needs.
   c. Suggest to Jimmy and his prescribing clinician that he be placed on a long-acting injectable form of antipsychotic medication to improve treatment nonadherence.

d. Encourage Jimmy's case manager to hold him responsible for the outcomes of his poor decisions by allowing periods of homelessness to serve as a natural consequence.

8. Individuals with SMI diagnoses can suffer from ineffective healthcare. Providers may be unaccustomed to working with this population or not comprehend obscure details described by the person seeking medical attention. This hurdle can be overcome by:
   a. Seeking medical attention at the emergency department.
   b. Having a community clinic in the area where individuals with SMI live.
   c. Medicate the patient before a medical examination.
   d. Integrating mental and physical health in one setting.

9. A female consumer with severe and recurrent mania argues with outpatient staff about her medication. She does not believe she has a mental illness. Although she takes medication during hospitalizations, she stops taking them after discharge. Which intervention is most helpful in promoting medication adherence?
   a. Assign a new outpatient staff to reduce the conflicts she is experiencing with her current providers.

b. Explain that the medications will help her and that all medications have side effects, but she can learn to live with these.
c. Involve her in a medication group that will teach her the types and names of psychotropic medications, their purpose, and possible side effects.
d. Explore her perceptions and experiences regarding medication and help her to connect taking medications with achieving her goals.

10. Isadora is a middle-aged woman living in a group home after being discharged from a psychiatric institution nearly 20 years ago. Isadora keeps to herself, stays in her room most of the day, and only ventures out for meals. Cassandra, the house manager, encourages Isadora to:
    a. Begin looking for a job
    b. Join a day program clubhouse
    c. Assist in the kitchen washing dishes
    d. Take on a roommate so as not to be alone

1. **b, c, d, e;** 2. **c;** 3. **c;** 4. **c;** 5. **a, b, c, d, e;** 6. **b;** 7. **b, c;** 8. **d;** 9. **d;** 10. **b**

Visit the Evolve website for a posttest on the content in this chapter: http://evolve.elsevier.com/Varcarolis

REFERENCES

Abrams, A. (2019). Medicaid dollars for housing? *ShelterForce: The Voice of Community Development.* Retrieved from https://shelterforce.org/2019/02/19/medicaid-dollars-for-housing/.

John, A., McGregor, J., Jones, I., Lee, S. C., Walters, J. T. R., Owen, M. J., et al. (2018). Premature mortality among people with severe mental illness—New evidence from linked primary care data. *Schizophrenia Research, 199,* 154–162.

Centers for Medicare and Medicaid Services. (2018). *Medicaid employment initiatives.* Retrieved from https://www.medicaid.gov/medicaid/ltss/employment/index.html.

Ghiasi, N., Azhar, Y., & Singh, J. (2019). *Psychiatric illness and criminality.* Treasure Island, FL: StatPearls. Retrieved from https://www.ncbi.nlm.nih.gov/books/NBK537064/.

Guth, M., Garfield, R., & Rudowitz, R. (2020). *The effects of Medicaid expansion under the ACA: Updated findings from a literature review.* Kaiser Family Foundation. Retrieved from https://www.kff.org/medicaid/issue-brief/the-effects-of-medicaid-expansion-under-the-aca-updated-findings-from-a-literature-review-august-2019/.

HelpGuide. (2019). *Substance use and mental health issues.* Retrieved from https://www.helpguide.org/articles/addictions/substance-abuse-and-mental-health.htm.

Khan, A. Y., Kalia, R., Ide, G. D., & Ghavami, M. (2017). Residual symptoms of schizophrenia: What are realistic treatment goals? *Current Psychiatry, 16*(3), 34–40.

Lipari, R., & Van Horn, S. (2017). *Smoking and mental illness among adults in the United States.* Retrieved from https://www.samhsa.gov/data/sites/default/files/report_2738/ShortReport-2738.html.

McKay, C., Nugent, K. L., Johnsen, M., Eaton, W. W., & Lidz, C. W. (2018). A systematic review of evidence for the clubhouse model of psychosocial rehabilitation. *Administration and Policy in Mental Health and Mental Health Services Research, 45*(1), 28–47.

Mueser, K. T. (2019). *Assertive community treatment for patients with severe mental illness.* UpToDate. Retrieved from https://www.uptodate.com/contents/assertive-community-treatment-for-patients-with-severe-mental-illness.

National Alliance on Mental Illness. (n.d.). Mental health conditions. Retrieved from https://www.nami.org/Learn-More/Mental-Health-Conditions.

National Alliance on Mental Illness. (2017). *Continuing disparities in access to mental and physical health care.* Retrieved from https://www.nami.org/parityreport.

National Alliance on Mental Illness. (2019a). *StigmaFree Me.* Retrieved from https://www.nami.org/Get-Involved/Take-the-stigmafree-Pledge/StigmaFree-Me.

National Alliance on Mental Illness. (2019b). *Learning to help your child and your family.* Retrieved from https://www.nami.org/Find-Support/Family-Members-and-Caregivers/Learning-to-Help-Your-Child-and-Your-Family.

National Institute of Mental Health. (2021). *Mental illness.* Retrieved from https://www.nimh.nih.gov/health/statistics/mental-illness.shtml.

Provincial System Support Program. (2017). *What is the effectiveness of cognitive behavioural therapy (CBT) for mental illnesses and substance use problems?.* Retrieved from https://eenet.ca/resource/what-effectiveness-cognitive-behavioural-therapy-cbt-mental-illness-and-substance-use.

Sherman, L. J., Lynch, S. E., Teich, J., & Hudock, W. J. (2017). *Availability of supported employment in specialty mental health treatment facilities and facility characteristics: 2014.* Substance Abuse and Mental Health Services Administration. Retrieved from https://www.samhsa.gov/data/sites/default/files/report_3071/ShortReport-3071.html.

Substance Abuse and Mental Health Services Administration. (2020). *Mental health and substance use disorders.* Retrieved from https://www.samhsa.gov/find-help/disorders.

Wang, P. W., Lin, H. C., Su, C. Y., Chen, M. D., Lin, K. C., Ko, C. H., et al. (2018). Effect of aerobic exercise on improving symptoms of individuals with schizophrenia: A single blinded randomized control study. *Frontiers in Psychiatry, 9,* 167.

Wojtalik, J., Keshavan, M., & Eack, S. (2017). Ten-year durability effects of cognitive enhancement therapy in early course schizophrenia. *Schizophrenia Bulletin, 43*(Suppl. 1), S56.

World Health Organization. (2018). *WHO guidelines: Management of physical health conditions of in adults with severe mental disorders.* Retrieved from https://www.who.int/mental_health/evidence/guidelines_severe_mental_disorders_web_note_2018/en/.

33

Forensic Nursing

L. Kathleen Sekula and Alison M. Colbert

Visit the Evolve website for a pretest on the content in this chapter: http://evolve.elsevier.com/Varcarolis

OBJECTIVES

1. Define forensic nursing, forensic psychiatric nursing, and correctional nursing.
2. Describe the educational preparation required for the forensic nurse generalist and the advanced practice forensic nurse.
3. Identify the functions of forensic nurses.
4. Discuss the specialized roles in forensic nursing.
5. Identify three roles of psychiatric nurses in the specialty of forensic nursing.
6. Discuss the roles of the forensic psychiatric nurse within the legal system.
7. Define correctional nursing and its role in reducing repeat incarcerations.

KEY TERMS AND CONCEPTS

advanced practice forensic nurse
competency evaluator
consultant
correctional nursing
criminal profiler
diminished capacity

expert witness
fact witness
forensic nurse examiner
forensic nurse generalist
forensic nursing
forensic psychiatric nurse

hostage negotiator
legal sanity
nurse coroner/death investigator
sexual assault nurse examiner
trauma-informed care

The rate of violent crime involving persons 12 years of age and older in the United States increased from 2.7 million in 2015 to 3.3 million in 2018, with rape/sexual assault increasing from 1.6 per 1000 in 2015 to 2.7 per 1000 in 2018 (Morgan & Oudekerk, 2019). Violent crimes are considered to comprise murder, rape, robbery, and aggravated assault. Both intentional injuries, including self-inflicted injuries, and those caused by acts of violence are among the top 15 killers of Americans of all ages and a leading cause of death among Americans between 1 and 44 years of age. The reduction of violence is a goal of *Healthy People 2030* (US Department of Health and Human Services, 2020). Box 33.1 identifies the specific goals of injury and violence prevention efforts.

Violence is a major focus of **forensics**, which is an abbreviation for *forensic science* and refers to the application of a broad spectrum of sciences to answer questions of interest to the legal system. Over the past 30 years, nurses have formalized a specialty of nursing called forensic nursing, which brings together traditional nursing practice and forensic knowledge to better serve victims and perpetrators of violence. This chapter explores a variety of roles that registered nurses assume within nursing that interface with the legal system.

FORENSIC NURSING

The definition of forensic nursing is:

Forensic nursing is specialized nursing care that focuses on patient populations affected by violence and trauma across the life span and in diverse practice settings. Forensic nursing includes education, prevention, and detection and treatment of the effects of violence in individuals, families, communities, and populations. Through leadership and interprofessional collaboration, the forensic nurse works to foster an understanding of the health effects, effective interventions, and prevention of violence and trauma in the United States and throughout the world (American Nurses Association [ANA] & International Association of Forensic Nurses [IAFN], 2017, p. 1).

Forensic nurses provide direct services to crime victims and perpetrators of crime and consultation services to colleagues in nursing, medicine, social work, rehabilitation, and the law. They can provide expert court testimony in cases related to their areas of practice and expertise and provide input on policy changes within forensic settings. They can also offer evaluation services regarding specific medical and psychiatric diagnoses for both victims and perpetrators.

BOX 33.1 Goals of *Healthy People 2030*: Injury and Violence Prevention

IVP-09	Reduce homicides
IVP-11	Reduce physical fighting among adolescents
IVP-12	Reduce gun carrying among adolescents
IVP-13	Reduce firearm-related deaths
IVP-14	Reduce nonfatal firearm-related injuries
IVP-16	Reduce nonfatal physical assault injuries
IVP-17	Reduce adolescent sexual violence by anyone
IVP-D04	Reduce intimate partner violence (i.e., contact sexual violence, physical violence, and stalking) across the life span
IVP-D05	Reduce contact sexual violence
IVP-AH-R11	Reduce the rate of adolescent and young adult victimization from crimes of violence

From US Department of Health and Human Services. (2020). *Healthy People 2030: Violence prevention*. Retrieved from https://health.gov/healthypeople/objectives-and-data/browse-objectives/violence-prevention.

The International Association of Forensic Nurses (IAFN) was formed in 1992, when 74 nurses—most of whom were sexual assault nurse examiners (SANEs)—came together to create an organization representing nurses whose practice overlapped with key areas of forensic science and the law (Lynch, 1997). A year after its creation, the organization had more than tripled in size; by 2019, the IAFN's membership had grown to well over 5000 nurses. The group now represents nurses who are forensic nurse generalists, SANEs, forensic psychiatric nurses, death investigators, risk managers, coroners, correctional nurse specialists, and others.

The American Nurses Association (ANA) officially recognized forensic nursing as a specialty practice area in 1995. The ANA then combined its efforts with those of the IAFN to develop and publish *Forensic Nursing: Scope and Standards of Practice*, which is currently in its third edition (2017). The goals of the IAFN are to do the following:

- Incorporate primary prevention strategies into our work at every level in an attempt to create a world without violence
- Establish and improve standards of evidence-based forensic nursing practice
- Promote and encourage the exchange of ideas and transmission of developing knowledge among its members and related disciplines
- Establish standards of ethical conduct for forensic nurses
- Create and facilitate educational opportunities for forensic nurses and related disciplines

Education

The IAFN recommends that forensic content be included at all levels of nursing education, both undergraduate and graduate. Specialty forensic nursing education is offered at all academic levels: baccalaureate (BSN), master's (MSN), doctor of nursing practice (DNP), and doctor of philosophy (PhD).

Forensic Nurse Generalist

A registered nurse who is employed in a forensic setting can be called a forensic nurse generalist if that nurse has completed further training through continuing education or graduate studies. The nurse may acquire additional knowledge and skills by completing a certificate program comprising continuing education in an area of forensic nursing. Nurses can also gain expertise by taking secondary education electives and/or pursuing a minor in forensic topics.

The role of the forensic nurse generalist may vary according to clinical settings, but consistent within this role is the need to be proficient in the assessment and treatment of victims and perpetrators of violence. With care of the patient at the forefront, the nurse may also become proficient in evidence collection and preservation, proper documentation, the legal system, and standards of care for both victims and perpetrators.

A forensic nurse generalist may work in a specialty area such as on a trauma team or in an emergency department, corrections, critical care department, outpatient women's health clinic, or may serve as a general resource person for colleagues in the clinical setting. The forensic nurse generalist often provides expertise as a resource for the care provider working with a patient who has been a victim or perpetrator of violence. In addition to addressing patients' physical and psychological needs, forensic nurses are prepared to identify and care for victims of violence, to offer trauma-informed care, and to know when to collect and preserve evidence.

Trauma-informed care stresses the impact that trauma has on the neuroendocrine system and variations that occur because of this impact. It is a practice that promotes a culture of safety, empowerment, and healing. It also requires that patient and provider both work toward mutually established goals and that providers are transparent about the care they provide. Nurses who engage in trauma-informed care strive to understand the patient's life experience. This understanding supports patient-centered care in which the patient actively participates in care decisions.

Patients may respond to acute or long-term trauma in various ways. Some may withdraw, whereas others exhibit behaviors that seem inappropriate, such as giggling or being strangely calm. Clinicians may read these behaviors differently, but we know that the trauma may take different forms in different patients. As such, nurses adjust their care in response to the patient's need. For example, allowing victims of sexual assault time to recover from the initial impact of violence, perhaps to complete a sleep cycle and to collect their thoughts, may allow them to provide a clearer picture of the actual events that occurred. Therefore, some police departments give victims a day or two before interviewing them in depth regarding their experience. All practicing nurses should be aware of trauma-informed care and how to develop their practice in a way that meets the needs of those whom they serve.

Advanced Practice Forensic Nursing

As of 2020, there was no credentialing for the forensic nurse who was prepared with a master's degree. However, master's-prepared forensic nurses are hired in various clinical and community settings as **advanced practice forensic nurses**. Typically, advanced practice forensic nurses have credentialing in another area, such as nurse practitioners in family, psychiatric, adult gerontological, and acute care.

Nurses in the advanced practice role have completed graduate education with a comprehensive focus on forensic nursing. Advanced practice forensic nurses may also have obtained credentials as nurse practitioners, clinical nurse specialists, or certified nurse-midwives. The education provides clinicians with nursing, medical, and legal content and focuses on collaboration among disciplines in the care of victims and perpetrators. The advanced practice registered nurse in forensics also has an educational background in psychiatric assessment and intervention, death investigation, forensic wound identification, evidence collection, family violence, sexual assault of all types and in varied populations, introductory law, and principles of criminal justice and forensic science.

Additional advanced training may take place after the completion of a master's degree. Individuals who are prepared with a DNP may evaluate and apply evidence-based forensic practice for the improvement of education, clinical practice, systems management, and nursing leadership. A PhD prepares nurses to initiate and conduct research in areas of forensics to advance nursing science and to ultimately enhance the practice of forensic nursing. Most forensic nurse researchers have completed a doctoral degree or another advanced degree.

Roles and Functions of Forensic Nurses

In forensic nursing, the nurse–patient relationship is based on the possibility that a crime has been committed. However, it is not the role of the forensic nurse to determine guilt or innocence or whether a victim is being candid in reporting what happened (Sekula, 2016). Forensic nurses are, most importantly, nurses. That means that they are expected to provide trauma-informed care in a way that focuses on the patient and the patient's needs. In addition to that care, the basic responsibilities of the forensic nurse include the following:

1. Identification and assessment of victims
2. Creation of treatment plans
3. Collection, documentation, and preservation of potential evidence
4. Follow-up referrals

Forensic nurses may have expertise in assessment and treatment related to competency, risk, and danger. They are educated in theories of violence and victimology, legal issues, and nursing science, which enable them to assess the circumstances of each case objectively.

An understanding of both the victim and the perpetrator enhances evidence collection. Forensic nurses may use general nursing skills in the care of victims and perpetrators or they may function primarily in the legal role as they collect evidence, testify in court, or collaborate with law practitioners regarding victims or perpetrators. The forensic nurse's role is to care for the patient—whether accuser or accused—and provide evidence collected as an expert while also providing excellent patient care.

Sexual Assault Nurse Examiner

The **sexual assault nurse examiner** (SANE) is also referred to as a sexual assault forensic examiner (SAFE) or forensic nurse examiner. This was the first specialized forensic role for nurses, and represents the largest subspecialty in forensic nursing. In this chapter, the acronym SANE is used. SANEs are forensic nurse generalists with advanced training in the care of adult and pediatric victims of sexual assault (SANE-A and SANE-P, respectively). The IAFN (2020) has established clear guidelines for the preparation of SANEs and provides certification for nurses, although not all nurses who work in this capacity have achieved certification.

A SANE training course typically lasts for 5 days (at least 40 contact hours) and is available online or in the classroom setting. After course completion, an expert SANE serves as a preceptor for the nurse until the nurse is proficient in conducting a patient examination. When the nurse has completed a required number of hours in SANE practice and has prepared adequately, the nurse can then achieve national certification through the IAFN or certification in those states where this is established. Chapter 29 addresses the role of the SANE nurse in more depth.

🌐 CONSIDERING CULTURE

A Web-Based Safety App: myPlan to ourCircle

Intimate partner violence is a critical public health issue that disproportionately affects black, indigenous, and people of color (BIPOC) populations. Native American women are victims of intimate partner violence at higher rates than all other ethnicities; they experience unique issues related to culture and social marginalization. Interventions meant to serve these populations are best guided by those needs and informed with input from the Native American community. myPlan is a nurse-developed, established, and evidence-based safety app used to address dating violence (Glass et al., 2015). Sabri and colleagues (2019) revised this app to better serve indigenous, refugee, and immigrant populations. An even more specific version of the app, ourCircle, was developed to meet the needs of the Native American population (Bagwell-Grey et al., 2020).

In order to develop ourCircle, researchers conducted focus groups and interviews with a sample that included Native American survivors of intimate partner violence and practitioners serving this population. Based on feedback, revisions to the app included a stronger focus on community and the addition of new resources. Edits were made to the terms used on the app. For example, "abuse/violence" was changed to "mistreatment" to better capture the terms endorsed by the survivors and practitioners. The next stage for the ourCircle developers will be to test the effectiveness of the intervention within those populations.

Adapted from Bagwell-Gray, M. E., Loerzel, E., Sacco, G. D., Messing, J., Glass, N., Sabri, B., et al. (2020). From myPlan to ourCircle: Adapting a web-based safety planning intervention for Native American women exposed to intimate partner violence. *Journal of Ethnic & Cultural Diversity in Social Work*, 1–18; Glass, N., Clough, A., Case, J., Hanson, G., Barnes-Hoyt, J., Waterbury, A., et al. (2015). A safety app to respond to dating violence for college women and their friends: The MyPlan study randomized controlled trial protocol. *BMC Public Health*, 15(1), 1–13; Sabri, B., Njie-Carr, V. P., Messing, J. T., Glass, N., Brockie, T., Hanson, G., et al. (2019). The weWomen and ourCircle randomized controlled trial protocol: A web-based intervention for immigrant, refugee and indigenous women with intimate partner violence experiences. *Contemporary Clinical Trials*, 76, 79–84.

Nurse Coroner/Death Investigator

The nurse coroner/death investigator role for nurses was created in the mid-1990s. Traditionally, the coroner is a public official primarily charged with the duty of determining how and why people die. Increasingly, nurses are prepared as death investigators or deputy coroners; they work as death investigators in medical examiners' or coroners' offices or independently in private offices. This expanding nursing role involves assessing the deceased through understanding, discovery, preservation, and use of evidence. An entry-level certification, death investigator, is available through the American Board of Medicolegal Death Investigation.

Nurses who work as nurse coroners or death investigators are prepared with medical knowledge that allows them to make expert judgments regarding the circumstances of death. These judgments are based on observations of history, symptomatology, autopsy results, toxicology, other diagnostic studies, and evidence revealed in other aspects of the case (Mitchell & Drake, 2016).

Nurses are able to expand the role of the coroner/death investigator and improve services provided to families, healthcare agencies, and communities by using basic principles of holistic nursing care. Knowledge of anatomy and physiology, pathophysiology, pharmacology, grief and grieving, growth and development, interviewing, outcome measurements, and other nursing knowledge strengthen the value of nurses in this setting.

FORENSIC PSYCHIATRIC NURSING

A forensic psychiatric nurse may be prepared as a generalist or at the advanced practice level. In the generalist role, nurses are prepared at the entry level with a university degree, associate degree, or diploma, which prepares them to function as direct care providers and patient advocates. At this level, a nurse who practices in a forensic psychiatric setting can gain advanced knowledge through continuing education or certificate programs that provide education in caring for the forensic patient.

At the advanced practice level, graduate education is required. This education prepares nurses to function as psychiatric nurse practitioners, and once prepared nurses to function as clinical nurse specialists. While the certification of clinical nurse specialist is no longer offered, individuals previously educated and certified still practice and function in the same way as nurse practitioners.

Additional graduate work in forensics at the master's and post–master's levels gives nurses the knowledge needed to practice with forensic populations. This specialty requires skills in psychiatric–mental health nursing assessment, evaluation, and the treatment of victims or perpetrators. The skills of both medical and psychiatric nursing combined with a thorough understanding of the criminal justice system result in individuals who are uniquely prepared for expert practice (Sekula & Amar, 2016).

A subspecialty in forensic psychiatric nursing is that of competency evaluator. In this role, the nurse carefully collects evidence by (1) evaluating the perpetrator's intent or (2) determining if the perpetrator had diminished capacity (impaired mental functioning) at the time of the crime. This evaluation aids in determining the degree of the crime and may later influence the

sentence. Forensic psychiatric nurses who work as competency evaluators collect evidence by spending many hours with a defendant and carefully documenting the dialogue. In this capacity, the role of the forensic psychiatric nurse is to provide assessment data that can help make a final diagnosis within the multidisciplinary forensic team (Sekula & Burgess, 2006).

The forensic psychiatric nurse is skilled in interpersonal communications and able to develop collegial relationships with people in other disciplines. A prerequisite communication skill is the ability to listen and accept others' values and motivations in a nonjudgmental way.

Forensic psychiatric nursing appeals to a particular type of nurse—one who thrives in a stimulating intellectual environment, seeks out opportunities to apply clinical skills to complex legal problems, and enjoys pushing the limits of traditional boundaries. Forensic psychiatric nurses are not completely understood within the legal system, mainly due to lack of knowledge regarding their roles. Professionalism in practice, research, and education are improving their visibility and credibility in this intersection between the healthcare and judicial system professions.

Roles and Functions of Forensic Psychiatric Nurses

The forensic psychiatric nurse may function as a psychotherapist, forensic nurse examiner, competency evaluator, fact or expert witness, consultant to law enforcement agencies or the criminal justice system, hostage negotiator, or criminal profiler. The roles of the forensic psychiatric nurse depend on the outcomes that the nurse is expected to achieve. The legal system may contract forensic psychiatric nurses to interface with the perpetrator for a variety of services. Correctional systems or a private organization may also employ forensic nurses to offer direct services to the perpetrator; they can also provide services to the victim in a variety of settings. A list of roles of forensic psychiatric nurses is provided in Box 33.2.

Psychotherapist

In addition to the competencies possessed by the generalist, the forensic advanced practice registered nurse in psychiatric–mental health may function as a psychotherapist, providing individual, family, and group therapy. Depending on educational preparation and individual state statutes, a psychiatric mental health nurse practitioner (PMH-NP) or a psychiatric mental health clinical nurse specialist who is board certified (PMHCNS-BC) has prescriptive privileges and initiates pharmacotherapy along with psychotherapy. Although this role is seriously limited within the corrections systems owing to procedural and economic

---

BOX 33.2 Roles of Forensic Psychiatric Nurses

- Psychotherapist
- Forensic nurse examiner
- Competency evaluator
- Fact or expert witness
- Consultant
- Hostage negotiator
- Criminal profiler

restrictions, it is often filled in the private sector for perpetrators with the necessary financial resources.

Forensic Nurse Examiner

The prosecution, defense, or judge may request an evaluation of a defendant. Evaluations are usually based on the defendant's history along with behavior at the scene of the crime, in jail, or in the courtroom. Important functions of the forensic nurse examiner include the following:

1. Conduct court-ordered evaluations regarding legal sanity or competency to proceed in a court case.
2. Respond to specific medicolegal questions as requested by the court.
3. Render an expert opinion in a written report or during courtroom testimony.

A comprehensive report is based on clinical data, observations of the defendant's behavior, forensic evidence contained in crime-scene reports or laboratory reports, a summary of psychological testing, and a thorough psychosocial history. The forensic nurse examiner interviews the defendant and notes her or his behavior, past diagnoses, personality traits, emotions, cognitive ability, symptoms of a psychiatric disorder, and the psychodynamics of interpersonal relationships.

The forensic psychiatric nurse examiner separates personal opinion from professional opinion. Personal opinion is based on one's background, upbringing, education, and value system. Professional opinion is based on scientific principle, advanced education in a specific field, and the unbiased standards set by research in that area. The forensic nurse examiner strives to remain neutral, objective, and detached while also providing patient-focused care within trauma-informed care principles.

Legal sanity is the individual's ability to distinguish right from wrong with reference to the act with which the individual is charged. Legal sanity is also characterized by the capacity to understand the nature and quality of the act and capacity to form the intent to commit the crime. Legal sanity is determined for the specific time of the act.

The forensic nurse examiner reconstructs the defendant's mental state by reviewing evidence left at the scene, witness statements, the self-report of the defendant's symptoms, and the defendant's motivation. Some of the issues addressed in the forensic nurse examiner's assessment and final report are (1) whether or not the defendant was using drugs, (2) whether a medical condition affected the defendant's reasoning ability, and (3) what the social context of the crime was.

In most states, the presence of a major mental disorder—usually referring to those disorders accompanied by psychoses with delusions, hallucinations, and disorganized thought (e.g., schizophrenia)—is a prerequisite for a ruling of *legal insanity*. However, a defendant who has a mental illness does not have to use this defense. It is the defendant's choice. The forensic nurse has a clear knowledge of which legal standard is being used and is able to articulate it to the court and jury. Legal tests of sanity may include use of the McNaughton rules, which include the terms *irresistible impulse* and *guilty but mentally ill*.

The *McNaughton rules* come from a trial in 1843 in which Daniel McNaughton was tried for the murder of a public official.

McNaughton believed that there was a conspiracy among the Tories of England to destroy him. In an attempt to assassinate the prime minister (who was the Tory leader), McNaughton mistakenly shot and killed the prime minister's secretary. McNaughton was judged to be criminally insane, acquitted of the murder, and institutionalized for life.

There was a public outcry over the leniency of this verdict. The House of Lords convened a special session of the judges to give an advisory opinion regarding the law of England governing the insanity defense. The judges advised that to be considered legally insane, the accused person with a mental disorder either must not know the nature and quality of the act or must not know whether the act is right or wrong. Whether or not the individual is responsible for his action is the underlying issue in the McNaughton rules.

Irresistible impulse was added to the McNaughton rules in 1929. This addition acknowledges that the person may have known the criminal act was wrong. However, it stipulates that if a person could not control one's behavior because of a psychiatric illness or a "mental defect," that person is not guilty.

Guilty but mentally ill is another insanity defense. Those who plead guilty but mentally ill are remanded (sent) to the correctional system, where they receive treatment for their mental disorder. They are then subject to the correctional system's parole decisions.

Whereas legal insanity is determined by the defendant's thinking at the time of the offense, *competence to proceed* is determined by the defendant's mental condition at the time of the trial. It is the capacity of the accused to assist the accused's attorney and to understand the legal proceedings. Because competence to proceed is a determination of mental capacity in the present, the defendant's competency must be determined each time a court hearing is held. A prior finding of incompetence, even if due to a developmental disability or mental illness, does not prevent a finding of competency in a future unrelated case.

Competency Evaluator

Under US federal law, no person may be tried if deemed legally incompetent. If this is the case, the defendant is sent to a suitable facility, usually a locked unit in a psychiatric facility, for a specified period of treatment to regain competency.

Roles of the competency evaluator include assessing mental health or illness, conducting a forensic interview, providing documentation, completing a formal report to the court, and testifying as an expert witness. Competency evaluators work with the defendant in one-on-one and group activities. For competency therapists, the patient is the court, not the defendant, and the products of their work are a competent defendant and a completed report. Becoming an advocate for the defendant rather than for the process is a breach of professional boundaries.

Fact or Expert Witness

There are three types of witnesses in a courtroom trial: (1) the principals (accusers/plaintiffs and accused/defendants), (2) fact witnesses, and (3) expert witnesses. Each witness has a specific role in the presentation of the case and in establishing the required burden of proof.

The court can subpoena any nurse to testify as a **fact witness**. A fact witness testifies regarding what was personally seen or heard, performed, or documented regarding a patient's care. The witness testifies as to firsthand experience only (Sekula & Burgess, 2006).

An expert witness is recognized by the court as having a certain level of skill or expertise in a designated area and as possessing superior knowledge because of one's education or specialized experience. The **expert witness** is used routinely in medical malpractice cases. Nurses functioning in this capacity are capable and qualified to summarize and explain complex and voluminous medical records and terminology to the jury.

A nurse may testify as a fact witness and an expert witness. For example, a SANE may testify regarding the facts of a case in which the SANE examined the victim and collected evidence and may also testify in the case because of expertise as a certified SANE-A.

Forensic nurses with advanced degrees are more likely to be called on as expert witnesses. To establish credibility as an expert witness and have one's opinion given equal weight to that of other professionals in court, the forensic nurse specialist maintains currency in clinical knowledge. In an expert witness, a thorough understanding of the current research literature, trustworthiness, and a professional presentation style are essential (Box 33.3). Professional credentials indicate clinical expertise. Trustworthiness is indicated by the degree of honesty and strength of opinion that is provided on the witness stand. A professional presentation style is important in setting a credible tone. Nurses who are expert witnesses must be able to communicate in a concise and convincing fashion. In addition, by conducting research and publishing the conclusions, such a nurse can show greater reliability of knowledge in specific areas.

Consultant

Over the past 5 decades, deinstitutionalization has created a need for interagency cooperation between mental health and law enforcement. This has occurred because many previously institutionalized individuals are now homeless and often, intentionally or unintentionally, become the focus of law enforcement.

BOX 33.3 Requirements for Expert Witness Testimony

Establishment of Expertise
- Academic preparation
- Professional training
- Practical working experience in the field
- Involvement in professional organizations
- Research and publications in the area of expertise

Establishment of Trustworthiness and Objectivity
- Comfortable with self
- Good presentation style
- Successful communication to jury
- Dress, manner, and performance that communicate professionalism

---

The forensic psychiatric nurse serving in a **consultant** role can provide advice to mental health agencies regarding the care of the individuals with legal issues. An entry-level certification is available—Legal Nurse Consultant—through the American Association of Legal Nurse Consultants. In this capacity, nurses may consult with law enforcement agencies regarding the status and suggested treatment of individuals with mental illness. The nurse may also act as an advocate for families and patients. The focus of the nurse who serves in this capacity is the perpetrator's well-being even if that results in civil detention and admission to a hospital.

A forensic psychiatric nurse may serve either side in a court case as a resource for education and information about mental illness. In this consultant role, the nurse may be asked to listen to witness testimony for the purpose of guiding further cross-examination or to assist in the preparation for trial by giving information about mental illnesses such as personality and paraphilic disorders. The nurse may testify about mental health treatment options, medications, and community resources.

Hostage Negotiator

In the late 1970s, the Federal Bureau of Investigation (FBI) began expanding the structure of its hostage-negotiating team by recommending the use of consultants who could address the mental state of perpetrators and recommend appropriate negotiating strategies. In the 1980s, local police agencies began to develop specialized teams that included consultants. When the forensic psychiatric–mental health nurse functions as a **hostage negotiator**, that role may include the following:

- Being on call around the clock to assist law enforcement officers on the scene
- Providing suggestions regarding negotiation techniques
- Assessing the mental status of the perpetrator
- Providing a link to mental health agencies
- Participating in a critique of the hostage incident
- Assessing released hostages
- Providing training in communication skills to law enforcement officers

The successful hostage negotiator thinks clearly under stress, communicates with persons from all socioeconomic classes, and demonstrates common sense and street smarts. Hostage negotiators must cope with uncertainty, accept responsibility without resorting to a higher authority, and be committed to the negotiation process.

Criminal Profiler

A **criminal profiler** attempts to provide law enforcement officials with specific information about the type of individual who may have committed a certain crime. This service is usually requested when the crime scene indicates psychopathology or when serial crime is suspected. Historically, criminal profilers came from a variety of backgrounds, including law enforcement, psychology, psychiatry, and criminal justice. The criminal profiler collects available data, attempts to reconstruct the crime, formulates a hypothesis, develops a profile, and tests it against the known data.

This is familiar territory for forensic psychiatric nurses, who are comfortable with the nursing processes of assessment, diagnosis (analysis), planning, implementation, and evaluation. Skilled profilers have the ability to reconstruct the crime using the criminal's reasoning process (Kocsis & Palermo, 2015). Although this requires time and thoughtful consideration, the insights gained are usually critical for diagnosis and treatment. Psychiatric mental health nurses offer special skills as profilers of perpetrators because of their knowledge of psychiatry and human behavior. Box 33.4 provides highlights regarding Ann Burgess, a founder of the AIFN and the first nurse criminal profiler with the FBI.

CORRECTIONAL NURSING

Correctional nursing refers to the care of people who are involved with the criminal justice system. Often, this presents challenges to the way nurses think about patients, especially when viewed within the limited context of "victim" and "perpetrator."

There is debate as to the terminology to be used when one is referring to forensic, correctional, and psychiatric–mental health nurses in correctional settings. Working in a correctional setting alone does not make a person a forensic nurse. Rather, it is advanced education and clinical practice that focuses on the unique needs of the population that differentiates a correctional nurse from a forensic nurse (Sekula, 2016).

It is difficult to estimate the total number of incarcerated individuals in the United States, as such an estimate would involve many different entities and institutions. However, around 2.3 million people are believed to be confined at any given time. This number includes individuals in state and federal prisons, juvenile correctional facilities, military prisons, immigration detention centers, state psychiatric hospitals, and other facilities in this country (Sawyer & Wagner, 2019). However, the number is actually higher, with another 4.5 million who are supervised in the community while on probation or on parole (Kaeble & Bonczar, 2017).

Incarcerated men and women have higher rates of serious and chronic physical and mental illnesses than individuals in the general population (Colbert et al., 2013). At least 14% of federal prison inmates and 26% of jailed individuals have serious mental illnesses as compared with 5% in the general population. Additionally, 37% of federal prisoners and 44% of those in jail have been told by a healthcare provider that they had a mental health disorder, usually major depressive disorder (Bronson & Berzofsky, 2017). The incidence of attention-deficit/hyperactivity disorder is 10 times greater among incarcerated individuals than in the general population (Young et al., 2015).

Alcohol and substance use are critical issues associated with incarceration. Approximately 25% of these individuals have an alcohol use disorder, with similar rates among men and women. More incarcerated women than men, 51% versus 30%

BOX 33.4   A Real-Life Mindhunter

Movies and television shows are full of stories about true crime. *Mindhunter*, a Netflix series from 2017 to 2019, tells the story of what is now known as the Behavioral Analysis Unit of the Federal Bureau of Investigation (FBI). What most people do not know is that the lead female character, Dr. Wendy Carr, a sociology professor, is actually based on the career of a forensic nurse.

This nurse is Ann Wolbert Burgess, who is considered a pioneer in forensic nursing. Her fascination with human behavior became evident during her nursing education and clinical experience on a psychiatric unit. Burgess subsequently received a doctor of nursing science (DNSc) degree and became a faculty member at both the University of Pennsylvania and Boston College. It was her seminal work, which culminated in the concept of rape trauma syndrome, that drew the attention of the FBI in the 1970s. In a profile written for the Boston College newspaper (Giacobbe, 2019), Burgess shared her experience of working at the FBI and being part of the team there. During that time, the bureau developed its methods of studying and learning from perpetrators.

Dr. Burgess currently teaches three forensic courses—victimology, forensic mental health, and forensic sciences—where students study the history, mindsets, and behaviors of people who have committed violent crimes. She emphasizes to her students that it was her training and experience as a nurse that gave her the unique perspective with which she views crime victims and perpetrators. This difference in perspective allowed her to help change the direction of crime investigation in a profound and meaningful way.

Dr. Burgess has published numerous journal articles and coauthored books on topics such as crime classification, rape investigation, and patterns of sexual violence. Her upcoming book, *A Killer by Design: How the FBI Academy's Behavioral Science Unit Learned to Hunt Serial Killers and Understand Criminal Minds*, is scheduled for publication in 2021.

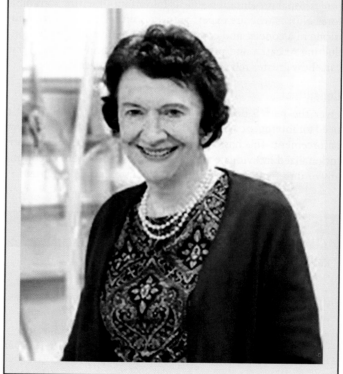

respectively, are believed to have a substance use disorder (Fazel et al., 2017). Despite the prevalence of these disorders, people rarely receive treatment in jail or prison. There is controversy over how to respond to people with substance use problems who commit crimes: Should they be diverted from incarceration and treated or should they be treated while incarcerated? These questions are related to an even more basic question of whether incarceration should constitute punishment or rehabilitation. There is significant evidence to support rehabilitation if the goal is to improve safety in communities and reduce crime. Drug courts and alcohol and substance treatment within correctional facilities result in decreased recidivism and increased abstinence from substance use after release.

Prisoners are the only group in the US population with a constitutional right to healthcare. Because most of their civil liberties are taken away from them and their movements are severely restricted, prisoners are unable to seek and secure healthcare services on their own. Therefore, correctional facilities must provide adequate health services to inmates, either directly or through community health providers. The question of whether nurses are providing *custody* or *caring* is a major issue in determining the role of the nurse in the corrections setting. This includes treatment for both mental and physical illnesses. The location of the work or the legal status of the patient, rather than the functions being performed, define the role of the correctional nurse.

Treatment and services for inmates with chronic psychiatric conditions are a significant part of the job for correctional staff. According to the US Department of Justice (2016), about one in three state prisoners, one in four federal prisoners, and one in six jail inmates receive psychiatric treatment during incarceration, which amounts to hundreds of thousands of incarcerated adults. Additionally, about one in four inmates with psychiatric disorders have been incarcerated three or more times.

Correctional nurses provide care for inmates with serious mental illnesses who are caught in a cycle of homelessness, psychiatric hospitalization, and imprisonment. Frequently, these individuals become incarcerated as a result of psychiatric emergencies that generally involve threats made to others. Because psychiatric facilities for the management of this type of emergency are scarce, these individuals often end up in jail. Once in jail, their psychiatric condition often worsens owing to lack of intervention. Some fortunate individuals end up in a secure treatment unit within their facility, where they receive proper medication and psychiatric–mental health nursing care.

Because of the long-term effects on recidivism (repeat offenders) and resource allocation, policy makers and legislators are beginning to recognize the importance of providing treatment for incarcerated individuals. In a US Department of Justice (2016) survey, the most common psychiatric symptoms in this population were insomnia, hypersomnia, and depressive symptoms. Psychotic symptoms of either or both delusions and hallucinations were identified in 25% of state inmates, 15% of federal inmates, and 10% of jail inmates. Especially critical within this population is a history of trauma or posttraumatic stress disorder (PTSD). However, the correctional setting is not conducive to the intensive therapy required to treat these issues adequately. Unfortunately, the needs of the vast majority of people in the correctional system with PTSD and/or a history of trauma are not adequately addressed.

VIGNETTE: Susan Barnes, 34 years old, was recently incarcerated after being arrested for public intoxication and retail theft.
Past History:
- Multiple incarcerations over the past 10 years for drug use and minor property crimes
- Previously diagnosed with bipolar I disorder, which was treated with multiple medications
- Past arrests associated with discontinuing medications and self-medicating with crack cocaine and other drugs

She reports having been off her medications "for a while." Correctional staff notes that she is behaving erratically, pacing the floor, and not sleeping. Her behavior is becoming more aggressive toward others, and the staff have threatened to put her in solitary confinement.

David, a forensic psychiatric nurse practitioner, interviews Ms. Barnes, who says she "feels great" and "the cops are just out to get me." Her speech is pressured and her tone is hostile. She is diagnosed with bipolar I in an acute manic phase. Her plan of care focuses on safety, stabilization, medications, patient education, and sleep hygiene. David orders her to be housed in the infirmary until she is stabilized, at which time she will be reevaluated for return to the general jail population.

Discharge planning is especially critical, since Ms. Barnes' involvement in the criminal justice system coincides with stopping her medications. She will be assessed for suitability in the forensic mental health court, which offers specialized services for offenders with severe mental illness. This program provides access to a variety of institutional and community-based services and allows the judge to require participation in treatment and follow-up as conditions for release from jail. The treatment plan includes intensive case management upon release to address needs such as housing, healthcare, and food. David knows that a key outcome for this patient is preventing a return to jail.

In addition to the needs of people living with mental illness while they are incarcerated, the nurse also addresses the needs of those same people when they are released and returning home. The reentry experience is more difficult for persons with mental illness because of factors such as physical health problems and both housing and employment difficulties (Colbert et al., 2013). To be effective, services for this population must include comprehensive discharge planning. Nurses working in this setting facilitate ongoing care for people living with chronic mental illness. This may include advocating for alternatives to incarceration because the prison systems are often poorly equipped to deal with the needs of people with severe mental illness. Moreover, it is not the role of incarceration to provide that kind of care. The alarmingly high rates of mental illness in the offender population, often referred to as the "criminalization of mental illness," has encouraged advocates to push for options other than jail or prison, such as treatment programs.

Correctional nurses working in facilities with comprehensive psychiatric services may provide psychiatric nursing care rather than forensic nursing activities. These functions include completing comprehensive mental status examinations and implementing psychiatric care plans. The following vignette illustrates the care provided by correctional psychiatric nurses.

VIGNETTE: Patrice, a 45-year-old woman incarcerated at a state facility, was convicted of assault with a deadly weapon after a confrontation. Her psychiatric diagnosis includes major depressive disorder and PTSD. She has a history of severe childhood abuse and intimate partner violence. Patrice sees Rosemary, the facility's psychiatric–mental health nurse practitioner, for medication management.

While she was watching television in the common area, Patrice attacked a fellow inmate for no apparent reason, screaming and clawing at anyone who approached her. Staff, unable to control her physically, placed her in solitary confinement with mechanical restraints.

Rosemary assesses Patrice and recognizes that she is having PTSD flashbacks, which are intensified by solitary confinement and restraints. Rosemary and the other staff were facing a common dilemma in correctional healthcare, namely custody versus caring.

While Rosemary's focus was on Patrice's needs, the correctional staff were focused on the goals of the facility related to violent offenders and protecting the environment. A successful correctional treatment team seeks to balance the two sides of this debate: that is, creating an environment where possible rehabilitation of offenders is possible without compromising the compulsory "punitive" aspects of incarceration.

EVIDENCE-BASED PRACTICE

Managing Highly Contagious Diseases in Prisons

Problem

Highly contagious diseases are especially dangerous in congregate settings such as correctional facilities.

Purpose of Study

The researchers sought to synthesize the best information available regarding outbreaks of disease in prison settings.

Methods

Seven electronic databases were searched for peer-reviewed articles and official reports published between January 1, 2000, and March 26, 2020, resulting in 27 relevant studies. These were then synthesized for common themes, scrutinized for gaps in the literature, and evaluated for effectiveness of containment strategies.

Key Findings/Themes
- Prisons require multiagency collaboration and health communication to best address contagious disease.
- Widespread screening for contagious diseases along with isolation, quarantine, and contact tracing are essential elements of disease containment.
- Immunization programs, surveillance, and prison-specific guidelines are useful in addressing outbreaks.

Implications for Nursing Practice

The themes identified in this study have become all too familiar. The pandemic of 2020 drove home the importance of public health measures in containing outbreaks to the public in general and to nurses specifically. Correctional nurses are the on-site experts and leaders in infection control, with basics based on Florence Nightingale's emphasis on handwashing, cleanliness, and fresh air.

Beaudry, G., Zhong, S., Whiting, D., Javid, B., Frater, J., & Fazel, S. (2020). Managing outbreaks of highly contagious diseases in prisons: A systematic review. *SSRN*. https://doi.org/10.2139/ssrn.3598874.

◼ KEY POINTS TO REMEMBER

- The IAFN was established in 1992 as the professional association representing this specialty. The IAFN offers certification for the SANE.
- Forensic nursing is a specialty area of practice that combines elements of traditional nursing, forensic science, and criminal justice.
- Forensic nurses may work as generalists or pursue additional education to work as advanced practice nurses.
- Forensic psychiatric nurses work in a variety of roles, including that of psychotherapist, forensic nurse examiner, competency evaluator, fact witness and expert witness, consultant, hostage negotiator, and criminal profiler.
- Forensic nursing brings together traditional nursing practice with forensic knowledge to better serve all persons within the healthcare system affected by violence in some way.

- The forensic nurse generalist is proficient in assessment and treatment of victims of violence, evidence collection and preservation, proper documentation, the legal system, and setting standards of care for victims and perpetrators.
- In contrast to other members of the treatment team on a forensic unit who can be supportive, accepting, and empathetic, the forensic nurse examiner remains neutral, objective, and detached.
- Correctional nursing is the care of incarcerated patients. Treatment of psychiatric disorders and alcohol and substance use are critical issues that are addressed in the prison population to decrease recidivism and promote a better quality of life.

◼ CRITICAL THINKING

1. Compare and contrast the roles of the forensic psychiatric nurse and the correctional nurse. How do their roles differ regarding their relationship with the patient?

2. Given the varied and complex roles within forensic psychiatric nursing, how does an advanced practice forensic psychiatric nurse prepare for these roles? What educational requirements should be considered?

3. All nurses are full partners with physicians and other health-care professionals in providing healthcare. How can a forensic psychiatric nurse prepare to be a part of that team?

4. As a forensic psychiatric nurse, describe circumstances under which you might be called to serve as a fact witness versus being called as an expert witness. What types of education and practice requirements are needed for each role?

CHAPTER REVIEW

1. The forensic nurse examiner is attempting to reconstruct the mental state of an individual accused of a hit-and-run automobile accident. Which question or questions would help to achieve that goal? *Select all that apply.*
   a. "Were you under the influence of illegal substances at the time of the accident?"
   b. "What were you feeling when you realized you had hit someone crossing the street?"
   c. "Have you ever been involved in a hit-and-run accident before?"
   d. "Can you remember the events leading up to the accident?"
   e. "Had you and your friends been drinking before the accident?"

2. A forensic nurse examiner is interviewing an individual accused of a homicide. Which question should the nurse ask in preparation for a possible legal insanity defense?
   a. "Have you ever been told that you are intellectually deficient?"
   b. "Do you ever hear voices that no one else can hear?"
   c. "What were you doing the day the crime was committed?"
   d. "Did you know the individual who was murdered?"

3. Which nurse would qualify as a fact witness in a case dealing with a physically abused young child?
   a. A psychiatric nurse
   b. A sexual assault nurse examiner nurse
   c. An emergency room nurse
   d. A pediatric intensive care unit nurse

4. Which intervention focused on children supports the *Healthy People 2030* goals related to injury and violence prevention? *Select all that apply.*
   a. Screening middle school–aged children for evidence of bullying
   b. Identifying risk-taking behaviors among high school students that often result in injury
   c. Holding a focus group discussion regarding the reasons why students bring weapons onto school property
   d. Holding a community forum to identify the main sources of violence to which children are exposed
   e. Screening to determine the prevalence of unprotected sex

5. Forensic nursing combines scientific knowledge and inquiry in an effort to serve
   a. Victims of crime
   b. Perpetrators of violence
   c. Victims and perpetrators of crime
   d. Families of crime victims

6. In understanding the role of victim and perpetrator, the act of evidence collection is enhanced. What knowledge base can be helpful in caring for the injured victim?
   a. Legal aspects
   b. Experience testifying in court
   c. Collaboration with law practitioners
   d. Medical-surgical nursing skills

7. For a competency hearing, the psychiatric forensic nurse has been asked to evaluate an incarcerated patient who has mental health problems. As the patient is being considered for sentencing, what is the psychiatric forensic nurse's role? *Select all that apply.*
   a. Assessing the patient for level of competency
   b. Determining whether the patient is guilty or innocent
   c. Helping to determine the length of the sentence
   d. Completing a formal report to the court
   e. Becoming an advocate for the incarcerated patient

8. To determine a patient's legal sanity or competency, the psychiatric forensic nurse must assess all of the following, *except*
   a. The patient's ability to distinguish right from wrong regarding the act committed
   b. The patient's capacity to understand the nature of the act committed
   c. The evidence with respect to the defendant's mental state at the time the act was committed
   d. The patient's social network

9. You are caring for Naomi, who has been arrested and is found to be at risk for alcohol and drug use. Which approach is the most useful in treating Naomi?
   a. Recommending that the patient receive treatment when released from jail
   b. Providing an immediate drug/alcohol treatment plan
   c. Immediately withdrawing all medications
   d. Isolating the patient until her withdrawal from drugs is complete

10. Which activity does a correctional nurse not fulfill within the corrections setting?
    a. Making nursing assessments
    b. Maintaining proper safety procedures
    c. Providing psychotherapy
    d. Documenting patient progress

1. **a, b, d, e**; 2. **b**; 3. **d**; 4. **b, c, d**; 5. **c**; 6. **d**; 7. **a, d**; 8. **d**; 9. **b**; 10. **c**

Visit the Evolve website for a posttest on the content in this chapter: http://evolve.elsevier.com/Varcarolis

REFERENCES

American Nurses Association & International Association of Forensic Nurses. (2017). *Forensic nursing: Scope and standards of practice* (3rd ed.). Silver Spring, MD. Nursesbooks.org.

Bronson, J., & Berzofsky, M. (2017). *Indicators of mental health problems reported by prisoners and jail inmates, 2011-12.* Retrieved from https://www.bjs.gov/content/pub/pdf/imhprpji1112.pdf.

Colbert, A. M., Sekula, L. K., Zoucha, R., & Cohen, S. M. (2013). Health care needs of women immediately post-incarceration: A mixed methods study. *Public Health Nursing, 30*(5), 409–419.

Fazel, S., Yoon, I. A., & Hayes, A. J. (2017). Substance use disorders in prisoners: An updated systematic review and meta-regression analysis in recently incarcerated men and women. *Addiction, 112*(10), 1725–1739.

Giacobbe, A. (2019). Mastermind. *BC News, 11*(4), 200–213. Retrieved from https://www.bc.edu/content/bc-web/bcnews/science-tech-and-health/nursing/mastermind.html.

International Association of Forensic Nurses. (2020). *Certification opportunities.* Retrieved from https://www.forensicnurses.org/page/CertOpportunities.

Kaeble, D., & Bonczar, T. P. (2017). *Probation and parole in the United States, 2015.* Retrieved from https://www.bjs.gov/content/pub/pdf/ppus15.pdf.

Kocsis, R. N., & Palermo, G. B. (2015). Disentangling criminal profiling: Accuracy, homology, and the myth of trait-based profiling. *International Journal of Offender Therapy and Comparative Criminology, 59*(3), 313–332.

Lynch, V. (1997). Forensic nursing. *Virginia Nurses Today, 5*(2), 27.

Mitchell, S. A., & Drake, S. A. (2016). Murder, assault and battery, stranger danger. In A. F. Amar, & L. K. Sekula (Eds.), *A practice guide to forensic nursing: Incorporating forensic principles into forensic practice* (pp. 243–261). Indianapolis, IN: Sigma Theta Tau International.

Morgan, R. E., & Oudekerk, B. A. (2019). *Criminal victimization, 2018.* United States Department of Justice. Retrieved from https://www.bjs.gov/index.cfm?ty=pbdetail&iid=6686.

Sawyer, W., & Wagner, P. (2019). *Mass incarceration: The whole pie 2019.* Northampton, MA: Prison Policy Initiative. Retrieved from https://www.prisonpolicy.org/reports/pie2019.html.

Sekula, L. K. (2016). What is forensic nursing? In A. F. Amar, & L. K. Sekula (Eds.), *A practice guide to forensic nursing: Incorporating forensic principles into forensic practice* (pp. 1–15). Indianapolis, IN: Sigma Theta Tau.

Sekula, K., & Amar, A. F. (2016). Forensic mental health nursing. In A. F. Amar, & L. K. Sekula (Eds.), *A practice guide to forensic nursing: Incorporating forensic principles into forensic practice* (pp. 225–242). Indianapolis, IN: Sigma Theta Tau.

Sekula, L. K., & Burgess, A. W. (2006). Forensic and legal nursing. In C. H. Wecht, & J. T. Rago (Eds.), *Forensic science and law: Investigative applications in criminal, civil, and family justice* (pp. 601–627). Boca Raton, FL: CRC Press.

US Department of Health and Human Services. (2020). *Healthy People 2030: Violence prevention.* Retrieved from https://health.gov/healthypeople/objectives-and-data/browse-objectives/violence-prevention.

US Department of Justice. (2016). *U.S. correctional population at lowest level since 2002.* Retrieved from https://www.bjs.gov/content/pub/press/cpus15pr.cfm.

Young, S., Moss, D., Sedgwick, O., Fridman, M., & Hodgkins, P. (2015). A meta-analysis of the prevalence of attention deficit hyperactivity disorder in incarcerated populations. *Psychological Medicine, 45*(2), 247–258.

34

Therapeutic Groups

Donna Rolin and Emily Fowler

🌐 Visit the Evolve website for a pretest on the content in this chapter: http://evolve.elsevier.com/Varcarolis

OBJECTIVES

1. Discuss Yalom's therapeutic factors of the group experience.
2. Differentiate between group content and process.
3. Identify the phases of group development and what is occurring during those phases.
4. Define task, maintenance, and individual roles of group members.
5. Discuss seven types of groups commonly led by registered nurses.
6. Describe three basic leadership styles that nurses may use when leading a therapeutic group.
7. Contrast professional confidentiality with individuals not bound to professional confidentiality and its ramifications for group work.
8. Describe a group intervention for (a) a monopolizing group member, (b) a member who is disruptive, and (c) a member who is silent.

KEY TERMS AND CONCEPTS

feedback
group content
group
group norms
group phases

group process
group psychotherapy
group work
individual roles
maintenance roles

task roles
therapeutic factors
therapeutic group

It takes people to make people sick, and it takes people to make people well again.

Harry Stack Sullivan (1953)

Humans are fundamentally social and are wired for attachment. We form groups because we are psychologically and physiologically dependent on one another. A group is an interconnected and interdependent set of individuals who come together for a shared purpose. Such purposes can vary as widely as becoming a married couple (a social group), inventing a cure for a virus (a scientific group), or building a house (a task group). Groups can be as large and complex as nations or as intimate as those who share our daily lives.

FROM GROUP TO THERAPEUTIC GROUP

The first and second World Wars are examples of the devastating destruction that can arise through human collaboration.

These two wars resulted in vast numbers of traumatized veterans and civilians. Psychotherapists, in an effort to help the large numbers of psychologically wounded veterans, began to treat individuals in groups after the wars. A therapeutic group is any group of people who meet for personal development and psychological growth.

Group settings provide an efficient method of addressing the needs of multiple individuals. However, there are drawbacks to this method, and group work may not suit every situation. See Box 34.1 for a list of the advantages and disadvantages of therapeutic groups.

Skilled group leaders can usually address and manage any issues that may arise. In fact, groups usually provide nurses with excellent opportunities to facilitate patients' growth. This chapter explores concepts central to group work, group leadership styles, evidence supporting the use of therapeutic groups, and various types of group treatment settings.

CONCEPTS COMMON TO ALL GROUPS

Therapeutic Factors

Irvin D. Yalom, an existential psychiatrist, developed an influential approach to group psychotherapy (Yalom & Leszcz, 2005). His framework encompasses themes of freedom and responsibility, isolation, meaninglessness, and death (Yalom, 1980). Yalom's widely used and well-regarded text, *Theory and Practice of Group Psychotherapy*, established existential therapy in the group therapy modality. He identified the core principles that make a group therapeutic. These therapeutic factors are aspects of the group experience that leaders and members have identified as curative (healing) and as crucial for therapeutic change. For example, within a therapeutic group, a member may recognize for the first time that she is not so different from those around her. Yalom calls this factor *universality*—a patient's recognition that other people feel the same way or have had the same experiences. When universality is discovered within a group, it helps to create a feeling of belonging and connection.

Group leaders can emphasize certain therapeutic factors that correlate with the desired outcome of the group. For example, many self-help groups—such as Alcoholics Anonymous—rely heavily on testimonials to foster the *instillation of hope*, whereas groups composed of members who have grappled with secrecy, such as patients with bulimia, often emphasize self-disclosure to promote *universality* (Yalom & Leszcz, 2005). The leader may also model some therapeutic behaviors during the initial phase of group development—for example, by *instilling hope* and *imparting information*. Table 34.1 summarizes the curative factors that may be beneficial to patients during group work.

BOX 34.1   Advantages and Disadvantages of Therapeutic Groups

Advantages

- Multiple members can be in treatment at the same time, thereby reaching more patients and reducing personnel costs.
- Members of a therapeutic group benefit from the knowledge, insights, and life experiences of both the leader and the participants.
- A therapeutic group can be a safe setting to learn new ways of relating to other people and to practice new communication skills.
- Groups can promote feelings of cohesiveness.

Disadvantages

- Individual members may feel cheated of participation time, particularly in large groups.
- Concerns over privacy.
- Disruptive group members reduce a group's effectiveness.
- Group norms may discourage personal opinions.
- Not all patients benefit from group treatment.

TABLE 34.1   Curative Factors in Group Work

Instillation of hope	The leader shares optimism about the successes of group treatment, and members share their improvements.	Testimonials from peers at Alcoholics Anonymous meetings provide firsthand stories of successfully dealing with recovery methods and inspire hope among members of the group.
Universality	Members realize that they are not alone with their problems, feelings, or thoughts.	Members of sexual abuse support groups may be struggling with shame. Being with peers who feel or have felt the same way makes them feel less alone and less ashamed.
Imparting of information	Participants receive formal teaching by the leader or advice from peers.	Leaders of groups for patients with HIV often incorporate medical material and information related to correcting fears and misconceptions about the transmission of infection.
Altruism	Members gain or profit from giving support to others, leading to improved self-esteem.	A patient says that she will never get over the loss of her husband. A second group member nods and responds, "I felt like that, too, after my husband died." The second group member feels pleased to have helped another person.
Corrective recapitulation of the primary family group	Members repeat patterns of behavior in the group that they learned in their families; from the safety of the group with feedback from the leader and peers, they learn about their own behavior.	A group member expresses frustration that other members are more appreciated, and she resents having to share time with the group. Group members note that she said the same thing about her siblings and suggest that she is appreciated.
Development of socializing techniques	Members learn new social skills based on others' feedback and modeling.	A man knew that others were avoiding social engagement with him but he was not sure why. Through a member's direct feedback, he learned that his tendency to obsessively insert irrelevant details in his communication created discomfort in others.
Imitative behavior	Members may copy the behavior of the leader or peers and thus can adopt healthier habits.	Patients with psychotic symptoms in a cognitive behavioral therapy group learn how to reduce the intensity of auditory hallucinations by watching the group leader and other members use cognitive behavioral strategies.
Interpersonal learning	The group itself is a laboratory for trying out new interpersonal skills. Members gain insight from others' feedback and from trying out new behaviors in the group.	Patients in the parent support group for children with attention-deficit/hyperactivity disorder role play responses to challenging behaviors of their children. Afterward, the group provides feedback to support the patients' learning.
Group cohesiveness	This factor arises in a mature group when members feels connected to one another, the leader, and the group as a whole.	A group develops norms that include nonjudgmental acceptance and inclusion, helping members learn to trust one another, disclose information about themselves, receive empathetic feedback, and feel accepted.
Catharsis	A genuine expression of feelings that can be interpreted by both the patient and the group. Overexpression of feelings can be detrimental to group processes.	Individuals in a group for women with early breast cancer are able to express emotions and needs within the context of the mutually supportive group.
Existential factors	Members examine aspects of life—such as loss, meaning, and mortality—that affect everyone in constructing meaning.	Individuals in a grief support group express positive thoughts and feelings in regard to the loss of a loved one and can also safely share negative thoughts and feelings.

Data from Yalom, I. D., & Leszcz, M. (2005). *The theory and practice of group psychotherapy* (5th ed.). New York, NY: Basic Books.

Group Content and Process

Group work consists of both group content and group process and involves recognizing what is happening on the surface versus what is going on underneath. If you were to tape record a group's interactions, type up what everyone says, and print it out, you would have a transcript of the group content. Minutes from meetings are also examples of group content.

Group process is the term used to describe everything else that goes on in the group. It refers to the way that group members interact with one another. They may, for example, be supportive, interruptive, judgmental, or silent. Their expressions may be concerned, hostile, open, closed, bored, or intense. Their speech may be rapid, loud, mumbled, or soft. The group process is the art of doing group work. For groups to be effective and helpful, the group process must be carefully managed and supported.

Groups tend to develop their own identities. Leaders are aware of these identities and may describe them positively, with terms such as *cohesive* and supportive, or negatively, with terms such as *codependent* or *disengaged*. This shared identity affects the development of group norms, which are established expectations or assumptions held by members of a group regarding the kind of behavior that is acceptable. Although group members rarely articulate these expectations spontaneously, they may do so if asked.

Group leaders pay careful attention to the development of cohesion within a group. Yalom identified cohesion as one of the curative factors of groups, and it continues to be a common focus of research around group efficacy and outcomes. The level of group cohesion reliably predicts group outcome, and group leaders attempt to routinely assess and improve group cohesion (Burlingame & Jensen, 2017). Outcomes are most strongly linked to cohesion when the leader focuses on member interactions and implements specific interventions—such as building a positive work relationship and handling conflict efficiently—to support a positive group environment and foster relationships among different members, members and the leader, and members and the group as a whole.

Other terms that are central to therapeutic groups are listed in Box 34.2.

> *Everybody is identical in their secret unspoken belief that way deep down they are different from everyone else.*
>
> **D. F. Wallace (1996)**

PHASES OF GROUP DEVELOPMENT

Group phases represent distinct periods or stages in the process of group development. All groups go through developmental phases similar to those identified for individual therapeutic relationships (refer to Chapter 8). In each phase of the therapeutic group, the group leader has specific roles and challenges to address in support of positive interaction, growth, and change.

Planning Phase

In developing a successful group, planning will include a description of specific characteristics. The group leader or leaders identify the following attributes:

- The name of the group
- Objectives of the group
- Types of individuals (e.g., diagnoses, age, gender) for inclusion
- Group schedule (frequency, times of meetings)
- Physical setting
- Seating configuration
- Description of leader and member responsibilities
- Methods or means of evaluating outcomes

Other decisions have to do with the type of group being planned. Some groups meet for a specific length of time to complete a certain task whereas others are open ended. Additional characteristics of groups are listed in Box 34.3.

When you are forming a group, it is important to consider group composition and patient selection, as these factors will ultimately affect the combination of personalities, interactive styles, and behavioral tendencies among the group's members. For an open group where members join and leave at different times, it is crucial to factor in how a new member will mesh with the existing members. Some common selection errors include adding a disruptive member to a young or inexperienced group or placing a withdrawn patient into an active, probing group (Kealy et al., 2016).

Planning and structure are especially important when group leaders are likely to change, as in inpatient settings, where staffing patterns vary. When several groups with a common goal are running simultaneously, as in a research study, consistency is crucial.

BOX 34.2   Terms Central to Therapeutic Groups

Terms Describing Group Work

Group content: All that is verbalized in the group (e.g., the group's topics).

Group process: The dynamics of interaction among the members (e.g., interaction, facial expressions, body language, and progression of group work).

Group norms: Expectations for behavior in the group that develop over time and provide structure (e.g., rules about starting on time, not interrupting).

Group themes: Members' expressed ideas or feelings that recur and share a common thread. The leader may clarify a theme to help members recognize it more fully.

Feedback: Providing group members with feedback about how they affect one another.

Conflict: Open disagreement among members. Positive conflict resolution within a group is key to successful outcomes.

BOX 34.3   Terms Describing Membership

Heterogeneous group: A group in which a range of differences exists among members.

Homogeneous group: A group in which members share central traits (e.g., men's group, individuals with bipolar disorder).

Closed group: A group in which membership is restricted; no new members are added even when others leave.

Open group: A group in which new members are added as others leave (e.g., inpatient group with transient membership).

Subgroup: Dyads or a small group within a larger group. Members of a subgroup may have greater loyalty, more similar goals, or more perceived similarities to one another than they do to the larger group.

Thoughtful consideration of the physical space is important. If possible, the size of the room should be based on the size of the group. A large room for a small group does not encourage intimacy, and an overcrowded room may cause discomfort and anxiety among members. Room temperature, lighting, external noise, and privacy are important comfort features to consider. Depending on the size of the group, organize the room and its physical boundaries with close, nonhierarchical seating. By arranging chairs in a circle, equality is communicated and members are able to see one another.

Inpatient groups tend to be somewhat different from outpatient groups. In general, inpatient groups require more structure owing to the acuity level of the hospitalized individuals as well as the turnover among group members. Table 34.2 compares outpatient and inpatient groups.

Orientation Phase

In the **orientation phase**, the group is forming. The group leader's role is active in structuring an atmosphere of respect, confidentiality, and trust. During the first session, the group leader begins by providing a personal introduction. The members are encouraged to get to know one another through their own introductions. The leader then describes the purpose of the group.

Initially, members may be overly polite, quiet, or anxious because they have not yet established trust with one another. Therapeutic interaction is supported when the directive group leader points out similarities among members, encourages them to talk directly to one another rather than to the leader, and reminds members of the ground rules for respectful, meaningful interaction.

Participants are urged to treat what happens in the group as confidential. Technology presents several challenges to confidentiality. Cellular phones and other electronic devices can be used to record voices and images or to make posts on social media. For this reason and also to reduce disruptive notifications, group members are instructed to turn off their electronic devices during group sessions.

Working Phase

During the **working phase**, the leader facilitates communication, the flow of group processes, and group conduct. The group leader's role is to encourage members to focus on problem solving consistent with the purpose of the group. As group members begin to feel safe within the group, conflicts may be expressed, which the group leader may view as a positive opportunity for group growth. It is important for the leader to guide and support conflict resolution. Through the successful resolution of conflicts, group members develop confidence in their problem-solving abilities and better support one another in their individual efforts to grow and change.

Tuckman's (1965) seminal work on group stages described steps within this working phase, which takes place after the "forming" phase. He called them the classic stages of "storming, norming, and performing" and identified them as natural and necessary in the development of a group.

- *Storming* refers to the disagreements, attempts at dominance, and personality clashes that are addressed in order for the work of the group to be done. The authority and legitimacy of the leader may be questioned in this phase.
- *Norming* occurs when personality clashes and disagreements are resolved and a spirit of cooperation emerges. Team members begin to settle into their respective roles.
- *Performing* groups have established norms and roles. Group members focus on achieving goals.

The sequence of these phases begins with the generation of group cohesion, followed by the completion of group tasks and resulting in the development of insight. Groups may revert to earlier stages when conflict arises. Leadership activities at different phases of group formation will require different approaches and strategies and ultimately yield team building.

Termination Phase

In the **termination phase**, the leader ensures that each member summarizes personal accomplishments, shares new insights, and identifies future goals. The leader encourages group members to provide both positive and negative feedback regarding the group experience. Feedback refers to information that group members get from other members about how they affect one another. Members may experience feelings of loss or anger about the group's ending. Sometimes, an individual may direct these feelings at other group members or the leader. It is important to address such feelings openly as part of the work toward successful group adjournment.

TABLE 34.2	Comparison of Outpatient and Inpatient Groups	
Group Component	**Outpatient Groups**	**Inpatient Groups**
Composition	The group has a stable composition.	The group is rarely the same for more than one or two meetings.
Membership selection	Members are carefully selected and prepared.	Patients are admitted to the group with little prior selection or preparation.
Level of functioning	Group members tend to have similar levels of functioning	Group members' functioning is variable.
Motivation	Motivated, self-referred patients make up the majority of outpatient groups. Some court-ordered participants may be less engaged.	Patients maybe ambivalent, since group work may be a condition of inpatient care.
Length of group treatment	Treatment may have predetermined number of sessions or continue indefinitely.	Treatment is limited to the period of hospitalization.
Distractions	There are few external influences within a dedicated group space.	Distractions are common in inpatient group work.
Cohesion	Group cohesion develops normally.	With short inpatient stays, cohesion may be limited.
Leadership	The leader may be less directive and peer leadership may play a role.	The group leader structures time and tends to be more directive.

Evaluation and Follow-up

Evaluation and follow-up are fundamental aspects of a therapeutic group. Feedback can be solicited periodically during the life of the group and also during termination. Objective measures are valuable in quantifying the group's effectiveness by identifying what patients found helpful or not helpful. The group questionnaire (Janis et al., 2018) may be used to evaluate patient perception of the group's relationships, quality, and structure.

ROLES OF THE GROUP MEMBERS

We each have a particular style of interacting with others. Some of us tend to sit back and observe, giving an opinion only after careful consideration. Others feel that it is important to keep everyone moving in a common direction, to help maintain order, or to actively urge people to continue working. The way we behave in groups is a function of our personalities (e.g., shy or outgoing), socialization (e.g., birth order, prior exposure to groups), and comfort/interest in the context of the group (e.g., topic, members, leader).

Studies of group dynamics have identified functional roles often assumed by group members that may either help or hinder the group's development. The classic descriptive categories for these roles are task, maintenance, and individual roles (Benne & Sheats, 1948):

- **Task roles** keep the group focused on its main purpose and getting the work done. For example, the information seeker requests clarification around the truthfulness of comments and appeals for reliable information relevant to the issue at hand.
- **Maintenance roles** keep the group together, help each person feel valuable and included, and create a sense of group cohesion. One such role is the harmonizer, who acts as a mediator between other members while trying to reconcile differences and relieve tension.
- **Individual roles** have nothing to do with helping the group but instead relate to specific personalities, personal agendas, and desires for having personal needs met. For example, a blocker throws up barriers to disrupt group progress or to avoid doing his own real work.

Awareness of roles that individual members assume can assist the group leader in identifying behaviors that may be reinforced or addressed. Members' growing self-awareness of their roles may encourage more deliberate and insightful group participation and growth.

Table 34.3 describes selected functional roles of group members.

THEORETICAL FRAMEWORKS FOR GROUPS

Psychiatric–mental health nurses are involved in a variety of therapeutic groups in acute care, long-term, and community treatment settings. All group leaders need a clear theoretical framework for analyzing their group's dynamics and progress. Table 34.4 describes common theoretical frameworks underlying group work.

TABLE 34.3 Functional Roles of Group Members

Role	Function	Example
Task roles	Elaborator	Gives examples and follows up the meaning of ideas
	Energizer	Encourages the group to make decisions or act
	Information giver	Provides facts or shares experience as an authority figure
	Opinion giver	Shares opinions, especially to influence group values
	Orienter	Notes the progress of the group toward goals
Maintenance roles	Compromiser	During conflict, yields to preserve group harmony
	Encourager	Praises and seeks input from others
	Follower	Agrees with the flow of the group
	Gatekeeper	Monitors the participation of all members to keep communication open and equal
	Standard setter	Verbalizes standards for the group
Individual roles	Aggressor	Criticizes and attacks others' ideas and feelings
	Blocker	Disagrees with and halts group issues; oppositional
	Help seeker	Excessively seeks sympathy from the group
	Recognition seeker	Seeks attention by boasting and discussing achievements
	Self-confessor	Verbalizes feelings or observations beyond the scope of the group topic

From Benne, K., & Sheats, P. (1948). Functional roles of group members. *Journal of Social Issues*, 4(2), 41–49.

TABLE 34.4 Theoretical Foundations of Group Work

Theoretical Base	Focus	Leader Practices
Humanism (patient centered, existential, experiential)	Self-actualization; awareness of subjective experience	Nondirective, active listening, Socratic dialogue
Cognitive behavioral	Specific maladaptive behaviors and thought patterns	Goal setting, planning, reinforcing, modeling, and monitoring
Psychodynamic (psychoanalytic, Gestalt)	Insight; resolution of intrapsychic conflict	Listening, interpreting, confronting, probing, working through, directing enactments
Educational	Information on specific topics; coping; emotional and practical support	Teaching, modeling, organizing, leading discussions, assessing
Systems (Adlerian, choice/reality, feminist, family, interpersonal)	Positive interaction with social and political milieu; balance between individual and society; social equality	Modeling, analyzing, strategizing, lifestyle investigation, activism

Virtual Groups

The COVID-19 pandemic that began in the spring of 2020 underscored the importance of having virtual options for group work (American Group Psychotherapy Association [AGPA], 2020). Legal challenges to providing electronic therapy quickly became apparent. For example, certain licensure regulations

TABLE 34.5   Types of Therapeutic Groups

Type	Purpose
PSYCHIATRIC-MENTAL HEALTH REGISTERED NURSE–LED GROUPS	
Educational	Educational groups help to increase knowledge or skills about a specific topic, such as symptoms management. These groups may be time limited or may be supportive for long-term treatment. Written handouts, PowerPoints, and video can supplement discussions.
Medication education	Nurses and pharmacists often lead medication education groups. A group setting will facilitate a helpful discussion among patients. For example, "Yes, I had a dry mouth when I first started taking that, but it got better. Hang in there."
Dual diagnosis	Dual-diagnosis groups discuss comorbid mental illness and substance use disorders. Since treatment issues for patients with dual diagnoses can be complex, group leaders must have competency in both areas.
Stress management	Stress management groups teach members about various relaxation techniques, including deep breathing, exercise, music, and spirituality. Mindfulness groups focus on developing awareness of the present moment with the intent of inducing relaxation and promoting insight into members' thoughts, emotions, and physical symptom responses.
Community meetings	The community meeting is the essential venue for information sharing and processing unit happenings. Patient governance and advocacy matters are ideally managed during these groups, and nurses are ideally suited to lead these groups because they model socially appropriate behavior; they are in close daily contact with patients and make frequent individual and unit assessments.
GROUPS LED BY ADVANCED PRACTICE PSYCHIATRIC–MENTAL HEALTH REGISTERED NURSES	
Group therapy	Group therapy is a specialized treatment led by professionals such as an advanced practice psychiatric–mental health registered nurse (PMH-APRN), psychologist, licensed professional counselor, or licensed clinical social worker. Groups may focus on specific topics such as depression, self-harm, substance use, or grieving. Group therapy aims to alleviate psychiatric symptoms and improve personal growth (APNA/ISPN/ANA, 2014).

will not allow clinicians to see out-of-state patients. Online groups must also comply with Health Insurance Portability and Accountability Act (HIPAA) standards, and practitioners may have to develop additional measures to make sure that members' confidentiality is protected in the online setting.

Practitioners who are used to seeing clients in person may find that the two-dimensional nature of online therapy can have a negative impact on the therapeutic relationship. Obstacles that clinicians encounter in online groups include losing control of the group setting (e.g., seating arrangements), the inability to read facial expressions and body language accurately, and the difficulty of being fully present in an online platform.

Although virtual therapy may be an imperfect replacement for in-person therapy, online therapy has resulted in positive outcomes (AGPA, 2020). Virtual group care may even provide a format to address issues the pandemic itself brought about, including isolation, grief, anger, increased depression, and even suicidal feelings and urges. Chen (2020) developed a study protocol to measure the efficacy of an online brief therapy group for adolescents with anxiety stemming from the pandemic. The protocol constitutes one of many that seek to better understand the effectiveness of online mental healthcare.

NURSES AS GROUP LEADERS

Registered nurses who have received a diploma, associate degree, or baccalaureate degree have holistic training and educational leadership skills to provide leadership in therapeutic groups in a variety of settings. Registered nurses may lead activity, educational, task, and support groups. Advanced practice registered nurses (APRNs) may lead these groups as well. APRNs are further qualified to facilitate other specialized group treatments, including group therapy, for which more advanced skills and training are required. Types of therapeutic groups are discussed in Table 34.5. Support and self-help groups are outlined in Box 34.4.

BOX 34.4   Support and Self-Help Groups

Support Groups
- Bereavement groups for those who have experienced the loss of a loved one
- Suicide survivor groups for those who have lost a loved one to suicide
- National Alliance on Mental Illness (NAMI) groups for patient/family support, education, and advocacy
- Cancer support groups for families and patients coping
- Virtual support groups for a growing number of people, providing online, synchronous interaction and support, which may be perceived as more private or anonymous
- Veterans support groups

Self-Help Groups
- Twelve-step groups that use a common model for recovery: Alcoholics Anonymous (AA) is the prototype for other 12-step groups
- Gamblers Anonymous (GA)
- Overeaters Anonymous (OA)
- Narcotics Anonymous (NA)
- Adult Children of Alcoholics (ACOA) and Al-Anon (friends and families of persons with alcohol use disorder)
- Recovery International for people who have had a mental illness
- National Mental Health Consumers Self-Help Clearinghouse, an information clearinghouse to guide consumers to the nearly 500 diverse types of self-help groups in operation.

An important aspect of the group leader's responsibility is modeling sensitivity and respect to both individual and larger cultural differences. The leader initially sets a foundation for open communication by defining the importance of shared respect for group conduct. As group members begin to engage with one another, the leader notes cultural differences that may affect efforts to maintain open, respectful communication. Diversity exists in many forms, including racial, ethnic, economic, and sexual orientation. By encouraging members to share and explore their cultural assumptions and beliefs, the leader promotes rich communication and provides the group with opportunities to explore similarities and differences in a safe environment.

Styles of Leadership

There are three basic styles of group leadership. All leaders have preferred methods of interacting that may range from directive to hands off. In group situations, however, leaders modify their approaches based on the group's goals. Ideally, a leader selects the style that is best suited to the therapeutic needs of a particular group.

- **Autocratic leaders** exert control over the group and do not directly encourage much interaction among members. For example, staff leading a daily community meeting for patients in a psychiatric hospital with a fixed, time-limited agenda may tend to be more autocratic.
- **Democratic leaders** support extensive group interaction in the process of problem solving. Psychotherapy groups most often employ this empowering leadership style.
- **Laissez-faire leaders** allow the group members to behave in any way they choose and do not attempt to control the direction of the group. In a creative group, such as an art or gardening group, the leader may choose a flexible laissez-faire style, directing the members only minimally to allow for a variety of responses and little productivity.
- In any relationship between nurses and patients, nurses use therapeutic communication techniques. When the nurse serves as group leader, that nurse's words have a tremendous impact on group content and process. Table 34.6 describes communication techniques frequently used and needed by group leaders.

Group Leader Supervision

Clinical supervision is important for registered nurse group leaders. It provides feedback about performance and enhances professional growth. Transference and countertransference issues occur in groups just as they do in therapeutic relationships during one-to-one work (refer to Chapter 8). These issues can be identified and managed effectively with the help of a trusted colleague or mentor. Clinical supervision also provides outside input and perspective while also supporting a focus on therapeutic goals.

Joint leadership of groups is a common practice and has several benefits, which include (1) providing training for less experienced staff, (2) allowing for immediate debriefing between leaders after sessions, and (3) offering two distinctive role models for teaching communication skills to members.

Yalom and Leszcz (2005) assert that working with a cotherapist offers unique advantages as well as potential risks. Cotherapists bring different points of view that may complement one another and generate additional strategies. Having more than one therapist also confers the advantage of activating more transference reactions, as clients will differ in their reactions to each leader. Having another leader can provide support in groups where strong countertransference reactions are likely, such as a trauma or cancer group. The risks that may arise with multiple leaders stem from problems that may arise in the relationship between the cotherapists, so it is important for coleaders to be comfortable and open with each other.

According to the *Psychiatric–Mental Health Nursing: Scope and Standards of Practice* (American Psychiatric Nurses Association [APNA], International Society of Psychiatric Nurses [ISPN], and the American Nurses Association, [ANA], 2014), APRNs are qualified to provide clinical supervision to other clinicians. The purpose of this supervision may be to meet professional requirements for peer supervision. In this role, the APRN may help group leaders to examine and improve their performance and effectiveness. APRN clinical supervisors extend confidentiality to the group leaders under their guidance. APRNs who lead group therapy also seek their own clinical supervision from experienced clinical psychiatric providers.

TABLE 34.6	Group Leader Communication Techniques
Technique	**Example**
Active listening	Eye contact; head nod, "Go on…"…
Ask questions	"Could you tell us the last time you did that?"
Giving information	"Antidepressants may take as long as four weeks or more to show full therapeutic effects."
Clarification	"What do you mean when you say 'I can't go back to work'?"
Confrontation	"Jane, you're saying 'nothing is wrong,' but you are crying."
Empathizing	"I can see how that experience was very painful."
Reflection	"I notice you're clenching your fists. What are you feeling right now?" "It sounds like that really upset you."
Summarizing	"We've talked about different types of cognitive distortions, and everyone identified at least one irrational thought that has influenced their behavior in a negative way. In the next session, we'll explore some strategies for correcting negative thinking."
Support	"It took a lot of courage to explore those painful feelings. You're really working hard on resolving this problem."

🌐 CONSIDERING CULTURE

Supporting LGBTQ Inclusion in Group Work

Group leaders are mindful of supporting all group members' participation. Leaders seek to eliminate barriers that might marginalize or silence members. Individuals of the lesbian, gay, bisexual, transsexual, and queer (LGBTQ) community are group members that are at risk for these barriers. One practice that is becoming increasingly common is for leaders to open a new group by sharing personal preferred pronouns and then asking the group members to do the same. A more formal approach targets the supervisory requirements for group leaders.

The LGBTQ Responsive Model for the Supervision of Group Work helps group leaders to gain the awareness, skills, and knowledge needed to work with LGBTQ individuals (Luke & Goodrich, 2013). This model was originally developed for use by school counselors, who often work without clinical supervision.

ETHICAL ISSUES IN GROUP THERAPY

The *Code of Ethics for Nurses with Interpretive Statements* (ANA, 2015) defines the professional ethical conduct of registered nurses. The nurse group leader has an ethical obligation to inform participants of risks and benefits of group participation (informed consent). They also discuss both confidentiality and exceptions to confidentiality. However, since a group is made up of individuals who are not bound by a professional code of ethics, there is no way to guarantee confidentiality. Other topics the group leader addresses include "Who is free to leave the group?" and "What are the rules about group members socializing outside the group?"

A member is removed from the group only as a last resort. One obvious reason for removal would be a member becoming violent or aggressive toward another member. This would necessitate temporary or permanent removal. Other reasons that might require temporary or permanent removal from the group include (1) a member's consistent unwillingness or inability to participate or (2) a member's violation of the agreed upon rules for group membership.

Group leaders obtain appropriate training or credentialing to practice and work within their defined scope of practice (APNA, ISPN, and ANA, 2014). Group leaders who are knowledgeable of the relevant guidelines and professional standards of practice are the most likely to help patients while also avoiding ethical quagmires (ANA, 2015).

To protect the integrity of the group therapy process, nurse clinicians use evidence-based practice. For instance, brief cognitive-behavioral therapy (CBT) has been demonstrated to be beneficial for major depressive disorder and anxiety disorders (Bernhardsdottir et al., 2013). Group CBT in conjunction with pharmacotherapy is another evidence-based treatment for reducing the symptoms of attention-deficit/hyperactivity disorder (ADHD) and functional impairment in the adolescent population (Vidal et al., 2015). Staying current with research helps nurse clinicians to select the best therapeutic modality for the target group. Evidence-based practice helps to ensure that the therapeutic group maximizes benefit and minimizes harm. See Table 34.7 for some examples of evidence-based groups.

DEALING WITH CHALLENGING MEMBER BEHAVIORS

Research into group dynamics has identified certain behaviors of individual members that are difficult to manage within a group. Many of patients' defensive behaviors interfere with their ability to function or achieve satisfaction in their lives. Group therapy is about working through problem behaviors and resistance, but some behaviors can be especially disruptive to the group process and difficult for the leader to manage.

In dealing with problematic behaviors and issues in groups, members may appreciate being helped to disclose their feelings and responses. The leader can encourage the use of statements that do not focus on "what" the other one did but on the "how," such as "When you speak this way, I feel …." The leader helps by noting that feelings are not right or wrong; they simply exist. People tend to feel less defensive when *I feel* statements rather than *you are* statements are used. This approach helps members feel that they are part of the group rather than alienated from it or threatened by it.

Patients who monopolize the group, those who complain but continue to reject advice, the patient who is disruptive, and

TABLE 34.7   Evidence-Based Group Treatment Methods

Population/Diagnosis	Group Modality	Evidence Source
Social anxiety disorder	Cognitive behavioral therapy	Meta-analysis of randomized-controlled trials (Barkowski et al., 2016)
Smoking cessation	Group program compared with self-help program, or brief support from healthcare provider	Cochrane Database of Systematic Reviews (Stead et al., 2017)
Major depressive disorder	Interpersonal therapy using an eight-session group protocol	World Health Organization (2016)
Adolescents with attention-deficit/hyperactivity disorder (ADHD)	Cognitive behavioral therapy	Randomized controlled trial (Vidal et al., 2015)
Irritability in children with severe mood dysregulation and ADHD	Joint parent–child group sessions	Randomized clinical trial (Waxmonsky et al., 2016)
Patients at risk for psychosis; early psychosis	Group- and family-based cognitive behavioral therapy	Pilot study (Landa et al., 2016); non-controlled study (Chung et al., 2013)
Bipolar disorder	Cognitive behavioral therapy	Randomized controlled trial (Costa et al., 2011)
Substance use disorder	Cognitive behavioral therapy, interpersonal therapy, and behavioral marital, modified psychodynamic, interactive, rational emotive, Gestalt, and psychodrama therapies	American Psychiatric Association Practice Guideline Treatment of Patients with Substance Use Disorders (Kleber et al., 2007)
Posttraumatic stress disorder (PTSD) and comorbid substance use disorders	"Seeking safety" model	Meta-analysis (Lenz et al., 2016)
Neurocognitive disorders	Group reminiscence therapy	Cochrane Database of Systematic Reviews (Woods et al., 2018)
Borderline personality disorder	Dialectical behavioral therapy	Cochrane Database of Systematic Reviews (Stoffers-Winterling et al., 2012)
Child conduct problems, parental mental health, and parenting skills	Behavioral and cognitive-behavioral therapy group-based parenting interventions	Cochrane Database of Systematic Reviews (Furlong et al., 2012)

the patient who stays silent are examples of challenging members who may benefit from specific group therapy interventions (Yalom & Leszcz, 2005).

Monopolizing Group Member

One subtle method in dealing with a monopolizing group member is to address the entire group. Provide them with a reminder that, during group work, everyone has an equal chance to contribute and members can evaluate whether or not anyone is dominating the group's time. It may be necessary to speak directly to the monopolizing group member, either privately or in the group setting. In private, you can share your observations and suggest that perhaps the individual's nervousness may be contributing to the talkativeness.

You may then ask the patient to limit contributions to a specific number of times, such as two or three. In the group setting, the leader may ask the group if they would like to share observations or feedback about other members, thereby offering a chance for self-reflection regarding the desired versus actual response the member is receiving from the group. This strategy is probably the most challenging but potentially the most rewarding in that members feel empowered and the real therapeutic forces of groups are utilized (Yalom & Leszcz, 2005).

Disruptive Group Member

Some members whose behavior is self-centered, angry, or attention-seeking may lack empathy, hope, or concern for other members of the group. They refuse to take any personal responsibility and can challenge the group leader and negatively affect the group process. They also tend to be unaware of the role they play in their own difficulties and their negative impact on the group.

When clients are angry, the group leader listens to the comments objectively. The leader may choose to speak to the group member in private and ask what is causing the anger. Sometimes, this simple exchange can make the patient feel more connected with the group leader and, more importantly, as a member of the group. This intervention will likely decrease hostile behavior and increase the group's benefit. Angry patients may be extremely vulnerable, and the practice of devaluing or demoralizing keeps others at a distance and maintains the patient's own precarious sense of safety. Leaders empathize with the patient in a matter-of-fact manner, such as, "You seem angry that the group wants to support you."

When clients seem out of touch with their emotions, the leader can encourage them to describe how their body is feeling physically or autonomically. The leader may ask these patients to focus on how such personal responses and emotions differ from those of members in the here in now. An additional request to help patients get in touch with their emotions is to invite them to imagine how other members may be feeling.

Members who display self-centered behavior often benefit from the direct feedback of other group members or may be able to gain insight from watching video from previous sessions. Some clients with narcissistic traits who feel undervalued can display explosive anger toward the group in an attempt at self-protection. The leader in these cases can play an important role in attempting to understand and advocate for these individuals when they feel hurt and hopefully prevent them from disrupting the group with outbursts or by leaving the group abruptly (Yalom & Leszcz, 2005).

Silent Group Member

Patients who are silent in the group may be observing intently until they decide that the group is safe for them. Other silent group members may believe that they are not as competent as other, more assertive group members. Such silence might or might not mean that the member is not engaged, but it is nevertheless addressed for several reasons. People who do not speak cannot benefit from others' feedback on their thoughts, and other group members are deprived of these group members' valuable insights. Furthermore, a silent group member may make others uncomfortable and create a sense of mistrust.

There are several techniques that may help, including allowing the person to have extra time to formulate thoughts before responding. One might say, "I'll give you a moment to think about that," and then waiting or coming back to the group member later. Another tactic is to make an assignment that every person in the group respond to a certain topic or question.

EXPECTED OUTCOMES

Expected outcomes of group participation vary depending on the type and purpose of the group. For education groups, such as a medication education group, the expected outcome would be the demonstration of precise knowledge, such as the following:

- Patient identifies three significant side effects of prescribed medication.
- Patient recognizes dangerous drug–drug and drug–food interactions for prescribed medications.
- Patient correctly identifies time of day and dose for each prescribed medication.

For therapy groups, the expected outcomes will focus more on insights, behavior changes, and reduction in symptoms. For example, in an alcohol use disorder treatment group, an expected outcome might be that the patient develops insight into the connection between drinking and negative consequences. An expected behavioral outcome would be abstinence from alcohol use or decreased risky use. In groups that focus primarily on emotional issues such as depression or anxiety, leaders can use standardized symptom surveys to measure symptom reduction as an outcome of group participation.

KEY POINTS TO REMEMBER

- A group format has advantages over individual therapy, including cost savings, increased feedback, an opportunity to practice new skills in a relatively safe environment, mutual learning, and instilling a sense of belonging.

- Yalom's therapeutic factors that operate in groups can lead to therapeutic change for members.
- Groups develop through predictable phases over time: planning phase, orientation phase, working phase, and

termination phase. Group leaders need to use specific skills depending upon the phase the group is in.

- For a group to continue and be productive, members fulfill specific functions known as task or maintenance roles. Individual roles are not productive and are based on individual personalities and needs. Nurse leaders reinforce productive group roles and confront non-productive individual roles.*taskmaintenance roles.*

- Clinical supervision is important, so that group leaders can analyze group interactions and characteristics as well as leadership techniques and countertransference experiences.

- Nurses have many opportunities to lead or colead therapeutic groups both in hospital and community settings.

- Psychoeducational groups, health teaching groups, and support groups are often led by registered nurses.

- Advanced practice mental health professionals such as APRNs may lead group therapy based on various theoretical models.

- Challenging member behaviors, such as monopolizing, being disruptive, and remaining silent, can be especially difficult. A variety of interventions are recommended to minimize such interference and maximize insight for the patient who is engaging in these behaviors.

CRITICAL THINKING

1. You are automatically a part of several groups during nursing education: your large cohort and also your smaller course and clinical practicum groups. Review Table 34.3 and think about your position and ways in which you tend to participate in your current groups at school.
   a. Which task role do you assume in your groups?
   b. Which maintenance role do you assume?
   c. Which individual group role (if any) is yours?
   d. In your class groups in general, how would you characterize the norms?

2. While you were participating in your nursing education groups, you may have noticed that some groups function better than others. Consider your current or a past clinical group and respond to the following questions:
   a. How would you describe the dynamics of the group?
   b. Which leadership styles have your instructors modeled?
   c. Were group members well prepared to participate in group sessions? If no, how did this affect the dynamic of the group?
   d. How did the instructor handle group monopolization, silence, complaining, or disruptive actions?

CHAPTER REVIEW

1. Which outcome would be appropriate for a group session on medication education? *Select all that apply.*
   a. Patient will identify three side effects of prescribed medication.
   b. Patient will verbalize the purpose of taking the medication.
   c. Patient will acknowledge and accept the financial cost of prescribed medications.
   d. Patient will correctly identify time of day and dose for each prescribed medication.
   e. Patient will list two potential drug–drug and drug–food interactions for prescribed medications.

2. What question by the nurse leader is helpful in managing a monopolizing member of a group?
   a. "You seem angry. Is there something you want to discuss with the group?"
   b. "Would it be helpful if you had time to think about the question?"
   c. "Would you tell us about experiences that have frightened you?"
   d. "Who else would like to share feelings about this issue?"

3. What advantages does group therapy have over individual therapy? *Select all that apply.*
   a. Groups are less expensive than one-on-one therapy.
   b. Groups provide an opportunity to learn from others.
   c. Groups are homogeneous in composition.
   d. Feedback is available from the group leader and group members.
   e. Interpersonal skills can be practiced in a safe environment.

4. What group would benefit most from a laissez-faire leader?
   a. Art group
   b. Grief group
   c. Social skills group
   d. Anger management group

5. The nurse describes the purpose of psycho-educational groups as providing group members with the knowledge and skills necessary to manage psychiatric symptoms. Which phase of group development is represented?
   a. Planning (formation) phase
   b. Orientation phase
   c. Working phase
   d. Termination phase

6. Group dynamics can vary widely, and sometimes members disrupt the group process. Which of the following participant traits may indicate a need for additional support for a new nurse facilitator? *Select all that apply.*
   a. A member with paranoid delusions
   b. A quietly tearful participant expressing suicidal thoughts
   c. An angry woman who raises her voice
   d. A calm but ineffective communicator

7. The advanced practice nurse is assigned a group of patients. Which patient would not be appropriate to consider for inpatient group therapy? *(Select all that apply.)* The patient who
   a. Has limited financial and social resources
   b. Is experiencing acute mania
   c. Has few friends on the unit

d. Is preparing for discharge tomorrow

e. Does not speak up often yet listens to others

8. Group members are having difficulty deciding what topic to cover in today's session. Which nurse leader response reflects autocratic leadership?

a. "We are talking about fear of rejection today."

b. "Let's go around the room and make suggestions for today's topic."

c. "I will let you come to a conclusion together about what to talk about."

d. "I'll work with you to find a suitable topic for today."

9. A patient continues to dominate the group conversation despite having been asked to allow others to speak. What is the group leader's most appropriate response?

a. "You are monopolizing the conversation."

b. "When you talk constantly, it makes everyone feel angry."

c. "You are supposed to allow others to speak also."

d. "When you speak out of turn, I am concerned that others will not be able to participate equally."

10. The nurse is planning the care of patients on her unit, which includes a dual-diagnosis group. Which patient would be appropriate for this group? The patient with

a. Major depression disorder and a history of recurrent suicidal ideation

b. Generalized anxiety disorder and frequent migraine headaches

c. Bipolar disorder and anorexia nervosa

d. Schizophrenia and alcohol use disorder

1. **a, b, d, e**; 2. **d**; 3. **a, b, d, e**; 4. **a**; 5. **b**; 6. **a, b**; 7. **b**; 8. **a**; 9. **d**; 10. **d**

Visit the Evolve website for a posttest on the content in this chapter: http://evolve.elsevier.com/Varcarolis

REFERENCES

American Group Psychotherapy Association. (2020). From the couch to the screen–Online (group) therapy. *Group Circle.* Retrieved from https://www.agpa.org/docs/default-source/practice-resources--group-circle/group-circle-winter2020-final.pdf?sfvrsn=1b0f98a9_2.

American Nurses Association. (2015). *Code of ethics with interpretive statements.* Retrieved from http://nursingworld.org/DocumentVault/Ethics-1/Code-of-Ethics-for-Nurses.html.

American Psychiatric Nurses Association, International Society of Psychiatric-Mental Health Nurses, & American Nurses Association. (2014). *Psychiatric-mental health nursing: Scope and standards of practice.* Silver Spring, MD: NurseBooks.org.

Barkowski, S., Schwartze, D., Strauss, B., Burlingame, G. M., Barth, J., & Rosendahl, J. (2016). Efficacy of group psychotherapy for social anxiety disorder: A meta-analysis of randomized-controlled trials. *Journal of Anxiety Disorders, 39,* 44–64.

Benne, K. D., & Sheats, P. (1948). Functional roles of group members. *Journal of Social Issues, 4*(2), 41–49.

Bernhardsdottir, J., Vilhjalmsson, R., & Champion, J. D. (2013). Evaluation of a brief cognitive behavioral group therapy for psychological distress among female Icelandic university students. *Issues in Mental Health Nursing, 34*(7), 497–504.

Burlingame, G. M., & Jensen, J. L. (2017). Small group process and outcome research highlights: A 25-year perspective. *International Journal of Group Psychotherapy, 67*(Suppl. 1), S194–S218.

Chen, S. (2020). An online solution focused brief therapy for adolescent anxiety during the novel coronavirus disease (COVID-19) pandemic: A structured summary of a study protocol for a randomised controlled trial. *Trials, 21,* 402.

Chung, Y. C., Yoon, K. S., Park, T. W., Yang, J. C., & Oh, K. Y. (2013). Group cognitive-behavioral therapy for early psychosis. *Cognitive Therapy and Research, 37*(2), 403–411.

Costa, R. T. D., Cheniaux, E., Rosaes, P. A. L., Carvalho, M. R. D., Freire, R. C. D. R., Versiani, M., & Nardi, A. E. (2011). The effectiveness of cognitive behavioral group therapy in treating bipolar disorder: A randomized controlled study. *Revista brasileira de psiquiatria, 33*(2), 144–149.

Furlong, M., McGilloway, S., Bywater, T., Hutchings, J., Smith, S. M., & Donnelly, M. (2012). Behavioural and cognitive–behavioural group–based parenting programmes for early–onset conduct problems in children aged 3 to 12 years. *Cochrane Database of Systematic Reviews, 2,* CD008225.

Janis, R. A., Burlingame, G. M., & Olsen, J. A. (2018). Developing a therapeutic relationship monitoring system for group treatment. *Psychotherapy, 50*(2), 105–115.

Kealy, D., Ogrodniczuk, J. S., Piper, W. E., & Sierra-Hernandez, C. A. (2016). When it is not a good fit: Clinical errors in patient selection and group composition in group psychotherapy. *Psychotherapy, 53*(3), 308–313.

Kleber, H. D., Weiss, R. D., Anton, R. F., George, T. P., Greenfield, S. F., Kosten, T. R., et al. (2007). Treatment of patients with substance use disorders: Second edition. *American Journal of Psychiatry, 164*(Suppl 4), 5–123.

Landa, Y., Mueser, K. T., Wyka, K. E., Shreck, E., Jespersen, R., Jacobs, M. A., et al. (2016). Development of a group and family-based cognitive behavioural therapy program for youth at risk for psychosis-. *Early Intervention in Psychiatry, 10*(6), 511–521.

Lenz, A. S., Henesy, R., & Callender, K. (2016). Effectiveness of seeking safety for co-occurring posttraumatic stress disorder and substance use-. *Journal of Counseling & Development, 94*(1), 51–61.

Luke, M., & Goodrich, K. M. (2013). Investigating the LGBTQ responsive model for supervision of group work. *Journal for Specialists in Group Work, 38*(2), 121–145.

Stead, O. F., Carroll, A. J., & Lancaster, T. (2017). Group behaviour therapy programmes for smoking cessation. *Cochrane Database of Systematic Reviews, 3*(3).

Stoffers-Winterling, J. M., Völlm, B. A., & Rücker, G., Timmer, A., Huband, N., & Lieb, K. (2012). Psychological therapies for people with borderline personality disorder. *Cochrane Database of Systematic Reviews, 8,* CD005652.

Tuckman, B. W. (1965). Developmental sequence in small groups. *Psychological Bulletin, 63,* 384–399.

Vidal, R., Castells, J., Richarte, V., Palomar, G., García, M., Nicolau, R., et al. (2015). Group therapy for adolescents with attention-deficit/hyperactivity disorder: A randomized controlled trial. *Journal of the American Academy of Child & Adolescent Psychiatry, 54*(4), 275–282.

Wallace, D. F. (1996). *Infinite jest: A novel.* Boston, MA: Little, Brown and Company.

Waxmonsky, J. G., Waschbusch, D. A., Belin, P., Li, T., Babocsai, L., Humphery, H., et al. (2016). A randomized clinical trial of an integrative group therapy for children with severe mood dysregulation. *Journal of the American Academy of Child & Adolescent Psychiatry, 55*(3), 196–207.

Woods, B., O'Philbin, L., Farrell, E. M., Spector, A. E., & Orrell, M. (2018). Reminiscence therapy for dementia. *Cochrane Database of Systematic Reviews, 18*(9), 715–727.

World Health Organization. (2016). *Group interpersonal therapy (IPT) for depression* (No. WHO/MSD/MER/16.4). Geneva, Switzerland: World Health Organization.

Yalom, I. D. (1980). *Existential psychotherapy.* New York, NY: Basic Books.

Yalom, I. D., & Leszcz, M. (2005). *The theory and practice of group psychotherapy* (5th ed.). New York, NY: Basic Books.

35

Family Interventions

Christina Fratena and Laura G. Leahy

🌐 Visit the Evolve website for a pretest on the content in this chapter: http://evolve.elsevier.com/Varcarolis

OBJECTIVES

1. Discuss the characteristics of a healthy family.
2. Identify the evolving nature of traditional family structures.
3. Differentiate family patterns of behavior as they relate to five family functions: management, boundaries, communication, emotional support, and socialization.
4. Compare and contrast models of modern family therapy.
5. Discuss the central concepts of the identified patient and triangulation.
6. Construct a genogram using a three-generation approach.
7. Recognize the significance of self-assessment to successful work with families.
8. Identify nursing diagnoses that provide a framework for nursing care.
9. Formulate outcome criteria for families.
10. Identify strategies for family intervention.
11. Distinguish between the nursing intervention strategies and counseling of a psychiatric-mental health registered nurse and those of a psychiatric-mental health advanced practice registered nurse with regard to psychotherapy.

KEY TERMS AND CONCEPTS

boundaries	enmeshment	genogram
clear boundaries	family therapy	identified patient
differentiation	family triangle	rigid boundaries
diffuse boundaries	flexibility	

In Western culture, the uniqueness of the individual and the search for autonomy are celebrated. Yet we are also defined and sustained by interwoven systems of human relationships, including the relationships developed with our family members. Families are the foundation and structure of most societies. Families are defined by reciprocal relationships in which persons are committed to one another.

Healthy family relationships support the well-being of individual family members. When children do not have family support—for instance, in cases of loss due to the ravages of war—they tend to respond with a range of adjustment difficulties and guilt reactions. These reactions can influence their health and well-being for years, if not a lifetime.

In other cases, the family remains physically intact, yet family members do not support one another. Emotional stress or trauma experienced by one family member, as well as complex life challenges faced by the family as a whole, can threaten interactions. For those families and for the members within them, family support and/or therapy are needed.

The family is the primary social system to which a person belongs and, in most cases, it is the most powerful system of which a person will ever be a member. The dynamics of the family subtly and significantly influence the beliefs and actions of individual members across the lifespan. Healthy families tend to deal better with developmental changes than less healthy families. However, even "normal" changes such as the birth of a child can test the strength of relationships even in the most resilient family.

FAMILY STRUCTURE

When Duvall (1957) described family functioning, she was referring to the nuclear family—mother, father, and children. Today, family structures are more complex. The following types of families that exist in the US include:

- **Nuclear family:** Children living with two parents who are married to each other and are each the biological or adoptive parents to all the children in the family.
- **Single-parent family:** Children living with a single adult of either gender.
- **Unmarried biological or adoptive family:** Children living with two unmarried parents who are the biological/adoptive parents to all the family's children.
- **Blended family/stepfamily:** Children living with one biological/adoptive parent and that parent's spouse.

- **Cohabitating family:** Children living with one biological/adoptive parent and that parent's unmarried cohabitating partner.
- **Extended family:** Children living with at least one biological/adoptive parent and at least one related nonparent adult (age 18 or older), such as a grandparent or adult sibling.
- **Grandparent family:** Children living with one or more grandparents.
- **Childless family:** Consists of partners living together and working together. They may have extensive involvement with pets and children of siblings and friends.
- **"Other" family:** Children living with related or unrelated adults who are not biological or adoptive parents. This includes children living with grandparents and foster families.

As the notion of family has broadened to incorporate nontraditional family structures, it has been a challenge for family therapists to recognize and incorporate similarly broad definitions of family in their work. Fig. 35.1 depicts the family structure of households in the United States by race and Hispanic origin.

FAMILY FUNCTIONS

A healthy family provides its members with tools to guide effective interactions within the family. The family also extends its influence when an individual functions in other intimate relationships, the workplace, culture, and society in general. The tools acquired through activities associated with family life include management activities, boundary delineation, communication patterns, emotional support, and socialization (Nichols, 2017).

Management

Every day in every family, decisions are made regarding issues of power, resource allocation (i.e., who gets what), rule-making, and the provision of financial support. These decisions contribute to adaptive family functioning. In healthy families, it is usually the adults who mutually agree on how to perform these management functions. In families with a single parent, these management functions may often become overwhelming. In chaotic families, an inappropriate member, such as a teenager, may be the one who makes management decisions.

Although children learn decision-making skills as they mature and increasingly make decisions and choices about their own lives, they should *not* be expected or forced to take on this responsibility for the family. A 12-year-old child, for example, should not be the one to decide whether to pay the gas bill or buy groceries.

Boundaries

Boundaries maintain distinctions between and among individuals in the family. They also distinguish between the family and individuals external to it. The establishment and maintenance of flexible and appropriate boundaries are essential to healthy family functioning.

Minuchin (1974) identified three types of boundaries within families: clear, diffuse, and rigid.

Clear Boundaries

Clear boundaries are adaptive and healthy. All members of the family understand these boundaries and they give family members a sense of self. They are firm, yet flexible, and provide a structure that responds and adapts to change. Clear boundaries allow family members to take on appropriate roles and to function without unnecessary or inappropriate interference from other members. They reflect structure while simultaneously supporting healthy family functioning and encouraging individual growth.

Diffuse Boundaries

Diffuse boundaries result in unclear boundaries and a lack of independence. Individuals in families with diffuse boundaries may have problems defining who they are. When boundaries are diffuse, individuals tend to become overly involved with one another. This overinvolvement is referred to as **enmeshment**.

When boundaries are diffuse, everyone, and thus no one, is in charge. It is not clear who is responsible for decisions and who has permission to act. Diffuse boundaries are particularly problematic when parent/child role enactment becomes blurry—for example, when a parent may be unemployed and one of the children takes responsibility for earning money to meet the family's basic needs.

In families with diffuse boundaries, individual members are discouraged from expressing their own views. **Differentiation,**

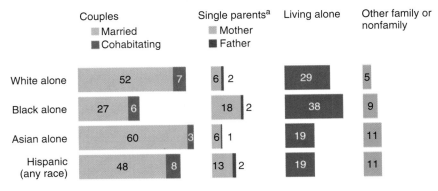

ᵃAt least one child of any age present

Fig. 35.1 Percentage of households by race and Hispanic origin of the householder. (US Census Bureau. [2019]. Current population survey, annual social and economic supplement. Retrieved from https://www.census.gov/content/dam/Census/library/visualizations/time-series/demo/families-and-households/hh-7a.pdf.)

or the ability to possess a strong identity and sense of self while maintaining an emotional connection with the family, is also discouraged. To an outsider, it may appear that family members are extremely close, and family members may believe that they are of one mind. They may take comfort that everyone thinks the same way. "No one in our family likes seafood." That sense is typically false, and deeper analysis often results in the discovery of suppressed frustrations, anger, and passive-aggressive behaviors.

Expression of separateness or independence is viewed as disloyalty to the family. Members are prone to psychological or psychosomatic symptoms, probably as a function of the individuals' inability to actually say or even to recognize how they feel. During times of change or crisis, whether the crisis is one of normal development (such as when a baby is born or an elderly grandparent dies) or one that is unanticipated (such as the loss of a pregnancy or serious debilitating injury to a family member), adaptation of both individuals and of the family as a whole is extremely difficult.

Rigid Boundaries

Families with **rigid boundaries** demand adherence to rules and roles—some apparent and some less so—regardless of circumstances or outcomes. Boundaries can be so firmly closed that family members are disengaged and avoid one another, resulting in little sense of family loyalty. In families in which rigid boundaries predominate, communication is minimal, and members rarely share thoughts and feelings. Isolation may be a marked feature in such family systems.

Disengaged family members lead highly separate and distinct lives. Because they do not learn intimacy in the family setting, individuals from disengaged families do not tend to develop insights into their own feelings and emotions. As a result, they may have a hard time bonding with others and participating in new family structures when they leave their families of origin and begin their lives as adults.

Communication

Communication patterns are extremely important in healthy families. Healthy communication patterns are characterized by clear and comprehensible messages (e.g., "I would like to go now" or "I don't like it when you interrupt what I'm saying"). Healthy communication within the family encourages members to ask for what they want and need and to share their feelings. Thoughts and feelings can be openly, honestly, and assertively expressed in families where communication is encouraged. Alternatively, those in legitimate positions of power within the family, typically the parents, are able to evaluate the appropriateness of family members' requests.

In healthy families, there is a necessary and natural hierarchy for the protection and socialization of younger family members. Parents are the leaders in the family and children are the followers. Despite this arrangement, children can voice their opinions and influence family decisions. In dysfunctional families, this seemingly simple hierarchy becomes unbalanced. When communication among family members is not clear and natural hierarchal roles become confused, communication cannot be used as a means to solve problems or to resolve conflict.

The cardinal rule for effective and functional communication in families is "Be clear and direct in stating what you want and need" whether you are in a powerful or a subordinate position. Speak from the "I" position as opposed to deferring to the "you." Clear communication is one of the hardest skills to cultivate in a family system. To be direct, individuals need to first have a sense that they are respected and loved and that it is safe to express personal thoughts and feelings. The consequences of being clear and direct may be unpleasant in a family system that does not tolerate openness. Box 35.1 offers examples of unhealthy family patterns of communication.

Emotional Support

All families, regardless of how healthy they are, encounter conflicts. In the most functionally healthy families, feelings of affection generally are paramount, and family members realize that bursts of anger and conflict reflect a short-term response. Anger and conflict do not dominate the family's pattern of interaction.

Healthy families are concerned with one another's needs, and family members' emotional and physical needs are met most of the time. When members' emotional needs are met, they feel support from those around them and are free to grow and explore new roles and facets of their personalities. A family dominated by conflict and anger alienates its members, leaving them isolated, fearful, and impaired emotionally.

Socialization

It is within families that individuals first learn social skills, such as how to interact in nonfamily venues, how to negotiate for personal needs, and how to plan. Children learn through parents' role modeling. Children learn through behavioral reinforcement about how to function effectively within the family and, when the system is successful, how to apply those skills in society.

BOX 35.1 Examples of Dysfunctional Communication

Manipulating
Instead of asking directly for what is wanted, family members manipulate others to get what they want. For example, a child starts a fight with a sibling to get attention. Another example is when a request is granted with "strings attached" so that the other person has a difficult time refusing the request: "If you clean my room for me, I won't tell Daddy you are getting bad grades in school."

Distracting
To avoid functional problem solving and resolving conflicts within the family, family members introduce irrelevant details into problematic issues.

Generalizing
Members use global statements such as "always" and "never" instead of dealing with specific problems and areas of conflict. Family members may state, "Harry is always angry," instead of exploring why Harry is upset.

Blaming
Family members blame others for failures, errors, or negative consequences of an action to deflect the focus from them.

Placating
Family members pretend to be well-meaning to keep peace in the family. "Don't yell at the children, dear. *I* put the shoes on the stairs."

Each developmental phase for family members and for the family as a whole brings new demands and requires new approaches to deal with changes. Parents are socialized into their family roles as they address the growth and developmental needs of each child. Parents' roles change when the children mature and leave home. This may necessitate partners' renegotiation of the patterning of their lives together. As time goes on, the parents may need their adult children's help if they become less able to care for their own needs.

It is not surprising that families have difficulty negotiating role change. Periods of change increase the overall stress within families. If the family is socialized to manage stress through open, direct communication, this period may be short-lived. However, if the family is not socialized to emotionally support its members or communicate effectively, the stress may linger, deteriorating the family's ability to function.

In response to the demands of change, healthy families demonstrate flexibility in adapting to new roles. Through well-organized management activities, firm but flexible boundary delineation, strong and appropriate communication patterns, ongoing provision of emotional support, and adept socialization, healthy families provide tools to their members to facilitate functioning for the present and into the future.

OVERVIEW OF FAMILY THERAPY

As a treatment approach, family therapy began to emerge in the 1920s as social psychologists recognized that behaviors among family members mutually influence the behaviors of individual members. The two major aims of family therapy are to:
1. Improve the skills of the individual members
2. Strengthen the functioning of the family as a whole

Family therapists are trained and practice at the advanced level. While you will not be conducting family therapy without an advanced degree, registered nurses often lead family groups for the purpose of education or support. Knowledge of basic family therapy skills will help you with group work. It will also provide you with information you can use for community referrals.

Family therapists use various strategies to assess a family's level of functioning. However, the following areas are almost always explored:

- Cohesiveness—how much time do members spend together as a family unit?
- Communication—do the members respectfully listen to one another's concerns and ideas and allow for open discussion when a disagreement arises?
- Appreciation—do the individual members contribute in meaningful ways to the functioning of the family and offer gratitude to one another that supports self-esteem?
- Commitment—do the individual members consider the impact of their actions on the family as a whole and in a manner that promotes unity?
- Coping—do the family members demonstrate the ability to support one another during times of crisis?
- Beliefs and values—does the family identify with or practice within a collective moral, ethical, or spiritual set of standards?

Specific approaches to therapy vary according to the philosophical viewpoint, education, and training of individual therapists. Family therapy's effectiveness is not tied to any particular theoretical approach. Table 35.1 lists specific therapies; identifies some of the therapists who contributed to their development and use; and highlights assumptions, concepts, and goals related to each therapy.

TABLE 35.1	**Models of Contemporary Family Therapy**			
Therapy	**Theorists**	**Assumptions**	**Concepts**	**Goals**
Contextual	Ivan Boszormenyi-Nagy (1987)	Values and ethics transcend generations and drive behaviors and relationships	Family problems arise from conflicts relating to loyalty, entitlement, legacy, and accounting	Gain insight into problematic relationships originating in the past to promote a "balanced ledger"
Family of origin	Murray Bowen (1978) Michael Kerr (1988)	Past issues influence present relationships; Anxiety inhibits change; Symptoms are indicators of stress and lower differentiation; Multigenerational transmission process	Family viewed as a system of emotional relationships; Triangulation and cutoff; Differentiation of self; Multigenerational transmission process; Sibling position matters	Foster differentiation and decrease emotional reactivity
Experiential-existential	Carl Whitaker (1978) Virginia Satir (1967)	Battle for structure, initiative, and self-worth; Growth occurs through shared experience	Symptoms express family pain; Use of nurturing to identify dysfunctional communication patterns	Guide the family to identify and develop their own solutions to dysfunctional behavior patterns
Structural	Salvador Minuchin (1974)	Inflexible structure leads to dysfunction; Restructuring leads to improved functioning	Identify patterns of enmeshment and disengagement; Clarify boundaries	Improve family relationships through restructuring the family hierarchy and boundaries
Strategic	Jay Haley (1967)	Family members perpetuate problems through their actions; People resist change	Symptoms are messages which serve functions in maintaining family homeostasis; Family rules are unspoken; Incongruous hierarchies	Realign family hierarchy through the use of rituals that change repetitive and maladaptive patterns of interaction
Cognitive-behavioral	Aaron Beck (2003)	Family relationships, cognitions, emotions, and behaviors mutually influence one another; Cognitive inferences evoke emotion and behavior	Focuses on negative cognitions; Uses learning theory to alter patterns leading to destructive behaviors; Use of "homework" assignments	Improve patterns of negative behaviors through changing thought patterns, which alleviates symptoms

Multiple-family group therapy is a useful therapeutic modality for families who are facing similar difficulties. By hearing other families discuss their problems, family members identify and gain insight into their own problems. New skills can be modeled and learned in the context of the group. In the case of multiple-family therapy, several families meet in one group with one or more therapists, usually once a week. A review of the literature showed multiple-family therapy as a best practice in schizophrenia and has shown promise in other psychiatric disorders, such as mood disorders, eating disorders, and substance use and addiction (Gelin et al., 2018).

CONCEPTS CENTRAL TO FAMILY THERAPY
The Identified Patient

When a family seeks treatment, the first task of the therapist is to address the presenting problem. That problem often belongs to the identified patient. The identified patient is an individual in the family typically regarded by family members as "the problem," the family member whose beliefs, perceptions, actions, and responses demand an immediate fix. Sometimes known as the family symptom-bearer, this person is generally the focus of most of the family system's concern.

From a therapeutic point of view, the identified patient may indeed be a problem. Yet this person may also serve to divert attention from other hidden problems of the family. The symptoms of the identified patient may actually serve as a stabilizing mechanism to bring about relatively cohesive behavior in a distressed family, at least in the short term. Identified patients may be aware, even on a remote level, of the role they serve in stabilizing the family. For example, adult children may sacrifice their autonomy by staying in the home to hold their parents together. This behavior demonstrates a violation of role boundaries.

The patient may or may not be the one who initially seeks help from inpatient or outpatient services. Some families will enter therapy on the recommendation of a clinician, as noted in the previous vignette with Diego's family. In other cases where criminal behavior is involved, a court may mandate family therapy. A family member other than the identified patient may initiate a request for therapy as well.

Triangulation

Dyads, consisting of two people, are often emotionally unstable. When tension in a dyad builds and communication fails, triangulation may be used to balance the relationship. **Triangulation** occurs when one family member does not communicate directly with another family member but will communicate with a third family member. This forces the third family member to be part of the triangle, and communication is then routed through the third person or even a pet.

For example, Charlotte is the youngest child of Amanda and Andrew. Charlotte has sensed increasing tension in her parents' marriage since her older siblings left home. When things get especially conflicted between Amanda and Andrew, Amanda vents her frustrations to Charlotte and even confided that Andrew had an affair. Charlotte is afraid that her parents will get a divorce when she goes away to college and is considering attending a local community college rather than her dream university. In this and many other cases, the family triangle (Fig. 35.2) serves to stabilize interpersonal relationships in the short term.

Triangulation can also be a form of splitting within the family system. One person may play a third family member against the one with whom he or she is upset. This splitting is accomplished through exaggeration, telling half-truths, or other manipulation of facts to present an untrue picture of the targeted person.

Although triangles within families tend to be structurally stable, the intensity of the triangulation process varies over time. During stressful times, triangulation may increase. Family triangles are destructive and may create emotional instability over the long-term family life-cycle.

Triangulating behavior occurs everywhere, not only in families but also in social situations among friends and in the workplace. You can monitor your own indirect communication and make an effort to communicate directly. Obviously, splitting behaviors are almost always emotionally unhealthy and should definitely be avoided.

Box 35.2 provides an overview of common terms used in discussions of family dynamics.

APPLICATION OF THE NURSING PROCESS

Nurses prepared at the basic level meet the needs of patients and families in inpatient and outpatient settings. Their work as part of the healthcare team can contribute significantly to the quality of intervention and patient outcomes. Psychiatric-mental health advanced practice registered nurses who have graduate or postgraduate training in family therapy may practice as nurse family therapists.

ASSESSMENT

A variety of assessment tools are available to help the nurse and nurse therapist assess how the family functions as a unit. These tools can also help to identify individual members' perceptions of how the family communicates and how they deal with

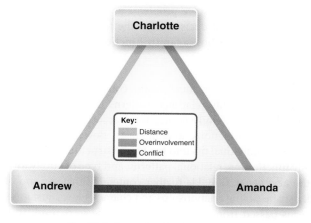

Fig. 35.2 Example of a family triangle.

BOX 35.2 Family Dynamics Terms

Boundaries: Clear boundaries are those that maintain distinctions between individuals within the family and between the family and the outside world. Clear boundaries allow for a balanced flow of energy between members. The roles of children and parent(s) are clearly defined. Diffuse or enmeshed boundaries are those in which there is a blending together of the roles, thoughts, and feelings of the individuals so that clear distinctions among family members fail to emerge. Rigid or disengaged boundaries are those in which the rules and roles are adhered to no matter what.

Differentiation: The ability to develop a strong identity and sense of self while at the same time maintaining an emotional connectedness with one's family of origin.

Double bind: Double binds occur between two or more people as a repeated experience. They involve two or more conflicting messages, a situation in which a positive command (often verbal) is followed by a negative command (often nonverbal). Double binds leave recipients confused, trapped, and immobilized because there is no appropriate way to act. A classic example is the command to "be spontaneous."

Family life cycle: The family's developmental process over time, which occurs in stages. Traditional stages include single young adult, newly married couple, a family with young children, a family with adolescents, launching children, and a family in later life. Needless to say, there are many different types of family life cycles, including single-parent families or families without children.

Hierarchy: The function of power and its structures in families, differentiating parental and sibling roles and generational boundaries.

Multigenerational issues (or intergenerational issues): Emotional patterns of interaction between family members that are passed down from previous generations. Examples of these patterns include the reenactment of fairly predictable and almost ritual-like patterns, repetition of themes or toxic issues, and repetition of reciprocal dyads, such as one person being the overfunctioner and another the underfunctioner.

Scapegoating: A form of displacement in which a family member, usually the least powerful or most different) is blamed for another family member's distress. The purpose is to keep the focus off the painful issues and the problems of the blamers. In a family, the blamers are often the parents and the scapegoat is a child. This child may continue to be scapegoated into adulthood.

Sociocultural context: The framework for viewing the family in terms of the influence of gender, race, ethnicity, religion, economic class, and sexual orientation.

Triangulation: Triangulation is used to balance anxiety, distance, and conflict in a two-person relationship by inserting a third person into the relationship.

The **genogram** is an efficient clinical summary and format for providing information and defining relationships across at least three generations. By creating a genogram, nurses and therapists are able to map the family structure and record family information that reflects both history and current functioning.

The information included on a genogram should include demographic data such as geographic location of family members, their respective occupations, and educational levels. You should also record functional information regarding medical, emotional, and behavioral status. Finally, note any critical events, such as important transitions, moves, job changes, separations, illnesses, and deaths. Females are represented in circles and males are represented in squares. Fig. 35.3 provides an example of a genogram based on information from the following vignette.

> **VIGNETTE:** Kate Smith is receiving therapy for major depressive disorder and cannabis use disorder. The psychiatric-mental health advanced practice registered nurse develops a genogram of the family based on the following information:
>
> Kate's parents, Hank and Catherine, are both college educated. Catherine, 35, has been treated for generalized anxiety disorder. Her mother, Sylvia, died by suicide at age 47 after a diagnosis of breast cancer. Catherine's family of origin never discusses the suicide. Catherine's brother Mike, 38, "drinks too much" and never finished high school. Her mother miscarried a female fetus before Catherine's birth. From an early age, many expectations were placed on her.
>
> Hank has a history of major depressive disorder. Hank is an only child whose father, Carl, died of a heart attack at age 43, Hank's present age. His mother, Cindy, is 65 years old and has chronic obstructive pulmonary disease.
>
> Hank and Catherine were married for 15 years before divorcing in 2013. Their two daughters, Kate and Jennifer, live with Hank. Kate, the identified patient, is 17 years old. She has been using marijuana. Jennifer is 14 years old and healthy. Kate and her mother have a conflicted relationship. Jennifer and her father are close. Kate often finds herself trying to "run interference" between her parents to shelter Jennifer from their parents' arguing.

Self-Assessment

Although nurse generalists do not provide family therapy, they do interact with patients and families. Most nurses come from families, and because no family is perfect, nurses may identify with certain family dynamics, which can trigger uncomfortable feelings. Nurses should be aware that their personal backgrounds, family of origin issues, and styles of interacting might affect their responses to patients and families.

As a nurse, you can even become triangulated into a patient's family system. You may notice that the patient is not speaking directly to his spouse but is speaking through you. A family member may attempt to bring you into a triangle by sharing negative information about the patient, particularly poor treatment by the patient toward this family member. Triangulation makes effective therapeutic intervention difficult. Having an anxiety level greater than the situation warrants is one indication that you are involved in triangulation. Direct communication on your part and encouraging the same in the patient and family members will help keep you out of unhelpful triangles.

NURSING DIAGNOSIS

Families often experience stress in times of anticipated developmental change, as well as in unanticipated change. Severe

emotional issues such as anger, conflict, and affection. You can even use some tools to show the family how they work together as a unit to plan and solve problems and to demonstrate how they make important decisions for the family. General assessment tools can show how a family functions.

Genograms

Bowen (1978) provided much of the conceptual framework for the analysis of family relational patterns using genograms. He proposed that the family is organized according to generation, age, sex, roles, functions, and interests. Bowen suggested that where each individual fits into the family structure influences the family functioning, relational patterns, and type of family formed in the next generation. He further contended that sex and birth order shape sibling relationships and characteristics, just as some patterns passed from one generation to the next result in persistent, interactive, emotional patterns, and triangulation.

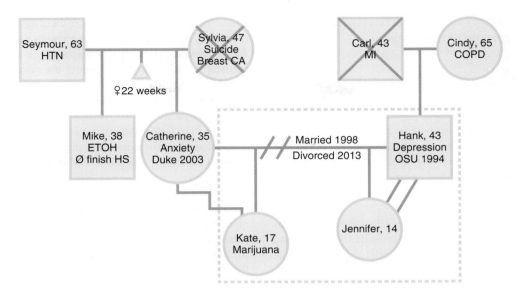

KEY: HTN = hypertension; COPD = chronic obstructive pulmonary disease;
MI = myocardial infarction; ETOH = alcohol; HS = high school
Fig. 35.3 The Smith family genogram.

BOX 35.3 Family-Related Nursing Diagnoses

- Risk for caregiver stress
- Caregiver stress
- Risk for impaired parenting
- Impaired parenting
- Readiness for effective parenting
- Risk for impaired caregiver child attachment
- Impaired caregiver child attachment
- Impaired family processes
- Readiness for positive family processes
- Sexual dysfunction
- Lack of resilience
- Risk for disturbed personal identity
- Disturbed personal identity
- Relationship problem
- Risk for chronic low self-esteem
- Chronic low self-esteem
- Impaired social interaction
- Risk for impaired family coping
- Impaired family coping

From International Council of Nurses. (2019). *International Classification for Nursing Practice catalog.* Retrieved from https://www.icn.ch/sites/default/files/inline-files/ICNP2019-DC.pdf.

---

dysfunctional patterns such as marked relational conflict, sexual misconduct, abuse, violence, and suicide exist within many families. These patterns can lead to physical or mental symptoms, at times requiring professional intervention, among its members. Psychiatric-mental health registered nurses' understanding of family dynamics within a context of broader sociocultural and personal variables assists in the identification of diagnoses.

Numerous nursing diagnoses are useful when working with families. Box 35.3 provides nursing diagnoses relevant to families and family functioning.

OUTCOMES IDENTIFICATION

Involving the family in the care of patients is often an essential outcome for patients who will require significant support. Outcomes should be developed with the input of both patients and families whenever possible.

Nurses provide family psychoeducation to support patients and families in understanding and coping with diagnoses. Through education, nurses reinforce strengths, help identify resources, and strengthen coping skills. Family teaching may include assisting members as they:

- Learn to accept the mental or physical illness of a family member.
- Learn to deal effectively with an ill member's symptoms, such as hallucinations, delusions, poor hygiene, physical limitations, and disfigurement.
- Develop an understanding of what medications can and cannot do and when the patient or family should seek advice from a professional.
- Learn what community resources are available and how to access them.
- Begin to feel less anxiety and regain or acquire a sense of control and balance in family life.

PLANNING

Nursing care for patients and their families usually occurs within the context of individual care planning. A planning priority is to address the safety needs of the family. For example, a member of the family may be at risk for acting in an aggressive or suicidal manner. A family member may be abusive or may be abused. If so, the nurse will need to determine whether to engage protective services for an abused family member or facilitate hospitalization to protect a suicidal or self-mutilating family member.

Nurses are adept at assisting family members to learn about the physical or mental illness of an afflicted family member; understand the effects, risks, and benefits of medications; and identify support groups and community resources. Planning and education are essential to help the family cope with crisis and improve the quality of life for all of its members. Identification of the extent of the family's knowledge deficit is equally important for organizing appropriate interventions.

INTERVENTION

Nurses prepared at the generalist level may provide counseling to family members utilizing a problem-solving approach. This approach addresses the immediate family conflict or crisis related to health or well-being. Developing and practicing effective listening skills and viewing family members in a non-judgmental manner are critically important qualities for nurses of all educational and training levels, regardless of the practice setting.

An important function for nurse generalists is to respond to cues from various family members that indicate the degree and amount of stress the family system is experiencing. Some indicators of stress in a family system are the following:

- Inability of the family or a family member to understand and act on treatments
- Somatic complaints among family members
- High degree of anxiety
- Depression or anger
- Problems in the school or work setting
- Substance use

Promoting and monitoring a family's mental health can occur in virtually any setting. Sometimes an informal conversation can have the greatest effect. For example, the question "Do you think you will help your mother taking the medications she's been prescribed?" would likely put the family member on the defensive. An invitation such as "Tell me your thoughts about the medication your mother has been prescribed" sets a collaborative tone between the nurse, patient, and family.

If extended family members are involved in the conversation, whether on the hospital unit or in a family session, the nurse should consider each member's view. How does the patient's medical regimen impact the way in which the family functions and what the individual members consider a possible solution?

Explain treatment plans in a clear and understandable manner, using language that is common to all family members, to help them make informed decisions. This is both a respectful and empowering way to work with families, indicating to them that *they* are the ones who are accountable and responsible for how they choose to use the information.

Elicit and listen to the perspective of each family member. It may seem surprising, but family members often hear the view of another member for the first time in this type of discussion. Personal perspectives may contribute to bewilderment or confusion among family members: "I didn't know you felt that way." The greater the family input, the more options exist for alternative ways of managing problematic situations.

Family Psychoeducation

Often, the most compelling family need is psychoeducation. This is particularly true for families who have a member with a severe mental illness. The primary goal of **family psychoeducation** is the sharing of mental healthcare information. Family education groups help family members better understand their member's illness, prodromal symptoms (symptoms that may appear before a diagnosis is reached or a relapse occurs), and medications needed to help reduce the symptoms.

Educational family meetings or multiple family meetings allow feelings to be shared and strategies for dealing with these feelings to be developed. Families can share painful issues of anger or loss, feelings of stigmatization or sadness, and feelings of helplessness. They can then put these feelings in a perspective that the family and individual members can deal with more satisfactorily.

An area in which family psychoeducation has been applied successfully is in the treatment of patients with schizophrenia. Families are extremely valuable and positive resources for patients, and family work promotes and supports families in coping with a member who has a severe psychiatric disorder. Psychoeducational groups also have proven helpful in parent management training, such as teaching a parent to work with a child with a conduct disorder.

🌐 CONSIDERING CULTURE

Family Interventions With Amish Patients

A waiting room full of family members is not unusual to see during the initial session with a patient from the Amish community. Clinicians may resort to asking, "Who is the patient?" Once the patient is engaged in care, family members may attend the appointment or expect a phone call in order to be involved.

In addition to family members' involvement in care, the church is extremely important. While most ministries request updates on the patient's progress, sometimes the patient requires the permission of church leaders to engage in treatment.

Amish patients in the psychiatric setting may also have a "support group" that is also considered an extension of the family. This support group is made up of two or three Amish couples who are responsible for checking in on the patient and the patient's family.

Boundaries within the Amish family tend to be both diffuse, resulting in overinvolvement, and rigid, resulting in demands for strict rules and roles. Differentiation and independence are discouraged. The family system is patriarchal. The husband is the head of the house and works outside the home. Once married, women manage the household and engage in child-rearing responsibilities.

Hard work is valued in the Amish community. Relaxation or taking a break is considered selfish or prideful. As a result, downtime is discouraged or even impossible—imagine having 8 children under the age of 10. Overwork may put vulnerable people at increased risk for psychiatric problems, such as anxiety disorders and major depressive disorder. Amish individuals may accept the advice to take better care of themselves and take breaks if it results in being better able to take care of others.

Adapted from Renee Bright, MEd, LPCC-S, SpringHaven Counseling Center, Ohio (personal communication, June 23, 2020).

EVALUATION

Both nurse generalists and psychiatric-mental health advanced practice registered nurses should evaluate the effectiveness of interventions. At the basic level, evaluation will address such issues as knowledge of therapeutic regimen, accessing outside support, and improved family coping. At the advanced level, evaluation focuses on the level of family members' individual and group functioning, whether conflicts are reduced or resolved, communication skills improved, coping methods strengthened, and whether family members have been better integrated into the broader societal system.

TREATMENT MODALITIES

Psychological Therapies

Psychiatric clinicians trained at an advanced level, including psychiatric-mental health advanced practice registered nurses, are qualified to conduct family therapy. This advanced treatment model has been applied to a variety of problems in children, adolescents, and adults. Treating the whole family appears to be particularly helpful in substance use disorders, child behavioral problems, marital relationship distress, and as an element of the treatment plan for schizophrenia (Deane et al., 2012).

Ma and colleagues (2019) conducted a systematic review and meta-analysis of cognitive-behavioral family intervention for patients with severe mental illness, specifically schizophrenia. This therapy shows promise in reducing delusions, delaying the first relapse episode, and reducing readmission rates.

Although therapists may adhere to different theories and use a wide variety of methods, the psychiatric advanced practice nurse aims to (Nichols, 2017):

- Reduce the dysfunctional behavior of individual family members
- Resolve or reduce intrafamily relationship conflicts
- Mobilize family resources and encourage adaptive family problem-solving behaviors
- Improve family communication skills
- Increase awareness and sensitivity to other family members' emotional needs and help family members meet their needs
- Strengthen the family's ability to cope with major life stressors and traumatic events, including chronic physical or psychiatric illness
- Improve integration of the family system into the societal system (e.g., school, medical facilities, workplace, and especially the extended family)
- Promote appropriate individual psychosocial development of each member of the family

Family therapy may not be helpful in some circumstances. For example, when the therapeutic environment is not safe and there is a risk for harm by information, uncontrolled anxiety, or hostility, a shared therapy session should be avoided. If the therapist is fairly sure that family members are not being honest, it is likely that the work being done will not be productive. If parental conflict involves issues of sexuality that are not appropriate for the children, these issues should be discussed in couples' counseling.

In most other situations, however, family therapy is useful. Family therapy is often combined with pharmacotherapy in the treatment of families who have a member with a psychiatric disorder, such as bipolar disorder, major depressive disorder, or schizophrenia. Other families may choose psychoeducational family therapy and/or self-help groups, which are good options that may be less costly and time-consuming.

EVIDENCE-BASED PRACTICE

Eating Disorders: Treating the Family

Problem
Eating disorders are complex, chronic, and affect every part of a person's being. Treatment is difficult and often includes integrating the family/caregivers. Emotion-focused family therapy (EFFT) has been shown to have positive short-term outcomes for caregivers but may have positive long-term outcomes as well.

Purpose of the Study
The purpose of this study was to identify if a 2-day EFFT workshop provided long-term benefits for caregivers of individuals with eating disorders.

Methods
Researchers used a two-phase, mixed methods style with 74 caregivers who participated in a 2-day EFFT workshop. In phase one, standard EFFT guidelines (psychoeducation, skill-building, and goal-setting) were used in a group format. In phase two, after 6 months of data collection, participants completed a semi-structured interview with questions related to the impact of the EFFT workshop.

Key Findings
- Caregivers experienced a reduction in fears and self-blame.
- Caregivers indicated an increase in confidence, behavioral skills, and emotional skills.
- Caregivers experienced a decrease in nonproductive enabling behaviors.
- Caregivers experienced improved self-efficacy.

Implications for Nursing Practice
This study demonstrated that EFFT may significantly improve long-term outcomes in caregivers of loved ones with an eating disorder. Nurses are important members of the multidisciplinary team in caring for patients with eating disorders and can provide patients with referrals and suggestions for such programs as EFFT.

From Nash, P., Renelli, M., Stillar, A., Streich, B., & LaFrance, A. (2020). Long-term outcomes of a brief emotion focused family therapy intervention for eating disorders across the lifespan: A mixed methods study. *Canadian Journal of Counselling and Psychotherapy, 54*(2), 130–149.

KEY POINTS TO REMEMBER

- Primary characteristics essential to healthy family functioning are flexibility and clear boundaries.
- The family structure has evolved from a nuclear family to a variety of combinations.
- The main functions of families are to provide management of the home, clear boundaries, clear communication based on a safe hierarchy, emotional support, and socialization through healthy role modeling.
- The aim of family therapy is to improve the skills of the individual family members and strengthen the functioning of the family as a whole.
- Concepts central to family therapy include the identified patient (who is usually regarded as the problem) and triangulation (a specific form of indirect communication).

- The nursing process provides an effective framework for assessing, diagnosing, planning, intervention, and evaluation of care that is based on family therapy concepts.
- The genogram is an efficient clinical summary and format for providing information and defining relationships across at least three generations.
- Registered nurses with basic training can interact and counsel families in most settings. Triangulation with patients and patients' families can be a challenge. Using direct communication and encouraging direct communication within families best address this problem.
- Along with other advanced practice psychiatric professionals, psychiatric-mental health advanced practice registered nurses who have specialized training may provide family therapy using a variety of theoretical approaches.

CRITICAL THINKING

1. Select a family with whom you have worked. Evaluate this family's status in terms of functionality with reference to the five family functions described in the text (i.e., management, boundaries, communication, emotional support, and socialization).
2. Create your own personal genogram, including at least three generations. Be sure to include the following:
   a. Location, occupation, and educational level
   b. Critical events, such as births, marriages, moves, job changes, separations, divorces, illnesses, and deaths
   c. Relationship patterns, including boundaries, enmeshment, triangulation, multigenerational issues, differentiation, and hierarchy
3. A family has just learned that their young son has a terminal illness. The parents have been fighting and blaming each other for ignoring the child's ongoing symptom of leg pain, which was diagnosed as advanced cancer. There are two other siblings in the family.
   a. How would you apply family concepts to help this family?
   b. What are some outcomes for this family? The family will:

CHAPTER REVIEW

1. Your 24-year-old patient is planning to leave the family to start a new job in a city 400 miles away. Which statement made by the patient best demonstrates a healthy sense of family support?
   a. "I've always been independent. That's how I was raised."
   b. "If I get in trouble financially, I know mom and dad will help me out."
   c. "I don't need anyone's help. Everyone has their own problems to deal with."
   d. "I'm going to miss everyone terribly, but I know they will support me in this decision."
2. A nurse works with patients whose families are attending family therapy. The nurse should recommend psychoeducational family therapy for which family?
   a. A family whose members have problems establishing and respecting boundaries.
   b. A family whose teenaged children are routinely making major family decisions.
   c. A family whose 18-year-old son has been diagnosed with schizophrenia.
   d. A family who communicates primarily using dysfunctional techniques.
3. A 10-year-old shares that he doesn't like spending weekends with his father "now that dad's girlfriend moved in." The nurse will discuss the issues with the child and parents based on an understanding of the stresses present in which type of family structure?
   a. Unmarried biological
   b. Cohabitating
   c. Blended
   d. Other
4. Which statement is an example of a parent demonstrating the dysfunctional communication technique of generalizing?
   a. "I want to be a good mother, but my husband just isn't involved with the kids."
   b. "I keep the peace by seldom asking any of the family to help with chores."
   c. "My wife's priorities are the kids, her parents, and then her job."
   d. "The kids never listen to me even when I threaten them."
5. Just before you escort the Juarez family in for a meeting, their 17-year-old son confides to you that he is gay. He says he has not told any other adult, including his parents. What is your best response to him?
   a. "Your parents have a right to know about this."
   b. "How do you think your parents would react if you told them?"
   c. "That's your decision, but you need to be careful about risky sexual behavior."
   d. "Lots of famous people are gay. You don't need to worry."
6. When performing an intake assessment on a family, you wish to map the family's structure and information that reflect both the family's history and current functioning. This assessment tool is called a:
   a. Mini-mental status exam
   b. Beck depression inventory
   c. Genogram
   d. Histogram

7. While you are working with a family whose son was admitted due to a psychotic break, you observe the mother say to her son, "What, no hug for your Mom?" As the son embraces his mother, she stiffens, which results in the young man backing away. She responds, "You only care about yourself." What behavior is this mother engaging in?
   a. Triangulation
   b. Scapegoating
   c. Double binding
   d. Differentiation

8. Which of the following family members should you refer to individual therapy rather than family therapy?
   a. A mother who has anxiety controlled by medication.
   b. A father who is questioning his sexuality.
   c. A son who is verbally abusive toward his parents.
   d. A daughter who has been treated for alcohol use disorder.

9. You are evaluating the family therapy experience. Which behavior would indicate that further family therapy is needed?
   a. Wife talks to her husband through their children.
   b. Son's grades have risen from a "D" average to a "C" average.
   c. Daughter's headaches have subsided.
   d. Mother has stopped using illicit substances.

10. Emotional support is an important family dynamic because it allows family members to:
   a. Feel secure enough to explore aspects of their personality.
   b. Feel isolated and fearful even though family members are near.
   c. Grow without boundaries within the family unit.
   d. Have bursts of anger without recourse or shame.

1. **d**; 2. **c**; 3. **b**; 4. **d**; 5. **b**; 6. **c**; 7. **c**; 8. **b**; 9. **a**; 10. **a**

Visit the Evolve website for a posttest on the content in this chapter: http://evolve.elsevier.com/Varcarolis

REFERENCES

Bowen, M. (1978). *Family therapy in clinical practice*. New York, NY: Jason Aronson.

Deane, F. R., Mercer, J., Talyarkhan, A., et al. (2012). Group cohesion and homework adherence in multi-family group therapy for schizophrenia. *Australian & New Zealand Journal of Family Therapy, 33*(2), 128–141.

Duvall, E. M. (1957). *Family development*. Oxford, UK: Lippincott.

Gelin, Z., Cooke-Darznes, S., & Hendrick, S. (2018). The evidence base for multiple family therapy in psychiatric disorders: A review (part 1). *Journal of Family Therapy, 40*(3), 302–325.

Ma, C. F., Chan, S. K. W., Chien, W. T., Bressington, D., Mui, E. Y. W., Lee, E. H. M., et al. (2019). Cognitive behavioral family intervention for people diagnosed with severe mental illness and their families. A systematic review and meta-analysis of randomized controlled trials. *Journal of Psychiatric Mental Health Nursing, 27*(2), 128–139.

Minuchin, S. (1974). *Families and family therapy*. Cambridge, MA: Harvard University Press.

Nichols, M. P. (2017). *Family therapy: Concepts and methods* (11th ed.). New York, NY: Pearson.

Integrative Care

Christina Fratena

Visit the Evolve website for a pretest on the content in this chapter: http://evolve.elsevier.com/Varcarolis

OBJECTIVES

1. Define complementary medicine, alternative medicine, and integrative care.
2. Identify trends in the use of nonconventional health treatments and practices.
3. Explore the classification of integrative care by domains: natural products, mind and body approaches, and other integrative approaches.
4. Discuss the techniques used in major complementary therapies and potential applications to psychiatric-mental health nursing practice.
5. Discuss the importance of educating the public in regards to research and safety of integrative modalities.

KEY TERMS AND CONCEPTS

acupuncture
aromatherapy
Ayurvedic medicine
chiropractic medicine
complementary and alternative
  medicine (CAM)

expressive therapies
healing touch
herbal therapy
holism
homeopathy
integrative care

naturopathy
Reiki
therapeutic touch
traditional Chinese medicine

Complementary and alternative medicine (CAM) is the conventional term for medical practices and products that are outside of standard medical care. Standard medical care refers to generally accepted treatments provided by healthcare professionals. CAM includes complementary medicine, alternative medicine, and integrative medicine. The distinctions between the three approaches can be seen in the following statements:

- Complementary medicine uses non-mainstream medicine in conjunction with standard medical care.
- Alternative medicine uses non-mainstream medicine instead of standard medical care.
- Integrative medicine uses non-mainstream medicine in conjunction with standard medical care in a coordinated way.

For the purposes of this nursing textbook, we discuss these approaches and replace the word *medicine* with the word *care*. Also, we will primarily refer to non-mainstream medicine as integrative care since this approach fits most closely with values in nursing. Integrative care places the patient at the center of care, focuses on prevention and wellness, and attends to the patient's holistic needs, including the physical, mental, and spiritual (Fontaine, 2019). The emphasis is on the body's ability to heal itself given the right tools and knowledge.

INTEGRATIVE CARE IN THE UNITED STATES

Conventional healthcare is a system of care in which healthcare professionals such as nurses, doctors, pharmacists, and therapists treat symptoms and diseases with drugs, surgery, and radiation. Other terms for mainstream medicine include allopathic medicine, biomedicine, conventional medicine, orthodox medicine, and Western medicine. Conventional healthcare has only been used for around 200 years, whereas CAM has been practiced worldwide for thousands of years (Fontaine, 2019). In the United States, up to two-thirds of individuals use nontraditional approaches to healthcare. The increased use may be due to a greater availability of CAM-prepared practitioners and practice facilities along with more public exposure to CAM through the media.

One of the essential differences between conventional and integrative healthcare is that conventional medicine focuses on what is done *to* the patient. Integrative practices are patient-centered, meaning that the patient participates *with* the provider to heal the body and mind. While Western medicine defines health as the absence of disease, integrative health views health by how well the physical, emotional, mental, environmental, spiritual, and societal components interrelate (Fontaine, 2019).

In 1998, the National Institutes of Health (NIH) established the National Center for Complementary and Alternative Medicine. In 2014, this center was renamed the National Center for Complementary and Integrative Health (NCCIH), making it one of 27 institutes and centers of the NIH. The strategic framework for NCCIH (2020) is based on three scientific and two cross-cutting objectives:

- Advance fundamental science and methods development regarding
  1. Basic biological mechanisms of action of natural products, including prebiotics and probiotics
  2. Mechanisms through which mind and body approaches affect health, resiliency, and well-being
  3. New and improved research methods and tools for conducting research studies of these health approaches
- Improve care for hard-to-manage symptoms by
  1. Developing and improving strategies for managing symptoms such as pain, anxiety, and depression
  2. Conducting studies in "real-world" settings to test the safety and efficacy of these health approaches

Trends in the use of integrative therapies were identified in the most recent report from the National Health Interview Survey, which is administered every 5 years (Clarke et al., 2018). This survey includes a supplemental complementary health questionnaire. Use of the top three complementary health modalities increased between 2012 and 2017, with a significant increase seen in the use of yoga and meditation and a modest increase in chiropractic care. Fig. 36.1 illustrates these changes.

Consumers and Integrative Care

Consumers are attracted to integrative care for a variety of reasons, including the following:

- A desire to actively participate in their healthcare and engage in holistic practices that can promote health and healing
- A desire to find therapeutic approaches that seem to carry lower risks than traditionally used medications
- Positive experiences with holistic integrative CAM practitioners, whose approach is supportive and inclusive

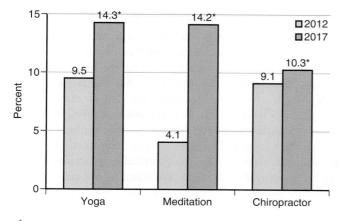

*Significantly different from 2012 (*P* < .05).

Fig. 36.1 Use of yoga, meditation, and chiropractors, 2012 and 2017. (From Clarke, T. C., Barnes, P.M., Black, L. I., Stussman, B. J., Barnes, P. M., & Nahin, R. L. [2018]. *Use of yoga, meditation, and chiropractors among U.S. adults aged 18 and over.* Retrieved from https://www.cdc.gov/nchs/data/databriefs/db325-h.pdf.)

- Dissatisfaction with the practice style of conventional medicine (e.g., rushed office visits, short hospital stays)

Other reasons individuals might try integrative approaches are listed in Box 36.1.

Integrative Nursing Care

The American Nurses Association (ANA) recognizes holistic nursing as an official specialty within the nursing profession. Along with the American Holistic Nurses Association (AHNA), the ANA publishes guidelines for this specialty in *Holistic Nursing: Scope and Standards of Practice* (ANA & AHNA, 2013). According to the AHNA, holistic nursing is "all nursing that has healing the whole person as its goal" (AHNA, 1998). More specifically, holism involves:

1. The identification of the interrelationships of the bio-psycho-social-spiritual dimensions of the person, recognizing that the whole is greater than the sum of its parts.
2. An understanding of the individual as a unitary whole in a mutual process with the environment.

The traditional psychiatric nursing assessment includes presenting problems, past psychiatric history, substance use, medical illnesses/surgeries, family psychiatric history, and social history. A holistic approach to assessment involves using open-ended questions to identify the patients' view of their experience and their concerns. Additional questions concerning nutrition, exercise, relationships, work, cultural, religious, and spiritual concerns, and the use of herbal supplements, should also be part of the assessment. Without prompting, patients are not as likely to disclose to healthcare providers what herbal remedies or supplements they are taking.

Nurses in any setting should have a basic knowledge of the treatments used in integrative care. Nursing programs often include basic integrative modalities, such as relaxation techniques and guided imagery. Some schools may include energy-based approaches, such as therapeutic touch. Inclusion of CAM information in nursing education is important because you will care for patients who use a variety of unconventional modalities. Activities such as assessment and patient education require a basic understanding of integrative approaches.

Consumers typically rely on health information obtained from friends, the internet, and social media. Based on these sources, they may be suspicious about some aspects of conventional healthcare. In fact, up to 72% of those searching the internet are doing so for a health-related purpose (Rew et al., 2018). Unfortunately, online sources have a high likelihood of inaccuracy of information. Helping consumers actively evaluate the quality of information available to them is an important nursing activity.

BOX 36.1 Factors Influencing Use of Complementary and Alternative Medicine

- One or more neuropsychiatric symptoms
- Recommendation by their provider
- Ineffective conventional treatment
- Financial cost of conventional treatment
- Non-symptomatic, general wellness, and prevention usage
- Recommendation by friends and family
- Use for improvement of energy and immune function

Integrative Care Education and Certification

Graduate programs in the United States that prepare nurses with a specialty in holistic nursing are increasing. Numerous post-master's certificate programs exist for advanced-practice registered nurses. Doctor of nursing practice (DNP) programs with an emphasis on integrative health are available.

The American Holistic Nurses Credentialing Corporation (AHNCC) offers two levels of certification for registered nurses. Both require 2000 hours or 1 year of full-time experience in holistic nursing within the past 5 years. They also require 48 hours of continuing nurse education in holistic care. The holistic nurse–board certified (HN-BC) certification is for diploma or associate degree–prepared nurses. The holistic baccalaureate nurse–board certified (HNB-BC) distinction is for baccalaureate-prepared nurses.

The AHNCC also offers two certificates for advanced practice registered nurses. In addition to meeting the hours of experience and continuing nurse education previously described for undergraduates, 500 hours of experience in the specialty is required. Registered nurses who have attained graduate status may sit for an examination, leading to the credential of advanced holistic nurse–board certified (AHN-BC). The other credential is based on the attainment of an advanced practice nursing degree (e.g., nurse practitioner) and prescriptive authority. This credential is referred to as advanced practice holistic nurse–board certified (APHN-BC).

Credentials are also available for other specific approaches, such as acupuncture, chiropractic medicine, naturopathy, and massage therapy. Regulation and licensing of CAM and healthcare providers vary from state to state. Efforts are underway to regulate integrative care through credentialing of integrative physicians and nonphysician practitioners, including nurses.

 HEALTH POLICY

Should Insurance Companies Provide Coverage for Integrative Medicine Treatment?

Some insurers provide coverage for certain modalities, such as chiropractic medicine, nutritional care, massage, mind-body approaches, and acupuncture. The covered benefits are narrowly defined, however. For instance, acupuncture can be used in some plans only as an alternative to anesthesia. This also leaves a wide range of approaches uncovered. In addition, licensed CAM providers are reimbursed less for their services than conventional providers.

In recent years, consumers in several states have lobbied to require insurance companies to reimburse for CAM. Proponents say enacting a law that requires third-party payers to provide coverage for CAM services would relieve a financial burden from consumers. Opponents argue that involving insurance companies could increase restrictions on the CAM. Oversight by the government would require providers to meet strict criteria that currently are not in place. They argue that this would lead to suffering on both the part of the business and the consumer. The amount and type of services could be limited.

Until federal or state laws are passed to require insurance coverage of CAM, there are other options for potential reimbursement. Consumers may attempt to petition their insurance companies to provide coverage based on medical necessity. This petitioning requires many steps, including a letter of medical necessity by a healthcare provider. Consumers who have health savings accounts (HSA) are also able to inquire about whether they can use this money to pay for CAM services. Recently, CAM providers began to provide consumers with itemized lists of diagnoses and codes that they can self-submit to their insurance companies. These methods have shown promise in at least part of the services being reimbursed.

CLASSIFICATION OF INTEGRATIVE CARE

Integrative care is classified into three domains: (1) natural products, (2) mind and body approaches, and (3) other CAM therapies (NCCIH, 2018).

Natural Products

Natural products include herbal medicine (botanicals) and also vitamins, minerals, and probiotics. With the proliferation of literature on herbal remedies and the accessibility of the products, increasing numbers of consumers are using these products to manage symptoms. A growing number of people in the United States are using herbal therapy for preventive and therapeutic purposes.

The American Association of Poison Control continues to show that most major classes of prescribed medications have significantly more adverse effects and fatalities than vitamins, dietary supplements, herbs, and homeopathic remedies (Gummin et al., 2018). In 2017, the number one cause of poisoning was pharmaceutical in 2314 (86.3%) of the 2682 fatalities.

Unfortunately, a major drawback to dietary supplements and herbs is that the current regulatory climate is not effective in managing these products. Given that use of herbal products has become more mainstream, the importance of better oversight of safety has been heightened. Bijaulija and colleagues (2017) propose seven guidelines to ensure product safety, quality, and efficacy of herbal products:

- Establishing methods of standardization, including specific testing to determine the quality of the herbal supplement
- Morphological or organoleptic evaluation, which evaluates the herb's size, color, odor, taste, touch, and texture
- Macroscopic and microscopic evaluation to determine the identity and degree of purity
- Physical evaluation to compare the herb in the supplement with visual documentation of the same properly identified material
- Chemical evaluation to determine quality and purity
- Biological evaluation, which includes screening for pesticide residues, arsenic, and heavy metals
- Stability testing for analysis of the product and proper shelf-life determination

While the majority of herbal supplements are generally safe, some herbs can have negative effects on certain individuals and interactions with other medications. For example, ginseng has anticoagulant effects. Drinking ginseng tea may increase the effects of prescription anticoagulants, and the consequences could seriously affect blood clotting. Although relatively rare, Kava used for anxiety or insomnia can be hepatotoxic. St. John's wort, which is used for major depressive disorder, can result in serotonin syndrome when combined with other serotonergic medications such as antidepressants, triptans, and methadone. It can also induce the metabolism of other medications, such as oral contraceptives, and some human immunodeficiency virus (HIV) medications.

We use caution with the term "natural" when discussing these products. This term may indicate that the chemicals in these medications are present in nature. The notion of naturalness suggests that alternative medications are harmless. However, even though something is called "natural," it may not be safe to use in or on the body.

Diet and Nutrition

Because psychiatric illness affects the whole person, it is not surprising that patients with psychiatric disorders often have nutritional disturbances. Their diets may be deficient in the proper nutrients, or they may eat too much or too little. In addition, metabolic syndromes accompanied by obesity, diabetes, and hyperlipidemia may occur *in response* to treatment with antipsychotic medications. Obesity and diabetes coexist at a greater-than-average rate in people with psychiatric disorders. Nutritional states may also *cause* psychiatric disturbances. Anemia, a common deficiency disease, is often accompanied by depression.

The influence of diet and nutrition on general health and mental health has been the subject of much research. The International Society for Nutritional Psychiatry Research (ISNPR, n.d.) identifies a mission to facilitate knowledge and grow the field of nutritional psychiatry research. Topics on their website include:

- The role of diet in psychotic disorders
- Fermented foods, microbiota, and mental health
- The connection between polyphenols and mental health
- Stress and emotional eating

The traditional Western diet tends to consist of highly processed food with little nutritional value. The link between inflammation and depression has been growing in recent years. A longitudinal study used the Dietary Inflammatory Index (DII) to identify if the diets of people with depression were anti-inflammatory or pro-inflammatory (Shivappa et al., 2018). They followed participants over 8 years and found that higher DII scores (pro-inflammatory diet) indicated a higher prevalence of depressive symptoms.

Another significant study looked at depressive symptoms in relation to diet and followed participants over 10 years (Le Port et al., 2012). This study indicated the following:

- Higher depressive symptoms in men occurred in those who ate a standard Western diet, increased snacking, and ate a large amount of food that was high in fat and sweets.
- Higher probability of depression in women is associated with greater amounts of snacking and larger consumption of foods low in fat.
- Reduced risk of depression was found in those eating regular meals that consisted of more fish, fruit, raw or cooked vegetables, and omega-3 fatty acids.
- Stress may increase unhealthy nutrition and cravings associated with emotional eating.

Megavitamin therapy, also called *orthomolecular therapy*, is a nutritional therapy that involves taking large amounts of vitamins, minerals, and amino acids. The theory is that the inability to absorb nutrients from a proper diet alone may lead to the development of illnesses. This type of therapy should be undertaken with caution because there is the potential for side effects.

Vitamin D. Vitamin D is a fat-soluble nutrient that is essential to bone health, cell growth, and immune function. This vitamin is absorbed primarily through sun exposure. Certain foods such as fatty fish (e.g., salmon, mackerel, and tuna), beef liver, cheese, and egg yolks are also sources of vitamin D. Specific serum blood screening is used to determine accurate results. The Endocrine Society recommends using the 25(OH)D test to screen for vitamin D levels (Smith et al., 2017).

Studies demonstrate a link between vitamin D and depression. In a recent meta-analysis (Vellekkat & Menon, 2019), researchers found that supplementation of vitamin D helped improve depressive symptoms. They speculate that this could be due to the role vitamin D has on lowering oxidative stress and inflammation, both of which have been theorized to worsen depression.

When ultraviolet light is converted to vitamin D in the body, there is no danger of overdose. However, when vitamin D is taken as an oral supplement, people could potentially take too much. The main consequence of toxicity is a buildup of calcium, a condition known as hypercalcemia. Symptoms of toxicity include:

- Nausea, vomiting
- Loss of appetite, increased thirst
- Frequent urination, constipation, diarrhea
- Muscle weakness
- Confusion
- Bone pain
- Kidney stones

Omega-3 fatty acids. Researchers continue to study the efficacy of omega-3 fatty acids in the treatment of depression and bipolar disorder. Supplementation was shown to be effective in a double-blind clinical trial for bipolar disorder (Shakeri et al., 2016). Another meta-analysis indicated a lower risk of depression in those who consumed more fish or omega-3 fatty acid (Yang et al., 2018).

Microbiomes. Human beings have up to 100 trillion microbial cells, primarily in the gut. The impact of the human microbiomes and chronic inflammatory states are both becoming more recognized as impacting mental health, particularly depression and anxiety. Healing the gut and body with proper nutrition, probiotics, and fermented foods has shown promise in treating these conditions and others (Selhub et al., 2014). Table 36.1 summarizes both herbal and dietary supplements used for psychiatric symptoms and disorders.

Mind and Body Approaches

Mind and body approaches are built on theories that focus on the continuous interaction between mind and body (Bartol, 2016). Most of these techniques emphasize the mind's capacity to affect bodily function and symptoms, but the reverse—the effects of bodily illness on mental health—is also part of the equation.

The significance of the mind-body relationship is well accepted in conventional medicine and probably is the domain most familiar to psychiatric-mental health nurses and nurses in general. Many of the mind-body interventions, such as cognitive behavioral therapy, relaxation techniques, guided imagery, and support groups, are now considered mainstream and have been the subject of considerable research.

Meditation and Mindfulness

Meditation is an extremely popular method recommended to reduce physical and emotional stress and to promote wellness. It can be most simply accomplished by concentrating on slow deep breathing and focusing on calming thoughts or the breath. Specific types of meditation include relaxation techniques (refer to Chapter

TABLE 36.1   Herbal/Dietary Supplements Used With Psychiatric Symptoms and Disorders

Herbal Supplement	Uses	Cautions
St. John's wort	Depression	• Interaction with other medications • Photosensitivity • Increased risk of serotonin syndrome when combined with pro-serotonergic medications such as antidepressants, triptans, and methadone
Kava (Kava kava)	Insomnia Fatigue Anxiety	• FDA warned against use due to the link to severe liver damage
Golden root (Rhodiola)	Anxiety Fatigue Depression	• Dizziness, dry mouth, and headaches may occur • Allergic reactions can occur
Valerian root	Insomnia Anxiety Depression	• Generally considered safe for short time periods • Mild side effects could include morning fatigue, headaches, dizziness, upset stomach
Chamomile	Sleeplessness Anxiety	• Allergic reactions can occur, particularly in those allergic to the daisy family of plants
Lavender	Anxiety Restlessness Insomnia Depression	• Topical use generally considered safe if diluted properly, although breast growth in young boys has been reported • Oil taken by mouth may be poisonous • Teas and extracts may cause side effects, including gastrointestinal complaints and headache • Use with medications with sedative properties may cause drowsiness to increase
Melatonin	Insomnia Jet lag Night shift	• May worsen mood in dementia • Side effects uncommon, but possibly drowsiness, dizziness, headache, nausea • Long-term use may affect the body's ability to produce melatonin on its own
SAMe	Depression	• May interact with certain medications • Increased risk of serotonin syndrome when combined with pro-serotonergic medications, such as antidepressants, triptans, and methadone • Side effects are uncommon
Fish oil (omega-3 fatty acids)	Depression Bipolar disorder	• Possible gastrointestinal effects, such as belching, indigestion • Caution with those having fish/shellfish allergies • May increase bleeding time

Source: National Center for Complementary and Integrative Health (NCCIH). Retrieved from https://nccih.nih.gov.

10) and mindfulness meditation by Kabat-Zinn, among others. Mindfulness-based interventions have been increasingly useful in conditions such as depression, anxiety, and chronic pain. The most recent systematic review indicated that mindfulness interventions were evidenced-based treatments for these conditions as well as in the prevention of illness (Gotink et al., 2015).

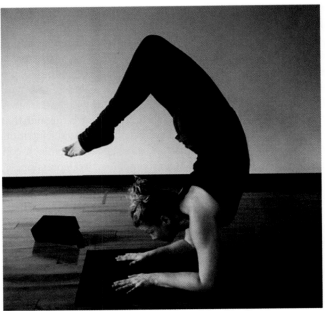

Fig. 36.2 Scorpion pose in yoga.

Yoga

Yoga is another popular method to both physically strengthen and emotionally relax people. It typically combines a variety of physical postures, meditation, and breathing techniques. Yoga may help, in part, by decreasing cortisol levels in the brain as well as helping to stabilize the hypothalamic-pituitary-adrenal (HPA) axis, thereby lowering the stress response (Pascoe et al., 2017; Fig. 36.2).

Exercise

Many patients with psychiatric disorders have low energy and motivation, leading them to become sedentary. This, in turn, can increase symptoms. including depression and anxiety. Exercise alters the levels of dopamine, serotonin, and norepinephrine and increases levels of brain-derived neurotrophic factor (BDNF). Exercise also increases cerebral blood flow; reduces oxidative stress levels; increases apoptosis in the brain, which can improve hippocampal function; and can turn on signaling pathways in the brain responsible for cognitive function and behavior (Hamilton & Rhodes, 2015). Extensive research with meta-analysis has been conducted on the positive benefits of exercise in a variety of mental health disorders, including the following:

- Exercise was effective in treating substance use disorders, including increasing the rate of abstinence, reducing withdrawal symptoms, and reducing symptoms of depression and anxiety (Wang et al., 2014).
- Exercise decreased psychiatric symptoms while enhancing cognition and cardiorespiratory fitness in individuals with schizophrenia (Stubbs et al., 2018).
- Physical exercise resulted in improved cognitive function—specifically, staying on task and completing tasks—in children and young adults with autism spectrum disorder and attention-deficit/hyperactivity disorder (Tan et al., 2016).
- Exercise—particularly, high-intensity exercise—can cause a decrease in anxiety levels (Aylett et al., 2018).

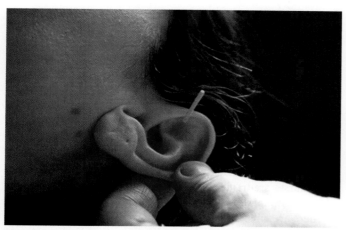

Fig. 36.3 "Shen men" area for acupuncture, which is used to relieve pain, stress, excessive sensitivity, anxiety, and insomnia.

Acupuncture

Acupuncture is becoming increasingly popular in the United States. A skilled therapist should perform it. Acupuncture involves placing needles into the skin at key points (meridians) to modulate the flow of qi. According to Taoists, qi is a life force that circulates throughout the universe and in our bodies in precise channels called meridians.

Sometimes, the needles are inserted and removed immediately; sometimes, they are twirled and even attached to stimulating electrodes. Another method is to leave them in place for a certain period of time. Following needle placement, patients describe feeling sensations such as rushing, warmth, tingling, or occasionally pain. Acupuncture acts by stimulating and altering patients' physical responses, including those affecting cardiac, endocrine, neurological, and immune function. It is commonly used in the treatment of pain and in some blood disorders, as well as for substance withdrawal and certain emotional disturbances (Fig. 36.3).

Guided Imagery

The use of **guided imagery** has been discussed in the nursing literature for decades. Imagery is used as a therapeutic tool for treating anxiety, pain, psychological trauma, and posttraumatic stress disorder (PTSD). Imagery may be combined with cognitive behavioral therapy to help war veterans and people who have survived natural disasters. Imagery enhances coping before childbirth or surgery, augments treatment, and minimizes the side effects of medications. It may help people cope with difficult times if they can imagine themselves as strong, coping, and eventually finding meaning in their experience.

Manipulative Practices

Manipulative, or body-based, practices relate to specific body systems and structures. These include joints and bones, circulation, and soft tissues. Two commonly used therapies—spinal manipulation and massage—fall within this category.

Spinal manipulation. **Spinal manipulation** is accomplished through chiropractic medicine, one of the most widely used integrative therapies. The term *chiropractic* comes from the Greek words *cheir* and *praxix*, meaning "treatment by hand" and "practice," respectively. Chiropractic medicine focuses on the relationship between structure and function and the way that relationship affects the preservation and restoration of health, using manipulative therapy as a treatment tool.

Daniel Palmer, a grocery store owner, developed the method in the late 1800s in an effort to heal others without drugs. Palmer developed a series of manipulative procedures to bring health to muscles, nerves, and organs that had gotten out of alignment. He referred to these misalignments as *subluxations*. He believed that subluxations were metaphysical and that they interfered with the flow through the body of "innate intelligence" (spirit or life energy).

Contemporary chiropractic medicine continues to be based on the theory that energy flows from the brain to all parts of the body through the spinal cord and spinal nerves. Manipulation of the spinal column, called *adjustment*, returns the vertebrae to their normal positions. Back pain is the most common reason people seek chiropractic treatment. Chiropractic manipulation treats a variety of other conditions, including general pain, headaches, allergies, and asthma. Manipulation is also helpful in reducing migraine, tension, or cervicogenic headache pain. Many chiropractors also treat patients with depression, anxiety, and chronic pain. Chiropractic treatment may be done in conjunction with herbs and supplements.

A comprehensive systematic review on the use of chiropractic medicine in disease showed that chiropractic care could improve conditions such as shoulder and neck pain and sports injuries (Salehi et al., 2015). Research also indicates chiropractic care may be an effective treatment for migraines (Rist et al., 2019).

Massage therapy. **Massage therapy** includes a broad group of medically valid therapies that involve rubbing or moving the skin. Massage therapists employ four basic techniques:
1. Effleurage—long gliding strokes over the skin
2. Pétrissage—kneading of the muscles to increase circulation
3. Vibration and percussion—a series of fine or brisk movements that stimulate circulation and relaxation
4. Friction or deep tissue massage—a technique used to increase circulation and release tight areas by applying deep pressure

Probably the best-known massage technique in the United States is **Swedish massage**, which provides soothing relaxation and increases circulation. Japanese **Shiatsu massage** was strongly influenced by traditional Chinese medicine (TCM) and developed from acupressure. It originated as a way to detect and treat problems in the flow of life energy (Japanese *ki*). The shiatsu practitioner uses fingers, thumbs, elbows, knees, or feet to apply pressure by massaging various parts of the body, known as *acupoints*.

Massage therapy has positive benefits in depression and stress. The most recent meta-analysis on this topic found depressive symptoms to be significantly lowered in those using massage therapy (Hou et al., 2010). Another systematic review by Smith and colleagues (2019) found that massage could be an effective tool in prenatal depression.

Other Complementary Therapies

Homeopathy and Naturopathy

Homeopathy is an example of Western alternative medicine. In homeopathy, small doses (dilutions) of specially prepared plant extracts, herbs, minerals, and other materials are used to stimulate the body's defense mechanisms and healing processes. Infinitely small doses of diluted preparations that produce symptoms mimicking those of an illness are used to help the body heal itself. Homeopathy is based on the law of similars, meaning like cures like. Dilutions are prescribed to match the patient's illness or symptom and personality profile. Healing occurs from the inside out, and symptoms disappear in the reverse order they appeared.

Homeopathic remedies are available over-the-counter. Consumers should have a full evaluation by a homeopathic practitioner before using any treatments. One study compared the outcomes of patients seeking help from general practitioners (GP) versus those who sought help from GP who also prescribed homeopathy (GP-Mx). The researchers found that those who sought help from the GP-Mx practitioners were less likely to use psychiatric medication and were slightly more likely to show improvement in symptoms (Grimaldi-Bensouda et al., 2016).

Naturopathy emphasizes health restoration rather than disease treatment, and a naturopathic physician may combine nutrition, homeopathy, herbal medicine, hydrotherapy, light therapy, therapeutic counseling, and other therapies. The underlying belief is that the individual is responsible for recovery.

EVIDENCE-BASED PRACTICE

Does Music Soothe Blood Draw Anxiety?

Problem

Nursing students often experience anxiety when performing procedures such as drawing blood for the first time. This anxiety may lead to poorer performance, decreased learning, and undue stress.

Purpose of Study

The purpose of the study was to determine if listening to music during drawing blood would decrease students' anxiety.

Methods

Researchers used a sample of 73 freshman nursing students enrolled in a fundamentals of nursing course. Participants were randomly assigned to either the control group with standard training or the experimental group that included the music intervention. Each group completed an anxiety scale along with measurements of their pulse rate and blood pressure.

Key Findings

- Students in the music intervention group experienced a significant reduction in anxiety.
- Students in the music intervention group had a better performance in the blood draw.
- Students in the music intervention group exhibited a decreased mean diastolic blood pressure.

Implications for Nursing Practice

This study demonstrated that listening to music may significantly improve symptoms of anxiety in nursing students during first-time blood draws. It also highlighted the nurse educator's role as being instrumental in using nonmainstream interventions to support nursing students' learning.

From Ince, S., & Cevik, K. (2017). The effect of music listening on the anxiety of nursing students during their first blood draw. *Nurse Education Today, 52,* 10–14.

Aromatherapy

Aromatherapy, the use of essential oils for enhancing physical and mental well-being and healing, is a popular therapy in the mainstream market. Essential oils, often derived from herbs and plants, may be applied topically, inhaled, or diffused into the atmosphere through a diffuser. You can find many essential oils in a variety of skin-care products, as well as used in baths and compresses. The sense of smell connects with the part of the brain that controls the autonomic (involuntary) nervous system. Depending on the essential oil used, the resulting effects are calming, pain-reducing, stimulating, sedating, or euphoria-producing. Some nurses are trained in this art and have introduced various oils into hospitals, nursing homes, and hospice situations.

There are anecdotal reports that aromatherapy is useful for pain relief, memory improvement, and wound healing. A systematic review suggests that aromatherapy, particularly lavender, improves postpartum problems such as nausea, baby blues, depression, mood lability, anxiety, stress, fatigue, pain, sleep, relaxation, healing, and prolactin levels (Rist et al., 2019). The researchers highlight the importance of these findings, since women are often drawn to more holistic approaches during pregnancy and postpartum.

The National Association for Holistic Aromatherapy (2019) provides guidelines for the use and safety of aromatherapy. The association also lists the most common essential oils used for mental health–related concerns (Table 36.2).

Safety guidelines for use of essential oils include becoming properly trained in their use, not taking oils by mouth, not using near the eye, keeping oils away from flames, storing in a cool, dark area, keeping oils away from children (use under age 2 is not recommended), knowing which essential oils cause photosensitivity, and using caution with undiluted application and in pregnancy (Buckle, 2016). Some individuals, particularly individuals with pulmonary disease, may be sensitive or allergic to essential oils when they come into contact with the skin or are inhaled. Before massaging any essential oil into the skin, check for an allergic reaction by diluting the oil, administering a small amount, and performing a 24-hour skin patch test.

TABLE 36.2 Essential Oils Used in Mental Health-Related Concerns

Essential Oil	Use
Roman chamomile	Relieving anxiety/stress
Clary sage	Relaxing, relieving anxiety/stress
Ginger	Emotionally and physically warming
Lavender	Calming, decreases anxiety
Lemon	Antistress
Mandarin	Calming
Neroli	Relieves and decreases anxiety; antidepressant, postpartum depression
Patchouli	Antidepressant
Rose	Relieves and decreases anxiety/stress
Vetiver	Calming, grounding
Ylang ylang	Antidepressant

National Association of Holistic Aromatherapy. (2019). *Most commonly used essential oils.* Retrieved from https://naha.org/explore-aromatherapy/about-aromatherapy/most-commonly-used-essential-oils.

Expressive Therapies: Music and Art

Many psychiatric treatment programs, including inpatient, partial hospitalization, intensive outpatient, and outpatient programs, are incorporating the use of expressive therapies. Both music and art therapists are trained in higher education programs and are licensed or certified in their fields. The American Music Therapy Association and the American Art Therapy Association provide guidelines for the care of people with a variety of medical illnesses, including mental illnesses. Their respective websites outline numerous research studies that have been conducted on the efficacy of these interventions. One meta-analysis showed music therapy to be one of the essential areas for the recovery process in individuals with mental illness (Solli et al., 2013).

Energy Therapies

Energy therapy is based on the belief that nonphysical bioenergy forces pervade the universe and people. Explanations vary as to the nature of this energy, the form of the therapies, and the rationale for how healing is believed to occur with its use. Some cultures believe the energy comes from God. Individuals who practice shamanic healing rituals believe the energy comes from various spirits through a priest or shaman. Therapeutic touch, healing touch, and Reiki are the most common energy therapies practiced by nurses.

Therapeutic touch. Therapeutic touch is a modality developed in the 1970s by Dolores Krieger, a nursing professor at New York University, and Dora Kunz, a Canadian healer. The premise for therapeutic touch is that balancing the body's energies promotes healing. In preparation for a treatment session, practitioners focus completely on the person receiving the treatment without any other distraction. Practitioners then assess the energy field, clear and balance it through hand movements, and/or direct energy in a specific region of the body. The therapist never physically touches the patient. Ideally, after undergoing a session of therapeutic touch, patients report a sense of deep relaxation.

Practitioners of therapeutic touch believe that the therapy is useful for many conditions, including pain relief, premenstrual syndrome, depression, complications in premature babies, and secondary infections associated with HIV infection. They believe that therapeutic touch can also lower blood pressure, decrease edema, ease abdominal cramps and nausea, resolve fevers, and accelerate the healing of fractures, wounds, and infections.

Healing touch. Healing touch is a derivative of therapeutic touch developed by a registered nurse, Janet Mentgen, in the early 1980s. Healing touch combines several energy therapies and is based on the belief that the body is a complex energy system that can be influenced by another through that person's intention for healing and well-being. Healing touch is related to therapeutic touch in the belief that working with people to achieve their highest level of well-being, not necessarily to relieve a specific symptom, is the goal.

Healing touch involves gentle laying on of hands on a clothed body or moving over the body in the energy field. The practitioner may focus on a specific problem area or the full body.

Reiki. The Japanese spiritual practice of Reiki has become a popular modality for nurses to learn and use. Reiki is an energy-based therapy in which the practitioner's energy is connected

CONSIDERING CULTURE

Amish Use of Natural Treatments

The Amish community relies heavily on what they describe as natural treatments. It is common to consult alternative providers, as well as lay providers and healers, for a variety of medical concerns, including psychiatric symptoms. Typical care includes natural supplements, special diets, chiropractic treatments, reflexology, iridology (diagnosis of illness by examination of the iris), and ridding the body of parasites.

Do these practices occur to reduce costs because most Amish do not have commercial insurance? Maybe in part. Yet members of the Amish community often spend a great deal of money on these treatments. For example, they may make a trip to Mexico to get chelation treatment or spend thousands of dollars on supplements.

The Amish often rely on word of mouth with regard to the treatments. If a close friend or relative quit taking his lithium in favor of natural pills and did well, another Amish individual with bipolar disorder might do the same. These practices often result in relapse, at which point the family is likely to seek conventional psychiatric care.

to a universal source (many interpret this as God or another sacred being) and is transferred to a recipient for physical or spiritual healing. Hospitals, hospices, cancer support groups, and clinics offer Reiki in complementary programs. A review of randomized trials suggested Reiki was effective for treating pain and anxiety (Thrane & Cohen, 2015).

Bioelectromagnetic-Based Therapies and Bright-Light Therapy

Bioelectromagnetic-based therapies involve the unconventional use of electromagnetic fields, such as pulsed fields, magnetic fields, or alternating-current or direct-current fields. Transcranial magnetic stimulation (TMS) and vagus nerve stimulation (VNS) treatments for depression are in this category and have US Food and Drug Administration approval. Chapter 14 provides more detail regarding TMS and VNS and their use for major depressive disorder.

Bright-light therapy has been shown as promising both in the treatment of seasonal affective disorder (SAD) and in nonseasonal depression. More studies are being done on the effectiveness of bright-light therapy in bipolar depression. A recent randomized controlled study indicated this therapy, given midday and in conjunction with antimanic treatment, was effective in achieving lower depression scores without the risk of inducing hypomania in bipolar depression (Shields & Wilson, 2016).

Prayer and Spirituality

Patients with psychiatric disorders often have significant spiritual needs. Some feel angry with God or another higher power for allowing them to suffer with disorders that affect every aspect of their lives. This anger can also be in relation to grief and loss. Some individuals harbor anger, for example, toward friends and family who may have rejected them or been judgmental. Other patients may wish to seek forgiveness because of the hurt they have caused others. Many patients rely on a higher power as their source of strength and maintain a deep abiding faith, despite the circumstances of their illnesses. Those dealing

TABLE 36.3 Complementary and Alternative Medicine Used for Psychiatric Disorders

Disorder	CAM Used (not all-inclusive)
Anxiety	Exercise, yoga, mindfulness-based stress reduction, music, acupuncture, homeopathy, Reiki
Bipolar disorder	Exercise, mindfulness/meditation, yoga
Major depressive disorder	Exercise, nutrition, chiropractic, bright-light therapy, music, Reiki, religious/spiritual, healing touch, qigong, massage
Posttraumatic stress disorder	Guided imagery, yoga, acupuncture
Schizophrenia/ psychosis	Exercise, yoga, acupuncture
Substance use disorder	Exercise, mindfulness/meditation, yoga, qigong

CAM, Complementary and alternative medicine.
Wynn, G. H. (2015). Complementary and alternative medicine approaches in the treatment of PTSD. *Current Psychiatry Reports, 17*(8), 600.

with substance use issues and attending a 12-step group are directed to identify a higher power.

Table 36.3 identifies CAM uses in psychiatric disorders.

Historical Notes Regarding CAM

Traditional Chinese Medicine

Traditional Chinese medicine provides the basic theoretical framework for many CAM therapies, including acupuncture, acupressure, transcendental meditation, tai chi, and qigong. TCM comes from the Eastern tradition, specifically the philosophy of Taoism, and emphasizes the promotion of harmony (health) or to bring order out of chaos (illness).

The main concept in TCM is the movement of life energy or essence, *qi*, which maintains an individual's health and wellness. If this life energy is disrupted, it can seriously impact the mind, body, and spirit (Shields & Wilson, 2016). TCM is a vast medical system based on a constellation of concepts, theories, laws, and principles of energy movement within the body. Therapy

addresses the patient's illness in relation to the complex interaction of mind, body, and spirit.

Adherents of TCM say that it addresses not only physiological and psychological symptoms but also cosmologic events that relate to the dynamics of the universe. These meridians become significant in the practice of acupuncture, touch therapy, and the more recent energy-based therapies used to treat emotional symptoms and promote mental health. Forms of movement such as qigong and tai chi may be used, as well as yoga. Viewed as a stressor itself, movement seems to mediate the effects of other stressors.

In TCM, health is the balance between *yin* and *yang*, and illness emanates from imbalances. The TCM practitioner uses the history and physical examination to understand the imbalances of mind, body, and spirit that have caused the patient's illness. Diagnosis involves both questioning and observing body structure, skin color, breath, body odors, nail condition, voice, gestures, mood, and pulse. Eastern goals, perspectives, and stages of healing are useful in treating mental illnesses, many of which are long term. The goals of healing in Eastern medicine include the following:

- Being in harmony with one's environment and with all of creation in mind, body, and spirit
- Reawakening the spirit to its possibilities
- Reconnecting with life's meaning

Ayurvedic Medicine

Ayurvedic (pronounced eye-yur-VEH-dik) medicine originated in India around 5000 BC and is one of the world's oldest medical systems. *Ayurveda* means "the science of life" and is a philosophy that emphasizes individual responsibility for health. Individuals are seen as consisting of the five elements of earth, water, fire, air, and space, which combine to regulate the mind, body, and spirit. Ayurveda views the body as *doshas* (vital energies), *dhatus* (tissues), and *malas* (waste products; Fontaine, 2019). Health is achieved when the doshas are in balance. Imbalance may be treated by nutrition, herbs, exercise, yoga, breathing, meditation, massage, aromatherapy, music, or purification with five procedures, called *panchakarma*.

KEY POINTS TO REMEMBER

- A philosophy of holism and promotion of therapeutic relationships are at the heart of psychiatric-mental health nursing and are important no matter what modality is used, conventional or integrative.
- Complementary, alternative, and integrative therapies are in demand as consumers seek a broader range of therapies than those offered by traditional medicine.
- Integrative care is classified as (1) natural products, (2) mind and body medicine, and (3) other complementary therapies.
- With the availability of information online, consumers are more likely to research their symptoms or condition and identify potential CAM treatments.

- An increasing amount of evidence-based research is available on the efficacy of the majority of CAM treatments used.
- Nurses are ideally positioned to guide patients to reliable resources, such as the NCCIH, that provide up-to-date information for healthcare practitioners and consumers.
- Nurses' knowledge of current research about major CAM therapies will assist in the purposeful and safe promotion of holistic integrative care.

CRITICAL THINKING

1. As a nurse, you may have patients who use integrative therapies in conjunction with the conventional therapies prescribed by the healthcare provider. Identify issues that are important to assess. Discuss how you would ask about the use of these nonconventional practices.
2. Discuss the role of exercise and nutrition in treating psychiatric illness. Given that many individuals are self-conscious about their weight, how would the nurse present this information to a patient in a nonjudgmental style?
3. How would a nurse educate a patient on the appropriate and safe use of aromatherapy?
4. By visiting their websites, determine how the NCCIH and other informational resources, such as the AHNA, provide information for the consumer and professionals.

CHAPTER REVIEW

1. Which statement made by the patient demonstrates an understanding of the foundational principle of integrative care?
   a. "My body has the ability to heal itself if we have the knowledge to give it the right tools."
   b. "The integrative care I'm getting is primarily a combination of complementary, alternative, and mainstream medicines."
   c. "Much of the knowledge that integrative care is based on comes from Western cultural traditions."
   d. "The most important focus of my integrative care is the cure of my cardiac illness."
2. When considering the goals of complementary and alternative medicines, which patient would be of particular interest to researchers studying advances in symptom management?
   a. One who experiences chronic pain related to a neck injury
   b. A patient diagnosed with an acute gastrointestinal infection
   c. A pregnant woman diagnosed with gestational diabetes
   d. A child requiring surgery for a clubbed foot
3. Which assessment question regarding a patient's report of pain demonstrates the nurse's attention to the principles of holistic nursing care?
   a. "When did your pain begin?"
   b. "Are you taking any herbal supplements for the pain?"
   c. "Has anyone else in your family ever experienced this kind of pain?"
   d. "How has the pain affected your daily ability to care for yourself?"
4. What medication education should the nurse provide to a patient who has expressed an interest in taking St. John's wort?
   a. Allergic reactions to this herb are common.
   b. Due to liver toxicity, regular liver function test should be conducted while taking it.
   c. St. John's wort should not be taken in combination with antidepressants.
   d. This medication results in gastrointestinal symptoms, including bleeding.
5. Which factor is likely to attract a patient to complementary and alternative medicine? *Select all that apply.*
   a. This nonmainstream approach is always less expensive than conventional medical treatment.
   b. A desire to choose personal healthcare practices.
   c. Using these approaches carries a lower risk than many pharmaceuticals.
   d. Traditional medicine has been unsuccessful in providing effective treatment.

   e. Integrative medication practices tend to produce desired results more quickly than conventional practices.
6. In contrast to most Western medicine, integrative care takes into consideration:
   a. The physician's diagnosis and the patient's response
   b. The nurse's ideas about healing in addition to the physician
   c. A whole-person perspective: body, mind, and spirit
   d. The diagnosis before beginning spirit work
7. A nursing student is experiencing increasing test anxiety. Her professor suggests the student try some integrative therapies. The student reported successful test anxiety reduction with which of the following therapies?
   a. Aromatherapy and breathing exercises
   b. Megavitamin therapy and yoga
   c. Naturopathy
   d. Reiki
8. The nurse is caring for a patient who has a question about the safety of an herbal supplement. Which nursing response is best?
   a. "Herbal supplements are regulated by the FDA."
   b. "Natural ingredients in herbal supplements are harmless."
   c. "Your primary care provider needs to be aware of any supplements you take."
   d. "Marketing for herbal supplements demonstrates that all supplements are safe."
9. A patient asks the nurse if exercise and what she eats can impact her mood. The nurse's best response is which of the following?
   a. "There is no need to be concerned about exercise and nutrition if you take your antidepressant."
   b. "Limited studies are available on exercise and nutrition and mood."
   c. "Exercise is helpful, but you don't need to worry about nutrition."
   d. "Extensive research has shown that exercise and proper nutrition greatly improve mood symptoms."
10. Reviewing prescription medications in the discharge instructions for a patient with a diagnosis of major depressive disorder, the nurse would caution the patient about which over-the-counter supplement(s)? *Select all that apply.*
    a. Fish oil
    b. SAMe
    c. St. John's wort
    d. Melatonin

1. a; 2. a; 3. b; 4. c; 5. b, c, d; 6. c; 7. a; 8. c; 9. d; 10. b, c

Visit the Evolve website for a posttest on the content in this chapter: http://evolve.elsevier.com/Varcarolis

REFERENCES

American Holistic Nurses Association. (1998). *Description of holistic nursing*. Retrieved from https://www.ahna.org/About-Us/What-is-Holistic-Nursing#:~:text=Holistic%20Nursing%20is%20defined%20as , Nurses'%20Association%2C%201998.

American Nurses Association & American Holistic Nurses Association. (2013). *Holistic nursing: Scope and standards of practice*. Silver Spring, MD: American Nurses Association.

Aylett, E., Small, N., & Bower, P. (2018). Exercise in the treatment of clinical anxiety in general practice—A systematic review and meta-analysis. *BMC Health Services Research, 18*(1), 1–18.

Bartol, G. (2016). The psychophysiology of body-mind healing. In B. M. Dossey, & L. Keegan (Eds.), *Holistic nursing: A handbook for practice* (7th ed.) (pp. 345–363). Burlington, MA: Jones & Bartlett.

Bijaulija, R. K., Alok, S., Chanchal, D. K., & Kumar, M. (2017). A comprehensive review of standardization of herbal drugs. *International Journal of Pharmaceutical Science and Research, 8*(9), 3663–3677.

Buckle, J. (2016). Aromatherapy. In B. M. Dossey, & L. Keegan (Eds.), *Holistic nursing: A handbook for practice* (7th ed.) (pp. 345–363). Burlington, MA: Jones & Bartlett.

Clarke, T. C., Barnes, P. M., Black, L. I., Stussman, B. J., & Nahin, R. L. (2018). *Use of yoga, meditation, and chiropractors among U.S. adults aged 18 and over*. Retrieved from https://www.cdc.gov/nchs/products/databriefs/db325.htm.

Fontaine, K. (2019). *Complementary and alternative therapies for nursing practice* (5th ed.). New York, NY: Pearson.

Gotink, R. A., Chu, P., Busschbach, J. J. V., Benson, H., Fricchoine, G. L., & Hunink, M. G. M. (2015). Standardised mindfulness-based interventions in healthcare: An overview of systematic reviews and meta-analysis of RCTs. *PLoS ONE, 10*(4), 1–17.

Grimaldi-Bensouda, L., Abenhaim, L., Massol, J., Guillemot, D., Avouac, B., Duru, G., et al. (2016). Homeopathic medical practice for anxiety and depression in primary care: The EPI3 cohort study. *BMC Complementary and Alternative Medicine, 16*(125), 1–10.

Gummin, D. D., Mowry, J. B., Spyker, D. A., Brooks, D. E., Osterthaler, K. M., & Banner, W. (2018). 2017 annual report of the American Association of Poison Control Centers' national poison control data system: 35th annual report. *Clinical Toxicology, 56*(12), 1213–1415.

Hamilton, G. F., & Rhodes, J. S. (2015). Exercise regulation of cognitive function and neuroplasticity in the healthy and diseased brain. *Progress in Molecular Biology and Translational Science, 135*, 381–406.

Hou, W. H., Chiang, P. T., Hsu, T. Y., Chiu, W. Y., & Yen, Y. C. (2010). Treatment effects of massage therapy in depressed people: A meta-analysis. *Journal of Clinical Psychiatry, 71*(7), 894–901.

International Society for Nutritional Psychiatry Research. (n.d.). Retrieved from http://www.isnpr.org.

Le Port, A., Gueguen, A., Kesse-Guyot, E., Melchoir, M., Lemogne, C., Nabi, H., et al. (2012). Association between dietary patterns and depressive symptoms over time: A 10-year follow-up study of The GAZEL cohort. *PLoS One, 7*(12), 1–8.

National Association for Holistic Aromatherapy. (2019). *Most commonly used essential oils*. Retrieved from https://naha.org/explore-aromatherapy/about-aromatherapy/most-commonly-used-essential-oils.

National Center for Complementary and Integrative Health. (2018). *Complementary, alternative, or integrative: What's in a name?* Retrieved from https://nccih.nih.gov/health/integrative-health.

National Center for Complementary and Alternative Medicine. (2020). *NCCIH facts at a glance and mission*. Retrieved from https://www.nccih.nih.gov/about/nccih-facts-at-a-glance-and-mission#:~:text=The%20mission%20of%20NCCIH%20is,improving%20health%20and%20health%20care.

Pascoe, M. C., Thompson, D. R., & Ski, C. F. (2017). Yoga, mindfulness-based stress reduction, and stress-related physiological measures: A meta-analysis. *Psychoneuroendocrinology, 86*, 152–168.

Rew, L. , Saenz, A., & Walker, L. O., Kowalski, M., Osypiuk, K., Vining, R. (2018). A systematic method for reviewing and analyzing health information on consumer-oriented websites. *Journal of Advanced Nursing, 74*(9), 2218–2226.

Rezaie-Keikhaie, K., Hastings-Tolsma, M., Bouya, S., Shad, S. F., Sari, M., Shoorvazi, M., et al. (2019). Effect of aromatherapy on post-partum complications: A systematic review. *Complementary Therapies in Clinical Practice, 35*(9), 290–295.

Rist, P. M., Hernandez, A., Bernstein, C., Kowalski, M., Osypiuk, K., Vining, R., et al. (2019). The impact of spinal manipulation on migraine pain and disability: A systematic review and meta-analysis. *Headache: Journal of Head and Face Pain, 59*(4), 532–542.

Salehi, A., Hashemi, N., Imanieh, M. H., & Saber, M. (2015). Chiropractic: Is it efficient in treatment of diseases? Review of systematic reviews. *International Journal of Community Based Nurse Midwifery, 3*(4), 244–254.

Selhub, E. M., Logan, A. C., & Bested, A. C. (2014). Fermented foods, microbiota, and mental health: Ancient practice meets nutritional psychiatry. *Journal of Physiological Anthropology, 33*(1), 1–12.

Shakeri, J., Khanegi, M., Golshani, S., Farnia, V., Tatari, F., Alikhani, M., et al. (2016). Effects of omega-3 supplement in the treatment of patients with bipolar I disorder. *International Journal of Preventive Medicine, 7*, 77.

Shields, D. A., & Wilson, D. R. (2016). Energy healing. In B. M. Dossey, & L. Keegan (Eds.), *Holistic nursing: A handbook for practice* (7th ed.) (pp. 345–363). Burlington, MA: Jones & Bartlett.

Shivappa, N., Hebert, J. R., Verone, N., Caruso, M. G., Notarnicola, M., Maggi, S., et al. (2018). The relationship between the dietary inflammatory index (DII) and incidence of depressive symptoms: A longitudinal cohort study. *Journal of Affective Disorders, 235*, 39–44.

Sit, D. K., McGowan, J., Wiltrout, C., Diler, R. S., Dills, J., Luther, J., et al. (2018). Adjunctive bright light therapy for bipolar depression: A randomized double-blind placebo-controlled trial. *American Journal of Psychiatry, 175*(2), 131–139.

Smith, L. M., Shewamene, Z., Galbally, M., Schmied, V., & Dahlen, H. (2019). The effect of complementary medicines and therapies on maternal anxiety and depression in pregnancy: A systematic review and meta-analysis. *Journal of Affective Disorders, 245*, 428–439.

Smith, L. M. (2017). *Estimation of the recommended daily allowance for vitamin intake using serum 25 hydroxyvitamin D level of 20ng/MI as the end point, may vary according to the analytical measurement technique used*. Retrieved from https://plan.core-apps.com/tristar_endo17/abstract/f7e437ee5c2d999047a0315444cbbebb.

Solli, H. P., Rolvsjord, R., & Borg, M. (2013). Toward understanding music therapy as a recovery-oriented practice within mental health care: A meta-synthesis of service users' experiences. *Journal of Music Therapy, 50*(4), 244–273.

Stubbs, B., Vancampfort, D., Hallgren, M., Firth, J., Veronese, N., Solmi, M., et al. (2018). EPA guidance on physical activity as a treatment for severe mental illness. *European Psychiatry, 54*(2018), 124–144.

Tan, B. W. Z., Pooley, J. A., & Speelman, C. P. (2016). A meta-analytic review of the efficacy of physical exercise interventions on cognition in individuals with autism spectrum disorder and ADHD. *Journal of Autism Developmental Disorders, 46*(9), 3126–3143.

Thrane, S., & Cohen, S. M. (2015). Effect of Reiki on pain and anxiety in adults: An in-depth literature review of randomized trials with effect size calculations. *Pain Management Nurse, 15*(4), 897–908.

Vellekkatt, F., & Menon, V. (2019). Efficacy of Vitamin D supplementation in major depression: A meta-analysis of randomized controlled trials. *Journal of Postgraduate Medicine, 65*(2), 74–80.

Wang, D., Wang, Y., Wang, Y., Rena, L., & Zhou, C. (2014). Impact of physical exercise on substance use disorders: A meta-analysis. *PLoS ONE, 9*(10), 1–15.

Yang, Y., Kim, Y., & Je, Y. (2018). Fish consumption and risk of depression: Epidemiological evidence from prospective studies. *Asia-Pacific Psychiatry, 10*(4), 1–11.

INDEX

Page numbers followed by *b, t,* and *f* indicate boxes, tables, and figures, respectively.